Handbook of Adolescent Health Psychology

William T. O'Donohue · Lorraine T. Benuto
Lauren Woodward Tolle
Editors

Handbook of Adolescent Health Psychology

Springer

Editors
William T. O'Donohue
Department of Psychology
University of Nevada
Reno, NV, USA

Lorraine T. Benuto
Department of Psychology
University of Nevada
Reno, NV, USA

Lauren Woodward Tolle
Licensed Clinical Psychologist
Project Manager, Integration Services
Aurora Mental Health Center
Aurora, CO, USA

ISBN 978-1-4614-6632-1 ISBN 978-1-4614-6633-8 (eBook)
DOI 10.1007/978-1-4614-6633-8
Springer New York Heidelberg Dordrecht London

Library of Congress Control Number: 2013932016

Printed on acid-free paper

Springer is part of Springer Science+Business Media (www.springer.com)

To our favorite adolescents, Anna and Izabel.
And to our favorite future adolescents Jorge, Jack, and Liam

Preface

Health psychology as a field is focused on the balance between physical and psychological health and disease. While literature on health psychology is not sparse, research on both mental and physical health intervention and outcome in adolescents has historically been neglected (Williams, Holmbeck, & Greenley, 2002). This comprehensive handbook seeks to fill this gap by covering a wide range of topics that fall under five general categories and constitute the organization of this handbook: General issues in adolescent health psychology, the developmental processes that occur during adolescence, treatment, and training of professionals as each relate to adolescent health psychology, mental health and adolescents, and physical health and adolescents. Each of these general categories translates to a section in this book, and each section contains several chapters that address topics that fall within each of the aforementioned categories. A description of each section follows.

General Issues Related to Adolescent Health Psychology

As indicated above, the field of health psychology is vast, and given the development processes that occur during adolescence, certain issues related to the field of adolescent health psychology merit a detailed discussion. In the first section of the book, general issues in adolescent health psychology are discussed. Specifically, a biopsychosocial perspective on adolescent health and disease is presented with an emphasis on risk-taking behaviors and the various biological, psychosocial, and environmental factors found to be associated with adolescent risk-taking behaviors. Next the influences that sociocultural and socioeconomic factors can have on adolescent health are explored. In this first section of this book, there are also chapters on public health approaches to adolescent health, epidemiology of adolescent health, disease prevention in adolescence, and determinants of health-related behaviors in adolescence. Other topics covered within this general section include stress, emotional regulation, and resilience in adolescence; mental health literacy; measurements and quality life instruments used with adolescents; the effects of physical activity on health; and sexual assault and intimate partner violence as each relates to the adolescent.

Adolescent Development

Adolescence is clearly a time during which much change occurs. These changes occur on multiple developmental levels including changes that are emotional, social, and physical. Naturally these changes can carry an impact on adolescent health both psychological and physical. Thus, the second section of this book focuses on adolescent development. Specifically, a discussion of continuity of behavior and parenting from childhood through adolescence is provided; school performance of the adolescent is discussed (with a discussion on factors that can influence school performance, e.g., chronic illness); brain development in the adolescent is reviewed; puberty and its role in adolescent maturation is explored; and the literature on adolescent sexuality and sexual behavior is reviewed.

Treatment

In fact, in this book, O'Donohue et al. emphasize how adolescents drivers of high health care costs in part due to their underuse of office visits and overuse of emergency department care (Newacheck, Wong, Galbraith, & Hung, 2003); how during the transition from childhood to adulthood, adolescents establish patterns of behavior and make lifestyle choices that affect both their current and future health; and how adolescence is a significant intervention point for behavior change (O'Donohue & Tolle, 2009). Therefore, a discussion on the treatment (both medical and behavioral) of the adolescent is warranted. Thus, in this book chapters relevant to intervention effectiveness research, training issues in adolescent health, delivery of interventions, confidentiality and care, and treatment adherence are included.

Mental Health

As indicated earlier in this chapter, the field of health psychology explores the intricate and complex associations between physical and psychological health and disease. Therefore, naturally, sections of this book relevant to medical and physical conditions as well as mental health conditions are necessary. Here we describe the chapters on mental health disorders and below we discuss medical/physical conditions. With regard to mental health disorders, our approach to determining which topics to cover was twofold. First we examined the Diagnostic and Statistical Manual of Mental Disorders 4th Edition Text Revision (DSM-IV-TR) (American Psychiatric Association, 2000) and determined which of the broad categories in the DSM-IV-TR were both relevant to the adolescent and merited a lengthy discussion. Second, we considered other circumstances or situations that arise during adolescence that are related to mental health. This process resulted in the inclusion of chapters on smoking, substance use, ADHD, antisocial behavior, personality disorders, self-harm, eating disorders, anxiety, depression and suicide-related behaviors, and intellectual disabilities.

Medical/Physical Conditions

With regard to physical and medical conditions, a review of the scientific literature, books that focus on adolescents that are related to health (physical or mental), and books that focus on health psychology (although not on adolescents) led us to determine which topics related to medical/physical conditions should be included in this handbook. The topics that we cover that are specific to medical/physical conditions are pregnancy, sexually transmitted infections, HIV, obesity, cardiovascular conditions, asthma, endocrine disorders, musculoskeletal injuries, and headaches.

Other Themes Present Throughout the Book

In addition to the sections of the book described above, certain themes present themselves throughout the book and are covered in greater detail in the introductory chapter of the handbook. The majority of these themes are largely related to prevention, which can be quite key in the health and well-being of the adolescent. In fact, extant research has indicated that wellness and periodic health checkups are instrumental in disease prevention and early diagnosis in primary care settings illustrating the importance of annual well-child (by child we also include adolescents) check-ups (Schor, 2012) which can include screening for mental health conditions (administered in primary care settings).

Other factors that are important to assess for when working with adolescents include emotion dysregulation and poor social skills as both have emerged as being primary contributors to adolescent psychological and behavior problems (e.g., Compas, Jaser, & Benson, 2009; Haynos & Fruzzetti, 2011; Hughes & Gullone, 2010). While the literature is lacking in empirically validated preventive interventions for this age group that focus on emotion regulation and social skills, we propose that a prevention program focusing on these areas would likely be effective in reducing adolescent psychopathology. Finally, a number of public health care crises uniquely affect adolescents, and their prevalence has shifted over the last decade. These include substance use; teenage pregnancy; and obesity. As are discussed in several chapters, prevention of the above can lead to positive health outcomes for the adolescent although unfortunately there is little empirical support for the prevention of these health crises to date.

Closing Comments

Clearly adolescence can be a challenging time, as the adolescent is faced with the task of dealing with biological and cognitive changes as well as with complex and interrelated sociopsychological tasks such as shifts in relationships with family, friends, the peer group, and the wider world (Coleman & Hagell, 2007; Seiffge-Krenke, 2009). As indicated at the outset of this preface, adolescents have historically been neglected in the health psychology research. Therefore, this handbook seeks to fill this gap and offer a comprehensive, up-to-date resource for mental health professionals, integrated care professionals, behavioral medicine professionals, and physicians and nurses written by leading authorities in the field. Last but certainly not least, this handbook emphasizes the importance of behavioral health and aligns with the changing perspective on mental health.

Reno, NV, USA William T. O'Donohue, Ph.D.
Reno, NV, USA Lorraine T. Benuto, Ph.D.
Aurora, CO, USA Lauren Woodward Tolle, Ph.D.

References

American Psychiatric Association. (2000). *Diagnostic and statistical manual of mental disorders* (4th ed., text rev.). Washington: Author.

Aruda, M., & Burke, P. (2012). Pregnancy in adolescence. In W. O'Donohue, L. Benuto, & L. Tolle (Eds.). *Handbook of adolescent health psychology*. New York: Springer.

Bethell C et al. (2002). *Partnering with parents to promote the healthy development of young children enrolled in Medicaid*. New York: The Commonwealth Fund.

Bethell C., Reuland C. P., Halfon, N., & Schor E. L. (2004). Measuring the quality of preventive and developmental services for young children: National estimates and patterns of clinicians' performance. *Pediatrics*, 113, 1973–1983.

Campbell, C., Hansen, D. J., & Nangle, D. W. (2010). Social skills and psychological adjustment. In D. W. Nangle, D. J. Hansen, C. A. Erdley, P. J. Norton (Eds.), *Practitioner's guide to empirically based measures of social skills*, (pp. 51–67). New York: Springer.

Chambers, C. V., & McManus, R. P. (2000). Childhood and adolescence. In R. Rakel (Ed.), *Textbook of family medicine,* (pp. 608–634). New York: W. B. Saunders.

Coleman, J., & Hagell, A., (2007). *Adolescence, risk and resilience: Against the odds*. West Sussex: Wiley.

Compas, B. E., Jaser, S. S., & Benson, M. A. (2009). Coping and emotion regulation: Implications for understanding depression during adolescence. In S. Nolen-Hoeksema, H. M. Lori (Eds.), *Handbook of depression in adolescents* (pp. 419–440). New York: Routledge/Taylor & Francis.

Havighurst, S. S., & Harley, A. (2007). *Tuning in to kids: Emotionally intelligent parenting: Program manual*. Melbourne: University of Melbourne.

Haynos, A. F., & Fruzzetti, A. E. (2011). Anorexia nervosa as a disorder of emotion dysregulation: Evidence and treatment implications. *Clinical Psychology: Science and Practice*. 18(3), 183–202.

Herman, K. C., Borden, L. A., Reinke, W. M., & Webster-Stratton, C. (2011). The impact of the incredible years parent, child, and teacher training programs on children's co-occurring internalizing symptoms. *School Psychology Quarterly*, 26(3), 189–201.

Hughes, E. K., & Gullone, E. (2010). Parent emotion socialisation practices and their associations with personality and emotion regulation. *Personality and Individual Differences*, 49(7), 694–699.

Kleve, L et al. (2011). Is the incredible years programme effective for children with neurodevelopmental disorders and for families with social services involvement in the "real world" of community CAMHS? *Clinical Child Psychology and Psychiatry*, 16(2), 253–264.

Koneru, B., Carone, E., Malatack, J. J., Esquivel, C. O., & Startzl, T. E. (1993). Missed opportunities in preventive pediatric health care. Immunizations or well-child care visits? *American Journal of Diseases of Children*, 147(10), 1081–1084.

Lavizzo-Mourey, R. (2009). The adolescent obesity epidemic. *Journal of Adolescent Health*, 45(3), S6–S7.

McGorry, P. D., Purcell, R., Goldstone, S., & Amminger, G. (2011). Age of onset and timing of treatment for mental and substance use disorders: Implications for preventive intervention strategies and models of care. *Current Opinion in Psychiatry*, 24(4), 301–306.

Miller, A. L., Smith, H. L., & Hashim, B. L. (2012). Dialectical behavior therapy with multiproblem adolescents. In P. C. Kendall (Ed.), *Child and adolescent therapy: Cognitive-behavioral procedures* (4th ed.), (pp. 398–410). New York: Guilford.

National Campaign to Prevent Teen and Unplanned Pregnancy. (2011). *Counting it up: The public costs of teen childbearing*. Accessed June 5, 2012 from: http://www.thenational-campaign.org/costs/pdf/counting-it-up/key-data.pdf.

National Center on Addiction and Substance Abuse at Colombia University. (2011). *Adolescent substance use: America's #1 public health problem*. Accessed June 1, 2012 from: http://www.casacolumbia.org/upload/2011/20110629adolescentsubstanceuse.pdf.

Newacheck, P. W., Wong, S. T., Galbraith, A. A., & Hung, Y. (2003). Adolescent health care expenditures: A descriptive profile. *Journal of Adolescent Health*, 32(6), 3–11.

Ogden C. L., Carroll, M. D., & Flegal, K. M. (2008). High body mass index for age among US children and adolescents, 2003–2006. *Journal of the American Medical Association*, 299(20), 2401–2405.

O'Donohue, W., & Tolle, L. W. (2009). Behavioral approaches to chronic disease in adolescence: A guide to integrative care. New York: Springer.

Schor, E. L. (2004). Rethinking well-child care. *Pediatrics*, 114(1), 210–216.

Scholer, S.J., Hudnut-Beumler, L., & Dietich, M.S. (2012). Why parents value a brief required primary care intervention that teaches discipline strategies. *Clinical Pediatrics*, 51(4), 1–8.

Seiffge-Krenke, I. (2009). Changes in stress perception and coping during adolescence: The role of situational and personal factors. *Child Development*, 80, 259–279.

Williams, P. G., Holmbeck, G. N., & Greenley, R. N. (2002) Adolescent health psychology. *Journal of Consulting and Clinical Psychology*, 70, 828–842.

Contents

Part I

General Issues in Adolescent Health Psychology

Introduction and the Wellness Imperative with Adolescent Behavioral Health

William T. O'Donohue, Lorraine T. Benuto, Lauren Woodward Tolle, Lucy Payne, and Roxy Davis

Health psychology as a field is focused on the intricate and complex balance between physical and psychological health and disease. While there is a large body of literature dedicated to the study of health psychology, research on both mental and physical health intervention and outcome in adolescents has historically been neglected (Williams, Holmbeck, & Greenley, 2002). This comprehensive handbook seeks to fill this gap by covering a wide range of topics that fall under five general categories: general issues in adolescent health psychology, the developmental processes that occur during adolescence, treatment and training of professionals as each relate to adolescent health psychology, mental health and adolescents, and physical health and adolescents. In this introductory chapter we focus on the following: child/adolescent well-visits as being health-promoting and preventative (both of which appear as themes throughout the book); screening in primary care; preventative interventions in adolescence; and public health crises affecting adolescents. The organization of the handbook is also reviewed.

W.T. O'Donohue, Ph.D. (✉) • L. Payne • R. Davis
Department of Psychology, University of Nevada, Reno, MS 0296, Reno, NV 89557, USA
e-mail: wto@unr.edu

L.T. Benuto, Ph.D.
Department of Psychology, Victims of Crime Treatment Center, University of Nevada, Reno, MS 0296, Reno, NV 89557, USA
e-mail: dr.benuto@gmail.com

L.W. Tolle, Ph.D.
Aurora Mental Health Center's Health Home, Aurora Mental Health Center, 11059 East Bethany Drive Suite 105, Aurora, CO 80014, USA
e-mail: lauren.tolle@gmail.com

Child/Adolescent Well-Visits

Wellness and periodic health checkups have long been instrumental in disease prevention and early diagnosis in primary care settings. Annual well-child (by child we also include adolescents) checkups specifically, have led to substantial reduction in many of the acute morbidities of the early twentieth century, increased survival from acute illness, and decrease childhood and infant mortality overall (Schor, 2012). These visits aim to achieve two primary goals: (1) promoting health and (2) preventing disease. The American Academy of Pediatrics (AAP) has created a set of guidelines for well-child visits, delineating what the physician should accomplish at each appointment. The Recommendations for Preventive Pediatric Health Care lists a series of tests, exams, screening, and immunizations that are appropriate for each visit. There are five basic areas of focus on the traditional well-child visit: (1) immunization for disease prevention, (2) monitoring and optimization of physical growth, (3) early detection of disease, (4) health promotion (safety and injury prevention, physics activity, nutrition), and (5) anticipatory guidance (eating, sleeping, self-control, discipline) (Talen, Stephens, Marik, & Buchholz, 2007).

W.T. O'Donohue et al. (eds.), *Handbook of Adolescent Health Psychology*,
DOI 10.1007/978-1-4614-6633-8_1, © Springer Science+Business Media New York 2013

These recommendations also include a developmental and behavioral assessment, that includes a developmental screening, autism screening, psychosocial/behavioral assessment, and alcohol and drug use assessment. In practice, however, well-child visits largely neglect aspects related to psychological and emotional health. What is most alarming is that the field of psychology has also failed to address this issue. Some efforts have been made to incorporate psychological screening and interventions during well-child visits. Scholer, Hudnut-Beumler and Dietrich (2012) implemented the use of a mandatory 10 min parenting video during the well-child visit. Participating parents reacted positively. More specifically, participating parents reported that they benefited from the instructional video on a personal level, indicating that the video was educational, reinforced their parenting and facilitated communication about parenting issues with their physicians. However, aside from a few isolated attempts, there is a large gap between parents' expressed interests, child and adolescent needs, and what actually happens in well-child visits. One survey (Bethell, Reuland, Halfon, & Schor, 2004) indicated that nearly all parents had at least one unmet need for psychosocial concerns. Another study indicated that 40 % of parents were asked about their children's learning, development, or behavior (Bethell et al., 2002). These data, although not surprising, certainly indicates that there is a gap between actual practice and ideal practice.

The general population has increasingly more information about the benefits of prevention and seeing a health care professional periodically. Cancer, heart disease, prenatal care, are just some of prevention and early detection efforts that can make a significant impact in the course and outcome of treatment. Dentistry is not much different. It is not uncommon for people to visit their dentist for a cleaning and checkup. When it comes to mental health care, the picture looks very different. Psychology has yet to fully join other fields when it comes to prevention. There are arguably several efforts to develop and implement prevention programs in schools and other settings. These programs are not yet widespread, and many lack adequate research and support from other agencies, including managed care organizations. Significant efforts are few and far between, and have adequately met the needs of population. Even when it comes to actual treatment a large portion of the population do not know that we have effective treatments for a variety of emotional difficulties, or that seeking help early before the problem leads to significant impairment in one's regular routine can help keep things from every getting that bad—or that there are several options for skills training (social skills, interpersonal skills, emotion regulation, etc.) that can be effective in helping people manage their difficulties. It can be said that part of the reason why psychological treatments are so unpopular is because of the dominance of the medical model and pharmacological treatments, as well as therapies that either harm or do not work (Lilienfeld, 2007; Whitaker, 2010). But that is hardly the whole story. What have we, as psychologists, really done to mainstream these effective treatments and make them a part of people's lives? One solution might come in the form of early and periodical intervention, such as with well-child checkups. Although the AAP guidelines are meant to encompass mental health checkups, the reality is much different. By bringing the responsibility of this important task to the field of psychology we would be able to provide more comprehensive and specialized services. In the remainder of this paper we discuss the model of a psychological well-child checkup and the overall goals. Then a detailed suggestion for three different age groups (adolescence, middle/late childhood, and early childhood) is provided.

As discussed above, the real picture of well-child visits in clinical practice is slightly different than what might have been intended by the AAP with its guidelines. Nonetheless, within its two primary goals of promoting health and disease prevention, well-child checkups can be said to focus on three main areas: (1) early detection of disease, (2) early intervention, and (3) immunization. The application of these same goals to a model of psychological well-child visits may cover an important gap in current practice. What would an annual psychological well-child checkup look like? We can begin exploring the ideas of a well-child checkup by applying the same main areas of focus within the medical model, namely, early detection, early intervention, and immunization. The primary goals of health promotion and disease prevention would also apply to the psychological model. First, early detection of psychopathology or problematic behavior can have great impact in treatment outcome. For example, early autism diagnosis is associated with more favorable treatment outcomes (e.g., Eikesth, Klintwall, Jahr, & Karlson, 2012). Similarly, detecting parenting difficulties early can potentially prevent significant common problems in later life—including adolescence—such as depression, suicidality, or delinquent behavior. If problems are detected, early intervention of course, would be implemented. For example, Linehan (1993) suggests that a pervasively invalidating environment for a child who is highly sensitive and highly reactive to emotions can lead to significant problematic behaviors later such as parasuicidal and suicidal behaviors. If such problems could be identified early on, before the pattern of problematic behavior emerges, it is likely that significant changes in family functioning can be achieved. Finally, a model of psychological well-child checkups can serve to teach skills and build resiliency in both parents and children. Social skills, emotion regulations kills, psychoeducation about bullying, effective problem solving, relationships, etc. could all be implemented in these regular visits in an age appropriate fashion.

Another benefit of annual well-child checkups would be the potential to reach more people, and intervene before impairment occurs. These can take place either during the annual well-child checkup at the pediatrician's office if an integrated care behavioral health person is co-located, or by an appropriately trained mental health professional in their office. The current model for psychological interventions utilizes the criterion of significant impairment in one or more life domains. Although this criterion makes sense in terms of making a diagnosis, it is less useful for intervention purposes. Most successful treatments we know, both in the medical and psychological fields, are those that are implemented early. Therefore, regular visits would allow the quick detection of problems as they first arise. Behavioral differences across time would be easily monitored and any developmental problems detected. For example, suppose a child comes for their well-child visit at age 6 and displays age appropriate social skills and behaviors. However, during the psychological checkup in the following year, this child appears withdrawn. It would be clear that a significant change occurred within the past year, and the psychologist would be prompted to further assess the child's difficulties. Clearly, we do not currently have an exhaustive list of evidence based prevention programs and treatments that could be easily implemented. Much still needs to be learned. However, the existence of periodic psychological checkup would set the occasion for further development of these programs and a wide range of materials such as parenting videos, self-help materials, Web sites.

Psychology faces other challenges that could be ameliorated by the implementation of well-child checkups. First, the scope and reach of our services is often limited to those that are experiencing significant distress. We have learned a great deal about human behavior, psychopathology, problematic behaviors, and treatment, but we are still limited to a simplified model of 50-min one-on-one sessions that fail to reach a broader public that could also benefit from our services. Many of these people we currently do not reach may even experience significant distress, but do not come to seek our services due a stigma about psychological treatment that is still prevalent in our society. Regular visits that start in childhood could potentially bring psychological treatments into the mainstream, making it more of a routine part of one's care, as it is going to the dentist when one has a cavity.

Adolescence is a period in which many of the high prevalence disorders of adulthood begin to emerge, such as anxiety, depression and substance abuse (McGorry et al., 2011). It is therefore critical for the availability of mental health prevention, early identification and intervention efforts in systems with which adolescents frequently come in contact. Accordingly, primary care screening for anxiety, depression and substance abuse is appropriate, however, complicated. Self-report measures of substance use in adolescence are notoriously unreliable (Harris et al., 2008); furthermore, some experimentation with drugs in adolescence is normative and perhaps even adaptive (Tucker et al., 2006), so subjecting all adolescents to drug screening in a routine psychological checkup would likely cause unnecessary stress for both the adolescents being screened and their parents. Screening for Oppositional Defiant Disorder and Conduct Disorder is also recommended at this age; although ODD symptoms usually develop by age 8, diagnosis of ODD tends to overlap significantly with CD, which more commonly emerges during adolescence (James & Campbell, 2006). Finally, eating disorders tend to emerge concurrently with the onset of puberty in early adolescence, so it is important to assess for them at this age as well (Moon & Campbell, 2006).

Screening in Primary Care

Depressive and anxiety disorders are typically diagnosed via self-report; scales exist that are specifically designed for late childhood and adolescence. Assessment of ODD and CD is excessively complicated and costly for a routine checkup, so clinicians should simply screen for indicators of problem behavior and refer for a more comprehensive evaluation when appropriate. Eating disorders are typically diagnosed through the use of a semi-structured interview called the Eating Disorders Examination; however, as the purpose of the psychological well-child assessment is not diagnosis, but rather preliminary screening and referral when necessary, conducting this interview in this setting would be inappropriate. Instead, the clinician should interview both child and parent about the child's eating behaviors, stress, and body image; it is important that these interviews be conducted separately, since adolescents with disordered eating are often unwilling to discuss these problems in front of their parents (Moon & Campbell, 2006).

Another approach might be to use the CBCL/6–18 and the Youth Self Report, a frequently used self-report questionnaire that is completed by the adolescent regarding his/her own behavior. The YSR possesses the same eight-syndrome scale structure as the CBCL/6–18, and is used to generate the same type of score report, in which the individual is compared to empirically determined norms. As with the other dimensional assessment instruments, the results from this scale may suggest a diagnosis if they are in the clinical range, or indicate that the adolescent would benefit from a preventive intervention if results are subclinical but elevated, or are trending towards clinical over time. The utility of the CBCL/6–18 and YSR in predicting long-term psychosocial outcomes among adolescents has been demonstrated empirically: Jaspers et al. (2012) found that emotional and behavioral problems as identified by the CBCL and YSR were highly stable from age 11 to 17. This also highlights the importance of prevention and early intervention for behavioral and emotional problems in adolescence.

Preventive Interventions in Adolescence

Two factors that emerge as being primary contributors to adolescent psychological and behavior problems are emotion dysregulation and poor social skills. In recent years a significant body of research has emerged identifying emotion dysregulation as a core feature across many behavior problems and psychopathology afflicting this age group, including depression, anxiety, aggression, eating disorders, and dating violence perpetration, (Compas, Jaser, & Benson, 2009; Haynos & Fruzzetti, 2011; Hughes & Gullone, 2011; McLaughlin et al., 2011; Shorey et al., 2011). Social competence is a key skill for successful functioning in adult life; adolescence is a time when social relationships become more complex and adult-like, so it is a crucial time to bolster social skills. Evidence shows that social skills deficits are implicated in many psychological disorders (Campbell, Hansen, & Nangle, 2010), and that social skills training programs, while not particularly effective on their own, are a valuable addition when incorporated into other treatment approaches (Spence, 2003).

While the literature is lacking in empirically validated preventive interventions for this age group that focus on emotion regulation and social skills, we propose that a prevention program focusing on these areas would likely be effective in reducing adolescent psychopathology. For example, Dialectical Behavior Therapy (DBT) is an integrative, largely skill-based treatment that incorporates both emotion regulation strategies and interpersonal effectiveness skills. Although no randomized controlled trials have been conducted with DBT for adolescents, it has been used as a treatment for suicidal and severely dysfunctional adolescents who have difficulty regulating their emotions and behavior, and the results so far are promising (Miller, Smith, & Hashim, 2012). Adaptation of the skills used in DBT into a more general prevention format could prove effective for prevention of adolescent psychopathology.

Public Health Crises Affecting Adolescents

A number of public health care crises uniquely affect adolescents, and their prevalence has shifted over the last decade. The National Center on Addiction and Substance Abuse at Colombia University identified adolescent substance use as America's #1 public health problem (CASA, 2011), despite evidence that adolescent substance use rates have been declining since 1999. In their report, it is identified that 75 % of high school students have tried an addictive substance (cigarettes, alcohol, marijuana, cocaine) and 50 % use them on an ongoing basis. It is also reported that these figures are likely an underestimation of adolescent substance use rates as this does not include adolescents who have dropped out of high school or who are incarcerated. Both the immediate and long-term consequences of adolescent substance use can be devastating. Impaired brain functioning, injuries, unintended pregnancies, criminal justice system involvement, chronic disease, addiction and death are just some of the potential consequences. CASA estimates that the cost for adolescent alcohol use is $68.0 billion, placing a significant burden on a number of systems, including juvenile and criminal justice, education, and health care (CASA, 2011). Adolescence is a time when experimenting with substances is frequently observed. At a developmental period when a host of mental health problems also surface, the potential for co-morbid substance use problems is enhanced by substances' perceived ability to help with coping, manage stress, look cool, or escape problems.

Rates of teen pregnancy have decreased significantly over the last decade, though 3 in 10 adolescent females will become pregnant at least once before the age of 20 (Aruda & Burke, 2013). These figures constitute significant costs both to the adolescent mother and the community at large. Specifically, teen childbearing in the USA cost taxpayers (federal, state, and local) at least $10.9 billion in 2008, according to an updated analysis by The National Campaign to Prevent Teen and Unplanned Pregnancy (2011). Most of the costs of teen childbearing are associated with negative consequences for the children of teen mothers, including increased costs for health care, foster care, incarceration, and lost tax revenue. At the individual level, teen mothers are at risk for lower educational attainment, school dropout, poverty and/or low income, poorer outcomes for their children, including higher risk for sons to be incarcerated and daughters to become teen mothers themselves (Aruda & Burke, 2013).

Adolescent obesity in the USA has tripled since 1970. An estimated one-third of adolescents age 12–19 are overweight or obese (Ogden, Carroll, & Flegal, 2008). Chronic diseases associated with obesity such as type 2 diabetes and hypertension, which are historically diagnosed in adults, are now being diagnosed in adolescence. Adolescents who are obese are also at higher risk for additional chronic illnesses, including heart disease, stroke, asthma, and some forms of cancer, in addition to having an 80 % chance of becoming an obese adult. Direct medical expenses attributed to childhood obesity are estimated at $14.0 billion per year (Lavizzo-Mourey, 2009).

These three public health epidemics facing adolescents are not new or emerging problems.

Rather, these problems have been consistent for decades and intervention efforts at a number of levels: individual, family, school, and community have been utilized. While trends for teen substance use and pregnancy have been decreasing, continued efforts are needed not only to treat the ongoing problem, but to push to prevent it and promote healthier alternatives. Service delivery of effective interventions need to be targeted to adolescents in a way that is acceptable to adolescents and meets them where they are. Innovative and upcoming prevention and intervention efforts such as hot spotting, or targeting areas identified at being at high risk, cross-age peer mentoring, and interventions using technology (online interventions, apps for smart phones, social networking) provide just a few applications for researchers and clinicians to consider. Interventions need to be designed to impact change not only at the micro- and meso-systems that adolescents interface with, including parents, peers, schools, community health care centers, and neighborhoods but also at the public policy level.

Organization of the Handbook

The field of health psychology explores the intricate and complex associations between physical and psychological health and disease. There is a vast amount of literature dedicated to the study of health psychology, although research on both mental and physical health intervention and outcome in adolescents has historically been neglected (Williams, Holmbeck, & Greenley, 2002). This book is a comprehensive volume that covers a wide range of topics that fall under five general categories: general issues in adolescent health psychology, the developmental processes that occur during adolescence, treatment and training of professionals as each relate to adolescent health psychology, mental health and adolescents, and physical health and adolescents. Each of these general categories translates to a section in this book and each section contains several chapters that address topics that fall within each of the aforementioned categories. The book has been organized in this manner as a review of the scientific literature, books that focus on adolescents that are related to health (physical or mental), and books that focus on health psychology (although not on adolescents) revealed several important topics that seemed to merit a discussion in the. A description of each book section follows.

General Issues Related to Adolescent Health Psychology

As indicated above, the field of health psychology is vast and given the development processes that occur during adolescence certain issues related to the field of adolescent health psychology merit a detailed discussion. In the first section of the book general issues in adolescent health psychology are discussed. Specifically a biopsychosocial perspective on adolescent health and disease is presented with an emphasis on risk-taking behaviors and the various biological, psychosocial, and environmental factors found to be associated with adolescent risk-taking behaviors. Next the influences that sociocultural and socioeconomic factors can have on adolescent health are explored. In this first section of this book there are also chapters on public health approaches to adolescent health, epidemiology of adolescent health, disease prevention in adolescence, and determinants of health-related behaviors in adolescence. Other topics covered within this general section include stress, emotional regulation and resilience in adolescence; mental health literacy; measurements and quality life instruments used with adolescents; the effects of physical activity on health; and sexual assault and intimate partner violence as each relates to the adolescent.

Adolescent Development

Adolescence is clearly a time during which much change occurs. These changes occur on multiple developmental levels including changes that are emotional, social, and physical. Naturally these changes can carry an impact on adolescent health both psychological and physical. Thus, the second section of this book focuses on adolescent development. Specifically, a discussion of continuity of behavior and parenting from childhood through adolescence is provided; school performance of the adolescent is discussed (with a discussion on factors that can influence school performance, e.g., chronic illness); brain development in the adolescent reviewed; puberty and its role in adolescent maturation is explored; and the literature on adolescent sexuality and sexual behavior is reviewed.

Treatment

O'Donohue et al. (in this book) emphasize how adolescents drivers of high health care costs in part due to their underuse of office visits and overuse of emergency department care (Newacheck, Wong, Galbraith, & Hung, 2003); how during the transition from childhood to adulthood, adolescents establish patterns of behavior and make lifestyle choices that affect both their current and future health (Centers for Disease Control and Prevention, 2011; O'Donohue & Tolle, 2009); and how adolescence is a significant intervention point for behavior change (O'Donohue & Tolle, 2009). Therefore, a discussion on the treatment (both medical and behavioral) of the adolescent is warranted. Therefore, in this book chapters relevant to intervention effectiveness research, training issues in adolescent health, delivery of interventions, confidentiality and care, and treatment adherence are included.

Mental Health

As indicated earlier in this chapter, the field of health psychology explores the intricate and complex associations between physical and psychological health and disease. Therefore, naturally sections of this book relevant to medical and physical conditions as well as mental health conditions are necessary. Here we describe the chapters on mental health disorders and below we discuss medical/physical conditions. With regard to mental health disorders, our approach to determining which topics to cover was twofold. First we examined the Diagnostic and Statistical Manual of Mental Disorders 4th Edition Text Revision (DSM-IV-TR: American Psychiatric Association, 2000) and determined which of the broad categories in the DSM-IV-TR were both relevant to the adolescent and merited a lengthy discussion. Second, we considered other circumstances or situations that arise during adolescence that are related to mental health. This process resulted in the inclusion of chapters on smoking, substance use, ADHD, anti-social behavior, personality disorders, self-harm, eating disorders, anxiety, depression and suicide-related behaviors, and intellectual disabilities.

Medical/Physical Conditions

With regard to physical and medical conditions, a review of the scientific literature, books that focus on adolescents that are related to health (physical or mental), and books that focus on health psychology (although not on adolescents) led us to determine which topics related to medical/physical conditions should be included in this handbook. The topics that we cover that are specific to medical/physical conditions are pregnancy, sexually transmitted infections, HIV, obesity, cardiovascular conditions, asthma, endocrine disorders, musculoskeletal injuries, and headaches.

References

American Psychiatric Association. (2000). *Diagnostic and statistical manual of mental disorders* (4th ed.). Washington, DC: American Psychiatric Association (Text revised).

Aruda, M., & Burke, P. (2013). Pregnancy in adolescence. In W. O'Donohue, L. Benuto, & L. Tolle (Eds.), *Handbook of adolescent health psychology*. New York: Springer.

Bethell, C., Peck, C., Abrams, M., Halfon, N., Sareen, H., & Collins, K. S. (2002). *Partnering with parents to promote the healthy development of young children enrolled in medicaid*. New York: The Commonwealth Fund.

Bethell, C., Reuland, C. P., Halfon, N., & Schor, E. L. (2004). Measuring the quality of preventive and developmental services for young children: National estimates and patterns of clinicians' performance. *Pediatrics, 113*, 1973–1983.

Compas, B. E., Jaser, S. S., & Benson, M. A. (2009). Coping and emotion regulation: Implications for understanding depression during adolescence. In S. Nolen-Hoeksema, L. M. Hilt, S. Nolen-Hoeksema, L. M. Hilt (Eds.), Handbook of depression in adolescents (pp. 419–440). New York, NY US: Routledge/Taylor & Francis Group.

Eikeseth, S., Klintwall, L., Jahr, E., & Karlsson, P. (2012). Outcome for children with autism receiving early and intensive behavioral intervention in mainstream preschool and kindergarten settings. *Research in Autism Spectrum Disorders, 6*, 829–835.

Harris, K. M., Griffin, B., McCaffrey, D. F., & Morral, A. R. (2008). Inconsistencies in self-reported drug use by adolescents in substance abuse treatment: Implications for outcome and performance measurements. *Journal of Substance abuse Treatment, 34*(3), 347–355.

Haynos, A. F., & Fruzzetti, A. E. (2011). Anorexia nervosa as a disorder of emotion dysregulation: Evidence and treatment implications. *Clinical Psychology: Science and Practice, 18*(3), 183–202.

Hughes, E. K., & Gullone, E. (2011). Emotion regulation moderates relationships between body image concerns and psychological symptomatology. *Body Image, 8*(3), 224–231.

James, C. L., & Campbell, J. M. (2006). Conduct disorder and oppositional defiant disorder. In R. W. Kamphaus, J. M. Campbell, R. W. Kamphaus, J. M. Campbell (Eds.), Psychodiagnostic assessment of children: Dimensional and categorical approaches (pp. 357–389). Hoboken, NJ US: John Wiley & Sons Inc.

Jaspers, M., de Winter, A. F., Huisman, M., Verhulst, F. C., Ormel, J., Stewart, R. E., & Reijneveld, S. A. (2012). Trajectories of psychosocial problems in adolescents predicted by findings from early well-child assessments. *Journal of Adolescent Health.*

Lavizzo-Mourey, R. (2009). The adolescent obesity epidemic. *Journal of Adolescent Health, 45*(3), S6–S7.

Lilienfeld, S. O. (2007). Psychological treatments that cause harm. *Perspectives on Psychological Science, 2*, 53–70.

Linehan, M. M. (1993). Skills Training Manual For Treatment of Borderline Personality Disorder. New York Guilford Press.

McGorry, P. D., Purcell, R., Goldstone, S., & Amminger, G. (2011). Age of onset and timing of treatment for mental and substance use disorders: Implications for preventive intervention strategies and models of care. *Current Opinion in Psychiatry, 24*(4), 301–306.

McLaughlin, K. A., Hatzenbuehler, M. L., Mennin, D. S., & Nolen-Hoeksema, S. (2011). Emotion dysregulation and adolescent psychopathology: A prospective study. *Behaviour Research And Therapy, 49*(9), 544–554.

Miller, A. L., Smith, H. L., & Hashim, B. L. (2012). Dialectical behavior therapy with multiproblem adolescents. In P. C. Kendall & P. C. Kendall (Eds.), *Child and adolescent therapy: Cognitive-behavioral procedures* (4th ed., pp. 398–410). New York: Guilford Press.

Moon, K. F., & Campbell, J. M. (2006). Eating and feeding disorders. In R. W. Kamphaus, J. M. Campbell, R. W. Kamphaus, J. M. Campbell (Eds.), Psychodiagnostic assessment of children: Dimensional and categorical approaches (pp. 283–317). Hoboken, NJ US: John Wiley & Sons Inc.

National Center on Addiction and Substance Abuse at Colombia University. (2011). *Adolescent substance use: America's #1 public health problem.* Retrieved June 1, 2012, from http://www.casacolumbia.org/upload/2011/20110629adolescentsubstanceuse.pdf.

Newacheck, P. W., Wong, S. T., Galbraith, A. A., Hung, Y. Y. (2003). Adolescent health care expenditures: a descriptive profile. *Journal of Adolescent Health 32*(6 Suppl), 3–11.

O'Donohue, W., & Tolle, L. W. (Eds.) (2009). Behavioral approaches to chronic disease in adolescence: A guide to integrative care. NY: Springer.

Ogden, C. L., Carroll, M. D., & Flegal, K. M. (2008). High body mass index for age among US children and adolescents, 2003–2006. *Journal of the American Medical Association, 299*(20), 2401–2405.

Scholer, S. J., Hudnut-Beumler, L., & Dietich, M. S. (2012). Why parents value a brief required primary care intervention that teaches discipline strategies. *Clinical Pediatrics, 51*(4), 1–8.

Schor, E. L. (2012). Rethinking well-child care. *Pediatrics, 114*(1), 210–216.

Shorey, R. C., Brasfield, H., Febres, J., & Stuart, G. L. (2011). An examination of the association between difficulties with emotion regulation and dating violence perpetration. *Journal of Aggression, Maltreatment & Trauma, 20*(8), 870–885.

Spence, S. H. (2003). Social skills training with children and young people: Theory, evidence and practice. *Child and Adolescent Mental Health, 8*(2), 84–96.

Talen, M. R., Stephens, L., Marik, P., & Buchholz, M. (2007). Well-child check-up revised: An efficient protocol for assessing children's social-emotional development. *Families, Systems, & Health, 25*(1), 23–35.

Tucker, J. S., Ellickson, P. L., Collins, R. L., & Klein, D. J. (2006). Are drug experimenters better adjusted than abstainers and users?: A longitudinal study of adolescent marijuana use. *Journal of Adolescent Health, 39*(4), 488–494.

The National Center on Addiction and Substance Abuse at Columbia University (2011). Adolescent Substance Abuse: America's #1 Public Health Problem. Downloaded June 2012 from: http://www.casacolumbia.org/upload/2011/20110629adolescentsubstanceuse.pdf.

National Campaign to Prevent Teen and Unplanned Pregnancy (2011). *Counting it up: The public costs of teen childbearing*. Retrieved June 5, 2012, from http://www.thenationalcampaign.org/costs/pdf/counting-it-up/key-data.pdf.

Whitaker, R. (2010). Anatomy of an epidemic: Magic bullets, psychiatric drugs, and the astonishing rise of mental illness in America. New York: Crown Publishers.

Williams, P. G., Holmbeck, G. N., & Greenley, R. N. (2002). Adolescent health psychology. *Journal of Consulting and Clinical Psychology, 70*, 828–842.

A Biopsychosocial Perspective of Adolescent Health and Disease

Jessica M. Sales and Charles E. Irwin Jr.

Adolescence is a developmental stage characterized by dramatic physical, cognitive, social and emotional changes. For most adolescents, it is a period marked by rapid physiological change, increased independence, a change in family relationships that is more interdependent, prioritizing peer affiliations, initiation of intimate partner relationships, identity formation, increased awareness of morals and values, and cognitive and emotional maturation. Despite the rapid change, the majority of adolescents cope successfully with the demands of physical, cognitive, and emotional development during this time period (Cicchetti & Rogosch, 2002). In addition to the "positive growth" seen during adolescence, it is also a developmental stage recognized for turmoil and challenges, partly due to increased exploration and risk-taking typical of adolescence. Although considered to be a normative part of adolescence, risk-taking behaviors are nonetheless concerning to parents, peers, teachers, clinicians, researchers, and society because these actions often endanger adolescents' current and future health and well-being (Sales & Irwin, 2009).

Risk is defined as a chance of loss and risk-taking is often defined as engaging in behaviors that may have harmful consequences, but simultaneously provide an outcome that can also be perceived as positive (Beyth-Marom & Fischoff, 1997). For example, driving too fast is considered a risk-taking behavior because it can result in a positive feeling (i.e., rush of adrenaline) while the action is occurring, but it also can result in serious harm to self or others (i.e., health-endangering). Examples of frequent health-endangering behaviors adolescents engage in include the use of tobacco and alcohol, experimentation with illicit and/or prescription drugs, unsafe sexual activities, poor eating habits, as well as delinquent actions (Centers for Disease Control and Prevention, 2010).

Adolescent risk-taking is concerning because of the immediate danger it poses, but also because research has demonstrated that the behaviors established during adolescence often persist into adulthood (Park, Mulye, Adams, Brindis, & Irwin, 2006). The potential long-term consequences of engaging in the most prevalent adolescent risk-taking behaviors include substance abuse, cancers associated with tobacco use, unwanted pregnancies, sexually transmitted infections (STIs) including HIV, obesity or other health problems caused by problem eating (i.e., eating disorders), and serious criminal activity (Sales & Irwin, 2009). For instance, in 2010 the *Monitoring the Future Study* found that

J.M. Sales, Ph.D. (✉)
Department of Behavioral Sciences and Health Education, Rollins School of Public Health, Emory University, 1518 Clifton Road Room 570, Atlanta, GA 30322, USA
e-mail: jmcderm@emory.edu

C.E. Irwin Jr., M.D.
Division of Adolescent Medicine, Department of Pediatrics, School of Medicine, University of California, San Francisco, Box 0503, LH 245, San Francisco, CA 94143, USA
e-mail: irwinch@peds.ucsf.edu

W.T. O'Donohue et al. (eds.), *Handbook of Adolescent Health Psychology*,
DOI 10.1007/978-1-4614-6633-8_2, © Springer Science+Business Media New York 2013

41 % of high school seniors had consumed alcohol in the past 30 days, and over 35 % had used marijuana in the past year, with 6.1 % using marijuana daily, and that the use of non-prescribed prescription-type drugs was high (21.6 % lifetime use) (Johnston et al., 2011). Specific to sexual behavior, after a decade of declining adolescent pregnancy rates, in 2006 the numbers inclined (Centers for Disease Control and Prevention (CDC), 2008), and in 2007 a report by the CDC indicated that one in four adolescent females have had an STI, with rates doubling in certain subgroups (Forhan et al., 2008). Finally, juveniles accounted for 17 percent of all arrests and 16 percent of all violent crime arrests in 1999 (Snyder, 2000). Adolescent female detainees are currently the fastest growing population of incarcerated adolescents. In 2008, female adolescents represented 30 % of total juvenile arrests. While the overall crime rate has declined in the past decade, the incarceration rate for girls, relative to boys, decreased less than males in most categories of crimes, including violent offenses (Puzzanchera, 2009).

Adolescent death is the ultimate consequence of risk-taking, with most cases of mortality in the USA during the adolescent period (approximately 75 %) resulting from preventable causes like motor vehicle crashes, unintended injuries, homicide and suicide (Fingerhut & Anderson, 2008). Thus, due to the immediate and long-term health consequences associated with adolescent risk-taking, identifying and understanding factors associated with adolescent risk-taking have become a public health priority. A variety of factors, including biological, psychosocial, and environmental, have been found to be associated with various adolescent risk-taking behaviors (Irwin & Millstein, 1986; Sales & Irwin, 2009). However, many studies, as well as theories, of risk-taking behavior are uni-dimensional and predominately focus on either biological, psychological, or environmental factors independently as they affect risk-taking.

Given the complexity of behavior, to provide a complete framework for examining the range of factors found to influence adolescent risk-taking behavior a theory or model must simultaneously take into account the role of biology, psychosocial influences, and the environment. In line with this ideology, the National Institute of Health (NIH) issued a report explicitly stating the need for a better understanding of the interaction between biology, environment, and behavior and stressed the utility of such an approach for advancing our understanding of behavior, particularly behaviors which place one at risk (Working Group of the NIH Advisory Committee, 2004). The biopsychosocial model of risk-taking (Irwin & Millstein, 1986) provides a framework in which social environmental factors as well as existing biological and psychological predispositions interact to influence risk-taking behavior.

In the remainder of this chapter, we (1) briefly review the studies or theories of risk-taking that focus predominately on one factor (i.e., biological, psychological, and environmental) as it related to risk-taking behavior; (2) describe the multi-dimensional biopsychosocial model of risk-taking; (3) provide empirical evidence supporting the utility of the biopsychosocial model for better understanding various adolescent health-endangering behaviors; and (4) suggest future directions for the utility of the biopsychosocial model of risk-taking for advancing our understanding of adolescent health.

The Biology of Adolescent Risk-Taking

Biological factors are thought to influence risk-taking behaviors through four sources: (1) genetic predispositions, (2) "direct" hormonal influences, (3) the influence of asynchronous pubertal timing (i.e., earlier or later timing than peers), and (4) brain/central nervous system development. Examples of each type of biological influence are presented in turn.

Genetic Predispositions

Long before the mapping of the human genome, the familial nature of health risk behaviors led some to speculate about the role of genetic predispositions in risk-taking behaviors. Early evidence from family studies demonstrated that risk-taking behaviors tended to cluster within families. Examples include substance abuse, criminal activity, and injury-related behavior. Specific to injury, Schor (1987) found that a small number of families accounted for a disproportionately large number of injury-related health care visits, and individual members of these "high injury" families had similar rates of unintentional injuries, with injury rates being stable over time. Moreover, many studies have demonstrated that children of alcoholics are nearly four times more likely than children of nonalcoholics to abuse alcohol as adults (Adger, 1991; Windle, 1997). Eloquently designed twin-adoption studies have been able to disentangle the effects of shared environment or learned behaviors from genetic predispositions, as children of alcoholic biological parents show a greater predisposition toward alcohol abuse even when raised by nonalcoholic adoptive parents (Cloninger, 1987).

Recent advances in genotyping techniques now allow the ability to further explore the role of genetic predispositions on adolescent risk-taking behaviors. For example, in regard to alcohol use, genetic studies support the Al allele of the D2 dopamine receptor gene (DRD2) as a risk marker for alcoholism and substance use disorders. Conner and colleagues (2005) found that male adolescents with the A1 (+) allele tried and got intoxicated on alcohol more often than boys without this genetic marker providing support for the DRD2 A1 allele as a marker identifying a subgroup of adolescent males at high risk for developing substance use problems.

Further, a genetic vulnerability factor in the promoter region of the serotonin transporter gene (5-HTTLPR) has been associated with both substance use and risky sexual behavior. One study conducted with adolescents found that substance use had a significant impact on the sexual risk behavior of youth with one or two copies of the short allele (the genetic variant associated with risk) at this site, but substance use had little effect on sexual behavior for youth without the short allele (Kogan et al., 2010).

These are only two examples of the current work in this emerging field. As the ability to affordably collect and analyze genetic data becomes more feasible, identifying other genetic markers that predispose adolescents towards other risk-taking behaviors is, certainly on the horizons.

Direct Hormonal Influences

Adolescence is a period also marked hormonal changes (increased reproductive/sex hormones, including estrogen, testosterone, etc.) (Spear, 2000). Puberty is associated with increases in gonadal sex hormones (Spear, 2000), and hormones have been postulated to play a role in brain development and in adolescent risk-taking (Irwin & Millstein, 1986; Shirtcliff, 2009; Steinberg, 2008). Hormones influence brain maturation of white matter (Asato, Terwilliger, Woo, & Luna, 2010; Perrin et al., 2008), and sex hormones contribute to the reorganization of dopaminergic neurons in the motivational system (Sisk & Zehr, 2005; Steinberg, 2008), which can then lead to behavioral manifestations in puberty (Shirtcliff, 2009; Sisk & Zehr, 2005; Steinberg, 2008). Hormones are necessary to activate neural circuitry dedicated to sexuality (Shirtcliff, 2009; Sisk & Foster, 2004), but are no longer necessary once individuals become sexually experienced (Shirtcliff, 2009). Stronger findings of the effects of sex hormones such as testosterone on sexual behavior are more commonly reported among females than males since small changes in testosterone are able to stimulate females' sex drive. According to Udry et al. (1986), the effects of androgens, such as testosterone, on sexual behavior of adolescent girls work directly on motivation for sexuality, libido, and possibly also personality. All these factors make adolescence and puberty particularly vulnerable periods, especially for young females in regard to sexual decision-making.

Influence of Asynchronous Pubertal Maturation

The timing of pubertal maturation is related to both genetics and hormonal fluctuations. For example, menarcheal age of mothers and daughters are usually significantly correlated, and physical pubertal development is preceded by elevations in respective sex steroid levels. There is recent evidence that pubertal timing in females is impacted by environmental factors as well, such as presence or absence of the father during childhood (Belsky, 2011; Deardorff et al., 2011).

Asynchronous pubertal maturation is maturation that occurs earlier or later than peers, and it has been hypothesized to be a factor in risk-taking (Irwin & Millstein, 1986). Physically mature-appearing adolescents, because of their older appearance, may be more apt to associate with older peers and engage in "adult" behaviors such as smoking, drinking, and sexual intercourse (Brooks-Gunn, 1988), and engaging in such behaviors may then be supported and imitated by peers. Research indicates that early maturing females are more likely to initiate sexual intercourse at younger ages (Phinney, Jensen, Olsen, & Cundick, 1990). Younger age at sexual debut is associated with less consistent contraception and increased numbers of lifetime sex partners, resulting in an increased risk for pregnancy and STIs (Ford et al., 2005; Kaestle, Halpern, Miller, & Ford, 2005; Manning, Longmore, & Giordano, 2000).

Brain and Central Nervous System Development

Recent advances in developmental neuroscience indicate that the brain continues to develop into adulthood. In fact, the cognitive-control system in the brain, which regulates impulse control, is a slow maturing system and makes adolescence a time of heightened vulnerability for risk-taking behavior (Steinberg, 2004). According to Steinberg (2007), adolescent risk-taking is the product of both logical reasoning and psychosocial factors. Logical reasoning abilities are mostly fully developed by the age of 15. However, the psychosocial capacities (i.e., impulse control, emotion regulation, delay of gratification, and resistance to peer influence) that facilitate decision-making and moderate risk-taking are guided by the cognitive-control systems in the brain and this system continues to mature well into young adulthood (Steinberg, 2004, 2007). The cognitive-control system, which mainly consists of outer regions of the brain such as the lateral prefrontal and parietal cortices and portions of the anterior cingulated cortex, is involved in executive function tasks like planning, thinking ahead, impulse control, and self-regulation (Giedd, 2008).

In addition, according to a recent review by Steinberg (2008), puberty is associated with the remodeling of dopaminergic pathways in the socioemotional brain system that influence reward salience and reward sensitivity, especially in social situations. This neural transformation is also accompanied by a significant increase in oxytocin receptors located within the socioemotional system, which is critical as oxytocin heightens adolescents' attentiveness to, and memory for, social information. Steinberg (2008) argues that the increase in oxytocin leads to an increase in the salience of peers, and this increase in the importance of peers and peer relations plays a role in encouraging risky behaviors. In sum, in comparison to younger youth, adolescents who have gone through puberty are more inclined to take risks in order to gain rewards, and this tendency is exacerbated by the presence of peers. Recent research from behavioral science is consistent with Steinberg's position. For instance, his laboratory-based research found that the presence of peers more than doubled the number of risks teenagers took in a video driving game and increased risk-taking by 50 % in college students, but had no effect among adults (Gardner & Steinberg, 2005).

Beyond Biology

Biological development during adolescence is accompanied by physiological changes in the ways in which adolescents perceive both themselves and the world around them. Cognitive development may occur in concert or asynchronously with physical development. When physical development precedes cognitive development (as often is the case with females experiencing early maturation) adolescents are at increased risk for engaging in health-endangering behaviors.

Further, although developmental neuroscience research has found that the brain is still developing into adulthood, the social world may have unrealistic e or unhealthy expectations of adolescents, especially those whom physically appear as adults. Thus, it is imperative to include the social environment in models exploring adolescent risk-taking. Indeed, when biological models are expanded to include "psychological" variables the combined effects of biological and psychological factors explains more of the variation in health-endangering behaviors (e.g., used cigarettes or marijuana) than either of these factors alone.

The Psychology of Adolescent Risk-Taking

Psychologically based studies of adolescent risk-taking behavior examine the roles of cognition, personality traits, and dispositional characteristics, such as self-esteem and depression, in risk-taking behavior. Examples of each are briefly presented and discussed in turn.

The Role of Cognition

Cognitive theories of risk-taking behavior explore how people perceive risk and make decisions about risk-taking. Specific to adolescents, risk perception theory has been guided by the premise that adolescents are "optimistically biased" or that they believe themselves invincible. The concept of invincibility has been frequently employed to explain or justify adolescent risk-taking behavior, although little evidence supports this assertion as people of all ages, not just adolescents, tend to underestimate the likelihood of experience adverse consequences of their actions (Reyna & Farley, 2006). For instance, Millstein and Halpern-Felsher (2002) demonstrated that increasing the salience of the risks associated with making a potentially dangerous decision had the same effect on adolescents and adults. Further, few age differences have been found in regard to individuals' evaluations of the risks inherent in a variety of dangerous behaviors, or in judgments about the seriousness of consequences resulting from risky behavior (Beyth-Marom, Austin, Fischoff, Palmgren, & Jacobs-Quadrel, 1993).

Research has also examined the role of decision-making on adolescent risk-taking. Fischoff (1992) identified five salient components of decision-making: (1) identify alternative options, (2) identify possible consequences, (3) evaluate the desirability of the potential consequences, (4) assess the likelihood of those consequences, and (5) combine the information to make a decision. According to Keating (1990), by middle adolescence (i.e., 14 or 15 years of age), most adolescents make decisions in a similar manner to adults. Although the decision-making process may be similar, the content of the aforementioned components may differ substantially between adults and adolescents. For instance, Beyth-Marom et al. (1993) found that adolescent and adult patterns of responses regarding risk-taking were similar, with both producing more negative consequences than positive ones. The difference was that adults reported more consequences overall than adolescents.

Another cognitive theory of adolescent is called fuzzy-trace theory (Reyna & Farley, 2006). Fuzzy-trace theory proposes that that adolescent decision-making is based on simple, gist mental representations of choices (i.e., "fuzzy" memory traces) as opposed to more detailed, verbatim representations or traces. Because of this, when adolescents attempt to rationally weigh costs and benefits (via the use of verbatim memory traces), risk-taking increases. However, risk-taking decreases when the core gist of a decision is processed and a decision is based on this gist information (Rivers, Reyna, & Mills, 2008).

The Role of Personality

Some evidence indicates that adolescent decision-making may reflect an overall tendency toward unconventional behavior. Jessor's Problem Behavior Theory links "unconventionality" in personality, among other things, with an increased likelihood of participating in problem behaviors such as risky sexual activity, substance use, and delinquency (Jessor, 2008; Jessor & Jessor, 1977).

Problem Behavior Theory has attempted to provide a theoretical framework for the connection observed between multiple problem behaviors. This theory suggests that multiple factors contribute to problem behaviors, defined as socially problematic, concerning, or undesirable behaviors usually eliciting some form of social or personal consequence (e.g., disapproval from others, incarceration, health compromise). The theoretical framework includes three major systems of explanatory variables: (1) the perceived-environment system, involving social controls, models, and support; (2) the personality system, involving values, expectations, beliefs, attitudes, and orientations toward self and society; and (3) the behavior system, encompassing both problem and conventional behaviors. Considering these explanatory systems, it is possible that engaging in health-compromising behaviors (i.e., smoking, sexual risk behaviors) may be related due to factors such as social support, depressive symptoms, self-esteem, and other factors underlying these risk behaviors and potentially accounting for the relationship among them.

The personality trait "sensation-seeking" has been used to explain adolescent risk-taking behavior. For example, Zuckerman (1979) states that sensation seeking is a "trait defined by the need for varied, novel and complex sensations and experiences and willingness to take physical and social risks for the sake of such experiences." Zuckerman developed a Sensation Seeking Scale to assess individual differences in optimal levels of arousal. Often high-sensation seekers tend to perceive less risk in many activities than low-sensation seekers. Even when the evaluation of the risk involved is equal between the two groups, high-sensation seekers are significantly more likely to anticipate more positive potential outcomes than low-sensation seekers. Sensation seeking has been associated with a variety of risk-taking behaviors including substance abuse, reckless driving, delinquent actions, and risky sexual behavior (Andrucci, Archer, Pancoast, & Gordon, 1989; Kalichman & Rompa, 1995; Newcomb & McGee, 1991; Tonkin, 1987). Further, an adolescent-specific sexual sensation-seeking scales has been recently developed (DiClemente et al., 2010), and adolescent females who endorsed high levels of sexual sensation seeking attitudes and behaviors also reported high levels of sexual risk-taking behaviors such as frequency of vaginal intercourse, number of sexual partners, and inconsistent condom use (Spitalnick et al., 2007). Not surprisingly perhaps, sensation seeking has also been linked to various biological markers including testosterone levels, electrodermal and heart rate responses, and cortical evoked potentials (Zuckerman, 1990).

The impulsivity seen among sensation-seekers may be seen in psychopathologic states that have been linked to an increased likelihood of risk-taking behaviors, primarily in male adolescents. Attention deficit hyperactivity disorder (ADHD) in males has been associated with an increased risk for delinquency. One study found that male youths with ADHD had arrest rates more than twice those of controls (Farrington, Loeber, & Van Kammen, 1990). Similarly, male youth with conduct disorders are at increased risk for alcohol and substance abuse (Kazdin, 1989).

The Role of Dispositional Characteristics

Self-esteem, depression and locus of control are often cited as theoretical or empirically supported predictors of risk-taking behavior. Lower self-esteem has been associated with age of sexual debut in adolescent females (Orr, Wilbrandt, Brack, Rauch, & Ingersoll, 1989). Depressive symptoms and stress have been related to the initiation and intensity of use of tobacco among adolescents (Covey & Tam, 1990), and more recently, to a various risky sexual behaviors in both adolescent males and females (Crepaz & Marks, 2001, Sales, Spitalnick, Crittenden, & DiClemente, 2009). Further, depression and external locus of control have been associated with substance use (Baumrind, 1987; Dielman et al., 1987). Kohler (1996) examined the relationship between locus of control, sensation-seeking, critical-thinking skills, and risk-taking among adolescents and found a significant correlation between risk-taking and gender, critical thinking, and locus of control. However, it should be noted that research has not supported a consistent role for any of these psychological factors in various risk-taking behaviors (Dryfoos, 1990; McCord, 1990; Sales, Spitalnick, Crittenden, & DiClemente, 2009).

Beyond the Psychological

In summary, cognitive factors such as risk perception and decision-making contribute to adolescent risk-taking. Although adolescents' decision-making processes appear to differ little from adults, adolescents lack adult experience interacting with the social/environmental world in general, and engaging in decision-making specifically. As articulated in fuzzy-trace theory, their judgments cannot reflect the influence of these experiences. Further, adolescent risk-related decision-making may reflect young people's tendencies toward unconventionality and/or sensation seeking. Sensation seeking is clearly related to increased rates of adolescent risk-taking behaviors, but not all risk-taking behavior can be construed as sensation seeking. Some clinical psychological difficulties such as excessive aggression, impulsivity, and attention deficit and conduct disorders increase the likelihood of adolescents engaging in risk-taking behavior. The role of depression, a highly prevalent issue facing adolescents, has been linked to substance abuse and risky sexual behaviors, but role of depressive mood in other types of risk behavior has yet to be established. Further, the evidence for a causal role for self-esteem and locus of control on risk-taking is unclear. Thus, biological and psychological factors are themselves important determinants of risk-taking behavior. They also are the personal filters through which social and environmental stimuli are interpreted and translated into action.

The Environment of Adolescent Risk-Taking

Environmental models of adolescent risk-taking behavior look at the roles of peers, family, and institutions (school, church, and/or social media) in risk-taking behaviors. These studies examine how the social/environmental context provides models, opportunities, and/or reinforcements for adolescent participation in risk-taking behaviors. The role of family, peers, and society in risk-taking behaviors are presented in turn.

The Role of Family

Although adolescence is a time of emerging autonomy and individuation from the family, most adolescents maintain close relationships with their parents (Steinberg, 1993) and parents continue to influence their children's behavior throughout adolescence. Parents play an important role in determining adolescent involvement in risk behaviors. Parental modeling of and permissive attitudes toward substance use have been implicated in the initiation of substance use in early adolescence (Hawkins & Fitzgibbon, 1993; Werner, 1991). Further, adolescents are less likely to abuse substances or to initiate sexual activity when parents provide emotional support and acceptance, and have a close relationship with their children (Turner, Irwin, Tschann, & Millstein, 1993).

In addition to modeling, parental monitoring has been widely studied as an important correlate of adolescent risk-taking behavior (Jaccard & Dittus, 1991). Monitoring and supervision incorporates both communication between parent and child, and supervision of the youth. Borawski and colleagues (2003) found that perceived parental monitoring, combined with trust, served as a significant protective factor against sexual activity for both males and females, and tobacco and marijuana use in females, and alcohol use in male adolescents. Less perceived parental monitoring has been associated with increased participation in antisocial activities, sexual risk-taking, and increased substance abuse or use (Chilcoat et al., 1995; Smith & Rosenthal, 1995; Steinberg, 1993).

Parental influence on adolescent behavior varies with the quality of the relationship between the adolescent and the parent (Bijur et al., 1991; Turner et al., 1993). Related to this, parental approaches to child rearing have also been associated with adolescents engaging in risk-taking behaviors. For instance, Baumrind (1991) found an association between adolescent substance use and parenting styles. Adolescents whose parents were "authoritative" (i.e., demanding and responsive) were less likely to use substances than either those with "authoritarian" (i.e., demanding but unresponsive) or those with "permissive" (i.e., nondemanding but responsive) parents. Adolescent with "neglecting and rejecting" parents were the most likely to engage in substance abuse.

In summary, family approval and modeling of risk behavior has been linked to adolescent risk-taking behavior. Parent–child relationships characterized by conflict, increased emotional distance, and non-responsiveness increase the likelihood of adolescents engaging in health endangering behaviors (see Chapter "Determinants of Health-Related Behaviors in Adolescence" by DiClemente, Brown, and Davis for a more thorough review).

Peers

According to Jessor and Jessor (1977) the relatively greater influence of peers compared to parents is associated with a greater tendency (or proneness) toward problem behaviors. As a result, parental impact on risk-taking behavior may wane as peer influences increase throughout adolescence. Consistent with this assertion, Jessor and colleagues (1980, 1983) found that peer influence more so than parental influence predicted marijuana use, problem drinking, and precocious sexual debut.

Peer influence has been a significant factor associated with adolescent substance use (Jessor, 1976; Kandel, 1985; Newcomb & Bentler, 1989), alcohol use (Urberg, Degirmencioglu, & Pilgram, 1997), delinquency (McCord, 1990) and sexual behaviors. Accordingly, peers have been identified as an important influence on the sexual behavior of adolescents in a wide range of populations (Buhi & Goodson, 2007; Pedlow & Carey, 2004). Also, adolescents are usually accompanied by one or more persons when committing crimes that range in seriousness from vandalism and drug use (Erickson & Jensen, 1977) to rape and homicide (Zimring, 1998). Further, social network analysis of smoking and drug-use behaviors among adolescents has found that both risk-taking and non-risk-taking behaviors (i.e., smoking and drug-use) are learned in the context of peer clusters, and risk-taking peer clusters execrate greater influence on those peers on the periphery of clusters than do non-risk-taking peer clusters (Pearson & Michell, 2000).

Traditionally "peer pressure" has been viewed as an etiologic factor in adolescent risk-taking behavior. If remains unclear if risk behaviors are initiated in order to conform to an existing peer group or if those prone to engage in risk-taking behaviors are drawn to those who are similarly inclined. Lashbrook (2000) provides one possible explanation for how peers exert their impact on adolescent risk-taking. Specifically, he demonstrated that older adolescents may attempt to avoid negative emotions, such as feelings of isolation and inadequacy, by participating in risky behaviors with peers. Recent findings suggest that the answer is not straightforward. Brady, Dolcini, Harper, and Pollack (2009) found that adolescents with low social support from peers maybe prone to engaging in sexual risk-taking as a response to stress, whereas adolescents with high peer support may engage in sexual risk-taking due to peer socialization of risk.

Society

Societal influences such as mass media and community norms may also influence risk-taking behavior. Role models and/or images portrayed in the media are regularly presented by the media engaging in various health-endangering behaviors (including unprotected sexual behavior and alcohol/substance use), though evidence for the influence of these models/images on actual behavior is lacking. A recent study conducted among adolescent African American girls found that those who watched rap music videos and who perceived more sexual stereotypes in the videos were more likely to engage in binge drinking, test positive for recent marijuana, have multiple sexual partners, and have a negative body image (Peterson, Wingood, DiClemente, Harrington, & Davis, 2007).

In addition to media, different communities and neighborhoods provide adolescents with opportunities and motivations to engage in risk-taking behavior. Peer norms reflected in local rates of substance use and teen pregnancy create expectancies of "typical" adolescent behavior (Crockett & Petersen, 1993). Local ordinances allowing cigarette vending machines, legalization of marijuana for medical purposes for adolescents, or lower ages to purchase alcohol provide opportunities for engaging in risk-taking behavior. Johnston and colleagues (1993) have reported that the perceived availability of marijuana in a community is not necessarily related to prevalence of use by teens. In fact, declines in marijuana use by high school seniors have been accompanied by unchanged or even increased perceived availability in recent years.

Cultural expectations may also influence adolescent risk-taking behavior. For instance, despite similar ages of sexual debut, the USA has the highest rates of adolescent childbearing and abortion in the developed world (Martin et al., 2006). This is speculated to be related to differing cultural attitudes toward adolescent sexuality and contraception (Geronimus, 2003). When looking within the USA only, contraception rates vary significantly by ethnicity and religious affiliation (Brewster, Cooksey, Guilkey, & Rindfuss, 1998; Santelli, Morrow, & Carter, 2004). Substance use and age of sexual debut also differ among different ethnic groups in the USA (Cavanagh, 2004; Guerra, Romano, Samuels, & Kass, 2000). (Note: Ethnicity associated differences may be confounded by factors related to socioeconomic status; See Chapter "Determinants of Health-Related Behaviors in Adolescence" by DiClemente, Brown, and Davis for further discussion.)

Beyond Environment

The studies presented demonstrate the complexity of the interaction between adolescents and their environment. The biopsychosocial model provides a framework in which environmental factors are brought to bear on existing biological and psychological predispositions to influence risk-taking behavior, and ultimately adolescent health.

The Biopsychosocial Model of Risk-Taking

The biopsychosocial model integrates two areas of research that have often been considered separately: (1) the relationship of biological development to psychosocial processing during adolescence, and (2) the relationship of risk-taking behaviors to psychosocial correlates of these behaviors (Sales & Irwin, 2009). According to this model, biological, psychological, and social or environmental factors influence adolescent risk-taking behaviors (Irwin & Millstein, 1986). Specifically the timing of biological maturation directly influences psychosocial functioning (i.e., cognition, perceptions of self and the social environment, and personal values). According to the model, biological, psychological, and social or environmental variables, mediated by perceptions of risk and peer-group characteristics, best predict adolescent risk-taking. Biological variables influencing adolescent risk-taking behavior include pubertal timing, hormonal effects, genetic predispositions, and brain maturation. Psychological variables associated with risk-taking include self-esteem, sensation seeking, and cognitive and affective states. Social influences on adolescent risk-taking include peers, parents, and school (see Fig. 1).

Given the framework of the biopsychosocial perspective, Irwin and colleagues (Irwin, 1990; Irwin & Millstein, 1986; Irwin & Ryan, 1989), have elaborated on the theory to include conditions that may increase the probability that a given adolescent will engage in risk-taking behaviors (see Fig. 2). Because of advances in our understanding of developmental neuroscience, a fourth biological factor has been added to the model. Now, the biological factors thought to predispose adolescents to risk-taking behaviors include male gender, genetic predispositions, hormonal influences, and prolonged brain

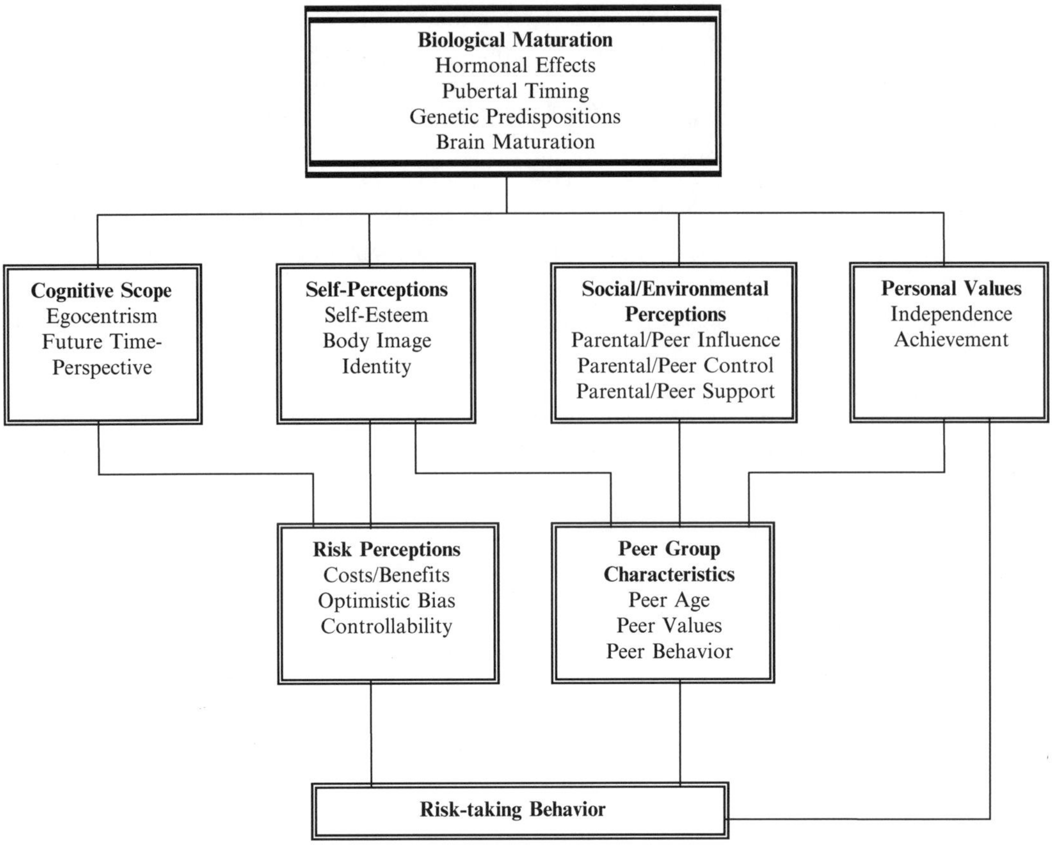

Fig. 1 Model based on the biopsychosocial causal model of risk-taking behavior (Irwin & Millstein, 1986)

maturation. Psychological predisposing factors include sensation seeking, risk perception, depression and low self-esteem. Social environmental predisposing factors include maladaptive parenting styles, parental modeling of risk behaviors, peer behaviors and socioeconomic status. Finally, adolescent vulnerability to risk-taking behaviors may be increased situationally by family disruption, school transitions, and substance use and peer initiation of risk-taking behaviors.

Research Supporting the Utility of the Biopsychosocial Model

A variety of studies provide support for the utility of the biopsychosocial model for examining adolescent risk-taking. For instance, Brooks-Gunn (1988) found that among female adolescents, early maturational timing was associated with a more negative self-image, and with earlier onset of sexual activity. For both males and females, early maturation is a risk factor for the initiation of substance use in adolescents (Tschann et al., 1994). Seminal work by Jessor and Jessor (1977) supports the roles of environment and personal values (i.e., psychosocial factors) in the onset of adolescent risk-taking behavior. Specifically, the predominance of peer influence over parental influence, along with adolescents placing a greater personal value on independence versus achievement resulted in an increased likelihood of adolescents engaging in risk-taking behavior. Moreover, Hughes et al. (1991) conducted a study with urban delinquent youth and concluded that alcohol/substance abuse during adolescence further added to biological predispositions, educational difficulties, and coercive family

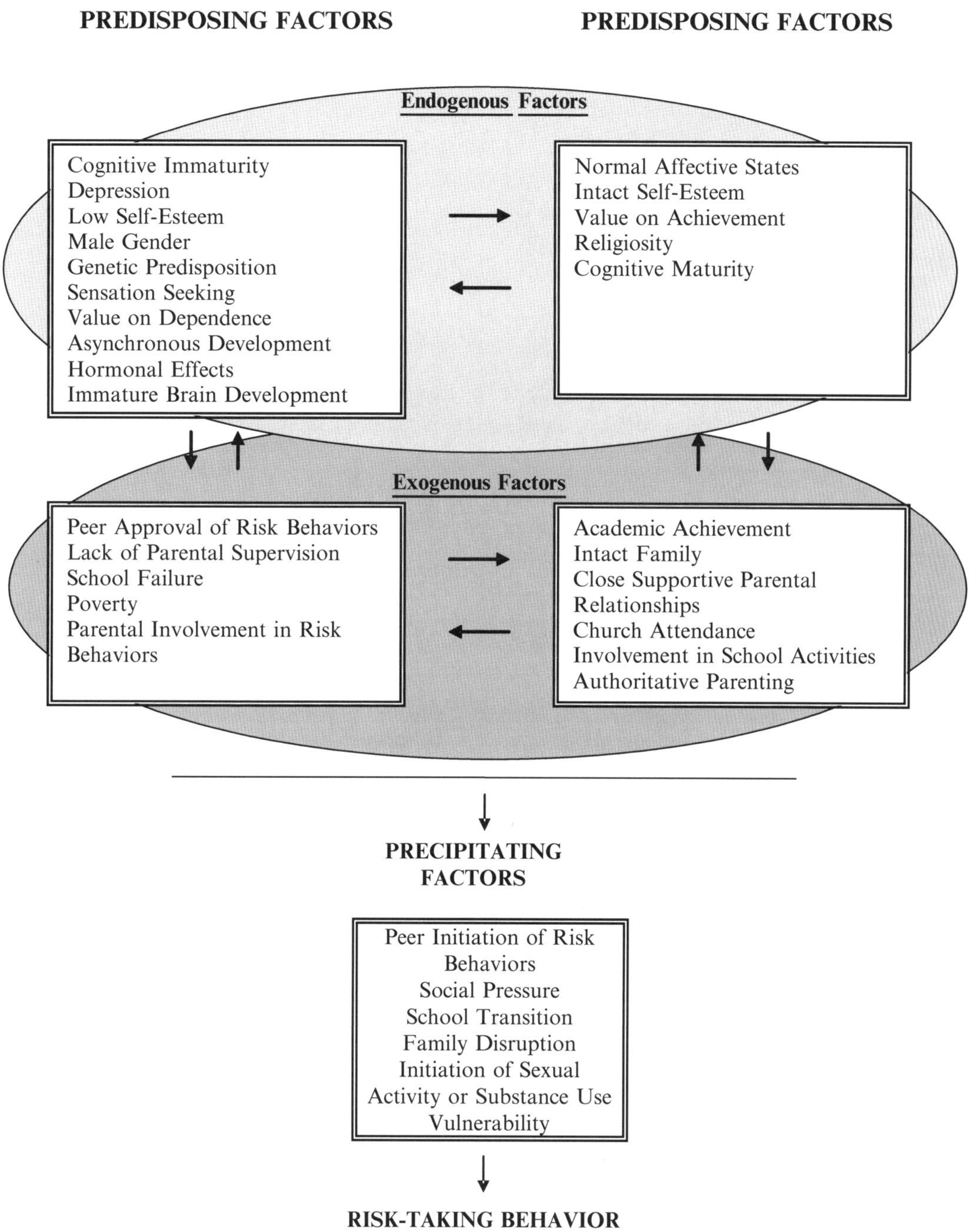

Fig. 2 Factors contributing to the onset of risk-taking behaviors during adolescence (Irwin & Millstein, 1986; Irwin & Ryan, 1989; Sales & Irwin, 2009)

environments, all of which contribute to their delinquent behavior. While most evidence supporting the biopsychosocial model stems from research in the USA, a study conducted with Japanese students, utilizing structural equation analysis, found that egocentrism contributes directly to health-endangering behaviors while influences of self-esteem and perceived social norms are mediated by risk perception (Omori & Ingersoll, 2005).

Often it is difficult for a single study to collect data for each area emphasized in the biopsychosocial model. Thus, articles which can overview and synthesize studies provide additional support for the utility of the biopsychosocial model. For example, a review by Ricciardelli and McCabe (2004), synthesized the literature and reported that among adolescent males, disordered eating and the pursuit of muscularity are consistently associated biological factors such as body mass index (BMI), psychological factors such as negative affect and self-esteem, and sociocultural factors such as perceived pressure to lose weight by parents and peers (Ricciardelli & McCabe, 2004). Further, Dodge and Pettit (2003) reviewed of the empirical literature pertaining to the development of chronic conduct problems in adolescence and conclude that reciprocal influences among biological dispositions, environments, and life experiences lead to recursive iterations across time which either worsen or diminish antisocial development. Additionally, their findings indicate that adolescents' cognitive and emotional processes mediate the relationship between life experiences and conduct problems. Finally, specific to aggression and delinquency in adolescent girls, a review by Celio, Karnik, and Steiner (2006) found that early maturation is a risk factor for aggression and delinquent behavior. However, the way in which early physical maturation is perceived and treated by others (family, peers, and society) also determines how adolescent girls behave.

Additional support for the biopsychosocial model comes from interventions designed to reduce adolescent risk-taking. For example, Brody et al. (2009) found that youth in the control group of their Strong African American Families (SAAF) intervention program with the polymorphism in the SCL6A4(5HTT) gene at 5-HTTLPR showed significant increases in risk behavior initiation (particularly substance use initiation) across 29 months of follow-up in comparison to youth in the SAAF program with the same genetic risk. These findings demonstrate that despite genetic predispositions, programs that work to intervene at the family level to build supportive family environments, along with increasing self-esteem and improving life skills of youth, can attenuate risk initiation among adolescents.

Thus, across various behavioral domains, research supports the utility of the biopsychosocial model for explaining adolescent risk-taking.

Future Directions for the Biopsychosocial Model

Give the complexity of human behavior, a model must encompass a variety of constructs to more fully explain and understand why some people opt to participate in health-endangering activities. Because the biopsychosocial approach includes various constructs empirically linked to adolescent, it is a more complex model, and until recently it has been incredibly difficult to empirically examine all of the factors comprising the model in one study. However, with recent advances in technology and a concerted effort by researchers (and funding agencies) to engage in interdisciplinary collaborations to more thoroughly examine health-compromising decisions and behaviors, future research may be able to do so more frequently.

For instance, the recent mapping of the human genome has allowed us to explore the biological underpinnings of behavior and cognition in ways not possible even a decade ago. Advances in gene mapping have lead to findings implicating particular genes in alcoholism and substance use disorders (Conner et al., 2005). Also, genetic markers for impulsivity (e.g., DRD4) and depressive symptomatology (e.g., 5HTT and MAOA) are currently being explored, and identifying a multitude of other genetic markers that predispose adolescents towards various risk-taking behaviors is on the horizon.

Advances in brain imaging science have allowed researchers to examine the brain across development and while engaging in problem solving. Many now believe, based upon neuroimaging studies, that mature decision making is composed of two networks: a highly interconnected cognitive-control network that biases decisions in favor of rational outcomes and a socioemotional network that biases decision making toward reward-based demands (Chein, 2008).

It is postulated that, in adults, the cognitive-control network can regulate the behavior of the socioemotional network, allowing for people to make rational, utilitarian decisions. However, neither of these systems is fully matured during adolescence, and each one develops along different timetables (Giedd, 2008). Thus, these two underdeveloped networks and their differing rates of development pave the way for heightened risk-taking during adolescence, which, as demonstrated by Gardner and Steinberg's (2005) work with teen drivers, may be further compounded by social and environmental factors, particularly the presence of peers. In the past decade great scientific advances have been made through neuroimaging studies, but understanding the relationship between neuroimaging findings and behavior is still in its infancy. Although this is an area of great academic interest and active research, demonstrating straight-forward relationships between the size of, neural activity in, or connectedness between particular brain regions and a specific behavior or ability has, to date, been challenging at best (DiFranza, 2011; Giedd, 2008; Rubinstein et al., 2011; Steinberg, 2008).

Technological advances have also bettered researchers' ability to assess adolescent risk-taking, as well as psychological and environmental influences on risk-taking. For example, it is now possible to detect through self-collected vaginal swab specimens, the presence of semen in vaginal fluid (Yc PCR). This can then be used as a nondisease marker of unprotected vaginal intercourse (Zenilman, Yuenger, Galai, Turner, & Rogers, 2005). Also, novel techniques, such as GeoCoding, allow researchers to spatially place participants in their physical neighborhoods, which are then mapped onto Census data to establish neighborhood profiles (Sales & Irwin, 2009). This provides an objective measure of neighborhood level social conditions including socioeconomic status, racial makeup, population density, as well as access to potentially health-compromising venues (such as fast-food restaurants and liquor stores) or health-promoting venues (such as grocery stories and green spaces). Further, the explosion of social media (e.g., Facebook, MySpace, YouTube) and mobile communication (e.g., cell-phones, iPhones, iPads, Netbooks) among adolescent populations in the USA and around the globe provide teens with nearly unlimited access to information (health promoting and health endangering) and social networks. These advances allow unique opportunities to access and assess adolescents, especially as it relates to decision-making, risk-taking, and health outcomes.

In the coming years it will be possible to explore biological influence on behavior and the interaction between biology, psychology, environment, adolescent risk-taking behavior, and health outcomes in ways never possible before. Thus, just as our society is becoming more and more complex, the utility of complex models of adolescent risk-taking like the biopsychosocial model will prove invaluable in guiding the next generation of adolescent health research.

References

Adger, H. (1991). Problems of alcohol and other drug abuse in adolescents. *Journal of Adolescent Health, 12*, 606–613.

Andrucci, G. L., Archer, R. P., Pancoast, D. L., & Gordon, R. A. (1989). The relationship of MMPI and sensation seeking scales to adolescent drug use. *Journal of Personality Assessment, 53*, 253–266.

Asato, M. R., Terwilliger, R., Woo, J., & Luna, B. (2010). White matter development in adolescence: A DTI study. *Cerebral Cortex, 20*, 2122–2131.

Baumrind, D. (1987). A developmental perspective on adolescent risk taking in contemporary America. In C. E. Irwin (Ed.), *Adolescent social behavior and health. New directions for child development* (Social and Behavioral Sciences Series, Vol. 37, pp. 93–125). San Francisco: Jossey Bass. Fall.

Baumrind, D. (1991). The influence of parenting style on adolescent competence and substance abuse. *Journal of Early Adolescence, 11*, 56–95.

Belsky, J. (2011). Family experience and pubertal development in evolutionary perspective. *Journal of Adolescent Health, 48*(5), 425–426.

Beyth-Marom, R., Austin, L., Fischoff, B., Palmgren, C., & Jacobs-Quadrel, M. (1993). Perceived consequences of risky behaviors: Adults and adolescents. *Developmental Psychology, 29*, 549–563.

Beyth-Marom, R., & Fischoff, B. (1997). Adolescents' decisions about risks: A cognitive perspective. In J. Schulenberg & J. L. Maggs (Eds.), *Health risks and developmental transitions during adolescence* (pp. 110–135). New York: Cambridge University Press.

Bijur, P. E., Kurzon, M., Hamelsky, V., & Power, C. (1991). Parent-adolescent conflict and adolescent injuries. *Journal of Developmental and Behavioral Pediatrics, 12*, 92–97.

Brady, S. S., Dolcini, M. M., Harper, G. W., & Pollack, L. M. (2009). Supportive friendships and community involvement moderate the association between stressful life events and sexual risk taking among African American adolescents. *Health Psychology, 28*(2), 238–248.

Brewster, K. L., Cooksey, E. C., Guilkey, D. K., & Rindfuss, R. R. (1998). The changing impact of religion on the sexual and contraceptive behavior of adolescent women in the United States. *Journal of Marriage and the Family, 60*, 493–504.

Broawski, E., Iefers-Landis, C. E., Lovegreen, L. D., & Trapl, E. S. (2003). Parental monitoring, negotiated unsupervised time, and parental trust: The role of perceived parenting practices in adolescent health risk behaviors. *Journal of Adolescent Health, 33*, 60–70.

Brody, G. H., Beach, S. R., Philibert, R. A., Chen, Y., & McBride Murray, V. (2009). Prevention effects moderate the association of 5-HTTLPR and youth risk behavior initiation: Gene x environment hypotheses tested via a randomized prevention design. *Child Development, 80*, 645–661.

Brooks-Gunn, J. (1988). Antecedents and consequences of variations in girls maturational timing. *Journal of Adolescent Health Care, 9*, 1–9.

Buhi, E. R., & Goodson, P. (2007). Predictors of adolescent sexual behavior and intention: A theory-guided systematic review. *Journal of Adolescent Health, 1*, 4–27.

Cavanagh, S. E. (2004). The sexual debut of girls in early adolescence: The intersection of race, pubertal timing, and friendship group characteristics. *Journal of Research on Adolescence, 14*, 285.

Celio, M., Karnik, N. S., & Steiner, H. (2006). Early maturation as a risk factor for aggression and delinquency in adolescent girls: A review. *International Journal of Clinical Practice, 60*, 1254–1262.

Centers for Disease Control and Prevention. (2008). Births: Preliminary Data for 2006. *National Vital Statistics Reports, 56*, 1–18.

Centers for Disease Control and Prevention. (2010). Youth risk behavior surveillance—United States, 2009. *MMWR, 59*(5), 1–142.

Chein, J. (2008). Linking risk-taking behavior and peer influence in adolescents. *Neuropsychiatry Reviews, 9*, 1.

Chilcoat, H. D., Dishion, T. J., & Anthony, J. C. (1995). Parent monitoring and the incidence of drug sampling in urban elementary school children. *American Journal of Epidemiology, 141*, 25–31.

Cicchetti, D., & Rogosch, F. A. (2002). A developmental psychopathology perspective on adolescence. *Journal of Consulting and Clinical Psychology, 70*, 6–20.

Cloninger, C. R. (1987). Neurogenetic adaptive mechanisms in alcoholism. *Science, 236*, 410–416.

Connor, B. T., Noble, E. P., Berman, S. M., Ozkaragoz, T., Ritchie, T., Antolin, T., et al. (2005). DRD2 genotypes and substance use in adolescent children of alcoholics. *Drug and Alcohol Dependence, 79*, 379–387.

Covey, L. S., & Tam, D. (1990). Depressive mood, the single-parent home and adolescent cigarette smoking. *American Journal of Public Health, 80*(11), 1330–1333.

Crepaz, N., & Marks, G. (2001). Are negative affective states associated with HIV sexual risk behaviors? A meta-analytic review. *Health Psychology, 20*(4), 291–299.

Crockett, L. J., & Petersen, A. C. (1993). Adolescent development: Health risks and opportunities for health promotion. In S. G. Millstein, A. C. Petersen, & E. O. Nightingale (Eds.), *Promoting the health of adolescents: New directions for the twenty-first century* (pp. 13–37). New York: Oxford University Press.

Deardorff, J., Ekwaru, J. P., Kushi, L. H., et al. (2011). Father absence, body mass index, and pubertal timing in girls: Differential effects by family income and ethnicity. *Journal of Adolescent Health, 48*, 441–447.

DiClemente, R. J., Milhausen, R. R., Salazar, L. F., Spitalnick, J., Sales, J. M., Crosby, R. A., et al. (2010). Development of the sexual sensation seeking scale for African American adolescent women. *International Journal of Sexual Health, 22*, 248–261.

Dielman, T. E., Campanelli, P. C., Shope, J. T., & Butchart, A. T. (1987). Susceptibility to peer pressure, self-esteem, and health locus of control as correlates of adolescent substance abuse. *Health Education Quarterly, 14*, 207–221.

DiFranza, J. R. (2011). Who are you going to believe? Adolescents and nicotine addiction. *Journal of Adolescent Health, 48*(1), 1–2.

Dodge, K. A., & Pettit, G. (2003). A biopsychosocial model of the development of chronic conduct problems in adolescence. *Developmental Psychology, 39*, 349–371.

Dryfoos, J. G. (1990). *Adolescents at risk*. Oxford: Oxford University Press.

Erickson, M., & Jensen, G. F. (1977). Delinquency is still a group behavior: Toward revitalizing the group premise of the sociology of deviance. *The Journal of Criminal Law and Criminology, 68*, 262–273.

Farrington, D. P., Loeber, R., & Van Kammen, W. (1990). *Cited in U.S. Congress Office of Technology Assessment Adolescent health-volume II: Background and the effectiveness of selected prevention and treatment services, OTA-H-466*. Washington, DC: U.S. Government Printing Office. November 1991.

Fingerhut, L. A., & Anderson, R. N. (2008). *The three leading causes of injury mortality in the United States, 1999–2005*. http://www.cdc.gov/nchs/products/pubs/pubd/hestats/injury99-05/injury99-05.htm#other_ages. Retrieved May 16, 2008, from http://www.cdc.gov/nchs/health-data-for-all-ages.htm.

Fischoff, B. (1992). Risk taking: A developmental perspective. In J. F. Yates (Ed.), *Risk-taking behavior* (pp. 132–162). New York: Wiley.

Ford, C. A., Pence, B. W., Miller, W. C., Resnick, M. D., Bearinger, L. H., Pettingell, S., et al. (2005). Predicting adolescents' longitudinal risk for sexually transmitted infection: Results from the National Longitudinal Study of Adolescent Health. *Archives of Pediatric and Adolescent Medicine, 159*(7), 657–664.

Forhan, S. E., Gottlieb, S. L., Sternberg, M. R., Xu, F., Datta, S. D., Berman, S., & Markowitz, L. E. (2008). *Prevalence of sexually transmitted infections and bacterial vaginosis among female adolescents in the United States: Data from the National Health and Nutrition Examination Survey (NHANES) 2003–2004.* Paper presented at the National STD Prevention Conference, Chicago, IL.

Gardner, M., & Steinberg, L. (2005). Peer influence on risk-taking, risk preference, and risky decision making in adolescence and adulthood: An experimental study. *Developmental Psychology, 41*, 625–635.

Geronimus, A. T. (2003). Damned if you do: Culture, identity, privilege, and teenage childbearing in the United States. *Social Science & Medicine, 57*, 881–893.

Giedd, J. N. (2008). The teen brain: Insights from neuroimaging. *Journal of Adolescent Health, 42*, 335–343.

Guerra, L. M., Romano, P. S., Samuels, S. J., & Kass, P. H. (2000). Ethnic differences in adolescent substance initiation sequences. *Archives of Pediatric Adolescent Medicine, 154*, 1089–1095.

Hawkins, J. D., & Fitzgibbon, J. J. (1993). Risk factors and risk behaviors in prevention of adolescent substance abuse. In M. Schydlower & P. D. Rogers (Eds.), *Adolescent medicine state of the art reviews: Adolescent substance abuse and addictions. 4*(2), 249–262.

Hughes, J. R., Zagar, R., Sylvies, R. B., Arbit, J., Busch, K. G., & Bowers, N. D. (1991). Medical, family, and scholastic conditions in urban delinquents. *Journal of Clinical Psychology, 47*, 448–464.

Irwin, C. E., Jr. (1990). The theoretical concept of at-risk adolescents. *Adolescent Medicine: State of the Art Reviews, 1*, 1–14.

Irwin, C. E., Jr., & Millstein, S. G. (1986). Biopsychosocial correlates of risk-taking behaviors during adolescence. *Journal of Adolescent Health Care, 7*, 82S–96S.

Irwin, C. E., Jr., & Ryan, S. A. (1989). Problem behaviors of adolescence. *Pediatrics in Review, 10*, 235–246.

Jaccard, J., & Dittus, P. (1991). *Parent-teen communication: Toward the prevention of unintended pregnancies*. New York: Springer.

Jessor, R. (1976). Predicting time of onset of marijuana use: A developmental study of high school youth. *Journal of Consulting and Clinical Psychology, 44*, 125–134.

Jessor, R. (2008). Description versus explanation in cross-national research on adolescence. *Journal of Adolescent Health, 43*(6), 527–528.

Jessor, R., Chase, C. A., & Donovan, J. E. (1980). Psychosocial correlates of marijuana use and problem drinking in a national sample of adolescents. *American Journal of Public Health, 70*, 604–613.

Jessor, R., Costa, F., Jessor, L., & Donovan, J. E. (1983). Time of first intercourse: A prospective study. *Journal of Personality and Social Psychology, 44*, 608–626.

Jessor, R., & Jessor, S. L. (1977). *Problem behavior and psychological development: a longitudinal study of youth.* New York, NY: Academic Press.

Johnston, L. D., O'Malley, P. M., & Bachman J. G. (1993). National survey results on drug use from the Monitoring the Future Study, 1975–1992. Rockville, MD: National Institute on Drug Abuse. U.S. Department of Health and Human Services, Public Health Service, National Institutes of Health. Washington, DC (NIH publication #93-3597).

Johnston, L. D., O'Malley, P. M., Bachman, J. G., & Schulenberg, J. E. (2011). *Monitoring the future national results on adolescent drug use: Overview of key findings, 2010.* Ann Arbor: Institute for Social Research, The University of Michigan.

Kaestle, C. E., Halpern, C. T., Miller, W. C., & Ford, C. A. (2005). Young age at first sexual intercourse and sexually transmitted infections in adolescents and young adults. *American Journal of Epidemiology, 161*(8), 774–780.

Kalichman, S. C., & Rompa, D. (1995). Sexual sensation seeking and sexual compulsivity scales: Reliability, validity, and predicting HIV risk behaviors. *Journal of Personality Assessment, 65*, 586–602.

Kandel, D. B. (1985). On processes of peer influences in adolescent drug use: A developmental perspective. *Advances in Alcohol & Substance Abuse, 4*(3–4), 139–163.

Kazdin, A. E. (1989). Developmental psychopathology: Current research, issues and directions. *American Psychologist, 44*, 180–187.

Keating, D. P. (1990). Adolescent thinking. In S. S. Feldman & G. R. Elliot (Eds.), *At the threshold: The developing adolescent* (pp. 54–89). Cambridge: Harvard University Press.

Kogan, S. M., Beach, S. R., Philibert, R. A., Brody, G. H., Chen, Y. F., & Lei, M. K. (2010). 5-HTTLPR status moderates the effect of early adolescent substance use on risky sexual behavior. *Health Psychology, 29*(5), 471–476.

Kohler, M. P. (1996). Risk-taking behavior: A cognitive approach. *Psychological Reports, 78*, 489–490.

Lashbrook, J. T. (2000). Fitting in: Exploring the emotional dimension of adolescent peer pressure. *Adolescence, 35*, 277–294.

Manning, W. D., Longmore, M. A., & Giordano, P. C. (2000). The relationship context of contraceptive use at first intercourse. *Family Planning Perspectives, 32*(2), 104–110.

Martin, J. A., Hamilton, B. E., Sutton, P. D., et al. (2006). Births: Final data for 2004. *National Vital Statistics Reports, 55*(1), 1–101.

McCord, J. (1990). Problem behaviors. In S. S. Feldman & G. R. Elliot (Eds.), *At the threshold: The developing adolescent* (pp. 414–429). Cambridge: Harvard University Press.

Millstein, S. G., & Halpern-Felsher, B. L. (2002). Perceptions of risk and vulnerability. *Journal of Adolescent Health, 31S*, 10–27.

Newcomb, M. D., & Bentler, P. M. (1989). Substance use and abuse among children and teenagers. *American Psychologist, 44*, 242–248.

Newcomb, M. D., & McGee, L. (1991). Influence of sensation seeking on general deviance and specific problem behaviors from adolescence to adulthood. *Journal of Personality and Social Psychology, 61*, 614–628.

Omori, M., & Ingersoll, G. M. (2005). Health-endangering behaviors among Japanese college students: A test of psychological model of risk-taking behaviors. *Journal of Adolescence, 28*, 17–33.

Orr, D. P., Wilbrandt, M. L., Brack, C. J., Rauch, S. P., & Ingersoll, G. M. (1989). Reported sexual behaviors and self-esteem among young adolescents. *American Journal of Diseases of Children, 143*, 86–90.

Park, M. J., Mulye, T. P., Adams, S. H., Brindis, C. D., & Irwin, C. E., Jr. (2006). The health status of young adults in the US. *Journal of Adolescent Health, 29*, 305–317.

Pearson, M. A., & Michell, L. (2000). Smoke Rings: Social network analysis of friendship groups, smoking and drug-taking. *Drugs: Education, Prevention and Policy, 7*(1), 21–37.

Pedlow, C. T., & Carey, M. P. (2004). Developmentally appropriate sexual risk reduction interventions for adolescents: Rationale, review of interventions, and recommendations for research and practice. *Annals of Behavioral Medicine, 27*(3), 172–184.

Perrin, J. S., Herve, P., Leonard, G., Perron, M., Pike, G. B., & Pitiot, A., et al. (2008). Growth of white matter in the adolescent brain: Role of testosterone and androgen receptor. *The Journal of Neuroscience, 28*(38), 9519–9524.

Peterson, S. H., Wingood, G. M., DiClemente, R. J., Harrington, K., & Davies, S. (2007). Images of sexual stereotypes in rap videos and the health of African American female adolescents. *Journal of Women's Health, 16*(8), 1157–1164.

Phinney, V. G., Jensen, L. C., Olsen, J. A., & Cundick, B. (1990). The relationship between early development and psychosexual behaviors in adolescent females. *Adolescence, 98*, 321–332.

Puzzanchera, C. (2009). *Juvenile arrests 2008. U.S. Department of Justice, Office of Juvenile Justice and Delinquency Prevention*. Retrieved from http://www.ncjrs.gov/pdffiles1/ojjdp/228479.pdf.

Reyna, V., & Farley, F. (2006). Risk and rationality in adolescent decision-making: Implications for theory, practice, and public policy. *Psychological Science in the Public Interest, 7*, 1–44.

Ricciardelli, L. A., & McCabe, M. P. (2004). A biopsychosocial model of disordered eating and the pursuit of muscularity in adolescent boys. *Psychological Bulletin, 30*, 179–205.

Rivers, S. E., Reyna, V. F., & Mills, B. A. (2008). Risk taking under the influence: A fuzzy-trace theory of emotion in adolescence. *Developmental Review, 28*, 107–144.

Rubinstein, M. L., Luks, T. L., Moscicki, A.-B., et al. (2011). Smoking-related cue-induced brain activation in adolescent light smokers. *Journal of Adolescent Health, 48*, 7–12.

Sales, J. M., & Irwin, C. E., Jr. (2009). Theories of adolescent risk-taking: A biopsychosocial model. In R. DiClemente & R. Crosby (Eds.), *Adolescent health: Understanding and preventing risk behaviors and adverse health outcomes* (pp. 31–50). San Francisco, CA: Jossey-Bass.

Sales, J. M., Spitalnick, J., Crittenden, C. P., & DiClemente, R. J. (2009). Depression and sexual risk-taking in adolescents. In F. Columbus (Ed.), *Sexual risk-taking*. Hauppauge, NY: Nova Science Publishers.

Santelli, J. S., Morrow, B., & Carter, M. (2004). Trends in contraceptive use among US high school students in the 1990s. *Journal of Adolescent Health, 34*, 140.

Schor, E. L. (1987). Unintentional injuries: Patterns within families. *American Journal of Disease of Children, 141*, 1280–1284.

Shirtcliff, E. (2009). Biological underpinnings of adolescent development. In R. DiClemente, J. S. Santelli, & R. A. Crosby (Eds.), *Adolescent health: Understanding and preventing risk behaviors*. Hoboken: Jossey-Bass.

Sisk, C. L., & Foster, D. L. (2004). The neural basis of puberty and adolescence. *Nature Neuroscience, 7*, 1040–1047.

Sisk, C. L., & Zehr, J. L. (2005). Pubertal hormones organize the adolescent brain and behavior. *Frontiers in Neuroendocrinology, 26*, 163–174.

Smith, A. M. A., & Rosenthal, D. A. (1995). Adolescents' perceptions of their risk environment. *Journal of Adolescence, 18*, 229–245.

Snyder, H.N. (2000). *Juvenile arrests, 1999*. Washington, DC: Office of Juvenile Justice and Delinquency Prevention, 1.

Spear, L. (2000). The adolescent brain and age-related behavioral manifestations. *Neuroscience and Behavioral Reviews, 24*, 417–463.

Spitalnick, J. S., DiClemente, R. J., Wingood, G. M., Crosby, R. A., Milhausen, R. R., Sales, J. M., et al. (2007). Brief report: Sexual sensation seeking and its relationship to risky sexual behavior among African American adolescent females. *Journal of Adolescence, 30*, 165–173.

Steinberg, L. (1993). Autonomy conflict and harmony in the family relationship. In S. S. Feldman & G. R. Elliot (Eds.), *At the threshold: The developing adolescent* (pp. 255–275). Cambridge: Harvard University Press.

Steinberg, L. (2004). Risk-taking in adolescence: What changes, and why? *Annals of the New York Academy of Sciences, 1021*, 51–58.

Steinberg, L. (2007). Risk taking in adolescence: New perspectives from brain and behavioral science. *Current Directions in Psychological Science, 16*, 55–59.

Steinberg, L. (2008). A social neuroscience perspective on adolescent risk-taking. *Developmental Review, 28*(1), 78–106.

Tonkin, R. S. (1987). Adolescent risk-taking behavior. *Journal of Adolescent Health Care, 8*, 213–220.

Tschann, J. M., Adler, N. E., Irwin, C. E., Jr., Millstein, S. G., Turner, R. A., & Kegeles, S. M. (1994). Initiation of substance use in early adolescence: The roles of pubertal timing and emotional distress. *Health Psychology, 13*, 326–333.

Turner, R. A., Irwin, C. E., Jr., Tschann, J. M., & Millstein, S. G. (1993). Health. *Psychology, 12*(3), 200–208.

Udry, J. R., Talbert, L. M., & Morris, N. M. (1986). Biosocial foundations for adolescent female sexuality. *Demography, 23*, 217–227.

Urberg, K. A., Degirmencioglu, S. M., & Pilgram, C. (1997). Close friends and group influence on adolescent cigarette smoking and alcohol use. *Developmental Psychology, 33*(5), 834–844.

Werner, M. J. (1991). *Adolescent substance abuse. Maternal and Child Health Technical Information Bulletin*. Cincinnati: National Center for Education in Maternal and Child Health.

Windle, M. (1997). Concepts and Issues in COA Research. *Alcohol Health and ResearchWorld, 21*(3), 185–191.

Working Group of the NIH Advisory Committee. (2004). Report of the working group of the NIH advisory committee to the director on research opportunities in the basic behavioral and social sciences. http://obssr.od.nih.gov/pdf/Basic%20Beh%20Report_complete.pdf.

Zenilman, J. M., Yuenger, J., Galai, N., Turner, C. F., & Rogers, S. M. (2005). Polymerase chain reaction detection of Y chromosome sequences in vaginal fluid: Preliminary studies of a potential biomarker for sexual behavior. *Sexually Transmitted Diseases, 32*(2), 90–94.

Zimring, F. E. (1998). *American youth violence*. Oxford, England: Oxford University Press.

Zuckerman, M. (1979). *Sensation seeking: Beyond the optimal level of arousal*. Hillsdale, NJ: Erlbaum.

Zuckerman, M. (1990). The psychophysiology of sensation seeking. *Journal of Personality, 58*, 313–341.

Issues of Diversity in Adolescent Health Psychology: Exploring Sociocultural Influences on Adolescent Health

Lorraine T. Benuto

The field of health psychology explores the intricate and complex balance between physical and psychological health and disease. There is a vast amount of literature dedicated to the study of health psychology although research on both mental and physical health intervention and outcome in adolescents has historically been neglected (Williams, Holmbeck, & Greenley, 2002) particularly in the case of adolescent ethnic minorities. According to the 2011 Statistical Abstract published by the US Census Bureau as of 2009 approximately 16 % of individuals aged 14–17 years were African American, 4 % were Asian, and 19 % were Hispanic. These numbers do not account for those individuals who endorsed more than one ethnic affiliation and therefore are likely an underestimate of the true diversity of the population. These data demonstrate the large portion of the US population that is comprised of ethnic minority adolescents and call upon the need for a thorough review of the scientific literature on adolescent cultural minorities and health psychology. Thus, this chapter aims to explore how culture, socioeconomic status (SES), ethnicity, acculturation, etc., impact physical and psychological health.

L.T. Benuto, Ph.D. (✉)
Department of Psychology, Victims of Crime Treatment Center, University of Nevada, Reno, MS 0296, Reno, NV 89557, USA
e-mail: dr.benuto@gmail.com

Key Constructs Related to This Chapter

While as a field we have evolved in terms of the ways in which we define constructs associated with the cultural sensitivity movement often times key constructs associated with this movement are left poorly defined (O'Donohue, 1995; Benuto & Leany, 2011). Thus, the first goal of this chapter is to provide operational definitions of the constructs that are discussed. The second goal of this chapter is to identify the most useful and/or common conceptual frameworks and models that are used to explore developmental processes as they pertain to adolescent development (to help organize our discussion on how sociocultural factors relate to adolescence). Finally the chapter uses these conceptual frameworks to understand sociocultural influences on adolescent health.

Constructs Related to the Cultural Sensitivity Movement

Acculturation

Acculturation has been defined as a process that includes cultural and psychological changes resulting from intercultural contact (Berry, 2003) including changes in customs, economic status, political life, social behavior (Berry, Phinney, Sam, & Vedder, 2006), attitudes toward

W.T. O'Donohue et al. (eds.), *Handbook of Adolescent Health Psychology*,
DOI 10.1007/978-1-4614-6633-8_3, © Springer Science+Business Media New York 2013

the acculturation process, and cultural identity (Phinney, 2003). While traditionally the acculturation process was considered to be unidimensional, more recently the concept of biculturalism (i.e., fusing elements of both cultures; Suárez-Orozco & Suárez-Orozco, 2001; Suárez-Orozco & Qin-Hilliard, 2004) has gained increased attention in the literature. While conventionally the negative impact of acculturation was the focus of researchers and theorists, this perspective has evolved such that biculturalism is now believed to serve as a protective factor against the problems associated with alienation and marginalization (Roth, 2004).

Race and Ethnicity

While historically race and ethnicity were viewed as separate entities, the current state of the science indicates that racial designations and ethnicity do not have scientific basis (Zwillich, 2001). Thus, for the purpose of this chapter, we use the term ethnicity to refer to the five major racial-ethnic groups identified by the US Census: White European Americans, African Americans, Asian Americans/Pacific Islanders, Native Americans, and Latino/Hispanics. While these groupings are traditionally used they are certainly accurately described as being too "lumpy" and are most likely not the best way to categorize ethnic groups as each of them encompasses many quite distinct cultures (from Indian to Japanese to Thai to Vietnamese to Korean, etc.: O'Donohue & Benuto, 2010). Nonetheless, the majority of research on sociocultural factors and health use these grouping, and therefore, for the sake of organization this chapter discusses research in the context of research that has been conducted on these groups.

Socioeconomic Status

Socioeconomic status (SES) has been conceptualized as an amalgam of economic, educational, racial, cultural and/or ethnic variables (Benuto & Leany, 2011). It is important to note that much of the research on socioeconomic status can be generalized to nonethnic minority adolescents who are come from poor economic or limited educational backgrounds although to a large extent the literature seems to confuse disadvantaged economic status with ethnic minority status (even though there are many Caucasians that can be categorized as economically disadvantaged and the reverse is also true—ethnic monitories can in fact be wealthy).

Conceptual Frameworks for Understanding Adolescent Development

Contexts for Adolescent Development

Holmbeck and Shapera (1999) have developed a framework for studying adolescence and have identified several contexts for adolescent development including the interpersonal context of adolescent development (family, peer, school, and work); primary developmental changes in adolescence (biological/puberty, psychological/cognitive, social redefinition); demography and interpersonal moderating variables (ethnicity, family structure, gender, individual response to developmental change, neighborhood/community factors, SES); and developmental outcomes of adolescence (achievement, autonomy, identity, intimacy, psychosocial adjustment, sexuality). In this chapter we use this model to illustrate the ways in with sociocultural factors can impact adolescent health both for the sake of organization and also because the various contexts described by Holmbeck and Shapera (1999) are consistently described in the scientific literature when adolescent development is discussed.

Ethnic Identity Models

While the context for adolescent development (Holmbeck & Shapera, 1999) discussed above is meant as a general model for understanding adolescent development, given this chapter's focus on sociocultural influences on adolescent health, it is worthwhile to discuss in detail the concept of ethnic identity. Atkinson, Morten, and Sue (1998) provide a conceptual framework to help understand the struggles individuals might face as they try and understand themselves in terms of their own culture, the dominant culture, and the sometimes oppressive relationship between the two cultures. The model is broken into five stages: (1) conformity (appreciating attitudes towards dominant group); (2) dissonance and appreciating (information and experiences are inconsistent with culturally held beliefs, attitudes and values); (3) resistance and immersion (the individual tends to endorse minority-held views completely and reject the dominant values of society and culture); (4) Introspection (discontent and discomfort toward rigid group views, no global negativism directed at his or her own group); (5) integrated awareness stage (belief that there are acceptable and unacceptable aspects in all cultures and that it is very important for the person to be able to examine and accept or reject those aspects of a culture that are not seen as desirable).

Using Conceptual Frameworks to Understand Sociocultural Influences on Adolescent Health

Contexts for Adolescent Development

Interpersonal Context of Adolescent Development

Family

First and foremost it is important to note that what is considered "family" can vary by culture. Among certain ethnic groups the family is mostly made up of immediate family members (as is portrayed in the media of the typical Caucasian family). In other cultures the family is made up of not only the immediate family members (mom, dad, and siblings) but also extended family members and in some instances multiple generations may be strongly present within the family unit (e.g., grandparents may live with their adult children and grandchildren; uncles, aunts, and cousins may live with or in very close proximity—e.g., within the sample apartment complex or next door—with the adolescent, their siblings and parents). And yet in other cultures, the single-parent family is the norm. As we discuss in a moment supervision carries a large impact on adolescent development and therefore those families that have multiple adults available for supervision may confer a great number of advantages for the adolescent in terms of outcome.

As mentioned above in some cultures the family unit will consist of a single mother (or even father) and there may or may not be a lot of contact and proximity with extended family members. In fact, nonmarital births accounted for 39.7 % of all US births in 2007 (Ventura, 2009) (although half of these were makeup of cohabitating parents: Kennedy & Bumpass, 2008), which is a substantial increase over the last 40 (or even 20) years (Martin et al., 2009). This has been observed to be the highest among African Americans, American Indians, and Hispanics (respectively) and the lowest among Asian Americans (Hummer & Hamilton, 2010).

As indicated above, family has been established as a context that carries an impact on adolescent health. For example, research has indicated that parental connectedness (i.e., feelings of warmth, love, and caring from parents) and perceived parental expectations for school completion predict multiple risk behaviors (e.g., alcohol, tobacco, and marijuana use and early sexual activity; Resnick et al., 1997). Furthermore, parental support influences health risk behavior through a variety of pathways (e.g., adaptive coping, academic competence, and fewer deviant peer affiliations; Wills & Cleary, 1996). Research has also indicated that the connection between the parent and the adolescent can influence health risk behavior (Resnick et al., 1997) as can the amount of parental monitoring (e.g., parental monitoring influences the degree of adolescent heavy drinking; Reifman, Barnes, Dintcheff, Farrell, & Uhteg, 1998).

Because parent-adolescent dynamics vary by culture, family dynamics and parent-adolescent relationships and their relationship to adolescent health may vary as well. For example, differential acculturation levels between the adolescent and the parent can carry a large impact on the adolescent. If the parents have not adapted to the host culture, the adolescent may be encouraged to stay within the ethnic community and not doing so may be perceived as a betrayal of the parents' cultural and traditional values. The adolescent may also be called upon to act as a navigator to his or her parents thus resulting in a dyad that contradicts traditional family values whereby the parents are expected to guide the children (Roth, 2004), e.g., the adolescent may be called upon to act as a translator, to guide the parent through the US school and/or health care system etc. This "parentification" of the adolescent can result in the adolescent later forming codependent relationships (Wells, Glickaf-Hughes, & Jones, 1999). Differential levels of acculturation have also been found to impact family stress and the use of effective parenting practices, i.e., a greater discrepancy in acculturation between parents and youth is associated with increases in family stress and decreases in effective parenting practices (Martinez, 2006). Finally, beyond creating complexities in the parent-adolescent relationship, differences in level of acculturation between parents and adolescents has actually been associated with the development of certain psychological disorders, e.g., conduct-disordered behavior, substance abuse (Martinez, 2006; Szapocznik, Ladner, & Scopetta, 1979; Szapocznik & Kurtines, 1989).

Peers

Simply put peers greatly impact adolescent development and research has indicated that adolescents tend to seek friendships based on racial-ethnic similarities (Crosnoe & Lopez-Gonzalez, 2005; Quillian & Campbell, 2003). Generally speaking, peer influence can be positive or negative. In terms of the former, peers are a critical form of social support (Brown, Dolcini, & Leventhal, 1997) and can carry a positive influence on the adolescent specifically with regard to academic achievement and school attachment (Crosnoe, Cavanagh, & Elder, 2003). In contrast peers can also carry a negative impact on adolescent behavior (e.g., substance use; Curran, Stice, & Chassin, 1997; sexual risk behavior; Black, Ricardo, & Stanton, 1997; Romer et al., 1994). For example, Williams, Holmbeck, and Greenley (2002) discuss how peer influence is related to risk behavior via cognitive variables such as perceived norms (e.g., perceiving the prevalence of substance use among peers to be high and thus interpreting this as being "normal"). Such perceived norms have been consistently related to adolescent substance use (Chassin, Presson, Sherman, Corty, & Olshavsky, 1984; Donaldson, Graham, & Hansen, 1994). If we consider that research has indicated that adolescent substance use varies by ethnic group (Johnston, O'Malley, & Bachman, 2001) as does number of sexual partners and age of sexual initiation (Kirby, 2001) we can see how perceived norms can vary by culture and result in negative outcomes for the cultural minority adolescent, i.e., if certain cultural groups perceive adolescent substance use or teenage pregnancy as the norm, adolescents that belong to these cultural groups are at a higher risk for engaging in these "normed" behaviors. On the contrary it is important to keep in mind that the reverse could also be true—that is if a cultural group creates norms that are positive (i.e., in the case of Asian cultures education is viewed as of utmost importance) the cultural minority adolescent is likely to increase their involvement in these positive, "normed" behaviors.

It is also important to note that to a large extent SES determines peer interactions, i.e., adolescents who come from economically advantaged backgrounds tend to develop friendships with other adolescents from economically advantaged backgrounds (e.g., wealthy adolescents are more likely to attend private schools, engage in extracurricular activities that have a cost associated with them etc.) whereas adolescents from economically *dis*advantaged backgrounds are more likely to attend schools with less resources and to develop friendships with other adolescents from economically *dis*advantaged backgrounds.

School

Connectedness with school has been found to be a protective factor in the development of risk behavior (Jessor, Van Den Bos, Vanderryn, Costa, & Turbin, 1995; Resnick et al., 1997), whereas academic difficulties and low commitment to school are predictive of higher levels of risk behavior (Bailey & Hubbard, 1990; Elliott, Huizinga, & Ageton, 1985; Jessor & Jessor, 1977) which may be a function of the quality of school the adolescent attend and thus related to SES. If we consider that there are ethnic differences in high school graduate rates (Rumberger & Rotermund, 2009), i.e., Asians have the highest school graduation rate (91.7 %) followed by Whites (79.7 %), Hispanics (60.3 %), and African Americans (59.4 %), we can expect risk behaviors to vary by ethnicity as well (which as we have established thus far, variations do exist). Also if we consider the perceived norm perspective discussed above, we can again see how varying graduation rates can either carry a positive impact on adolescent behavior (as in the case of Asians the norm is a high school diploma) or a negative impact on behavior (as might be the case in Hispanics and African Americans whereby a large number of adolescents from these cultural groups do not graduate).

It is also worth mentioning that the type of school the adolescent attends can carry an impact on their performance, success etc. which brings into play other components of socioeconomic status. Compared to suburban schools, inner-city schools are usually overcrowded and understaffed thus offering an inferior level of education (Orfield & Yun, 1999), which does not promote success for the adolescents who attend these schools. This may be in part related to the disparities noted in college enrollment as 62.3 % of students enrolled in a degree-granting institution in 2009 were White, 14.3 % were Black, 12.5 % were Hispanic, 6.5 % were Asian/Pacific Islander, and 1 % were American Indian/Alaskan Native (US Department of Education, 2011).

Work

The majority of the literature has indicated that negative outcomes for the employed adolescent are few so long as the adolescent works less than 15 h/week (Hirschman & Voloshin, 2007). In fact when time spent working is less than 15 h per week better educational outcomes are observed in student workers than in those students who do not work at all (Carr, Wright, & Brody, 1996). However, working more than 20 h per week is a consistent predictor of risk behavior (Resnick et al., 1997) and employment at high levels of intensity reduces time spent on school-related activities resulting in poor educational outcomes (Lillydahl, 1990). While generally speaking, ethnic differences in student employment are small (Hirschman & Voloshin, 2007) these results may be slightly confounded by the higher high school graduation rates of Whites. In fact, Fuligni and Pedersen (2002) explored changes in the sense of obligation to assist, support, and respect the family among an ethnically diverse sample and found that Filipino and Latin American families reported the strongest sense of familial duty during young adulthood, which partially explained their tendency to live with and contribute financially to their families.

Primary Developmental Changes in Adolescence (Biological/Puberty, Psychological/Cognitive, Social Redefinition)

While certainly the biological changes that occur during adolescence do not vary in terms of the physiological processes, ethnic differences in pubertal timing have been shown to exist as do psychological implications for these differences. Specifically, Hispanic, Asian/Pacific Island, and African-American girls are more likely to experience menarche slightly earlier (4–7 months) than non-Hispanic White girls (Koprowski, Ross, Mack, Henderson, & Bernstein, 1999) and early-maturing girls are more likely to experience an adverse psychological impact as a result of early maturation, e.g., deviant behavior (Stattin & Magnusson, 1990) substance use (Lanza & Collin, 2002), concerns with weight and body image (Halpern, Udry, Campbell, & Suchindran, 1999), and psychological distress/depressive symptoms (e.g., Ge, Conger, & Elder, 2001; Graber, Lewinsohn, Seeley, & Brooks-Gunn,

1997). In terms of adolescent boys, research has indicated that the onset of puberty (as assessed by Tanner pubic-hair stage) occurs at age 11.2, 12.0, and 12.3 years for White, Black, White, and Mexican-American boys, respectively (Reiter & Lee, 2001), indicating that Black males mature at the earliest age. In terms of outcome research has indicated that there is an initial social advantage for early maturing boys, but also more adjustment problems (Cobb, 2010).

Demography and Interpersonal Moderating Variables

Here most certainly (in fact by definition) cultural factors are relevant. A discussion on the key constructs related to the cultural sensitivity movement (acculturation, ethnicity/race, and socioeconomic status) follows.

Acculturation and Ethnicity: Is the Impact Positive or Negative?

Acculturation

Generally speaking adolescence is a time during which social acceptance is highly sought. If adolescents are rejected by their peers etc. consequences can ensue. Further complications for the ethnic minority adolescent may develop as he or she may be seeking acceptance from two distinct cultural groups (i.e., the culture of origin and the host culture). If the ethnic minority adolescent feels rejected on both ends or observes his or her culture to be devalued and denigrated, he or she may identify and internalize these negative perceptions, leading to ethnic self-hate (Vega, Hough, & Romero, 1983). Roth (2004) discusses how the adolescent (specifically the Hispanic adolescent) may respond by being passive and thus developing depression and substance abuse. On the other hand, the adolescent may decide to defy the majority culture, which can lead to poor social and financial outcomes and marginalization. If the adolescent is unable to embrace their culture of origin and also rejects the host culture they may join gangs, which may provide a sense of belonging, solidarity, protection, discipline, and warmth.

While the above outlines the negative impact that acculturation or biculturalism can have on the adolescent, research has also suggested that a multicultural context can carry a positive impact by aiding in the development of flexibility, adaptability, and empathy for others—these personality characteristics can be beneficial to social relationships (Ramirez, 1983). In fact research has shown that a diverse ethnic context can reduce peer victimization, promote feelings of safety, and improve intergroup relations among ethnic minority youth (Graham, 2006; Juvonen, Nishina, & Graham, 2006); can be positively related to academic motivation (Tan, 1999); and foster an appreciation of diverse viewpoints (Kurlaender & Yun, 2002). Furthermore, ethnic composition of the class, status of the group, and social norms, have been found to affect children's positive evaluations of other groups (Kinket & Verkuyten, 1999). The above can promote a greater sense of belonging (Tan, 1999) and greater ethnic identity (Martinez & Dukes, 1997) which has been associated with the development of better coping skills and decreased aggression (McMahon & Watts, 2002) and higher levels of self-esteem, self- confidence, and purpose in life (Dukes & Martinez, 1994).

While a large body of literature has suggested ethnic differences in terms of behaviors that we typically perceive as "risk" behaviors in adolescence (e.g., substance use, unprotected sex etc.) one group of researchers have found that the combination of race or ethnicity, SES, and family structure together actually predict a relatively small amount of variance in adolescent risk behaviors (Blum et al., 2000). Specifically Blum and colleagues (2000) collected data from a nationally representative sample of 7th to 12th graders and a resident parent. Results from this study indicated that White adolescents were actually more likely to smoke cigarettes, drink alcohol, and attempt suicide in the younger years than were Black and Hispanic youths. Black youths were more likely to have had sexual intercourse and both Black and Hispanic youths were more likely than White teens to engage in violence. However, when gender, race/ethnicity, income, and family structure were controlled for the combination of these demographics explained no more than 10 % of the variance in each of the five risk behaviors among younger adolescents and no more than 7 % among older youths. These findings suggest that when taken together, race/ethnicity, income, and family structure provide only limited understanding of adolescent risk behaviors.

Language

Language has long since been conceptualized as a marker of acculturation and whereby bilingualism was previously perceived as an obstacle to assimilation and a cognitive disadvantage, it is now regarded as the opposite. In fact Suárez-Orozco & Suárez-Orozco (2001) discussed how higher degrees of bilingualism appear to be related to higher cognitive attainment (Hakuta & Garcia, 1989). Nonetheless, one would be hard-pressed to argue that learning a second language in adolescence would be an easy feat (particularly as compared to learning a second language early in childhood). In fact, in the context of adolescent development it is important to note that adolescents who are in the process of learning a second language (e.g., English) are usually over-represented in learning-disabled classes and linguistic problems represent one of the most frequent reasons for psychiatric school referrals. Experts have identified that difficulty with verbal expression frequently results in frustration and acting-out behaviors in these students (Suárez-Orozco & Suárez-Orozco, 2001). Nonetheless, the issue of bilingualism is rarely considered as a contributory factor to the development of such issues (Canino & Spurlock, 1994).

SES

As previously mentioned, issues related to SES are not so much directly related to ethnicity, acculturation etc. but more so to poverty and therefore this portion of this chapter can be generalized to nonethnic minorities who are poor. Nonetheless, it is important to note that specific to cultural minorities (specifically immigrants) most Hispanics who immigrate to the USA to escape poverty tend to be low-skilled workers from the rural areas of Latin America and may be semiliterate in their own languages. The end result of this is the immigrant ends up working low-paying jobs with limited ability towards upward mobility (Roth, 2004).

Generally speaking, the adolescent psychiatry literature indicates that poverty alone is not sufficient to cause problems in development (Canino & Spurlock, 1994) and factors such as family discord and disruption of attachment carry a stronger influence on the development of mental health problems in children and adolescents (Roth, 2004).

Furthermore, as indicated above SES contributes to adolescent outcome and development in a number of indirect ways (e.g., residing in crime-ridden neighborhoods, interactions with peers, etc.). Additional factors related to SES that substantially influence health (both in adolescence and beyond) are largely related to access to resources. For example, the percentage of adolescent and child citizens with no medical insurance are as follows: 33.4 % Hispanic, 21.2 % African American, and 14.2 % white non-Hispanic children and adolescents have no medical insurance (US Census Bureau, 2002) and are generalizable to adults and children as well.

Developmental Outcomes of Adolescence (Achievement, Autonomy, Identity, Intimacy, Psychosocial Adjustment, Sexuality) Including Ethnic Identity Development

Certainly autonomy and identity are often discussed in the literature on culture. In fact collectivism vs. individualism is an often-cited difference between certain cultural groups and racial or ethnic identity is often discussed as a large component of who one is and the achievement of such an identity is considered to be a huge developmental milestone. A recent report titled "Understanding Adolescents" discusses how young people tend to adapt to the values and ways of the new culture more readily than their parents do in some instances this causes a rift between the family's expectations of the adolescent to maintain the values and customs of their 'old' culture and the norms of the new culture (which must be ascribed to so that the adolescent can fit in with their peers). Generally speaking adolescents who come from inter-cultural relationships or who are being raised by a parent (or parents) who do not ascribe to North American cultural values face the typical challenges associated with adolescence combined with having to integrate knowledge of both their in-home (the culture of origin) and back-yard culture (their host culture), e.g., two languages, two sets of behavioral and social expectations, etc. In fact there may be a large variability in terms of the cultural values and norms as they pertain to the central tasks of adolescence (e.g., developing a sense of identity, autonomy etc.). We only need to look to popular media to see this conflict portrayed on the big screen. The movie *Real Women have Curves*:

> Freshly graduated from high school, Ana receives a full scholarship to Columbia University. Her very traditional, old-world parents feel that now is the time for Ana to help provide for the family, not the time for college. Torn between her mainstream ambitions and her cultural heritage she agrees to work with her mother at her sister's downtown LA sewing factory. Over the summer she learns to admire the hardworking team of women who teach her solidarity and teamwork. Still at odds with what her mother expects of her, Ana realizes that leaving home to continue her education is essential to finding her place proudly in the world as an American and Chicana.

Ethnic/racial identity is discussed in further detail momentarily and specific ethnic differences in psychosocial related variables are discussed later in the chapter.

Discussing Specific Ethnic Differences in Epidemiology

Experts have discussed how people use health care and how patients make decision about whether to follow medical advice is influenced by individual beliefs and perceptions in combination with environmental resources or barriers (Rodriguez-Gomez & Salas-Serrano, 2006). Furthermore, epidemiological research has clearly indicated ethnic differences in physical and mental disease. For example, Hispanic adolescents have been found to have higher prevalence rates of asthma (e.g., Wickrama, Elder, & Abraham, 2007) than Caucasians (Wickrama et al., 2007), Asians (Flores, & Tomany-Korman, 2008), and Blacks (Laditka, Laditka, & Probst, 2006). Almost twice as many Hispanic and Black adolescents are overweight than White adolescents (Ogden, Flegal, Carroll, & Johnson, 2002) and according to the CDC (2011) Type 2 Diabetes appears to be increasing among both girls and boys, particularly in some racial and ethnic minority groups.

Ethnic differences in adolescent health-risk behaviors have also been identified, e.g., White adolescents are more likely to smoke heavily than non-whites (Centers for Disease Control & Prevention, 2010c) although the literature on substance use is mixed in terms of whether or not Whites use substance at a greater rate than ethnic minority adolescents. Finally, there are also ethnic differences in terms of diagnoses of mental health conditions. For example, Whites and Hispanics are more commonly diagnosed with eating disordered behavior (Davis & Yager, 1992) and depression appears to be far more prevalent in White adolescents than ethnic minority adolescents (Keller, Salazar, & Courtney, 2010).

Discussing Cultural Differences by Ethnicity

African Americans

Generally speaking, African Americans tend to show poorer health than Caucasians, tend to underutilize services or drop out of services at higher rates (Kar, Kramer, Skinner, & Zambrana, 1995), are more often misdiagnosed, and more likely to be diagnosed as having a severe mental illness (US Department of Health and Human Services, 2001). Kazarian (2001) discusses several factors that are associated with the health inequalities of African Americans (e.g., research has indicated that African Americans show health disadvantages relative to Caucasians) including genetic predisposition to certain diseases; low levels of income, education, occupation, and wealth; high general stress, acculturative stress, or race-related stress; high-fat diets, smoking, unprotected sex; failure to use safety belts, sedentary lifestyle, high levels of alcohol consumption, use of illicit drugs; exposure to toxic chemicals and other environmental hazards; fatalistic or helpless attitude, strong sense of the present but not the future, underutilization of formal health care system, delay in seeking heath care; and issues related to access to health care.

Asian Americans

Research has indicated that both Asian adolescents and adults do experience psychological and psychiatric problems (Kim, 1978; Leong, 1986; Sue et al., 1994) and some research has indicated that Asian immigrants are less likely to rate their health as excellent then other Americans (10 % vs. 40 % respectively) (Loo, 1998). Some experts have suggested that this may be related to the stress of acculturation, fewer socioeconomic resources, language barriers, issues related to access, and the biomedical model that pervades in the USA which contradicts traditional Asian health beliefs, i.e., explanations for illness drive health and illness behavior and satisfaction with health care, and compliance (Kirscht, 1977). Nonetheless, Asians are thinner (Centers for Disease Control & Prevention, 2009) and have lower rates of cancer than most other groups (Centers for Disease Control & Prevention 2010a, 2010b, 2011), suggesting that they may actually have superior health than other ethnic groups.

Specific to Asian adolescents researchers have found that emotional and behavioral difficulties tend to be more prevalent when the adolescent's acculturation level differs from that of their parents (Lee, 1996). Asians have also been found to underutilize mental health services (e.g., Loo, 1998; Sue et al., 1994) and even terminate therapy prematurely (Zane & Sue, 1996) both of which can have deleterious consequences on health.

Hispanic/Latino

A number of factors have been found to impact Latinos' use of health-related services (e.g., mental health services). In fact Latinos often perceive mental health services as unnecessary, unwelcoming, or not useful; are likely to use services mostly when in crisis; and have high dropout rates and undesirable treatment outcomes (US DHHS, 2001). Lack of insurance coverage can also contribute to underutilization of services (Iniguez & Palinkas, 2003) although certainly this is not specific to Latinos and applies to all who lack coverage.

Summary and Conclusions

In this chapter information regarding the operational definitions associated with the concept of culture have been defined, contexts for adolescent development and their relationship to sociocultural factors have been explored, and ethnic differences with regard to conditions that impact health have been provided. Generally speaking, it is evident that sociocultural factors can be health-promoting, health-demoting, or a combination of both. While not a large focus of this chapter, the most problematic sociocultural factor is poverty as poverty largely impacts access to health services and access is an often-cited health-demoter. Overall, it is apparent that the ethnic minority adolescent is faced with the same trials and tribulations as the nonethnic minority adolescent and may experience some culture-specific complications that can impact health.

In terms of practical implications, those who work with adolescent ethnic minorities are well-advised to be aware of differences in prevalence rates in certain mental and physical diseases and to examine how cultural factors may impact the larger occurrences of such diseases and how these cultural factors can be changed to reduce such occurrences. Ethnic differences in prevalence rates aside, minority status should not be used as an excuse to administer sub-par treatments on the premise that evidence-based treatments have not been specifically tested with a specific cultural group. In the realm of research, it is imperative that researchers begin to disentangle the impact of economic status on health from the cultural characteristics that constitute an ethnic group. As it stands issues related to access (which are a function of economic status) are often confused and lumped together with ethnic minority status and certainly one can be economically disadvantaged and not be an ethnic minority and vice versa.

References

Atkinson, D. R., Morten, G., & Sue, D. W. (1998). *Counseling American minorities* (5th ed.). Boston: McGraw-Hill.

Bailey, S., & Hubbard, R. L. (1990). Developmental variation in the context of marijuana initiation among adolescents. *Journal of Health and Social Behavior, 31*(1), 58–70.

Benuto, L., & Leany, B. D. (2011). Reforms for ethnic minorities and women. In N. A. Cummings & W. T. O'Donohue (Eds.), *Understanding the behavioral healthcare crisis: The promise of integrated care and diagnosis* (pp. 367–394). New York: Routledge.

Berry, J. W. (2003). Acculturation: Advances in theory, measurement, and applied research. In K. M. Chun, P. Organista, & G. Marin (Eds.). Washington, DC: American Psychological Association.

Berry, J. W., Phinney, J. S., Sam, D. L., & Vedder, P. (2006). *Immigrant youth in cultural transitions: Acculturation, identity, and adaptation across national contexts*. Mahwah: Erlbaum Associates Publisher.

Black, M. M., Ricardo, I. B., & Stanton, B. (1997). Social and psychological factors associated with AIDS risk behavior among low-income, urban, African American adolescents. *Journal of Research on Adolescence, 7*(2), 173–195.

Blum, R. W., Beuhring, T., Shew, M. L., Bearinger, L. H., Sieving, R. E., & Resnick, M. D. (2000). The effects of race/ethnicity, income, and family structure on adolescent risk behavior. *American Journal of Public Health, 90*(12), 1879–1884.

Brown, B. B., Dolcini, M. M., & Leventhal, A. (1997). Transformations in peer relationships in adolescence: Implications for health-related behavior. In J. Schulenberg, J. L. Maggs, & K. Hurrelmann (Eds.), *Health risks and developmental transitions during adolescence* (pp. 161–189). NewYork: Cambridge University Press.

Canino, I. A., & Spurlock, J. (1994). *Culturally diverse children and adolescents: Assessment, diagnosis, and treatment*. New York: Guilford Press.

Carr, R. V., Wright, J. D., & Brody, C. J. (1996). Effects of high school work experience a decade later: Evidence from the national longitudinal survey. *Sociology of Education, 69*(1), 66–81.

CDC. (2011). Children & Diabetes. Retrieved from http://www.cdc.gov/diabetes/projects/diab_children.htm.

Centers for Disease Control & Prevention. (2009). *Minority health surveillance—Reach U.S. 2009*. Retrieved from http://www.cdc.gov/Features/dsREACHUS/.

Centers for Disease Control & Prevention. (2010a). *Breast cancer rates by race and ethnicity*. Retrieved from http://www.cdc.gov/cancer/breast/statistics/race.htm.

Centers for Disease Control & Prevention. (2010b). *Lung cancer rates by race and ethnicity*. Retrieved from http://www.cdc.gov/cancer/lung/statistics/race.htm.

Centers for Disease Control & Prevention. (2010c). Youth risk behavior surveillance—United States, 2009. *Morbidity and Mortality Weekly Report, 59*(SS5), 1–13.

Centers for Disease Control & Prevention. (2011). *Prostate cancer rates by race and ethnicity*. Retrieved from http://www.cdc.gov/cancer/prostate/statistics/race.htm.

Chassin, L., Presson, C. C., Sherman, S. J., Corty, E., & Olshavsky, R. O. (1984). Predicting the onset of cigarette smoking in adolescents: A longitudinal study. *Journal of Applied Social Psychology, 14*, 224–243.

Cobb, N. J. (2010). Adolescence: Continuity, change, and diversity (7th ed.). In E. O. Reiter, & P. A. Lee. Have the onset and tempo of puberty changed? *Archives of Pediatrics & Adolescent Medicine, 155*, 988–989.

Crosnoe, R., Cavanagh, S., & Elder, G. H. (2003). Adolescent friendships as academic resource: The intersection of friendship, race, and school disadvantage. *Sociological Perspectives, 46*(1), 331–352.

Crosnoe, R., & Lopez-Gonzalez, L. (2005). Immigration from Mexico, school composition, and adolescent functioning. *Sociological Perspectives, 48*, 1–24.

Curran, P. J., Stice, R., & Chassin, L. (1997). The relation between adolescent alcohol use and peer alcohol use: A longitudinal random coefficient model. *Journal of Consulting and Clinical Psychology, 65*(1), 130–140.

Davis, C., & Yager, J. (1992). Transcultural aspects of eating disorders: A critical literature review. *Culture, Medicine and Psychiatry, 16*(3), 377–394.

Donaldson, S. I., Graham, J. W., & Hansen, W. B. (1994). Testing the generalizability of intervening mechanism theories: Understanding the effects of adolescent drug use prevention interventions. *Journal of Behavioral Medicine, 17*(2), 195–216.

Dukes, R. L., & Martinez, R. (1994). The impact of Ethgender on self-esteem among adolescents. *Adolescence, 29*, 105–115.

Elliot, D. S., Huizinga, D., & Ageton, S. (1985). *Explaining delinquency and drug use*. Beverly Hills, CA: Sage.

Flores, G., & Tomany-Korman, S. C. (2008). Racial and ethnic disparities in medical and dental health, access to care, and use of services in US children. *Pediatrics, 121*(2), e286–e298.

Fuligni, A. J., & Pedersen, S. (2002). Family obligation and the transition to young adulthood. *Psychology, 38*(5), 856–868.

Ge, X., Conger, R. D., & Elder, G. H. (2001). Pubertal transition, stressful life events, and the emergence of gender differences in adolescent depressive symptoms. *Developmental Psychology, 37*(3), 404–417.

Graber, J. A., Lewinsohn, P. M., Seeley, J. R., & Brooks-Gunn, J. (1997). Is psychopathology associated with the timing of pubertal development? *Journal of the American Academy of Child and Adolescent Psychiatry, 36*(12), 1768–1776.

Graham, S. (2006). Peer victimization in school. *Current Directions in Psychological Science, 15*, 317–321.

Hakuta, K., & Garcia, E. E. (1989). Bilingualism and education. *American Psychologist, 44*(2), 374–379.

Halpern, C. T., Udry, J. R., Campbell, B., & Suchindran, C. (1999). Effects of body fat on weight concerns, dating, and sexual activity: A longitudinal analysis of Black and White adolescent girls. *Developmental Psychology, 35*(3), 721–736.

Hirschman, C., & Voloshin, I. (2007). The structure of teenage employment: Jobs held by high school seniors. *Research in Social Stratification and Mobility, 25*(3), 189–203.

Holmbeck, G. N., & Shapera, W. E. (1999). Research methods with adolescents. In P. C. Kendal, J. N. Butcher, & G. N. Holmbeck (Eds.). *Handbook of research methods in clinical psychology*. New York: Wiley.

Hummer, R. A., & Hamilton, E. R. (2010). Race and ethnicity in fragile families. *The Future of Children, 20*(2), 113–131.

Iniguez, E., & Palinkas, L. A. (2003). Varieties of health services utilization by underserved Mexican American women. *Journal of Health Care for the Poor and Underserved, 14*, 52–69.

Jessor, R., & Jessor, S. L. (1977). *Problem behavior and psychosocial development: A longitudinal study of youth*. New York: Academic Press.

Jessor, R., Van Den Bos, J., Vanderryn, J., Costa, F., & Turbin, M. (1995). Protective factors in adolescent problem behavior: Moderator effects and developmental change. *Developmental Psychology, 31*, 923–933.

Johnston, L. D., O'Malley, P. M., & Bachman, J. G. (2001). *Monitoring the future national survey results on drug use, 1975–2000. Volume I: Secondary school students* (NIH Publication No. 01-4924). Bethesda, MD: National Institute on Drug Abuse, p. 492.

Juvonen, J., Nishina, A., & Graham, S. (2006). Ethnic diversity and perceptions of safety in urban middle schools. *Psychological Science, 17*(5), 393–400.

Kar, S., Kramer, J., Skinner, J., & Zambrana, R. E. (1995). Panel VI: Ethnic minorities, health care systems, and behavior. *Health Psychology, 14*, 641–646.

Kazarian, S. S. (2001). Health issues in North American people of African heritage. In S. S. Kararian & D. R. Evans (Eds.), *Handbook of cultural health psychology*. San Diego, CA: Academic Press.

Keller, T. E., Salazar, A. M., & Courtney, M. E. (2010). Prevalence and timing of diagnosable mental health, alcohol, and substance use problems among older adolescents in the child welfare system. *Child and Youth Services Review, 32*(4), 626–634.

Kennedy, S., & Bumpass, L. (2008). Cohabitation and children's living arrangements: New estimates from the United States. *Demographic Research, 19*, 1663–1692.

Kim, B. C. (1978). *The Asian Americans, changing patterns, changing needs*. Montclair, NJ: Association of Koran Christian Scholars in North America.

Kinket, B., & Verkuyten, M. (1999). Intergroup evaluation and social context: A multilevel approach. *European Journal of Social Psychology, 29*(2–3), 219–237.

Kirby, D. (2001). *Emerging answers: Research findings on programs to reduce teen pregnancy*. Retrieved from http://eric.ed.gov/ERICWebPortal/search/detailmini.jsp?_nfpb=true&_&ERICExtSearch_SearchValue_0=ED456171&ERICExtSearch_SearchType_0=no&accno=ED456171.

Kirscht, J. P. (1977). Communication between patients and physicians. *Annals of Internal Medicine, 86*(4), 499–500.

Koprowski, C., Ross, R. K., Mack, W. J., Henderson, B. E., & Bernstein, L. (1999). Diet, body size and menarche in a multiethnic cohort. *British Journal of Cancer, 79*(11–12), 1907–1911.

Kurlaender, M., & Yun, J. T. (2002). *The impact of racial and ethnic diversity on educational outcomes: Cambridge, MA school district*. Cambridge, MA: The Civil Rights Project, Harvard University.

Laditka, S. B., Laditka, J. N., & Probst, J. C. (2006). Racial and ethnic disparities in potentially avoidable delivery complications among pregnant medicaid beneficiaries in South Carolina. *Maternal and Child Health Journal, 10*(4), 339–350.

Lanza, S. T., & Collins, L. M. (2002). Pubertal timing and the stages of substance use in females during early adolescence. *Prevention Science, 3*, 69–82.

Lee, J. (1996). *Unraveling the "Model Minority" stereotypes: Listening to Asian American youth*. New York, NY: Teachers College Press.

Leong, F. T. L. (1986). Counseling and psychotherapy with Asian Americans: Review of the literature. *Journal of Counseling Psychology, 33*, 196–206.

Lillydahl, J. H. (1990). Academic achievement and part-time employment of high school students. *The Journal of Economic Education, 21*(3), 307–316.

Loo, C. M. (1998). *Chinese America: Mental health and quality of life in the inner city*. Thousand Oaks, CA: Sage.

Martin, J. A., Hamilton, B. E., Sutton, P. D., Ventura, S. J., Menacker, F., Kirmeyer, S., et al. (2009). *Births: Final date for 2006*. Retrieved from http://www.cdc.gov/nchs/products/nvsr.htm#vol48.

Martinez, C. R., Jr. (2006). Effects of differential family acculturation on Latino adolescent substance use. *Family Relation, 55*(3), 306–317.

Martinez, R. O., & Dukes, R. L. (1997). The effects of ethnic identity, ethnicity, and gender on adolescent well-being. *Journal of Youth and Adolescence, 26*, 503–516.

McMahon, S. D., & Watts, R. J. (2002). Ethnic identity in urban African American youth: Exploring links with self-worth, aggression, and other psychosocial variables. *Journal of Community Psychology, 30*, 411–431.

O'Donohue, W. T (1995). Cultural sensitivity: A critical examination. In R. H. Wright & N. A. cummings (Eds.), *Destructive trends in mental health* (pp. 29–44). New York, NY: Routledge.

O'Donohue, W., & Benuto, L., (2010). The many problems with cultural sensitivity. *Scientific Review of Mental Health Practice*, *7*(2), 34–37.

Ogden, C. L., Flegal, K. M., Carroll, M. D., & Johnson, C. L. (2002). Prevalence and trends in overweight among use children and adolescents, 1999–2000. *Journal of the American Medical Association, 288*(12), 1728–1732.

Orfield, G., & Yun, J. T. (1999). *Resegregation in American schools*. Cambridge, MA: The Civil Rights Project, Harvard University.

Phinney, J. S. (2003). Ethnic identity and acculturation. In K. M. Chun, P. Balls Organista, & G. Marin (Eds.). *Ethnic identity and acculturation*. Washington, DC: American Psychological Association.

Quillian, L., & Campbell, M. E. (2003). Beyond black and white: The present and future of multiracial friendship segregation. *American Sociological Review, 68*(4), 540–566.

Ramirez, M. (1983). *Psychology of the Americas: Mestizo perspectives on personality and mental health*. New York: Pergamon.

Reifman, A., Barnes, G. M., Dintcheff, B. A., Farrell, M. P., & Uhteg, L. (1998). Parental and peer influences on the onset of heavier drinking among adolescents. *Journal of Studies on Alcohol, 59*, 311–317.

Reiter, E. O., & Lee, P. A. (2001). Have the onset and tempo of puberty changed? *Archives of Pediatrics & Adolescent Medicine, 155*(9), 1022–1028.

Resnick, M. D., Bearman, P. S., Blum, R. W., Bauman, K. E., Harris, K. M., Jones, J., et al. (1997). Protecting adolescents from harm: Findings from the National Longitudinal Study on Adolescent Health. *Journal of the American Medical Association, 278*(10), 823–832.

Rodriguez-Gomez, J. R., & Salas-Serrano, C. C. (2006). Treatment adherence in ethnic minorities: Particularities and alternatives. In W. T. O'Donohue & E. R. Levensky (Eds.), *Promoting treatment adherence: A practical handbook for health care providers* (pp. 393–400). California: Sage.

Romer, D., Black, M., Ricardo, I., Feigelman, S., Kaljee, L., Galbraith, J., et al. (1994). Social influences on the sexual behavior of youth at risk for HIV exposure. *American Journal of Public Health, 84*(6), 977–985.

Roth, E. M. (2004). Hispanic adolescents and their families sociocultural factors and treatment considerations. *Adolescent Psychiatry, 28*, 251–278. 28.

Rumberger, R. W., & Rotermund, S. (2009). *Ethnic and gender differences in California high school graduation rates*. Retrieved from http://www.hewlett.org/uploads/files/CDRP_EthnicandGenderDifferences Graduation_Rates.pdf.

Stattin, H., & Magnusson, D. (1990). *Pubertal maturation in female development. Paths through life* (Vol. 2). Hillsdale, England: Lawrence Erlbaum Associates.

Suárez-Orozco, M., & Qin-Hilliard, D. B. (Eds.). (2004). *Globalization: Culture and education in the new millennium*. California: University of California Press.

Suárez-Orozco, C., & Suárez-Orozco, M. M. (2001). *Children of immigration*. Cambridge, MA: Harvard University Press.

Sue, S., Nakamura, C. Y., Chi-Ying Chung, R., & Yee-Bradbury, C. (1994). Mental health research on Asian Americans. *Journal of Community Psychology, 22*(2), 61–67.

Szapocznik, J., & Kurtines, W. M. (1989). *Breakthroughs in family therapy with drug abusing and problem youth*. New York: Springer.

Szapocznik, J., Ladner, R., & Scopetta, M. (1979). Youth drug abuse and subjective distress in a Hispanic population. In G. M. Beschner & A. S. Friedman (Eds.), *Youth drug abuse* (pp. 463–511). Lexington, MA: Heath.

Tan, G. (1999). Perceptions of multiculturalism, academic achievement, and intent to stay in school among Mexican American students. *Journal of Research and Development in Education, 33*, 1–14.

U.S. Census Bureau. (2002). *Health insurance coverage 2001* (USCB). Washington, DC: U.S. Department of Commerce.

U.S. Department of Education, National Center for Education Statistics. (2011). Higher Education General Information Survey (HEGIS). Retrieved from http://nces.ed.gov/programs/digest/d11/tables/dt11_237.asp.

U.S. Department of Health and Human Services. (2001). *Mental health: Culture, race, and ethnicity – A supplement to mental health: A report of the Surgeon General*. Rockville, MD: U.S. Department of Health and Human Services, Office of the Surgeon General.

Vega, W. A., Hough, R., Hough, R., & Romero, A. (1983). Family life patterns among Mexican Americans. In G. Powell et al. (Eds.), *The psychosocial development of minority children*. New York: Bruner-Mazel.

Ventura, S. J. (2009). *Changing patterns of nonmarital childbearing in the United States*. Hyattsville, MD: National Center for Health Statistics.

Wells, M., Glickauf-Hughes, C., & Jones, R. (1999). Co-dependency: A grass roots construct's relationship to shame-proneness, low self-esteem, and childhood parentification. *American Journal of Family Therapy, 27*, 63–71.

Wickrama, K. A. S., Elder, G. H., Jr., & Abraham, T. (2007). Rurality and ethnicity in adolescent physical illness: Are children of the growing Latino population at excess health risk? *The Journal of Rural Health, 23*(3), 228–237.

Williams, P. G., Holbeck, G. N., & Neff, R. (2002). Adolescent health psychology. *Journal of Consulting and Clinical Psychology, 70*(3), 828–842.

Wills, T. A., & Cleary, S. D. (1996). How are social support effects mediated: A test with parental support and adolescent substance use. *Journal of Personality and Social Psychology, 71*, 937–952.

Zane, N., & Sue, S. (1996). Health issues of Asian Pacific American adolescents. In M. Kagawasinger, P. A. Katz, D. A. Taylor, & J. H. M. Vanderryn (Eds.), *Health issues for minority adolescents* (pp. 142–167). Lincoln: University of Nebraska Press.

Zwillich, T. (2001). *Human genome project director peers into the future*. Washington, DC: Reuters Medical News. Retrieved March 10, 2001, from http://medformation.com/mf/news.

Socioeconomic Influences on Health and Health Behavior in Adolescents

Julia Dmitrieva

A substantial amount of research has linked socioeconomic status (SES) to health among adults (Adler et al., 1994). As such, individuals placed at a lower SES gradient are at higher risk for mortality and morbidity across a wide range of physical and mental health outcomes (Illsley & Baker, 1991; McDonough, Duncan, Williams, & House, 1997). Relatively less is known about the effects of SES on children's health, although, some evidence suggests that SES begins to impact health in-utero (contributing to, for example, low birth weight and birth defects) and its effects last throughout lifespan, manifesting in neurological problems, complications of bacterial and viral infections, and behavioral problems (Aber, Bennett, Conley, & Li, 1997; Bradley & Corwyn, 2002). Compared to literature investigating adults and children, research on SES disparities in health among adolescents is scarcer. Furthermore, a significant proportion of findings do not differentiate among children and adolescents, failing to investigate the unique nature of adolescence –a developmental period that is marked by prominent changes in physical and psychological development (Yurgelun-Todd, 2007). The following chapter reviews current empirical literature linking SES and health among adolescents, pointing out similarities and differences in the role of SES for children vs. adolescents' health.

Adolescents and Social Context

The period of adolescence is arguably the healthiest and most resilient of the entire life span. The typical adolescent enjoys peak performance in a number of physiologic indicators of health, including muscular strength, flexibility of joints, and increased resistance to colds. Yet, the overall morbidity and mortality rates increase as much as 200 % during middle childhood and adolescence. Moreover, adolescence is a time of biological and social transitions, with youth continuing to undergo a number of profound neurological, hormonal, and psychosocial changes that make them potentially vulnerable to factors such as poverty and low SES. As they mature, adolescents experience sustained growths in planning, reasoning abilities, problem-solving, and inhibitory control (Luna, Padmanabhan, & O'Hearn, 2010). These changes take place as the adolescent brain undergoes the second wave of overproduction of gray matter (Giedd et al., 1999), followed by synaptic pruning and increases in white matter (Gogtay & Thompson, 2010). With pubertal initiation of hormonal changes, adolescents exhibit greater risk-taking and novelty-seeking (Steinberg, 2008), an increase in emotional intensity, and an

J. Dmitrieva, Ph.D. (✉)
Department of Psychology, University of Denver,
2155 South Race Street, Denver, CO 80208-3500, USA
e-mail: jdmitrieva@psy.du.edu

W.T. O'Donohue et al. (eds.), *Handbook of Adolescent Health Psychology*,
DOI 10.1007/978-1-4614-6633-8_4,

increased likelihood of being diagnosed with affective disorders (Pine, 2003). These changes point to adolescence as a time of considerable brain plasticity, with particular adolescence-limited vulnerabilities to psychosocial stress. In fact, research indicates that adolescents are more sensitive to the effects of stressors and negative life events than children or adults are (Walker, Sabuwalla, & Huot, 2004). Furthermore, socioeconomic disadvantage, a context associated with detriments in health among adults, may be even more harmful to adolescents, as it can set a stage for vulnerabilities that alter trajectories of health and health-associated behaviors throughout adulthood.

At the psychosocial level, adolescence is the time of increasing autonomy and self-determination. As parental influence gradually declines, youths begin to turn to their peers for social support, romantic involvements, and information relevant for identity and self (Steinberg & Silverberg, 1986). These changes may contribute to a decline in the importance of family context for adolescent adjustment and increasing roles of peer, school, and neighborhood contexts. However, the effects of parental SES continue to exert an influence on health, as it is an important determinant of access to good schools, safe neighborhood environments, and high-quality health care.

Understanding the effects of SES on youth health is critical, given the recent history of economic changes. Economic conditions have declined for many families in the USA, over the past decade. For the first time since the Great Depression, the housing prices have followed a sustained decline (Organisation for Economic Co-operation & Development, 2010). Combined with subprime mortgage practices, this trend has started an avalanche of mortgage foreclosures that has forced millions of families out of their homes. Although no official information is available on the number of completed foreclosures in the past years, some estimate that 2.5 million households have lost their home to foreclosure in the short period between January 2007 and the end of 2009 (Bocian, Li, Ernst, & Center for Responsible Lending, 2010). The housing crisis has, in turn, triggered a shortage of liquidity in the US banking system, leading to the wide-spread economic consequences. As a result, the unemployment rate among individuals aged 16 years and older increased from 3.9 % in 2000 to 10.5 % in 2010 (US Bureau of Labor Statistics, 2011). Similarly, the real median household income for full-time workers has declined by 4.2 % between 2007 and 2009, and approximately 31.6 % of the population has had at least one episode of poverty that lasted 2 or more months between 2004 and 2007 (DeNavas-Walt, Proctor, Smith, & US Census Bureau, 2010). The impact of the economic crisis has not been experienced to the same extend by some segments of the population. For example, the average household income has dropped for families with children, whereas families without children have experienced an increase in income (DeNavas-Walt et al., 2010). Most importantly, income inequalities have expanded over the past decade, with the 5 and 9 % declines in the real income among households in the 50th and 10th income percentiles, respectively. This drop in income corresponded to no significant changes in real income of households in the 90th percentile for income.

These trends are especially troubling given that the effects of SES go beyond the effects of severe poverty (e.g., a level of poverty where individuals are not able to meet basic nutritional or health care needs). In contrast, the effects of SES are monotone, with higher levels of SES providing extra health advantage at every level of the hierarchy (Adler et al., 1994; Backlund, Sorlie, & Johnson, 1996; Ecob & Davey Smith, 1999; Marmot et al., 1991). Thus, even relatively modest negative changes in the economic conditions of today's youths can precipitate measurable declines in health.

History and Definitions

There is a history of disagreements among social scientists regarding the precise definition of the SES (e.g., McLoyd, 1997). Most would agree that SES should embody the idea of capital, including financial capital (e.g., material resources and assets), human capital (e.g., education), and social capital (e.g., resources available through social networks) (Bradley & Corwyn, 2002). The core of the disagreement emerges from various strategies that are available to assess these aspects of capital. For example, financial capital is often measured by income. However, current earnings may not be the best indicator of financial resources available to an individual. Compared to this, a measure that includes income, occupational status, and financial assets (e.g., housing tenure) provides a better estimate of the financial resources and opportunities (Ostrove, Feldman, & Adler, 1999; Williams & Collins, 1995).

Notwithstanding this debate, social scientists often employ a composite measure of SES that comprises of income, social status (e.g., education), and occupational status (Adler et al., 1994). Whereas some researchers combine the three indicators into a single measure, others use one of these indicators as a measure of SES. This chapter considers the effects of both the broadly defined combined indicator SES and its specific facets.

Although there is an unequivocal link between SES and health among adults and children, this association is less unambiguous among adolescents. Goodman (1999) reports that SES is related to increased depression, greater obesity, and lower self-rated overall health. However, among adolescents, SES is not associated with asthma prevalence and is inconsistently related to suicide attempts (Goodman, 1999).

During the late 1980s and early 1990s, the existence of SES disparities in health during adolescence has been questioned by several investigators who observed a lack of the expected SES-to-health associations among youth. Most notably, West (West, 1988; West, Macintyre, Annandale, & Hunt, 1990) hypothesized that the effects of SES on health during adolescence should be evident within the domain of chronic illnesses, because chronic illnesses are likely to have been acquired as a consequence of childhood exposure to low SES conditions. In contrast, acute and adolescent-onset conditions should not be affected by SES because of the increasing influences of school, peer group, and youth culture during this period of life. His analysis of data for youth in the UK through mid-1990s revealed a pattern that is consistent with this theory (West, 1997). Since then, several other researchers (e.g., Pensola & Valkonen, 2000; Vuille & Schenkel, 2001; Williams, Currie, Wright, Elton, & Beattie, 1997) have found supporting evidence for West's (1988, 1990) hypothesis. Thus, these researchers came to view adolescence as the time of equalization, when adolescent autonomy and youth culture has an equalizing effect on youth from families with different SES standings.

A more recent analysis of health inequalities in the UK, however, suggests that the attenuation in SES health disparities among adolescents is only evident when considering some measures of health but not others. For example, Spencer's (2006) analysis of 15,756 children and adolescents from 8,541 British households found that there is an attenuation of SES differences for youth-reported health outcomes, but not parent-reported health outcomes of 12- to 14-year old adolescents. Furthermore, adolescents between the ages of 14 and 18 years old do not exhibit the hypothesized attenuation in SES-to-health differences. Likewise, Chen, Matthews, and Boyce (2002) reviewed seven large-scale studies of SES effects on children and adolescents, concluding that SES is linked to all-cause mortality and morbidity in a monotonic fashion in both of these age groups. More specifically, youths of lower SES were more likely to die from chronic conditions, such as asthma, cancers, congenital abnormalities, and heart disease, as well as from acute conditions, such as pneumonia or injuries. Similarly, youths of lower SES also had higher rates of chronic and acute conditions, and experienced greater impairment in association with their illnesses.

SES and Specific Health Problems

Physical Health

Cardiovascular Health

Cardiovascular disease is the leading cause of death in the USA (Heron et al., 2009). Although cardiovascular problems are often diagnosed late in the disease process, research indicates that the precursors of heart disease start in adolescence (McCarron & Davey Smith, 2003). The atherosclerotic lesions, for example, begin to form during childhood and are present in the arteries of more than half of young adolescents (McGill et al., 2000b). Given the infrequent nature of cardiovascular diseases among adolescents, there are no studies linking the effects of SES on adolescent cardiovascular disease. However, the effects of SES can be seen on the risk factors that are strongly linked with future development of coronary heart disease. As such, lower SES youths have higher rates of cigarette smoking, higher adiposity, shorter height, higher consumption of fat, and lower consumption of fiber (Batty & Leon, 2002). Furthermore, the effects of SES can be seen on adolescents' ratings of the indices of subclinical cardiovascular disease (Thurston & Matthews, 2009).

Obesity

The rise of obesity is a major health problem, with adolescent obesity rates increasing worldwide (Kohn et al., 2006; Yoon et al., 2006). Currently, about one-third of US adults and approximately 17 % of children and adolescents are obese (Centers for Disease Control and Prevention, 2011a). There is a well-established link between SES and obesity among adults (see McLaren for a review, 2007) and research on adolescents finds a similar link. For example, Goodman (1999) analyzed the effects of SES on adolescent obesity for 15,483 adolescents participating in the National Longitudinal Study of Adolescent Health. She found that income and education are two independent predictors of adolescent obesity. In the follow-up analyses, Goodman, Slap, and Bin (2003) report that 32 % of cases of adolescent obesity are attributable to lower income and 39 % are attributable to parental education. Physical inactivity, inequalities in access to health care, and differences in diet are the probable mechanisms that link obesity and SES.

Asthma

Asthma is the third-ranking cause of hospitalizations for youth under 15 years old (DeFrances, Cullen, & Kozak, 2007), with about one out of every ten school-aged children suffering from asthma (Centers for Disease Control and Prevention, 2011b). The association between asthma and SES among children is quite clear—children of lower SES have a higher prevalence of asthma and respiratory conditions, and suffer from more sever and frequent symptoms (Chen et al., 2002). On the other hand, the findings for adolescents are strikingly less certain. For example, of fourteen studies reviewed by Chen et al. (2002), none found an inverse association between SES and asthma prevalence. Instead, four studies found a positive association, with higher SES placing youth at a higher risk for asthma and wheezing, eight did not find a significant association, and two had mixed results with positive associations found for some measures of income but not for others. Results from other, more recent, studies also support previous work by finding a positive association between SES and asthma prevalence (e.g., Farfel, Tirosh, Derazne, Garty, & Afek, 2010). Results for symptom severity are more consistent, with lower SES being linked to greater symptom severity and hospitalizations rates. Consistent with these findings, low SES predicts greater impairment, as measured by rescue inhaler use and school absences, among 9–18 year old youth over the 6-month period (Chen, Fisher, Bacharier, & Strunk, 2003). Thus, the pattern of findings for asthma prevalence is consistent with the hygiene hypothesis, whereby improved quality of life removes protective factors that prevent the development of asthma. In contrast, the findings for symptom severity follow a more traditional pattern of associations, where SES-related exposure to neighborhood pollutants, parental smoking, and high family stress exacerbate the frequency and severity of asthma symptoms.

Mental Health

Many of the mental health problems have their onset during adolescence (Benes, 2003; Kessler et al., 2005; Walker & Bollini, 2002) and adolescent psychopathology is associated with future impairments and mental health problems (Heijmens Visser, Van der Ende, Koot, & Verhulst, 2002; Hofstra, Van de Ende, & Verhulst, 2001).

Youth of low SES are more likely to live in dangerous neighborhoods, be exposed to family stress and poor parenting, and have parents who suffer from psychopathology. Thus, low SES confers a risk for the development of internalizing and externalizing problems (Leventhal, & Brooks-Gunn, 2000; Loeber et al., 1998; Marmorstein, & Iacono, 2004; Schneiders et al., 2003). Indeed, there is a substantial support for the link between SES and children and adolescent psychopathology (Bolger et al., 1995; Brooks-Gunn & Duncan, 1997; Lahey et al., 1995; McCoy et al., 1999; McLeod & Shanahan, 1993).

Depression

There is a history of research linking lower SES with a greater likelihood of major depression and a greater number of depressive symptoms among adults (Adler et al., 1994, Lynch et al., 1997). This link between SES and depression begins to surface during adolescence (Lempers, Clark-Lempers, & Simons, 1989; McLoyd, 1997), at the time when many affected individuals begin to experience depressive symptoms for the first time. As such, Goodman et al. (2003) reported that 26 % of cases of adolescent depression are attributable to income and 40 % are attributable to parental education. The association between SES and depression has been hypothesized to be partially mediated by the contextual risk factors that are associated with living in the lower SES conditions—e.g., greater economic hardship and material disadvantages, greater family stress, and lower availability of social support. However, it is important to note that the effects of SES on adolescent depressed mood remain significant even after taking into account adolescent self-esteem, stress exposure, health behaviors (e.g., smoking cigarettes and drinking alcohol), and social ties with parents, peers, and school (Call & Nonnemaker, 1999).

Although the link between SES and depression is important in and of itself, it has additional implications for other physical health problems. Depression is a known risk factor for other health conditions, potentially serving as a mediating mechanism that connects lower SES to other illnesses. Compared to other psychological predictors, depression has the strongest association with the coronary heart disease (Booth-Kewley & Friedman, 1987), with major depressive disorder predicting a twofold increase in the rates of major cardiac events (e.g., myocardial infarction) among the adult patients with coronary heart disease (Chen et al., 2002). In addition, depression has been linked to asthma, arthritis, and ulcers (Friedman & Booth-Kewley, 1987) and dysregulated immune function (Miller, Cohen, & Herbert, 1999). Thus, lower socioeconomic standing may lead to depression in adolescence and young adulthood, which in turn may lead to further depression and other chronic conditions in adulthood. However, whether depression accounts for the link between SES and these conditions remains to be investigated.

Externalizing Problems

Externalizing behavior is chiefly a disorder of childhood and adolescence. Although for some children externalizing problems begin as early as age four, the rate and variety of externalizing problems increase throughout adolescence for the majority of affected youth (Bongers, Koot, van der Ende, & Verhulst, 2004). In fact, criminologists commonly refer to the age-crime curve that depicts a sharp adolescent rise in various criminal offenses, followed by a decline in criminal behavior throughout young and middle adulthood (e.g., FBI Uniform Crime Report, 2001). The association between SES and externalizing problems begins to emerge in early childhood and becomes relatively stable by middle through early adolescence (Achenbach et al., 1990, McLeod & Shanahan, 1993; McLoyd, 1997). By adolescence, the SES–behavior link is well established and a large number of studies report a greater propensity for antisocial behavior among lower-SES youths (e.g., Agnew, Matthews, Bucher, Welcher, & Keyes, 2008; Elliott & Ageton, 1980; Jarjoura, Triplett, & Brinker, 2002; Wright, Caspi, Moffitt, Miech, & Silva, 1999). However, it is important to note that SES has the strongest link with moderate to serious problem behaviors, and little relationship with minor behavioral problems (Agnew et al., 2008).

Several theories have been proposed to explain the SES–externalizing behavior link. According to strain theory (Agnew, 1999; Greenberg, 1977), low-SES adolescents experience economic problems, and it is their inability to achieve immediate economic goals or a loss of valued goods that drive adolescents toward delinquent behavior. The family process theories, on the other hand, maintain that economic hardships disrupt parent-child relationships, increase family conflict, and undermine parents' ability to effectively discipline their children. This disruption of the family system is responsible for adolescent externalizing behavior (e.g., Conger & Conger, 2002). Finally, peer researchers note that, compared to children, adolescents spend more time with their peers and adolescents who associate with deviant peers are more likely to be involved in delinquent behavior (e.g., Vitaro, Tremblay, Kerr, Pagani, & Bukowski, 1997). Research shows support for all three theories—adolescents' inability to reach economic goals (Agnew, 1994; Baron, 2004; Cernkovich, Giordano, & Rudolph, 2000), family conflict (Conger, Ge, Elder, Lorenz, & Simons, 1994; Wadsworth & Compas, 2002), and affiliation with antisocial peers (Sampson & Groves, 1989) mediate the path between SES and externalizing behavior.

Substance Abuse

Adolescence is the time when problems with nicotine dependence and alcohol and drug use begin to surface. Most smokers, for example, are introduced to their first cigarette during adolescence and begin habitual smoking before the age 18 (Giovino, Henningfield, Tomar, Escobedo, & Slade, 1995). Accordingly, the SES assessed in childhood and adolescence has an effect on adolescent and adult rates of cigarette smoking (Adler et al., 1994; Chen et al., 2002). The nature of the association between SES and cigarette smoking changes with age. Individuals of lower SES are more likely to begin smoking at an earlier age, with no SES differences in the initiation rates during adolescence (Chassin, Presson, Sherman, & Edwards, 1992). However, there is substantial evidence that adolescents of low SES have higher rates of smoking (due to newly initiated and established smokers combined together) (e.g., Melotti et al., 2011). Thus, during adolescence, SES does not appear to contribute to the adolescent onset of cigarette smoking, but it does contribute to smoking rates.

Furthermore, there is conflicting data regarding the direction of the effects of SES on substance use, with many studies reporting a negative association, but some studies reporting a positive association. For example, some found that the rates of smoking are negatively associated with SES (Escobedo, Anda, Smith, Remington, & Mast, 1990) and the risk of smoking for low-SES youth increases. In contrast, different studies find a negative SES–smoking association, low-SES standing elevates the risk of smoking from 1.4 to 2.5 times for children under 12 and from 1.6 to 4.5 times for youths who are older than 12 (Chen et al., 2002). Similarly, Melotti et al. (2011) report a higher rate of binge drinking among low-SES youth. However, other researchers found that the risk of substance use is also elevated among the affluent youth (Ennett, Flewelling, Lindrooth, & Norton, 1997; Hanson & Chen, 2007). Taken together, the findings of both negative and positive effects suggest a curvilinear effect of SES (Chassin, Beltran, Lee, Haller, & Villalta, 2010), with elevated rates of substance use at both the low and high ends of the SES distribution. Whereas the effects of low SES can be attributed to classic low-SES factors, such as higher levels of stress and lower parental supervision, mechanisms that transmit the effects of high SES on substance use include greater availability of financial resources (Hanson & Chen, 2007) and higher achievement pressures (Luthar & Latendresse, 2005).

Theories of SES and Health

Historically, two major theories have been advanced to explain the association between SES and health—i.e., the social causation and the social selection theories. The social causation theory asserts that poverty is responsible for the environmental adversity and stress that are, in turn, implicated in the etiology of the physical and mental problems experienced by the low-SES youths (e.g., Conger & Conger, 2002; Haas, 2006). The social selection (also known as the drift) theory proposes that those with physical and mental disorders drift into lower SES or fail to rise out of low SES (e.g., McLeod & Kaiser, 2004; Wender, Rosenthal, Kety, Schulsinger, & Welner, 1973). According to this theory, positive psychological adjustment and good physical health are the adaptive qualities that allow an individual to better adjust to their environment and, consequently, be more successful in the social and economic realm. Both, socioeconomic advantage and these positive qualities could be further transmitted to the offspring generation, either via social (e.g., cultural transmission of the value of persistence in the face of adversity or of good health habits) or genetic modes of transmission.

Elements of both theories have been supported by research. Longitudinal studies provide support for the social causation theory, demonstrating that loss of income predicts deterioration in mental health (Catalano, Dooley, Wilson, & Hough, 1993; Dodge, Pettit, & Bates, 1994; Link & Phelan, 1995; Loeber, Green, Keenan, & Lahey, 1995; Shaw, Winslow, Owens, & Hood, 1998). On the other hand, there is also evidence for the social selection theory. It is known, for example, that psychiatric disorders predict poor educational and occupational outcomes (Miech, Caspi, Moffitt, Wright, & Silva, 1999). There is also evidence that childhood externalizing problems diminish youth chances of receiving a high school degree, and of subsequent college enrollment (McLeod & Kaiser, 2004). However, this model does not provide a complete picture of the SES–health association because SES shows prospective effects on health (Adler et al., 1994).

Thus, a more complete theory of SES-to-health association requires specification of both social causation and social selection patterns. Conger and Donnellan (2007) proposed the Interactionist Perspective, combining the social causation and social selection theories. This model suggests a reciprocal process by which childhood SES predicts children's and adolescents' personal characteristics that further influence their SES during adulthood. In support of the model, recent studies find that childhood family SES is predictive of mental and physical problems among youth, in turn predicting economic problem during young adulthood (Conger, Conger, & Martin, 2010). Similarly, Martin et al. (2010) report that parental SES predicts adolescent problem behaviors, which in turn are associated with subsequently lower SES and greater family stress when adolescents reach adulthood. The lower SES and higher family stress were further associated with the offspring antisocial behavior, providing a compelling picture of intergenerational transmission of the socioeconomic standing and antisocial behavior.

In a different attempt to reconciliate the social selection and social causation theories, each of the two patterns of association can be seen as better suited for explaining some disease processes than others. Indeed, Johnson, Cohen, Dohrenwend, Link, and Brook (1999) investigated multigenerational associations among SES and health measures in a sample 736 families. Their results provide some support for the social causation hypothesis, indicating that low parental SES is associated with higher likelihood of offspring anxiety, depression, disruptive disorders, and personality disorders, over and beyond the effects of parental psychopathology, single-parent status, and IQ. Offspring alcohol and marijuana abuse were not predicted by parental SES. The social selection hypothesis was also supported for some outcomes: adolescents who were diagnosed with disruptive disorders or substance abuse disorders were twice as likely to drop out of high school and almost four times more likely to discontinue education after completing high school than youth not diagnosed with these disorders. However, the social selection hypothesis was not supported for anxiety, depression, and personality disorders. Thus, the direction of association between SES and health can vary across different adolescent health outcomes. Further multigenerational investigations would be required to test the combined propositions of the social selection and social causation theories across different health outcomes.

Finally, the application of the social selection theory to adolescents requires a slight reconceptualization. Children's and adolescents' health is not likely to influence their SES. Thus, it is more reasonable to assume that illness on the part of the parents (or members of a prior generation) is responsible for the family drift in SES. Youth demonstrate a correlation between SES and illness because of the hereditary nature of the illnesses they have inherited from their parents. If propositions of the social selection theory are correct, we can expect a lower correspondence between the parental SES and youth health than between the parental SES and parental health. This proposition has not been empirically tested; however, the greater amount of inconsistencies in the SES disparities in health among youth than adults provides a descriptive rationale for testing this assertion.

Mediating Mechanisms

Part of the complexity of SES effects on health is in the multi-causality and multi-finality of the processes involved in the link between SES and health. The effects of SES are broad, influencing a wide range of domains of functioning, such as a person's physical environment (e.g., exposure to pathogens, toxic hazards, and carcinogens), social environment (e.g., exposure to violence, stress, and access to social capital), and health behaviors. (e.g., cigarette smoking, alcohol drinking). Theoretical literature linking SES and health proposes a variety of mechanisms from these domains as potential mediators of the link between SES and health. Many of these mechanisms have not been formally tested among adolescents (as is the case where there is evidence for the SES effects on the proposed mediating variable and of mediating variable on the health outcome, but no formal tests of the mediation pathway) or have been tested in some age groups but not others. Nonetheless, these mediating models provide theoretical background to guide future research and offer promise of clarifying mechanisms explaining SES and health associations.

Access to Resources

Access to resources is the most obvious mechanism linking SES and health. Inability to purchase goods, poor nutrition, and lower access to health care are associated with poorer immune functioning, greater nutritional deficiencies, and higher rates of infectious and chronic diseases among children (Bradley & Corwyn, 2002). Families with lower SES have lower rates of visiting the doctor than families with higher socioeconomic standing (Chen et al., 2002). When families of lower SES receive care, it is of lower quality than care received by higher SES families (Williams, 1990). However, access to health care alone does not explain health disparities of the low vs. high SES individuals in their entirety (Adler, Boyce, Chesney, Folkman, & Syme, 1993), and SES differences in health remain among individuals with universal health coverage (e.g., Bradley & Corwyn, 2002).

Psychosocial Mechanisms

Stress

The strain of low SES is felt by all family members, overwhelming their coping resources and leading to negative emotional states such as anxiety, depression, and hostility. These emotions, in turn, are known to lead to poor health (Ewart, Elder, Smyth, Sliwinski, & Jorgensen, 2011; Gallo & Matthews, 1999). The Family Stress Model (FSM; Conger, Ge, Elder, Lorenz, & Simons, 1994) has been proposed to explain how economic problems lead to poor marital relationship quality and marital instability. According to this model, the stress of economic hardship and economic pressures on family resources contribute to parents' emotional and behavioral problems (e.g., depression, anxiety, anger, substance use, and antisocial behavior), which, in turn, lead to interparental conflict and poor parenting quality, ultimately increasing the likelihood of emotional and behavioral problems on the part of the child (Conger & Conger, 2002; Conger & Donnellan, 2007). The model has received extensive support across different ethnic groups and geographic locations, predicting emotional and behavioral problems among youth (see Conger et al., 2010 for a review). There is also evidence that the impact of family stress that is associated with low SES extends throughout adolescence and into adult years (Sobolewski & Amato, 2005).

As a result, stress is responsible for much of the effect of SES on health (Adler et al., 1999; McLoyd, 1998a). In addition to higher interparental stress, low-SES families also experience more uncontrollable stressful life events (Bradley & Corwyn, 2002).These uncontrollable stressful life events place an individual at a greater risk for a heart attack (Theorell, 1974), infectious disease, heart disease, stroke, gastrointestinal problems, and depression (Adler et al., 1999; Bradley & Corwyn, 2002). Some of these associations are also confirmed for children and adolescents, with a positive relation between greater exposure to stressful life events and an elevated risk for psychopathology (Chen et al., 2002; Pine, 2003). Finally, the impact of stress exposure on emotional functioning is greater for persons of lower than higher SES (McLeod & Kessler, 1990). Thus, SES increases the likelihood of exposure to life events stress, as well as reduces an individual's capacity to cope with that stress.

One of the factors helping to explain the effects of stress on health is the construct of allostatic load, or the cumulative physiological demands that are placed on an organism in order to adapt (i.e., achieve allostasis) to the demands imposed by environmental stressors. Greater demands create greater allostatic load that can contribute to chronic physiological changes such as a persistent elevated blood pressure. There is mounting evidence for the link between SES and allostatic load (Johnston-Brooks et al., 1998). Specifically, there is some evidence for the disregulation of the serotonergic function, hypothalamic-pituitary-adrenal (HPA) axis activity, and immune system functioning in relation to poverty and lower SES. Along the same lines, other studies report that harsh parenting, exposure to violence, and frequent negative life events are associated with muted cardiovascular reactivity (Boyce & Chesterman, 1990; Krenichyn, Saegert, & Evans, 2001; Murali & Chen, 2005)—a measure of the organism's ability to mobilize in response to stress. Thus, there appears to be an accumulated wear and tear on the cardiovascular stress response in relation to chronic exposure to stressors that are commonly experienced by youth of lower SES.

Emotional Processing

Some researchers have noted that SES may influence health through its effects on emotional processing (Adler, et al., 1994; Chen et al., 2002). As has already been noted above, economic deprivation is associated with depression, which in turn is linked to other diseases such cardiovascular disease and ulcers. In addition to depression, dispositional hostility (measured by anger-proneness; cynical view of others, and antagonistic behavior), low sense of control, and low optimism have been linked to both SES and physical health. For example, Barefoot et al. (1991) studied a national sample of US adults and found higher hostility among less educated participants. Similar findings are reported by other researchers (Chen et al., 2002). Hostility, in turn, has been prospectively linked to coronary heart disease and premature mortality (Barefoot, Dahlstrom, & Williams, 1983; Dembroski, MacDougall, Costa, & Grandits, 1989; Siegman, Dembroski, & Ringel, 1987). However, these mediating pathways have not been formally tested and it remains to be seen whether depression, hostility, sense of control, and optimism explain the link between SES and physiological health. Furthermore, it is not known whether the associations among emotional processing, SES, and physiological health are present during adolescence. Given that adolescence is the time of rapid development in each of the four measures of emotional processing, it stands to reason that socioeconomic deprivation during adolescence may have the most profound effect on their levels and developmental trajectories.

Health Behaviors

Substance Abuse

As has been noted above, smoking, drug use, and binge drinking are associated with lower SES. And, it is well-known that substance use is associated with a myriad of health problems.

Therefore, it makes theoretical sense that smoking and substance abuse would mediate the link between SES and adolescent health. However, few studies have examined that possibility. Surprisingly, those that explored this research question do not find evidence that these health behaviors explain the link between SES and health (Adler et al., 1999; Harrell et al., 1998; Wohlfarth & Van den Brink, 1998). Further research is needed to examine the role of substance abuse as a mediator of the SES–health link among adolescents.

Physical Inactivity

It is a well-established fact that the lack of physical activity is linked to obesity (Bouchard, Shepard, Stephens, Sutton, & McPherson, 1990) and, consequently, coronary heart disease (McGill et al., 2000a). The exercise habits are established early in the life and often persist into adulthood. In one study, for example, 71 % of 14-year-old adolescents who engaged in weekly exercise continued to exercise regularly by the age of 24 (Pietila et al., 1995 from Chen). A number of studies have found an inverse link between SES and physical activity among adults (Adler et al., 1994). Similar findings are reported for adolescents (Gottlieb & Chen, 1985; Tuinstra, Groothoff, van den Heuvel, & Post, 1998; Toftegaard-Støckel, Nielsen, Ibsen, & Andersen, 2011).

Various factors could help account for the SES–physical inactivity link. Low-SES families experience more stress, leaving parents strapped for time and psychological resources. In this circumstance, parents may serve as poor role models for physical activity and healthy lifestyle. Likewise, low-SES parents are more likely to suffer from depression, which would also prevent them from engaging in physical exercise. Furthermore, low-SES families have a more limited access to the facilities that promote exercise. A number of studies have found a disparity in the distribution of parks and playgrounds (Wolch, Wilson, & Fehrenback, 2005) and fewer free facilities in the low SES areas as compared to higher SES areas (Estabrooks, Lee, & Gyurcsik, 2003; Moore et al., 2008). Finally, factors such as facility safety, gangs, drug abuse, and crime rates in the low-SES parks and neighborhoods prevent many youths from utilizing the existing facilities (Sobal & Stunkard, 1989).

Exposure to Risky Social Environments

The peer context is especially important as a mediating mechanism for the transmission of SES effects on health during adolescent years. Youth of lower SES often live in dangerous neighborhoods, where they are exposed to higher rates of violence (McLoyd, 1998a) and stressful life events (Attar, Guerra, & Tolan, 1994). Adolescents living in impoverished neighborhoods are also more likely to be exposed to antisocial peers, and this exposure is particularly relevant for adolescent problems behaviors and substance use. Given that adolescents engage in antisocial behavior and substance use in the company of peers (Chassin et al., 2004), peer behavior is one of the key predictors of adolescent outcomes. In one experimental study of youth performance on a risk-taking task, middle adolescents doubled the amount of risky behavior when accompanied by peers, as compared to when they were completing the task alone (Gardner & Steinberg, 2005). Indeed, resistance to peer pressure undergoes development between the ages of 14 and 18, with no significant developmental changes prior or after that age range (Steinberg & Monahan, 2007).

Biological Mechanisms

Exposure to Pollution and Toxic Substances

The housing conditions of adolescents living in poverty are often substandard, exposing them to dangerous conditions, such as unprotected stairwells, pests, and unsafe heating appliances; thus, predisposing those youth to greater risks of illness and injuries (Bradley & Corwyn, 2002). Research shows that children of low SES are more likely to live in houses with lead paint and to have elevated blood levels of lead (Pamuk et al., 1998). Furthermore, living in crowded housing conditions has been linked to elevated resting blood pressure in boys (Evans, Lepore,

Shejwal, & Palsane, 1998). Beyond the effects of poverty-stricken households, exposure to pollution and toxic substances outside the home can also serve as the mediators of the SES–health link. Indeed, children of lower SES are exposed to air with higher carbon monoxide levels, which in turn has a significant effect on asthma severity (Neidell, 2004).

Inflammation

Another biological pathway connecting SES to health outcomes is through inflammation (Chen & Miller, 2007). Low SES is associated with elevated systemic inflammatory profiles among adults (Hemingway et al., 2003; Panagiotakos et al., 2005) and children (Chen et al., 2006; Chen, Fisher, Bacharier, & Strunk, 2003). Elevated inflammation, in turn, is associated with a wide range of illness. For example, inflammation is implicated it the growth and rupturing of atherosclerotic plaques (Libby, 2001; Ross, 1999) as well as depression, anorexia, and social withdrawal (Dantzer, O'Connor, Freund, Johnson, & Kelley, 2008; Miller, Maletic, & Raison, 2009). Furthermore, there is evidence that children of low SES grow up to have elevated inflammation profiles (Chen, Miller, Kobor, & Cole, 2011). Future research needs to investigate the degree to which inflammation explains the connection between SES and health, and test which specific health outcomes are particularly well-explained by this process.

Cortisol

The effects of stress on health may be also mediated by the HPA axis. Cortisol is one of the most-studied glucocorticoid hormones that is involved in energy metabolism and coping with stress (e.g., Dickerson & Kemeny, 2004). Adult normal cortisol levels follow a circadian rhythm with the highest levels peaking at 30 min after morning awakening, a sharp decline over the first 2 h after awakening, and a gradual decline over the remainder of the day and night (Kirschbaum et al., 1990). This cortisol rhythm is not inborn and continues to evolve during infancy and early childhood, and its development is dependent on environmental factors (Watamura et al., 2004). Research on the developmental changes in the HPA axis functioning during adolescence is sparse, the study of SES effects on adolescent HPA axis are sparser still. Recent studies report higher basal cortisol levels for children of lower SES, with the strength of this association increasing between the ages of 6 and 10 (Lupien, King, Meaney, and McEwen, 2000). This association, however, disappears by the time youth begin their transition into high school (Lupien, King, Meaney, and McEwen, 2001). There is also emerging evidence supporting the view that cortisol is a mediator of the effects of socioeconomic stress on health (Flinn & England, 1997).

Blood Pressure

Although not formally tested as a mediator, high blood pressure is one of the primary pathways that are suspected to link SES and cardiovascular disease. First, blood pressure tends to track over age—i.e., with childhood high blood pressure being a risk factor for high blood pressure during adulthood (Chen et al., 2002). Furthermore, high blood pressure is an important risk factor for cardiovascular disease (McGill et al., 2000b). Finally, there is an association between high blood pressure and SES in childhood (Chen et al., 2002). Chen et al. (2002) reviewed all studies of SES and blood pressure through year 2002. They concluded that the association between SES and blood pressure is not present during the adolescent years. However, a more recent study has suggested that there may be an association between the neighborhood SES and individual's blood pressure, with low SES being associated with an increase in systolic blood pressure (McGrath, Matthews, & Brady, 2006).

Summary and Future Directions

Based on the reviewed literature, it can be concluded without a doubt that socioeconomic standing has an effect on adolescent health. Specifically, lower SES can be linked to elevated risk for coronary heart disease, obesity, asthma severity, depression, externalizing problems, and substance use. Access to resources, stress, health behaviors, affiliation with antisocial peers, and environmental pollution appear to be the key correlates of low SES, which may help explain the SES disparities in health among adolescents. Furthermore, disregulation of the inflammatory, HPA, and cardiovascular systems may serve as biological mediators between these correlates of low SES and adolescent health.

Despite this extensive evidence, there is substantial room for future research. Research shows that risk exposure in a greater number of domains (e.g., in the family stress, peer, and health behavior domains) is associated greater likelihood of negative health outcomes. However, it is less clear which specific factors are more strongly predictive of which specific outcomes. Such knowledge can only be obtained from studies that test a wide range of mediating variables across a wide range of health outcomes. Unfortunately, most previous studies have focused on a limited number of outcomes and mediating variables. Toward the same goal, there is a need for theories that would predict differential mediating pathways for the SES-to-health association. Such theories would also need to take into account that the same environmental conditions can change their meaning over age—living in a poverty-stricken neighborhood may be associated with fewer educational and recreational resources among younger children but result in affiliation with deviant peers among adolescents (Bradley & Corwyn, 2002). Finally, there is a need for models that can predict the combined effects of various components of SES and their synergistic interaction with each other or with other measures of family, neighborhood, and peer context (McLoyd, 1998a).

Future research will also need to expand the search for potential moderators of the SES-to-health link. For example, emerging research suggests that social support and effective coping can help buffer the effects of SES on psychological and physical health (Chen & Miller, 2007; Leinonen et al., 2003). Studies that examine a wide range of protective factors will help determine optimal intervention strategies for youth at risk for specific health outcomes.

Our growing knowledge of the genetic risk factors that influence health and psychological adjustment can help improve our understanding of the nature of the SES–health association. SES and genetic risk may follow a diathesis-stress pattern of associations for some outcomes, with greatest risk present for those who are at risk in both the socioeconomic and genetic domains. For example, a recent study reports that the negative effect of the rs3809508 neuromedin B gene polymorphism on adolescent obesity is exacerbated by lower maternal education (Pigeyre et al., 2010). Under a different model of associations (Belsky, 2005; Boyce & Ellis, 2005), genetic markers may serve as risk factors among low-SES youth and as protective factors among high-SES youth. For example, a genetic predisposition for novelty-seeking may be associated with substance use and externalizing problems in low-SES environments and to creativity and intellectual curiosity in an enriched medium-through-high SES environments.

Finally, additional attention should be paid to the dynamic nature of some of the socioeconomic variables. Several researchers note that the effects of poverty may depend on the duration and age of onset of the low-SES conditions (Duncan & Brooks-Gunn, 1997, Miller & Korenman, 1994). Along similar lines, there may be differential effects of slow versus sudden or rapid deterioration of the socioeconomic conditions. New analytic techniques that allow for a group-based modeling of different developmental trajectories can be especially useful for addressing this set of questions. For example, a recent study by Marin, Chen, and Miller (2008) identified four distinct trajectories of SES changes during childhood and linked these trajectories to adolescent blood pressure. Their findings indicate that early SES (as compared to later changes in SES) is the most powerful predictor of adolescent blood pressure. Finally, future research should also employ creative research designs, for example semi-experimental designs where a subsample of participants is undergoing a rapid change in SES and a subsample does not experience a change in SES or experiences a gradual change.

References

Aber, J. L., Bennett, N. G., Conley, D. C., & Li, J. (1997). The effects of poverty on child health and development. *Annual Review of Public Health, 18*, 463–483.

Achenbach, T., Bird, H., Canino, G., Phares, V., Gould, M., & Rubio-Stipec, M. (1990). Epidemiological comparisons of Puerto Rican and U.S. mainland children: Parent, teacher and self reports. *Journal of the American Academy of Child Adolescent Psychiatry, 29*, 84–93.

Adler, N. E., Boyce, W. T., Chesney, M. A., Folkman, S., & Syme, S. L. (1993). Socioeconomic inequalities in health. No easy solution. *JAMA, 269*, 3140–3145.

Adler, N.E., Boyce, T., Chesney, M.A., Cohen, S., Folkman, S., Kahn, R. L., & Syme, S. L. (1994). Socioeconomic status and health: the challenge of the gradient. *American Psychologist, 49*, 15–24.

Adler, N. E., Marmot, M., McEwen, B. S., & Stewart, J. (1999). *Socioeconomic status and health in industrialized nations*. New York: New York Academy of Science.

Agnew, R. (1994). Delinquency and the desire for money. *Justice Quarterly, 11*, 411–427.

Agnew, R. (1999). A general strain theory of community differences in crime rates. *Journal of Research in Crime and Delinquency, 36*, 123–155.

Agnew, R., Matthews, S. K., Bucher, J., Welcher, A. N., & Keyes, C. (2008). Socioeconomic status, economic problems, and delinquency. *Youth and Society, 40*, 159–181.

Backlund, E., Sorlie, P. D., & Johnson, N. J. (1996). The shape of the relationship between income and mortality in the United States: Evidence from the National Longitudinal Mortality Study. *Annals of Epidemiology, 6*, 12–20.

Barefoot, J. C., Dahlstrom, W. G., & Williams, R. B. (1983). Hostility, CHD incidence, and total mortality: A 25-year follow-up study of 255 physicians. *Psychosomatic Medicine, 45*, 59–64.

Barefoot, J. C., Peterson, B. L., Dahlstrom, W. G., Siegler, I. C., Anderson, N. B., & Williams, R. B. (1991). Hostility patterns and health implications: Correlates of Cook–Medley Hostility Scale scores in a national survey. *Health Psychology, 10*, 18–24.

Baron, S. W. (2004). General strain, street youth and crime: A test of Agnew's revised theory. *Criminology, 42*, 457–483.

Batty, G. D., & Leon, D. A. (2002). Socio economic position and coronary heart disease risk factors in children and young people Evidence from UK epidemiological studies. *European Journal of Public Health, 12*, 263–272.

Belsky, J. (2005). Differential susceptibility to rearing influence: An evolutionary hypothesis and some evidence. In B. Ellis & D. Bjorklund (Eds.), *Origins of the social mind: Evolutionary psychology and child development* (pp. 139–163). New York: Guilford.

Benes, F. M. (2003). Why does psychosis develop during adolescence and early adulthood? *Current Opinion in Psychiatry, 16*, 317–319.

Bocian, D. G., Li, W., Ernst, K. S., & Center for Responsible Lending. (2010). *Foreclosures by race and ethnicity: The demographics of a crisis*. Retrieved August 28, 2011, from http://www.responsiblelending.org/mortgage-lending/research-analysis/foreclosures-by-race-and-ethnicity.pdf.

Bolger, K. E., Patterson, C. J., Thompson, W. W., & Kupersmidt, J. B. (1995). Psychosocial adjustment among children experiencing persistent and intermittent family economic hardship. *Child Development, 66*, 1107–29.

Bongers, I. L., Koot, H. M., van der Ende, J., & Verhulst, F. C. (2004). Developmental trajectories of externalizing behaviors in childhood and adolescence. *Child Development, 75*, 1523–1537.

Booth-Kewley, S., & Friedman, H. S. (1987). Psychological predictors of heart disease: A quantitative review. *Psychological Bulletin, 101*, 343–362.

Bouchard, C., Shepard, R. J., Stephens, T., Sutton, J. R., & McPherson, B. D. (1990). *Exercise, Fitness and Health*. Champaign, IL: Human Kinetics.

Boyce, W. T., & Chesterman, E. (1990). Life events, social support, and cardiovascular reactivity in adolescence. *Developmental and Behavioral Pediatrics, 11*, 105–111.

Boyce, W. T., & Ellis, B. J. (2005). Biological sensitivity to context: I An evolutionary-developmental theory of the origins and functions of stress reactivity. *Development and Psychopathology, 17*, 271–301.

Bradley, R. H., & Corwyn, R. E. (2002). Socioeconomic status and child development. *Annual Review of Psychology, 53*, 371–399.

Brooks-Gunn, J., & Duncan, G. J. (1997). The effects of poverty on children. *Future of Children, 7*, 55–71.

Call, K. T., & Nonnemaker, J. (1999). Socioeconomic disparities in adolescent health: Contributing factors. *Annals of the New York Academy of Sciences, 896*, 352–355.

Catalano, R., Dooley, D., Wilson, G., & Hough, R. (1993). Job loss and alcohol abuse: a test using data from the Epidemiologic Catchment Area project. *Journal of Health and Social Behavior, 34*, 215–225.

Centers for Disease Control and Prevention. (2011a). *Obesity and overweight*. Retrieved from http://www.cdc.gov/nchs/fastats/overwt.htm.

Centers for Disease Control and Prevention. (2011b). *Vital signs*. Retrieved May, 2011, from http://www.cdc.gov/vitalsigns/asthma/.

Cernkovich, S. A., Giordano, P. C., & Rudolph, J. L. (2000). Race, crime, and the American dream. *Journal of Research in Crime and Delinquency, 37*, 131–170.

Chassin, L., Beltran, I., Lee, M., Haller, M., & Villalta, I. (2010). Vulnerability to substance use disorders in childhood and adolescence. In R. E. Ingram & J. M. Price (Eds.), *Vulnerability to psychopathology: Risk across the lifespan* (2nd ed., pp. 113–140). New York, NY, US: Guilford Press.

Chassin, L., Hussong, A., Barrera, M., Jr., Molina, B., Trim, R., & Ritter, J. (2004). Adolescent substance use. In R. Lerner & L. Steinberg (Eds.), *Handbook of adolescent psychology* (2nd ed., pp. 665–696). New York: Wiley.

Chassin, L., Presson, C. C., Sherman, S. J., & Edwards, D. (1992). The natural history of cigarette smoking and young adult social roles. *Journal of Health and Social Behavior, 33*, 328–347.

Chen, E., Fisher, E. B., Jr., Bacharier, L. B., & Strunk, R. C. (2003). Socioeconomic status, stress, and immune markers in adolescents with asthma. *Psychosomatic Medicine, 65*, 984–992.

Chen, E., Hanson, M. D., Paterson, L. Q., Griffin, M. J., Walker, H. A., & Miller, G. E. (2006). Socioeconomic status and inflammatory processes in childhood asthma: The role of psychological stress. *Journal of Allergy and Clinical Immunology, 117*, 1014–1020.

Chen, E., Matthews, K. A., & Boyce, W. T. (2002). Socioeconomic differences in children's health: How and why do these relationships change with age? *Psychological Bulletin, 128*, 295–329.

Chen, E., & Miller, G. E. (2007). Social context as an individual difference in psychoneuroimmunology. In M. R. Irwin (Ed.), *Psychoneuroimmunology* (4th ed., pp. 497–508). Boston, MA: Elsevier.

Chen, E., Miller, G. E., Kobor, M. S., & Cole, S. W. (2011). Maternal warmth buffers the effects of low early-life socioeconomic status on pro-inflammatory signaling in adulthood—adults with retrospective reports of maternal warmth and SES (during first 5 years of life). *Molecular Psychiatry, 16*, 729–737.

Conger, R. D., & Conger, K. J. (2002). Resilience in Midwestern families: Selected findings from the first decade of a prospective, longitudinal study. *Journal of Marriage and Family, 64*, 361–373.

Conger, R. D., Conger, K. J., & Martin, M. J. (2010). Socioeconomic status, family process, and individual development. *Journal of Marriage and Family, 72*, 685–704.

Conger, R. D., & Donnellan, M. B. (2007). An interactionist perspective on the socioeconomic context of human development. *Annual Review of Psychology, 58*, 175–199.

Conger, R. D., Ge, X., Elder, G. H., Jr., Lorenz, F. O., & Simons, R. L. (1994). Economic stress, coercive family process, and developmental problems of adolescents. *Child Development, 65*, 541–561.

Dantzer, R., O'Connor, J. C., Freund, G. G., Johnson, R. W., & Kelley, K. W. (2008). From inflammation to sickness and depression: When the immune system subjugates the brain. *Nature Reviews Neuroscience, 9*, 46–56.

DeFrances, C. J., Cullen, K. A., & Kozak, L. J. (2007). National Hospital Discharge Survey: 2005 annual summary with detailed diagnosis and procedure data. National Center for Health Statistics. *Vital Health Statistics 12*, 1–209.

Dembroski, T. M., MacDougall, J. M., Costa, P. T., Jr., & Grandits, G. A. (1989). Components of hostility as predictors of sudden death and myocardial infarction in the multiple risk factor intervention trial. *Psychosomatic Medicine, 51*, 514–522.

DeNavas-Walt, C., Proctor, B. D., Smith, J. C., & U.S. Census Bureau. (2010). Current population reports, P60-238, *Income, poverty, and health insurance coverage in the United States*: *2009*, Washington, DC: U.S. Government Printing Office.

Dickerson, S. S., & Kemeny, M. E. (2004). Acute stressors and cortisol responses: A theoretical integration and synthesis of laboratory research. *Psychological Bulletin, 130*, 355–391.

Dodge, K. A., Pettit, G. S., & Bates, J. E. (1994). Socialization mediators of the relation between socioeconomic status and child conduct problems. *Child Development, 65*, 649–665.

Duncan, G. J., & Brooks-Gunn, J. (1997). *Consequences of growing up poor*. New York: Russell Sage Found.

Ecob, R., & Davey Smith, G. (1999). Income and health: What is the nature of the relationship? *Social Science and Medicine, 48*, 693–705.

Elliott, D., & Ageton, S. S. (1980). Reconciling race and SES differences in self-reported and official estimates of delinquency. *American Sociological Review, 45*, 95.

Ennett, S., Flewelling, R., Lindrooth, R., & Norton, E. (1997). School and neighborhood characteristics associated with school rates of alcohol, cigarette, and marijuana use. *Journal of Health and Social Behavior, 38*, 55–71.

Escobedo, L. G., Anda, R. F., Smith, P. F., Remington, P. L., & Mast, E. E. (1990). Sociodemographic characteristics of cigarette smoking initiation in the United States. *Journal of the American Medical Association, 264*, 1550–1555.

Estabrooks, P. A., Lee, R. E., & Gyurcsik, N. C. (2003). Resources for physical activity participation: Does availability and accessibility differ by neighborhood socioeconomic status? *Annals of Behavioral Medicine, 25*, 100–104.

Evans, G. W., Lepore, S. J., Shejwal, B. R., & Palsane, M. N. (1998). Chronic residential crowding and children's well being: An ecological perspective. *Child Development, 69*, 1514–1523.

Ewart, C. K., Elder, G. J., Smyth, J. M., Sliwinski, M. J., & Jorgensen, R. S. (2011). Do agonistic motives matter more than anger? Three studies of cardiovascular risk in adolescents. *Health Psychology, 30*, 510–524.

Farfel, A., Tirosh, A., Derazne, E., Garty, B. Z., & Afek, A. (2010). Association between socioeconomic status and the prevalence of asthma. *Annals of Allergy Asthma and Immunology, 104*, 490–495.

Flinn, M. V., & England, B. G. (1997). Social economics of childhood glucocorticoid stress response and health. *American Journal of Physical Anthropology, 102*, 33–53.

Friedman, H. S., & Booth-Kewley, S. (1987). The "disease-prone" personality: A meta-analytic review of the construct. *American Psychologist, 42*, 539–555.

Gallo, L. C., & Matthews, K. A. (1999). Do negative emotions mediate the association between socioeconomic status and health? In N. E. Adler, M. Marmot, B. S.

McEwen, & J. Stewart (Eds.), *Socioeconomic status and health in industrialized nations* (pp. 226–245). New York: New York Academy of Science.

Gardner, M., & Steinberg, L. (2005). Peer influence on risk taking, risk preference, and risky decision making in adolescence and adulthood: An experimental study. *Developmental Psychology, 41*, 625–635.

Giedd, J., Blumenthal, J., Jeffries, N., Castellanos, F., Liu, H., Zijdenbos, A., et al. (1999). Brain development during childhood and adolescence: A longitudinal MRI study. *Nature Neuroscience, 2*, 861–863.

Giovino, G. A., Henningfield, J. E., Tomar, S. L., Escobedo, L. G., & Slade, J. (1995). Epidemiology of tobacco use and dependence. *Epidemiologic Reviews, 17*, 48–65.

Gogtay, N., & Thompson, P. M. (2010). Mapping gray matter development: Implications for typical development and vulnerability to psychopathology. *Brain and Cognition, 72*, 6–15.

Goodman, E. (1999). The role of socioeconomic status gradients in explaining differences in US adolescents' health. *American Journal of Public Health, 89*, 1522–1528.

Goodman, E., Slap, G. B., & Bin, H. (2003). The public health impact of socioeconomic status on adolescent depression and obesity. *American Journal of Public Health, 93*, 1844–1850.

Gottlieb, N. H., & Chen, M. S. (1985). Sociocultural correlates of childhood sporting activities: Their implications for heart health. *Social Science Medicine, 21*, 533–539.

Greenberg, D. F. (1977). Delinquency and the age structure of society. *Contemporary Crises, 1*, 189–223.

Haas, S. A. (2006). Health selection and the process of social stratification: The effect of childhood health on socioeconomic attainment. *Journal of Health and Social Behavior, 47*, 339–354.

Hanson, M. D., & Chen, E. (2007). Socioeconomic status and substance use behaviors in adolescents: The role of family resources versus family social status. *Journal of Health Psychology, 12*, 32–35.

Harrell, J. S., Bangdiwala, S. I., Deng, S., Webb, J. P., & Bradley, C. (1998). Smoking initiation in youth: The roles of gender, race, socioeconomics, and developmental status. *Journal of Adolescent Health, 23*, 271–79.

Heijmens Visser, J. H., Van der Ende, J., Koot, H. M., & Verhulst, F. C. (2002). Predictors of psychopathology in young referred to mental health services in childhood or adolescence. *British Journal of Psychiatry, 177*, 59–65.

Hemingway, H., Shipley, M., Mullen, M. J., Kumari, M., Brunner, E., Taylor, M., et al. (2003). Social and psychosocial influences on inflammatory markers and vascular function in civil servants (The Whitehall II study). *American Journal of Cardiology, 92*, 984–987.

Heron, M. P., Hoyert, D. L., Murphy, S. L., Xu, J. Q., Kochanek K. D., & Tejada-Vera. B. (2009). Deaths: Final data for 2006. *National Vital Statistics Reports, 57*(14). Hyattsville, MD: National Center for Health Statistics.

Hofstra, M. B., Van de Ende, J., & Verhulst, F. C. (2001). Adolescent's self-reported problems as predictors of psychopathology in adulthood: 10 year follow up study. *British Journal of Psychiatry, 179*, 203–209.

Illsley, R., & Baker, D. (1991). Contextual variations in the meaning of health inequality. *Social Science and Medicine, 32*, 359–365.

Jarjoura, G. R., Triplett, R. A., & Brinker, G. P. (2002). Growing up poor: Examining the link between persistent childhood poverty and delinquency. *Journal of Quantitative Criminology, 18*, 159–187.

Johnson, J. G., Cohen, P., Dohrenwend, B. P., Link, B. G., & Brook, J. S. (1999). A longitudinal investigation of social causation and social selection processes involved in the association between socioeconomic status and psychiatric disorders. *Journal of Abnormal Psychology, 108*, 490–499.

Johnston-Brooks, C. H., Lewis, M. A., Evans, G. W., & Whalen, C. K. (1998). Chronic stress and illness in children: The role of allostatic load. *Psychosomatic Medicine, 60*, 597–603.

Kessler, R. C., Berglund, P., Demler, O., Jin, R., Merikangas, K. R., & Walters, E. E. (2005). Life-time prevalence and age-of-onset distributions of DSM-IV disorders in the National Comorbidity Survey Replication. *Archives of General Psychiatry, 62*, 593–602.

Kirschbaum, C., Steyer, R., Eid, M., Patalla, U., Schwenkmezger, P. & Hellhammer, D. H. (1990). Cortisol and behavior: Application of a latent state-trait model to salivary cortisol. *Psychoneuroendocrinology, 15*, 297–307.

Kohn, M., Rees, J. M., Brill, S., Fonseca, H., Jacobson, M., Katzman, D. K., et al. (2006). Preventing and treating adolescent obesity: A position paper of the Society for Adolescent Medicine. *Journal of Adolescent Health, 38*, 784–787.

Krenichyn, K., Saegert, S., & Evans, G. W. (2001). Parents as moderators of psychological and physiological correlates of inner-city children's exposure to violence. *Journal of Applied Developmental Psychology, 22*, 581–602.

Lahey, B. B., Loeber, R., Hart, E. L., Frick, P. J., Applegate, B., Zhang, Q., et al. (1995). Four-year longitudinal study of conduct disorders in boys: Patterns and predictors of persistence. *Journal Abnormal Psychology, 104*, 83–93.

Leinonen, J. A., Solantaus, T. S., & Punamäki, R. (2003). Social support and the quality of parenting under economic pressure and workload in Finland: The role of family structure and parental gender. *Journal of Family Psychology, 17*, 409–418.

Lempers, J. D., Clark-Lempers, D., & Simons, R. L. (1989). Economic hardship, parenting, and distress in adolescence. *Child Development, 60*, 25–39.

Leventhal, T., & Brooks-Gunn, J. (2000). The neighbourhoods they live in: Effects of neighborhood residence upon child and adolescent outcomes. *Psychological Bulletin, 126*, 309–337.

Libby, P. (2001). Current concepts of the pathogenesis of the acute coronary syndromes. *Circulation, 104*, 365–372.

Link, B. G., & Phelan, J. (1995). Social conditions as fundamental causes of disease. *Journal of Health and Social Behavior, 35*, 80–94.

Loeber, R., Green, S. M., Keenan, K., & Lahey, B. B. (1995). Which boys will fare worse? Early predictors of the onset of conduct disorder in a six-year longitudinal study. *Journal of the American Academy of Child and Adolescent Psychiatry, 34*, 499–509.

Loeber, R., Farrington, D. P., Stouthamer-Loeber, M., & Van Kammen, W. B. (1998). *Antisocial behavior and mental health problems: Explanatory factors in childhood and adolescence*. Mahwah, NJ: Lawrence Erlbaum.

Luna, B., Padmanabhan, A., & O'Hearn, K. (2010). What has fMRI told us about the development of cognitive control through adolescence? *Brain and Cognition, 72*, 101–113.

Lupien, S. J., King, S., Meaney, M. J., & McEwen, B. S. (2000). Child's stress hormone levels correlate with mother's socioeconomic status and depressive state. *Biological Psychiatry, 48*, 976–980.

Lupien, S. J., King, S., Meaney, M. J., & McEwen, B. S. (2001). Can poverty get under your skin? Basal cortisol levels and cognitive function in children from low and high socioeconomic status. *Development and Psychopathology, 13*, 653–676.

Luthar, S. S., & Latendresse, S. J. (2005). Children of the affluent: Challenges to well-being. *Current Directions in Psychological Science, 14*, 49–53.

Lynch, J. W., Kaplan, G. A., & Salonen, J. T. (1997). Why do poor people behave poorly? Variation in adult health behaviors and psychosocial characteristics by stages of the socioeconomic lifecourse. *Social Science and Medicine, 44*, 809–819.

Marin, T. J., Chen, E., & Miller, G. E. (2008). What do trajectories of childhood socioeconomic status tell us about markers of cardiovascular health in adolescence? *Psychosomatic Medicine, 70*, 152–159.

Marmorstein, N. R., & Iacono, W. G. (2004). Major depression and conduct disorder in youth: Associations with parental psychopathology and parent-child conflict. *Journal of Child Psychology and Psychiatry, 45*, 377–386.

Marmot, M. G., Smith, G. D., Stansfeld, S., Patel, C., North, F., Head, J., et al. (1991). Health inequalities among British civil servants: The Whitehall II study. *Lancet, 337*, 1387–1393.

Martin, M. J., Conger, R. D., Schofield, T. J., Dogan, S. J., Widaman, K. F., Donnellan, M. B., et al. (2010). Evaluation of the interactionist model of socioeconomic status and problem behavior: A developmental cascade across generations. *Development and Psychopathology, 22*, 695–713.

McCarron, P., & Davey Smith, G. (2003). Physiological measurements in children and young people, and risk of coronary heart disease in adults. In A. Gates (Ed.), *A lifecourse approach to coronary heart disease prevention scientific and policy review* (pp. 49–78). London, England: The Stationery Office.

McCoy, M. B., Frick, P. J., Loney, B. R., & Ellis, M. L. (1999). The potential mediating role of parenting practices in the development of conduct problems in a clinic-referred sample. *Journal of Child and Family Studies, 8*, 477–94.

McDonough, P., Duncan, G. J., Williams, D., & House, J. (1997). Income dynamics and adult mortality in the United States, 1972 through 1989. *American Journal of Public Health, 87*, 1476–1483.

McGill, H. C., McMahan, C. A., Herderick, E. E., Malcom, G. T., Tracy, R. E., Strong, J. P., et al. (2000). Origin of atherosclerosis in childhood and adolescence. *American Journal of Clinical Nutrition, 72*, 1307S–1315S.

McGill, H. C., McMahan, C. A., Zieske, A. W., et al. (2000). Associations of coronary heart disease risk factors with the intermediate lesion of atherosclerosis in youth. The Pathobiological Determinants of Atherosclerosis in Youth (PDAY) Research Group. *Arteriosclerosis, Thrombosis, and Vascular Biology, 20*, 1998–2004.

McGrath, J. J., Matthews, K. A., & Brady, S. S. (2006). Individual versus neighborhood socioeconomic status and race as predictors of adolescent ambulatory blood pressure and heart rate. *Social Science and Medicine, 63*, 1442–1453.

McLaren, L. (2007). Socioeconomic status and obesity. *Epidemiologic Reviews, 29*, 29–48.

McLeod, J. D., & Kaiser, K. (2004). Childhood emotional and behavioral problems and educational attainment. *American Sociological Review, 69*, 636–658.

McLeod, J. D., & Kessler, R. C. (1990). Socioeconomic status differences in vulnerability to undesirable life events. *Journal of Health and Social Behavior, 31*, 162–172.

McLeod, J., & Shanahan, M. (1993). Poverty, parenting, and children's mental health. *American Sociologic Review, 58*, 351–66.

McLoyd, V. C. (1997). The impact of poverty and low socioeconomic status on the socioemotional functioning of African-American children and adolescents: Mediating effects. In R. D. Taylor & M. Wang (Eds.), *Social and emotional adjustment and family relations in ethnic minority families* (pp. 7–34). Mahwah, NJ: Erlbaum.

McLoyd, V. (1998a). Socioeconomic disadvantage and child development. *American Psychologist, 53*, 185–204.

Melotti, R., Heron, J., Hickman, M., Macleod, J., Araya, R., & Lewis, G. (2011). Adolescent alcohol and tobacco use and early socioeconomic position: The ALSPAC birth cohort. *Pediatrics, 127*, 948–955.

Miech, R. A., Caspi, A., Moffitt, T. E., Wright, B. R. E., & Silva, P. A. (1999). Low socio-economic status and mental disorders: A longitudinal study of selection and causation during young adulthood. *American Journal of Sociology, 104*, 1096–1131.

Miller, G. E., Cohen, S., & Herbert, T. B. (1999). Pathways linking major depression and immunity in ambulatory female patients. *Psychosomatic Medicine, 61*, 850–860.

Miller, J. E., & Korenman, S. (1994). Poverty and children's nutritional status in the United States. *American Journal of Epidemiology, 140*, 233–42.

Miller, A. H., Maletic, V., & Raison, C. L. (2009). Inflammation and its discontents: The role of cytokines in the pathophysiology of major depression. *Biological Psychiatry, 65*, 732–741.

Moore, L. V., Diez Roux, A. V., Evenson, K. R., McGinn, A. P., & Brines, S. J. (2008). Availability of recreational resources in minority and low socioeconomic status areas. *American Journal of Preventive Medicine, 34*, 16–22.

Murali, R., & Chen, E. (2005). Exposure to violence and cardiovascular and neuroendocrine measures in adolescents. *Annals of Behavioral Medicine, 30*, 155–163.

Neidell, M. J. (2004). Air pollution, health, and socioeconomic status: The effect of outdoor air quality on childhood asthma. *Journal of Health Economics, 23*, 1209–1236.

Organisation for Economic Co-operation & Development. (2010). *OECD economic surveys: United States 2010*. Retrieved August 25, 2011, from http://www.oecd.org/document/43/0,3746,en_2649_34569_46023275_1_1_1_1,00.html.

Ostrove, J. M., Feldman, P., & Adler, N. E. (1999). Relations among socioeconomic indicators and health for African-Americans and whites. *Journal of Health Psychology, 4*, 451–63.

Pamuk, E., Makuc, D., Heck, K., Reuben, C., & Lochner, K. (1998). *Socioeconomic Status and Health Chartbook. Health United States, 1998*. Hyattsville, MD: National Center for Health Statistics.

Panagiotakos, D. B., Pitsavos, C., Manios, Y., Polychronopoulos, E., Chrysohoou, C. A., & Stefanadis, C. (2005). Socio-economic status in relation to risk factors associated with cardiovascular disease, in healthy individuals from the ATTICA study. *European Journal of Cardiovascular Prevention and Rehabilitation, 12*, 68–74.

Pensola, T. H., & Valkonen, T. (2000). Mortality differences by parental social class from childhood to adulthood. *Journal of Epidemiology and Community Health, 54*, 525–529.

Pietila, A. M., Hentinen, M., & Myhrman, A. (1995). The health behavior of northern Finnish men in adolescence and adulthood. *International Journal of Nursing Studies, 32*, 325–338.

Pigeyre, M., Bokor, S., Romon, M., Gottrand, F., Gilbert, C. C., Valtueña, J., et al. (2010). Influence of maternal educational level on the association between the rs3809508 neuromedin B gene polymorphism and the risk of obesity in the HELENA study. *International Journal of Obesity, 34*, 478–486.

Pine, D. S. (2003). Developmental psychobiology and response to threats: Relevance to trauma in children and adolescents. *Biological Psychiatry, 53*, 796–808.

Ross, R. (1999). Atherosclerosis—an inflammatory disease. *New England Journal of Medicine, 340*, 115–126.

Sampson, R. J., & Groves, W. B. (1989). Community structure and crime: Testing social disorganization theory. *The American Journal of Sociology, 94*, 774–802.

Schneiders, J., Drukker, M., Van der Ende, J., Verhulst, F. C., van Os, J., & Nicolson, N. A. (2003). Neighbourhood socioeconomic disadvantage and behavioural problems from late childhood into early adolescence. *Journal of Epidemiology and Community Health, 57*, 699–703.

Shaw, D. S., Winslow, E. B., Owens, E. B., & Hood, N. (1998). Young Children's Adjustment to Chronic Family Adversity: A Longitudinal Study of Low-Income Families. *Journal of the American Academy of Child and Adolescent Psychiatry, 37*, 545–553.

Siegman, A. W., Dembroski, T. M., & Ringel, N. (1987). Components of hostility and the severity of coronary heart disease. *Psychosomatic Medicine, 49*, 127–135.

Sobal, J., & Stunkard, A. J. (1989). Socioeconomic status and obesity: A review of the literature. *Psychological Bulletin, 105*, 260–75.

Sobolewski, J. M., & Amato, P. R. (2005). Economic hardship in the family of origin and children's psychological well-being in adulthood. *Journal of Marriage and Family, 67*, 141–156.

Steinberg, L. (2008). A social neuroscience perspective on adolescent risk-taking. *Developmental Review, 28*, 78–106.

Steinberg, L., & Monahan, K. (2007). Age differences in resistance to peer influence. *Developmental Psychology, 43*, 1531–1543.

Steinberg, L., & Silverberg, S. (1986). The vicissitudes of autonomy in early adolescence. *Child Development, 57*, 841–851.

Theorell, T. (1974). Life events before and after the onset of a premature myocardial infarction. In B. S. Dohrenwend & B. P. Dohrenwend (Eds.), *Stressful life events: Their nature and effects* (pp. 101–117). New York: Wiley.

Thurston, R. C., & Matthews, K. A. (2009). Racial and socioeconomic disparities in arterial stiffness and intima media thickness among adolescents. *Social Science and Medicine, 68*, 807–813.

Toftegaard-Støckel, J., Nielsen, G. A., Ibsen, B., & Andersen L. B. (2011). Parental, socio and cultural factors associated with adolescents' sports participation in four Danish municipalities. *Scandinavian Journal of Medicine and Science in Sports, 21*, 606–611.

Tuinstra, J., Groothoff, J. W., van den Heuvel, W. J., & Post, D. (1998). Socio-economic differences in health risk behavior in adolescence: Do they exist? *Social Science and Medicine, 47*, 67–74.

U.S. Bureau of Labor Statistics. (2011). *Labor force statistics from the current population survey employment status of the civilian population*. Retrieved August 25, 2011, from http://www.bls.gov/data.

Vitaro, F., Tremblay, R. E., Kerr, M., Pagani, L., & Bukowski, W. M. (1997). Disruptiveness, friends' characteristics, and delinquency in early adolescence: A test of two competing models of development. *Child Development, 68*, 676–689.

Vuille, J.-C., & Schenkel, M. (2001). Social equalization in health of youth. *European Journal of Public Health, 11*, 287–293.

Wadsworth, M. E., & Compas, B. E. (2002). Coping with family conflict and economic strain: The adolescent perspective. *Journal of Research on Adolescence, 12*, 243–274.

Walker, E., & Bollini, A. M. (2002). Pubertal neurodevelopment and the emergence of psychotic symptoms. *Schizophrenia Research, 54*, 17–23.

Walker, E., Sabuwalla, Z., & Huot, R. (2004). Pubertal neuromaturation, stress sensitivity, and psychopathology. *Development and Psychopathology, 16*, 807–824.

Watamura, S. E., Donzella, B., Kertes, D. A., & Gunnar, M. R. (2004). Developmental changes in baseline cortisol activity in early childhood: Relations with napping and effortful control. *Developmental Psychobiology, 45*, 125–133.

Wender, P.H., Rosenthal, D., Kety, S.S., Schulsinger, F., & Welner, J. (1973). Social class and psychopathology in adoptees. A natural experimental method for separating the roles of genetic and experimential factors. *Archives of General Psychiatry, 28*, 318–325.

West, P. (1988). Inequalities? Social class differentials in health in British youth. *Social Science Medicine, 27*, 291–296.

West, P. (1997). Health inequalities in the early years: Is there equalisation in youth? *Social Science Medicine, 44*, 833–858.

West, P., Macintyre, S., Annandale, E., & Hunt, K. (1990). Social class and health in youth: Findings from the west of Scotland twenty-07 study. *Social Science Medicine, 30*, 665–73.

Williams, D. R. (1990). Socioeconomic differentials in health: A review and redirection. *Social Psychology Quarterly, 53*, 81–99.

Williams, D. R., & Collins, C. (1995). U.S. socioeconomic and racial differentials in health: Patterns and explanations. *Annual Review of Sociology, 21*, 349–386.

Williams, J. M., Currie, C. E., Wright, P., Elton, R. A., & Beattie, T. F. (1997). Socioeconomic status and adolescent injuries. *Social Science Medicine, 44*, 1881–1891.

Wohlfarth, T., & Van den Brink, W. (1998). Social class and substance use disorders: The value of social class as distinct from socioeconomic status. *Social Science and Medicine, 47*, 51–68.

Wolch, J., Wilson, J., & Fehrenback, J. (2005). Parks and park funding in Los Angeles: An equity-mapping analysis. *Urban Geography, 25*, 4–35.

Wright, B. R., Caspi, A., Moffitt, T. E., Miech, R. A., & Silva, P. A. (1999). Reconsidering the relationship between SES and delinquency: Causation but not correlation. *Criminology, 37*, 175–194.

Yoon, K. H., Lee, J. H., Kim, J. W., Cho, J. H., Choi, Y. H., Ko, S. H., et al. (2006). Epidemic obesity and type 2 diabetes in Asia. *Lancet, 368*, 1681–1688.

Yurgelun-Todd, D. (2007). Emotional and cognitive changes during adolescence. *Current Opinions in Neurobiology, 17*, 251–257.

Public Health Approaches to Adolescent Health Beyond Disease and Illness

Richard E. Kreipe

Introduction

Two seminal events provide a frame for public health approaches to adolescent disease and illness: the formation of the United States Public Health Service (USPHS) and the establishment of the World Health Organization (WHO). Within this framework, this chapter addresses contemporary public health approaches for adolescents beyond disease and illness. Next, contemporary public health efforts in the United States, now guided by a comprehensive set of goals and objectives called *Healthy People* including adolescent-specific content, are explored. Adolescent health issues, the unique needs of adolescents to improve their health, and the importance of adolescent public health are then outlined. Within that context, practical issues in public health practice focused on adolescents are detailed. Emphasis is placed on positive youth development, a youth-oriented strategy involving active youth participation as a public health approach.

Partially supported by MCHB Grant #T71MC00012.

R.E. Kreipe, M.D. (✉)
Division of Adolescent Medicine,
Department of Pediatrics, Golisano Children's Hospital,
601 Elmwood Avenue, Box 690, Rochester,
NY 14642, USA
e-mail: Richard_Kreipe@URMC.Rochester.Edu

Historical Framework to Public Health and Adolescent Health Psychology

The formation of the USPHS can be traced back to the *Act for the Relief of Sick and Disabled Seamen* of 1798 authorizing government-operated marine hospitals to care for American merchant seamen (U.S. Department of Health and Human Services, 2011). Although subsequent legislation broadened the scope of USPHS, it is important to note that the majority of seamen in 1798 were adolescents. At that time, sailors generally went to sea as boys, and by the time they were 16 years old they could be rated as seamen, but most left the sea in young adulthood (Lambert, 2011). With respect to adolescent psychology, Lambert noted, "the idea of being single, free of responsibilities and well paid would have made a career at sea obviously alluring" (Lambert, 2011). Thus, the earliest federal public health activity was largely a response to the health care needs of this population of adolescents. As noted in Box 1 the field of public health relevant to adolescents now includes seven essential activities (Centers for Disease Control and Prevention, 2011).

The WHO, established in 1948 as the international public health arm of the United Nations, defines health as "a state of complete physical, mental and social well-being and not merely the absence of disease or infirmity" (World Health Organization, 2011a). Thus, any discussion of

W.T. O'Donohue et al. (eds.), *Handbook of Adolescent Health Psychology*,
DOI 10.1007/978-1-4614-6633-8_5,

Box 1 Seven Essential Public Health Activities Relevant to Adolescent Populations (Centers for Disease Control and Prevention, 2011)

1. Monitoring their health status
2. Mobilizing community partnerships to identify and solve health problems
3. Developing policies and plans that support individual and community health efforts to improve adolescent health
4. Enforcing laws and regulations that protect health and ensure safety of adolescents
5. Assuring a competent public adolescent health care workforce
6. Evaluating the effectiveness, accessibility, and quality of personal and population-based health services
7. Conducting research related to new insights and innovative solutions to health problems

adolescent health and adolescent health psychology must move beyond disease and illness to comprehensive well-being. The WHO defines adolescents as youth between 10 and 19 years old, accounting for 20 % of the world population, with 85 % of all adolescents living in developing countries (Global Health Council, 2011). As noted in Box 2, nearly two-thirds of premature deaths and one-third of disease burden in adults can be traced to conditions or behaviors that began in youth. Promoting healthy practices among youth that protect them from health risks is critical to the future of every country's health and social infrastructure and to the prevention of health problems in adulthood (World Health Organization, 2011b). In 2002, the UN General Assembly Special Session on Children recognized the need for the "development and implementation of national health policies and programmes for adolescents, including goals and indicators, to promote their physical and mental health" (World Health Organization, 2011b).

Box 2 World Health Organization: 10 Facts on Adolescent Public Health Issues

1. 20 % of people in the world are adolescents, and 85 % of them live in developing countries. Nearly 2/3 of premature deaths and 1/3 of the total disease burden in adults are associated with modifiable conditions or behaviors that began in youth, including tobacco use, a lack of physical activity, unprotected sex, or exposure to violence.
2. Young people 15–24 years old accounted for an estimated 45 % of new HIV infections worldwide in 2007.
3. About 16 million girls 15–19 years old give birth every year—roughly 11 % of all births worldwide—with the vast majority to adolescents in developing countries. Pregnancy-related death rates are much higher for adolescents than for older women.
4. Many children in developing countries enter adolescence undernourished, making them more vulnerable to disease and early death. Conversely, overweight and obesity—another form of malnutrition with serious health consequences—is increasing among young people in developed countries.
5. More than 20 % of adolescents experience some form of mental illness, such as depression, mood disturbances, substance abuse, suicidal behaviors, or eating disorders.
6. The vast majority of tobacco users worldwide begin during adolescence. More than 150 million adolescents use tobacco, and this number is increasing globally.
7. Alcohol consumption among young people reduces self-control, increases risky behaviors, and is a primary cause of injuries (including those due to road traffic accidents), violence (especially domestic violence), and premature deaths.
8. Among 15–19-year-olds, suicide is the second leading cause of death,

followed by violence in the community and the family.

9. Unintentional injuries are a leading cause of death and disability in adolescents, with road traffic injuries, drowning, and burns the most common types. Injury rates among adolescents are highest in developing countries, and within countries, they are more likely to occur among adolescents from poorer families.
10. Many adolescent health challenges are closely interrelated and successful interventions in one area can lead to positive outcomes in other areas.

(Modified from www.who.int/features/factfiles/adolescent_health/facts/en/index.html Accessed August 28, 2011.)

Healthy People: US National Adolescent Public Health Goals, Objectives, and Strategies

Healthy People 1990: Under the leadership of the Surgeon General Julius B. Richmond, *Healthy People* was established as a blueprint to improve the health of all Americans over a decade. With core concepts now considered axiomatic, it laid out a US national public health policy for the first time. Described as a document "to encourage a second public health revolution," it reflected the first consensus among key stakeholders to focus on health promotion and disease prevention (CDC, 1989). A 1980 Surgeon General's companion Report *Promoting Health, Preventing Disease: Objectives for the Nation* for the first time included an adolescent and young adult outcome—mortality reduction (Public Health Service, 1980). A pediatrician who appreciated the special needs of adolescents, Dr. Richmond, presciently wrote, "achievement of these objectives by 1990 is a shared responsibility, requiring a concerted effort not only by the health community, but also by leaders in education, industry, labor, community organizations and many others" (Public Health Service, 1980).

Healthy People 2000 and 2010: In its second iteration, *Healthy People 2000*, there was a focus to reduce disparities among populations, such as the higher rates of sexually transmitted infections (STIs) in adolescents and young adults compared to older adults. The third iteration, *Healthy People 2010*, shifted from reducing to *eliminating* disparities, especially as they existed within a population, such as the higher rates of STIs among African-American compared to White adolescents in the same age-group. In addition, for the first time, *Healthy People 2010* included 21 "critical" national health objectives (CNHOs) across six domains for youth 10–24 years old: (1) mortality, (2) unintentional injury, (3) violence, (4) substance use and mental health, (5) reproductive health, and (6) prevention of chronic disease during adulthood. Following the end of the 2000–2010 decade, the first comprehensive study of the 21 CNHOs in *Healthy People 2010* was recently published, with both encouraging and discouraging findings (Jiang, Kolbe, Seo, Kay, & Brindis, 2011; Kreipe, 2011).

Although mortality for 10–24-year-olds in the United States was reduced compared to baseline, disparities in deaths continued to exist, based on sex, age, race, and ethnicity in a consistently troubling pattern, with males exceeding females, older groups exceeding younger groups, and Blacks exceeding both Whites and Hispanics in mortality. With respect to mortality rates, White and Hispanic 10–14-year-olds and females 10–19 years old all met *Healthy People 2010* targets, but 20–24-year-old mortality increased from baseline. This disturbing trend emphasizes the importance of focusing on young adults as an often overlooked population (Park, Mulye, Adams, Brindis, & Irwin, 2006).

The "Other" race/ethnic mortality category contains two small subgroups that reflect extremes of mortality rates. American Indian/Alaskan Native youth have the highest same-age mortality rate among all racial/ethnic groups for both males and females, while Asian/Pacific Islanders have the lowest (National Adolescent Health Information Center, 2006). Among American Indian/Alaskan

Native youth, death rates due to motor vehicle crashes or to suicide are twofold greater than rates for the next highest group, non-Hispanic Whites (National Adolescent Health Information Center, 2006). On the other hand, as a group Asian/Pacific Islander youth have relatively low rates of substance and alcohol use (National Adolescent Health Information Center, 2006), providing possible insight into alcohol-related MVC death reduction. Researchers have identified cultural factors including an emphasis on family reputation, humility, keeping a low profile, negative community sanctions on excessive drinking and behavior, and the impact of moderate parental drinking practices in the Asian/Pacific Islander population (Williams, 1984/1985). Although such protective influences may be mitigated as families accommodate to and are assimilated into mainstream culture, studying low-risk populations may suggest specific interventions for high-risk populations.

Outcomes for two other objectives deserve special attention because they worsened over time. Rates for the STI *Chlamydia* and for overweight/obesity worsened markedly from baseline to 2010 targets. Among 15–24-year-olds, females attending family planning clinics experienced a −125 % deviation from the 2010 target to reduce *Chlamydia* rates, while females and males at STI clinics had a −34 % and −52 %, respectively, deviation (Jiang et al., 2011). Overweight or obesity in 12–19-year-olds increased by 62 %, representing a −115 % deviation from the 2010 target (Jiang et al., 2011).

In *Healthy People 1990*, smoking was the major target of health promotion and disease prevention, and obesity was only mentioned in relation to hypertension and cardiovascular disease in adults (Public Health Service, 1980). Gonorrhea was the primary STI; *Chlamydia* was noted as an agent causing newborn illness and did not become a reportable STI until 1995. Obesity has replaced tobacco as a public health priority for preventable mortality and morbidity among adolescents and young adults (Ogden, Carroll, & Flegal, 2008), and *Chlamydia* is now the most common STI in 15–24-year-olds, and becoming ever more so (Centers for Disease Control and Prevention, 2010a). Disparities are evident in both of these domains as well: obesity is higher among males than females, and among Blacks and Hispanics than Whites, and increases with age (Eaton et al., 2010).

Healthy People 2020: As a tribute to Dr. Richmond's visionary leadership, *Healthy People*, now in its fourth iteration for the years 2010–2020, includes a new goal: "to improve the healthy development, health, safety, and well-being of adolescents and young adults," (Healthy, 2020a) and two new topic areas: adolescent health and lesbian, gay, bisexual, and transgender health (Healthy, 2020b), each with special relevance to adolescent health. Another feature of *Healthy People 2020* with respect to adolescent health psychology is a new focus on identifying, measuring, and tracking health disparities by examining the determinants of health, with a goal of achieving health equity by eliminating disparities and improving the health of all groups. Health disparity exists if, for any reason, a health outcome occurs to a greater or lesser extent between populations of adolescents. Because databases such as those analyzed for the comprehensive study of 2010 outcomes are limited to a narrow range of individual characteristics, such as sex, race, and ethnicity, other potential dimensions of disparity (e.g., sexual identity, disability, socioeconomic status, or geographic location) that may foster or impair an individual's ability to achieve good health have had limited inclusion in public health policy development. These features are more difficult to measure, but compared to the standard individual demographics may be more responsive to interventions and have an even greater impact on adolescent health psychology.

Thus, a range of personal, social, economic, and environmental factors affect adolescent health status. To that end, *Healthy People 2020* encourages the development of objectives that address the relationship between health status and biology, individual behavior, health services, social factors, and policies. An ecological approach—in which adolescents are seen to affect the environment and the environment affects the adolescent—requires a dual focus at both individual and population levels of adolescents (Kreipe, 2011). Because the determinants of health are interactive and dynamic, effective public health interventions must mirror these qualities. For example, the adolescent population is becoming increasingly ethnically diverse, with recent dramatic increases in the numbers of Hispanic and Asian American youth. The adolescent and young adult population is not only more diverse than the adult population, but becoming so more rapidly (National Adolescent Health Information Center, 2008). This is important because family structure both varies by racial/ethnic group (National Adolescent Health Information Center, 2008) and influences health outcomes. Meeting the goal of improving the healthy development, health, safety, and well-being of adolescents in the context of rapidly expanding diversity will require culturally effective public health practices and increased attention to disparate health and academic outcomes known to correlate highly with poverty, especially among adolescents from minority racial and ethnic groups (Healthy, 2020a).

The collaborative entity that has been responsible for overseeing national efforts to address adolescent health deserves mention. The National Initiative to Improve Adolescent Health (NIIAH, www.cdc.gov/HealthyYouth/AdolescentHealth/NationalInitiative) is led by two federal agencies collaborating with a variety of partner organizations and key stakeholders to mobilize activity directed at the adolescent health objectives in *Healthy People*. NIIAH has a national, state, and community focus and commitment to the health, safety, positive development, and well-being of adolescents, young adults, and their families. To improve health and safety outcomes, NIIAH addresses access to quality health, safety education, and health care, with attention to social determinants of, and the elimination of disparities in, health, safety, and well-being of adolescents and young adults and their families (CDC, 2011). Leaders in adolescent health have noted that emerging data indicate a "clear, sustained, and appropriately-supported national mandate for relevant agencies to collaboratively pursue a new National Initiative to Improve the Health of Adolescents and Young Adults by the Year 2020" (Jiang et al., 2011).

Thus, adolescent health psychology and public health activities intersect at both the individual and the population level. Readers are referred to the chapters in this book by Clements-Nolle (epidemiology), DiClemente (determinants of health-related behaviors), Leany (brain development), Dmitrieva (socioeconomical influences), and Coleman (processes of risk and resilience) for a more in-depth discussion of factors that must be appreciated to develop effective public health interventions with respect to adolescent health psychology.

Adolescent Health, Disease, and Illness Responsive to Public Health Approaches

A federal monograph on adolescent health services emphasizes that adolescent patterns of behavior determine young people's health status both in the present and the future (National Research Council and Institute of Medicine, 2009a). Contemporary public health and social problems in America that either start or peak between 10 and 24 years of age include (1) homicide, especially among urban minority youth; (2) suicide, especially among suburban or rural youth; (3) motor vehicle crashes, including those caused by drinking and driving; (4) substance use and abuse; (5) smoking; (6) STIs, including human immunodeficiency virus (HIV), with the highest risk group being adolescent and young adult males who have sex with males; (7) teenage unplanned pregnancies; and (8) homelessness (Healthy, 2020a). Although these health threats are largely preventable, adolescents are in a developmental transition (no longer children but not yet adults) and sensitive to environmental influences (Mulye et al., 2009). As previously noted regarding the ecological nature of adolescent heath, disease, and illness, environmental factors, including family, peer group, school, neighborhood, policies, and societal cues, can either support or challenge young people's health and well-being (National Research Council, 1993).

As documented throughout this book, adolescence is a critical life-course phase, with a variety of developmental tasks that must be successfully negotiated for an individual to transition to healthy adulthood (Kreipe, 2008). Also, many conditions linked to multiple environmental risks, as well as protective factors, covary with each other. Thus, adolescents who have good communication and connection with an adult are less likely to engage in risky behaviors (Resnick et al., 1997). Likewise, risky behavior is less likely in adolescents whose parents monitor their activities and provide safe opportunities for development (Aufseeser, Jekielek, & Brown, 2006). On the other hand, adolescents who live in poverty have poorer health and less access to health care (Larson & Halfon, 2010). With respect to school, academic skills are associated with higher rates of healthy behavior (Centers for Disease Control and Prevention, 2010b); high school graduation lowers the risk of health problems (Muennig & Woolf, 2007), incarceration, and financial instability (Sum, Khatiwada, & McLaughlin, 2009). Neighborhoods provide an important ecological context in adolescent health, with youth from areas with concentrated poverty being at particular risk for mental health problems, delinquency, and unhealthy sexual behaviors (Leventhal & Brooks-Gunn, 2004). An environmental factor of increasing concern, due to our lack of complete understanding regarding its potential for good or harm, is the media, with an increased risk of adolescents who are exposed to media violence, sexual content, smoking, and drinking alcohol engaging in them (Roberts, Henriksen, & Foehr, 2004).

Effective Public Health Policies and Programs Targeting Adolescent Health Problems

There are numerous examples of public health interventions targeting adolescents with specific health problems, each with a slightly different approach.

Graduated Driver Licensing and Tobacco Reduction Programs: Legislative approaches such as state-graduated driver licensing programs are highly effective (D'Angelo, Halpern-Felsher, & Abraham, 2010), while those limiting the sale of tobacco products are probably not as effective as media campaigns, such as "Reality Check" or the "Truth Campaign," to reduce youth tobacco use by emphasizing that the tobacco industry manipulates adolescents to become addicted to nicotine with devious marketing and advertising strategies (American Legacy Foundation, 2011). See also the chapter in this book by Brook, Pahl, Brook, and Brown (smoking).

Adolescent Pregnancy Prevention Programs: Despite an overall decrease in US teen pregnancy rates over the past two decades, the rates continue to far exceed those in other developed countries. In 2010, the federal government established the Office of Adolescent Health within the Department of Health and Human Services, which is funding a broad, long-term research effort related to evidence-based teen pregnancy prevention programs across the country. This initiative supports replication of extant evidence-based programs as well as the study of promising programs to establish a firm scientific foundation of evidence of effectiveness in the real world. A thorough scientific review of interventions with an evidence-base of effectiveness is available at the Office of Adolescent Health website devoted to this topic (Department of Health and Human Services, 2010). Also see the chapter by Aruda (pregnancy) in this book for more information.

Violence Prevention Programs: Effective public health violence prevention programs generally fall into community-based or school-based interventions. Community-based strategies include those that focus on (1) parents and family designed to improve family relations by combining training in parenting skills, education about development and the factors that predispose youth to violent behavior, and exercises to help parents develop skills for communicating with their children and for resolving conflict in nonviolent ways; (2) home-visitation which brings community resources to at-risk families in their homes during regularly scheduled home visits, including providing psychological support and other services to help parents function more effectively; (3) social-cognitive skills development to equip adolescents with the skills they need to deal effectively with difficult social situations; or (4) mentoring, in which a young person is paired with an adult who acts as a supportive, nonjudgmental role model, has been shown to significantly improve school attendance and performance, reduce violent behavior, decrease the likelihood of drug use, and improve relationships with friends and parents (Thornton, Craft, Dahlberg, Lynch, & Baer, 2002).

School-based violence prevention programs fall into two categories: universal, in which programs designed to reduce or prevent violent behavior are delivered to all students in a classroom, or targeted, in which programs are delivered to all students in a grade or school in high-risk areas (e.g., with low socioeconomic status or high rates of violence or crime). A comprehensive review of such programs and independent meta-analysis found strong evidence that universal school-based programs decrease rates of violence and aggressive behavior among students at all grade levels, leading the federal Task Force on Community Preventive Services to recommend universal school-based programs to prevent or reduce violent behavior (Centers for Disease Control and Prevention, 2007).

Mental, Emotional, and Behavioral Disorder Prevention: Recognizing that mental disorders are among the most common causes of disability, *Healthy People 2020* has an expanded focus on this issue with respect to adolescents (Healthy, 2020b). The current model framing these disorders emphasizes the interaction of social, environmental, and genetic factors across the lifespan, so that prevention efforts must entail an interdisciplinary, multipronged approach. Balancing risk factors that predispose youth to mental illness are protective factors that increase the likelihood of mental health. Highly informative is emerging evidence regarding brain development in adolescents and young adults (see Lany's chapter on brain development) that provides a biopsychosocial framework to understand phenomenon in this domain. See also chapters in this book by Donohue, Urgelles, and Fayeghi (substance use); O'Mara, Lee, and King (depression and suicide); Grant (anxiety); and Gazke-Kopp, DuPuis, and Nix (behavior problems) for more details.

A recent National Research Council and Institute of Medicine comprehensive review of the prevention of mental disorders and substance abuse among youth identified multiple strategies shown to enhance their psychological and emotional well-being (National Research Council and Institute of Medicine, 2009b). Research including meta-analyses and numerous randomized trials demonstrate the value of the following:

- *Strengthening families* by targeting problems (e.g., substance use or aggressive behavior); teaching effective parenting skills; improving communication; and helping families deal with disruptions (e.g., divorce or death) or adversities (e.g., parental mental illness or poverty).
- *Strengthening individuals* by building resilience skills, cognitive processes, and behaviors (National Research Council and Institute of Medicine, 2009b).
- *Preventing specific disorders* (e.g., anxiety or depression) by screening individuals at risk and offering cognitive training or other preventive interventions. Given the 20 % prevalence of mental health conditions in adolescents, many of which are undiagnosed and untreated, an alternative approach could be to screen all adolescents at primary care visits (Columbia University Teen Screen®, 2011; National Research Council and Institute of Medicine, 2009b).
- *Promoting mental health in schools* by offering support to youth who are under serious stress; modifying the school environment to promote pro-social behavior; developing students' skills at decision making, self-awareness, and conducting relationships; and targeting violence, aggressive behavior, and substance use (National Research Council and Institute of Medicine, 2009b; University of California Center for Mental Health in Schools, 2011).
- *Promoting mental health through health care and community programs* by promoting and supporting pro-social behavior, teaching coping skills, and targeting modifiable lifestyle factors that can affect behavior and emotional health, such as

sleep, diet, activity and physical fitness, sunshine and light, and television viewing (National Research Council and Institute of Medicine, 2009b).

Positive Youth Development Approach to Adolescent Health and Wellness

Background on Positive Youth Development (PYD): As noted above, past public health interventions have largely centered on early identification and treatment, or the prevention, of problems. This perspective focuses on harm reduction rather than health promotion. *Healthy People 2020* identifies PYD as an emerging issue to prevent risk behaviors, but from the perspective of promoting healthy youth development (Healthy, 2020a). PYD interventions are intentional processes that provide all youth with the support, relationships, experiences, resources, and opportunities that lead to positive outcomes needed to become successful and competent adults (Bernat & Resnick, 2006). Addressing the positive development of young people facilitates their adoption of healthy behaviors and helps to ensure a healthy and productive future adult population (McNeely & Blanchard, 2009).

PYD is grounded in work related to resilience (see chapter by Williams in this book), enabling youth to have positive outcomes despite adversity. Characteristic features of such "resilient" youth include having a close relationship with an adult role model or caregiver, an "easy" temperament, pro-social friends and interests, and good language and reasoning skills (Werner & Smith, 2001). Once considered an intrinsic trait, research has demonstrated that resilience can be enhanced by externally applied interventions, and therefore an opportunity for a public health approach. Damon notes that the PYD approach envisions young people as resources rather than as problems for society, with an emphasis on manifest potentialities rather than supposed incapacities of young people (Damon, 2004). PYD acknowledges adversities and challenges, but resists viewing development as an effort to overcome deficits and risk. Thus, it aims to understand, educate, and engage youth in productive activities rather than to correct, cure, or treat them (Damon, 2004).

Definition and Key Features of PYD: Although many youth activities may be considered as "positive youth development" programming, there are several characteristic features, outlined in Box 3, that define key elements of PYD (Seligman, 2005). Positive youth development is a framework that guides communities in the way that they organize services, opportunities, and supports to help youth develop to their full potential (Dotterweich, 2011). Pittman notes that PYD emphasizes that problem-free is not fully prepared, and the need to move from "beating the odds" to "changing the odds" for youth to achieve well-being as an adult (Pittman, Irby, & Ferber, 2000). Effective PYD enhances the "5 Cs" of individual Competence, Connection, Confidence, Caring, and Character. From a public health perspective, PYD moves beyond disease treatment or prevention to optimal health and wellness.

Box 3 Characteristic Features of Positive Youth Development Programming (Seligman, 2005)

1. *Promote bonding*: youth emotional attachment and commitment to social relationships in the family, peer group, school, community, or culture
2. *Foster resiliency*: youth capacity to adapt to stressful events in healthy and flexible ways
3. *Promote competencies*: social, emotional, cognitive, behavioral, and moral
4. *Encourage self-determination*: youth ability to think for oneself and act consistent with those thoughts, related to the need for competence, autonomy, and relatedness
5. *Foster spirituality*: youth moral reasoning or commitment, or belief in a moral order

6. *Develop self-efficacy*: youth perception that goals can be achieved by one's own action
7. *Nurture clear and positive identity*: youth internal organization of coherent sense of self
8. *Foster belief in the future*: youth internalization of hope and optimism about possibilities
9. *Recognize positive behavior*: positive social response to desired youth behaviors
10. *Provide opportunities for meaningful pro-social involvement*: youth presented with events and activities across social environments to encourage pro-social interactions
11. *Establish pro-social norms*: encourage youth to adopt healthy beliefs and clear standards for behavior through a range of approaches

Models of PYD: Three models of PYD deserve mention regarding reducing risks and promoting health. Communities That Care (CTC® www.sdrg.org/CTCInterventions.asp) is a coalition-building program designed to help a broad-based group of community stakeholders to gather and process information about their community and apply PYD interventions to address their specific youth issues. Involving research findings from numerous disciplines, the CTC® model establishes priorities with measurable, strength-based outcomes for a whole community. Although initially focused on reducing or preventing substance use, other positive outcomes have been noted (Catalano, Gavin, & Markham, 2010). A commentary by the CTC® group in a recent Journal of Adolescent Health supplement framed PYD as a means to promote adolescent sexual and reproductive health (Hawkins et al., 1992).

The Search Institute (www.search-institute.org) was established to provide leadership, knowledge, and resources to promote healthy youth and communities. It focuses on cultivating 40 developmental assets® associated with a young person thriving, dichotomized into 20 internal and 20 external assets, each divided into four categories that have 4–6 anchor points (Search Institute, 2011). Internal asset categories include commitment to learning, positive values, social competencies, and positive identity. A youth who is optimistic about her or his personal future is an example of a positive identity item. External assets, related to domains in which adults can play an important role, are grouped into the following categories: support, empowerment, boundaries and expectations, and constructive use of time. A youth perceiving that adults in the community value youth is an example of an empowerment external asset. Extensive research has shown that assets correlate positively with health-promoting behaviors, while the lack of assets correlates with a variety of risky health behaviors (Mannes, 2006). Not all assets have the same influence on health, however. The internal assets of being motivated to do well in school and of caring about one's own school have a very powerful positive correlation with healthy behaviors and attitudes.

Finally, a PYD intervention deserving mention is Assets Coming Together (ACT) for Youth, a statewide academic-public health collaborative launched in 2000. With funding from the New York State Department of Health (NYS DOH) and its AIDS Institute, the initial focus of ACT for Youth was to reduce violence, abuse, and high-risk sexual behavior among youth through the creation of 11 Community Development Partnerships (later 12 Collaborations for Community Change). Two academic Centers of Excellence (COE) provided technical assistance, training, and other support to both the community partnerships and the NYS DOH. One COE, composed of four partners, now provides academic support and technical assistance about PYD to the NYS DOH, and evaluation and training for communities funded by the NYS DOH. In so doing, the COE connects PYD research to public health practice. Modeling a basic tenet of PYD that adults need to partner with youth in developing programs, ACT for Youth maintains an online presence (www.actforyouth.net), as well as a linked site for and by youth with input from PYD leaders in NYS DOH (www.nysyouth.net). This academic-public health-youth partnership is considered a "big picture" PYD-public health model for other states (Pittman, Martin, & Yohalem, 2006).

ACT for Youth: ACT for Youth is grounded in principles and practical issues detailed in the National Research Council/Institute of Medicine's monograph *Community Programs to Promote Youth Development* (National Research Council and Institute of Medicine, 2002), and the subsequent *Youth Development Handbook*: *Coming of Age in American Communities*, edited by ACT for Youth leaders (Hamilton & Hamilton, 2004). It is one of the first sustained statewide PYD initiatives framed as a public health intervention (Birkhead, Riser, Mesler, Tallon, & Klein, 2006) in which social policy is translated into adolescent public health practice (Kreipe, 2006). Several features of ACT for Youth are notable: a formal Youth Development Team (YDT is a public-private, statewide partnership of leading agencies) providing early leadership grounded in a common, holistic vision (Carter et al., 2006); an emphasis on meaningful "youth engagement" (Schulman, 2006); policy-level support for PYD assuring that all youth-oriented programs funded by NYS have an evidence-based PYD orientation (Riser, Mesler, Tallon, & Birhhead, 2006); a long-standing mutually supportive relationship among the COE, NYS DOH and AIDS Institute, and communities; and a commitment to applying cutting-edge research to practice in the field.

NYS Youth Development Team: The vision of the YDT is for families, schools, and communities to partner in support of the development of healthy, capable, and caring youth. In the spirit of the WHO definition of health, the ultimate outcome is for young people to become healthy, caring, competent, and contributing adults, fully prepared to be parents, workers, leaders, entrepreneurs, and citizens of the future (Carter et al., 2006). Because transforming this vision into statewide practice requires committed actions (policy, funding, and training) at both the state and community levels, meeting this goal requires key stakeholders at all levels to address positive youth health outcomes through effective partnerships. Challenges to the process include ongoing consistent leadership, adequate resources to sustain efforts, marketing strategies, engaging ever-changing membership, buy-in and ownership of PYD, long-term integration of PYD into the fabric of organizations and agencies, positive local involvement, and maintaining collaborations with PYD a high priority for all stakeholders (Carter et al., 2006). Key elements and lessons learned from the first 5 years of the YDT guiding ACT for Youth (Carter et al., 2006) are adapted and detailed in Box 4.

Box 4 Key Elements and Lesson Learned from Statewide PYD Partnerships (Carter et al., 2006)

- Shared vision and leadership modeling PYD principles
- Common goals, definitions, and language unifying all activities
- Broad range of strategic partnerships, with authentic buy-in and minimal hierarchal structure
- Nonexclusive, diverse group of stakeholders who are also decision-makers
- Sustained commitment to PYD at all levels, requiring new connections, linkages, and resources
- Adaptability to approaches while maintaining fidelity to evidence-based public health models
- Partners recognize the relevance of PYD to their organization as well as the "big picture"
- PYD institutionalized at all levels as an evidence-based effective public health intervention

Youth Engagement: An essential, but often overlooked, element of PYD is the active engagement of youth by adults. As noted by Schulman—herself an adolescent when she authored an article on the concept—the terms "youth voice," "participation," "partnerships," and "engagement" are often used interchangeably, but the underlying concepts are hierarchical (Schulman, 2006). Obtaining *youth voice* represents the lowest level of PYD interaction: the opinions of youth are sought, often after decisions have been made by adults, so that youth are asked to choose among a few preconceived ideas with little reciprocity. When youth are more valued as team members and become more actively involved in PYD, *participation* occurs as youth allocate their time and energy to community, school, and family activities (Schulman, 2006). As reciprocity deepens, participation transforms into *partnerships* when consistent, mutual relationships between youth and adults are formed, and values and power are shared. *Engagement*, the ultimate level of involvement, occurs when youth-adult partnerships feature a belief in, and commitment to, mutually meaningful, collective action, emanating from shared feelings of passion, excitement, and focus (Schulman, 2006).

A study of the outcomes of ACT for Youth related to youth participation concluded that (1) the Collaborations for Community Change modeled effective youth engagement, and through those efforts, youth participation was both visible and became a community-wide expectation. The voices of youth were reflected in local policy and programmatic agendas; (2) as youth participation became a visible norm in communities, ACT for Youth supported organizations creating youth engagement opportunities in community health; and (3) ACT for Youth built the capacity of adults (community leaders, practitioners, and citizens) to partner with local youth. By providing training, technical assistance, and logistical support, the collaborations helped communities involve youth in community planning and implementation of initiatives (Zeldin, Petrokubi, Collura, Camino, & Skolaski, 2009).

ACT for Youth: A Statewide Approach to Effect Community Change

An important and active public-private partnership bridging many sectors, the NYS YDT was created in 1998 by the NYS DOH and the NYS Office of Children and Family Services to promote PYD principles and strategies throughout health, human service, education, and other sectors across NYS. Within the NYS DOH, the Center for Community Health's Bureau of Child and Adolescent Health and the AIDS Institute's Bureau of Special Populations joined together to promote PYD in communities throughout NYS by supporting ACT for Youth with public health funds from a variety of federal and state sources (Riser et al., 2006). Redirecting these funds, all of which targeted ACT for Youth goals, into a single stream focused on PYD resulted in highly leveraged, efficient, and effective use of resources.

By bringing together partners who might not otherwise collaborate—but who experienced synergies in working together for a common adolescent health goal—ACT for Youth modeled PYD principles at the level of state government. That is, the NYS DOH provided services, opportunities, and supports emphasizing (1) positive outcomes, (2) individual development, (3) youth engagement with strategies aimed to involve all youth, (4) long-term commitment, (5) community involvement, and (6) collaboration (Whitlock, 2011). The sustained commitment to PYD by the

Box 5 Guidelines to Integrate PYD into Health Department Programs (Whitlock, 2011)

- Base program goals on a PYD approach
- Assure that everyone involved has a core knowledge base about PYD
- Offer practical assistance in putting the principles of PYD into action
- Promote PYD through funding decisions
- Encourage programs to offer meaningful opportunities and roles for young people
- Facilitate opportunities for programs to share successful strategies
- Integrate YD into prevention programs with the support of academic and research institutions
- Include YD outcomes in program evaluation activities

NYS DOH has been demonstrated for more than 11 years in statewide policy and program development, supported by funding and other resources. The NYS DOH compiled guidelines for integrating PYD into Health Department Programs, outlined in Box 5 (Whitlock, 2011).

Trusting, Long-Standing, Mutual Relationships: An important element of ACT for Youth has been the commitment of resources, policies, and programs to PYD, as well as the presence of strong cross-sector relationships at the leadership level for more than a decade. The NYS DOH Adolescent Health Coordinator (also a leader at the Bureau of Child and Adolescent Health) in collaboration with the Director of the ACT for Youth COE (a developmental psychologist and social scientist based at Cornell University) and the Directors of the other partner organizations in the COE (the Division of Adolescent Medicine at the University of Rochester, the NYS Center for School Safety, and the Cornell Cooperative Extension of New York City) have developed trusting, mutual relationships that model the core elements of PYD programming. Having the same individuals lead this effort over time has required creative responses to challenges, such as three changes in NYS administration and two economic downturns. However, responding successfully to challenges with a commitment to disseminating and diffusing messages regarding PYD in a variety of ways (e.g., online messaging, webinars, publications, conferences, and trainings) has led to continued integration of PYD into statewide youth services, programming, policy, and funding, with national public health implications (Healthy, 2020a).

Commitment to Translating Research into Practice: Public health practice needs to be grounded by models with demonstrated effectiveness. Such evidence-based models are not stagnant, but require ongoing adaptations that maintain fidelity with the core features of a model. This translation is sometimes difficult for youth-serving agencies in the field that might be more action oriented than science driven. Early in ACT for Youth, a community group asked the COE for a program that could be taken "off the shelf and put to use." The COE response was a quote from Bronfenbrenner (who coined the term *human ecology*): "the purpose of social science is not to answer questions, but to question answers."

Academic partners at Cornell University and the University of Rochester, as well as leaders at NYS DOH, are guided by the scientific evidence base for PYD as they work with community groups focused on PYD public health interventions in real-world settings across the state. The resulting practical implementation of evidence-based models with fidelity in communities is evaluated by the academic partners focused on the same goals. Thus, ACT for Youth has included the creation of a PYD outcome tool for youth (Sabaratnam & Klein, 2006), the evaluation of community partnerships themselves (Surko, Lawson, Gaffney, Claiborne, 2006), and youth in participatory research and evaluation (Powers & Tiffany, 2006). The strength of these horizontal, cross-sector, practice-oriented partnerships informed by research regarding best-practices may explain the success of ACT for Youth as a public health approach (Zeldin et al., 2009).

Summary

The USPHS was founded more than 200 years ago largely to address the diseases and illnesses of adolescent seaman. Over the subsequent years, increasing public health attention in America was directed at the promotion of health and wellness, beyond the treatment or prevention of disease or illness. Worldwide there has also been increasing public health attention to adolescents, with the recognition of the tremendous burden borne by societies for adolescent morbidity and mortality—largely related to behaviors and therefore theoretically preventable. Due to the limited success of campaigns targeted at specific conditions, PYD has gained traction as a public health approach to adolescent issues. By combining an emphasis on positive features of youth within a developmental framework, the provision of what youth need to thrive, the involvement of broad-based coalitions of key stakeholders, and the active engagement of youth as partners in the process rather than mere recipients, this public health approach holds great promise, as noted previously (Whitlock, 2011) and in Healthy People 2020 (Healthy People, 2011a, 2011b). Continued research is needed to determine the elements of success in a variety of applications.

References

American Legacy Foundation. (2011). Retrieved August 29, 2011, from www.legacyforhealth.org.

Aufseeser, D., Jekielek, S., & Brown, B. (2006). *The family environment and adolescent well-being: Exposure to positive and negative family influences*. Washington: Child Trends; and San Francisco: National Adolescent Health Information Center, University of California. Retrieved August 29, 2011, from www.childtrends.org/Files/Child_Trends-2006_06_01_FR_FamilyEnvironmen.pdf.

Bernat, D. H., & Resnick, M. D. (2006). Healthy youth development: Science and strategies. *Journal of Public Health Management and Practice, 12*(Suppl 6), S10–S16. Retrieved August 30, 2011, from http://journals.lww.com/jphmp/Fulltext/2006/11001/Healthy_Youth_Development__Science_and_Strategies.4.aspx.

Birkhead, G. S., Riser, M. H., Mesler, K., Tallon, T. C., & Klein, S. J. (2006). Youth development is a public health approach. *Journal of Public Health Management Practice* (Suppl):S1–S3.

Carter, T. P., Spitalny, K. C., & Marsh, N. R., et al. (2006). Comprehensive statewide approach to improve youth outcomes: Experience of the New York State Youth Development Team. *Journal of Public Health Management Practice*, (Suppl), S32–S40.

Catalano, R. F., Gavin, L. E., & Markham, C. M. (2010). Future directions for positive youth development as a strategy to promote adolescent sexual and reproductive health. *Journal of Adolescent Health, 46*, S92–S96.

CDC. (1989). Health objectives for the Nation. *Morbidity and Mortality Weekly Report, 38*(37), 629–633.

CDC. (2011). *National initiative to improve adolescent health*. Retrieved August 28, 2011, from www.cdc.gov/healthyyouth/adolescenthealth/nationalinitiative/index.htm.

Centers for Disease Control and Prevention. (2007). The effectiveness of universal school-based programs for the prevention of violent and aggressive behavior: A report on recommendations of the Task Force on Community Preventive Services. *Morbidity and Mortality Weekly Report. 56*(RR-7), 1–12. Retrieved August 29, 2011, from www.cdc.gov/mmwr/PDF/rr/rr5607.pdf.

Centers for Disease Control and Prevention. (2010a). *Sexually transmitted disease surveillance, 2009*, Atlanta, GA: U.S. Department of Health and Human Services, November 2010. Retrieved August 28, 2011, from www.cdc.gov/std/stats09/surv2009-Complete.pdf.

Centers for Disease Control and Prevention. (2010b). *National Center for Chronic Disease Prevention and Health Promotion. Healthy youth! Student health and academic achievement*. Atlanta: CDC. Retrieved August 29, 2011, from http://www.cdc.gov/HealthyYouth/health_and_academics/index.htm#2.

Centers for Disease Control and Prevention. (2011). *National Public Health Performance Standards Program. Essential Public Health Services*. Retrieved August 28, 2011, from http://www.cdc.gov/nphpsp/essentialServices.html.

Columbia University Teen Screen®. (2011). *National Center for Mental Health Checkups*. Retrieved August 30, 2011, from http://www.teenscreen.org.

D'Angelo, L. J., Halpern-Felsher, B. L., & Abraham, A. (2010). Society for Adolescent Health and Medicine. Adolescents and driving: A Position Paper of the Society for Adolescent Health and Medicine. *Journal of Adolescent Health, 47*, 212–214.

Damon, W. (2004). What is positive youth development? *Annals of American Academy of Political and Society Science, 591*, 13–24.

Department of Health and Human Services (HHS). (2010). *Office of Public Health and Science, Office of Adolescent Health. Overview of the teen pregnancy prevention research evidence review*. Washington: HHS. Retrieved August 29, 2011, from www.hhs.gov/ash/oah/prevention/research/index.html.

Dotterweich, J. (2011). *Principles of youth development. ACT for Youth website*. Retrieved August 31, 2011, from www.actforyouth.net/youth_development/development.

Eaton, D. K., Kann, L., & Kinchen, S., et al. (2010). Youth risk behavior surveillance—United States, 2009. Methodology of the youth risk behavior surveillance system. *Morbidity and Mortality Weekly Report* June 4, 2010/Vol. 59/No. SS-5 4:53(No RR-12).

Global Health Council. (2011) *Adolescent health*. Retrieved August 28, 2011, from www.globalhealth.org/child_health/adolescent.

Hamilton, S. F., & Hamilton, M. A. (Eds.). (2004). *The youth development handbook: Coming of age in American communities*. Thousand Oaks, CA: Sage Publications.

Hawkins, J. D., Catalano, R. F., & Associates. (1992). *Communities that care: Action for drug abuse prevention*. San Francisco: Jossey-Bass, Inc.

Healthy People 2020. (2011a). *Adolescent health*. Retrieved August 28, 2011, from www.healthypeople.gov/2020/topicsobjectives2020/overview.aspx?topicid=2.

Healthy People 2020. (2011b). *New topic areas*. Retrieved August 28, 2011, from http://www.healthypeople.gov/2020/about/new2020.aspx.

Jiang, N., Kolbe, L. J., Seo, D.-C., Kay, N. S., & Brindis, C. D. (2011). Health of adolescents and young adults: Trends in achieving the 21 Critical National Health Objectives by 2010. *Journal of Adolescent Health, 49*(2), 124–132.

Kreipe, R. E. (2006). Adolescent health and youth development: Turning social policy into public health practice. *Journal of Public Health Management Practice*, (Suppl), S4–S6.

Kreipe, R. E. (2008). Introduction to interviewing: The art of communicating with adolescents. In A. Joffe (Ed.), *Evaluation and management of adolescent issues. Adolescent Medicine: State of the Art Reviews. 19*(1), 1–17.

Kreipe, R. E. (2011). Focusing on populations to improve the health of individual adolescents and young adults. *Journal of Adolescent Health, 49*(2), 111–112.

Lambert A. (2011). *Life at sea in the Royal Navy of the 18th century*. Updated February 17, 2011. Retrieved August 28, 2011, from www.bbc.co.uk/history/british/empire_seapower/life_at_sea_01.shtml.

Larson, K., & Halfon, N. (2010). Family income gradients in the health and health care access of US children. *Matern and Child Health Journal, 14*(3), 332–342.

Leventhal, T., & Brooks-Gunn, J. (2004). Diversity in developmental trajectories across adolescence: Neighborhood influences. In R. M. Lerner & L. Steinberg (Eds.), *Handbook of adolescent psychology* (2nd ed., pp. 451–486). Hoboken, NJ: Wiley.

Mannes, M. (2006). Research on and evidence for the developmental assets model (appendix B). In D. Fisher, D. Imm, M. Chinman, & A. Wandersman, (Eds.), *Getting to outcomes with developmental assets: Ten steps to measuring success in youth programs and communities* (pp 275–299). Minneapolis: The Search Institute.

McNeely, C., & Blanchard, J. (2009). *The teen years explained: A guide to healthy adolescent development*. Baltimore: Johns Hopkins Bloomberg School of Public Health, Center for Adolescent Health. Retrieved August 27, 2011, from www.jhsph.edu/adolescenthealth.

Muennig, P., & Woolf, S. H. (2007). Health and economic benefits of reducing the number of students per classroom in US primary schools. *American Journal of Public Health., 97*(11), 2020–2027.

Mulye, T. P., Park, M. J., Nelson, C. D., et al. (2009). Trends in adolescent and young adult health in the United States. *Journal of Adolescent Health, 45*(1), 8–24.

National Adolescent Health Information Center. (2006). *Fact sheet on mortality: Adolescents and young adults*. San Francisco, CA: Author, University of California. Retrieved August 28, 2011, from http://nahic.ucsf.edu//downloads/Mortality.pdf.

National Adolescent Health Information Center. (2008). *Fact sheet on demographics: Adolescents and young adults*. San Francisco, CA: Author, University of California. Retrieved August 28, 2011, from http://nahic.ucsf.edu//downloads/Demographics08.pdf.

National Research Council. (1993). *Panel on high-risk youth, Commission on behavioral and social sciences and education. Losing generations: Adolescents in high-risk settings*. Washington: National Academies Press. Retrieved August 29, 2011, from www.nap.edu/openbook.php?record_id=2113&page=1.

National Research Council and Institute of Medicine. (2002). *Community programs to promote youth development*. Washington, DC: National Academy Press.

National Research Council and Institute of Medicine. (2009). Committee on adolescent health care services and models of care for treatment, prevention, and healthy development. In R. S. Lawrence, J. A. Gootman, & L. J. Sim (Eds.), *Adolescent health services: Missing opportunities*. Washington: National Academies Press.

National Research Council and Institute of Medicine. (2009). Committee on the prevention of mental disorders and substance abuse among children, youth, and young adults. In M. E. O'Connell, T. Boat, K. E. Warner (Eds.), *Preventing mental, emotional, and behavioral disorders among young people: Progress and possibilities*. Washington: National Academies Press. Retrieved August 30, 2011, from www.iom.edu/Reports/2009/Preventing-Mental-Emotional-and-Behavioral-Disorders-Among-Young-People-Progress-and-Possibilities.aspx.

Ogden, C. L., Carroll, M. D., & Flegal, K. M. (2008). High body mass index for age among US children and adolescents, 2003–2006. *Journal of the American Medical Association, 299*, 2401–2405. Retrieved August 28, 2011, from www.cdc.gov/chronicdisease/overview/index.htm#ref4.

Park, M. J., Mulye, T. P., Adams, S. H., Brindis, C. D., & Irwin, C. E., Jr. (2006). The health status of young adults in the United States. *Journal of Adolescent Health, 39*(3), 305–317.

Pittman, K., Irby, M., & Ferber, T. (2000). *Unfinished business: Further reflections on a decade of promoting youth development*. Washington, DC: The Forum for Youth Investment. Retrieved August 31, 2011, from www.ppv.org/ppv/publications/assets/74_sup/ydv_1.pdf.

Pittman, K. J., Martin, S., & Yohalem, N. (2006). Youth development as a "Big Picture" public health strategy. *Journal of Public Health Management Practice*; (Suppl), S23–S25.

Powers, J. L., & Tiffany, J. S. (2006). Engaging youth in participatory research and evaluation. *Journal of Public Health Management Practice* (Suppl), S79–S87.

Public Health Service. (1980). *Promoting health/preventing disease: Objectives for the Nation*. Washington, DC: U.S. Department of Health and Human Services, Public Health Service.

Resnick, M. D., Bearman, P. S., Blum, R. W., et al. (1997). Protecting adolescents from harm: Findings from the National Longitudinal Study on adolescent health. *Journal of the American Medical Association, 278*(10), 823–832.

Riser, M. H., Mesler, K., Tallon, T. C., & Birhhead, G. S. (2006). New York State's "Assets Coming Together (ACT) for Youth": A statewide approach effects community change. *Journal of Public Health Management Practice* (Suppl), S41–S47.

Roberts, D. F., Henriksen, L., & Foehr, U. G. (2004) Adolescents and media. In R. M. Lerner & L. Steinberg (Eds.), *Handbook of adolescent psychology* (2nd ed.). (pp. 487–521) Hoboken, NJ: Wiley.

Sabaratnam, P., & Klein, J. D. (2006). Measuring youth development outcomes for community program evaluation and quality improvement: Findings from

dissemination of the Rochester Evaluation of Asset Development for Youth (READY) tool. *Journal of Public Health Management Practice* (Suppl), S88–S94.
Schulman, S. (2006). Terms of engagement: Aligning youth, adults, and organizations toward social change. *Journal of Public Health Management Practice* (Suppl), S26–S31.
Search Institute. (2011). *Developmental assets*. Retrieved August 31, 2011, from www.search-institute.org/developmental-assets/lists.
Seligman, M. E. P. (2005). The positive perspective on youth development. In D. L. Evans, E. B. Foa, R. E. Gur, H. Hendin, C. P. O'Brien, M. E. P. Seligman, B. T. Walsh (Eds.), *Treating and preventing adolescent mental health disorders: What we know and what we don't know* (pp. 497–527). New York: Oxford University Press. Retrieved August 30, 2011, from http://amhi-treatingpreventing.oup.com/anbrg/private/content/mentalhealth/9780195173642/p127.html.
Sum, A., Khatiwada, I., & McLaughlin, J. (2009). The consequences of dropping out of high school: Joblessness and jailing for high school dropouts and the high cost for taxpayers. Boston: Center for Labor Market Studies, Northeastern University.
Surko, M., Lawson, H. A., Gaffney, S., Claiborne, N. (2006). Targeting evaluations of youth development-oriented community partnerships. *Journal of Public Health Management Practice* (Suppl), S95–S107.
Thornton, T. N., Craft, C. A., Dahlberg, L. L., Lynch, B. S., & Baer, K. (2002). *Best practices of youth violence prevention: A sourcebook for community action (rev.)*. Atlanta: Centers for Disease Control and Prevention, National Center for Injury Prevention and Control. Retrieved August 29, 2011, from www.cdc.gov/violenceprevention/pub/YV_bestpractices.html.
U.S. Department of Health and Human Services. (2011). *Historical highlights*. Retrieved August 28, 2011, from www.hhs.gov/about/hhshist.html.
University of California Center for Mental Health in Schools. (2011). Retrieved August 30, 2011, from http://smhp.psych.ucla.edu/.
Werner, E. E., & Smith, R. S. (2001). *Journeys from childhood to midlife: Risk, resilience, and recovery*. Ithaca: Cornell University Press.
Whitlock J. (2011). *Understanding youth development principles and practices. ACT for youth research facts and findings 2004, September 1–4*. Retrieved August 28, 2011, from www.actforyouth.net/resources/rf/rf_understandyd_0904.pdf.
Williams M. (1984/1985). Alcohol and ethnic minorities: Asian/Pacific Americans—An update. *Alcohol Health and Research World*, *9*(2), 64–66, winter 1984/1985.
World Health Organization. (2011a). *Frequently asked questions. What is the WHO definition of health?* Retrieved August 28, 2011, from www.who.int/suggestions/faq/en/.
World Health Organization. (2011b). Media centre. *Young people: Health risks and solutions*. Retrieved August 28, 2011, from www.who.int/mediacentre/factsheets/fs345/en/index.html.
Zeldin, S., Petrokubi, J., Collura, J., Camino, L., & Skolaski, J. (2009). *Strengthening communities through youth participation: Lessons learned from the ACT for youth initiative*. Ithaca, NY: ACT for Youth Center of Excellence.

The Epidemiology of Adolescent Health

K. Clements-Nolle and C.M. Rivera

Introduction

The transition from childhood to adulthood (adolescence) is a period of rapid physical, emotional, and developmental change. While most adolescents in the United States are healthy (Centers for Disease Control and Prevention [CDC] 2010a), adolescence is a time when many health problems are first identified. Rates of adolescent obesity, diabetes, and asthma have all increased dramatically over the past several decades signifying likely increases in adult chronic disease in the future (Perrin, Bloom, & Gortmaker, 2007). Furthermore, new population-level data suggests that the majority of mental disorders among adults emerge during adolescence (Merikangas et al., 2010). Adolescence is also a time when peer influence becomes very important, and many young people begin to experiment with alcohol, tobacco, and other drugs and explore their own sexuality. The behavioral risk taking that occurs during adolescence can profoundly impact immediate and long-term health outcomes.

To accurately describe the health of adolescents, it is important to review mortality and morbidity data as well as a range of behavioral health indicators. This chapter provides a summary of adolescent health epidemiology in five major areas: (1) chronic disease, (2) mental health and suicide, (3) substance use, (4) sexual health, and (5) injury and violence. While adolescence is generally defined as the period from puberty to maturity (typically 10–19 years) (National Research Council and Institute of Medicine, 2009), surveillance systems and national surveys use varying age groups. Therefore, the specific age range and definition of adolescence will be presented whenever possible. In addition, gender and racial and ethnic variation in adolescent health will be reported when the data sources allow for such comparison. This is critical as biological and behavioral risk factors differ for adolescent males and females and the US adolescent population is increasingly becoming more diverse (U.S. Census Bureau, 2011). Finally, it is important to note that most nationally representative data sources and ongoing behavioral surveillance systems do not assess sexual orientation and many measures of socioeconomic vulnerability. Therefore, the disproportionate burden of physical, mental, and behavioral health problems experienced by gay, lesbian, bisexual, and transgender adolescents and other subpopulations such as homeless adolescents, adolescents involved in foster care and juvenile justice systems, and recent immigrants is not adequately reflected.

K. Clements-Nolle, Ph.D., M.P.H. (✉)
C.M. Rivera, M.P.H.
School of Community Health Sciences, University of Nevada, Reno, Mailstop 274, Reno, NV 89557-0036, USA
e-mail: clements@unr.edu

W.T. O'Donohue et al. (eds.), *Handbook of Adolescent Health Psychology*,
DOI 10.1007/978-1-4614-6633-8_6, © Springer Science+Business Media New York 2013

Chronic Disease

The number of adolescents in the United States living with a chronic health condition has increased significantly in the past four decades (Perrin et al., 2007). Most of this growth reflects an increase in the incidence of asthma, obesity, and diabetes (Perrin et al., 2007). Adolescents living with chronic illness lead complicated lives and struggle with medication adherence, frequent medical visits, and internalized stress as a result of feeling different from other adolescents. Increasing rates of chronic health conditions among adolescents also imply increased rates in the US adult population in the next few decades. This will likely contribute to higher health care costs, decreased productivity of the workforce, and poor quality of life among affected individuals (Perrin et al., 2007).

Asthma

Asthma has more than doubled since the 1980s and is currently the leading chronic illness among adolescents (American Lung Association, 2010; Perrin et al., 2007). However, it is important to note that one of the primary surveys used to track asthma, the National Health Interview Survey (NHIS), was redesigned in 1997 and much of the difference in the pre-1997 and post-1997 rates may be attributable to changes in the questionnaire and rates have been relatively stable since 1997 (Akinbami, Moorman, Garbe, & Sondik, 2009). According to the 2009 National Health Interview Survey (NHIS), 17.2 % of adolescents (12–17 years) have ever been diagnosed with asthma and 11.2 % still have asthma (CDC, 2010a). Asthma rates among high school students in 2009 were consistent with NHIS findings with 22 % reporting a history of asthma and 10.8 % reporting current asthma (Eaton et al., 2010).

According to the NHIS, childhood asthma rates were consistently higher among males compared to females; however, at 16–17 years of age current asthma prevalence is similar for males and females (Akinbami et al., 2009) and the YRBS reported higher rates for females (Eaton et al., 2010). Black adolescents had higher lifetime and current asthma prevalence compared to those who are Hispanic or white (Eaton et al., 2010; CDC, 2010a). Furthermore, Akinbami and Schoendorf (2002) found that black adolescents were more likely to be hospitalized due to asthma and were four times more likely to die from asthma than Hispanic or white adolescents (Akinbami & Schoendorf, 2002). Income inequality appears to be associated with asthma rates with the highest lifetime and current rates reported among children and adolescents who relied on Medicaid and other forms of public insurance and those who were living in poverty (CDC, 2010a).

Asthma morbidity contributes to significant personal and societal costs. Children and adolescents have higher rates of asthma-related use of health care services than adults (Akinbami, Moorman & Liu, 2011). Asthma is also the most common cause of school absenteeism due to chronic conditions. In 2008, it was estimated that children and adolescents with asthma missed 10.5 million school days in a year and 5.5 % had an activity limitation due to asthma (Akinbami et al., 2011).

Obesity

Adolescent obesity (BMI for age at or above the 95th percentile) has more than tripled in the past 30 years. The prevalence of obesity among US adolescents aged 12–19 years increased from 5.0 % in 1980 to 18.1 % in 2008 (Ogden, Carroll, Curtin, Lamb, & Flegal, 2010) and in 2009, 12 % of high school students were classified as obese (Eaton et al., 2010).

Adolescent obesity disproportionately affects minority youth. The prevalence of obesity among high school students was higher among black and Hispanic than white students (Eaton et al., 2010). Similarly, the National Health and Nutrition Examination Survey (NHANES) found that in 2008 the prevalence of obesity was significantly higher among Mexican-American adolescent males than among non-Hispanic white adolescent males. Among girls, non-Hispanic black adolescents were significantly more likely to be obese compared with non-Hispanic white adolescents (Ogden et al., 2010). Bethell and colleagues (2010) also found that obesity rates were higher among publicly insured adolescents (10–17 years) compared to those who are privately insured (Bethell, Simpson, Stumbo, Carle, & Gombojav, 2010).

Specific causes for the increase in childhood obesity are not clearly established as longitudinal research in this area is limited and the factors associated with obesity are highly correlated (U.S Department of Health and Human Services, 2011). However, adolescent obesity is directly influenced by exercise and diet. The CDC recommends that young people (ages 6–17) participate in at least 60 min of physical activity daily (CDC, 2011a). However, in 2009, only 18 % of high school students had participated in at least 60 min per day of physical activity and only 33 % attended physical education class daily. Furthermore, a quarter (24.9 %) of students played video or computer games or used a computer for something that was not schoolwork for 3 or more hours per day and 32.8 % watched television 3 or more hours per day on an average school day. Only 22.3 % of high school students had eaten fruits and vegetables five or more times per day during the 7 days before the survey (Eaton et al., 2010).

Obese adolescents experience a number of physical and emotional health problems. One recent study found that 39 % of obese children and adolescents had two or more risk factors for cardiovascular disease such as high cholesterol, blood pressure, or lipid levels (Freedman, Zuguo, Srinivasan, Berenson, & Dietz, 2007). Adolescent obesity is also associated with increased risk for type 2 diabetes (Fagot-Campagna, Narayan, & Imperatore, 2001), sleep problems (Mallory, Fiser, & Jackson, 1989), and earlier maturation, particularly among females (Adar & Gorden-Larson, 2001). Furthermore, many obese adolescents suffer from poor self-esteem, depression, and low quality of life (Swartz & Puhl, 2003; Schwimmer, Burwinkle, & Varni, 2003; U.S. Surgeon General, 2001).

As obese adolescents age, they are at increased risk for becoming overweight or obese during adulthood (Patten et al., 2011; Supinya & Biro, 2011; Whitaker, Wright, Pepe, Seidel, & Dietz, 1997). For example, one study found that 80 % of adolescents (10–15) who were overweight were obese adults at age 25 (Whitaker et al., 1997). This contributes to adverse health outcomes during adulthood such as cardiovascular disease, hypertension, type 2 diabetes, and osteoarthritis (Reilly & Kelly, 2011; Adar & Gorden-Larson, 2001; U.S. Surgeon General, 2001; Dietz, 1998; Whittaker et al., 1997).

Diabetes

Historically, type 1 diabetes was the most common type of diabetes diagnosed among adolescents in the United States; however, in the last two decades, type 2 diabetes, formerly known as adult-onset diabetes, has increasingly been reported among adolescents (CDC, 2011b). The increase in adolescent type 2 diabetes is likely a result of dramatic increases in child and adolescent obesity and physical inactivity (CDC, 2011b). According to estimates from the largest surveillance study of diabetes among adolescents to date, in 2001 there were 121,509 adolescents (10–19 years) who had physician-diagnosed diabetes in the United States (2.80 cases per 1,000 adolescents) (SEARCH for Diabetes in Youth Study Group, 2006).

Overall, diabetes was more prevalent among females than males and black and white adolescents had the highest rates, followed by Hispanic, American Indian, and Asian and Pacific Islander adolescents. While type 1 diabetes accounted for most diagnosed diabetes cases, type 2 diabetes was more prevalent among minority populations. Type 2 diabetes accounted for 6 % of the white adolescent diabetes cases compared to 22 % of Hispanic cases, 33 % of black cases, 40 % of Asian and Pacific Islander cases, and 76 % of American Indian cases (SEARCH for Diabetes in Youth Study Group, 2006). The extremely high rate of type 2 diabetes found among American Indian adolescents in the SEARCH study supports previous research (Fagot-Campagna et al., 2000).

Adolescents with diabetes have an increased risk of developing health complications during adulthood such as heart disease, stroke, kidney disease, nervous system disease, and blindness (CDC, 2011b). Obesity is common among adolescents with type 2 diabetes and many adolescents with type 2 diabetes have multiple cardiovascular risk factors (Liu et al., 2010). Furthermore, adolescents with type 2 diabetes experience lower quality of life compared to those with type 1 diabetes (Naughton et al., 2008).

Mental Health and Suicide

Almost half of the US adolescent population (13–18) is affected by a mental health disorder (Merikangas et al., 2010). Due to a complex interaction of biological, cognitive, social, and environmental factors there are clear gender differences in adolescent mental health disorders. Anxiety, mood, and eating disorders are more common among female adolescents while behavioral disorders are more common among male adolescents (Zahn-Waxler, Shirtcliff, & Marceau, 2008). Poor mental health during adolescence may contribute to school dropout, family dysfunction, juvenile delinquency, substance use, risky sexual behaviors, and intentional and unintentional injuries (Glied & Pine, 2002; Angold et al., 1988; Ellickson, Saner, & McGuigan, 1997). Furthermore, approximately 8.9 billion dollars are spent on the treatment of child and adolescent mental health conditions annually (Soni, 2009).

Epidemiologic surveillance of mental health among adolescents has historically been limited to local and regional surveys using different methodologies, adult recall of mental health issues during adolescence, and national assessment of the symptoms of mental health disorders. However, the National Comorbidity Survey Replication (NCS-R) was recently enhanced to assess a broad range of DSM-IV disorders in a nationally representative sample of adolescents aged 13–18 years (NCS-A) (Merikangas, Avenevoli, Costello, Koretz, & Kessler, 2009). These results were first published in 2010 and represent the first national estimates of mental health disorders among adolescents in the United States. The adolescent mental health disorder estimates in the NCS-A are similar to those for adults in the NCS-R suggesting that the majority of disorders among adults emerge during adolescence (Merikangas et al., 2010).

Anxiety Disorders

There are several subtypes of anxiety disorders, including general anxiety, phobias, panic disorder, and post-traumatic stress disorder (PTSD). Chen and colleagues found that 40 % of adolescents (12–17 years) had symptoms of anxiety disorder (Chen, Killeya-Jones, & Vega, 2005) and the NCS-A demonstrated that nearly one third (31.9 %) of adolescents (13–18) suffered from an anxiety disorder based on DSM-IV classification (Merikangas et al., 2010).

According to the NCS-A, all anxiety disorder subtypes were more frequent in females compared to males, with the greatest gender difference found for PTSD. Overall, the prevalence of anxiety disorders was similar for different age groups, but there were several anxiety subtypes that demonstrated increasing prevalence with age (general anxiety, PTSD, panic disorder, and social phobia). It is also important to note that the median age of onset for anxiety was the earliest of any mental health disorder (6 years). Higher rates of anxiety disorders were found among black adolescents compared to white adolescents (Merikangas et al., 2010).

Mood Disorders

The NCS-A found that 14.3 % of adolescents (13–18) experienced mood disorders with 11.7 % meeting the criteria for major depressive disorder (MDD) or dysthymia (Merikangas et al., 2010). This supports findings from the National Survey on Drug Use and Health (NSDUH) demonstrating that 12.8 % of adolescents (12–17) reported at least one major depressive episode (MDE) in their lifetime and 7.9 % experienced a MDE during the past year (Substance Abuse and Mental Health Administration [SAMHSA], 2007). Only

38.9 % of adolescents who experienced MDE in the past year received treatment for depression (saw or talked to a medical doctor or other professional or used prescription medication) (SAMHSA, 2007).

Both the NCS-A and NSDUH found that females were approximately twice as likely to experience depression compared to males and prevalence of depression steadily increased with age (SAMHSA, 2007; Merikangas et al., 2010). According to the NCS-A, the median age of onset of mood disorders was 13 years (Merikangas et al., 2010), supporting prospective studies that demonstrated that the age of onset of depression is between 11 and 14 years (Lewinsohn, Rohde, & Seeley, 1998). Mood disorders were slightly higher among Hispanic adolescents compared to white adolescents in the NCS-A (Merikangas et al., 2010).

Behavior Disorders

According to NCS-A findings, 19.6 % of adolescents (13–18) had any behavior disorder, with 12.6 % meeting the diagnostic criteria for oppositional defiant disorder (ODD), 6.8 % for conduct disorder (CD), and 8.7 % for attention-deficit/hyperactivity disorder (ADHD) (Merikangas et al., 2010). The ADHD rates in the NCS-A confirm previous estimates from 2005 that found that 8.9 % of adolescents (12–17 years) had ever been told they had ADHD (Bloom, Dey, & Freeman, 2006).

According to the NCS-A, all conduct disorders were more prevalent among males compared to females with the greatest gender difference found for ADHD. The median age of onset for behavior disorders was 11 years and while the prevalence of ADHD and ODD remained relatively stable by age group, rates of CD increased as age increased. Racial/ethnic differences in behavioral disorders were not apparent (Merikangas et al., 2010)

Substance Use Disorders

Substance use is highly prevalent among adolescents and early initiation of substance use increases the likelihood of developing substance abuse or dependence during adolescence and into adulthood (Guttmannova et al., 2011). According to the NCS-A, 11.4 % of adolescents (13–18 years) met the criteria for a substance use disorder, with 8.9 % of adolescents diagnosed with drug abuse/dependence and 6.4 % with alcohol abuse/dependence (Merikangas et al., 2010). The median age of onset for substance abuse disorders was 15 years and substance use disorders increased with age with 22.3 % of adolescents 17–18 classified as having a substance use disorder. The NSDUH represents a younger adolescent population (12–17 years) and found that in 2009, 7 % of adolescents in the United States had abused or been dependent on alcohol or illicit drugs in the past year (SAMHSA, 2010).

Substance abuse disorders were somewhat higher among male adolescents in the NCS-A; however the prevalence of substance dependence or abuse among males was similar to females according to NSDUH findings (6.7 % vs. 7.4 %, respectively). Black adolescents in the NCI-A were less likely to have a substance abuse disorder compared to white adolescents (Merikangas et al., 2010).

Despite high rates of adolescent substance abuse disorders, receipt of treatment is low. In 2009, it was estimated that 1.8 million adolescents (7.2 %) needed treatment for a substance use disorder; however, only 8.4 % of those who needed treatment received it at an appropriate specialty clinic (hospitals [inpatient only], drug or alcohol rehabilitation facilities [inpatient or outpatient], or mental health centers) (SAMHSA, 2010).

Eating Disorders and Unhealthy Weight Loss Behaviors

According to NCS-A findings, lifetime prevalence of any eating disorder (anorexia nervosa, bulimia nervosa, and binge eating disorder) was 2.7 %. These disorders were twice as prevalent among females compared to males and increased with age (Merikangas et al., 2010). In addition to eating disorders, there is concern about unhealthy weight loss behaviors among adolescents such as fasting, vomiting, or taking laxatives. The 2009 YRBS found that nationwide, 10.6 % of high school students did not eat for 24 or more hours; 5 % had taken diet pills, powders, or liquids without a doctor's advice; and 4 % had vomited or taken laxatives to lose weight or keep from gaining weight in the past 30 days.

Overall, the prevalence of these unhealthy weight loss behaviors was higher among female compared to male students; no clear racial or ethnic differences were identified (Eaton et al., 2010).

Suicide

In 2007, suicide was the third leading cause of death for adolescents (12–17 years) (National Center for Injury Prevention and Control, 2011). Furthermore, many youth think about or attempt suicide. In 2009, 13.8 % of high school students seriously considered attempting suicide, 10.9 % made a suicide plan, and 6.3 % attempted suicide at least one time in the past year (Eaton et al., 2010).

While suicide ideation and attempts were higher for females compared to males (Eaton et al., 2010), completion rates were higher for males (National Center for Injury Prevention & Control, 2011) who often use more lethal methods such as firearms (Moscicki, 2001). In 2008, completed suicide rates among American Indian/ Alaska Native adolescents (12–17) were four times higher the rates of any other racial/ethnic group (National Center for Injury Prevention and Control, 2011). According to YRBS findings, attempted suicide was higher among black and Hispanic than white students and suicide ideation was higher among Hispanic than white and black students (Eaton et al., 2010). However, it is important to note that YRBS results for American Indian/Alaska Native students were not published.

Substance Use

Adolescent substance use is a leading cause of morbidity and mortality both during adolescence and into adulthood. While widespread public health intervention has contributed to a steady decline in adolescent alcohol, tobacco, and other drug use in the past two decades, rates have stabilized or increased in recent years. Early initiation of substance use is linked with greater likelihood of developing a substance use disorder (Guttmannova et al., 2011) and long-lasting neurophysiological changes in brain development (Ehlers & Criado, 2010; Mata et al., 2010). Substance use is associated with mental health disorders (Kandel et al., 1997), sexual risk taking (Connell et al., 2009), motor vehicle crashes (Dunlop & Romer, 2010), and violence (SAMHSA, 2010; Brady, Tschann, Pasch, Flores, & Ozer, 2008).

There are a number of ongoing substance use surveillance systems that monitor trends in adolescent substance use. The National Survey on Drug Use and Health (NSDUH) collects data on adolescents age 12–17 years; the Monitoring the Future (MTF) survey assesses 8th, 10th, and 12th grade students; and the Youth Risk Behavior Survey (YRBS) samples students in the 9th through 12th grades. Alcohol and drug use prevalence is consistently lower in the NSDUH compared to the MTF and the YRBS. Such differences are likely the result of sampling a younger population and differences in survey methodology, such as surveying in the home instead of at school (Harrison, 2001).

Alcohol Use

Both NSDUH and MTF findings demonstrate a steady decline in current (past month) alcohol use since the mid 1990s; however, prevalence did not change from 2008 to 2009 (SAMHSA, 2010; Johnston, O'Malley, Bachman, & Schulenberg, 2011). Substantial declines in binge drinking and age of initiation have also been observed (SAMHSA, 2010; Eaton et al., 2010). Despite such declines, alcohol remains the most commonly used drug among adolescents. In 2009, the prevalence of alcohol use in the past month ranged from 14.7 % according to the NSDUH to 41.8 % for high school students (SAMHSA, 2010; Eaton et al., 2010). Binge drinking (5 or more drinks in one sitting) in the past month ranged from 8.8 % (NSDUH) to

24.2 % (YRBS) (SAMHSA, 2010; Eaton et al., 2010). The YRBS also reported that 21.1 % of high school students began consuming alcohol before the age of 13 years (Eaton et al., 2010).

Overall, rates of current drinking, binge drinking, and initiation before the age of 13 were higher among males than females (SAMHSA, 2010; Eaton et al., 2010). The prevalence of current alcohol use and binge drinking was greatest for white adolescents, followed by Hispanic, and then black adolescents (Eaton et al., 2010; SAMHSA, 2010; Johnston et al., 2011). However, according to the YRBS, Hispanic adolescents were more likely to report drinking before the age of 13 (Eaton et al., 2010).

Tobacco Use

Current smoking among adolescents has also declined since the 1990s, but remained steady from 2008 to 2009 (Johnston et al., 2011; SAMHSA, 2010). In 2009, current cigarette use ranged from 8.9 % (NSDUH) to 19.5 % (YRBS) and daily cigarette use was between 2.1 % (NSDUH) and 11.2 % (YRBS) (SAMHSA, 2010; Eaton et al., 2010). According to the YRBS, 10.7 % of high school students have smoked a whole cigarette by the age of 13. Current smoking and smoking initiation were higher for males compared to females (SAMHSA, 2010; Eaton et al., 2010). Current smoking prevalence was highest among American Indian and Alaska Native adolescents followed by white, Hispanic, and black adolescents (SAMHSA, 2010; Eaton et al., 2010).

Despite declines in smokeless tobacco use since 1990s, both the MTF and NSDUH found that smokeless tobacco use increased in the last year measured (Johnston et al., 2011; SAMHSA, 2010). In 2009, current smokeless tobacco use ranged from 2.3 % (NSDUH) to 8.9 % (YRBS) (SAMHSA, 2010; Eaton et al., 2010). Current use of smokeless tobacco was greater among males than females (Eaton et al., 2010; SAMHSA, 2010; Johnston et al., 2011) and white adolescents, followed by Hispanic adolescents, and then black adolescents (Eaton et al., 2010).

Marijuana and Other Illicit Drug Use

Overall, the percentage of adolescents who reported current (past month) illicit drug use (with or without marijuana) gradually declined during the last decade, but has started to increase in the last couple of years (SAMHSA, 2010; Johnston et al., 2011). In 2009, the prevalence of current illicit drug use, including marijuana, ranged from 10 % (NSDUH) to 15.8 % (MTF) (SAMHSA, 2010; Johnston et al., 2011). Current marijuana use ranged from 7.3 % (NSDUH) to 20.8 % (YRBS) and 7.5 % of high school students reported using marijuana before the age of 13 (SAMHSA, 2010; Eaton et al., 2010). Current use of illicit drugs other than marijuana was lower, ranging from 1 % to 2.5 % for inhalants, 0.9 % to 1.3 % for hallucinogens, and 0.3 % to 1 % for cocaine according to NSDUH and MTF, respectively (SAMHSA, 2010; Johnston et al., 2011).

Males reported higher rates of current marijuana and other illicit drug use as well as early initiation of use compared to females (SAMHSA, 2010; Eaton et al., 2010). Racial/ethnic comparisons of current illicit drug use among adolescents were not systematically reported; however, the YRBS found that current use of marijuana is highest among black students (Eaton et al., 2010).

Nonmedical Prescription Drug Use

Overall, nonmedical prescription drug use among adolescents peaked in the early to mid 2000s and has stabilized since this time (SAMHSA, 2010; Johnston et al., 2011). In 2009, 20.2 % of high school students reported having ever taken a prescription drug without a prescription from a doctor (Eaton et al., 2010). The MTF study found that 9.7 % of adolescents reported narcotic drug use other than heroin (Oxycontin and Vicodin) in the past 12 months (Johnston et al., 2011) and NSDUH found that 3.1 % of adolescents reported current (past month) nonmedical prescription drug use (taking pain relievers, tranquilizers, stimulants, and sedatives without a prescription and taken for the intent of feeling the drug's effects) (SAMHSA, 2010).

Nonmedical prescription drug use is unique in that use is higher among females than males (SAMHSA, 2010). Furthermore, prevalence of prescription drug use appears to vary by geographic location. According to 2008 NSDUH findings, nonmedical prescription drug use was 26 times higher among rural adolescents compared to urban adolescents (Havens, Young, & Havens, 2011). Lifetime use of nonmedical prescription drugs was highest among white high school students, followed by Hispanic and black students (Eaton et al., 2010).

Sexual Health

The proportion of US adolescents who are sexually active has declined and birth control rates have increased during the past two decades (Eaton et al., 2011). Despite such improvements, adolescents and young adults account for nearly half the new sexually transmitted infections (STI) each year (Weinstock, Berman & Cates, 2004) and the USA continues to have one of the highest teen pregnancy rates in the developed world (McKay & Barrett, 2010).

Recent data suggests that acquisition of STIs occurs soon after sexual activity begins (Forhan et al., 2009). While adolescent STI infection may be benign, some common STIs contribute to long-term health problems. According to the CDC, half of new gonorrhea cases and more than half of new chlamydia cases are undiagnosed (CDC, 2010b). If left untreated, chlamydia and gonorrhea can cause pelvic inflammatory disease (PID) and infertility (CDC, 2010b). In addition, persistent infection with high-risk human papillomavirus (HPV) contributes to the development of cervical and anal cancer (Bosch & de Sanjosé, 2003; CDC, 2010b).

Teen pregnancy also has negative consequences for the mother, the child, and society. Preterm birth, low birth weight, and infant mortality rates are higher for births to teen mothers compared to births to adult women (Gilbert, Jandial, Field, Bigelow, & Danielsen, 2004). Furthermore, teen mothers are less likely to finish high school and their children are more disadvantaged compared to children of older mothers (Manlove, Terry-Humen, Mincieli, & Moore, 2008; Perper, Peterson, & Manlove, 2010). Each year, teen childbearing costs the United States at least $9 billion dollars for additional services and reduced tax revenue (Hoffman, 2006).

Sexual Behaviors

In 2009, almost half (46 %) of high school students reported ever having sex and 13.8 % had more than four sexual partners. While sexual activity increases with age, it is important to note that 5.9 % of high school students had sex before the age of 13. Over one third (34.2 %) of high school students had sex in the past 3 months (sexually active). Among students who were sexually active, 21.6 % drank alcohol or used drugs before their last sexual intercourse and 61.1 % reported using a condom the last time they had sex. Other forms of birth control used during last sexual intercourse included birth control pills (19.8 %) and Depo-Provera (3.1 %) (Eaton et al., 2010).

Males and females were equally likely to report ever having sex, but females were slightly more likely to report recent sexual activity. Males were more likely than females to report having sex before the age of 13, having four or more partners, and using alcohol or drugs before last sex (Eaton et al., 2010). Black students reported higher rates of lifetime and recent sexual activity, having sex before the age of 13, and having multiple partners than white and Hispanic students. However, the prevalence of having used a condom during last sexual intercourse was higher among white and black students compared to Hispanic students (Eaton et al., 2010).

Sexually Transmitted Infections

Data from the nationally representative National Health and Nutrition Examination Survey (NHANES) found that 37.7 % of sexually experienced female adolescents (14–19) were infected with one or more of the five most common STIs (chlamydia, gonorrhea, herpes simplex virus type 2,

HPV, and trichomonas) and the prevalence of STI infection increased to 53.5 % among female adolescents who reported three or more partners (Forhan et al., 2009). HPV infection accounted for nearly three quarters of the overall STI prevalence among female adolescents (Forhan et al., 2009), supporting sentinel surveillance in six US cities that found that 35 % of adolescents (14–19) were infected with a high-risk HPV subtype (CDC, 2010b).

Reportable STI surveillance has also demonstrated high rates of infection among adolescents. In 2009, adolescent females (15–19) had the highest rate of chlamydia (3,329.3 cases per 100,000 population) compared with any other age or sex group. Chlamydia infection rates among adolescent females increased 1.8 % from 2008 to 2009. Among adolescent males, chlamydia infection rates were much lower (735.5 per 100,000), but increased 5 % from 2008 to 2009 (CDC, 2010b). Chlamydia rates were much higher among black adolescents compared to other racial and ethnic groups, primarily due to the extremely high rates of chlamydia infection among black females (CDC, 2011c).

Adolescent females also had the highest rate of gonorrhea infection (568.8 cases per 100,000) in 2009, a 10.5 % decrease from 2008. Gonorrhea rates among adolescent males were more than 50 % lower than female rates (250.0 cases per 100,000) and decreased 10 % from 2008 to 2009 (CDC, 2010b). Gonorrhea rates were highest among black adolescents and while there has been a steady decline in gonorrhea rates for all racial ethnic groups since 2006, the decrease has been lower for blacks (CDC, 2011c).

Unlike other STIs, syphilis rates are higher among young adults (20–24) than adolescents. However, syphilis rates among female adolescents increased from 1.5 cases per 100,000 in 2004 to 3.3 cases per 100,000 in 2009 and adolescent male infection increased from 1.3 cases per 100,000 to 6.0 cases per 100,000 in 2009 (CDC, 2010b). Syphilis rates are highest among black adolescents and over the past 5 years, primary and secondary syphilis rates among young black men (15–24) have increased more than 150 %; much of this increase has been among young men who have sex with men (CDC, 2011c).

The disproportionate rate of STI among black adolescents is the result of many factors including limited access to testing and treatment and a higher pool of infection in low-income communities (CDC, 2011c).

HIV/AIDS

In 2008, almost 2,000 new diagnoses of HIV infection were reported among adolescents (13–19) (CDC, 2011d). However, it is important to note that only 12.7 % of high school students reported being tested for HIV in 2009 (Eaton et al., 2010) and the average period of time from HIV infection to the development of AIDS is 10 years. Therefore, a proportion of HIV cases diagnosed among young adults represent infection that occurred during adolescence.

Most (89 %) adolescent HIV diagnoses in 2008 were among young men who have sex with men; however, females accounted for 29 % of adolescent infection compared with 20 % of infection for young adults (20–24). Black adolescents have been disproportionately affected by the HIV epidemic. In 2008, 17 % of adolescents (13–19) in the United States were black, yet an estimated 75 % of adolescent diagnoses of HIV infection were among black adolescents. Furthermore, the disproportionate rate of infection among black adolescents was greater than that observed for older populations. Hispanic adolescents represented the second largest percentage of adolescent HIV infection (13 %), followed by white adolescents (11 %) (CDC, 2011d).

Pregnancy

A decline in sexual activity and improved contraceptive use have contributed to a 41 % drop in teen (15–19) pregnancy rates since the peak in 1990 (Kost, Henshaw, & Carlin, 2010; Santelli, Lindberg, Finer, & Singh, 2007). Despite such progress, teenage pregnancy and birthrates in the USA remain high and the vast majority of teen pregnancies are unwanted (Finer & Henshaw, 2006). In 2006 (the most recent data available), 750,000 female teens (15–19) became pregnant (approximately 7 % of this age group) (Kost et al., 2010). Teen pregnancy rates in 2006 were more than twice as high among black and Hispanic teens compared to white teens (Kost et al., 2010).

Following a consistent decline since 1990, the US teen birthrate increased slightly between 2005 and 2007, and then resumed declining. In 2009, 410,000 female adolescents (15–19) gave birth, representing the lowest teen birthrate ever recorded (39.1 births per 1,000 females) (Pazol et al., 2011). From 1990 to 2009 the adolescent birthrate decreased 50 % among black, 41 % among white, and 33 % among Hispanic adolescents. In 2009, birthrates for black adolescents and Hispanic adolescents were more than double the rate for white teens (Pazol et al., 2011).

Injury and Violence

Unintentional injury is the leading cause of death among adolescents in the United States (National Center for Injury Prevention and Control, 2011) costing society $69 billion in lifetime medical expenses and productivity loss for injuries occurring during adolescence (10–19) (Miller, Finkelstein, Zaloshnja, & Hendrie, 2006). In addition, there is concern about the high rates of adolescent fighting, bullying, and dating violence among high school students (Eaton et al., 2010). Adolescent victims of interpersonal violence and bullying are at increased risk for substance use and mental health problems, including suicidal behavior (Brooks, Harris, Thrall, & Woods, 2002; CDC, 2006a; Hanson, 2002; Carlyle & Steinman, 2007).

Motor Vehicle Injuries and Deaths

Motor vehicle accidents was the number one cause of death among adolescents, accounting for 68.8 % of unintentional injury deaths in 2007 (National Center for Injury Prevention and Control, 2011). Overall, risky behaviors contributing to motor vehicle injuries and deaths have decreased in the last decade (Eaton et al., 2010). Research suggests that changes in licensing requirements, seat belt laws, and enforcement have decreased adolescent motor vehicle injuries and deaths (Sivak & Schoettle, 2010; Carpenter & Stehr, 2008). Despite such reductions, 9.7 % of high school students reported that they rarely or never wore a seat belt and among those who rode a motorcycle, 31.9 % did not wear a helmet in the past 12 months (Eaton et al., 2010). In the past month, 28.3 % of high school students rode in a car with someone who had been drinking alcohol and 9.7 % had driven after drinking alcohol at least once (Eaton et al., 2010).

All behaviors contributing to motor vehicle injuries and deaths were higher among males than females and motor vehicle death rates are more than twice as high among males compared to females (CDC, 2011e). Such gender differences may be the result of greater risk taking behavior among males (Turner & McClure, 2003). Most behaviors contributing to unintentional injury and motor vehicles were highest among black adolescents, followed by Hispanic, and then white adolescents except for riding in a car with someone who had been drinking which was highest among white adolescents (Eaton et al., 2010).

Homicide

In 2007, homicide was the second leading cause of death among adolescents (12–17) (National Center for Injury Prevention and Control, 2011). The homicide death rate for male adolescents was six times greater than that for female adolescents. Homicide is the leading cause of death for black male adolescents. The risk of dying from homicide among black male adolescents is more than twice that of Hispanic males and about 15 times that of white males (CDC, 2010c).

Fighting

In 2009, nearly one third (31.5 %) of US high school students reported that they had been in a fight and 3.8 % had been injured in a fight to the extent that they needed to be treated by a doctor or nurse in the past 12 months (Eaton et al., 2010). Furthermore, 14.4 % of adolescents (12–17) had participated in a group-against-group fight and 7.2 % had attacked someone with the intent to harm or seriously hurt them in the past 12 months (SAMHSA, 2010). In the past month, 17.5 % of high school students carried a weapon and 5.9 % carried a gun at least once (Eaton et al., 2010). Overall, fighting and weapon-carrying behaviors among high school students were higher for males than females. Among males, fighting and being injured in a fight were more frequently reported by black students, followed by Hispanic, and then white students. Black students were also more likely to report carrying a gun, followed by white, and then Hispanic students (Eaton et al., 2010).

Bullying

Bullying has historically included physical bullying and verbal bullying. However, technology bullying has become of increasing concern as the prevalence of adolescents who are victims of electronic aggression has risen (Wolak, Mitchell, & Finkelhor, 2006). In 2009, 19.9 % of high school students reported having been bullied on school property in the past 12 months and 5 % reported missing at least 1 day of school in the past month because they felt unsafe at school or on their way to or from school (Eaton et al., 2010). A nationally representative study with 16,000 students (grades 6–10) found that 10.6 % of students reported bullying sometimes and 8.8 % did so once a week or more. Prevalence of bullying victimization was similar, with 8.5 % of students reporting that they were sometimes bullied and 8.4 % stating that they were bullied once a week or more (Nansel et al., 2001). Co-occurrence of being the perpetrator and the victim of bullying was not common (Nansel et al. 2001; Carlyle & Steinman, 2007).

Overall, bullying victimization and perpetration decreased as grade level increased and these behaviors were more frequently reported by males compared to females (Eaton et al., 2010; Nansel et al., 2001; Carlyle & Steinman, 2007). Racial and ethnic differences in bullying across studies are inconsistent. While the YRBS found that bullying victimization was highest among white adolescents, followed by Hispanic, and then black adolescents (Eaton et al., 2010), Carlyle and Steinman (2007) found that both perpetration and victimization were highest among American Indian followed by black adolescents.

Dating Violence

In 2009, 9.8 % of high school students reported having been hit, slapped, or physically hurt on purpose by a boyfriend or girlfriend in the past 12 months (Eaton et al., 2010). Though not specific to dating relationships, 7.4 % of high school students reported that in their lifetime they had been forced to have sexual intercourse when they did not want to (Eaton et al., 2010). A recent national survey of adolescents (13–18) found that dating violence was common, including sexual abuse (25 %), physical abuse (15 %), repeated verbal abuse (11 %), and threats of physical or sexual abuse (18 %) from a partner. Furthermore, the majority of adolescents knew someone their age experiencing some form of dating violence (Teen Research Unlimited, 2009).

Both males and females report being the victim of dating violence, while sexual violence victimization is higher among females (Eaton et al., 2010), possibly due to a power imbalance (Barter, 2009). The prevalence of having been intentionally hurt by a boyfriend or girlfriend or forced to sexual intercourse was both higher among black students, followed by Hispanic, and white students (Eaton et al., 2010).

Summary

While most adolescents are healthy, dramatic increases in asthma, obesity, and diabetes have been observed in the past few decades suggesting significant individual and societal costs in the future (Perrin et al., 2007). Moreover, almost half of the US adolescent population meets the criteria for a mental health disorder (Merikangas,

2010) and suicide remains a leading cause of death for this age group (National Center for Injury Prevention & Control, 2011). Overall, there have been improvements in adolescent substance use and sexual risk taking since the 1990s (Eaton et al., 2011; SAMHSA, 2010; Johnston et al., 2011); however, there is evidence that such improvements have leveled off in recent years and the impact of such behaviors (e.g., automobile crashes, STI infection, teen pregnancy, interpersonal violence) remains unacceptably high. Furthermore, data continue to demonstrate socioeconomic and racial/ethnic disparities in most adolescent health indicators.

The most common adolescent health problems presented in this chapter are preventable. There is an urgent need for policies, strategies, and interventions that promote healthy behaviors and resilience among adolescents, while improving their access to care and support services.

References

Adar, L. S., & Gorden-Larson, P. (2001). Maturational timing and overweight prevalence in US adolescent girls. *American Journal of Public Health, 91*, 642–644.

Akinbami, L. J., & Schoendorf, K. C. (2002). Trends in childhood asthma: Prevalence, health care utilization, and mortality. *Pediatrics, 110*(2), 315–322.

Akinbami, L. J., Moorman, J. E., Garbe, P. L., & Sondik, E. J. (2009). Status of childhood asthma in the United States, 1980–2007. *Pediatrics, 123*, s131–s145.

Akinbami, L. J., Moorman, J. E., & Liu, X. (2011). Asthma prevalence, health care use and mortality: United States, 2005–2009. *National Health Statistics Reports, 32*, 1–15.

American Lung Association. (2010). *Trends in asthma morbidity and mortality*. Retrieved April 28, 2011, from http://www.lungusa.org/finding-cures/our-research/trend-reports/asthma-trend-report.pdf.

Angold, A., Messer, S. C., Stangl, D., Farmer, E. M., Costello, E. J., & Burns, B. J. (1988). Perceived parental burden and service use for child and adolescent psychiatric disorders. *American Journal of Public Health, 88*, 75–80.

Barter, C. (2009). In the name of love: Partner abuse and violence in teenage relationships. *British Journal of Social Work, 39*, 211–233.

Bethell, C., Simpson, L., Stumbo, S., Carle, A. C., & Gombojav, N. (2010). National, state, and local disparities in childhood obesity. *Health Affairs, 29*(3), 347–356.

Bloom, B., Dey, A. N., & Freeman, G. (2006). Summary health statistics for U.S. children: National Health Interview Survey, 2005. *Vital Health and Statistics, 10*(231), 1–84.

Bosch, F. X., & de Sanjosé, S. (2003). Human papillomavirus and cervical cancer—Burden and assessment of causality. *Journal of the National Cancer Institute. Monographs, 31*, 3–13.

Brady, S. S., Tschann, J. M., Pasch, L. A., Flores, E., & Ozer, E. J. (2008). Violence involvement, substance use and sexual activity among Mexican-American and European-American adolescents. *Journal of Adolescent Health, 43*, 285–295.

Brooks, T. L., Harris, S. K., Thrall, J. S., & Woods, E. R. (2002). Association of adolescent risk factors with mental health symptoms in high school students. *Journal of Adolescent Health, 31*, 240–246.

Carlyle, K. E., & Steinman, K. J. (2007). Demographic differences in the prevalence, co-occurrence, and correlates of adolescent bullying at school. *Journal of School Health, 77*(9), 623–629.

Carpenter, C. S., & Stehr, M. (2008). The effects of mandatory seat belt laws on seat belt use, motor vehicle fatalities, and crash-related injuries among youths. *Journal of Health Economics, 27*, 642–662.

Centers for Disease Control and Prevention. (2006a). Physical dating violence among high school students—United States, 2003. *Morbidity and Mortality Weekly Report, 55*, 532–535.

Centers for Disease Control and Prevention. (2010a). *Summary health statistics for U.S. children: National Health Interview Survey, 2009*. National Center for Health Statistics (PHS)-2011-1575, Series 10, Number 247.

Centers for Disease Control and Prevention. (2010b). *Sexually transmitted disease surveillance 2009*. Retrieved April 28, 2011, from http://www.cdc.gov/std/stats09/default.htm.

Centers for Disease Control and Prevention. (2010c). *Mortality among teenagers aged 12–19 years: United States, 1999–2006*. Retrieved April 28, 2011, from http://www.cdc.gov/nchs/data/databriefs/db37.htm.

Centers for Disease Control and Prevention. (2011a). *How much physical activity do children and adolescents need*? Retrieved April 28, 2011, from http://www.cdc.gov/physicalactivity/everyone/guidelines/children.html.

Centers for Disease Control and Prevention. (2011b). *Diabetes public health resource. Children and diabetes: More information*. Retrieved April 28, 2011, from http://www.cdc.gov/diabetes/projects/cda2.htm.

Centers for Disease Control and Prevention. (2011c). *African Americans and sexually transmitted diseases*. Retrieved April 28, 2011, from http://www.cdc.gov/nchhstp/newsroom/docs/AAs-and-STD-Fact-Sheet-042011.pdf.

Centers for Disease Control and Prevention. (2011d). *HIV/AIDS surveillance in adolescents and young adults (through 2008)*. Retrieved April 28, 2011, from http://www.cdc.gov/hiv/topics/surveillance/resources/slides/adolescents/index.htm.

Centers for Disease Control and Prevention. (2011e). *Health, United States, 2010: With special feature on death and dying. Hyattsville, MD. 2011*. Retrieved April 28, 2011, from http://www.cdc.gov/nchs/data/hus/hus10.pdf#specialfeature.

Chen, K. W., Killeya-Jones, L. A., & Vega, W. (2005). Prevalence and co-occurrence of psychiatric symptom clusters in the U.S. adolescent population using DISC predictive scales. *Clinical Practice and Epidemiology in Mental Health, 1*, 22.

Connell, C. M., Gilreath, T. D., & Hansen, N. B. (2009). A multiprocess latent class analysis of the co-occurrence of substance use and sexual risk behavior among adolescents. *Journal of Studies on Alcohol and Drugs, 70*, 943–951.

Dietz, W. H. (1998). Health consequences of obesity in youth: childhood predictors of adult disease. *Pediatrics, 101*(3 pt2), 518–525.

Dunlop, S. M., & Romer, D. (2010). Adolescent and young adult crash risk: Sensation seeking, substance use propensity, and substance use behaviors. *Journal of Adolescent Health, 46*, 90–92.

Eaton, D. K., Kann, L., Kinchen, S., Shanklin, S., Ross, J., Hawkins, J., et al. (2010). Youth risk behavior surveillance–United States, 2009. *Morbidity and Mortality Weekly Report, 59*, 1–142.

Eaton, D. K., Lowry, R., Brener, N. D., Kann, L., Romero, L., & Wechsler, H. (2011). Trends in human immunodeficiency virus- and sexually transmitted disease-related risk behaviors among U.S. High school students, 1991–2009. *American Journal of Preventive Medicine, 40*(4), 427–433.

Ehlers, C. L., & Criado, J. R. (2010). Adolescent ethanol exposure: Does it produce long-lasting electrophysiological effects? *Alcohol, 44*, 27–37.

Ellickson, P., Saner, H., & McGuigan, K. A. (1997). Profiles of violent youth: Substance use and other concurrent problems. *American Journal of Public Health, 87*, 985–991.

Fagot-Campagna, A., Narayan, K. M. V., & Imperatore, G. (2001). Type 2 diabetes in children: exemplifies the growing problem of chronic diseases [Editorial]. *British Medical Journal, 322*, 377–378.

Fagot-Campagna, A., Pettitt, D. J., Engelgau, M. M., Burrows, N. R., Geiss, L. S., Valdez, R., et al. (2000). Type 2 diabetes among North American children and adolescents: An epidemiologic review and a public health perspective. *Journal of Pediatrics, 136*(5), 664–672.

Finer, L. B., & Henshaw, S. K. (2006). Disparities in rates of unintended pregnancies in the US. *Perspectives on Sexual and Reproductive Health, 38*(2), 90–96.

Forhan, S. E., Gottlieb, S. L., Sternberg, M. R., Xu, F., Datta, S. D., McQuillan, G. M., et al. (2009). Prevalence of sexually transmitted infections among female adolescents aged 14 to 19 in the United States. *Pediatrics, 124*(6), 1505–1512.

Freedman, D. S., Zuguo, M., Srinivasan, S. R., Berenson, G. S., & Dietz, W. H. (2007). Cardiovascular risk factors and excess adiposity among overweight children and adolescents: The Bogalusa Heart study. *Journal of Pediatrics, 150*(1), 12–17.

Gilbert, W., Jandial, D., Field, N., Bigelow, P., & Danielsen, B. (2004). Birth outcomes in teenage pregnancies. *The Journal of Maternal-Fetal & Neonatal Medicine, 16*(5), 265–270.

Glied, S., & Pine, D. S. (2002). Consequences and correlates of adolescent depression. *Archives of Pediatrics & Adolescent Medicine, 156*, 1009–1014.

Guttmannova, K., Bailey, J. A., Hill, K. G., Lee, J. O., Hawkins, J. D., Woods, M. L., et al. (2011). Sensitive periods for adolescent alcohol use initiation: Predicting the lifetime occurrence and chronicity of alcohol problems in adulthood. *Journal of Studies on Alcohol and Drugs, 72*, 221–231.

Hanson, R. F. (2002). Adolescent dating violence: prevalence and psychological outcomes. *Child Abuse & Neglect, 26*, 447–451.

Harrison, L. (2001). Understanding the differences in youth drug prevalence rates produced by the MTF, NHSDA, and YRBS studies. *Journal of Drug Issues, 31*(3), 665–694.

Havens, J. R., Young, A. M., & Havens, C. E. (2011). Nonmedical prescription drug use in a nationally representative sample of adolescents: Evidence of greater use among rural adolescents. *Archives of Pediatrics & Adolescent Medicine, 165*(3), 250–255.

Hoffman, S. D. (2006). *By the numbers—The public costs of teen childbearing*. Retrieved April 28, 2011, from http://www.thenationalcampaign.org/resources/pdf/pubs/btn_full.pdf.

Johnston, L. D., O'Malley, P. M., Bachman, J. G., & Schulenberg, J. E. (2011). *Monitoring the Future national results on adolescent drug use: Overview of key findings, 2010*. Ann Arbor: Institute for Social Research, University of Michigan.

Kandel, D. B., Johnson, J. B., Bird, H. R., Canino, G., Goodman, S. H., Lahey, B. B., et al. (1997). Psychiatric disorders associated with substance use among children and adolescents: Findings from the Methods for the Epidemiology of Child and Adolescent Mental Disorders (MECA) study. *Journal of Abnormal Child Psychology, 25*(2), 121–132.

Kost, K., Henshaw, S., & Carlin, L. (2010). *U.S. teenage pregnancies, births and abortions: National and State Trends and Trends by Race and Ethnicity*. Retrieved April 28, 2011, from http://www.guttmacher.org/pubs/USTPtrends.pdf.

Lewinsohn, P. M., Rohde, P., & Seeley, J. R. (1998). Major depressive disorder in older adolescents: Prevalence, risk factors, and clinical implications. *Clinical Psychology Review, 18*, 765–794.

Liu, L. L., Lawrence, J. M., Davis, C., Liese, A. D., Pettitt, D. J., Pihoker, C., et al. (2010). Prevalence of overweight and obesity in youth with diabetes in USA: the SEARCH for Diabetes in Youth study. *Pediatric Diabetes, 11*(1), 4–11.

Mallory, G. B., Fiser, D. H., & Jackson, R. (1989). Sleep-associated breathing disorders in morbidly obese children and adolescents. *Journal of Pediatrics, 115*, 892–897.

Manlove, J., Terry-Humen, E., Mincieli, L., & Moore, K. (2008). Outcomes for children of teen mothers from kindergarten through adolescence. In S. Hoffman & R. Maynard (Eds.), *Kids having kids: Economic costs and social consequences of teen pregnancy*. Washington, DC: The Urban Institute Press.

Mata, I., Perez-Iglesias, R., Roiz-Santianez, R., Tordesillas-Gutierrez, D., Pazos, A., Gutierrez, A., et al. (2010). Gyrification brain abnormalities associated with adolescence and early-adulthood cannabis use. *Brain Research, 1317*, 297–304.

McKay, A., & Barrett, M. (2010). Trends in teen pregnancy rates from 1996–2006: A comparison of Canada, Sweden, USA, and England/Whales. *The Canadian Journal of Human Sexuality, 19*(1–2), 43–52.

Merikangas, K., Avenevoli, S., Costello, J., Koretz, D., & Kessler, R. C. (2009). National comorbidity survey replication adolescent supplement (NCS-A): I. Background and measures. *Journal of the American Academy of Child and Adolescent Psychiatry, 48*, 367–369.

Merikangas, K. R., He, J., Burstein, M., Swanson, S. A., Avenevoli, S., Cui, L., et al. (2010). Lifetime prevalence of mental disorders in U.S. adolescents: Results from the National Comorbidity Survey Replication-Adolescent Supplement (NCS-A). *Journal of the American Academy of Child and Adolescent Psychiatry, 49*(10), 980–989.

Miller, T. R., Finkelstein, A. E., Zaloshnja, E., & Hendrie, D. (2006). The cost of child and adolescent injuries and the savings from prevention. In K. D. Liller (Ed.), *Injury prevention for children and adolescents: Research, practice, and advocacy*. Washington, DC: APHA Press.

Moscicki, E. K. (2001). Epidemiology of completed and attempted suicide: Toward a framework for prevention. *Clinical Neuroscience Research, 1*(5), 310–323.

Nansel, T. R., Overpeck, M., Pilla, R. S., Ruan, W. J., Simons-Morton, B., & Scheidt, P. (2001). Bullying behaviors among US youth: Prevalence and association with psychosocial adjustment. *Journal of the American Medical Association, 285*(16), 2094–2100.

National Center for Injury Prevention and Control. (2011). *WISQARS injury mortality reports, 1999–2008*. Retrieved April 28, 2011, from http://www.cdc.gov/injury/wisqars/index.html.

National Research Council and Institute of Medicine. (2009). *Adolescent health services: Missing opportunities*. Washington, DC: National Academy Press.

Naughton, M. J., Ruggiero, A. M., Lawrence, J. M., Impetore, G., Klingensmith, G. J., Waitzfelder, B., et al. (2008). Health-related quality of life of children and adolescents with type 1 or type 2 diabetes mellitus: SEARCH for Diabetes in Youth Study. *Archives of Pediatrics & Adolescent Medicine, 162*(7), 649–657.

Ogden, C. L., Carroll, M. D., Curtin, L. R., Lamb, M. M., & Flegal, K. M. (2010). Prevalence of high body mass index in US children and adolescents, 2007–2008. *Journal of the American Medical Association, 303*(3), 242–249.

Patton, G. C., Coffey, C., Carlin, J. B., Sawyer, S. M., Williams, J., Olsson, C. A., et al. (2011). Overweight and obesity between adolescence and young adulthood: A 10-year prospective cohort study. *Journal of Adolescent Health, 48*(3), 275–280.

Pazol, K., Warner, L., Gavin, L., Callaghan, W. M., Spitz, A. M., Anderson, J. E., et al. (2011). Vital signs: Teen pregnancy–United States, 1991–2009. *Morbidity and Mortality Weekly Report, 60*, 1–8.

Perper, K., Peterson, K., & Manlove, J. (2010). *Child trends fact sheet: Diploma attainment among teen mothers*. Retrieved April 28, 2011, from http://www.childtrends.org/files//child_trends-2010_01_22_fs_diplomaattainment.pdf.

Perrin, J. M., Bloom, S. R., & Gortmaker, S. L. (2007). The increase of childhood chronic conditions in the United States. *Journal of the American Medical Association, 297*(4), 2755–2759.

Reilly, J. J., & Kelly, J. (2011). Long-term impact of overweight and obesity in childhood and adolescence on morbidity and premature mortality in adulthood: Systematic review. *International Journal of Obesity, 35*(7), 891–898.

Santelli, J. S., Lindberg, L. D., Finer, L. B., & Singh, S. (2007). Explaining recent declines in adolescent pregnancy in the United States: The contribution of abstinence and improved contraceptive use. *American Journal of Public Health, 97*(1), 150–156.

Schwimmer, J. B., Burwinkle, T. M., & Varni, J. W. (2003). Health-related quality of life of severely obese children and adolescents. *Journal of the American Medical Association, 289*(14), 1813–1819.

SEARCH for Diabetes in Youth Study Group. (2006). The burden of diabetes mellitus among US youth: Prevalence estimates from the SEARCH for diabetes in youth study group. *Pediatrics, 118*, 1510–1518.

Sivak, M., & Schoettle, B. (2010). Toward understanding the recent large reductions in U.S. road fatalities. *Traffic Injury Prevention, 11*(6), 561–566.

Soni, A. (2009). *The five most costly children's conditions, 2006: Estimates for the U.S. civilian noninstitutionalized children, ages 0–17*. Agency for Healthcare Research and Quality. Statistical Brief #242.

Substance Abuse and Mental Health Services Administration. (2007). *Results from the 2006 National Survey on Drug Use and Health: National findings*. Office of Applied Studies, NSDUH Series H-32, DHHS Publication No. SMA 07-4293.

Substance Abuse and Mental Health Services Administration. (2010). *Results from the 2009 National Survey on Drug Use and Health: Volume I. Summary of National findings*. Office of Applied Studies, NSDUH Series H-38A, DHHS Publication No. SMA Findings.

Supinya, I., & Biro, F. M. (2011). Adolescent women and obesity. *Journal of Pediatric and Adolescent Gynecology, 24*, 58–61.

Swartz, M. B., & Puhl, R. (2003). Childhood obesity: A societal problem to solve. *Obesity Reviews, 4*(1), 57–71.

Teen Research Unlimited. (2009). *Teen dating abuse report 2009: Impact of the economy and parent/teen dialogue on dating relationships and abuse*. Retrieved April 28, 2011, from http://loveisnotabuse.com/c/document_library/get_file?p_l_id=45693&folderId=72612&name=DLFE-202.pdf

Turner, C., & McClure, R. (2003). Age and gender differences in risk-taking behaviour as an explanation for high incidence of motor vehicle crashes as a driver in young males. *International Journal of Injury Control and Safety Promotion, 10*(3), 123–130.

U.S. Census Bureau. (2011). *U.S. interim projections by age, sex, race, and Hispanic origin: 2000–2050*. Retrieved from http://www.census.gov/population/www/projections/usinterimproj/.

U.S. Department of Health and Human Services. (2011). *Childhood obesity*. Retrieved April 28, 2011, from http://aspe.hhs.gov/health/reports/child_obesity/#_ftn14.

U.S. Surgeon General. (2001). *Overweight and obesity: Health consequences*. Retrieved April 28, 2011, from http://www.surgeongeneral.gov/topics/obesity/calltoaction/fact_consequences.htm.

Weinstock, H., Berman, S., & Cates, W., Jr. (2004). Sexually transmitted diseases among American youth: Incidence and prevalence estimates, 2000. *Perspectives on Sexual and Reproductive Health, 36*(1), 6–10.

Whitaker, R. C., Wright, J. A., Pepe, M. S., Seidel, K. D., & Dietz, W. H. (1997). Predicting obesity in young adulthood from childhood and parental obesity. *The New England Journal of Medicine, 37*(13), 869–873.

Wolak, J., Mitchell, K., & Finkelhor, D. (2006). *Online victimization: 5 years later*. Alexandria, VA: National Center for Missing and Exploited Children. Retrieved April 28, 2011, from http://www.missingkids.com/en_US/publications/NC167.pdf.

Zahn-Waxler, C., Shirtcliff, E. A., & Marceau, K. (2008). Disorders of childhood and adolescence: Gender and psychopathology. *Annual Review of Clinical Psychology, 4*, 275–303.

Disease Prevention in Adolescence

Lorraine T. Benuto

Prevention in Adolescent Health Psychology: A Historical Perspective on Adolescent Prevention Programs

Prevention efforts with adolescents are not a new endeavor and actually have a long history within the scientific literature. Catalano and colleagues (2002) have provided a nice review of the history of prevention efforts for children and adolescents. Specifically, they have noted how early in the 1950s increases in juvenile crime prompted prevention efforts with federal funding initiatives and later with the development of settlement houses for character development geared at troubled youth. Later the emphasis became focused on supporting families, schools, and communities before problem behaviors emerged in children and circumstances of children's lives thought to be responsible for producing problem behaviors became the focus.

Many early prevention programs were not based on theory or outcome or process research (Catalano et al., 2002), and results from earlier outcome studies suggested questionable efficacy of prevention programs geared at reducing problem behaviors such as drug use, pregnancy, sexually transmitted disease, dropping out of school, or engaging in violent or delinquent behavior (Ennett, Tobler, Ringwalt, & Flewelling, 1994; Kirby, Harvey, Claussenius, & Novar, 1989; Snow, Gilchrist, & Schinke, 1985; Thomas et al., 1992). Fortunately prevention strategies have since evolved (although the effect sizes for outcome studies remain small) and the emphasis on a single factor being the cause of problem behavior has shifted to an emphasis on interrupting the processes that lead to problem behaviors; the identification of proximal (i.e., the more closely related) predictors (e.g., peer influence to engage in problem behaviors) of problem behaviors; the co-occurrence of problem behaviors within a single child; addressing environmental predictors and individual-environmental interactions in seeking to change behavior; and promoting healthy development (Catalano et al., 2002). The result of this shift has been a focus on two paradigms consisting of positive youth development and prevention science (emphasis on reducing risk factors and enhancing protective factors). Prevention efforts are typically discussed in the context of primary, secondary, and tertiary prevention (Constantine, 2012—see Table 1 for definitions and examples).

Do Behavioral Health Prevention Efforts Parallel Medical Ones?

Historically speaking (prior to socially based prevention efforts) the medical field has long since focused on prevention. As early as the 1800s

L.T. Benuto, Ph.D. (✉)
Department of Psychology, Victims of Crime Treatment Center, University of Nevada, Reno, MS 0296, Reno, NV 89557, USA
e-mail: dr.benuto@gmail.com

W.T. O'Donohue et al. (eds.), *Handbook of Adolescent Health Psychology*,
DOI 10.1007/978-1-4614-6633-8_7, © Springer Science+Business Media New York 2013

Table 1 Defining prevention

Type of prevention	Definition (Constantine, 2012)	Example
Primary prevention	Focused on avoiding the development of new health problems (e.g., positive health promotion, healthy development interventions)	Attempts to prevent or reduce health risk behaviors, for example, tobacco use, unsafe sex, or sedentariness
Secondary prevention	Provide early identification and treatment of existing health problems or established harmful health behaviors	Routine screening for sexually transmitted infections and partner notification where necessary
Tertiary prevention	Focuses on the management and treatment of chronic diseases and conditions, and of diseases with long-lasting consequences	Diet management for individuals diagnosed with diabetes to prevent the development of other diseases that can result from diabetes (e.g., high blood pressure, nephropathy)

vaccination efforts began with the use of the smallpox vaccine and in 1905 the United States Supreme Court ruled that the state could enact compulsory laws to protect the public in the event of a communicable disease (Albert, Ostheimer, & Breman, 2001). As is implied by the Supreme Court's ruling, at the outset of the use of vaccines was much controversy and disagreement regarding their use (Wolfe & Sharpe, 2002). Nonetheless, vaccinations have been described as one of the top ten achievements of public health in the twentieth century (CDC, 1999), and the efficacy of vaccines has been duly noted via a dramatic decrease in disease rates (e.g., polio: CDC, 2005) as well as via controlled research studies (e.g., Belshe et al., 2001; Vu, Farish, Jenkins, & Kelly, 2002).

Therefore, from a medical perspective prevention can be good if follow-through exists and the causal mechanisms are well understood. Certainly with vaccinations behavioral components are minimal, as this type of prevention only requires that the patient presents himself or herself at a medical center to receive the vaccination. Nonetheless, behavioral-type interventions have been used in conjunction with such efforts via the administration of educational brochures, videos, and even in-person presentations (e.g., in the hospital after a baby is born, during a routine medical exam, in specialized programs such as WIC [woman-infant-child]). More recently large-scale media campaigns have also been used to promote vaccinations and to deliver information to potential consumers about their benefits (e.g., the HPV vaccine which prevents the acquisition of a specific type of genital wart virus believed to cause cervical cancer). Furthermore, behavioral interventions often play a large role in other typically thought of as medical prevention efforts (e.g., prevention of diabetes often involves behavioral components related to healthy eating and exercise).

Prevention Aims for Adolescents

Certainly the number of prevention domains is vast as one could focus on the prevention of just about anything, particularly with regard to adolescents. In this chapter we will review those prevention domains that have received the largest focus. A review of hits in Google using the terms "prevention" and "adolescent" revealed a large focus on prevention for specific domains. These include sexual risk, substance use, obesity, suicide, and severe behavioral problems. A discussion of programs related to these domains follows.

Sexual Risk

In terms of prevention, using a broad perspective to reduce high-risk sexual behavior including the reduction of STIs is one of CDC's top six priorities and because it is a "winnable battle" such prevention is of paramount importance to health and quality of life for youth (CDC, 2013). Vaccines are currently available for the prevention of hepatitis B and the human papilloma virus and vaccines for other sexually transmitted infections are in development (Mast et al., 2005;

Stanberry et al., 2002) and can be used as a primary prevention strategy. Secondary prevention efforts can also be useful in terms of sexually transmitted infections and two means of accomplishing this are via routine screening and partner notification (Auslander, Catallozzi, & Rosenthal, 2012) so that early treatment for infection can be obtained. In terms of the efficacy of vaccinations as a primary prevention strategy, a meta-analysis conducted by Lu, Kumar, Castellsague, and Giuliano (2011) revealed that prophylactic HPV vaccines are safe, well tolerated, and highly efficacious in preventing persistent infections and cervical diseases associated with vaccine-HPV types among young females. The authors did note that research on the long-term efficacy and safety does need to be addressed.

Beyond vaccinations and the secondary prevention strategies mentioned above, a large number of prevention efforts have been made in the sexual risk domain. In the chapter of this text on sexually transmitted infections, Auslander et al. (2012) discuss extensively strategies to reduce adolescent exposure to and acquisition of sexually transmitted infections. They review the literature on routine screening and partner notification, interventions to delay sexual initiation and promote condom use in those choosing to have intercourse, and uptake of other biomedical strategies, including vaccines and microbicides.

Results from an extant review of the literature indicate that the most effective programs address social influences; are grounded within social learning theory (Kirby, 1992); and provide information about STIs, motivational training, and behavior skills for negotiation of abstinence and condoms (Johnson, Scott-Sheldon, Huedo-Medina, & Carey, 2011). Such programs tend to be carried out in community or school settings over multiple sessions in a group-format (Underhill, Operario, & Montgomery, 2007b). Despite that these ingredients appear to be key in achieving higher success, the effect sizes remain small.

Relevant to this discussion is the debate on comprehensive vs. abstinence-only sex education programs. Critics of comprehensive sex education programs have suggested that such programs will increase sexual behavior (Kirby, Laris, & Rolleri, 2007; Underhill et al., 2007b) although research has clearly demonstrated that sex education about abstinence and birth control is associated with healthier sexual behaviors and outcomes. In fact, research on comprehensive sex education programs has indicated that they are successful at delaying sexual initiation, increasing condom use, and reducing unprotected intercourse (Auslander et al., 2012). Conversely, abstinence-only programs (that teach abstinence until marriage) have not been shown to be effective at reducing adolescents' sexual risk behaviors (Trenholm et al., 2007; Underhill, Operario, & Montgomery, 2007a) as while certainly abstaining from sex certainly reduces exposure and acquisition of sexually transmitted infections, such methods have very high failure rates (Fortenberry, 2005).

In sum, with regard to the prevention of sexually transmitted infections in adolescence there are medical interventions (i.e., vaccinations) that can act well as a primary prevention strategy at least in the short term (longitudinal research examining efficacy is lacking). From a behavioral/medical perspective the use of condoms can also be helpful in preventing the acquisition of sexually transmitted infections. To some extent both of these efforts require prevention strategies that are behavioral in nature and research on sex education programs has indicated relatively small effect sizes for abstinence-only programs (Silva, 2002) with superior outcomes for comprehensive sex education programs (Auslander et al., 2012; DiCenso, Guyatt, Willan, & Griffith, 2002).

Pregnancy

Alongside sexual risk for sexually transmitted diseases is unintended pregnancy among adolescents. Aruda and Burke (2012) outline statistics for pregnancy among teenagers noting that the birthrate for teenagers aged 15–17 has fallen since 1991; in 2009 was the lowest it has ever been in nearly 70 years; three in ten girls become pregnant at least once by age 20; one in five pregnancies is to a teen mother; 82 % of pregnancies among 15–19-year-olds are unplanned; and large disparities persist in race and ethnicity. These statistics indicate that even though teenage pregnancy rates have decreased teenage pregnancy remains to be a societal problem.

In terms of prevention, one of the CDC's top six priorities is teen pregnancy prevention (CDC, 2013). Aruda and Burke (2012) discuss how in the early to mid twentieth century there was a eugenics movement (based on the belief that the wrong people were having children and being unmarried constituted being a "wrong" person) and sexually active young women were seen as unfit. This prompted the introduction of prevention as it relates to teenage pregnancy with the aim being to ensure that poverty and delinquency were not passed from one generation to another. During the post-World War I era there was a focus on "unwed mothers" and "illegitimate children" (with less emphasis placed on age) and during this time, unmarried teenagers who became pregnant were considered to be delinquents or to have emotional or psychological problems. Despite the above, because prior to the 1960s, most teenage pregnancies led to marriage, teenage pregnancy was a societal nonissue (Aruda & Burke, 2012). In the past four decades we have seen even more historical shifts with the availability of birth control and abortion as an option for teenagers. Nonetheless, the teen parent has been portrayed as a "perpetrator of poverty" (Furstenberg, 2003) and teen pregnancy has been established to be a social problem that does carry stigma despite the media's attempts to glamorize the pregnant teenager (Aruda & Burke, 2012).

Currently the most commonly employed pregnancy prevention programs are educational in nature and are often referred to as family life education and include components of sexuality, reproduction, decision-making, and sexual relationship issues (Nitz, 1999). Kirby (1992, 1999) has established that prevention approaches can be divided into five groups:

1. Programs that increase knowledge and emphasize the risks and consequences of pregnancy
2. Programs that clarify values and provide skills, especially decision-making and communication skills
3. Abstinence-only curricula
4. HIV/AIDS education
5. Theoretically based programs building on the successes and failures of previous programs, with more rigorous evaluation

Of importance is the large political debate that has ensued over the use of abstinence-only vs. abstinence-plus (aka comprehensive sex education) curricula. While a discussion on such programs was provided above with regard to sexually transmitted infections there is a separate body of literature that examines the impact of such programs on teenage pregnancy.

Approximately 10 years ago a research article on the outcome of interventions to reduce unintended pregnancies among adolescents (DiCenso et al., 2002) indicated that interventions did not delay initiation of sexual intercourse in women or men, they did not improve birth control use by either women or men, and they did not reduce pregnancy rates in women (although there were significantly fewer pregnancies in women who received multifaceted program). This publication prompted a media heyday and subsequently experts in the field pointed to some of the flaws in the study that may account for the poor findings (McKay, Fisher, Maticka-Tyndale, & Barrett, 2001).

More recently Bennett and Nassim (2005) systematically reviewed school-based teenage prevention programs and found that the majority of abstinence-plus programs increase rates of contraceptive use in teens for up to 30 months. Hoyt and Broom (2002) discuss that programs that share the most improvements in teen pregnancy rates share the following nine characteristics:

1. They focus on reducing sexual behaviors that lead to unintended pregnancy or STD.
2. They include behavioral goals, teaching methods, and materials that are age and culturally appropriate so that the problem is always seen through the eyes of the students whom the programs seek to serve.
3. They are based on theoretical approaches, such as social learning theories, which have been demonstrated to be effective in influencing health-related risky behaviors.
4. They are of appropriate length to allow participants to complete important activities.

For example, a program does not merely consist of an assembly, but includes multiple components with sufficient time for follow-up.
5. They provide accurate and basic information about the risks of unprotected sex and methods of avoiding unprotected sex.
6. They use teaching methods that are designed to actively involve the participants so as to personalize the information
7. They include activities that address social pressures related to sex.
8. They provide models of and practice in communication, negotiation, and refusal skills.
9. They provide training and practice sessions to teacher or peer program leaders who are selected because they believe in the program.

While a large number of prevention programs have been created and tested (for a detailed review of school-based programs please see Hoyt and Broom, 2002, and for a detailed review of general interventions and programs see Nitz, 1999) the consensus seems to be that while lowering teenage pregnancy rates has been somewhat successful there is still a lack of well-established prevention programs with good outcome (as is the case with programs aimed at preventing exposure to and acquisition of sexually transmitted diseases). Most recently, the Teen Pregnancy Prevention Initiative (TPPI) funded by the CDC for 2010–2015 has targeted nine communities nationally with high teen pregnancy rates and is looking for a 10 % decrease through four key components: implementation of evidence-based programs, quality community linkages, education, and sustainability (CDC, 2013).

Sexual and Intimate Partner Violence

Chu, Sundermann, and DePrince (2012) have covered quite extensively the scientific literature on prevention of sexual and intimate partner violence and readers are encouraged to see the relevant chapter of this text for a more detailed overview. In sum the literature (see Whitaker et al., 2006) has indicated superior efficacy for two programs titled Safe Dates (Foshee et al., 1998, 2004) and Youth Relationships Project (Wolfe et al., 2003, 2009). Safe Dates consists of school and community components and activities are geared at changing norms of dating violence and improving prosocial skills. Alternatively the Youth Relationships Project is designed to be carried out in community agencies and targets high-risk adolescents.

Smoking

Prevention of adolescent smoking programs is similar to those programs used to prevent other adolescent substance use. Many programs have been developed and tested and meta-analyses have been conducted to compare the efficacy rates of such programs. For example, Rooney and Murray (1996) conducted a meta-analysis in which they examined 90 studies with 131 interventions that used school-based, peer-led, and social influence programs aimed at the prevention of tobacco use. Results from this meta-analysis indicated a small effect size for such programs at posttest (1 year out). Effect sizes were larger for programs targeting sixth graders, programs that were concentrated in a short period or that offered booster sessions, and programs that included a trained teacher and an untrained same-age peer leader.

Readers are encouraged to see the chapter of this text on smoking (Brook, Pahl, Brook, & Brown, 2012) for an elaborate review of the various prevention programs for smoking that exist. Suffice to say, prevention interventions at the individual level should focus on general problem-solving and coping skills, social competence, behavioral self-management, life skills, and specific cigarette refusal skills (Dierker, Merikangas, & Essau, 1997). At the contextual level (1) adolescents should be provided with the opportunity to engage in alternative activities; (2) aims should be made for organizational changes in schools; and (3) community leaders should be trained to organize smoking and drug use prevention task forces (Dierker et al., 1997). A comprehensive approach focusing on different sources of social influence, as well as individual-level factors, seems the most promising (Brook et al., 2012).

Alcohol and Other Substance Use

It is no secret that substance use among adolescents is a continual problem. In fact research has indicated that an astounding near 50 % of teenagers in the United States have used an illicit drug by the 8th grade (Johnston, O'Malley, Bachman, & Schulenberg, 2010). Generally speaking scientific research has indicated that school-based drug prevention programs have the *potential* to reduce drug use in adolescents (Tobler et al., 2000) although unfortunately most drug prevention programs are not effective (White & Pitts, 1998). These findings have prompted efforts to determine what specifically must be included in such prevention efforts to achieve efficacy.

Results from an extensively well-conducted meta-analysis on school-based prevention programs (Tobler et al., 2000) included 144 studies of 207 school-based drug prevention programs indicated that certain programs did reduce substance use whereas others did not. Programs that reduced substance use employed *interactive* methods (these programs provide contact and communication opportunities for the exchange of ideas among participants; encourage the learning of drug refusal skills; are focused on social influence approach to drug prevention; and include generic skills training, e.g., assertiveness, coping, communication), while the less effective programs used *noninteractive* methods (these programs focus only on knowledge of substances, helping the adolescent develop insight into personal feelings and behaviors and on the adolescent's problem-solving skills regarding personal drug use).

Cuijpers (2002) has attempted to identify "effective ingredients" of school-based drug prevention programs by conducting a systematic review of the literature (he reviewed meta-analyses, studies examining mediating variables of interventions, and studies directly comparing prevention programs with or without specific characteristics). This review resulted in the identification of seven evidence-based quality criteria that programs should incorporate:

1. Proven effects: the effects of a program should have been proven using well-designed scientific research procedures.
2. Interactive delivery methods are superior.
3. The "social influence model" is the best we have.
4. Focus should be on norms (social prevalence knowledge, social acceptability knowledge, normative expectations, friends' reactions to drug use), commitment of students to not use substances, and intentions not to use.
5. Adding community interventions (e.g., family interventions, mass media campaigns, and community mobilizing committees) increases effects.
6. The use of peer leaders may strengthen the short-term effects of prevention program and programs should peer leaders either in lieu of or in conjunction with adult leaders.
7. Adding life-skills training to social influence programs may strengthen the effects of prevention programs.

More recently Lemstra et al. (2010) conducted a systematic review of the literature to determine if school-based marijuana and alcohol prevention programs were effective in preventing marijuana and alcohol use in adolescents between the ages of 10 and 15 years. Results from this extensive review indicated that the most effective primary prevention programs for reducing marijuana and alcohol use among adolescents in the long term were comprehensive programs that included antidrug information combined with refusal skills, self-management skills, and social skills training.

Obesity and Related Conditions

The World Health Organization (2013) has asserted that obesity is an escalating global epidemic. Because childhood and adolescent obesity are strong predictors of adult obesity and there is a host of problems that develop as a result of obesity (e.g., type 2 diabetes insulin resistance, hypertension: Spruikt-Metz, 2011) prevention efforts are an absolute must. Despite the strong interest and dedication of resources to prevention efforts childhood and adolescent obesity remain high. In fact, the CDC (Ogden & Carroll, 2010) has indicated that in 2007–2008 19.3 % of male adolescents and 16.8 % of female adolescents aged 12–19 were obese.

The *Handbook of Pediatric and Adolescent Obesity Treatment* (O'Donohue, Moore, & Scott, 2008) offers an extensive overview of etiological, diagnostic, and sociocultural considerations; relevant process variables; treatment approaches (with an emphasis on stepped care); and nutritional approaches with regard to obesity in children and adolescents. Prevention efforts with regard to obesity can come in many forms including the prevention of further weight gain; the prevention of health conditions associated with obesity; or alternatively prevention of obesity in the first place (i.e., preventing normal weight or overweight children and adolescents from becoming obese). Within this handbook a specific discussion on prevention is provided (Story & Kaphinger, 2008) and will be reviewed here, as will be other relevant literature.

Because more than 95 % of children and adolescents (aged 5–17) are enrolled in school, school-based interventions make sense given the magnitude of continuous and intensive contact that academic institutions have with school-aged children and adolescents (Story & Kaphinger, 2008). That being said, school-based interventions have been demonstrated to improve obesity-related behaviors and reduce obesity (Gortmaker et al., 1999) although with limited success (Dobbins, De Corby, Robeson, Husson, & Tirilis, 2009). Recently, Stice, Shaw, and Marti (2006) conducted a meta-analysis to review obesity prevention programs. Their study included 64 prevention programs that aimed to produce weight gain prevention efforts. Of these programs 21 % produced significant prevention effects but these were typically pre-to-post effects (programs that have succeeded at preventing weight gain tend not to have long-term staying power: Spruikt-Metz, 2011). Effects were greatest for programs targeting children and adolescents (as opposed to preadolescents) and females. Programs that were relatively brief, programs solely targeting weight control vs. other health behaviors (e.g., smoking), programs evaluated in pilot trials, and programs wherein participants must self-select into the intervention had the greatest effects and factors such as mandated improvements in diet and exercise, sedentary behavior reduction, delivery by trained interventionists, and parental involvement were not associated with significantly larger effects (Stice et al., 2006).

With further regard to school-based prevention efforts and future directions, Story and Kaphingst (2008) discuss how school-based interventions appear to hold promise but future research is needed with a focus on strengthening physical activity and healthy eating. They also discuss how programs should target different levels such as the school environment, behavioral curricula, and parent involvement. Finally, they discuss the need for the field to establish whether certain types of interventions are more successful with children of different ages, gender/sex, and/or ethnic background. Furthermore, Spruikt-Metz (2011) discusses the need for multifactorial theoretical approaches that consider the impact of system, environment, and organizational issues; the need for programs that address individual as well as group behavior change; and the necessity of stakeholders (families, schools, policy-makers) being included in the decision-making process about intervention strategies to be implemented (Summerbell et al., 2005).

Suicide

Three terms are often used in the literature that focuses on suicide: suicidal ideation (defined as thoughts of killing oneself without regard to intention to act on the thoughts); suicide attempt (a self-inflicted, potentially injurious behavior with a nonfatal outcome where there was intent to die); and death by suicide (a self-inflicted death) (Silverman et al., 2007). Such behaviors are often referred to as suicide-related behaviors (O'Mara, Lee, & King, 2012). Suicide is the third leading cause of death among adolescents and young adults in the United States and prevalence rate for suicide deaths in the United States among adolescents (13–19 years old) was 6.03 per 100,000 (Center for Disease Control, 2010a) from 2000 to 2007. Rates for suicide-related behaviors in adolescents are substantially higher and 13.8 % of high school students report seriously having considered attempting suicide in the past year, 10.9 % made a plan for how they would attempt suicide, 6.3 % attempted suicide, and 1.9 % made a suicide attempt that required medical attention (Center for Disease Control, 2010b). Unfortunately, experts have noted that there is a paucity of studies demonstrating empirical effectiveness of suicide prevention programs (Cooper, Clements, & Holt, 2011).

High school-based suicide prevention programs can be separated into four general categories: enhancing protective factors, curriculum-based programs, gatekeepers, and screening programs (Cooper et al., 2011). A recent review of suicide prevention programs has indicated that such programs have demonstrated post-improvements in knowledge, attitudes, and help-seeking behavior. Specifically, in a systemic review of the literature on the effectiveness of middle and high school-based suicide prevention programs for adolescents, Cusimano and Sameem (2011) reviewed 36 relevant studies. Of these 36 studies, eight studies were identified as being well-performed, controlled, and assigned intervention and control strategies to students in middle school or high schools and five of these studies demonstrated significant improvements in knowledge (these studies were as follows: Portzky & van Heeringen, 2006; Aseltine & DeMartino, 2004; Aseltine et al., 2007; Kalafat & Elias, 1994).

Beyond school-based programs other interventions can help to reduce suicide behavior and ultimately prevent suicide. Tarrier, Taylor, and Gooding (2008) conducted a systematic review and meta-analysis of cognitive-behavioral interventions to reduce suicide behavior. Ultimately their work included a review of 28 studies and results from this work indicated a highly significant effect for cognitive-behavioral therapies (CBTs) for reducing suicide behavior. However, of these 28 studies, seven utilized adolescents as participants and stratified results indicated that CBT appears effective with adult populations but not with adolescents.

A methodological problem in the study of suicide prevention programs is the lack of longitudinal research. Such studies are necessary as are comparisons between groups who have received prevention efforts and those who have not with the aim being to determine whether or not suicide-related behaviors are present to a lesser extent among those adolescents who have partaken in a suicide prevention program. Research as described above is necessary to truly determine the efficacy of suicide prevention programs. The majority of outcome research on suicide prevention programs focuses on the acquisition of knowledge and follow-up assessment is typically short term.

Severe Behavioral Problems

The literature on adolescent health is replete with discussions on how adolescence is a time of experimentation, risk, and opportunity (Schwartz et al., 2010) of which delinquency can result. Delinquency is most common in adolescence beginning in early adolescence (age 11–13) and peaking at age 17 (Li et al., 2011) and research has indicated that delinquency in early adolescence is predictive of poor outcome in life (e.g., engagement in serious antisocial behavior: Loeber & Le Blanc, 1990).

Research on prevention efforts with regard to delinquent behavior is plenty. For example, research has indicated that higher degrees of behavioral and emotional school engagement predict a significantly lower risk of involvement in delinquency (Li et al., 2011). Furthermore, research on the effects of therapeutic foster care on violent outcomes among juveniles indicates >70 % reduction for felony assaults during the first year after completion of the program (Hahn et al., 2005). Research has also focused on recidivism in terms of delinquent behavior. For example, Genovés, Morales, and Sánchez-Meca (2006) reviewed the outcomes of best available empirical research regarding the effectiveness of treatment programs implemented in secure corrections to prevent the recidivism of serious (violent and chronic) juvenile offenders (from 12 to 21 years old). Results from this review indicated that a relatively low effective size ($r=0.07$) with cognitive-behavioral methods of treatment was the most effective in decreasing recidivism.

A Fiscal Perspective

In this chapter thus far, we have reviewed the literature on prevention of sexual risk, substance use, obesity, suicide, and severe behavioral problems. While certainly from a theoretical perspective prevention efforts make fiscal sense (if you can prevent any of the above in adolescents there are many potential financial gains, e.g., if an adolescent does not engage in risky sexual behavior he/she has a low chance of catching an STD which can require treatment), our review of the literature has elucidated that the efficacy of most prevention programs is limited. Some experts have written on this very topic exploring the cost-effectiveness of prevention programs and many have cited difficulties in terms of the assessment of cost-effectiveness due to methodological differences in research studies, i.e., making programs and outcome difficult to compare (Kilian et al., 2011). Nonetheless, as indicated above the fairly limited levels of efficacy achieved via the prevention programs described within this chapter make prevention efforts a hard sell from a money-saving perspective. Despite this, a large number of experts have attempted to outline why promotion and prevention makes fiscal sense.

Proponents of fiscal savings from prevention programs have illustrated the high cost of mental health diagnosis like depression (due to missed days of work, premature retirement, and long-term unemployment) and schizophrenia (McDaid, 2011), both due to the disorders themselves and also because people with poor mental health have a higher probability of being physically unhealthy compared to those without mental health problems (Harris & Barraclough, 1998). Furthermore, researchers have demonstrated the astronomical savings that can occur for the prevention of even one case of conduct disorder ($3,481,433) (Foster & Jones, 2005) and on a smaller scale research has indicated that the cost-effectiveness per unit of change on the Child Behavior Checklist is $337 over a 3-month period (DePanilis & Zlotnik, 2008). Nonetheless, even proponents of prevention as a cost-saver have noted that there is a huge research gap in terms of the costs and cost-effectiveness of mental disorder prevention or mental health promotion programs and the types of treatment for mental disorder that provides the greatest social benefit for the invested money in children and adolescents (Kilian, Losert, Park, McDaid, & Knapp, 2010). In sum, the verdict is still out in terms of whether or not prevention programs actually have us money (given the very small effect sizes observed in the outcome research) and if they do to what extent.

Summary, Conclusions, and Next Steps

In this chapter we have provided a historical perspective on adolescent prevention programs and we discussed the parallel between medical prevention efforts and behavioral health prevention efforts. With regard to the specific literature on prevention efforts employed in adolescence we provided a review of the literature on prevention programs aimed at reducing sexual risk, substance use, obesity, suicide, and severe behavioral problems. We concluded with a discussion on the fiscal aspects of prevention programs.

In the behavioral health literature, Gordon Paul's question, "What treatment, by whom, is most effective for this individual with that specific problem, under which set of circumstances?" (Paul, 1967, p. 111) is often cited. Certainly this question illustrates the complexities involved in selecting and administering an intervention. prevention interventions are not exempt from such complexities and as illustrated by our review of the literature, we do not know the answer to the question posed by Paul. In fact, experts have indicated that we do not have a specific list of effective ingredients when it comes to prevention and the less-than-desirable effect sizes for prevention programs demonstrate that as a field we are not experts in terms of designing and implementing prevention programs that are highly effective. Clearly, across the board research demonstrating large effect sizes for prevention programs is lacking. This has prompted a discussion on whether or not prevention programs make fiscal sense and the verdict is still out in terms of whether or not prevention programs save money and if so how much (after all the design and implementation of prevention programs are hardly free).

Nonetheless, we can at least attempt to answer a portion of Paul's question. In terms of the "whom" our literature review has indicated that the delivery of prevention should be conducted by both experts and peers as at least some research has demonstrated superior effect sizes when peers are involved as leaders. The individuals we have discussed in this chapter have of course been adolescents although the literature has indicated that some programs seem to work better with specific age groups and at times effects have been demonstrated to be greater among females. In terms of "specific problems," there are seemingly endless things to prevent and we didn't attempt to address them all (we didn't discuss depression, school dropout, etc.) and instead we focused on those that seemed to be the greater focus of our field.

The last portion of Paul's question "under what circumstances" is quite difficult to address. To a large extent it seems that school is where the majority of prevention efforts take place. Perhaps this is in part the problem and if such efforts were more profuse (e.g., there was a home-based component, a web component) the effect sizes for these programs would be larger. There also seems to be a lack of research in terms of what dosage is needed. Clearly in the medical field, it is possible to determine the precise dose necessary to achieve the desired result, e.g., in the case of vaccination for some vaccinations a single does is all that is needed whereas for others booster follow-ups are necessary. In the behavioral health arena it does not appear that we have adequately studied the extent to which each component of prevention programs contributes to the overall effect and we have also not examined the amount necessary (i.e., a single administration vs. a yearly administration vs. a monthly administration) to achieve the desired results. Lastly, it seems that nobody has focused on a complete curriculum and instead across the board it appears that everyone simply focuses on a small portion of a much larger landscape (e.g., instead of having a pregnancy prevention program why not simply have a program that addresses pregnancy prevention, sexual risk, suicide risk, substance use, etc.).

In terms of directions the field should go with regard to adolescent health prevention efforts, it seems that more research is needed to determine what exactly works with regard to prevention from a behavioral health perspective. Most notably an examination perhaps via regression analysis to determine which components seem to carry the biggest impact and certainly an examination of "dosing" need to be carried out. To some extent research supports that using social learning theory to guide the development of programs may prove fruitful. Other components that seem to be at least somewhat effective include the use of interactive methods to delivery information and the incorporation of skills training (e.g., social skills) into prevention programs.

References

Albert, M., Ostheimer, K. G., & Breman, J. G. (2001). The last smallpox epidemic in Boston and the vaccination controversy. *The New England Journal of Medicine, 344*, 375–9.

Aruda, M. M., & Burke, P. (2012). Pregnancy in adolescence. In W. O'Donohue, L. Benuto, & L. Woodward-Tolle (Eds.), *Handbook of adolescent health psychology*. New York: Springer.

Aseltine, R. H., & DeMartino, R. (2004). An outcome evaluation of the SOS suicide prevention program. *American Journal of Public Health, 94*(3), 446–451.

Aseltine, R. H., Jr., James, A., Schilling, E. A., & Glanovsky, J. (2007). Evaluating the SOS suicide prevention program: A replication and extension. *BMC Public Health, 7*, 161.

Auslander, B. A., Catallozzi, M., & Rosenthal, S. L. (2012). Sexually transmitted infections (STIs) and the developing adolescent: Influences of and strategies to reduce STI acquisition. In W. O'Donohue, L. Benuto, & L. Woodward-Tolle (Eds.), *Handbook of adolescent health psychology*. New York: Springer.

Belshe, R. B., et al. (2001). Safety, efficacy and effectiveness of the influenza virus vaccine, trivalent, types A and B, live, cold-adapted (CAIV-T) in healthy children and healthy adults. *Vaccine, 19*(17–19), 2221–2226.

Bennett, S. E., & Nassim, N. P. (2005). School-based teenage pregnancy prevention programs: A systematic review of randomized controlled trials. *Journal of Adolescent Health, 36*(1), 72–81.

Brook, J. S., Pahl, K., Brook, D. W., & Brown, E. N. (2012). Smoking in Adolescence. In W. O'Donohue, L. Benuto, & L. Woodward-Tolle (Eds.), *Handbook of Adolescent Health Psychology*. New York: Springer.

Catalano, R., Berglund, M. L., Ryan, G. A. M., Lonczak, H. S., & Hawkins, J. D. (2002). Positive youth development in the United States: Research findings on evaluations of positive youth development programs. *Prevention & Treatment, 5*(15).

CDC (2013). *Winnable Battles*. Retrieved from http://www.cdc.gov/winnablebattles/.

Centers for Disease Control and Prevention (CDC). (1999). Ten great public health achievements—United States, 1900–1999 *MMWR*. Atlanta, GA: Centers for Disease Control and Prevention (CDC), 1999;48(12):241–243. Accessed April 25, 2010.

Centers for Disease Control and Prevention. (2005). Summary of notifiable diseases—United States, 2003. *Morbidity and Mortality Weekly Report, 52*(54).

Centers for Disease Control and Prevention. (2010a). *Web-based injury statistics query and reporting system (WISQARS)*. Retrieved from http://www.cdc.gov/ncipc/wisqars.

Centers for Disease Control and Prevention. (2010b). Youth risk behavior surveillance—United States. *Morbidity and Mortality Weekly Report, 59*, SS-5.

Chu, A. T., Sundermann, J. M., & DePrince, A. P. (2012). Intimate partner violence in adolescent romantic relationships. In W. O'Donohue, L. Benuto, & L. Woodward-Tolle (Eds.), *Handbook of adolescent health psychology*. New York: Springer.

Constantine, N. A. (2012). Intervention effectiveness research in adolescent health psychology: Methodological issues & strategies. In W. O'Donohue, L. Benuto, & L. Woodward-Tolle (Eds.), *Handbook of adolescent health psychology*. New York: Springer.

Cooper, G. D., Clements, P. T., & Holt, K. E. (2011). Examining childhood bullying and adolescent suicide: Implications for school nurses. *The Journal of School Nursing*. doi:10.1177/1059840512438617.

Cuijpers, P. (2002). Effective ingredients of school–based drug prevention programs. A systematic review. *Addictive Behaviors, 27*, 1009–1023.

Cusimano, M., & Sameem, M. (2011). The effectiveness of middle and high school based suicide prevention programs for adolescents: A systematic review. *Injury Prevention, 17*, 43–49.

DePanilis, D., & Zlotnik, J. L. (2008). Retention of frontline staff in child welfare: A systematic review of research. *Children and Youth Services Review, 30*(9), 995–1008.

DiCenso, A., Guyatt, G., Willan, A. A., & Griffith, L. L. (2002). Interventions to reduce unintended pregnancies among adolescents: Systematic review of randomized controlled trials. *British Medical Journal, 324*(7351), 1426–1430. doi:10.1136/bmj.324.7351.1426.

Dierker, L., Merikangas, K. R., & Essau, C. A. (1997). Substance use disorders. In C. A. Essau & F. Petermann (Eds.), *Developmental psychopathology: Epidemiology, diagnostics and treatment* (pp. 311–344). Australia: Harwood Academic.

Dobbins, M., De Corby, K., Robeson, P., Husson, H., Tirilis, D. (2009). School-based physical activity programs for promoting physical activity and fitness in children and adolescents aged 6–18. *Cochrane Database of Systematic Reviews, 1*, CD007651. doi: 10.1002/14651858.CD007651.

Ennett, S. T., Tobler, N. S., Ringwalt, C. L., & Flewelling, R. L. (1994). How effective is drug abuse resistance education? A meta-analysis of Project DARE outcome evaluations. *American Journal of Public Health, 84*, 1394–1401.

Fortenberry, D. (2005). The limits of abstinence-only in preventing sexually transmitted infections. *Journal of Adolescent Health, 36*, 269–270.

Foshee, V., Bauman, K. E., Arriaga, X. B., Helms, R. W., Koch, G. G., & Linder, G. F. (1998). An evaluation of safe dates, an adolescent dating violence prevention program. *American Journal of Public Health, 88*, 45–50.

Foshee, V. A., Bauman, K. E., Ennett, S. T., Linder, G., Benefield, T., & Suchindran, C. (2004). Assessing the long-term effects of the safe dates program and a booster in preventing and reducing adolescent dating violence victimization and perpetration. *American Journal of Public Health, 94*, 619–624.

Foster, E. M., & Jones, D. E. (2005). The high costs of aggression: Public expenditures resulting from conduct disorder. *American Journal of Public Health, 95*(10), 1767–1772.

Furstenberg, F. (2003). Teenage childbearing as a public issue and private concern. *Annual Review of Sociology, 29*, 23–39.

Genovés, V., Morales, L., & Sánchez-Meca, J. (2006). What works for serious juvenile offenders? A systematic review. *Psicothema, 18*(3), 611–619.

Gortmaker, S. L., et al. (1999). Impact of a school-based interdisciplinary intervention on diet and physical activity among urban primary school children: Eat well and keep moving. *Archives of Pediatric Adolescent Medicine, 153*(9), 975–983.

Hahn, R. A., et al. (2005). The effectiveness of therapeutic foster care for the prevention of violence: A systematic review. *American Journal of Prevention Medicine, 28*, 72–90.

Harris, E. C., & Barraclough, B. (1998). Excess mortality of mental disorders. *The British Journal of Psychiatry, 173*, 11–53.

Hoyt, H. H., & Broom, B. L. (2002). School-based teen pregnancy prevention programs: A review of the literature. *The Journal of School Nursing, 18*(1), 11–17. doi:10.1177/10598405020180010401.

Johnson, B. T., Scott-Sheldon, L. A. J., Huedo-Medina, T. B., & Carey, M. P. (2011). Interventions to reduce sexual risk for HIV in adolescents, 1985–2008.

Archives of Pediatrics & Adolescent Medicine, 175(1), 77–84. doi:10.1001/archpediatrics.2010.251.

Johnston, L. D., O'Malley, P. M., Bachman, J. G., & Schulenberg, J. E. (2010). *Monitoring the future national survey results on drug use, 1975-2009: Vol. I, Secondary school students* (NIH Publication No.10–7584). Bethesda, MD: National Institute on Drug Abuse.

Kalafat, J., & Elias, M. (1994). An evaluation of adolescent suicide intervention classes. *Suicide & Life-Threatening Behavior, 24*, 224–233.

Kilian, R., Losert, C., McDaid, D., Park, A.-La., & Knapp, M. (2011). Cost-effectiveness analysis in child and adolescent mental health problems: An updated review of the literature. *Psychiatrische praxis, 38* (S 01). S03_4_EC. ISSN 0303-4259.

Kilian, R., Losert, C., Park, A., McDaid, D., & Knapp, M. (2010). Cost-effectiveness analysis in child and adolescent mental health problems: An updated review of literature. *International Journal of Mental Health Promotion, 12*(4), 45–57.

Kirby, D. (1992). School-based programs to reduce sexual risk-taking behaviors. *Journal of School Health, 62*, 280–286.

Kirby, D. (1999). Reducing adolescent pregnancy: Approaches that work. *Contemporary Pediatrics, 16*, 83–94.

Kirby, D., Harvey, P., Claussenius, D., & Novar, M. (1989). A direct mailing to teenage males about condom use: Its impact on knowledge, attitudes and sexual behavior. *Family Planning Perspectives, 21*, 12–18.

Kirby, D., Laris, B. A., & Rolleri, L. A. (2007). Sex and HIV education programs: Their impact on sexual behavior of young people throughout the world. *Journal of Adolescent Health, 40*, 206–217.

Lemstra, M., Bennett, N., Nannapaneni, U., Neudorf, C., Warren, L., Kershaw, T., et al. (2010). A systematic review of school-based marijuana and alcohol prevention programs targeting adolescents aged 10–15. *Addiction Research & Theory, 18*(1), 84–96. doi:10.3109/16066350802673224.

Li, Y., Zhang, W., Liu, J., Arbeit, M. R., Schwartz, S. J., Bowers, E. P., et al. (2011). The role of school engagement in preventing adolescent delinquency and substance use: A survival analysis. *Journal of Adolescence, 34*(6), 1181–1192.

Loeber, R., & Le Blanc, M. (1990). Toward a developmental criminology. *Crime and Justice, 12*, 375–473.

Lu, B., Kumar, A., Castellsague, X., & Giuliano, A. R. (2011). Efficacy and safety of prophylactic vaccines against cervical HPV infection and diseases among women: A systematic review & meta-analysis. *BMC Infectious Disease, 11*(13), 1–16.

Mast, E., Weinbaum, C., Fiore, A., Alter, M., Bell, B., Finelli, L., et al. (2005). A comprehensive immunization strategy to eliminate transmission of hepatitis B virus infection in the United States recommendations of the Advisory Committee on Immunization Practices (ACIP) part 1: Immunization of infants, children, and adolescents. *Morbidity and Mortality Weekly Report, 54*(16), 1–23.

McDaid, D. (2011). Making the long-term economic case for investing in mental health to contribute to sustainability. Retrieved from http://www.vleva.be/sites/www.vleva.eu/files/nieuws/bijlages/long_term_sustainability_en.pdf.

McKay, A., Fisher, W., Maticka-Tyndale, E., & Barrett, M. (2001). Adolescent sexual health education: Does it work? Can it work better? An analysis of recent research and media reports. *Canadian Journal Of Human Sexuality, 10*(3–4), 127–135.

Nitz, K. (1999). Adolescent pregnancy prevention: A review of interventions and programs. *Clinical Psychology Review, 19*(4), 457–471. doi:10.1016/S0272-7358(98)00087-7.

O'Donohue, W. T., Moore, B., & Scott, B. J. (2008). *Handbook of pediatric & adolescent obesity*. New York: Routledge.

O'Mara, R. M., Lee, A., & King, C. A. (2012). Depression and suicide-related behaviors in adolescence. In W. O'Donohue, L. Benuto, & L. Woodward-Tolle (Eds.), *Handbook of adolescent health psychology*. New York: Springer.

Ogden, C., & Carroll, M. (2010). *Prevalence of obesity among children and adolescents: United States, trends 1963–1965 through 2007–2008*. Retrieved from http://www.cdc.gov/nchs/data/hestat/obesity_child_07_08/obesity_child_07_08.htm.

Paul, G. L. (1967). Outcome research in psychotherapy. *Journal of Consulting and Clinical Psychology, 31*, 109–118.

Portzky, G., & van Heeringen, K. (2006). Suicide prevention in adolescents: A controlled study of the effective psycho-educational program. *Journal of Child Psychology and Psychiatry, 47*(9), 910–918.

Rooney, B. L., & Murray, D. M. (1996). A meta-analysis of smoking prevention programs after adjustment for the errors in the unit of analysis. *Health Education Quarterly, 23*(1), 48–64.

Schwartz, J., Phelps, E., Lerner, J. V., Huang, S., Brown, C. H., & Lewin-Bizan, S. (2010). Promotion as prevention: Positive youth development as protective against tobacco, alcohol, illicit drug, and sex initiation. *Applied Developmental Science, 14*, 1–15.

Sieving, R. E., McMorris, B. J., Beckman, K. J., Pettingell, S. L., Secor-Turner, M., Kugler, K., et al. (2011). Prime time: 12-month sexual health outcomes of a clinic-based intervention to prevent pregnancy risk behaviors. *Journal of Adolescent Health, 49*(2), 172–179.

Silva, M. (2002). The effectiveness of school-based sex education programs in the promotion of abstinent behavior: A meta-analysis. *Health Education Research, 17*(4), 471–481. doi:10.1093/her/17.4.471.

Silverman, M., Berman, A. L., Sanddal, N. D., O'Carroll, P. W., & Joiner, T. E., Jr. (2007). Rebuilding the Tower of Babel: A revised nomenclature for the study of suicide and suicidal behaviors: Part 2: Suicide-related ideations, communications, and behaviors. *Suicide & Life-Threatening Behavior, 37*(3), 264–277.

Snow, W. H., Gilchrist, L. D., & Schinke, S. P. (1985). A critique of progress in adolescent smoking prevention. *Children and Youth Services Review, 7*, 1–19.

Spruikt-Metz, D. (2011). Etiology, treatment, and prevention of obesity in childhood and adolescence: A decade in review. *Journal of Research on Adolescence, 21*(1) 129–152.

Stanberry, L. R., Spruance, S. L., Cunningham, A. L., Bernstein, D. I., Mindel, A., & Sacks, S., et al. (2002). Glycoprotein-D-adjuvant vaccine to prevent genital herpes. *The New England Journal of Medicine, 347*, 1652–1661.

Stice, E., Shaw, H., & Marti, C. N. (2006). A meta-analytic review of obesity prevention programs for children and adolescents: The skinny on interventions that work. *Psychological Bulletin, 132*(5), 667–691.

Story, M., & Kaphinger, K. M. (2008). School-based prevention of child & adolescent obesity. In W. T. O'Donohue, B. Moore, & B. J. Scott (Eds.), *Handbook of pediatric & adolescent obesity*. New York: Routledge.

Summerbell, C. D. et al. (2005). Interventions for preventing obesity in children. *Cochrane Database of Systematic Reviews, 3*, 1–70.

Tarrier, N., Taylor, K., & Gooding, P. (2008). Cognitive-behavioral interventions to reduce suicide behavior: A systematic review and meta-analysis. *Behavior Modification, 32*(1), 77–108.

Thomas, B., Mitchell, A., Devlin, M., Goldsmith, C., Singer, J., & Watters, D. (1992). Small group sex education at school: The McMaster Teen Program. In B. C. Miller, J. J. Card, R. L. Paikoff, & J. L. Peterson (Eds.), *Preventing adolescent pregnancy* (pp. 28–52). Newbury Park, CA: Sage Publications.

Tobler, N. S., Roona, M. R., Ochshorn, P., Marshall, D. G., Streke, A. V., & Stackpole, K. M. (2000). School-based adolescent drug prevention programs: 1998 meta-analysis. *Journal of Primary Prevention, 20*, 275–337.

Trenholm, C., Devaney, B., Fortson, K., Quay, L., Wheeler, J., & Clark, M. (2007). *Impacts of Fourt Title V, Section 510 Abstinence Education Programs, Final Report*. Princeton, N: Matematica Policy Research.

Underhill, K., Operario, D., & Montgomery, P. (2007a). Abstinence-only programs for HIV infection prevention in high-income countries (Review). *Cochrane Database System Review, 4*, CD005421.

Underhill, K., Operario, D., & Montgomery, P. (2007b). Systematic review of abstinence-plus HIV prevention programs in high-income countries. *PLoS Medicine, 4*, 1471–1485.

Vu, T., Farish, S., Jenkins, M., & Kelly, H. (2002). A meta-analysis of effectiveness of influenza vaccine in persons aged 65 years and over living in the community. *Vaccine, 20*(13–14), 1831–1836.

Whitaker, D. J., Morrison, S., Lindquist, C., Hawkins, S. R., O'Neil, J. A., Nesius, A. M., et al. (2006). A critical review of interventions for the primary prevention of perpetration of partner violence. *Aggression and Violent Behavior, 11*, 151–166.

White, D., & Pitts, M. (1998). Educating young people about drugs: A systematic review. *Addiction, 93*(10), 1475–1487.

Wolfe, R. M., & Sharpe, L. K. (2002). Anti-vaccinationists past and present. *British Medical Journal, 325*, 430–432.

Wolfe, D. A., Wekerle, C., Scott, K., Straatman, A., Grasley, C., & Reitzel-Jaffe, D. (2003). Dating violence prevention with at-risk youth: A controlled outcome evaluation. *Journal of Consulting and Clinical Psychology, 71*, 279–291.

Wolfe, D. A., Crooks, C. C., Chiodo, D., & Jaffe, P. (2009). Child maltreatment, bullying, gender-based harassment, and adolescent dating violence: Making the connections. *Psychology of Women Quarterly, 33*, 21–24.

World Health Organization. (2013). *Controlling the global obesity epidemic*. Retrieved from http://www.who.int/nutrition/topics/obesity/en/.

Determinants of Health-Related Behaviors in Adolescence

Ralph J. DiClemente, Jennifer L. Brown, and Teaniese Latham Davis

Introduction

Adolescence is a developmental stage characterized by significant physical, intellectual, emotional, and social changes. During adolescence, youth establish behavioral patterns and make lifestyle choices that affect both their current and future health (CDC, 2011). Although adolescence can sometimes be a turbulent developmental period fraught with potential threats to mental and physical health, many adolescents traverse this period unscathed (DiClemente, Santelli, & Crosby, 2009). Others, unfortunately, adopt health risk behaviors that significantly compromise their mental and physical well-being, thus limiting achievement of their full potential (DiClemente et al., 2009). Risk behaviors are not, however, random, inevitable, or uncontrollable. Indeed, there is accumulating evidence identifying determinants of adolescents' health risk behaviors that in turn may increase the likelihood of experiencing adverse health outcomes. Furthermore, there is ample empirical evidence indicating that risk behaviors are preventable and amenable to change through interventions.

R.J. DiClemente, Ph.D. (✉) • J.L. Brown, Ph.D.
T.L. Davis, Ph.D., M.P.H.
Department of Behavioral Sciences and Health Education, Rollins School of Public Health and Center for AIDS Research, Emory University, 1518 Clifton Road NE, Atlanta, GA 30322, USA
e-mail: ridclem@emory.edu; jennifer.brown@emory.edu; tlatham@emory.edu

Healthy People 2010 is part of an ongoing national initiative summarizing critical objectives that should be attained in order to improve the health of all United States citizens (Park, Brindis, Chang, & Irwin, 2008; U.S. Department of Health and Human Services, 2000a, 2000b). Within *Healthy People 2010*, the Centers for Disease Control and Prevention (CDC) Division of Adolescent and School Health outlined critical health objectives for adolescents and young adults between the ages of 10 and 24 (Centers for Disease Control and Prevention, 2004; Park et al., 2008). These objectives focus on individual health outcomes and associated behaviors that pose the greatest threat to the health of adolescents and subsequently to adult health and well-being (Centers for Disease Control and Prevention, 2004). *Healthy People 2010* identified the following six areas as posing the greatest health threats to adolescents: (a) mortality, (b) unintentional injury, (c) violence, (d) mental health and substance abuse, (e) reproductive health, and (f) chronic disease. Within each of these six domains, the initiative articulates specific desired behavioral outcomes to be attained; for example, the violence domain of the plan seeks to reduce homicides, physical fighting, and weapon carrying on school property among adolescents (Centers for Disease Control and Prevention, 2004; Park et al., 2008).

Public health interventions seek to improve the health of adolescents across these critical domains. In order to design the most effective behavior change interventions, one must first identify key determinants for each health outcome and related

W.T. O'Donohue et al. (eds.), *Handbook of Adolescent Health Psychology*,
DOI 10.1007/978-1-4614-6633-8_8, © Springer Science+Business Media New York 2013

health behaviors. Within the fields of health psychology and public health, numerous health behavior theories have identified important determinants of health outcomes, focusing primarily on individual-level factors. In contrast, socio-ecological models of health behavior illustrate that an individual's behavior occurs within a larger social context (Bronfenbrenner, 1979, 1994; DiClemente, Salazar, Crosby, & Rosenthal, 2005). As such, socio-ecological models of adolescent health consider individual, peer, familial, relational, community, and societal factors that influence health behavior engagement and subsequent health outcomes (DiClemente et al., 2005).

In this chapter, we first provide an overview of a socio-ecological model of adolescent health behavior determinants, highlighting some of the key individual, family, peer, relational, community, and societal determinants of health outcomes. We then provide illustrative examples of interventions designed to address important health determinants and associated behaviors at each level within the socio-ecological model. It is our goal to provide representative research examples focusing on the key health outcomes as outlined by the Critical Health Objectives for adolescent health in *Healthy People 2010* (Park et al., 2008; U.S. Department of Health and Human Services, 2000a, 2000b). Specifically, we will provide an overview of important determinants and interventions designed to address adolescents' health across the following domains: (a) mortality, (b) unintentional injury, (c) violence, (d) mental health and substance abuse, (e) reproductive health, and (f) chronic disease. Thus, this chapter will synthesize findings from discrete but related levels of research, as each of these levels represents important determinants of adolescent health.

Socio-Ecological Model

Overview of Individual-Level Interventions

Individual-level interventions represent a prominent approach to improving the health outcomes of adolescents by promoting health behavior change. Such intervention approaches focus on targeting relevant intrapsychic or psychological influences (e.g., impulsivity, self-esteem) without addressing pervasive contextual influences that directly or indirectly influence health outcomes (DiClemente et al., 2005). While there is evidence to suggest individual-level intervention approaches are effective in promoting health behavior change, they may not be sufficient to produce sustained behavior change over protracted periods of time or in the presence of countervailing influences (DiClemente et al., 2005). Additionally, addressing behavior change solely at the individual level may lack sufficient breadth to reach large segments of the at-risk adolescent population (DiClemente et al., 2005).

Overview of the Socio-Ecological Model

A socio-ecological perspective involves examining the behaviors of individuals within the context of their social and physical environment. Socio-ecological factors include cultural influences, familial influences, peer influences, and societal influences (Bronfenbrenner, 1979, 1994). The model presented in Fig. 1 is an adaptation of Bronfenbrenner's ecological model (DiClemente et al., 2005). It depicts five concentric spheres of influence that correspond to varying levels of analysis. The innermost sphere represents the individual and includes psychological characteristics and individual behaviors. The family/peer, relational, and community spheres suggest that interactions between adolescents, family members, and peers have a strong influence on adolescents' behaviors. The outermost sphere indicates that characteristics of the society at large (e.g., cultures, values, norms, health care policies, media, gender, and racial/ethnic discrimination) provide a broader context in which adolescents, institutions, and communities are embedded, and thus may have a potent effect on adolescents' behaviors. The multiplicity of influences among spheres ultimately shapes adolescents' behaviors and related health outcomes.

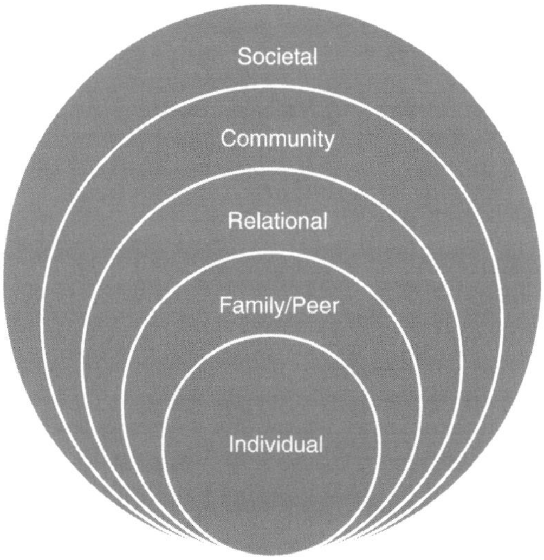

Fig. 1 A socio-ecological model of risk and protective factors for adolescents' health behaviors

Health-Related Behaviors: Risk and Protective Factors

Overview of Risk and Protective Factors

Determinants of adolescent health can be classified as factors that either increase or decrease the probability of a particular outcome or behavior occurring. Risk factors refer to behaviors or characteristics of individuals that increase the probability of a future negative health outcome or disease in one group relative to a comparable group without or with different levels of the behavior or characteristic (Rothstein, 2003). Risk factors may be either directly or indirectly related to a particular health outcome or disease (Rothstein, 2003). For example, smoking cigarettes is a behavioral risk factor that increases the likelihood of experiencing negative health outcomes (e.g., emphysema, increased blood pressure) and disease (e.g., cancer). Additional examples of risk factors on an individual level include sexual risk behavior, substance use, engaging in violent behavior, and suicidal ideation (Wang, Hsu, Lin, Cheng, & Lee, 2010).

In contrast, protective factors increase the likelihood of health-promoting behaviors and positive health outcomes (Jessor, Turbin, & Costa, 1998; Keeler & Kaiser, 2010). As such, protective factors are associated with decreased engagement in health risk behaviors and fewer negative health consequences (Keeler & Kaiser, 2010; Resnick et al., 1997). Further, protective factors may also buffer the negative influence of risk exposure (Jessor et al., 1998). For instance, parental monitoring of adolescents' activities may serve as a protective factor decreasing adolescents' engagement in health risk behaviors including use of alcohol or drugs (Barnes, Welte, Hoffman, & Dintcheff, 2005; Martins, Storr, Alexandre, & Chilcoat, 2008; Rai et al., 2003; Tobler & Komro, 2010). Other examples of individual-level protective factors include self-esteem, self-efficacy to engage in health-promoting behaviors, and effective emotion regulation (Wang et al., 2010). On a relational level, examples of protective factors include family connectedness, support or perceived caring from family members, and high perceived safety at school (Saewyc et al., 2009). Thus, determinants of adolescent health may be classified as either risk or protective factors for engaging in a particular health behavior and subsequently experiencing a given health outcome or disease.

While, for heuristic purposes, we have linked specific risk behaviors with specific adverse health outcomes, for instance, our example of smoking (risk behavior) and emphysema (adverse health outcome), a particular risk behavior may be related to a host of adverse outcomes. For illustrative purposes, non-condom-protected sexual behavior (risk behavior) may be related to HIV infection, infection with other sexually transmitted infections (e.g., chlamydia, gonorrhea, trichomoniasis, herpes simplex virus type 2), and, for women, unintended pregnancy. Each of these adverse outcomes, in turn, may be associated with further adverse conditions. For example, chlamydial infections may result in ectopic pregnancy or pelvic inflammatory disease; HIV infection may lead to a host of other opportunistic infections. Thus, while there is some specificity between risk behaviors and adverse health outcomes, it is worth bearing in mind that some risk behaviors, while certainly associated with specific adverse outcomes, may also be related to a host of other adverse health outcomes. Perhaps the best example is that of cigarette smoking. While we often think immediately of the association between cigarette smoking and cancer, particularly lung cancer, it is important to note that cigarette smoking is related to diverse cancers, including oral pharyngeal as well as heart disease, and other lung diseases (i.e., emphysema). Thus, preventing or reducing the likelihood of adolescents' engagement in risk behaviors actually affects the probability of developing a wide array of health adverse outcomes. Of course, the number of preventable adverse outcomes will vary by the type of risk behavior.

Individual Characteristics

Individual-level determinants of adolescent health include a multitude of risk factors. Unfortunately, the developmental period of adolescence is associated with greater engagement in some health risk behaviors including delinquency and crime. Indeed, Mash and Barkley suggested girls' problems with delinquency increase from mid-adolescence to adulthood (2003). Delinquency is at its height during adolescence, marked by alcohol, tobacco, and other drug use. Teenaged adolescents and young adults also commit most crimes, with a peak during ages 15–17 years. The age-crime curve holds true for many countries, including the United States. Crime decreases with age; however there are not clear evidence-based explanations for this decline as adolescents age (Smith, 1995). Additionally, school engagement diminishes as adolescents lose interest or experience disciplinary problems with authority figures (Robins, 1995). Collectively, an individual's age (i.e., the developmental period during adolescence) may serve as an important predisposing determinant for health risk practices and subsequent negative health outcomes.

Adolescents' engagement in health risk behaviors tends to cluster such that individuals engaging in one risk behavior may be more likely to engage in other health risk practices. For instance, participating in physical fights, carrying weapons, and non-seat belt use are individual risk behaviors significantly associated with the leading causes of death among young people, namely, motor vehicle crashes, homicide, and suicide (CDC, 2010b). Research has also established that aggression and violent crime are strongly associated with drug use and a range of other criminal and delinquent behaviors (Farhat, Simons-Morton, & Luk, 2011; Smith, 1995). Substance use has also been identified as a risk factor for risky sexual behavior. In one study, African American adolescent girls with biologically confirmed marijuana use were more than three times more likely to test positive for an STD, two times more likely to report non-condom use in the recent past, and more than three times more likely to report a history of inconsistent condom use (Liau et al., 2002). Additionally, reporting a sex partner who was high or drunk during sex has been associated with STD transmission (Crosby et al., 2008; Doherty, Adimora, Schoenbach, & Aral, 2007).

Adolescents experiencing elevated psychological distress or mental illness may also be more prone to risky health behaviors and experience associated negative health outcomes. In a study examining the relationship between psychological functioning and sexual behaviors, young women with high psychological distress were significantly more likely to have a diagnosed STD, report inconsistent condom use, have sex while high or drunk, and report perceived partner concurrency (Seth, Raiji, DiClemente, Wingood, & Rose, 2009). Psychological distress has also been related to psychosocial mediators of condom use, including lower partner sexual communication, lower condom use self-efficacy, lower refusal self-efficacy, and higher fear of communicating with partners (Seth et al., 2009). High levels of depressive symptoms among adolescent girls have been associated with increased number of lifetime partners and having an external locus of control (Rubin, Gold, & Primack, 2009). These examples, among others from the adolescent health literature, point to the deleterious impact of psychological distress on adaptive health behavior engagement.

There are individual characteristics among adolescents that are protective against risky and unhealthy behaviors. When examining factors facilitating nonsmoking, adolescents cited self-confidence and concerns about their personal appearance as two of the most important reasons for not smoking (Kulbok et al., 2008). Prospective research has also shown optimistic thinking style as protective against depressive symptoms among adolescents (Patton et al., 2011). In one study, adolescents with high levels of optimism were half as likely to have depressive symptoms, compared to adolescents with low levels of optimism. Optimistic thinking was protective against substance use among girls, but not boys (Patton et al., 2011). Overall, life satisfaction among adolescents may also serve as a protective factor reducing risk practices. For instance, adolescents with high levels of life satisfaction were less likely to report current marijuana use or former marijuana experimentation (Farhat et al., 2011).

Cognitive risk appraisals allow adolescents to examine the advantages and disadvantages of engaging in a particular behavior. As such, adolescents are more likely to engage in healthy behaviors if perceived benefits exist. When examining tobacco use patterns, nonsmoking adolescents cited reasons of wanting to live longer, less worry about being addicted, better breathing, and easier participation in athletic activities as protective against their tobacco use (Kulbok et al., 2008). Additionally, likelihood of engaging in healthy behaviors increases when few perceived disadvantages exist. In one study, most nonsmoking adolescents agreed there was not anything bad about being a nonsmoker (Kulbok et al., 2008). Collectively, these studies point to adaptive psychological health and well-being as protective factors associated with reductions in health risk behaviors.

Unfortunately, adolescence is a period typically associated with greater engagement in some health risk practices relative to later in adulthood. Furthermore, individual health risk behaviors are likely to co-occur with other risk practices. While a review of all individual-level determinants of adolescent health is beyond the scope of this chapter, psychological functioning can serve as an important risk or protective factor for subsequent health outcomes. Additionally, cognitive strategies to appraise risk and evaluate the advantages and disadvantages of a particular behavior may serve to either increase or decrease engagement in these practices.

Family and Peer Characteristics

The roles of parents and family are critical in keeping adolescents safe (DiClemente et al., 2005). Perceived family support, parent-family connectedness, family structure, family cohesiveness, parental monitoring, and parent-adolescent communication may help prevent adolescents from engaging in many health risk behaviors as well as improve management of chronic illness or disease (DiClemente et al., 2005). For adolescents with chronic diseases, such as asthma, familial characteristics and interactions play an important role in the effective management of asthma symptoms and adherence to medication and other medical protocols (Fiese, Wamboldt, & Anbar, 2005; Fiese, 2008; Fiese, Winter, Anbar, Howell, & Poltrock, 2008; Fiese, Winter, & Botti, 2011). Indeed, established family medication management routines have been associated with greater asthma treatment adherence and effective health care utilization by adolescents and their caregivers (Fiese et al., 2005).

Monitoring of adolescents' activities by parents or caregivers typically serves as a protective factor against adverse health outcomes. Indeed, greater parental monitoring has been associated with lower substance use among adolescents (Barnes et al., 2005; Farhat et al., 2011; Martins et al., 2008; Rai et al., 2003; Tobler & Komro, 2010). Parental monitoring may also mitigate the consequences associated with witnessing violent acts including externalizing behaviors and mental health difficulties (e.g., depressive symptoms; Bacchini, Miranda, & Affuso, 2011; Copeland-Linder, Lambert, & Ialongo, 2010; Sullivan, Kung, & Farrell, 2004). Additional evidence suggests that adolescents who report their parents know where they are and who they are with are substantially less likely to engage in sexual risk behaviors or have an STI (Crosby et al., 2006; DiClemente,

Crosby, & Wingood, 2002; DiClemente et al., 2005; Voisin, DiClemente, Salazar, Crosby, & Yarber, 2006). Collectively, these studies point to parental monitoring as a protective factor against engaging in health risk behaviors and may buffer against negative consequences associated with experiencing adverse events.

Adolescents' parental relationships are commonly in transition along with usually experiencing at least one transition into middle or junior high school (Alsaker, 1995; Rice & Dolgin, 2002). The influence of the parent-adolescent relationship is based on the frequency of their interaction. Parents' communication with their adolescent children affords the possibility to impart health knowledge and promote health behavior engagement. Unfortunately, parents and caregivers may not discuss important health information before risk behavior occurs (Beckett et al., 2010). However, better communication between adolescents and their parents or caregivers may serve as a protective factor against engaging in risk behaviors. For example, adolescents who discuss sexual health topics with their parents have demonstrated greater confidence negotiating safer sexual practices with their partners including more consistent condom use (Buzi, Smith, & Weinman, 2009; DiClemente et al., 2001; Hadley et al., 2009; Shoop & Davidson, 1994; Whitaker, Miller, May, & Levin, 1999).

Family structure characteristics are often associated with adolescents' health outcomes and behaviors. For example, family structure has been related to an adolescents' STD status (Sionean et al., 2001). In one study, having unemployed parents more than doubled the likelihood of having a history of gonorrhea, relative to adolescents living with employed parents (Sionean et al., 2001). Additionally, the absence of a parent may adversely impact an adolescent's moral development (Rice & Dolgin, 2002). Some research also suggests the association between family structure and adolescent risk behaviors occurs due to an interaction between protective and risk factors (Wang et al., 2010). Adolescents' perception regarding their mother's risk behavior has been a statistically significant factor explaining adolescent risk behavior (Wang et al., 2010). Family networks can also serve as a protective factor. African American adolescent girls living with their mothers who report a supportive family have endorsed fewer sexual risk behaviors, including being more likely to use condoms during sex, less likely to report emotional abuse from sex partners, reporting fewer partner barriers to engaging in safe sex, having less fear of condom negotiation, and having higher self-efficacy to negotiate condoms with partners (Crosby, DiClemente, Wingood, & Harrington, 2002). Thus, a supportive, cohesive family may be a protective factor while family structures characterized by greater distress may be a risk factor for health risk behaviors and negative health outcomes.

Another developmental aspect of adolescence is the increasing importance of peer influences (DiClemente et al., 2005). Perceived norms regarding peers' engagement in health risk behaviors exert a strong influence on use of alcohol, tobacco, drugs, initiation of sexual intercourse, and sexual risk practices among adolescents (Andrews, Hampson, & Peterson, 2010; DiClemente et al., 2005; Kumar, O'Malley, Johnston, Schulenberg, & Bachman, 2002; Pandina, Johnson, & White, 2010; Schinke, Fang, & Cole, 2008; Sieving, Eisenberg, Pettingell, & Skay, 2006; Verkooijen, de Vries, & Nielsen, 2007). Consequently, adolescents may adopt the perceived high-risk practices of their peers. For instance, if adolescents believe that their peers are not using condoms and engaging in other sexual risk behaviors, they may be more likely to engage in these behaviors themselves (Bachanas et al., 2002; Boyer, Tschann, & Shafer, 1999; Doljanac & Zimmerman, 1998; Millstein & Moscicki, 1995; Salazar et al., 2011). In contrast, perceived peer norms may also serve as a protective factor when adolescents perceive that risk behaviors are not normative among their peers (DiClemente, 1991; Maxwell, 2002). For example, in a nationally representative sample of 8th, 10th, and 12th grade students, greater schoolwide disapproval of substance use was associated with lower rates of tobacco, alcohol, and drug use by adolescents (Kumar et al., 2002). In an incarcerated sample, adolescents who perceived peer norms supportive of condom use were more likely to report consistent condom use (DiClemente, 1991). Research has also indicated that peer norms combined with self-efficacy to engage in safer sexual behaviors mediate the relationship between media exposure to sexual content and adolescents' initiation of sexual behaviors (Martino, Collins, Kanouse, Elliott, & Berry, 2005).

Adolescents' risk practices may be more directly influenced by the behaviors of their friends and peers (Pandina et al., 2010; Schinke et al., 2008). Peer pressure to engage in risk behavior increases during adolescence. There is greater pressure by peers to smoke, drink alcohol, and engage in sexual intercourse during this developmental period (Eicher, Clasen, & Brown, 1986). Indeed, one study found that alcohol and drug use by an adolescent girl's best friend was predictive of her own substance use (Schinke et al., 2008). Among African American adolescent girls an association between reporting that less than half of their girlfriends used condoms consistently predicted youth's own risky sexual behavior across six measures of condom use (Crosby et al., 2003). Adolescents have a propensity to select peer groups similar to them and seek out peer groups to assist with identity formation and consolidation (Eccles & Barber, 1999; Eccles & Gootman, 2002). Thus, associating with a peer group engaging in health risk practices may increase adolescents' own health behaviors.

The structure of the peer network may also impact health outcomes among adolescents. Haynie assessed whether characteristics of the peer network were related to an adolescent's delinquent behavior (2001). Results indicated an association between friends' delinquency and an adolescent's delinquent behavior (Haynie, 2001). Second, the delinquency-peer association was moderated by the structure of the peer networks (Haynie, 2001). The association was stronger when the peer network had high density, the adolescent was more popular, and the adolescent was more central in the friendship network. Thus, the level of network cohesion places more controls on network members to align with the network's behavioral disposition (Haynie, 2001).

Relational Characteristics

Relationship characteristics play an important role in influencing adolescents' engagement in risk behaviors and likelihood of experiencing negative health outcomes. Characteristics of adolescents' relationships are particularly prominent determinants of sexual health and influence adolescents' risky behavior and their likelihood of acquiring an STI. There are also important gender differences in relationship features associated with STI transmission. Among adolescent females, lack of relationship control (Crosby et al., 2000), longer length of relationship (Catania et al., 1989; Crosby et al., 2000; Fortenberry, Tu, Harezlak, Katz, & Orr, 2002), fear of condom use negotiation (Sionean et al., 2002), less frequent partner communication about sexually related topics (Begley, Crosby, DiClemente, Wingood, & Rose, 2003; Catania et al., 1989; Sieving et al., 1997), and having older sexual partners (Begley et al., 2003; DiClemente, Crosby, et al., 2002; Miller, Clark, & Moore, 1997) have all been associated with greater likelihood of engaging in STI risk behaviors or STI transmission. Other relational risk factors associated with increased STI transmission risk include perceptions of partner control over STI acquisition (Rosenthal et al., 1999), perception of low partner support of condoms (Weisman et al., 1991), being a date rape victim (Valois et al., 1999), and being a victim of dating violence or abuse (Silverman, Raj, Mucci, & Hathaway, 2001; Valois et al., 1999; Wingood & DiClemente, 1997; Wingood, DiClemente, McCree, Harrington, & Davies, 2001). Similar associations have been found for having a new partner and having a risky sexual partner (Bunnell et al., 1999; Katz, Fortenberry, Tu, Harezlak, & Orr, 2001). Having greater partner-dependence has also been associated with less condom use (Senn, Carey, Vanable, & Coury-Doniger, 2010). Economic dependence on a sexual partner impacts the relationship's power dynamics and subsequently prevents the dependent partner from engaging in risk reduction or protection strategies (Gorbach & Holmes, 2003).

The progression of adolescents' romantic relationships also influences behavior practices and related health outcomes. Kaestle and Halpern examined the nature of adolescents' relationships prior to engaging in romantic partnerships (Kaestle & Halpern, 2005). A majority of adolescent women, 51.8 %, reported being acquaintances with their partner before getting into a relationship, 42.6 % reported being friends, while 5.7 % reported not knowing their partner before getting into a relationship (Kaestle & Halpern, 2005). Adolescent women in this study who were friends before engaging in a romantic relationship were significantly less likely to have sex (Kaestle & Halpern, 2005). In contrast, adolescent women who had not met their partner before getting into a romantic relationship were more likely to have sex (Kaestle & Halpern, 2005). According to Andrinopoulos, Kerrigan, and Ellen (2006), young women may seek out romantic partnerships to fulfill a desire for emotional support, security, and intimacy in sexual partnerships. Furthermore, romantic relationships help young women cope with other problems and may subsequently affect their sexual behaviors (Andrinopoulos et al., 2006). For instance, one young woman discussed the process of "catching feelings" or developing emotional ties after having sex with a romantic partner (Andrinopoulos et al., 2006). Collectively, these studies highlight the important role that adolescents' relationships play in shaping their behaviors which may in turn impact their short- and long-term health.

Community Characteristics

Community characteristics and involvement with community organizations can also influence adolescents' adoption of protective health behaviors. Adolescents' affiliations with social organizations, adolescents who perceive that they have higher levels of social support, and positive school environments may serve as protective factors (St. Lawrence, Brasfield, Jefferson, & Allyene, 1994). For example, among a nationally representative sample of adolescents, a sense of belonging to a school was associated with delaying sexual intercourse (Resnick et al., 1997). School connectedness and environment impact health outcomes for adolescents as well. In one study, having a positive academic climate was associated with lower risk for marijuana experimentation among girls (Farhat et al., 2011). In contrast, experiences of being bullied increased the risk for marijuana experimentation and other substance use among girls (Carlyle & Steinman, 2007; Farhat et al., 2011). Being bullied was also associated with depressive affect and substance use among adolescents (Carlyle & Steinman, 2007).

An emerging line of inquiry suggests that social capital, another community characteristic, may influence adolescents' risk behaviors. Social capital is an index comprised of trust, reciprocity, and cooperation among members of a social network (Putnam, 2000). A recent study demonstrated that social capital was inversely correlated with AIDS cases and STI incidence including chlamydia, gonorrhea, and syphilis among adults (Holtgrave & Crosby, 2003). More recent research has shown that adolescents residing in states with greater levels of social capital were less likely to engage in certain sexual risk behaviors (Crosby, Holtgrave, DiClemente, Wingood, & Gayle, 2003). Greater levels of social capital, however, may not be protective for adolescents if the social network involved is antisocial in nature, such as a gang. It has been suggested that gangs are a community problem with underlying neighborhood factors such as the need for protection from crime and/or abusive families, peer pressures, and lack of money-making opportunities serving as major risk factors for gang involvement (Curry & Thomas, 1992; Walker-Barnes & Mason, 2001). When adolescents choose to join a gang, they put themselves at greater risk for engaging in a diverse array of health-compromising behaviors such as violence, risky sexual behaviors, antisocial behaviors, and alcohol/drug use (Deschenes & Esbensen, 1999; Esbensen, Peterson, Taylor, & Freng, 2009; Hunt, Joe-Laidler, & MacKenzie, 2000). One study of high-risk African American adolescent females found gang involvement to be related to school expulsion, binge drinking, using marijuana, engaging in physical fights, and positive diagnoses of *Trichomonas vaginalis* and *Neisseria gonorrhoeae* (Wingood et al., 2002).

Societal Characteristics

Sociological constructs of race and gender influence adolescents' health (DiClemente et al., 2005). Despite efforts to reduce health disparities, ethnic minority adolescents continue to experience poorer health outcomes. For example, epidemiological data indicate African American female adolescents experience disproportionate rates of sexually transmitted infections (STI) and HIV relative to other racial/ethnic groups and males (CDC, 2010a). The apparent influences of race/ethnicity may be confounded by a host of environmental factors (DiClemente et al., 2005). Indeed, disparities existing in the availability of preventative services and access to necessary medical care (Elster, Jarosik, VanGeest, & Fleming, 2003; Flores & Tomany-Korman, 2008). Poverty may be a risk factor where its direct association with race/ethnicity exerts an indirect influence on health outcomes (DiClemente et al., 2005). With regard to sexual health, it has been suggested that higher STI/HIV rates among African American adolescents may be linked to living in geographic clusters characterized by lower socioeconomic status, low educational attainment, compromised family structures, and poverty (DiClemente et al., 2005; Fullilove, 1998).

Sociological constructs of race and gender may also interact with adolescents' peer network to heighten risk for adverse health outcomes. For example, high-risk sexual networks among Black women are a primary concern in STI transmission. Population patterns of exposure are fundamental determinants of health at the population level (Adimora & Schoenbach, 2005). Considering that the individual risk behaviors (i.e., number of sex partners, condom use) of young Black women are not significantly different than young White women, other larger societal factors are associated with increased risk for negative sexual health outcomes (Hallfors, Iritani, Miller, & Bauer, 2007). The pool of available sexual partners within which Black young women have sex is a higher risk network of partners. Black young women's sexual networks have been negatively impacted by racial segregation, low sex ratios in the Black population, drugs, incarceration, as well as economic adversity operating alongside the low sex ratio (Adimora & Schoenbach, 2005). As an example, research indicates a strong correlation between incarceration and chlamydia and gonorrhea rates (Thomas & Sampson, 2005). Thus, the interaction between societal features and other levels within the socio-ecological model serves as an important determinant of adolescent health outcomes.

With widespread availability of media from a growing number of sources, adolescents are exposed to increasing amounts of media that can influence their health behavior choices (Strasburger & Hogan, 2009). For example, in a recent large cross-sectional survey of adolescents, youth reported being exposed to tobacco-promoting messages from a number of media outlets including television, movies, ads in magazines, and from numerous sources on the Internet (Duke et al., 2009). Unfortunately, positive media portrayals of risk behavior practices may increase engagement in these behaviors by adolescents (Media power-for good and for ill, 2010). For instance, studies point to an association between increased exposure to tobacco-promoting media and use of tobacco among adolescents (Primack, Land, & Fine, 2008; Villanti, Boulay, & Juon, 2011; Weiss et al., 2006). More broadly, a recent review of the impact of media exposure found a consistent association between increased media consumption and use of tobacco, alcohol, and other substances (Nunez-Smith et al., 2010). Therefore, frequent exposure to media messaging that normalizes risk behaviors may in turn promote adolescents engagement in those behaviors.

Implementation of policies and regulations to promote health behavior engagement at the societal level can serve as a protective factor for adolescents' health. Legislation can modify health behavior via a variety of channels. For example, states with stricter tobacco control laws (e.g., clean air laws) have lower rates of adolescent tobacco use (Botello-Harbaum et al., 2009). Additionally, policies that increase the price associated with tobacco have been linked to decreased tobacco purchases and use by adolescents (Liang & Chaloupka, 2002; Tworek et al., 2010). Professional medical organizations also have the potential to promote adolescent health through their organization's policy statements. For instance, the American Academy of Pediatrics now recommends banning all tobacco advertisements in the media given the role media can play to promote health risk behaviors (Strasburger, 2010). Thus, policy has great potential to improve the health of adolescents by enacting legislation or altering societal structures to prevent disease or adverse health consequences and decrease risk behavior engagement among adolescents.

Health-Related Behavior Change Intervention Approaches: Levels of Change

While the socio-ecological model of health behavior suggests a multifaceted approach to intervention development and design, behavior change interventions typically intervene at a particular level within the model. In what follows, we provide an overview of individual-, relational-, family-, community-, and society-level interventions designed to promote health behavior adaptation among adolescents. Because describing all health promotion interventions for adolescents is not feasible, we instead strive to provide representative intervention examples that typify strategies to modify health behaviors at each of the levels of the model.

Individual Level

Multiple individual-level interventions exist targeting a wide range of health behaviors among adolescents, including preventing pregnancy (Blank, Baxter, Payne, Guillaume, & Pilgrim, 2010), increasing STD screening (Tebb, Wibbelsman, Neuhaus, & Shafer, 2009), improving birth outcomes for adolescent mothers (Koniak-Griffin, Anderson, Verzemnieks, & Brecht, 2000), improving medication adherence (Dean, Walters, & Hall, 2010), reducing tobacco and substance use (Tait & Hulse, 2003), promoting weight loss for overweight adolescents (Stuart, Broome, Smith, & Weaver, 2005), reducing risky driving (Farrow, 1989), and treating depression (David-Ferdon & Kaslow, 2008) and anger (Eyberg, Nelson, & Boggs, 2008). These interventions use strategies such as increasing knowledge via education (Savage, Farrell, McManus, & Grey, 2010), self-efficacy to engage in behaviors, skills building (Savage et al., 2010), emotion regulation, role-plays, case management (Savage et al., 2010), and cognitive behavioral therapy (Forman & Barakat, 2011).

As an example, individual-level weight-loss interventions for overweight adolescents often focus on diet and exercise programs. Many of these programs target the individual (Krzystek-Korpacka et al., 2011), while some also tailor intervention messages to the adolescent's specific needs or individual behaviors (Elloumi et al., 2009). Some weight-loss interventions are implemented face-to-face with a counselor or trainer (Elloumi et al., 2009; Krzystek-Korpacka et al., 2011). However, one study used an Internet-based approach to target individual-level weight loss strategies in conjunction with access to an online case manager. Intervention activities included setting nutrition and physical activity goals, self-monitoring, problem solving, creating a behavioral contract, and relapse prevention (White et al., 2004). Thus, individual-level interventions seek to improve individuals' health knowledge while building skill and promoting self-efficacy to engage in behavior change. Such interventions offer the potential to address an individual's unique needs and tailor intervention content.

Relational Level

Relational-level interventions target relationship factors (e.g., communication skills) within adolescents' relationships to promote behavior change. Relational-level interventions are particularly important to consider when designing sexual health interventions. Such relational-level interventions directly address salient influences associated with STI risk and protective behaviors while also transferring the burden to initiate STI-protective behaviors from one person to the dyad. This is particularly important for adolescent females who are in power-imbalanced relationships with their male partners (Begley et al., 2003; DiClemente, Wingood, et al., 2002; Ellen, Aral, & Madger, 1998; Gollub & Stein, 1993). Additionally, this type of intervention holds great promise for enhancing not only the adoption of STI-preventive behaviors by the dyad but also, in the event of dissolution, the generalization of recently adopted STI-preventive behaviors to new relationships. In the same vein, existing strategies often fail to recognize the unique dilemmas that adolescents confront when disclosing positive STI diagnoses to sexual partners. Thus, "adolescent-friendly" partner services represent an approach that may promote disclosure and care-seeking behavior of partners. Specifically, "adolescent friendly" signifies an approach that is developmentally appropriate and incorporates activities designed to teach adolescents how to effectively communicate positive diagnoses to sexual partners and promote care-seeking among those partners (Fortenberry, Brizendine, Katz, & Orr, 2002). The use of partner-delivered medication for treating STIs could also be used as an adjunct to the adolescent-friendly services, thereby preventing subsequent reinfection and transmission (Kissinger et al., 1998).

Family Level

Family-level interventions have been effective intervention approaches to improve adolescents' mental health, reduce risk behavior engagement, and manage chronic illness. Family therapy approaches have demonstrated improvement among adolescents with mental health conditions including depressive disorders (Diamond & Siqueland, 1995; Diamond et al., 2010; Kolko, Brent, Baugher, Bridge, & Birmaher, 2000), anxiety disorders (Bögels & Siqueland, 2006; Kendall, Hudson, Gosch, Flannery-Schroeder, & Suveg, 2008; Storch et al., 2010), eating disorders (Doyle, Le Grange, Loeb, Doyle, & Crosby, 2010; Eisler, Simic, Russell, & Dare, 2007; le Grange, Crosby, Rathouz, & Leventhal, 2007; Lock et al., 2010; Schmidt et al., 2007), and substance use disorders (Liddle, Rowe, Dakof, Henderson, & Greenbaum, 2009; Rowe, 2010). Family-based interventions have also been developed to improve the management of chronic illnesses such as diabetes among adolescents (Anderson, Brackett, Ho, & Laffel, 1999; Keogh et al., 2007; Nansel et al., 2009; Satin, La Greca, Zigo, & Skyler, 1989; The TODAY Study Group, 2010). In one such trial of an intervention to manage type I diabetes, the family intervention was conducted during routine medical visits and provided youth and their parents with information regarding glucose management and sought to improve parental involvement with insulin injections and glucose monitoring (Anderson et al., 1999). This intervention also provided participants with skills to manage conflict and improve communication skills (Anderson et al., 1999). Results indicated that adolescents who received the family-based intervention had improved glucose levels and more consistent parental involvement with insulin injections, and decreased conflict (Anderson et al., 1999). Findings from this study and other family-level interventions highlight the important role families can play in working collaboratively to manage illness and also prevent negative health outcomes. In particular, such interventions typically seek to improve familial communication and to promote strategies to effectively manage conflict and manage disease.

Family-level interventions have also been effective in reducing risk behavior engagement. A recent meta-analysis of family interventions found that such interventions were efficacious in delaying initiation of alcohol use and frequency of drinking among adolescents (Smit, Verdurmen, Monshouwer, & Smit, 2008). Additionally, family interventions have resulted in decreased substance use and externalizing behaviors (e.g., aggression) among at-risk adolescents (Connell, Dishion, Yasui, & Kavanagh, 2007; Spoth, Redmond, Shin, & Azevedo, 2004; Stormshak et al., 2011). For example, one family intervention conducted ecological assessments in the home and schools and utilized motivational interviewing to promote parenting skills and provide caregivers and youth with feedback (Stormshak et al., 2011). Findings from this study suggest that adolescents receiving the family intervention, relative to the control condition, had decreased engagement in antisocial behaviors, alcohol use, marijuana use, and tobacco use (Stormshak et al., 2011). This study illustrates that intervening with caregivers and their children can be efficacious in reducing risk behaviors during adolescence.

Community Level

Community-level health promotion interventions target entire communities or specific community structures (e.g., schools, community organizations) to improve health outcomes within an adolescent population. In such studies whole communities may be randomized to receive the treatment or to be a comparison community. As such, cities with similar characteristics (e.g., population density, prevalence of a given health outcome) are selected to ensure comparability of results across communities. Thus, the goal of this study design is to evaluate the efficacy of public health interventions to improve health outcomes community-wide. For example, to curb adolescents' use of tobacco, several community-level interventions have been implemented and evaluated (Altman, Wheelis, McFarlane, Lee, & Fortmann, 1999; Biglan, Ary, Smolkowski, Duncan, & Black, 2000; Johnson et al., 1990; Pentz et al., 1989; Perry, Kelder, Murray, & Klepp, 1992). In one such study, eight Kansas City communities were randomized either to a comprehensive tobacco prevention intervention involving schools, parents, mass media, and community organizations or a control condition consisting of only media and community organization approaches (Johnson et al., 1990). Over a 3-year period there were significant reductions in adolescent tobacco use among those receiving the more comprehensive community-level intervention (Johnson et al., 1990). This study highlights the impact that interventions targeting multiple community structures can have on adolescent health promotion.

Alternatively, community-level interventions may target specific community structures or organizations to improve health behavior outcomes. To reduce adolescent tobacco use, a number of studies have sought to enforce stricter penalties for merchants selling to adolescents or alter adolescents' access to tobacco products (Bowen, Orlandi, Lichtenstein, Cummings, & Hyland, 2002, 2003; Chen & Forster, 2006; Feighery, Altman, & Shaffer, 1991; Forster et al., 1998; Rigotti et al., 1997). One intervention sought to reduce merchants' sales of tobacco-related products to minors (Rigotti et al., 1997). Across the communities that received the intervention there was significant improvement in business compliance with tobacco sales to adolescents (Rigotti et al., 1997). Thus, addressing specific community structures that contribute to negative health outcomes may be an efficacious approach to promote positive health behavior change. Such interventions also offer the potential to reach a larger number of adolescents.

Delivering behavior change interventions within school settings has also been an effective community-level approach. For examples, schools can play a role in reducing sexual risk-taking by making condoms available. Adolescents who have better accessibility and availability of condoms tend to have higher rates of condom use without an increase in overall rates of sexual activity (Bunnell et al., 1999; Wingood & DiClemente, 1997; Wingood et al., 2001). The link between better accessibility and availability and increased condom use may be explained by related research which showed that those who carry condoms are more likely to use condoms than those who do not always carry condoms (Katz et al., 2001). The Coordinated School Health Programs (CSHP) are another key strategy to increase opportunities to engage in physical activity and offer greater access to nutritious options for adolescents in school (CDC, 2008). The Centers for Disease Control and Prevention (CDC) also suggests strengthening schools' physical activity and nutrition policies for students and programs for staff (CDC, 2008). This is an example of using coordinated efforts on multiple levels to impact the individual.

Societal Level

Societal level interventions have great potential to reach a large audience. Mass media campaigns can be an effective tool for reaching adolescents who may not otherwise be exposed to interventions (DiClemente et al., 2005). Mass media campaigns have been utilized to improve adolescents' sexual health with messages to decrease behaviors that put youth at risk for negative health outcomes including STI and HIV and promote increased condom use (de Vroome et al., 1990; Hausser & Michaud, 1994; Kennedy, Mizuno, Seals, Myllyluoma, & Weeks-Norton, 2000; Romer et al., 2009; Zimmerman et al., 2007). A recent media campaign utilizing culturally sensitive HIV prevention messages targeted to African American adolescents found that the media intervention resulted in behavior change (e.g., increased condom use) and also positive changes in related psychosocial constructs (e.g., sex refusal self-efficacy; Romer et al., 2009). Another media campaign among sexually active 14–18-year-old adolescents study used radio ads, promotional materials, a telephone information line, and peer outreach and found that such an approach• increased adolescents' condom use (Kennedy et al., 2000).

Changes on a societal level can also increase access and acceptability of preventative health services for adolescents (DiClemente et al., 2005). With respect to adolescents' sexual health and STI/HIV prevention, health care organizations that provide greater incentives for reproductive health practitioners to screen, counsel, and educate adolescents at risk for or diagnosed with an STI may reduce STI/HIV transmission (DiClemente et al., 2005). Furthermore, changing the incentive structure to provide such services offers the potential to reduce the rate of new and repeat STI (DiClemente et al., 2005). Greater availability of reproductive health services will ensure that adolescents receive STI prevention education, testing, and treatment despite income disparities and in turn can improve their sexual health (DiClemente et al., 2005). Additionally, these services should exempt adolescents from obtaining parental consent for treatment (DiClemente et al., 2005). Thus, improving medical care access and provision of comprehensive STI prevention, testing, and treatment have the potential to reduce STI/HIV transmission among adolescents' sexual networks community-wide.

Changes to existing laws or policies have the potential to significantly impact the health practices of adolescents society-wide. Unfortunately, motor vehicle accidents continue to be a leading cause of adolescent mortality in the United States (Irwin, 2005). However, policy changes have been linked to decreased adolescent fatalities from motor vehicle accidents (Irwin, 2005; Maupin et al., 2004). Policies to increase use of graduated licensing programs for teenagers in conjunction with harsher penalties for driving under the influence of substances have been associated with fewer motor vehicle accidents among adolescents (Irwin, 2005). Furthermore, policies to increase the price of alcohol have been linked to fewer drunken driving incidents by adolescents (Adrian, Ferguson, & Her, 2001; Grossman, Chaloupka, Saffer, & Laixuthai, 1994). Thus, policies may seek to directly target a particular behavior (e.g., by increasing the age required to get a driver's license) or may indirectly affect health behaviors (e.g., by changing overall drinking patterns and in turn reducing drunk driving incidents). Such policies have enormous potential to promote adolescent health and decrease risk behavior engagement among this vulnerable population.

A Social-Ecological Approach to Health-Related Behavior Change

The central premise of the socio-ecological model is that none of its levels should function in isolation from the others. Indeed, we suggest that designing effective health promotion interventions can best be achieved by taking full advantage of the "synergy" among the five levels that comprise the model (DiClemente et al., 2005). Prevention approaches should capitalize on the cumulative reinforcement of messages using coordinated, diverse interactive channels and resources. This coordinated approach can amplify and complement isolated approaches, thereby optimizing and sustaining favorable intervention effects. Thus, although this approach requires intensified efforts and resources, its returns warrant implementation to improve adolescents' health. However, it is critical to note that implementation of this framework necessitates the ability to influence policies; thus, policy can be considered as a cornerstone of the socio-ecological approach.

Conclusions

Healthy People 2010 established a road map to improve the health of all US citizens. This initiative highlighted critical health domains to be addressed among adolescents. Across all of these domains, there are a multitude of determinants that either directly or indirectly impact health behavior engagement and related health outcomes. A socio-ecological model categorizes health determinants of an individual across social and environmental levels. Understanding the contextual determinants of health allows health psychologists to design effective interventions and improve the health outcomes of adolescents. Health behavior change interventions targeting multiple system levels afford great potential both to improve adolescents' immediate health and also impact their long-term health and well-being.

Acknowledgments This research was supported by a grant from the National Institute of Mental Health (5R01 MH070537) to the first author. Additional support was provided by the Emory Center for AIDS Research (P30 AI050409). Jennifer L. Brown was supported by K12 GM000680 from the National Institute of General Medical Sciences.

References

Adimora, A. A., & Schoenbach, V. J. (2005). Social context, sexual networks, and racial disparities in rates of sexually transmitted infections. *The Journal of Infectious Diseases, 191*(Suppl 1), S115–S122.

Adrian, M., Ferguson, B. S., & Her, M. (2001). Can alcohol price policies be used to reduce drunk driving? Evidence from Canada. *Substance Use & Misuse, 36*(13), 1923–1957.

Alsaker, F. D. (1995). Timing of puberty and reactions to pubertal changes. In M. Rutter (Ed.), *Psychosocial disturbances in young people: Challenges for prevention* (pp. 37–82). New York, NY: Cambridge University Press.

Altman, D. G., Wheelis, A. Y., McFarlane, M., Lee, H., & Fortmann, S. P. (1999). The relationship between tobacco access and use among adolescents: A four community study. *Social Science & Medicine (1982), 48*(6), 759–775.

Anderson, B. J., Brackett, J., Ho, J., & Laffel, L. M. (1999). An office-based intervention to maintain parent-adolescent teamwork in diabetes management. Impact on parent involvement, family conflict, and subsequent glycemic control. *Diabetes Care, 22*(5), 713–721.

Andrews, J. A., Hampson, S., & Peterson, M. (2010). Early adolescent cognitions as predictors of heavy alcohol use in high school. *Addictive Behaviors*. doi:10.1016/j.addbeh.2010.12.011.

Andrinopoulos, K., Kerrigan, D., & Ellen, J. M. (2006). Understanding sex partner selection from the perspective of inner-city black adolescents. *Perspectives on Sexual and Reproductive Health, 38*(3), 132–138.

Bacchini, D., Miranda, M. C., & Affuso, G. (2011). Effects of parental monitoring and exposure to community violence on antisocial behavior and anxiety/depression among adolescents. *Journal of Interpersonal Violence, 26*(2), 269–292. doi:10.1177/0886260510362879.

Bachanas, P. J., Morris, M. K., Lewis-Gess, J. K., Sarett-Cuasay, E. J., Sirl, K., Ries, J. K., et al. (2002). Predictors of risky sexual behavior in African American adolescent girls: Implications for prevention interventions. *Journal of Pediatric Psychology, 27*(6), 519–530. doi:10.1093/jpepsy/27.6.519.

Barnes, G. M., Welte, J. W., Hoffman, J. H., & Dintcheff, B. A. (2005). Shared predictors of youthful gambling, substance use, and delinquency. *Psychology of Addictive Behaviors, 19*(2), 165–174. doi:10.1037/0893-164x.19.2.165.

Beckett, M. K., Elliott, M. N., Martino, S., Kanouse, D. E., Corona, R., Klein, D. J., et al. (2010). Timing of parent and child communication about sexuality relative to children's sexual behaviors. *Pediatrics, 125*(1), 34–42.

Begley, E., Crosby, R. A., DiClemente, R. J., Wingood, G. M., & Rose, E. (2003). Older partners and STD prevalence among pregnant African American teens. *Sexually Transmitted Diseases, 30*(3), 211–213.

Biglan, A., Ary, D. V., Smolkowski, K., Duncan, T., & Black, C. (2000). A randomised controlled trial of a community intervention to prevent adolescent tobacco use. *Tobacco Control, 9*(1), 24–32.

Blank, L., Baxter, S. K., Payne, N., Guillaume, L. R., & Pilgrim, H. (2010). Systematic review and narrative synthesis of the effectiveness of contraceptive service interventions for young people, delivered in educational settings. *Journal of Pediatric and Adolescent Gynecology, 23*(6), 341–351. doi:10.1016/j.jpag.2010.03.007.

Bögels, S. M., & Siqueland, L. (2006). Family cognitive behavioral therapy for children and adolescents with clinical anxiety disorders. *Journal of the American Academy of Child and Adolescent Psychiatry, 45*(2), 134–141. doi:10.1097/01.chi.0000190467.01072.ee.

Botello-Harbaum, M. T., Haynie, D. L., Iannotti, R. J., Wang, J., Gase, L., & Simons-Morton, B. (2009). Tobacco control policy and adolescent cigarette smoking status in the United States. *Nicotine & Tobacco Research, 11*(7), 875–885.

Bowen, D. J., Orlandi, M. A., Lichtenstein, E., Cummings, K. M., & Hyland, A. (2002). Intervention effects on youth tobacco use in the community intervention trial (COMMIT). *Tobacco Control, 11*(4), 382.

Bowen, D. J., Orlandi, M. A., Lichtenstein, E., Cummings, K. M., & Hyland, A. (2003). Intervention effects on youth tobacco use in the community intervention trial (COMMIT). *Journal of Epidemiology and Community Health, 57*(2), 159–160.

Boyer, C. B., Tschann, J. M., & Shafer, M.-A. (1999). Predictors of risk for sexually transmitted diseases in ninth grade urban high school students. *Journal of Adolescent Research, 14*(4), 448–465. doi: 10.1177/0743558499144004.

Bronfenbrenner, U. (1979). *The ecology of human development*. Cambridge, MA: Harvard University Press.

Bronfenbrenner, U. (1994). Ecological models of human development. In M. Gauvain & M. Cole (Eds.), *Readings on the development of children* (2nd ed., pp. 37–43). New York: Freeman.

Bunnell, R. E., Dahlberg, L., Rolfs, R., Ransom, R., Gershman, K., Farshy, C., et al. (1999). High prevalence and incidence of sexually transmitted diseases in urban adolescent females despite moderate risk behaviors. *The Journal of Infectious Diseases, 180*(5), 1624–1631.

Buzi, R. S., Smith, P. B., & Weinman, M. L. (2009). Parental communication as a protective factor in increasing condom use among minority adolescents. *International Journal of Adolescent Medicine and Health, 21*(1), 51–59.

Carlyle, K. E., & Steinman, K. J. (2007). Demographic differences in the prevalence, co-occurrence, and correlates of adolescent bullying at school. *Journal of School Health, 77*(9), 623–629. doi: 10.1111/j.1746-1561.2007.00242.x.

Catania, J. A., Coates, T. J., Greenblatt, R. M., Dolcini, M. M., Kegeles, S. M., Puckett, S., et al. (1989). Predictors of condom use and multiple partnered sex among sexually-active adolescent women: Implications for AIDS-related health interventions. *Journal of Sex Research, 26*(4), 514.

CDC. (2008, August 20). *Make a difference at your school: Key strategies to prevent obesity*. Retrieved April 30, 2011, from http://www.cdc.gov/healthyyouth/keystrategies/index.htm.

CDC. (2010a). *Sexually transmitted disease surveillance 2009*. Atlanta: U.S. Department of Health and Human Services.

CDC. (2010b). Youth risk behavior surveillance—United States, 2009. *MMWR. Morbidity and Mortality Weekly Report, 59*(SS-5), 1–142.

CDC. (2011). *Adolescent health*. Retrieved April 10, 2011, from http://www.cdc.gov/HealthyYouth/adolescenthealth/index.htm.

Centers for Disease Control and Prevention. (2004). *Improving the health of adolescents & young adults: A guide for states and communities*. Atlanta, GA: Division of Adolescent and School Health, Health Resources and Services Administration, M. A. C. H. B., Office of Adolescent Health, & National Adolescent Health Information Center, U. O. C., San Francisco.

Chen, V., & Forster, J. L. (2006). The long-term effect of local policies to restrict retail sale of tobacco to youth. *Nicotine & Tobacco Research, 8*(3), 371–377. doi:10.1080/14622200600670249.

Connell, A. M., Dishion, T. J., Yasui, M., & Kavanagh, K. (2007). An adaptive approach to family intervention: Linking engagement in family-centered intervention to reductions in adolescent problem behavior. *Journal of Consulting and Clinical Psychology, 75*(4), 568–579. doi:10.1037/0022-006x.75.4.568.

Copeland-Linder, N., Lambert, S. F., & Ialongo, N. S. (2010). Community violence, protective factors, and adolescent mental health: A profile analysis. *Journal of Clinical Child and Adolescent Psychology, 39*(2), 176–186. doi:10.1080/15374410903532601.

Crosby, R. A., DiClemente, R. J., Wingood, G. M., & Harrington, K. (2002). HIV/STD prevention benefits of living in supportive families: A prospective analysis of high risk African-American female teens. *American Journal of Health Promotion, 16*(3), 142–145.

Crosby, R. A., DiClemente, R. J., Wingood, G. M., Salazar, L. F., Harrington, K., Davies, S. L., et al. (2003). Identification of strategies for promoting condom use: A prospective analysis of high-risk African American female teens. *Prevention Science, 4*(4), 263–270.

Crosby, R. A., Diclemente, R. J., Wingood, G. M., Salazar, L. F., Lang, D., Rose, E., et al. (2008). Co-occurrence of intoxication during sex and sexually transmissible infections among young African American women: Does partner intoxication matter? *Sexual Health, 5*(3), 285–289.

Crosby, R. A., DiClemente, R. J., Wingood, G. M., Sionéan, C., Cobb, B. K., & Harrington, K. (2000). Correlates of unprotected vaginal sex among African American female adolescents: Importance of relationship dynamics. *Archives of Pediatrics & Adolescent Medicine, 154*(9), 893–899.

Crosby, R. A., Holtgrave, D. R., DiClemente, R. J., Wingood, G. M., & Gayle, J. A. (2003). Social capital as a predictor of adolescents' sexual risk behavior: A state-level exploratory study. *AIDS and Behavior, 7*(3), 245–252.

Crosby, R., Voisin, D., Salazar, L. F., DiClemente, R. J., Yarber, W. L., & Caliendo, A. M. (2006). Family influences and biologically confirmed sexually transmitted infections among detained adolescents. *The American Journal of Orthopsychiatry, 76*(3), 389–394. doi:10.1037/0002-9432.76.3.389.

Curry, G. D., & Thomas, R. W. (1992). Community organization and gang policy response. *Journal of Quantitative Criminology, 8*(4), 357–374. doi:10.1007/bf01093640.

David-Ferdon, C., & Kaslow, N. J. (2008). Evidence-based psychosocial treatments for child and adolescent depression. *Journal of Clinical Child and Adolescent Psychology, 37*(1), 62–104. doi:10.1080/15374410701817865.

de Vroome, E. M., Paalman, M. E., Sandfort, T. G., Sleutjes, M., de Vries, K. J., & Tielman, R. A. (1990).

AIDS in The Netherlands: The effects of several years of campaigning. *International Journal of STD & AIDS, 1*(4), 268–275.

Dean, A. J., Walters, J., & Hall, A. (2010). A systematic review of interventions to enhance medication adherence in children and adolescents with chronic illness. *Archives of Disease in Childhood, 95*(9), 717–723.

Deschenes, E. P., & Esbensen, F.-A. (1999). Violence and gangs: Gender differences in perceptions and behavior. *Journal of Quantitative Criminology, 15*(1), 63–96. doi:10.1023/a:1007552105190.

Diamond, G., & Siqueland, L. (1995). Family therapy for the treatment of depressed adolescents. *Psychotherapy: Theory, Research, Practice, Training, 32*(1), 77–90. doi:10.1037/0033-3204.32.1.77.

Diamond, G. S., Wintersteen, M. B., Brown, G. K., Diamond, G. M., Gallop, R., Shelef, K., et al. (2010). Attachment-based family therapy for adolescents with suicidal ideation: A randomized controlled trial. *Journal of the American Academy of Child and Adolescent Psychiatry, 49*(2), 122–131. doi:10.1097/00004583-201002000-00006.

DiClemente, R. J. (1991). Predictors of HIV-preventive sexual behavior in a high-risk adolescent population: The influence of perceived peer norms and sexual communication on incarcerated adolescents' consistent use of condoms. *The Journal of Adolescent Health, 12*(5), 385–390. doi:10.1016/0197-0070(91)90052-n.

DiClemente, R. J., Crosby, R. A., & Wingood, G. M. (2002). Enhancing STD/HIV prevention among adolescents: The importance of parenteral monitoring. *Minerva Pediatrica, 54*(3), 171–177.

DiClemente, R. J., Salazar, L. F., Crosby, R. A., & Rosenthal, S. L. (2005). Prevention and control of sexually transmitted infections among adolescents: The importance of a socio-ecological perspective–a commentary. *Public Health, 119*(9), 825–836.

DiClemente, R. J., Santelli, J. S., & Crosby, R. A. (2009). Adolescent risk behaviors and adverse health outcomes: Future directions for research, practice, and policy. In R. J. DiClemente, J. S. Santelli, & R. A. Crosby (Eds.), *Adolescent health: Understanding and preventing risk behaviors* (pp. 549–560). San Francisco, CA: John Wiley & Sons.

DiClemente, R. J., Wingood, G. M., Crosby, R., Cobb, B. K., Harrington, K., & Davies, S. L. (2001). Parent-adolescent communication and sexual risk behaviors among African American adolescent females. *The Journal of Pediatrics, 139*(3), 407–412.

DiClemente, R. J., Wingood, G. M., Crosby, R. A., Sionean, C., Cobb, B. K., Harrington, K., et al. (2002). Sexual risk behaviors associated with having older sex partners: A study of Black adolescent females. *Sexually Transmitted Diseases, 29*(1), 20–24.

Doherty, I. A., Adimora, A. A., Schoenbach, V. J., & Aral, S. O. (2007). Correlates of gonorrhoea among African Americans in North Carolina. *International Journal of STD & AIDS, 18*(2), 114–117.

Doljanac, R. F., & Zimmerman, M. A. (1998). Psychosocial factors and high-risk sexual behavior: Race differences among urban adolescents. *Journal of Behavioral Medicine, 21*(5), 451–467.

Doyle, P. M., Le Grange, D., Loeb, K., Doyle, A. C., & Crosby, R. D. (2010). Early response to family-based treatment for adolescent anorexia nervosa. *The International Journal of Eating Disorders, 43*(7), 659–662.

Duke, J. C., Allen, J. A., Pederson, L. L., Mowery, P. D., Xiao, H., & Sargent, J. D. (2009). Reported exposure to pro-tobacco messages in the media: Trends among youth in the United States, 2000-2004. *American Journal of Health Promotion, 23*(3), 195–202.

Eccles, J. S., & Barber, B. L. (1999). Student council, volunteering, basketball, or marching band: What kind of extracurricular involvement matters? *Journal of Adolescent Research, 14*(1), 10.

Eccles, J., & Gootman, J. A. (Eds.). (2002) *Community programs to promote youth development*. (Y. Board on Children, and Families, Division of Behavioral and Social Sciences and Education, Trans.). Committee on Community-Level Programs for Youth. Washington, DC: National Academy Press.

Eicher, S. A., Clasen, D. R., & Brown, B. B. (1986). Perceptions of peer pressure, peer conformity dispositions, and self-reported behavior among adolescents. *Developmental Psychology, 22*(4), 521–530.

Eisler, I., Simic, M., Russell, G. F. M., & Dare, C. (2007). A randomised controlled treatment trial of two forms of family therapy in adolescent anorexia nervosa: A five-year follow-up. *Journal of Child Psychology and Psychiatry, 48*(6), 552–560.

Ellen, J. M., Aral, S. O., & Madger, L. S. (1998). Do differences in sexual behaviors account for the racial/ethnic differences in adolescents' self-reported history of a sexually transmitted disease? *Sexually Transmitted Diseases, 25*(3), 125–129.

Elloumi, M., Ben Ounis, O., Makni, E., Van Praagh, E., Tabka, Z., & Lac, G. (2009). Effect of individualized weight-loss programmes on adiponectin, leptin and resistin levels in obese adolescent boys. *Acta Paediatrica, 98*(9), 1487–1493. doi:10.1111/j.1651-2227.2009.01365.x.

Elster, A., Jarosik, J., VanGeest, J., & Fleming, M. (2003). Racial and ethnic disparities in health care for adolescents: A systematic review of the literature. *Archives Of Pediatrics & Adolescent Medicine, 157*(9), 867–874.

Esbensen, F.-A., Peterson, D., Taylor, T. J., & Freng, A. (2009). Similarities and differences in risk factors for violent offending and gang membership. *Australian and New Zealand Journal of Criminology, 42*(3), 310–335. doi:10.1375/acri.42.3.310.

Eyberg, S. M., Nelson, M. M., & Boggs, S. R. (2008). Evidence-based psychosocial treatments for children and adolescents with disruptive behavior. *Journal of Clinical Child and Adolescent Psychology, 37*(1), 215–237. doi:10.1080/15374410701820117.

Farhat, T., Simons-Morton, B., & Luk, J. W. (2011). Psychosocial correlates of adolescent marijuana use: Variations by status of marijuana use. *Addictive Behaviors, 36*(4), 404–407. doi:10.1016/j.addbeh.2010.11.017.

Farrow, J. A. (1989). Evaluation of a behavioral intervention to reduce DWI (driving while intoxicated) among adolescent drivers. *Alcohol, Drugs & Driving, 5*(1), 61–72.

Feighery, E., Altman, D. G., & Shaffer, G. (1991). The effects of combining education and enforcement to reduce tobacco sales to minors. A study of four northern California communities. *Journal of the American Medical Association, 266*(22), 3168–3171.

Fiese, B. H. (2008). Breathing life into family processes: Introduction to the special issue on families and asthma. *Family Process, 47*(1), 1–5. doi:10.1111/j.1545-5300.2008.00235.x.

Fiese, B. H., Wamboldt, F. S., & Anbar, R. D. (2005). Family asthma management routines: Connections to medical adherence and quality of life. *The Journal of Pediatrics, 146*(2), 171–176.

Fiese, B., Winter, M., Anbar, R., Howell, K., & Poltrock, S. (2008). Family climate of routine asthma care: Associating perceived burden and mother-child interaction patterns to child well-being. *Family Process, 47*(1), 63–79. doi:10.1111/j.1545-5300.2008.00239.x.

Fiese, B. H., Winter, M. A., & Botti, J. C. (2011). The ABCs of family mealtimes: Observational lessons for promoting healthy outcomes for children with persistent asthma. *Child Development, 82*(1), 133–145. doi:10.1111/j.1467-8624.2010.01545.x.

Flores, G., & Tomany-Korman, S. C. (2008). Racial and ethnic disparities in medical and dental health, access to care, and use of services in US children. *Pediatrics, 121*(2), e286–e298.

Forman, S. G., & Barakat, N. M. (2011). Cognitive-behavioral therapy in the schools: Bringing research to practice through effective implementation. *Psychology in the Schools, 48*(3), 283–296. doi:10.1002/pits.20547.

Forster, J. L., Murray, D. M., Wolfson, M., Blaine, T. M., Wagenaar, A. C., & Hennrikus, D. J. (1998). The effects of community policies to reduce youth access to tobacco. *American Journal of Public Health, 88*(8), 1193–1198.

Fortenberry, J. D., Brizendine, E. J., Katz, B. P., & Orr, D. P. (2002). The role of self-efficacy and relationship quality in partner notification by adolescents with sexually transmitted infections. *Archives of Pediatrics & Adolescent Medicine, 156*(11), 1133–1137.

Fortenberry, J. D., Tu, W., Harezlak, J., Katz, B. P., & Orr, D. P. (2002). Condom use as a function of time in new and established adolescent sexual relationships. *American Journal of Public Health, 92*(2), 211–213. doi:10.2105/ajph.92.2.211.

Fullilove, R. E. (1998). Race and sexually transmitted diseases, Editorial, *Sexually Transmitted Diseases*, 130. Retrieved from https://login.proxy.library.emory.edu/login?url=http://search.ebscohost.com/login.aspx?direct=true&db=hch&AN=350528&site=ehost-live.

Gollub, E. L., & Stein, Z. A. (1993). Commentary: The new female condom–item 1 on a women's AIDS prevention agenda. *American Journal of Public Health, 83*(4), 498.

Gorbach, P. M., & Holmes, K. K. (2003). Transmission of STIs/HIV at the partnership level: Beyond individual-level analyses. *Journal of Urban Health: Bulletin of the New York Academy of Medicine, 80*(4 Suppl 3), iii15–iii25.

Grossman, M., Chaloupka, F. J., Saffer, H., & Laixuthai, A. (1994). Effects of alcohol price policy on youth: A summary of economic research. *Journal of Research on Adolescence, 4*(2), 347–364. doi:10.1207/s15327795jra0402_9.

Hadley, W., Brown, L. K., Lescano, C., Kell, H., Spalding, K., DiClemente, R. J., et al. (2009). Parent-adolescent sexual communication: Associations of condom use with condom discussions. *AIDS and Behavior, 13*(5), 997–1004.

Hallfors, D. D., Iritani, B. J., Miller, W. C., & Bauer, D. J. (2007). Sexual and drug behavior patterns and HIV and STD racial disparities: The need for new directions. *American Journal of Public Health, 97*(1), 125. doi:10.2105/ajph.2005.075747.

Hausser, D., & Michaud, P. A. (1994). Does a condom-promoting strategy (the Swiss STOP-AIDS campaign) modify sexual behavior among. *Pediatrics, 93*(4), 580.

Haynie, D. L. (2001). Delinquent peers revisited: Does network structure matter? *The American Journal of Sociology, 106*(4), 1013.

Holtgrave, D. R., & Crosby, R. A. (2003). Social capital, poverty, and income inequality as predictors of gonorrhoea, syphilis, chlamydia and AIDS case rates in the United States. *Sexually Transmitted Infections, 79*(1), 62–64.

Hunt, G., Joe-Laidler, K., & MacKenzie, K. (2000). 'Chillin', being dogged and getting buzzed': Alcohol in the lives of female gang members. *Drugs: Education, Prevention & Policy, 7*(4), 331–353. doi:10.1080/713660126.

Irwin, C. E., Jr. (2005). Driving in America: A convergence of public policy and science. *The Journal of Adolescent Health, 36*(6), 452–453. doi:10.1016/j.jadohealth.2005.03.013.

Jessor, R., Turbin, M. S., & Costa, F. M. (1998). Protective factors in adolescent health behavior. *Journal of Personality and Social Psychology, 75*(3), 788–800. doi:10.1037/0022-3514.75.3.788.

Johnson, C. A., Pentz, M. A., Weber, M. D., Dwyer, J. H., Baer, N., MacKinnon, D. P., et al. (1990). Relative effectiveness of comprehensive community programming for drug abuse prevention with high-risk and low-risk adolescents. *Journal of Consulting and Clinical Psychology, 58*(4), 447–456. doi:10.1037/0022-006x.58.4.447.

Kaestle, C. E., & Halpern, C. T. (2005). Sexual activity among adolescents in romantic relationships with friends, acquaintances, or strangers. *Archives of Pediatrics & Adolescent Medicine, 159*(9), 849–853.

Katz, B. P., Fortenberry, J. D., Tu, W., Harezlak, J., & Orr, D. P. (2001). Sexual behavior among adolescent women at high risk for sexually transmitted infections. *Sexually Transmitted Diseases, 28*(5), 247–251.

Keeler, H. J., & Kaiser, M. M. (2010). An integrative model of adolescent health risk behavior. *Journal of Pediatric Nursing, 25*(2), 126–137.

Kendall, P. C., Hudson, J. L., Gosch, E., Flannery-Schroeder, E., & Suveg, C. (2008). Cognitive-behavioral therapy for anxiety disordered youth: A randomized clinical trial evaluating child and family modalities. *Journal of Consulting and Clinical Psychology, 76*(2), 282–297. doi:10.1037/0022-006x.76.2.282.

Kennedy, M. G., Mizuno, Y., Seals, B. F., Myllyluoma, J., & Weeks-Norton, K. (2000). Increasing condom use among adolescents with coalition-based social marketing. *AIDS, 14*(12), 1809–1818.

Keogh, K. M., White, P., Smith, S. M., McGilloway, S., O'Dowd, T., & Gibney, J. (2007). Changing illness perceptions in patients with poorly controlled type 2 diabetes, a randomised controlled trial of a family-based intervention: Protocol and pilot study. *BMC Family Practice, 8*, 36.

Kissinger, P., Brown, R., Reed, K., Salifou, J., Drake, A., Farley, T. A., et al. (1998). Effectiveness of patient delivered partner medication for preventing recurrent Chlamydia trachomatis. *Sexually Transmitted Infections, 74*(5), 331–333.

Kolko, D. J., Brent, D. A., Baugher, M., Bridge, J., & Birmaher, B. (2000). Cognitive and family therapies for adolescent depression: Treatment specificity, mediation, and moderation. *Journal of Consulting and Clinical Psychology, 68*(4), 603–614. doi:10.1037/0022-006x.68.4.603.

Koniak-Griffin, D., Anderson, N. L. R., Verzemnieks, I., & Brecht, M. (2000). A public health nursing early intervention program for adolescent mothers: Outcomes from pregnancy through 6 weeks postpartum. *Nursing Research, 49*(3), 130–138.

Krzystek-Korpacka, M., Patryn, E., Kustrzeba-Wojcicka, I., Chrzanowska, J., Gamian, A., & Noczynska, A. (2011). The effect of a one-year weight reduction program on serum uric acid in overweight/obese children and adolescents. *Clinical Chemistry and Laboratory Medicine, 49*(5), 915–921. doi:10.1515/cclm.2011.130.

Kulbok, P. A., Rhee, H., Botchwey, N., Hinton, I., Bovbjerg, V., & Anderson, N. L. R. (2008). Factors influencing adolescents' decision not to smoke. *Public Health Nursing, 25*(6), 505–515. doi:10.1111/j.1525-1446.2008.00737.x.

Kumar, R., O'Malley, P. M., Johnston, L. D., Schulenberg, J. E., & Bachman, J. G. (2002). Effects of school-level norms on student substance use. *Prevention Science, 3*(2), 105–124. doi:10.1023/a:1015431300471.

le Grange, D., Crosby, R. D., Rathouz, P. J., & Leventhal, B. L. (2007). A randomized controlled comparison of family-based treatment and supportive psychotherapy for adolescent bulimia nervosa. *Archives of General Psychiatry, 64*(9), 1049–1056.

Liang, L., & Chaloupka, F. J. (2002). Differential effects of cigarette price on youth smoking intensity. *Nicotine & Tobacco Research, 4*(1), 109–114.

Liau, A., Diclemente, R. J., Wingood, G. M., Crosby, R. A., Williams, K. M., Harrington, K., et al. (2002). Associations between biologically confirmed marijuana use and laboratory-confirmed sexually transmitted diseases among African American adolescent females. *Sexually Transmitted Diseases, 29*(7), 387–390.

Liddle, H. A., Rowe, C. L., Dakof, G. A., Henderson, C. E., & Greenbaum, P. E. (2009). Multidimensional family therapy for young adolescent substance abuse: Twelve-month outcomes of a randomized controlled trial. *Journal of Consulting and Clinical Psychology, 77*(1), 12–25. doi:10.1037/a0014160.

Lock, J., Le Grange, D., Agras, W. S., Moye, A., Bryson, S. W., & Jo, B. (2010). Randomized clinical trial comparing family-based treatment with adolescent-focused individual therapy for adolescents with anorexia nervosa. *Archives of General Psychiatry, 67*(10), 1025–1032. doi:10.1001/archgenpsychiatry.2010.128.

Martino, S. C., Collins, R. L., Kanouse, D. E., Elliott, M., & Berry, S. H. (2005). Social cognitive processes mediating the relationship between exposure to television's sexual content and adolescents' sexual behavior. *Journal of Personality and Social Psychology, 89*(6), 914–924. doi:10.1037/0022-3514.89.6.914.

Martins, S. S., Storr, C. L., Alexandre, P. K., & Chilcoat, H. D. (2008). Adolescent ecstasy and other drug use in the National Survey of Parents and Youth: The role of sensation-seeking, parental monitoring and peer's drug use. *Addictive Behaviors, 33*(7), 919–933. doi:10.1016/j.addbeh.2008.02.010.

Mash, E. J., & Barkley, R. A. (2003). *Child psychopathology* (2nd ed.). New York, NY: The Guilford Press.

Maupin, J. E., Jr., Schlundt, D., Warren, R., Miller, S., Goldzweig, I., & Warren, H. (2004). Reducing unintentional injuries on the nation's highways: Research and program policy to increase seat belt use. *Journal of Health Care for the Poor and Underserved, 15*(1), 4–17.

Maxwell, K. A. (2002). Friends: The role of peer influence across adolescent risk behaviors. *Journal of Youth and Adolescence, 31*(4), 267–277. doi: 10.1023/a:1015493316865.

Miller, K. S., Clark, L. F., & Moore, J. S. (1997). Sexual initiation with older male partners and subsequent HIV risk behavior among female adolescents. *Family Planning Perspectives, 29*(5), 212.

Millstein, S. G., & Moscicki, A. B. (1995). Sexually-transmitted disease in female adolescents: Effects of psychosocial factors and high risk behaviors. *The Journal of Adolescent Health, 17*(2), 83–90.

Nansel, T. R., Anderson, B. J., Laffel, L. M. B., Simons-Morton, B. G., Weissberg-Benchell, J., Wysocki, T., et al. (2009). A multisite trial of a clinic-integrated intervention for promoting family management of pediatric type 1 diabetes: Feasibility and design. *Pediatric Diabetes, 10*(2), 105–115.

Nunez-Smith, M., Wolf, E., Huang, H. M., Chen, P. G., Lee, L., Emanuel, E. J., et al. (2010). Media exposure and tobacco, illicit drugs, and alcohol use among children and adolescents: A systematic review. *Substance Abuse, 31*(3), 174–192. doi:10.1080/08897077.2010.495648.

Pandina, R. J., Johnson, V. L., & White, H. R. (2010). Peer influences on substance use during adolescence and emerging adulthood. In P. L. Scheier (Ed.), *Handbook of drug use etiology: Theory, methods, and empirical findings* (pp. 383–401). Washington, DC US: American Psychological Association.

Park, M. J., Brindis, C. D., Chang, F., & Irwin, C. E., Jr. (2008). A Midcourse review of the healthy people 2010: 21 critical health objectives for adolescents and young adults. *The Journal of Adolescent Health, 42*(4), 329–334.

Patton, G. C., Tollit, M. M., Romaniuk, H., Spence, S. H., Sheffield, J., & Sawyer, M. G. (2011). A prospective study of the effects of optimism on adolescent health risks. *Pediatrics, 127*(2), 308. doi:10.1542/peds.2010-0748.

Pentz, M. A., MacKinnon, D. P., Flay, B. R., Hansen, W. B., Johnson, C. A., & Dwyer, J. H. (1989). Primary prevention of chronic diseases in adolescence: Effects of the midwestern prevention project on tobacco use. *American Journal of Epidemiology, 130*(4), 713–724.

Perry, C. L., Kelder, S. H., Murray, D. M., & Klepp, K. I. (1992). Communitywide smoking prevention: Long-term outcomes of the minnesota heart health program and the class of 1989 study. *American Journal of Public Health, 82*(9), 1210–1216.

Primack, B. A., Land, S. R., & Fine, M. J. (2008). Adolescent smoking and volume of exposure to various forms of media. *Public Health, 122*(4), 379–389.

Putnam, R. D. (2000). *Bowling alone: The collapse and revival of American community*. New York, NY: Touchstone Books/Simon & Schuster.

Rai, A. A., Stanton, B., Wu, Y., Li, X., Galbraith, J., Cottrell, L., et al. (2003). Relative influences of perceived parental monitoring and perceived peer involvement on adolescent risk behaviors: An analysis of six cross-sectional data sets. *The Journal of Adolescent Health, 33*(2), 108–118. doi:10.1016/s1054-139x(03)00179-4.

Resnick, M. D., Bearman, P. S., Blum, R. W., Bauman, K. E., Harris, K. M., Jones, J., et al. (1997). Protecting adolescents from harm: Findings from the National Longitudinal Study on Adolescent Health. *Journal of the American Medical Association, 278*(10), 823–832. doi:10.1001/jama.278.10.823.

Rice, F. P., & Dolgin, K. G. (2002). *The adolescent: Development, relationships, and culture* (10th ed.). Boston, MA: Allyn and Bacon.

Rigotti, N. A., DiFranza, J. R., Chang, Y., Tisdale, T., Kemp, B., & Singer, D. E. (1997). The effect of enforcing tobacco-sales laws on adolescents' access to tobacco and smoking behavior. *The New England Journal of Medicine, 337*(15), 1044–1051. doi:10.1056/nejm199710093371505.

Robins, L. N. (1995). Sociocultural trends affecting the prevalence of adolescent problems. In M. Rutter (Ed.), *Psychosocial disturbances in young people: Challenges for prevention* (pp. 367–384). New York, NY: Cambridge University Press.

Romer, D., Sznitman, S., DiClemente, R., Salazar, L. F., Vanable, P. A., Carey, M. P., et al. (2009). Mass media as an HIV-prevention strategy: Using culturally sensitive messages to reduce HIV-associated sexual behavior of at-risk African American youth. *American Journal of Public Health, 99*(12), 2150–2159. doi:10.2105/ajph.2008.155036.

Rosenthal, S. L., Cohen, S. S., DeVellis, R. F., Biro, F. M., Lewis, L. M., Succop, P. A., et al. (1999). Locus of control for general health and STD acquisition among adolescent girls. *Sexually Transmitted Diseases, 26*(8), 472–475.

Rothstein, W. G. (2003). *Public health and the risk factor*. Rochester, NY: University of Rochester Press.

Rowe, C. L. (2010). Multidimensional family therapy: Addressing co-occurring substance abuse and other problems among adolescents with comprehensive family-based treatment. *Child and Adolescent Psychiatric Clinics of North America, 19*(3), 563–576.

Rubin, A. G., Gold, M. A., & Primack, B. A. (2009). Associations between depressive symptoms and sexual risk behavior in a diverse sample of female adolescents. *Journal Of Pediatric And Adolescent Gynecology, 22*(5), 306–312.

Saewyc, E. M., Homma, Y., Skay, C. L., Bearinger, L. H., Resnick, M. D., & Reis, E. (2009). Protective factors in the lives of bisexual adolescents in North America. *American Journal of Public Health, 99*(1), 110. doi:10.2105/ajph.2007.123109.

Salazar, L. F., Head, S., Crosby, R. A., DiClemente, R. J., Sales, J. M., Wingood, G. M., et al. (2011). Personal and social influences regarding oral sex among African American female adolescents. *Journal of Women's Health, 20*(2), 161–167. doi:10.1089/jwh.2010.2247.

Satin, W., La Greca, A. M., Zigo, M. A., & Skyler, J. S. (1989). Diabetes in adolescence: Effects of multifamily group intervention and parent simulation of diabetes. *Journal of Pediatric Psychology, 14*(2), 259–275.

Savage, E., Farrell, D., McManus, V., & Grey, M. (2010). The science of intervention development for type 1 diabetes in childhood: Systematic review. *Journal of Advanced Nursing, 66*(12), 2604–2619. doi:10.1111/j.1365-2648.2010.05423.x.

Schinke, S. P., Fang, L., & Cole, K. C. A. (2008). Substance use among early adolescent girls: Risk and protective factors. *The Journal of Adolescent Health, 43*(2), 191–194. doi:10.1016/j.jadohealth.2007.12.014.

Schmidt, U., Lee, S., Beecham, J., Perkins, S., Treasure, J., Yi, I., et al. (2007). A randomized controlled trial of family therapy and cognitive behavior therapy guided self-care for adolescents with bulimia nervosa and related disorders. *The American Journal of Psychiatry, 164*(4), 591–598.

Senn, T. E., Carey, M. P., Vanable, P. A., & Coury-Doniger, P. (2010). Partner dependence and sexual risk behavior among STI clinic patients. *American Journal of Health Behavior, 34*(3), 257–266.

Seth, P., Raiji, P., DiClemente, R., Wingood, G., & Rose, E. (2009). Psychological distress as a correlate of a biologically confirmed STI, risky sexual practices, self-efficacy and communication with male sex partners in African-American female adolescents. *Psychology, Health & Medicine, 14*(3), 291–300.

Shoop, D. M., & Davidson, P. M. (1994). AIDS and adolescents: The relation of parent and partner communication to adolescent condom use. *Journal of Adolescence, 17*(2), 137–148. doi:10.1006/jado.1994.1014.

Sieving, R. E., Eisenberg, M. E., Pettingell, S., & Skay, C. (2006). Friends' influence on adolescents' first sexual intercourse. *Perspectives on Sexual and Reproductive Health, 38*(1), 13–19.

Sieving, R., Resnick, M. D., Bearinger, L., Remafedi, G., Taylor, B. A., & Harmon, B. (1997). Cognitive and behavioral predictors of sexually transmitted disease risk behavior among sexually active adolescents. *Archives of Pediatrics & Adolescent Medicine, 151*(3), 243–251.

Silverman, J. G., Raj, A., Mucci, L. A., & Hathaway, J. E. (2001). Dating violence against adolescent girls and associated substance use, unhealthy weight control, sexual risk behavior, pregnancy, and suicidality. *Journal of the American Medical Association, 286*(5), 572.

Sionean, C., DiClemente, R. J., Wingood, G. M., Crosby, R., Cobb, B. K., Harrington, K., et al. (2001). Socioeconomic status and self-reported gonorrhea among African American female adolescent. *Sexually Transmitted Diseases, 28*(4), 236.

Sionean, C., DiClemente, R. J., Wingood, G. M., Crosby, R., Cobb, B. K., Harrington, K., et al. (2002). Psychosocial and behavioral correlates of refusing unwanted sex among African-American adolescent females. *The Journal of Adolescent Health, 30*(1), 55–63.

Smit, E., Verdurmen, J., Monshouwer, K., & Smit, F. (2008). Family interventions and their effect on adolescent alcohol use in general populations: A meta-analysis of randomized controlled trials. *Drug and Alcohol Dependence, 97*(3), 195–206. doi:10.1016/j.drugalcdep. 2008.03.032.

Smith, D. J. (1995). Towards explaining patterns and trends in youth crime. In M. Rutter (Ed.), *Psychosocial disturbances in young people: Challenges for prevention* (pp. 166–211). New York, NY: Cambridge University Press.

Spoth, R., Redmond, C., Shin, C., & Azevedo, K. (2004). Brief family intervention effects on adolescent substance initiation: School-level growth curve analyses 6 years following baseline. *Journal of Consulting and Clinical Psychology, 72*(3), 535–542. doi:10.1037/0022-006x.72.3.535.

St. Lawrence, J. S., Brasfield, T. L., Jefferson, K. W., & Allyene, E. (1994). Social support as a factor in African-American adolescents' sexual risk behavior. *Journal of Adolescent Research, 9*(3), 292–310. doi:10.1177/074355489493002.

Storch, E. A., Lehmkuhl, H. D., Ricketts, E., Geffken, G. R., Marien, W., & Murphy, T. K. (2010). An open trial of intensive family based cognitive-behavioral therapy in youth with obsessive-compulsive disorder who are medication partial responders or nonresponders. *Journal of Clinical Child and Adolescent Psychology, 39*(2), 260–268.

Stormshak, E. A., Connell, A. M., Véronneau, M. H., Myers, M. W., Dishion, T. J., Kavanagh, K., et al. (2011). An ecological approach to promoting early adolescent mental health and social adaptation: Family centered intervention in public middle schools. *Child Development, 82*(1), 209–225. doi:10.1111/j.1467-8624.2010.01551.x.

Strasburger, V. C. (2010). Policy statement–children, adolescents, substance abuse, and the media. *Pediatrics, 126*(4), 791–799.

Strasburger, V. C., & Hogan, M. J. (2009). Media exposure and adolescents' health behavior. In R. J. DiClemente, J. S. Santelli, & R. A. Crosby (Eds.), *Adolescent health: Understanding and preventing risk behaviors* (pp. 411–446). San Francisco, CA: Jossey-Bass.

Stuart, W. P., Broome, M. E., Smith, B. A., & Weaver, M. (2005). An integrative review of interventions for adolescent weight loss. *The Journal of School Nursing, 21*(2), 77–85.

Sullivan, T. N., Kung, E. M., & Farrell, A. D. (2004). Relation between witnessing violence and drug use initiation among rural adolescents: Parental monitoring and family support as protective factors. *Journal of Clinical Child and Adolescent Psychology, 33*(3), 488–498. doi:10.1207/s15374424jccp3303_6.

Tait, R. J., & Hulse, G. K. (2003). A systematic review of the effectiveness of brief interventions with substance using adolescents by type of drug. *Drug and Alcohol Review, 22*(3), 337. doi:10.1080/09595230 31000154481.

Tebb, K. P., Wibbelsman, C., Neuhaus, J. M., & Shafer, M.-A. (2009). Screening for asymptomatic chlamydia infections among sexually active adolescent girls during pediatric urgent care. *Archives of Pediatrics & Adolescent Medicine, 163*(6), 559–564.

The TODAY Study Group. (2010). Design of a family-based lifestyle intervention for youth with type 2 diabetes: The TODAY study. *International Journal of Obesity, 34*, 217–226.

Thomas, J. C., & Sampson, L. A. (2005). High rates of incarceration as a social force associated with community rates of sexually transmitted infection. *The Journal of Infectious Diseases, 191*, S55–S60.

Tobler, A. L., & Komro, K. A. (2010). Trajectories or parental monitoring and communication and effects on drug use among urban young adolescents. *The Journal of Adolescent Health, 46*(6), 560–568. doi:10.1016/j.jadohealth.2009.12.008.

Tworek, C., Yamaguchi, R., Kloska, D. D., Emery, S., Barker, D. C., Giovino, G. A., et al. (2010). State-level tobacco control policies and youth smoking cessation measures. *Health Policy, 97*(2–3), 136–144.

U.S. Department of Health and Human Services. (2000a). *Healthy people 2010, 2nd ed. understanding and improving health and objectives for improving health.*

Washington, D.C: U.S. Government Printing Office. Retrieved from http://www.healthypeople.gov/document/tableofcontents.htm.

U.S. Department of Health and Human Services. (2000b). *Tracking healthy people 2010*. Washington, DC: U.S. Government Printing Office. Retrieved from http://www.healthypeople.gov/document/tableofcontents.htm.

Valois, R. F., Oeltmann, J. E., Waller, J., & Hussey, J. R. (1999). Relationship between number of sexual intercourse partners and selected health risk behaviors among public high school adolescents. *The Journal of Adolescent Health, 25*(5), 328–335.

Verkooijen, K. T., de Vries, N. K., & Nielsen, G. A. (2007). Youth crowds and substance use: The impact of perceived group norm and multiple group identification. *Psychology of Addictive Behaviors, 21*(1), 55–61. doi:10.1037/0893-164x.21.1.55.

Villanti, A., Boulay, M., & Juon, H.-S. (2011). Peer, parent and media influences on adolescent smoking by developmental stage. *Addictive Behaviors, 36*(1–2), 133–136. doi:10.1016/j.addbeh.2010.08.018.

Voisin, D. R., DiClemente, R. J., Salazar, L. F., Crosby, R. A., & Yarber, W. L. (2006). Ecological factors associated with STD risk behaviors among detained female adolescents. *Social Work, 51*(1), 71–79.

Walker-Barnes, C. J., & Mason, C. A. (2001). Perceptions of risk factors for female gang involvement among African American and Hispanic women. *Youth & Society, 32*(3), 303.

Wakefield, M. A., Loken, B., Hornik, R. C. (2010). Use of mass media campaigns to change health behavior. *Lancet, 376*, 1261–1271.

Wang, R.-H., Hsu, H.-Y., Lin, S.-Y., Cheng, C.-P., & Lee, S.-L. (2010). Risk behaviours among early adolescents: Risk and protective factors. *Journal of Advanced Nursing, 66*(2), 313–323. doi:10.1111/j.1365-2648.2009.05159.x.

Weisman, C. S., Plichta, S., Nathanson, C. A., Ensminger, M., & Robinson, J. C. (1991). Consistency of condom use for disease prevention among adolescent users of oral contraceptives. *Family Planning Perspectives, 23*(2), 71.

Weiss, J. W., Cen, S., Schuster, D. V., Unger, J. B., Johnson, C. A., Mouttapa, M., et al. (2006). Longitudinal effects of pro-tobacco and anti-tobacco messages on adolescent smoking susceptibility. *Nicotine & Tobacco Research, 8*(3), 455–465.

Whitaker, D. J., Miller, K. S., May, D. C., & Levin, M. L. (1999). Teenage partners' communication about sexual risk and condom use: The importance of parent-teenager discussions. *Family Planning Perspectives, 31*(3), 117–121.

White, M. A., Martin, P. D., Newton, R. L., Walden, H. M., York-Crowe, E. E., Gordon, S. T., et al. (2004). Mediators of weight loss in a family-based intervention presented over the internet. *Obesity Research, 12*(7), 1050–1059.

Wingood, G. M., & DiClemente, R. J. (1997). The effects of an abusive primary partner on the condom use and sexual negotiation practices of African-American women. *American Journal of Public Health, 87*(6), 1016–1018.

Wingood, G. M., DiClemente, R. J., Crosby, R., Harrington, K., Davies, S. L., & Hook, E. W., 3rd. (2002). Gang involvement and the health of African American female adolescents. *Pediatrics, 110*(5), e57.

Wingood, G. M., DiClemente, R. J., McCree, D. H., Harrington, K., & Davies, S. L. (2001). Dating violence and the sexual health of black adolescent females. *Pediatrics, 107*(5), E72.

Zimmerman, R. S., Palmgreen, P. M., Noar, S. M., Lustria, M. L. A., Lu, H.-Y., & Horosewski, M. L. (2007). Effects of a televised two-city safer sex mass media campaign targeting high-sensation-seeking and impulsive-decision-making young adults. *Health Education & Behavior, 34*(5), 810–826. doi:10.1177/1090198107299700.

Psychosocial Stress, Emotion Regulation, and Resilience in Adolescence

Sheila E. Crowell, Chloe R. Skidmore, Holly K. Rau, and Paula G. Williams

Introduction

Adolescence is a crucial developmental period in which to examine relations between emotion regulation, psychosocial stress, and resilience. A central task facing adolescents is to acquire effective emotion regulation strategies without the level of adult support afforded in childhood (Cicchetti & Rogosch, 2002). Simultaneously, heightened peer contact introduces countless sources of stress and associated opportunities for emotion regulation (e.g., romantic relationships, substance exposure, academic and athletic competition). Although many teenagers navigate these years effectively, for those who do not the health consequences can be enormous. During adolescence, risk for psychopathology increases dramatically (Paus, Keshavan, & Giedd, 2008), accidental injuries and suicide are leading causes of death (National Center for Injury Prevention and Control, 2009), and risk behaviors with a lasting influence on health begin to emerge (Eaton et al., 2008).

A goal of adolescent health research is to better predict which youth will adapt successfully to the task demands of this stage and which youth will struggle. For example, certain individual traits (e.g., high intelligence) and contextual factors (e.g., supportive adult relationships) are associated consistently with competent functioning across development (Luthar, Cicchetti, & Becker, 2000). These factors often emerge as correlates of successful adaptation for youth in both low- and high-risk contexts. This suggests that resilient outcomes for high-risk youth may emerge from some of the same features that promote typical, healthy development (Masten, 2001). Researchers hypothesize that strong emotion regulation skills are foundational to both healthy and resilient outcomes (Buckner, Mezzacappa, & Beardslee, 2003). However, there are very few developmental studies that examine emotion regulation, resilience, and health among youth exposed to adversity.

With this chapter, we review the definitions and conceptual challenges associated with research on psychosocial stress, emotion regulation, and resilience. We examine the intersection of these three distinct literatures and their relevance to health research and treatment. Advances in intervention and prevention will follow from an improved understanding of the mechanisms by which adaptive emotion regulation strategies emerge, develop, and contribute to healthy outcomes. This requires careful attention to the definition of key constructs, how samples were selected and defined, and the interpretation of data acquired at different levels of analysis.

S.E. Crowell, Ph.D. (✉) • C.R. Skidmore, B.S.
H.K. Rau, M.S. • P.G. Williams, Ph.D.
Department of Psychology, University of Utah, 380 South 1530 East, Room 502, Salt Lake City, UT 84112-0251, USA
e-mail: sheila.crowell@psych.utah.edu; chloe.skidmore@psych.utah.edu; holly.rau@psych.utah.edu; paula.williams@psych.utah.edu

W.T. O'Donohue et al. (eds.), *Handbook of Adolescent Health Psychology*,
DOI 10.1007/978-1-4614-6633-8_9,

Definitions and Concepts

Defining Stress

Stress can be defined as any real or perceived threat to a person's well-being or homeostasis. This is often divided into two broad categories of stressors: *physiologic* and *psychogenic* (e.g., Morilak et al., 2005). Physiologic stress follows from any real and imminent threat that requires physical adaptations in order to meet environmental demands and restore homeostasis (e.g., attack or injury). The bodily response to physiologic stress is present regardless of whether a person perceives or is consciously aware of the stimulus. In contrast, psychogenic stress relies upon a person's perception and interpretation in order to attribute a stressful quality to the stimulus. There is considerable variability in response to psychogenic stressors, or whether an event is interpreted as stressful at all. Many physiologic stressors are also compounded by psychogenic interpretations of the event.

Historically, researchers viewed psychogenic stress as the primary source of individual differences in the stress response. It is now clear that personality and personal history can also influence the likelihood and frequency of exposure to physiologic stressors (Hammen, 1991, 2005). Furthermore, people vary widely in their exposure to stress, the magnitude of their physiological and emotional responses to adverse circumstances, the duration of their recovery following a stressor, the length of time needed to recover following negative life events, and whether there is adequate restoration during or between times of stress (Williams, Smith, Gunn, & Uchino, 2010). Examination of individual differences across these four component processes—exposure, reactivity, recovery, and restoration—may inform our understanding of the mechanisms by which adversity is associated with negative health consequences (Hawkley & Cacioppo, 2003; Uchino, Smith, Holt-Lunstead, Campo, & Reblin, 2007; Williams et al., 2010).

There are many mechanisms that appear to account for the lasting effects of stress on health and well-being. These mechanisms can be best understood within a conceptual framework that differentiates between those stressors that lead to temporary disruptions in homeostasis versus those that produce more lasting biological adaptations. This second process is termed allostasis—the process by which the body achieves stability through change (e.g., Sterling & Eyer, 1988). Whereas *homeostatic* processes promote stability via brief, temporary adjustments within the typical operating ranges of physiological systems, *allostatic* processes produce long-term alterations within these operating ranges and are invoked to maintain stability in the face of extreme or prolonged stress (Beauchaine, Neuhaus, Zalewski, Crowell, & Potapova, 2011; Lupien et al., 2006; McEwen, 1998).

In this review, we examine some of the biological adaptations (i.e., allostasis) that are associated with protracted distress. We also discuss how individual variability in the four primary stress processes: exposure, reactivity, recovery, and restoration could contribute to the emergence of adaptive or maladaptive emotion regulation strategies. There is strong evidence to suggest that adverse experiences, particularly in early development, can produce lasting alterations to the limbic-hypothalamic-pituitary-adrenal axis (LHPA), neurotransmitter and neuropeptide functioning, brain structure, and gene expression (e.g., de Kloet, Joels, & Holsboer, 2005; Mead, Beauchaine, & Shannon, 2010). In turn, these biological adaptations can affect emotion regulation and health.

Defining Emotion Regulation

Emotions are automated, rapid, and dynamic response tendencies that have been preserved across evolution to promote survival behaviors (Cole, Martin, & Dennis, 2004; Ekman, 1992; Ekman & Friesen, 1976; Gross, 1998b). Understanding emotional processes is important to the study of adolescent health, given that many behavioral problems are characterized by poor modulation of affect (e.g., Beauchaine, Gatzke-Kopp, & Mead, 2007). However, assessing the *regulation* of emotion presents conceptual and measurement challenges, because most regulatory efforts are internal and unobservable. In contrast, emotion *dysregulation* is often reflected in quantifiable behaviors. Accordingly, we give considerable attention to the construct of emotion dysregulation, which captures "patterns of emotion regulation that have acquired a maladaptive quality, such that emotions seem to interfere with functioning" (Cole & Hall, 2008, p. 266).

There is a growing literature on emotion dysregulation, psychopathology, and health behaviors (Davidson, 2000; Oshri, Rogosch, Burnette, & Cicchetti, 2011). However, there are inconsistencies across studies in terminology, measurement, and level of analysis (e.g., behavioral, physiological; Adrian, Zeman, & Veits, 2011; Cole et al., 2004; Goldsmith & Davidson, 2004; Gross, 2007). According to one conceptualization, dysregulated emotion can be distinguished from typical emotional responses by four key characteristics (Cole & Hall, 2008). First, dysregulated emotions are prolonged, and regulatory attempts are ineffective (e.g., anxiety, depressed mood, irritability, and anger can be difficult to modulate for adolescents with certain psychiatric diagnoses). Second, dysregulated emotions interfere with appropriate social and goal-directed behaviors (e.g., attending school). Third, dysregulated emotions are often expressed in inappropriate social contexts or when the emotion is unshared by others. Finally, the onset of dysregulated emotions can be too abrupt and/or recovery is too slow. Poor emotional recovery (e.g., dysphoria that does not respond to situational changes) and emotional lability (e.g., unpredictable and quick changes of mood) are common among adolescents with psychological problems.

Consistent with this framework, emotion regulation and dysregulation have almost always been defined as individual processes. Regulation is thought to occur internally, when a person influences which emotion is felt, when the emotion occurs, or how it is experienced and expressed behaviorally (Gross, 1998a). Similarly, emotion dysregulation is viewed as a person's failure to modify emotions in any or all of these ways, often leading to context-inappropriate affect and/or behavior (Gratz & Roemer, 2004). Thus, most researchers operate on the assumption that emotion regulation and dysregulation occur within, rather than between individuals.

We suggest that emotion regulation is better understood as an individual *and* interpersonal process (Hughes, Crowell, Uyeji, & Coan, 2012). Because we are a social species, humans are adapted to use social proximity as the default strategy for all metabolically intensive activities, including emotion regulation. This hypothesis has been articulated within social baseline theory (SBT), which suggests that all people are "hard-wired to assume close proximity to conspecifics, and to utilize social proximity as a baseline affect regulation strategy" (Coan, 2008; Coan, 2010, p. 213). From this perspective, healthy and resilient outcomes may also be due to effective *co-regulation* across the life span, rather than individual regulatory efforts alone. This may be particularly true for adolescents who are transitioning from adult to mostly peer sources of co-regulation (Hughes et al., 2012).

Defining Resilience

Resilience has also been defined and measured variably across studies. However, nearly all definitions emphasize adaptive or competent functioning across one or more domains, despite significant adversity or trauma (Cicchetti & Blender, 2006; Curtis & Cicchetti, 2003; Luthar et al., 2000; Shannon, Beauchaine, Brenner, Neuhaus, & Gatzke-Kopp, 2007). This has been operationalized as a dynamic developmental process where a person achieves "desirable outcomes in spite of significant challenges to adaptation or development" (Masten & Coatsworth, 1995, p. 737). Such challenges are often operationalized by experiences of neglect, poverty, or exposure to severe or prolonged abuse (Cicchetti & Blender, 2006).

Positive adaptation and competence are often measured at the individual level and can include positive developmental outcomes in spite of stressful life circumstances (e.g., academic success, strong social skills, effective emotion regulation strategies), or a surprising absence of problems (e.g., lack of psychopathology despite a strong familial loading; Shannon et al., 2007). Because such outcomes are often assessed within the child or adolescent, it is tempting to view resilience as constellation of personality traits or innate abilities. However, resilient functioning is a dynamic, collaborative, and fluctuating product of biology–environment interactions across development (Masten, 2004).

A challenge of resilience research is that adaptive functioning is often discussed in relation to an expected—but hypothetical—negative outcome. For this reason, resilience can only be understood properly when there is significant risk exposure. Without such adversity, resilience is difficult to distinguish from a wide range of typical outcomes and the construct loses much of its meaning (see Shannon et al., 2007). Although resilience is often defined broadly, our focus here is on the development of emotion regulation skills or the absence of psychopathology, when clinical problems characterized by emotion dysregulation could be expected.

Conceptualizing Stress, Resilience, and Emotion Regulation

The literatures on stress, resilience, and emotion regulation have partially independent traditions. Yet there are clear advantages to conceptualizing these phenomena within a unified framework. The term resilience often implies that a person has acquired at least some emotion regulation skills in spite of significant stress exposure (Buckner et al., 2003). More importantly, resilience and emotion regulation are both complex developmental processes that can be altered subtly or dramatically through stress exposure (Charney, 2004). There are many common themes across these three constructs. However, we find an interpersonal understanding of stress, emotion regulation, and resilience to be well suited for understanding how these three processes interact and develop across time. By adolescence, interpersonal stressors are key precipitants of depression, anxiety, aggression, and suicidality (Clarke, 2006; Hilt, Cha, & Nolen-Hoeksema, 2008; Johnson et al., 2002). Similarly, both resilience and emotion regulation can be conceptualized more effectively as transactional, rather than solely individual processes (Masten, 2001).

An interpersonal perspective has advantages over a strictly individual-differences approach and is more consistent with the current understanding of resilience (Cicchetti & Blender, 2006). Early work on resilience implied that some children had an innate capacity to withstand adversity (see Masten, 2001 for a review). This innate capacity was hypothesized to emerge through a combination of high intelligence and an easy disposition. Criticisms of this perspective are twofold. First, there are no public heath interventions that can readily affect these highly heritable aspects of early infant temperament. Second, personality characteristics are neither inherently problematic nor beneficial. Rather, the same trait could confer vulnerability or resilience depending upon contextual risk and/or protective factors. More recent definitions of resilience assume that interactive processes shape adaptive outcomes and, therefore, neither risk nor resilience can be attributed to purely heritable or environmental sources of transmission (Shannon et al., 2007).

As alluded to above, a similar conceptual shift can be identified in the literature on emotion dysregulation. Over the past two decades research on emotion regulation/dysregulation has increased exponentially (e.g., Cole et al., 2004; Cole, Michel, & Teti, 1994). However, there are inconsistencies across studies in the assessment and interpretation of emotion regulation/dysregulation. By and large, developmental researchers have examined emotional processes within dyadic or other complex family systems (e.g., Crowell et al., 2008; Deater-Deckard & Petrill, 2004; Fosco & Grych, 2008; Sroufe, Duggal, Weinfield, & Carlson, 2000). Researchers studying older adolescents or adults have traditionally pursued an individual-differences approach to evaluating regulatory successes and failures, often paying minimal tribute to the interpersonal context in which regulation or dysregulation occur (e.g., John & Gross, 2007).

From a life span development perspective, emotion regulation and resilience can be viewed as transactional, interpersonal processes that emerge initially within early attachments and continue through peer relationships and pair bonding. Stress or threat within key childhood attachment relationships can produce lasting alterations to the biological systems involved in stress reactivity, recovery, and restoration (Schore, 2001). Across development these biological adaptations may also affect internal working models of key relationships, alter peer bonding behavior, and may lead to insecure expectations of co-regulation by adolescence or adulthood (Diamond, 2001; Hughes et al., 2012). Even though attachments are often viewed as noncentral to the daily functioning of adults, it is well established that healthy relationships in adulthood can reduce cardiovascular arousal, lower glucocorticoid levels, attenuate threat-related brain activation, and promote health and longevity (see Coan, 2008 for a review). In contrast, interpersonal stressors may shape and maintain problems with emotion regulation and health from infancy through adulthood.

Interpersonal Stress and the Development of Emotion Dysregulation

In a landmark study, Weaver et al. (2004) found that the licking, grooming, and nursing behavior of rat mothers had a lasting effect on the stress reactivity of their pups. Mothers who engaged in a higher rate of these behaviors produced pups that were less fearful and had more modest HPA responses to stress when compared with the offspring of mothers that engaged in lower rates of licking, grooming, and nursing. In this study, variability in early rearing environments shaped later behavioral phenotypes via two biological mechanisms—increased serotonin ($5HT_7$) receptor density in the hippocampus and higher glucocorticoid receptor (GR) expression—systems involved in mood regulation, behavioral impulsivity, and stress reactivity. Similar mechanisms appear to explain the links between early stress, physiology, and behavior in humans as well (Hyman, 2009).

Animal research comprises much of the literature linking early stress exposure to later difficulties with self-regulation and health. However, findings from animal studies are not translated easily to humans (Beauchaine et al., 2011). Animals can be randomly assigned to stressors, exposed to adverse conditions in a dose-dependent fashion, or have the effects of certain genes activated or silenced. In contrast, human research is necessarily correlational and stressors are rarely independent. Adolescents who are exposed to interparental conflict, for example, may also suffer the consequences of neighborhood violence, exposure to environmental toxins, or peer rejection (Guerra, 1997). Moreover, certain heritable vulnerabilities, such as trait impulsivity, are often correlated with environmental risk exposure (Gatzke-Kopp, 2011). This makes it difficult to determine whether allostatic effects can be attributed to adverse experiences, other third variables, gene–environment interactions, or gene–environment correlations.

Regardless, evidence from both animal and human studies reveals that there are lasting biological sequelae of early adversity (Mead et al., 2010). A thorough review of such biological adaptations is beyond the scope of this chapter. Thus, we focus on some of the structural and functional alterations that may contribute to emerging differences in stress *reactivity*, *recovery*, and *restoration* across early development. These biological changes may also shape key aspects of adolescent and young adult personality, which, in turn, can affect the frequency, intensity, and duration of stress *exposure* in a dynamic, feed-forward fashion. Profound distress, particularly during sensitive periods of development, can effectively alter the human experience—producing lasting changes to biological systems and the basic capacity for self-regulation (see, e.g., studies of children reared in extreme deprivation; Nelson, 2007). Similar mechanisms may explain the link between more widespread forms of stress exposure and later variability in emotion regulation skills.

Stress Reactivity

Stress reactivity is the rapid cascade of physiological, cognitive, emotional, and/or behavioral responses that follow a stressor and shift an organism into a heightened state of biological and behavioral preparedness (Williams et al., 2010). A common assumption is that heightened stress reactivity represents a maladaptive "holdover" from a period of our evolutionary past when stressors were more frequent and lethal (see Boyce & Ellis, 2005, for a review). In our present context this vulnerability is often viewed as problematic, leading to psychopathology and health problems for highly reactive individuals.

Yet, accumulating evidence reveals that, among children, heightened reactivity alone is not associated consistently with poor health. Rather, highly reactive children may experience greater *or fewer* health problems depending on their developmental context. In one study, high-reactive children reared in stressful home or childcare environments also experienced the highest levels of respiratory illness. However, the high-reactive children who were in protective environments were the healthiest of all. Across both high- and low-risk settings, the low-reactive youth showed no effect of context on their health (Boyce et al., 1995). Such findings suggest that high reactivity in children can confer risk or benefit depending upon environmental factors.

Further complicating matters, the relation between reactivity and psychological outcomes may depend upon the timing and number of biological assessments. For example, children with high salivary cortisol early in the school year (when peer groups are forming) but normal levels later in the year (when peer groups were established) were rated as outgoing, well liked, and socially competent; those children who maintained high cortisol reactivity or who changed from low/normal to high levels were rated as solitary and had greater negative affectivity (Gunnar, Tout, de Haan, Pierce, & Stanbury, 1997). These findings imply that heightened reactivity may be beneficial initially, but problematic if sustained—especially when the environmental context is no longer novel or threatening. Stressors, such as starting school, likely elicit strong homeostatic responses. However, if sustained, allostatic processes may be invoked, leading to long-term biological adaptations in stress response systems.

There are also differences in stress reactivity that emerge in studies that include repeated assessments across early development. A common pattern is one in which neurobiological systems are initially *hyper*-reactive to extreme stressors (e.g., maternal separation, chronic exposure to a dominant male) then, following prolonged stress, shift to a chronically *hypo*-reactive baseline state (Mead et al., 2010; Miller, Chen, & Zhou, 2007; Susman, 2006). Abused monkey infants, for example, display elevated levels of cortisol during the first month of life, the period when infants receive the harshest treatment from mothers. Over time, the abused infants have low levels of cortisol, particularly in the morning (see Loman & Gunnar, 2010). A similar down-regulation has been found in studies of rodents who were separated repeatedly from their mothers (Meaney, Brake, & Gratton, 2002) or who lost in an aggressive interaction with a dominant male (Covington & Miczek, 2005). In both studies, decreased dopamine transporter binding led to biobehavioral differences in the stress response and enhanced behavioral sensitivity to drugs of abuse (i.e., the stress-exposed rodents also self-administered greater amounts of cocaine). Taken together, these studies reveal a pattern of hypo-reactivity to prolonged stress exposure. Such dampened responses may reflect allostatic adaptations to chronic adversity.

Unfortunately, the direction of biological adaptations to stress is not consistent across studies, and chronic hyperactivation is also a common pattern (e.g., Sanchez et al., 2010). This may be because measurements are affected by the time of day the assessments are administered, the length of time post-stressor, the nature of the stressor, the developmental timing of adversity, the genetic vulnerabilities of the stress-exposed individual, the contextual factors that either exacerbate or buffer against adversity, and the measure of "reactivity" itself (see Cicchetti, Rogosch, Gunnar, & Toth, 2010). Furthermore, child temperament can also affect the direction of biological responses to adversity. In one study, toddlers were coded as either inhibited/vigilant (i.e., "doves") or bold/aggressive (i.e., "hawks"; Davies, Sturge-Apple, & Cicchetti, 2011).

For dove children, interparental aggression predicted greater cortisol reactivity over a 1-year period. Conversely, hawk children showed diminished cortisol reactivity over the year. Dove children also showed increased internalizing symptoms but decreases in attention/hyperactivity problems whereas hawk children were more likely to develop problems with attention/hyperactivity.

Thus, the research linking stress exposure to stress reactivity and then to subsequent health problems paints a complicated developmental picture. Although several unifying theories are beginning to emerge (e.g., Miller et al., 2007), a life span theory is premature due to inconsistencies in the definition and measurement of key constructs, differences in samples, and a paucity of life span longitudinal studies. The research reviewed here suggests a developmental trajectory in which high reactivity can confer risk or benefit depending upon both infant temperament and the environmental context (Boyce & Ellis, 2005; Davies et al., 2011). At typical levels of adversity, there appears to be a linear relation with health outcomes—higher reactivity often predicts greater health risk. At either end of the distribution, however, the findings are less consistent. Youth who have been exposed to extreme adversity often show a down-regulation across biological measures of reactivity, which may be due to hypervigilance or orienting (which lowers heart rate; Porges, 1995), or it could be due to the nature of laboratory stress paradigms, which are often mild when compared with the stressors of daily life. In contrast, youth raised in exceptionally protective environments may show high reactivity to laboratory stressors. However, this reactivity could show no relation or a negative association with health problems (Boyce et al., 1995). It is clear that researchers will need to examine the moderating effects of temperament on reactivity for youth raised in both high- and low-risk environments.

Stress Recovery

Stress recovery typically refers to (1) emotional or physiological arousal immediately following stress exposure, or (2) the length time required for a person to return to a baseline emotional or physiological state. Researchers examining stress processes among adults have argued that effective recovery from a stressful event is important for health and well-being (Brosschot, Gerin, & Thayer, 2006; Schwartz et al., 2003). Indeed, rapid physiological recovery is presumed to mark adaptive strategies for energy conservation when an active response to a stimulus is no longer required. Following acute stress, parasympathetic nervous system (PNS) activity can facilitate cardiac recovery via inhibitory inputs to the heart (e.g., Porges, 2001). Thus, researchers often describe increases in PNS activity (measured peripherally as respiratory sinus arrhythmia; RSA) as one index of effective physiological recovery.

Some researchers have broadened the construct of recovery to include both stress anticipation (i.e., worry) and response (i.e., rumination; Brosschot, Pieper, & Thayer, 2005). From this perspective, poor recovery is better conceptualized as an inability to achieve optimal physiological functioning, even when not engaging with a stressor. This concept is consistent with the literature on allostatic load—chronic exposure to stress fundamentally alters the set point for physiological responses, affecting both baseline and recovery levels. However, this poses a challenge for measuring poor recovery, which is often operationalized as post-task change from baseline (i.e., delta).

Relative to stress reactivity, recovery has received less attention in the developmental literature (Santucci et al., 2008). This may be due to the inherent limitations of laboratory assessments, in which stressors are necessarily mild and recovery, therefore, tends not differ from baseline levels (Crowell et al., 2005; Evans & Kim, 2007). However, some studies support the theory that rapid physiological recovery is associated with resiliency during stress. For example, children with higher time-one RSA (ages 4–5) showed greater reactivity to maternal criticism at time-two (age 8) but a faster recovery (Gottman & Katz, 2002). These children also scored higher on mother-reports of their ability to down-regulate negative emotion. Thus, higher baseline RSA and faster physiological recovery appear to be associated with more effective and rapid self-soothing.

The developmental literature would benefit from a greater focus on stress recovery. Although there are relatively few reports of poor physiological recovery among children, the adult literature may generalize to adolescents. In one meta-analysis of cortisol recovery among adults, there were very few tasks that produced lasting cortisol elevations (Dickerson & Kemeny, 2004). Indeed, only the uncontrollable, social-evaluative stressors were associated with persistent cortisol elevations up to 60 min post-stressor. Other tasks showed a return to baseline levels by 21–40 min after the stressor. Studies with adolescents that have used social-evaluative stress have not found a consistent pattern characterized by a slow return to baseline (see Westenberg et al., 2009, p. for a review). This may be due to strong physiological anticipation effects or developmental differences between adolescents and adults. The prefrontal cortex reaches maturation late in adolescence or early adulthood (e.g., Toga, Thompson, & Sowell, 2006). Because maturation of the prefrontal cortex results in enhanced self-regulation of feelings (e.g., through increased use of verbalization) and the ability to exercise inhibitory cognitive and behavioral control (Diamond & Aspinwall, 2003), brain development may contribute to observed differences in stress recovery.

Stress Restoration

Restoration refers to the collection of processes that operate to "refresh, buttress, and repair various forms of cellular damage" and to return a true baseline level of physiologic activity (Cacioppo & Berntson, 2007). Frequent exposure to stress may actually impede the restoration process, particularly sleep, resulting in decreased ability to cope (Leffert & Petersen, 1996; Petersen, Kennedy, & Sullivan, 1991). Without adequate restoration, the adolescent is ill prepared to face the task-demands of school, extracurricular activities, and maintaining key relationships.

The need for rest and restoration appears to increase during adolescence, as this developmental stage is associated with higher metabolic activity and appetitive drive (Ganji & Betts, 1995; Post & Kemper, 1993). Despite growth and increased nutritional demands, adolescents tend to sleep *less*, as indicated by both total time spent sleeping (Levy, Gray-Donald, Leech, Zvagulis, & Pless, 1986) and time spent in slow wave, restorative sleep (Dahl & Lewin, 2002). Adolescents also exhibit delays in sleep phase (i.e., going to bed and waking later than other age groups). These changes in sleep patterns are often at odds with socio-educational demands for both early-morning and evening activities (Carskadon, Vieira, & Acebo, 1993).

A thorough review of sleep and recovery during adolescence is beyond the scope of this review. However, sleep deprivation among adolescents has a profound negative effect on behavioral, emotional, and attentional control (Dahl & Lewin, 2002). Poor sleep quality is associated with a compromised ability to identify facial emotion expressions in a laboratory task (Soffer-Dudek, Sadeh, Dahl, & Rosenblat-Stein, 2011). Sleep problems among adolescents are also related to psychopathology, suicidal ideation, self-harm behaviors, and suicide attempts (Liu & Buysse, 2006; Wong, Brower, & Zucker, 2009). Researchers have also found that adolescent insomnia predicts depression in young adulthood (Baglioni et al., 2011). As with the other stress component processes, individual differences stress restoration—the extent to which an adolescent obtains adequate sleep in the face of stressful circumstances—can be considered an indicator of resilience.

The Effects of Stress on Emotion Regulation and Resilience

Children who face chronic adversity often show delays across multiple markers of self-regulation (Curtis & Cicchetti, 2003), including emotion regulation (e.g., proactive coping, altering affective responses to meet situational demands, emotional awareness, and other skills; see Gratz & Roemer, 2004). In a sample of extremely impoverished youth, those who were categorized as resilient (lower externalizing/internalizing problems and higher functioning) also had experienced fewer uncontrollable negative life events, scored lower on chronic strain (e.g., hunger, cold, danger), were less likely to have a history of abuse, and had higher self-esteem, better parental monitoring, and greater self-regulation skills (Buckner et al., 2003). In turn, better self-regulation skills predicted the use of proactive coping strategies in response to controllable and uncontrollable stress scenarios (Buckner, Mezzacappa, & Beardslee, 2009).

This line of research raises interesting questions about stress, resilience, and emotion regulation. Although resilient and non-resilient children were similar across many variables—level of poverty, single or dual parent household, sex, race, IQ, and history of homelessness—there were clear differences in both the quantity and quality of stressors (Buckner et al., 2003, 2009). It appears as though resilient children were buffered against chronic stress, in part, by a parent whose functioning was less impaired. Even in the face of extreme poverty, children fared better when parent(s) were vigilant and not abusive. One hypothesis is that such parents can serve as more effective sources of emotional co-regulation, which may promote a developmental pathway characterized by healthier peer relationships, better coping, lower impulsivity, and more adaptive emotion regulation strategies (Hughes et al., 2012). Unfortunately, these researchers did not assess physiological or neuroendocrine markers of stress reactivity. If they had, it would be possible to evaluate how stress reactivity relates to resilience and whether temperament or gene-environment correlations account for the relations between better parenting, less stress exposure, lower reactivity, and resilient outcomes.

Emotion Regulation, Resilience, and Adolescent Health

Adolescence is a period characterized by profound life changes. For many youth, the teenage years are characterized by higher rates of both interpersonal and uncontrollable stressors. However, there is substantial variability in the experience of stress. For example, adolescents vary in the type, frequency, and duration of stressful events, and in their perceptions of adverse events. As we have highlighted in this chapter, it is not possible to consider stress exposure without also attending to the contextual and interpersonal factors that shape emotion regulation and resilience. Factors such as temperament, family context, and the quantity/quality of stress exposures may affect which adolescents are resilient in the face of adversity and which will go on to develop lasting psychological and health problems.

Over the past several decades, resilience research has become more sophisticated. Whereas resilience was once defined as a constellation of impressive character strengths, the construct is now viewed as complex, transactional, and context-dependent. Increasingly, scientists have come to view resiliency, in one or more domains, as an achievable goal for many youth. Yet there are obstacles to achieving this goal. Childhood trauma can be quite different from the stressors that many adults face. For many youth, stressors occur within the most important attachment relationships. Furthermore, adversity in childhood is nearly always chronic, which means that few children are able to achieve adequate restoration between negative life events.

As highlighted above, future research on resilience would benefit from a thorough evaluation of child temperament, contextual factors, and biological assessments of stress reactivity, recovery, and restoration. Ideally, such research will follow children into adolescence and beyond, establishing key biological vulnerabilities early in the course of development and assessing biological adaptations to extreme adversity. Allostatic adaptations to stress—both behavioral and physiological—are often adaptive within high-risk contexts, while also contributing to psychopathology, morbidity, and early mortality. Ultimately interventions that reduce strain on care-providers have the potential to increase resiliency, self-regulation, and health among children and adolescents.

References

Adrian, M., Zeman, J., & Veits, G. (2011). Methodological implications of the affect revolution: A 35-year review of emotion regulation assessment in children. *Journal of Experimental Child Psychology, 110*, 171–197.

Baglioni, C., Battagliese, G., Feige, B., Spiegelhalder, K., Nissen, C., Voderholzer, U., et al. (2011). Insomnia as a predictor of depression: A meta-analytic evaluation of longitudinal epidemiological studies. *Journal of Affective Disorders, 135*, 10–19.

Beauchaine, T. P., Gatzke-Kopp, L., & Mead, H. K. (2007). Polyvagal theory and developmental psychopathology: Emotion dysregulation and conduct problems from preschool to adolescence. *Biological Psychology, 74*, 174–184.

Beauchaine, T. P., Neuhaus, E., Zalewski, M., Crowell, S. E., & Potapova, N. (2011). The effects of allostatic load on neural systems subserving motivation, mood regulation, and social affiliation. *Development and Psychopathology, 23*, 975–999.

Boyce, W. T., Chesney, M., Alkon, A., Tschann, J. M., Adams, S., Chesterman, B., et al. (1995). Psychobiologic reactivity to stress and childhood respiratory illnesses: Results of two prospective studies. *Psychosomatic Medicine, 57*, 411–422.

Boyce, W. T., & Ellis, B. J. (2005). Biological sensitivity to context: I. An evolutionary-developmental theory of the origins and functions of stress reactivity. *Development and Psychopathology, 17*, 271–301.

Brosschot, J. F., Gerin, W., & Thayer, J. F. (2006). The perseverative cognition hypothesis: A review of worry, prolonged stress-related physiological activation, and health. *Journal of Psychosomatic Research, 60*, 113–124.

Brosschot, J. F., Pieper, S., & Thayer, J. F. (2005). Expanding stress theory: Prolonged activation and perseverative cognition. *Psychoneuroendocrinology, 30*, 1043–1049.

Buckner, J. C., Mezzacappa, E., & Beardslee, W. R. (2003). Characteristics of resilient youths living in poverty: The role of self-regulatory processes. *Development and Psychopathology, 15*, 139–162.

Buckner, J. C., Mezzacappa, E., & Beardslee, W. R. (2009). Self-regulation and its relations to adaptive functioning in low income youths. *American Journal of Orthopsychiatry, 79*, 19–30.

Cacioppo, J. T., & Berntson, G. G. (2007). The brain, homeostasis, and health: Balancing demands of the internal and external milieu. In H. S. Friedman & R. C. Silver (Eds.), *Foundations of health psychology* (pp. 73–91). New York: Oxford University Press.

Carskadon, M. A., Vieira, C., & Acebo, C. (1993). Association between puberty and delayed phase preference. *Sleep, 16*, 258–262.

Charney, D. S. (2004). Psychobiological mechanisms of resilience and vulnerability: Implications for successful adaptation to extreme stress. *Focus, 2*, 368–391.

Cicchetti, D., & Blender, J. A. (2006). A multiple-levels-of-analysis perspective on resilience. *Annals of the New York Academy of Sciences, 1094*, 248–258.

Cicchetti, D., & Rogosch, F. A. (2002). A developmental psychopathology perspective on adolescence. *Journal of Consulting and Clinical Psychology, 70*, 6–20.

Cicchetti, D., Rogosch, F. A., Gunnar, M. R., & Toth, S. L. (2010). The differential impacts of early physical and sexual abuse and internalizing problems on daytime cortisol rhythm in school-aged children. *Child Development, 81*, 252–269.

Clarke, A. (2006). Coping with interpersonal stress and psychosocial health among children and adolescents: A meta-analysis. *Journal of Youth and Adolescence, 35*, 10–23.

Coan, J. A. (2008). Toward a neuroscience of attachment. In J. Cassidy & P. R. Shaver (Eds.), *Handbook of attachment: Theory, research and clinical applications* (2nd ed., pp. 241–264). The Guilford Press, New York, NY.

Coan, J. A. (2010). Adult attachment and the brain. *Journal of Social and Personal Relationships, 27*, 210–217.

Cole, P. M., & Hall, S. E. (2008). Emotion dysregulation as a risk factor for psychopathology. In T. P. Beauchaine & S. P. Hinshaw (Eds.), *Child and adolescent psychopathology* (pp. 265–299). Hoboken, NJ: Wiley.

Cole, P. M., Martin, S. E., & Dennis, T. A. (2004). Emotion regulation as a scientific construct: Methodological challenges and directions for child development research. *Child Development, 75*, 317–333.

Cole, P. M., Michel, M. K., & Teti, L. O. D. (1994). The development of emotion regulation and dysregulation: A clinical perspective. *Monographs of the Society for Research in Child Development, 59*, 73–100.

Covington, H., & Miczek, K. (2005). Intense cocaine self-administration after episodic social defeat stress, but not after aggressive behavior: Dissociation from corticosterone activation. *Psychopharmacology, 183*, 331–340.

Crowell, S. E., Beauchaine, T. P., McCauley, E., Smith, C., Stevens, A. L., & Sylvers, P. D. (2005). Psychological, physiological, and serotonergic correlates of parasuicidal behavior among adolescent girls. *Development and Psychopathology, 17*, 1105–1127.

Crowell, S. E., Beauchaine, T. P., McCauley, E., Smith, C., Vasilev, C., & Stevens, A. L. (2008). Parent-child interactions, peripheral serotonin, and intentional self-injury in adolescents. *Journal of Consulting and Clinical Psychology, 76*, 15–21.

Curtis, W. J., & Cicchetti, D. (2003). Moving research on resilience into the 21st century: Theoretical and methodological considerations in examining the biological contributors to resilience. *Development and Psychopathology, 15*, 773–810.

Dahl, R. E., & Lewin, D. S. (2002). Pathways to adolescent health sleep regulation and behavior. *Journal of Adolescent Health, 31*, 175–184.

Davidson, R. J. (2000). Affective style, psychopathology, and resilience: Brain mechanisms and plasticity. *American Psychologist, 55*, 1196–1214.
Davies, P. T., Sturge-Apple, M. L., & Cicchetti, D. (2011). Interparental aggression and children's adrenocortical reactivity: Testing an evolutionary model of allostatic load. *Development and Psychopathology, 23*, 801–814.
de Kloet, E. R., Joels, M., & Holsboer, F. (2005). Stress and the brain: From adaptation to disease. *Nature Reviews Neuroscience, 6*, 463–475.
Deater-Deckard, K., & Petrill, S. A. (2004). Parent–child dyadic mutuality and child behavior problems: An investigation of gene–environment processes. *Journal of Child Psychology and Psychiatry, 45*, 1171–1179.
Diamond, L. M. (2001). Contributions of psychophysiology to research on adult attachment: Review and recommendations. *Personality and Social Psychology Review, 5*, 276–295.
Diamond, L. M., & Aspinwall, L. G. (2003). Emotion regulation across the life span: An integrative perspective emphasizing self-regulation, positive affect, and dyadic processes. *Motivation and Emotion, 27*, 125–156.
Dickerson, S. S., & Kemeny, M. E. (2004). Acute stressors and cortisol responses: A theoretical integration and synthesis of laboratory research. *Psychological Bulletin, 130*, 355–391.
Eaton, D. K., Kann, L., Kinchen, S., Shanklin, S., Ross, J., Hawkins, J., et al. (2008). Youth risk behavior surveillance—United States, 2007. *MMWR Surveillance Summaries, 57*, 1–131.
Ekman, P. (1992). An argument for basic emotions. *Cognition and Emotion, 6*, 169–200.
Ekman, P., & Friesen, W. V. (1976). Measuring facial movement. *Environmental Psychology and Nonverbal Behavior, 1*, 56–75.
Evans, G. W., & Kim, P. (2007). Childhood poverty and health. *Psychological Science, 18*, 953–957.
Fosco, G. M., & Grych, J. H. (2008). Emotional, cognitive, and family systems mediators of children's adjustment to interparental conflict. *Journal of Family Psychology, 22*, 843–854.
Ganji, V., & Betts, N. (1995). Fat, cholesterol, fiber and sodium intakes of US population: Evaluation of diets reported in 1987–1988 Nationwide Food Consumption Survey. *European Journal of Clinical Nutrition, 49*, 915–920.
Gatzke-Kopp, L. M. (2011). The canary in the coalmine: The sensitivity of mesolimbic dopamine to environmental adversity during development. *Neuroscience and Biobehavioral Reviews, 35*, 794–803.
Goldsmith, H. H., & Davidson, R. J. (2004). Disambiguating the components of emotion regulation. *Child Development, 75*, 361–365.
Gottman, J. M., & Katz, L. F. (2002). Children's emotional reactions to stressful parent-child interactions: The link between emotion regulation and vagal tone. *Marriage and Family Review, 34*, 265–283.
Gratz, K. L., & Roemer, L. (2004). Multidimensional assessment of emotion regulation and dysregulation: Development, factor structure, and initial validation of the difficulties in emotion regulation scale. *Journal of Psychopathology and Behavioral Assessment, 26*, 41–54.
Gross, J. J. (1998a). Antecedent- and response-focused emotion regulation: Divergent consequences for experience, expression, and physiology. *Journal of Personality and Social Psychology, 74*, 224–237.
Gross, J. J. (1998b). The emerging field of emotion regulation: An integrative review. *Review of General Psychology, 2*, 271–299.
Gross, J. J. (2007). *Handbook of emotion regulation*. New York: Guilford Press.
Guerra, N. G. (1997). Intervening to prevent childhood aggression in the inner city. In J. McCord (Ed.), *Violence and childhood in the inner city* (pp. 256–312). New York: Cambridge University Press.
Gunnar, M. R., Tout, K., de Haan, M., Pierce, S., & Stanbury, K. (1997). Temperament, social competence, and adrenocortical activity in preschoolers. *Developmental Psychobiology, 31*, 65–85.
Hammen, C. (1991). Generation of stress in the course of unipolar depression. *Journal of Abnormal Psychology, 100*, 555–561.
Hammen, C. (2005). Stress and depression. *Annual Review of Clinical Psychology, 1*, 293–319.
Hawkley, L. C., & Cacioppo, J. T. (2003). Loneliness and pathways to disease. *Brain, Behavior, and Immunity, 17*, 98–105.
Hilt, L. M., Cha, C. B., & Nolen-Hoeksema, S. (2008). Nonsuicidal self-injury in young adolescent girls: Moderators of the distress-function relationship. *Journal of Consulting and Clinical Psychology, 76*, 63–71.
Hughes, A. E., Crowell, S. E., Uyeji, L., & Coan, J. A. (2012). A developmental neuroscience of borderline pathology: Emotion dysregulation and social baseline theory. *Journal of Abnormal Child Psychology, 40*, 21–33.
Hyman, S. E. (2009). How adversity gets under the skin. *Nature Neuroscience, 12*, 241–243.
John, O. P., & Gross, J. J. (2007). Individual differences in emotion regulation. In J. J. Gross (Ed.), *Handbook of emotion regulation* (pp. 351–372). New York: The Guilford Press.
Johnson, J. G., Cohen, P., Gould, M. S., Kasen, S., Brown, J., & Brook, J. S. (2002). Childhood adversities, interpersonal difficulties, and risk for suicide attempts during late adolescence and early adulthood. *Archives of General Psychiatry, 59*, 741–749.
Leffert, N., & Petersen, A. C. (1996). Biology, challenge, and coping in adolescence: Effects on physical and mental health. In M. H. Bornstein & J. L. Genevro (Eds.), *Child development and behavioral pediatrics* (pp. 129–154). Mahwah, NJ: Lawrence Erlbaum and Associates.
Levy, D., Gray-Donald, K., Leech, J., Zvagulis, I., & Pless, I. B. (1986). Sleep patterns and problems in adolescents. *Journal of Adolescent Health Care, 7*, 386–389.

Liu, X., & Buysse, D. J. (2006). Sleep and youth suicidal behavior: A neglected field. *Current Opinion in Psychiatry, 19*, 288–293.

Loman, M. M., & Gunnar, M. R. (2010). Early experience and the development of stress reactivity and regulation in children. *Neuroscience and Biobehavioral Reviews, 34*, 867–876.

Lupien, S. J., Ouellet-Morin, I., Hupbach, A., Tu, M. T., Buss, C., Walker, D., et al. (2006). Beyond the stress concept: Allostatic load—a developmental biological and cognitive perspective. In D. Cicchetti & D. J. Cohen (Eds.), *Developmental psychopathology, Vol 2: Developmental neuroscience* (2nd ed., pp. 578–628). Hoboken, NJ: Wiley.

Luthar, S. S., Cicchetti, D., & Becker, B. (2000). The construct of resilience: A critical evaluation and guidelines for future work. *Child Development, 71*, 543–562.

Masten, A. S. (2001). Ordinary magic: Resilience processes in development. *American Psychologist, 56*, 227–238.

Masten, A. S. (2004). Regulatory processes, risk, and resilience in adolescent development. *Annals of the New York Academy of Sciences, 1021*, 310–319.

Masten, A. S., & Coatsworth, J. D. (1995). Competence, resilience, and psychopathology. In D. Cicchetti & D. Cohen (Eds.), *Developmental psychopathology* (Risk, disorder, and adaptation, Vol. 2, pp. 715–752). New York: Wiley.

McEwen, B. S. (1998). Stress, adaptation, and disease: Allostasis and allostatic load. *Annals of the New York Academy of Sciences, 840*, 33–44.

Mead, H. K., Beauchaine, T. P., & Shannon, K. E. (2010). Neurobiological adaptations to violence across development. *Development and Psychopathology, 22*, 1–22.

Meaney, M. J., Brake, W., & Gratton, A. (2002). Environmental regulation of the development of mesolimbic dopamine systems: A neurobiological mechanism for vulnerability to drug abuse? *Psychoneuroendocrinology, 27*, 127–138.

Miller, G. E., Chen, E., & Zhou, E. S. (2007). If it goes up, must it come down? Chronic stress and the hypothalamic-pituitary-adrenocortical axis in humans. *Psychological Bulletin, 133*, 25–45.

Morilak, D. A., Barrera, G., Echevarria, D. J., Garcia, A. S., Hernandez, A., Ma, S., et al. (2005). Role of brain norepinephrine in the behavioral response to stress. *Progress in Neuro-Psychopharmacology and Biological Psychiatry, 29*, 1214–1224.

National Center for Injury Prevention and Control. (2009). *CDC Injury Research Agenda, 2009–2018*. Retrieved from http://www.cdc.gov/injury/ResearchAgenda/index.html

Nelson, C. A. (2007). A neurobiological perspective on early human deprivation. *Child Development Perspectives, 1*, 13–18.

Oshri, A., Rogosch, F. A., Burnette, M. L., & Cicchetti, D. (2011). Developmental pathways to adolescent cannabis abuse and dependence: Child maltreatment, emerging personality, and internalizing versus externalizing psychopathology. *Psychology of Addictive Behaviors, 25*, 634–644.

Paus, T., Keshavan, M., & Giedd, J. N. (2008). Why do many psychiatric disorders emerge during adolescence? *Nature Reviews Neuroscience, 9*, 947–957.

Petersen, A. C., Kennedy, R. E., & Sullivan, P. (1991). Coping with adolescence. In M. E. Colten & S. Gore (Eds.), *Adolescent stress: Causes and consequences* (pp. 93–110). New York: Aldine de Gruyter.

Porges, S. W. (1995). Orienting in a defensive world: Mammalian modifications of our evolutionary heritage. A polyvagal theory. *Psychophysiology, 32*, 301–318.

Porges, S. W. (2001). The polyvagal theory: Phylogenetic substrates of a social nervous system. *International Journal of Psychophysiology, 42*, 123–146.

Post, G. B., & Kemper, H. C. (1993). Nutrient intake and biological maturation during adolescence. The Amsterdam growth and health longitudinal study. *European Journal of Clinical Nutrition, 47*, 400–408.

Sanchez, M. M., Mccormack, K., Grand, A. P., Fulks, R., Graff, A., & Maestripieri, D. (2010). Effects of sex and early maternal abuse on adrenocorticotropin hormone and cortisol responses to the corticotropin-releasing hormone challenge during the first 3 years of life in group-living rhesus monkeys. *Development and Psychopathology, 22*, 45–53.

Santucci, A. K., Silk, J. S., Shaw, D. S., Gentzler, A., Fox, N. A., & Kovacs, M. (2008). Vagal tone and temperament as predictors of emotion regulation strategies in young children. *Developmental Psychobiology, 50*, 205–216.

Schore, A. N. (2001). The effects of early relational trauma on right brain development, affect regulation, and infant mental health. *Infant Mental Health Journal, 22*, 201–269.

Schwartz, A. R., Gerin, W., Davidson, K. W., Pickering, T. G., Brosschot, J. F., Thayer, J. F., et al. (2003). Toward a causal model of cardiovascular responses to stress and the development of cardiovascular disease. *Psychosomatic Medicine, 65*, 22–35.

Shannon, K. E., Beauchaine, T. P., Brenner, S. L., Neuhaus, E., & Gatzke-Kopp, L. (2007). Familial and temperamental predictors of resilience in children at risk for conduct disorder and depression. *Development and Psychopathology, 19*, 701–727.

Soffer-Dudek, N., Sadeh, A., Dahl, R. E., & Rosenblat-Stein, S. (2011). Poor sleep quality predicts deficient emotion information processing over time in early adolescence. *Sleep, 34*, 1499–1508.

Sroufe, L. A., Duggal, S., Weinfield, N., & Carlson, E. (2000). Relationships, development, and psychopathology. In A. J. Sameroff, M. Lewis, & S. M. Miller (Eds.), *Handbook of developmental psychopathology* (2nd ed., pp. 57–74). New York: Kluwer Academic.

Sterling, P., & Eyer, J. (1988). Allostasis: A new paradigm to explain arousal pathology. In S. Fisher & J. Reason (Eds.), *Handbook of life stress, cognition and health* (pp. 629–649). Oxford, England: Wiley.

Susman, E. J. (2006). Psychobiology of persistent antisocial behavior: Stress, early vulnerabilities and the attenuation hypothesis. *Neuroscience and Biobehavioral Reviews, 30*, 376–389.

Toga, A. W., Thompson, P. M., & Sowell, E. R. (2006). Mapping brain maturation. *Trends in Neurosciences, 29*, 148–159.

Uchino, B. N., Smith, T. W., Holt-Lunstead, J., Campo, R. A., & Reblin, M. (2007). Stress and illness. In J. T. Cacioppo, L. G. Tassinary, & G. G. Berntson (Eds.), *Handbook of psychophysiology* (pp. 608–632). New York: Cambridge University Press.

Weaver, I. C. G., Cervoni, N., Champagne, F. A., D'Alessio, A. C., Sharma, S., Seckl, J. R., et al. (2004). Epigenetic programming by maternal behavior. *Nature Neuroscience, 7*, 847–854.

Westenberg, P. M., Bokhorst, C. L., Miers, A. C., Sumter, S. R., Kallen, V. L., van Pelt, J., et al. (2009). A prepared speech in front of a pre-recorded audience: Subjective, physiological, and neuroendocrine responses to the Leiden Public Speaking Task. *Biological Psychology, 82*, 116–124.

Williams, P. G., Smith, T. W., Gunn, H. E., & Uchino, B. N. (2010). Personality and stress: Individual differences in exposure, reactivity, recovery, and restoration. In R. Contrada & A. Baum (Eds.), *Handbook of stress science: Biology, psychology, and health* (pp. 231–245). New York: Springer.

Wong, M. M., Brower, K. J., & Zucker, R. A. (2009). Childhood sleep problems, early onset of substance use and behavioral problems in adolescence. *Sleep Medicine, 10*, 787–796.

Health Literacy, Mental Health, and Adolescents

Jennifer A. Manganello, Tetine Sentell, and Terry C. Davis

Introduction

Health literacy is a growing field with a continuously expanding body of research and a growing number of practice and policy guidelines (Wolf et al., 2009).[1] Given the increasing attention to this topic, it is surprising that there has been little research focused on adolescents (Manganello, 2008). There is also limited research in the USA about health literacy and mental health. This chapter will address the intersection of health literacy and mental health, including mental health literacy, with a focus on adolescents. We will give a summary of definitions of health literacy and mental health literacy, and provide a brief overview of research that has focused on both health literacy, including its relationship to mental health outcomes, and mental health literacy. We will highlight research in these areas that has been conducted with adolescents, and propose ideas for future work.

Health Literacy

Definitions

Health literacy is commonly defined as "the degree to which individuals have the capacity to obtain, process, and understand basic health information and services needed to make appropriate health decisions" (Ratzan & Parker, 2000). More recently, there has been a shift to also focus on the demands of health information and services. A newer definition states that health literacy is when "the skills and ability of those requiring health information and services are aligned with the demand and complexity of information and services" (p. 28) (Parker & Ratzan, 2010).[2] This approach emphasizes that information and services provided by various sources should be easily understandable, "accurate, and actionable" (p. 1) (U.S. Department of Health and Human Services, 2010). This is especially important given that the National Action Plan states that "nearly 9 out of 10 adults have difficulty

[1] A detailed overview of the history of research and policy related to health literacy can be found in Parker and Ratzan (2010) (Parker & Ratzan, 2010).

[2] Two papers provide a useful discussion of health literacy definitions (Berkman, Davis, & McCormack, 2010; Peerson & Saunders, 2009).

J.A. Manganello, Ph.D., M.P.H. (✉)
Department of Health Policy, Management and Behavior, University at Albany School of Public Health, One University Place, #165, Rensselaer, NY 12144, USA
e-mail: jmanganello@albany.edu

T. Sentell, Ph.D.
Office of Public Health Studies, University of Hawai'i at Manoa, 1960 East-West Road, Biomed D104G, Honolulu, HI 96822, USA

T.C. Davis, Ph.D.
Departments of Medicine and Pediatrics, Louisiana State University Health Sciences Center-Shreveport, 1501 Kings Highway, Shreveport, LA 71130, USA

W.T. O'Donohue et al. (eds.), *Handbook of Adolescent Health Psychology*,
DOI 10.1007/978-1-4614-6633-8_10, © Springer Science+Business Media New York 2013

using the everyday health information that is routinely available in our health care facilities, retail outlets, media, and communities" (p. 1) (U.S. Department of Health and Human Services, 2010).

Summary of Knowledge

Health literacy research has assessed health literacy skills, studied the relationship of health literacy with service use and health outcomes, investigated measurement options, and evaluated services, programs, and health information materials. Regarding research related to prevalence, many adults in the USA lack the health literacy skills needed to function in a complex health care system. Assessment of health literacy skills varies based on the population studied and instruments used to measure health literacy, but in general, "limited health literacy affects people of all ages, races, incomes, and education levels" (p. 1) (U.S. Department of Health and Human Services, 2010). A useful estimate comes from the 2003 National Assessment of Health Literacy, which found that 36 % of adults have limited health literacy (*basic* or *below basic* health literacy levels) (Kutner, Greenberg, Jin, & Paulsen, 2006). Rates of low health literacy are higher for minorities, people over 65, those with less than a GED or high school diploma, and individuals living below the poverty level (Kutner et al., 2006). Studies specific to mental health settings have found a high prevalence of low literacy among patients in a "psychiatric emergency service" (Currier, Sitzman, & Trenton, 2001) and in an "indigent psychiatric population" (Christensen & Grace, 1999).

For adolescents, the prevalence of low health literacy is not as well understood as that of adults. In one study, 46 % of adolescents ages 10–19 from clinics, schools, and summer programs in North Carolina and Louisiana were reading below grade level (Davis et al., 2006). Although little research has quantified health literacy levels for adolescents, education research suggests high rates of low literacy in general among US school children. For instance, the 2009 National Assessment of Educational Progress (NAEP) found that only 38 % of twelfth graders and 32 % of eighth graders read proficiently at grade level (National Center for Education Statistics, 2009). Black and Hispanic students had an increased likelihood of poor reading skills compared to other groups including Whites and Asians, as did students from city, town, or rural environments compared to those from suburban environments (National Center for Education Statistics, 2009).

Apart from studying prevalence, there has been an increasing focus on the impact of low health literacy on outcomes. Studies have found health literacy is associated with a variety of negative health outcomes, with a recent review of the literature (95 articles) stating that "differences in health literacy level were consistently associated with increased hospitalizations, greater emergency care use, lower use of mammography, lower receipt of influenza vaccine, poorer ability to demonstrate taking medications appropriately, poorer ability to interpret labels and health messages, and, among seniors, poorer overall health status and higher mortality" (p.v.) (Berkman et al., 2011).

While there has been wide agreement that low health literacy has a negative impact on health outcomes for adults, there is limited research concerning health literacy and youth outcomes, both for adolescents and children (Manganello, 2008; Sanders et al., 2009). A growing body of literature has focused on the health literacy of parents, especially those with small children, with findings suggesting that "low caregiver literacy is common and is associated with poor preventive care behaviors and poor child health outcomes" (p. 131) (Sanders et al., 2009). While parents play a significant role in the health care of adolescents, this age group differs from children in that they are beginning to make their own choices about health behaviors and can be more involved with treatment, communicate directly with providers, and administer their own medication.

Regardless of age group, less research has considered the impact of health literacy on mental health outcomes compared to physical health outcomes in the USA (Lincoln et al., 2006). Only ten journal articles were identified in a recent review of health literacy research (Berkman et al., 2011), and findings to date are mixed. Some studies have found that low literacy is associated with greater depression symptoms (Berkman et al., 2011; Lincoln et al., 2006), while others have not observed an association (Berkman et al., 2011). For example, In a sample of Medicare enrollees, Gazmararian found the association of low health literacy and depression went away when controlling for health status (Gazmarian, Baker, Parker, & Blazer, 2000). Other research suggests there is a link between low health literacy and psychiatric disorders (Lincoln, 2008) and poor mental health (Wolf, Gazmararian, & Baker, 2005). Sentell and Shumway (2003) showed that literacy was independently associated with mental health status in a national sample (Sentell & Shumway, 2003). One report using education level as a predictor found that people with more education were more likely to use behavioral health services (Smith, Armstrong, & Davis, 2006), and were less likely to have acute care visits.

Another area of health literacy research includes the study of measurement. Multiple tools can assess literacy skills specific to medical settings, including the Rapid Estimate of Adult Literacy in Medicine (REALM) (Davis et al., 1993), the Test of Functional Health Literacy in Adults (TOFHLA) (Parker, Baker, Williams, & Nurss, 1995), and the Newest Vital Sign (NVS) (Weiss et al., 2005). Tools that have been validated with adolescents include the REALM-Teen (Davis et al., 2006), TOFHLA (Chisolm & Buchanan, 2007), and one based on comprehension of health information provided in passages (Wu et al., 2010). The measurement of health literacy is a particularly active area of research in this field with a number of tools currently in development.[3]

Research related to interventions has also been conducted, although there is a need for more work in this area (U.S. Department of Health and Human Services, 2010), especially with adolescents. The interventions to date have mainly focused on designing and testing materials and ways to make information easier to understand for those with low health literacy. Findings have been mixed, but some recommendations have resulted from the work, including the use of picture-based instructions (Berkman et al., 2011; U.S. Department of Health and Human Services, 2010). Additional interventions include the development and evaluation of programs designed to enhance health literacy skills for those with low health literacy (Berkman et al., 2011), redesigning materials for those with low literacy (Berkman et al., 2011; Pignone, DeWalt, Sheridan, Berkman, & Lohr, 2005), raising awareness of health literacy issues among providers (Kripalani & Weiss, 2006), improving provider communication (Connelly, 2007; Ferreira et al., 2005; Kripalani & Weiss, 2006), and making organizational changes (U.S. Department of Health and Human Services, 2010). However, little information about interventions for adolescent populations exists, with the exception of discussion of health education classes and school programs (Brey et al., 2007; St Leger, 2001).

Mental Health Literacy

Definitions

The term health literacy takes a general approach to understanding health information, and has been applied to a variety of health topics. However, in recent years, professionals have also developed terms that reflect specific skills related to subareas of health including nutrition (Zoellner, Connell, Bounds, Crook, & Yadrick, 2009) and oral health (Jones, Lee, & Rozier, 2007).

A specific definition for mental health literacy was published in 1997 by Anthony Jorm, who stated that mental health literacy is "the knowledge and beliefs about mental disorders which aid their recognition, management, or prevention" (p. 2) (Jorm et al., 1997). Jorm considered mental health literacy to include the ability to identify disorders, understand risk factors and causes of disorders, be familiar with both self and professional help that is available to treat disorders, to

[3]For more information on measurement, see a recent report from the Institute of Medicine (Hernandez, 2009).

know how to obtain information about mental health, and to have attitudes that lead a person to seek help if needed. Since then, a majority of the work related to mental health literacy has relied upon this definition.

Summary of Knowledge

Limited work has been done concerning mental health literacy in the USA for either adults or youth. A recent review identified only 12 studies of adults between the years of 1987 and 2007 (Cabassa, 2009). Studies related to youth are even less common. Coles and Coleman (2010), using Jorm's definition, studied undergraduate students in a psychology course. After reviewing a series of vignettes, fewer than half correctly identified panic disorder and generalized anxiety disorder, and there seemed to be a relationship between perception of cause of the disorder and whether help should be sought for that disorder (Coles & Coleman, 2010). Olsson and Kennedy (2010), using Jorm's definition, found students in Virginia in grades 6 through 12 ($n=281$) had difficulty identifying mental disorders, and those who reported they would seek help for treatment were more likely to be those who had an easier time identifying disorders (Olsson & Kennedy, 2010).

While little research on this topic has taken place in the USA, there has been considerable action around this work outside the USA, with research occurring most often in Australia (Jorm et al., 2006). However, mental health literacy research specifically focusing on adolescents even internationally is rare (Burns & Rapee, 2006). The handful of adolescent studies suggest that adolescents have mixed abilities to identify depression when reading vignettes ($N=202$, ages 15–17, Australia) (Burns & Rapee, 2006) and are unlikely to respond to a friend experiencing problems in a way that would assist them with getting treatment ($n=1,137$, school years 8–10, Australia) (Kelly, Jorm, & Rodgers, 2006). Some research has also found that girls have higher mental health literacy than boys (Burns & Rapee, 2006; Cotton, Wright, Harris, Jorm, & McGorry, 2006). For instance, a study of youth ($n=1,207$, ages 12–25, Australia) discovered that girls were more likely to recognize symptoms of depression when reading a vignette (although no differences were noted for the psychosis vignette) (Cotton et al., 2006). Much of the work done has focused on assessing rates and characteristics of mental health literacy, with a focus on recognition of symptoms and knowledge about treatment options, as opposed to studying the relationship between mental health literacy skills and outcomes.

Some work has established methods to measure mental health literacy. A majority of published studies have relied on providing vignettes with follow-up questions (Bapat, Jorm, & Lawrence, 2009; Coles & Coleman, 2010; Cotton et al., 2006; Lauber, Nordt, Falcato, & Rossler, 2003; Marie, Forsyth, & Miles, 2004), including the Mental Health Literacy Questionnaire (Jorm et al., 1997) and the Friend in Need Questionnaire (Burns & Rapee, 2006), while some have used self-report questions about attitudes, beliefs, and knowledge (Farrer, Leach, Griffiths, Christensen, & Jorm, 2008; Lauber et al., 2003). There do not appear to be any word recognition tests similar to those seen in the health literacy field, but work has been done to develop a 28-item scale to assess mental health literacy for caregivers of children with mental health problems (Smith et al., 2007).

Researchers have also examined interventions designed to enhance mental health literacy, with mass media campaigns being one of the main strategies studied that appear to be effective (Francis, Pirkis, Dunt, Blood, & Davis, 2002). School-based programs for adolescents have had some limited success, and programs for caregivers of people with mental illness have had some positive results (Francis et al., 2002). A literature review specific to adolescents and young adults provides an overview of intervention programs that have enhanced mental health literacy and recommends campaigns targeting entire communities as well as specific campaigns for adolescents, and school-based educational programs, as useful intervention options (Kelly, Jorm, & Wright, 2007). For example, an Australian depression program called *beyondblue* has a youth component called Ybblue. An evaluation of that program found that youth who were familiar with it were better able to identify depression symptoms and were more likely to rate professional treatment options as helpful (Morgan & Jorm, 2007). Also in Australia, a media campaign called The Compass Strategy targeting 12–25-year-olds was successful in increasing self-identified depression and addressing barriers related to seeking help (Wright, McGorry, Harris, Jorm, & Pennell, 2006). In another study of 472 secondary school students in England, researchers found that attitudes toward people with mental health problems became more positive after an education intervention involving educational workshops (Pinfold et al., 2003). They also found that female students and those students who knew someone with a mental illness were more likely to experience an attitude change (Pinfold et al., 2003). One USA study suggested that a program called *In Our Own Voice* did not increase mental health literacy for adolescents 1 week after the intervention, but did show an improvement at 4 and 8 weeks after the intervention (Pinto-Foltz, Logsdon, & Myers, 2011).

Implications for Adolescents

The existing literature suggests that both health literacy and mental health literacy have implications for the diagnosis and treatment of mental health issues for youth. First, low health literacy and low mental health literacy could impact the ability of adolescents and their parents to obtain reliable information about mental health. Knowing how to search for information, understanding information obtained, and assessing reliability and credibility of information are all critical to recognizing symptoms of mental health problems, when treatment should be sought, and what treatment options are available.

Less than a third of adolescents seek help for mental health issues (Gulliver, Griffiths, & Christensen, 2010). "The ability to correctly recognize mental disorders has been found to be associated with better help-seeking preferences in young people aged 12–25 years" (p. 359) (Scott & Chur-Hansen, 2008), suggesting that that mental health literacy, especially the ability to identify symptoms, can play an important role in whether youth seek treatment or not (Cotton et al., 2006). Low health literacy could also impact an individual's ability to access and navigate the mental health system, understand treatment options, and know whether or not one has insurance coverage and how it works. Recent studies suggest that enhancing mental health literacy can help youth seek treatment early (Kelly et al., 2007) and know how and where to access treatment (Burns & Rapee, 2006). Several barriers to seeking mental health treatment for adolescents were identified in a recent literature review of 22 studies from various countries including youth ages 12–25 (Gulliver et al., 2010). Stigma was the most significant barrier adolescents faced in seeking mental health care, a barrier that has been identified in much of the literature on adults as well (Barney, Griffiths, Jorm, & Christensen, 2006; Gorman, Blow, Ames, & Reed, 2011; Ward, Clark, & Heidrich, 2009). Other barriers for youth included concerns about confidentiality and preference to rely on self, limited knowledge about services, and a failure to recognize symptoms, which the authors considered to be related to low mental health literacy (Gulliver et al., 2010). Given these barriers, programs to improve the mental health literacy of adolescents would likely be useful in ensuring that adolescents are aware of symptoms of mental health problems and know how to seek treatment.

For those adolescents who do make it into treatment, low health literacy may limit adherence to treatment. Many therapies may include a complex schedule of medications and/or psychotherapy that could demand high health literacy skills, including math skills. Low health literacy may also influence the ability to communicate with mental health providers and clearly understand information given by providers. Among adult patients with low health literacy, poor oral communication with providers has been noted, including problems understanding the explanation of conditions and process of care or treatment plans (Schillinger, Bindman, Wang, Stewart, & Piette, 2004; Williams, Davis, Parker, & Weiss, 2002), which can have an effect on compliance

(Williams et al., 2002). Some therapies might demand homework activities, which would be challenging for an adolescent with limited health literacy. In addition to helping with compliance, improved mental health literacy might also help adolescents be able to make informed decisions about which treatments are the safest, most effective, and appropriate ones for their condition.

For adolescents, obtaining treatment for a mental health problem is not just important from a medical perspective. Identifying and treating mental health issues among adolescents can have an impact on their success in school, and the ability to succeed in school is critically important for adolescents given the significant role education plays in predicting one's future life trajectory for health and other factors (Cutler & Lleras-Muney, 2006). Depression and anxiety, for instance, can impact school performance (Charvat, 2008), and "poor academic functioning and inconsistent school attendance were identified as early signs of emerging or existing mental health problems during childhood and adolescence" (p. 1) (DeSocio & Hootman, 2004).

Finally, as adolescents are at a gateway between receiving parental supervision for medical care and achieving independence, they are likely taking on new responsibilities related to health care management. They may be responsible for making their own health decisions, including being responsible for taking their own medications and choosing which medications to take (Manganello, 2008; Sanders et al., 2009), as well as getting to and from treatment. At the same time, parents/guardians typically still play a role in health care. Thus, the health literacy and mental health literacy of parents is also important to consider.

Conclusions

We believe there is much work to be done concerning health literacy, adolescents, and mental health, especially in the United States. Given the potential implications that health literacy may have on the mental health of adolescents, more research on adolescent health literacy, especially as it relates to mental health, is needed, and issues unique to adolescents' mental health care needs and concerns will need to be better understood and addressed specifically.

Research should address predictors of mental health literacy for adolescents as well as outcomes for adolescents with low mental health literacy. Investigation into how health providers should best communicate about mental health issues to adolescents with low mental health literacy is also warranted. In addition, further study of the measurement of health literacy and mental health literacy for adolescents is important, and studies should continue to evaluate programs to enhance health literacy and mental health literacy for adolescents. Can interventions for adolescents improve their mental health literacy, and what are the most optimal interventions to do so? Information about mental health should be easy to understand for adolescents and should be provided in a way that is both appealing to and captures the attention of this age group. Thus, future work should evaluate what information should be given and how to best provide that information to adolescents. Other issues to address include the role of media in influencing adolescent mental health literacy, as well as interpersonal influences, such as family and friends.

Adolescence is a critical period in a life course in which the cumulative experiences of childhood can not only contribute to current health status but can also lead to choices about pathways and behaviors that may last through adulthood. Poor health literacy and mental health literacy, and poor mental health, can be particularly disruptive to this path. These two factors together may be worse in a nonadditive way, particularly among adolescents experiencing distress who, due to poor mental health literacy, may not know what they are experiencing, how to describe it, or where and how to get help for it. Further, if their caregivers also have low health literacy and/or low mental health literacy, this may exacerbate the problem by creating additional barriers to diagnosis and treatment. There is a need to better understand the role of health literacy and mental health literacy for the mental health of adolescents, and how these relationships may be distinct from patterns seen in adults and children. We hope this overview will inspire future work and consideration of this important topic.

Acknowledgements We would like to thank Mark Duheme for his assistance with the literature review for this chapter.

References

Bapat, S., Jorm, A., & Lawrence, K. (2009). Evaluation of a mental health literacy training program for junior sporting clubs. *Austalian Psychiatry, 17*(6), 475–479.

Barney, L. J., Griffiths, K. M., Jorm, A. F., & Christensen, H. (2006). Stigma about depression and its impact on help-seeking intentions. *The Australian and New Zealand Journal of Psychiatry, 40*, 51–54.

Berkman, N., Davis, T., & McCormack, L. (2010). Health literacy: What is it? *Journal of Health Communication, 15*(S2), 9–19.

Berkman, N., Sheridan, S., Donahue, K., Halpern, D., Viera, A., Crotty, K., et al. (2011). *Health literacy interventions and outcomes: An updated systematic review*. Retrieved from http://www.ahrq.gov/clinic/tp/lituptp.htm.

Brey, R. A., Clark, S. E., & Wantz, M. S. (2007). Enhancing health literacy through accessing health information, products, and services: An exercise for children and adolescents. *Journal of School Health, 77*(9), 640–644.

Burns, J., & Rapee, R. (2006). Adolescent mental health literacy: Young people's knowledge of depression and help seeking. *Journal of Adolescence, 29*(2), 225–239.

Cabassa, L. (2009). *Mental health literacy in the United States: A systematic review of population based studies*. Paper presented at the Society for Social Work and Research, New Orleans, LA.

Charvat, J. (2008). *Research on the relationship between mental health and academic achievement*. Retrieved from http://www.nasponline.org/advocacy/Academic-MentalHealthLinks.pdf.

Chisolm, D. J., & Buchanan, L. (2007). Measuring adolescent functional health literacy: A pilot validation of the test of functional health literacy in adults. *Journal of Adolescent Health, 41*(3), 312–314.

Christensen, R. C., & Grace, G. D. (1999). The prevalence of low literacy in an indigent psychiatric population. *Psychiatric Services, 50*, 262–263.

Coles, M., & Coleman, S. (2010). Barriers to treatment seeking for anxiety disorders: Initial data on the role of mental health literacy. *Depression and Anxiety, 27*, 63–71.

Connelly, R. (2007). *A process evaluation of a health literacy intervention targeting pediatric providers' communication skills at the Texas Children's Health Plan*. Unpublished Dissertation, Texas Medical Center.

Cotton, S., Wright, A., Harris, M., Jorm, A., & McGorry, P. (2006). Influence of gender on mental health literacy in young Australians. *Australian and New Zealand Journal of Psychiatry, 40*, 790–796.

Currier, G., Sitzman, R., & Trenton, A. (2001). Literacy in the psychiatric emergency service. *Journal of Nervous and Mental Disease, 189*(1), 56–58.

Cutler, D., & Lleras-Muney, A. (2006). *Education and health: Evaluating theories and evidence*. Retrieved from http://www.nber.org/papers/w12352.

Davis, T. C., Long, S., Jackson, R. H., Mayeaux, E. J., Jr., George, R., Murphy, P. W., et al. (1993). Rapid estimate of adult literacy in medicine: A shortened screening instrument. *Family Medicine, 25*(6), 256–260.

Davis, T. C., Wolf, M. S., Arnold, C. L., Byrd, R. S., Long, S. W., Springer, T., et al. (2006). Development and validation of the Rapid Estimate of Adolescent Literacy in Medicine (REALM-Teen): A tool to screen adolescents for below-grade reading in health care settings. *Pediatrics, 118*(6), e1707–e1714.

DeSocio, J., & Hootman, J. (2004). Children's mental health and school success. *The Journal of School Nursing, 20*(4), 189–196.

Farrer, L., Leach, L., Griffiths, K., Christensen, H., & Jorm, A. (2008). Age differences in mental health literacy. *BMC Public Health, 8*(1), 125.

Ferreira, M. R., Dolan, N. C., Fitzgibbon, M. L., Davis, T. C., Gorby, N., Ladewski, L., et al. (2005). Health care provider-directed intervention to increase colorectal cancer screening among veterans: Results of a randomized controlled trial. *Journal of Clinical Oncology, 23*(7), 1548–1554.

Francis, C., Pirkis, J., Dunt, D., Blood, R., & Davis, C. (2002). *Improving mental health literacy: A review of the literature*. Melbourne: Centre for Health Program Evaluation.

Gazmarian, J., Baker, D., Parker, R., & Blazer, D. (2000). A multivariate analysis of factors associated with depression. *Arch Internal Medicine, 160*, 3307–3314.

Gorman, L., Blow, A., Ames, B., & Reed, P. (2011). National guard families after combat: Mental health, use of mental health services, and perceived treatment barriers. *Psychiatric Services, 62*(1), 28–34.

Gulliver, A., Griffiths, K., & Christensen, H. (2010). Perceived barriers and facilitators to mental health help-seeking in young people: A systematic review. *BMC Psychiatry, 10*, 113.

Hernandez, L. (2009). *Measures of health literacy: A workshop summary*. Retrieved from http://www.nap.edu/catalog.php?record_id=12690.

Jones, M., Lee, J. Y., & Rozier, R. G. (2007). Oral health literacy among adult patients seeking dental care. *The Journal of the American Dental Association, 138*(9), 1199–1208.

Jorm, A., Barney, L., Christensen, H., Highet, N., Kelly, C., & Kitchener, B. (2006). Research on mental health literacy: What we know and what we still need to know. *Australian and New Zealand Journal of Psychiatry, 40*(1), 3–5.

Jorm, A., Korten, A., Jacomb, P., Christensen, H., Rodgers, B., & Pollitt, P. (1997). "Mental health literacy": A survey of the public's ability to recognise mental disorders and their beliefs about the effectiveness of treatment. *The Medical Journal of Australia, 166*(4), 182–186.

Kelly, C., Jorm, A., & Rodgers, B. (2006). Adolescents' responses to peers with depression or conduct disorder. *Australian and New Zealand Journal of Psychiatry, 40*, 63–66.

Kelly, C., Jorm, A., & Wright, A. (2007). Improving mental health literacy as a strategy to facilitate early intervention for mental disorders. *The Medical Journal of Australia, 187*(7), S26–S30.

Kripalani, S., & Weiss, B. D. (2006). Teaching about health literacy and clear communication. *Journal of General Internal Medicine, 21*(8), 888–890.

Kutner, M., Greenberg, E., Jin, Y., & Paulsen, C. (2006). *The health literacy of America's adults: Results from the 2003 National Assessment of Adult Literacy (NCES 2006–483)*. Washington, DC: U.S. Department of Education, National Center for Education.

Lauber, C., Nordt, C., Falcato, L., & Rossler, W. (2003). Do people recognise mental illness? *European Archives of Psychiatry and Clinical Neuroscience, 253*(5), 248–251.

Lincoln, A. (2008). Limited literacy and psychiatric disorders among users of an urban safety net hospital's mental health outpatient clinic. *Journal of Nervous and Mental Disease, 196*(9), 687–693.

Lincoln, A., Paasche-Orlow, M., Cheng, D., Lloyd-Travaglini, C., Caruso, C., Saitz, R., et al. (2006). Impact of health literacy on depressive symptoms and mental health-related quality of life among adults with addiction. *Journal of General Internal Medicine, 21*, 818–822.

Manganello, J. (2008). Health literacy and adolescents: A framework and agenda for future research. *Health Education Research, 23*(5), 840–847.

Marie, D., Forsyth, D., & Miles, L. (2004). Categorical ethnicity and mental health literacy in New Zealand. *Ethnicity and Health, 9*(3), 225–252.

Morgan, A., & Jorm, A. (2007). Awareness of beyondblue: The national depression initiative in Australian young people. *Australasian Psychiatry, 15*(4), 329–333.

National Center for Education Statistics, U. S. D. O. E. (2009). *The Nation's Report Card: Reading*. Retrieved from http://nationsreportcard.gov/reading_2009/.

Olsson, D., & Kennedy, M. (2010). Mental health literacy among young people in a small US town: Recognition of disorders and hypothetical helping responses. *Early Intervention in Psychiatry, 4*(4), 291–298.

Parker, R. M., Baker, D. W., Williams, M. V., & Nurss, J. (1995). The test of functional health literacy in adults (TOFHLA): A new instrument for measuring patients' literacy skills. *Journal of General Internal Medicine, 10*, 537–541.

Parker, R. M., & Ratzan, S. (2010). Health literacy: A second decade of distinction for Americans. *Journal of Health Communication, 15*(1), 20–33.

Peerson, A., & Saunders, M. (2009). Health literacy revisited: What do we mean and why does it matter? *Health Promotion International, 24*(3), 285–296.

Pignone, M., DeWalt, D. A., Sheridan, S., Berkman, N., & Lohr, K. N. (2005). Interventions to improve health outcomes for patients with low literacy: A systematic review. *Journal of General Internal Medicine, 20*(2), 185–192.

Pinfold, V., Toulmin, H., Thornicroft, G., Huxley, P., Farmer, P., & Graham, T. (2003). Reducing psychiatric stigma and discrimination: Evaluation of educational interventions in UK secondary schools. *British Journal of Psychiatry, 182*, 342–346.

Pinto-Foltz, M., Logsdon, M., & Myers, J. (2011). Feasibility, acceptability, and initial efficacy of a knowledge-contact program to reduce mental illness stigma and improve mental health literacy in adolescents. *Social Science and Medicine, 72*(12), 2011–2019.

Ratzan, S., & Parker, R. (2000). Introduction. In C. Selden, M. Zorn, S. Ratzan, & R. Parker (Eds.), *National library of medicine current bibliographies in medicine: Health literacy*. Bethesda, MD, USA: National Institutes of Health, Department of Health and Human Services.

Sanders, L., Steven Federico, S., Klass, P., Abrams, M., & Dreyer, B. (2009). Literacy and child health: A systematic review. *Archives of Pediatrics and Family Medicine, 163*(2), 131–140.

Schillinger, D., Bindman, A., Wang, F., Stewart, A., & Piette, J. (2004). Functional health literacy and the quality of physician-patient communication among diabetes patients. *Patient Education and Counseling, 52*(3), 315–323.

Scott, L., & Chur-Hansen, A. (2008). The mental health literacy of rural adolescents: Emo subculture and SMS texting. *Australasian Psychiatry, 16*(5), 359–362.

Sentell, T., & Shumway, M. (2003). Low literacy and mental illness in a nationally representative sample. *Journal of Nervous and Mental Disease, 191*(8), 549–552.

Smith, R., Armstrong, M., & Davis, C. (2006). *The effect of health knowledge and literacy on utilization, cost, service quality, and quality of life in children and adult medicaid mental health consumers*. Retrieved from http://home.fmhi.usf.edu/common/file/ahca/ahca2006/220-69.pdf.

Smith, R., Armstrong, M., Davis, C., Massey, O., McNeish, R., & Smith, R. (2007). *Development and testing of an instrument to measure mental health literacy*. Retrieved from http://home.fmhi.usf.edu/common/file/ahca/ahca2007/220-99.pdf.

St Leger, L. (2001). Schools, health literacy and public health: Possibilities and challenges. *Health Promotion International, 16*(2), 197–205.

U.S. Department of Health and Human Services, O. O. D. P. A. H. P. (2010). *National Action Plan to improve health literacy*. Retrieved from http://www.health.gov/communication/hlactionplan/.

Ward, E., Clark, L. O., & Heidrich, S. (2009). African American women's beliefs, coping behaviors, and barriers to seeking mental health services. *Qualitative Health Research, 19*(11), 1589–1601.

Weiss, B. D., Mays, M. Z., Martz, W., Castro, K. M., DeWalt, D. A., Pignone, M. P., et al. (2005). Quick assessment of literacy in primary care: The Newest Vital Sign. *Annals of Family Medicine, 3*(6), 514–522.

Williams, M., Davis, T., Parker, R., & Weiss, B. (2002). The role of health literacy in patient-physician communication. *Family Medicine, 34*(5), 383–389.

Wolf, M. S., Gazmararian, J. A., & Baker, D. W. (2005). Health literacy and functional health status among older adults. *Archives of Internal Medicine, 165*, 1946–1952.

Wolf, M. S., Wilson, E. A. H., Rapp, D. N., Waite, K. R., Bocchini, M. V., Davis, T. C., et al. (2009). Literacy and learning in health care. *Pediatrics, 124*(Suppl 3), S275–S281.

Wright, A., McGorry, P. D., Harris, M. G., Jorm, A. F., & Pennell, K. (2006). Development and evaluation of a youth mental health community awareness campaign—The Compass Strategy. *BMC Public Health, 6*, 215–213.

Wu, A. D., Begoray, D. L., MacDonald, M., Wharf Higgins, J., Frankish, J., Kwan, B., et al. (2010). Developing and evaluating a relevant and feasible instrument for measuring health literacy of Canadian high school students. *Health Promotion International, 25*(4), 444–452.

Zoellner, J., Connell, C., Bounds, W., Crook, L., & Yadrick, K. (2009). Nutrition literacy status and preferred nutrition communication channels among adults in the Lower Mississippi Delta. *Preventing Chronic Disease, 6*(4), A128.

Advances in the Measurement and Utilization of Health-Related Quality of Life Instruments

Alexandra L. Quittner, Ivette Cejas, and Laura S. Blackwell

Introduction

Adolescents with chronic illnesses have unique and important perspectives on how their illness affects their daily lives. Obtaining this information directly from them in a standardized way represents a significant shift in health outcomes research and is particularly relevant for adolescents with chronic diseases, in which a more collaborative model of care is required. As adolescents are transitioning toward more independent care, measuring their symptoms and the effects of a disease on their daily functioning should be utilized to optimize disease management. Patient-reported outcomes (PROs) form the larger umbrella under which measures, such as health-related quality of life (HRQOL), are positioned.

A PRO is defined as "any report of the status of a patient's health condition that comes directly from the patient, without interpretation of the patient's response by a clinician or anyone else" (FDA, p. 2). PROs include HRQOL instruments that measure four core domains: (1) disease state and physical symptoms, (2) functional status (e.g., performing daily activities), (3) psychological and emotional functioning, and (4) social functioning. Additionally, they may include observable (e.g., coughing) or non-observable outcomes known only to the patient (e.g., perceptions of pain, feelings of depression).

Importance of Patient Perspective

There are several advantages to utilizing HRQOL measures. First, in most cases, only the patient is able to report how he or she is functioning and feeling on a daily basis. Both younger children and adolescents are keenly aware of their symptoms and are able to provide reliable and valid estimates if measured in a developmentally appropriate way (Modi & Quittner, 2003; Riley, 2004). For example, intensity and relief of pain symptoms is best measured by asking the patient, and there is a long tradition of using PROs in this context to evaluate the efficacy of new pain medications (Stinson & McGrath, 2011). This is also true for many physical and emotional symptoms, such as chest congestion and tightness, and anxiety and depression, which cannot be measured "objectively."

Second, PROs are important because they standardize the patient's report of symptoms and response to treatment elicited during a physical exam. Physicians typically ask patients informally about their current symptoms, recent changes in

A.L. Quittner, Ph.D. (✉) • L.S. Blackwell, M.A.
Department of Psychology, University of Miami, 5665 Ponce de Leon Blvd, Coral Gables, FL 33146, USA
e-mail: aquittner@miami.edu; l.blackwell@umiami.edu

I. Cejas, Dr.
Department of Otolaryngology, University of Miami Miller School of Medicine, 1120 NW 14 Street, CRB 5th floor, Miami, FL 333136, USA
e-mail: icruz@med.miami.edu

W.T. O'Donohue et al. (eds.), *Handbook of Adolescent Health Psychology*,
DOI 10.1007/978-1-4614-6633-8_11,

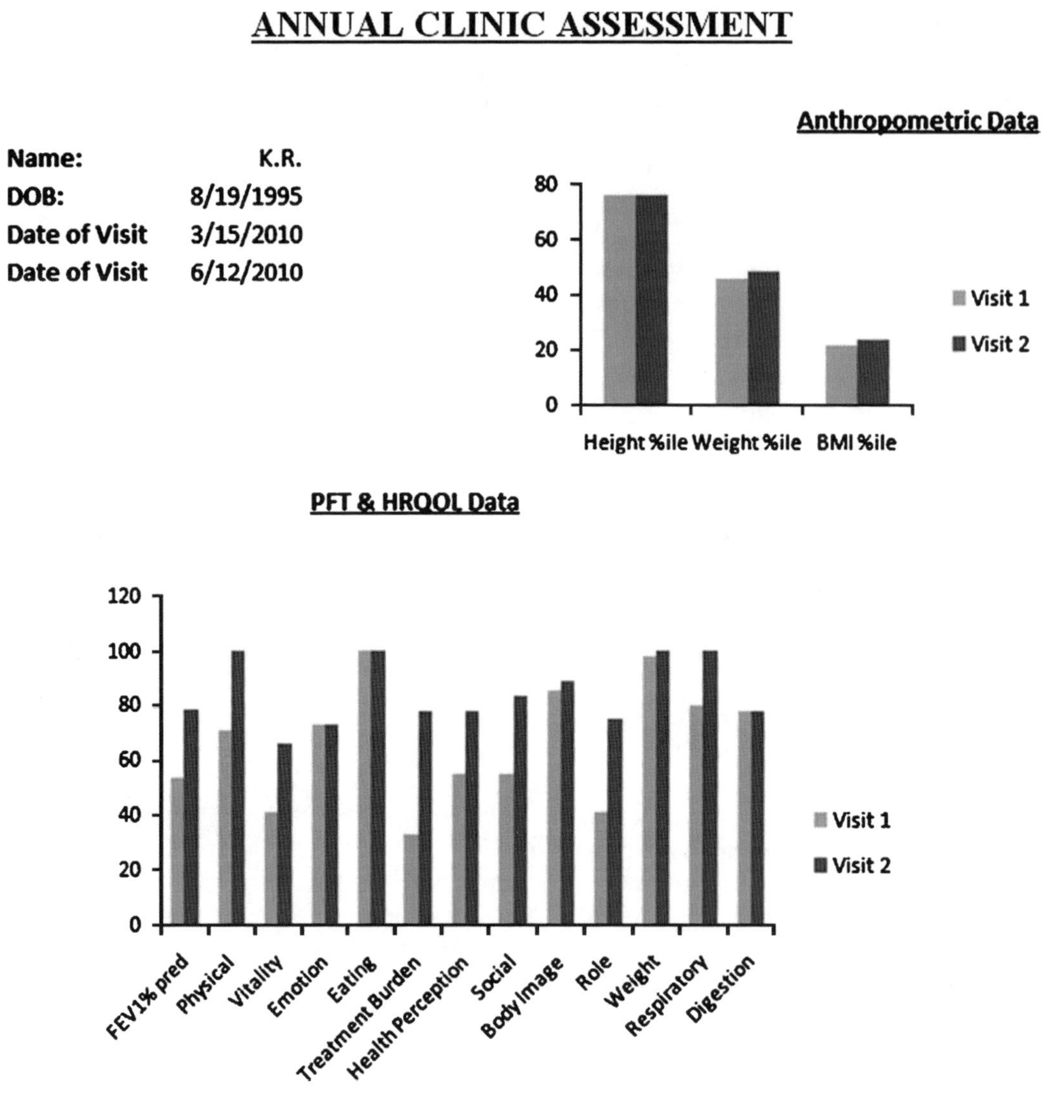

Fig. 1 Example of how to use HRQOL measures at annual clinic visits. Comparisons of HRQOL and medical data

those symptoms, and the efficacy of their current treatment regimen. Although these data strongly influence clinical decision-making, this informal approach has drawbacks: information may be incomplete, there are inconsistencies across physicians in how these questions are asked, and there is the potential for measurement error in either the patient's report or in the physician's interpretation and recording of this information. In contrast, use of a standardized PRO can directly capture the information that is needed without introducing respondent and recall biases, such as the patient's desire to "please" the physician, different time frames for recall (e.g., symptoms over past week vs. past month), or different interpretations of what the patient has said. Standardizing this process also increases the reliability of the assessment and allows health care providers to compare a patient's scores across visits or to a larger, normative database (see Fig. 1).

Finally, if developed using modern measurement techniques (FDA, 2009; Schwarz & Sudman, 1996), PROs can be used as primary or secondary outcomes in clinical trials of new medications or behavioral interventions (Goss & Quittner, 2007; Retsch-Bogart et al., 2009; Turner, Quittner, Parasuraman, Kallich, & Cleeland, 2007). In the context of clinical trials, PROs can also add unique information to physiological outcomes (e.g., pulmonary functioning) and capture both the side effects of new medications and the burden of adhering to a new treatment (Sawicki et al., 2011). For adolescents with chronic conditions, adherence to prescribed medications is quite low, and linking improvement in patient-reported symptoms to their treatment regimen could improve adherence behaviors (Barker & Quittner, 2010; Robinson, Callister, Berry, & Dearing, 2008).

PRO in Clinical Trials

Recently, the Food and Drug Administration (FDA) has recognized the importance of PROs for evaluating new medications and treatments, and has released a "guidance" which outlines criteria for their development and use in clinical trials (FDA, 2009). Currently, 14 % of registered clinical trials report using a PRO; however, this ranges from 5 to 22 % based on the disease (Scoggins & Patrick, 2009). Efforts to develop reliable and valid PROs have been very successful, leading to their use for several different purposes: (1) as primary or secondary outcomes in clinical trials; (2) to evaluate new pharmaceutical, surgical, and behavioral interventions; (3) to describe the impact of illness on patient functioning; (4) to document the natural history of the disease; (5) to analyze the costs and benefits of medical interventions; and (6) to aid in clinical decision-making. Recently, an inhaled antibiotic was approved using a PRO, the Cystic Fibrosis Questionnaire-Revised (CFQ-R; Quittner et al., 2005) as a primary endpoint. Respiratory symptoms improved significantly, with concomitant increases in pulmonary function, as measured by the respiratory symptoms scale of the CFQ-R (McCoy et al., 2008; Oermann et al., 2010; Retsch-Bogart et al., 2009).

In general, the FDA encourages investigators and/or clinicians to determine whether an adequate PRO instrument already exists, because of the intensive effort required to develop and validate a new one (Turner et al., 2007). The FDA reviews every step in the PRO development process, including the adequacy of content validity (e.g., patient interviews, focus groups) and instrument's psychometric properties. Specific steps for PRO development include (1) hypothesizing a conceptual framework (e.g., linking concepts to product claim); (2) adjusting conceptual framework and drafting a preliminary instrument (e.g., obtaining patient input through qualitative interviews); (3) confirming conceptual framework and other measurement properties (e.g., reliability, validity); (4) collecting, analyzing, and interpreting data (e.g., determining the minimal important difference [MID]); and (5) modifying instrument (see Fig. 2).

Regardless of the measure's structure or complexity, to utilize a PRO in a clinical trial, the instrument must meet rigorous psychometric criteria, including documentation of several types of reliability and validity. Reliability indices include internal consistency (Cronbach's alpha), test–retest reliability, and cross-informant consistency. Construct validity includes predictive (associations between the PRO and other outcomes), convergent (correlations between the PRO and a similar measure), divergent (PRO is not correlated with unrelated constructs), and discriminate (PRO differentiates between patients with differing levels of disease severity). These analyses combine to produce evidence that the "construct" being targeted is measured by the instrument. In addition, the MID, which establishes the smallest change that can be detected by respondents, must be determined (Guyatt, Osoba, Wu, Wyrwich, & Norman, 2002; Quittner, Modi et al., 2009; Wyrwich, Tierney, Babu, Kroenke, & Wolinsky, 2005). The MID provides an empirical method for interpreting the *clinical significance* of the observed effects (Quittner, Modi et al., 2009).

Health-Related Quality of Life

HRQOL measures are a distinct type of PRO which yield multidimensional profile scores across several areas of functioning. There are both

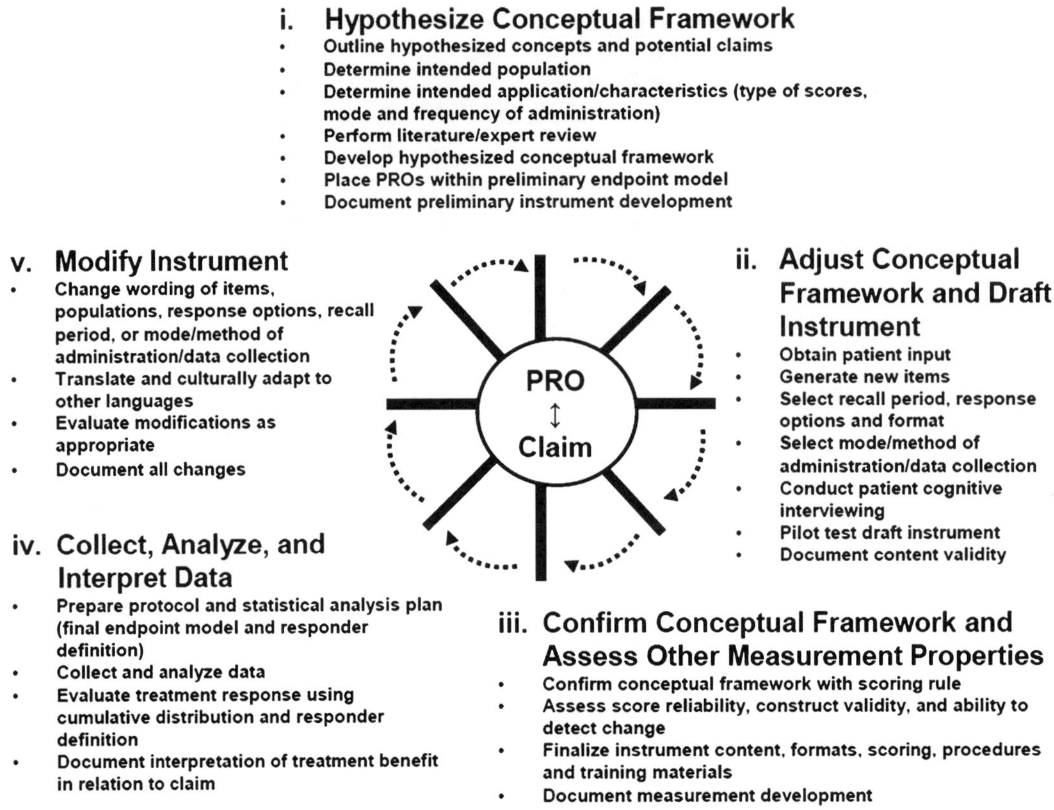

Fig. 2 Development of a PRO Instrument: An Iterative Process, U.S. Department of Health and Human Services, Food and Drug Administration (2009) (Copyright 2009, Food and Drug Administration)

generic and disease-specific HRQOL measures. Generic measures utilize general items that are applicable to both healthy populations and those with chronic conditions. Several generic instruments are well-established, including the Pediatric Quality of Life Inventory (Varni, Seid, & Rode, 1999), the Child Health and Illness Profile (Starfield et al., 1995), and the Youth Quality of Life (Edwards, Huebner, Connell, & Patrick, 2002). These measures have been shown to correlate with disease severity, discriminate between healthy and chronically ill populations, and can be used to compare adolescents with different conditions. However, because they are general, they lack precision and sensitivity to change, and often do not provide specific information for intervention. In addition, these instruments are not accepted by the FDA for approval of new drugs or devices.

In contrast, disease-specific HRQOL measures focus on the domains of functioning most relevant for a particular disease and its treatment. These measures are able to detect small, but clinically meaningful changes and often identify important targets for clinical intervention. Several disease-specific HRQOL measures have been developed for adolescents with chronic diseases including diabetes, obesity, cystic fibrosis, cancer, asthma, epilepsy, and HIV/AIDS (see Table 1). However, disease-specific instruments do not currently exist for a number of conditions, including irritable bowel syndrome (IBS), sickle cell disease, thalassemia, solid organ transplant, and cardiovascular disease, among others. Future research should focus on the development of HRQOL measures in these diseases.

To ensure the use of high-quality measures, an evidenced-based categorization system was

Table 1 Disease-specific health related quality of life measures for adolescents with chronic diseases

Instrument	Age range	Respondent	EBA rating	ePRO
Diabetes				
Audit of diabetes-dependent QoL—teen	13–18 years	Adolescent	Well-established	
Diabetes self-management profile	6–15 years	Child/adolescent	Well-established	
Diabetes quality of life measure	13–17 years	Adolescent	Well-established	
PedsQL—diabetes module	5–18 years	Child/adolescent	Well-established	
	2–18 years	Parent	Well-established	
Obesity				
Impact of weight on quality of life—kids	11–19 years	Adolescent	Well-established	
Sizing them up	5–18 years	Parent	Approaching	
Cystic fibrosis				
Cystic fibrosis quality of life questionnaire	14 years–adult	Adolescent/adult	Well-established	
Cystic fibrosis questionnaire—revised (CFQ-R)	6 years–adult	Child/adolescent/ adult	Well-established	
Questions on life satisfaction—cystic fibrosis	16 years–adult	Adolescent/adult	Well-established	
Asthma				
About my asthma (AMA)	6–12 years	Child	Approaching	
Adolescent asthma quality of life questionnaire (AAQOL)	12–17 years	Child	Well-established	
Childhood asthma questionnaires	4–7 years	Child	Well-established	
	8–11 years	Child/adolescent	Well-established	
	12–16 years	Adolescent	Well-established	
Children's health survey for asthma (CHSA)	7–16 years	Child	Well-established	
	5–12 years	Parent	Well-established	
Pediatric asthma quality of life questionnaire	7–17 years	Child/adolescent	Well-established	✔
Pediatric asthma caregiver's quality of life questionnaire	7–17 years	Parent	Well-established	✔
Asthma-related quality of life scale (ARQOLS)	6–13 years	Child	Well-established	
TACQOL-asthma	8–16 years	Child and parent	Approaching	
PedsQL—asthma module	5–18 years	Child	Well-established	
	2–18 years	Parent	Well-established	
Life activities questionnaire for childhood asthma	5–17 years	Child/adolescent	Approaching	
How are you?	8–12 years	Child	Promising	
	8–12 years	Parent	Promising	
Integrated therapeutics group child asthma short form	2–17 years	Parent	Well-established	
Headaches				
24-h adolescent migraine questionnaire	12–18 years	Adolescent and parent	Promising	
PedMIDAS	6–18 years	Child	Well-established	
Quality of life headache in youth	12–18 years	Adolescent and parent	Well-established	
Epilepsy				
Quality of life in epilepsy inventory for adolescents (QOLIE-AD-48)	11–17 years	Adolescent	Well-established	
The child self-report scale and parent-proxy response scale	8–15+ years	Child/adolescent	Promising	
	6–15 years	Parent	Promising	
US version—quality of life in childhood epilepsy questionnaire	4–18 years	Parent	Approaching	

(continued)

Table 1 (continued)

Instrument	Age range	Respondent	EBA rating	ePRO
Cancer				
Behavioral affective and somatic experiences scale (BASES)	2–20 years	Child, parent, and nurse	Well-established	
The Miami pediatric quality of life questionnaire	1–18 years	Child and parent	Approaching	
The Minneapolis–Manchester quality of life	8–12 years	Child/adolescent	Approaching	
	13–18 years	Adolescent	Approaching	
The pediatric cancer quality of life inventory (PCQL)	8–18 years	Child and parent	Well-established	
The pediatric oncology quality of life scale	5–17 years	Parent	Well-established	
PedsQL—cancer module	8–12 years	Child	Well-established	
	13–18 years	Adolescent	Well-established	
Play performance scale for children	6 months–16 years	Parent	Promising	
Quality of life—cancer survivors questionnaire	16–29 years	Adolescent/adult	Well-established	
The Royal Marsden Hospital pediatric oncology quality of life questionnaire	3–19 years	Youth and parents	Promising	
Juvenile rheumatoid arthritis				
Juvenile arthritis quality of life questionnaire	2–18 years	Child/adolescent	Well-established	
PedsQL—rheumatoid arthritis module	5–18 years	Child/adolescent	Well-established	
	2–18 years	Parent		
HIV/AIDS				
Multidimensional quality of life questionnaire for HIV/AIDS	12–20 years	Child/adolescent	Well-established	
Chronic pain				
McGill pain questionnaire	10–adult	Child/adolescent/adult	Well-established	
Quality of life questionnaire for adolescents with chronic pain CLA-CP	12–18 years	Adolescent	Approaching	
PedsQL—pain module	5–18 years	Child/adolescent	Well-established	
	2–18 years	Parent		

designed to assist clinicians and investigators in selecting the best measure and to foster greater integration of science and practice (Cohen et al., 2008; Palermo et al., 2008). Measures have been classified into three categories: (a) well-established, (b) approaching well-established, and (c) promising. To be classified as "well-established," the measure must have good psychometric properties and be published in at least two peer-reviewed articles by more than one investigative team. "Approaching well-established" requires that the measure have moderate or unclear psychometric properties and be utilized in at least two peer-reviewed articles by the same research group. "Promising" requires moderate or unclear psychometrics and publication in one peer-reviewed article. Across all of these categories, sufficient detail about the measure is necessary to allow critical evaluation and replication of results (e.g., measure and manual provided upon request) (Cohen et al., 2008). For a detailed review of the psychometric properties of available HRQOL measures for adolescents with chronic illnesses see Quittner, Cruz, Modi, and Marciel (2009).

Use of Proxy Measures of HRQOL

Although self-report is the preferred mode of assessment for HRQOL instruments, there are situations in which this is not possible. This includes infants and toddlers who cannot complete an instrument, children with developmental delays or severe communication deficits (e.g., mental retardation), or adolescents who are in the terminal stages of an illness. In these cases, proxy respondents provide a critical window into the child or adolescents' functioning. Proxy respondents in these cases are often parents, but could include teachers or other caregivers. In the pediatric literature, parent-proxy measures are frequently used (Eiser & Morse, 2001; Quittner, Modi, & Roux, 2003; Turner et al., 2007). In studies comparing patient and parent-proxy HRQOL scores, evidence of convergence between child/adolescent and parent responses is mixed, with better agreement on domains of functioning that are more observable (e.g., coughing, walking up stairs) and poor agreement on domains that are less accessible to parents (e.g., emotional and peer functioning) (Haverman, Vreys, Proesmans, & De Boeck, 2006; Modi & Quittner, 2003; Verrips, Vogels, den Ouden, Paneth, & Verloove-Vanhorick, 2000). The FDA guidance strongly discourage the use of proxy measures for those who are capable of reporting themselves, but allow proxy responses for events or behaviors that are easily observable. In an effort to adhere to these guidelines, HRQOL measures are now being developed for younger populations. For example, a preschool version of the Cystic Fibrosis Questionnaire-Revised (CFQ-R) is being developed for children ages 3–6 years using a forced choice paradigm, with pictures illustrating each item (Cruz et al., 2009).

Using PROs in Clinical Practice

New efforts are being made to incorporate PROs into clinical practice. Given the growing number of well-established HRQOL measures and the recommendation by the American Academy of Pediatrics to involve children in their own health care (American Academy of Pediatrics, 1997), it would be useful to assess HRQOL during routine clinic visits. For example, children and adolescents could complete the CFQ-R prior to their laboratory tests (e.g., lung function) and physical exam so that data on their symptoms and daily functioning could be integrated with their spirometry and exam results to provide a more comprehensive evaluation of their current health status (see Fig. 1). Changes in patient symptoms might even precede a change in lung function, providing an "early warning" system for earlier intervention. A complete assessment of the patients' HRQOL can also be completed during annual clinic visits to determine how their disease and/or treatments are affecting their daily life (e.g., physical, emotional, and social functioning). Data on their symptoms could then be integrated to facilitate a discussion between the patient and physician about the efficacy of their current regimen and increase shared decision-making in relation to newly prescribed medications. Given the extensive data indicating that adherence to chronic medications for asthma, CF, epilepsy, and diabetes is quite poor (Hood, Peterson, Rohan, & Drotar, 2009; Modi & Quittner, 2006; Modi, Rausch, & Glauser, 2011), utilizing patient-reported data and involving the patient in discussions of their regimen is one way to address this problem. A recent longitudinal study of pediatric and adult patients with CF found that changes in respiratory symptoms and weight were significantly correlated with changes on relevant CFQ-R scores (respiratory symptoms, weight), indicating that this PRO is sensitive to changes in health status over time (Sawicki et al., 2011).

Electronic Patient-Reported Outcomes

The use of PROs in clinical trials has increased dramatically over the past decade, and with the publication of the FDA Guidance on PROs, this trend is likely to continue. As the demand and utilization of these measures increase, so does the need for effective and efficient methods of data collection. Electronic patient-reported outcomes (ePROs) have become an increasingly popular method to collect information on health outcomes, particularly in clinical trials.

A variety of platforms for ePROs have been developed, including automated telephone systems, conventional computers, computers with touch screens, tablet PCs, personal digital assistants (PDAs), and smartphones (Coons et al., 2009). Identifying the most appropriate platform depends on the specific trial and study conditions, including the nature of the outcome, patient population, trial design, frequency of data collection, and complexity of the measure being used. Typically, the best solution may be a combination of these assessment platforms. To date, no guidelines have been developed for selecting the most appropriate platform for administration of an ePRO or which platforms should be used together to obtain the best results (Bausch & Goldfarb, 2009).

Electronic assessment methods offer a number of advantages over paper–pencil methods (Gwaltney, Shields, & Shiffman, 2008). The use of ePROs reduces missing and inconsistent data, which can improve data quality and integrity. Thus, data management is simplified because manual data entry is eliminated, which reduces errors and personnel effort. Data security and privacy issues can be easily managed with modern network and data encryption methods. Complex skip patterns, which often are confusing for patients and lead to incomplete or invalid data, can be automatized for simple administration. Studies have also identified improved adherence when using ePROs in comparison to paper–pencil methods (Stone et al., 2002). In many cases the cost of implementing an ePRO is less than the cost of paper. While the up-front costs for software development and purchase of devices may be higher than the paper methods, the real cost of implementing ePROs is often less than or similar to the overall cost of paper–pencil administration (Gwaltney, Shields, & Shiffman, 2008).

Furthermore, utilization of ePROs may be particularly beneficial for adolescent populations. Information and communication technology has become a central part of the everyday life of adolescents, with more than 85 % of American youth, ages 12–17, using the Internet and nearly half logging on daily (Lenhart, Madden, & Hitlin, 2005). An overwhelming majority of all teenagers, 84 %, report owning at least one personal media device, such as a desktop or laptop computer, a cell phone, or a personal digital assistant (PDA), with 44 % reporting owning two or more devices (Lenhart et al., 2005). They use these devices for studying, playing games, and seeking information on the Internet, and they communicate via mobile phones, social networking, and video games. Given that information technology plays a pivotal role in adolescents' everyday lives, it seems that ePROs are most applicable to this technologically sophisticated population.

An additional advantage of ePROs is their ability to use voice software to read text information. This is particularly important for younger adolescents and those who have reading difficulties or visual impairments. This not only eliminates the need for an assistant to administer the measure but allows for standardization of administration to increase its reliability and validity.

Despite the numerous benefits of ePROs, there are several limitations that warrant discussion. The recent FDA Guidance specifically addressed concerns with ePROs. One primary concern was the risk that the investigator does not have control over data collection. For example, direct control over the data may be maintained by a sponsor or a contracted organization rather than the principle investigator. Furthermore, additional security controls and system maintenance plans that ensure data integrity are critical, particularly during network failures or software updates. This type of risk management could lead to costly quality control strategies.

The FDA indicated an openness to the use of ePROs in clinical trials, although they will be subject to the same strict standards as paper-based PROs mentioned in the guidance. An ePRO measure that has been adapted from a paper-based measure ought to produce data that are equivalent or superior to the data produced from the original version. Although the FDA does not make a distinction between minor, moderate, or substantial modifications, the guidance indicates that additional validation is required when "an instrument is altered in item content or format" (Coons et al., 2009; FDA, 2009). Therefore, it is still important to test and validate an ePRO measure once modifications have been made to ensure its equivalence to the original measure.

Collaborative Medicine

In addition to increased attention to PROs, there has been a movement toward family-centered care for patients with chronic conditions. Collaborative care is a paradigm in which the patient and physician make critical health decisions together (Berwick, 2003; Bodenheimer, Lorig, Homan, & Grumbach, 2002). Although the physician is considered the "expert" on the disease process, the patient is viewed as the expert on how their disease and its treatments affect his/her daily life (i.e., school functioning, treatment burden, side effects of medications). This model emphasizes the patient's responsibility for managing his/her condition and empowers the patient to communicate more directly with providers, problem-solve issues related to adherence, and participate in medical decision-making (Gawande, 2004; Leape et al., 2009; Safran, 2003).

This is particularly important for adolescents with chronic illnesses for whom rates of adherence typically decline, leading to worse health outcomes (Spencer, Cooper, & Milton, 2010; Zemanick et al., 2010; Zindani, Streetman, Streetman, & Nasr, 2006). During this developmental period, adolescents seek greater autonomy and independence from their parents, which can lead to worse adherence and more frequent conflict about daily treatments (Modi, Marciel, Slater, Drotar, & Quittner, 2008). Integrating adolescents earlier and more fully into the health care process is likely to increase their motivation to adhere to their treatments and more successfully transition to adult care.

Recommendations and Future Directions

Although significant progress has been made over the last 20 years in defining and measuring HRQOL using patient input, there is still considerable room for improvement. Efforts to develop reliable and valid PROs have been highly successful, with several instruments reaching the "well-established" designation (Palermo et al., 2008). This interest reflects a shift in health care toward inclusion of patients in shared decision-making and more collaborative relationships between patients with chronic conditions and health care providers. It also dovetails with the movement toward evidence-based practice and assessment. To date however, several chronic diseases have no validated PRO available. In addition, the focus has primarily been on the development of paper–pencil measures, with few ePRO instruments currently available (see Table 1). As the use of technology increases among adolescents, more focus should be placed on modifying and evaluating existing, well-established measures to the ePRO platform.

In a recent "vision" workshop held at the National Institute of Child Health and Human Development, the committee determined that the development of PROs, particularly for children and adolescents with chronic illnesses, should be a funding priority (Barkovich, Szefler, Olson, & Rymer, 2011). It will be particularly important to include PROs in clinical and behavioral trials, in addition to integrating them into family-centered care. Psychologists, who have a strong background in psychometrics and assessment, are in an ideal position to contribute to these developments.

References

American Academy of Pediatrics. (1997). Guidelines for child health supervision III. Vol III. Elf Groce, IL: American Academy of Pediatrics.

Barker, D. H., & Quittner, A. L. (2010). A biopsychosocial model of CF: Social and emotional functioning, adherence and quality of life. In J. Allen, H. Panitch & R. Rubenstein (Eds.), *Lung biology in health and disease series: Cystic fibrosis* (pp. 468–481). New York: Informa Healthcare.

Barkovich, A. J., Szefler, S. J., Olson, E., Rymer, W. (2011). *Scientific vision workshop on diagnostics and therapeutics [white paper]*. Retrieved from National Institute of Child Health and Human Development http://www.nichd.nih.gov/vision/comments/whitepapers/Diag_Therp_White_Paper_040311.pdf.

Bausch, E., & Goldfarb, S. (2009). Electronic patient-reported outcomes for collecting sensitive information from patients. *The Journal of Supportive Oncology, 7*(3), 98–99.

Berwick, D. M. (2003). Disseminating innovations in health care. *Journal of the American Medical Association, 289*, 1969–1975.

Bodenheimer, T., Lorig, K., Homan, H., & Grumbach, K. (2002). Patient self-management of chronic disease in primary care. *Journal of American Medicine Association, 288*(19), 2469–2475.

Cohen, L., La Greca, A. M., Blount, R. L., Kazak, A. E., Holmbeck, G. N., & Lemanek, K. L. (2008). Introduction: Evidence-based assessment in pediatric psychology. *Journal of Pediatric Psychology, 33*, 2.

Coons, S. J., Gwanltney, C. J., Hays, R., Lundy, J. L., Sloan, J. A., Revicki, D. A., et al. (2009). Recommendations on evidence needed to support measurement equivalence between electronic and paper-based patient-reported outcome (PRO) measures: ISPOR ePRO Good Research Practices Task Force Report. *Value in Health, 12*(4), 419–429.

Cruz, I., Marciel, K. K., Cheney, J., Wainwright, C., Campbell, M., & Quittner, A. L. (2009). The preschool cystic fibrosis questionnaire revised: Initial validation results. *Pediatric Pulmonology, 32*(Suppl), 421 [Abstract].

Edwards, T. C., Huebner, C. E., Connell, F. A., & Patrick, D. L. (2002). Adolescent quality of life, part I: Conceptual and measurement framework. *Journal of Adolescence, 25*(3), 275–286.

Eiser, C., & Morse, R. (2001). Quality-of-life measures in chronic diseases of childhood. *Health Technology Assessment, 5*(4), 1–157.

Gawande, A. (2004, December 4). The Bell curve: What happens when patients find out how good their doctors really are? *The New Yorker*, 82–91.

Goss, C. H., & Quittner, A. L. (2007). Patient-reported outcomes in cystic fibrosis. *Proceedings of the American Thoracic Society, 4*, 378–386.

Guyatt, G. H., Osoba, D., Wu, A. W., Wyrwich, K. W., Norman, G. R., & Clinical Significance Consensus Meeting Group. (2002). Methods to explain the clinical significance of health status measures. *Mayo Clinic Proceedings, 77*, 371–383.

Gwaltney, C. J., Shields, A. L., & Shiffman, S. (2008). Equivalence of electronic and paper-and pencil administration of patient-reported outcome measures: A meta-analytic review. *Value in Health, 11*, 322–333.

Havermans, T., Vreys, M., Proesmans, M., & De Boeck, C. (2006). Assessment of agreement between parents and children on health-related quality of life in children with cystic fibrosis. *Child: Care, Health and Development, 32*(1), 1–7.

Hood, K. K., Peterson, C. M., Rohan, J. M., & Drotar, D. (2009). Association between adherence and glycemic control in pediatric type 1 diabetes: A meta-analysis. *Pediatrics, 124*, e1171–e1179.

Leape, L., Berwick, D., Clancy, C., Conway, J., Gluck, P., Guest, J., et al. (2009). Transforming healthcare: A safety imperative. *Quality & Safety in Health Care, 18*, 424–428.

Lenhart, A., Madden, M., & Hitlin, P. (2005, July 27). *Teens and technology: You are leading the transition to a fully wired and mobile nation.* Retrieved from www.pewInternet.org/pdfs/PIP_Teens_Tech_July2005web.pdf.

Stinson, J. N., & McGrath, P. J. (2011). Measurement and assessment of pain in pediatric patients. In M. E. Lynch, K. D. Craig, & P. W. H. Peng (Eds.), *Clinical pain management: A practical guide* (pp. 64). Oxford, UK: Wiley-Blackwell.

McCoy, K. S., Quittner, A. L., Oermann, C. M., Gibson, R. L., Retsch-Bogart, G. Z., & Montgomery, A. B. (2008). Inhaled aztreonam lysine for chronic airway pseudomonas aeruginosa in cystic fibrosis. *American Journal of Respiratory and Critical Care Medicine, 178*, 921–928.

Modi, A. C., Marciel, K. K., Slater, S. K., Drotar, D., & Quittner, A. L. (2008). The influence of parental supervision on medical adherence in adolescents with cystic fibrosis: Developmental shifts from early to late adolescence. *Children's Health Care, 37*, 78–92.

Modi, A. C., & Quittner, A. L. (2003). Validation of a disease-specific measure of health-related quality of life for children with cystic fibrosis. *Journal of Pediatric Psychology, 28*, 535–546.

Modi, A. C., & Quittner, A. L. (2006). Barriers to treatment adherence for children with cystic fibrosis and asthma: What gets in the way? *Journal of Pediatric Psychology, 31*, 846–858.

Modi, A. C., Rausch, J. R., & Glauser, T. A. (2011). Patterns of nonadherence to antiepileptic drug therapy in children with newly diagnosed epilepsy. *Journal of the American Medical Association, 305*(16), 1669–1676.

Oermann, C. M., Retsch-Bogart, G. Z., Quittner, A. L., Gibson, R. L., McCoy, K. S., Montgomery, A. B., et al. (2010). An 18-month study of the safety and efficacy of repeated courses of inhaled aztreonam lysine in cystic fibrosis. *Pediatric Pulmonology, 45*(11), 1121–1134.

Palermo, T. M., Long, A. C., Lewandowski, A. S., Drotar, D., Quittner, A. L., & Walker, L. S. (2008). Evidence based assessment of health related quality of life and functional impairment in pediatric psychology. *Journal of Pediatric Psychology, 33*, 983–996.

Quittner, A. L., Buu, A., Messer, M. A., Modi, A. C., & Watrous, M. (2005). Development and validation of the cystic fibrosis questionnaire (CFQ) in the United States: A health related quality of life measure for cystic fibrosis. *Chest 128*, 2347–2354.

Quittner, A. L., Cruz, I., Modi, A. C., & Marciel, K. K. (2009). Health-related quality of life instruments for adolescents with chronic diseases. In W. O'Donohue & L. Tolle (Eds.), *Behavioral approaches to chronic disease in adolescence: A guide to integrative care* (pp. 311–327). New York: Springer.

Quittner, A. L., Modi, A. C., & Roux, A. L. (2003). Psychosocial challenges and clinical interventions for children with cystic fibrosis: A developmental approach. In R. Brown (Ed.), (pp. 333–361), *Handbook of pediatric psychology in school settings*. New Jersey: Lawrence Erlbaum Associates.

Quittner, A. L., Modi, A. C., Wainwright, C., Otto, K., Kirihara, J., & Montgomery, A. B. (2009). Determination of the minimal clinically important difference (MCID) scores for the Cystic Fibrosis Questionnaire-Revised (CFQ-R) Respiratory Symptom scale in two populations of patients with CF and chronic Pseudomonas aeruginosa airway infection. *Chest, 135*, 1610–1618.

Retsch-Bogart, G. Z., Quittner, A. L., Gibson, R. L., Oermann, C. M., McCoy, K. S., Montgomery, A. B., et al. (2009). Efficacy and safety of inhaled aztreonam lysine for airway Pseudomonas in cystic fibrosis. *Chest, 135*, 1223–1232.

Riley, A. W. (2004). Evidence that school-age children can self-report on their health. *Ambulatory Pediatrics, 4S*, 371–376.

Robinson, J. H., Callister, L. C., Berry, J. A., & Dearing, K. A. (2008). Patient-centered care and adherence: Definitions and applications to improve outcomes. *Journal of the American Academy of Nurse Practitioners, 20*, 600–607.

Safran, C. (2003). The collaborative edge: Patient empowerment for vulnerable populations. *International Journal of Medical Informatics, 69*(2–3), 185–190.

Sawicki, G. S., Rasouliyan, L., McMullen, A. H., Wagener, J. S., McColley, S. A., Pasta, D. J., et al. (2011). Longitudinal assessment of health-related quality of life in an observational cohort of patients with cystic fibrosis. *Pediatric Pulmonology, 46*(1), 36–44.

Schwarz, N., & Sudman, S. (1996). *Answering questions: Methodology for determining cognitive and communicative processes in survey research.* San Francisco: Jossey-Bass.

Scoggins, J. F., & Patrick, D. L. (2009). The use of patient-reported outcomes instruments in registered clinical trials: Evidence from ClinicalTrials.gov. *Contemporary Clinical Trials, 30*(4), 289–292.

Spencer, J., Cooper, H., & Milton, B. (2010). Qualitative studies of type 1 diabetes in adolescence: A systematic literature review. *Pediatric Diabetes, 11*(5), 364–375.

Starfield, B., Riley, A. W., Green, B. F., Ensminger, M. E., Ryan, S. A., Kelleher, K., et al. (1995). The adolescent child health and illness profile: A population-based measure of health. *Medical Care, 33*, 553–66.

Stone, A. A., Shiffman, S., Schwartz, J. E., et al. (2002). Patient non-compliance with paper diaries. *British Medical Journal, 324*, 1193–1194.

Turner, R. R., Quittner, A. L., Parasuraman, B. M., Kallich, J. D., & Cleeland, C. S. (2007). Patient-reported outcomes: Instrument development and selection issues. *Value in Health, 10*(s2), S86–S93.

U.S. Department of Health and Human Services, Food and Drug Administration. (2009). Guidance for industry, patient-reported outcome measures: Use in medical product development to support labeling claims. Federal Registration.

Varni, J. W., Seid, M., & Rode, C. A. (1999). The PedsQL: Measurement model for the pediatric quality of life inventory. *Medical Care, 37*, 126–39.

Verrips, G. H., Vogels, A. G., den Ouden, A. L., Paneth, N., & Verloove-Vanhorick, S. P. (2000). Measuring health-related quality of life in adolescents: Agreement between raters and between methods of administration. *Child: Care, Health and Development, 26*(6), 457–469.

Wyrwich, K. W., Tierney, W. M., Babu, A. N., Kroenke, K., & Wolinsky, F. D. (2005). A comparison of clinically important differences in health-related quality of life for patients with chronic lung disease, asthma or heart disease. *Health Services Research, 40*(2), 577–92.

Zemanick, E. T., Harris, K., Conway, S., Konstan, M. W., Marshall, B., Quittner, A. L., et al. (2010). Measuring and improving respiratory outcomes in cystic fibrosis lung disease: Opportunities and challenges to therapy. *Journal of Cystic Fibrosis, 9*(1), 1–16.

Zindani, G. N., Streetman, D. D., Streetman, D. S., & Nasr, S. Z. (2006). Adherence to treatment in children and adolescent patients with cystic fibrosis. *Journal of Adolescent Health, 38*, 13–17.

The Effects of Physical Activity on the Physical and Psychological Health of Adolescents

Erika M. Shearer and Brie A. Moore

The Effects of Physical Activity on the Physical and Psychological Health of Adolescents

Adolescence offers a unique opportunity for establishing positive health behaviors that can persist into adulthood. One such health behavior is engaging in increased levels of physical activity. During adolescence physical activity dramatically decreases, with children and teens demonstrating a 50 % reduction in their total daily expenditure of energy per body weight (Kemper, 2002). Decreased physical activity has been linked not only to obesity but also to depression and greater risk of hypertension and cardiovascular disease in adulthood (Lobstein, Baur, & Uauy, 2004). Increasing physical activity, in conjunction with appropriate dietary modifications, is a well-established means for controlling obesity (Hayman, 2002). Given the striking increase in prevalence of adolescent overweight and obesity, it is imperative that effective interventions are developed for the adolescent population.

From the 1980s to the early 2000s, the prevalence of obesity (defined as a body mass index at least in the 95th percentile, CDC, 2004) among adolescents has increased dramatically. According to a 2003–2004 Centers for Disease Control and Prevention (CDC) survey, the prevalence of obesity increased from 11 % to 19 % among 6- to 11-year-olds and increased from 11 % to 17 % among 12- to 19-year-olds (CDC, 2004). These recent increases have been particularly evident among non-Hispanic black and Mexican-American adolescents (Zametkin, Zoon, Klein, & Munson, 2003). The current estimates of adolescent obesity in the United States suggest the presence of racial disparities, with 21.5 % of African-Americans, 21.8 % of Hispanics, and 12.3 % of non-Hispanic whites being overweight (Strauss & Pollack, 2001). The CDC has labeled these increases in obesity prevalence as an epidemic that is linked not only to the overconsumption of foods but also to sedentary lifestyle behaviors (Clemmens & Hayman, 2004).

Childhood and adolescent obesity can have physical, psychological, and social consequences and can contribute to future complications in adulthood. For example, type 2 diabetes, which was formerly thought of as an adult disease, is now becoming more prevalent among children and adolescents (Baranowski et al., 2000). Childhood- and adolescent-onset obesity may be associated with higher rates of death and cardiovascular mortality than adult-onset obesity. Adults who were obese as children have been

E.M. Shearer, M.A. (✉)
Department of Psychology, University of Nevada, 298, Reno, NV 89557, USA
e-mail: erikamshearer@gmail.com

B.A. Moore, Ph.D.
University of Nevada, 6490 S. McCarran Blvd. Street D1-28, Reno, NV 89509, USA
e-mail: brieamoore@yahoo.com

W.T. O'Donohue et al. (eds.), *Handbook of Adolescent Health Psychology*,
DOI 10.1007/978-1-4614-6633-8_12,

found to have increased morbidity and mortality regardless of adult weight (Riddoch, 1998; Styne, 2001). Obesity increases the risk of cardiovascular disease, insulin resistance, diabetes, hypertension, cancer, gall bladder disease, and atherosclerosis (Styne, 2001). There are psychological ramifications of obesity as well. It has been found that obese children as young as 5 years old report feeling decreased self-esteem due to their obesity (Bradford, 2009). Furthermore, nearly half of obese adolescents report moderate to severe depressive symptoms and a third report feelings of anxiety (Bradford, 2009).

Traditionally, overweight and obesity have been framed in a biopsychosocial framework in which genetic and biologic, psychological, and environmental factors overlap. It has been estimated that genetic factors contribute to a third of obesity (Bradford, 2009). These genetic factors include the hundreds of genes and genetic markers that have been linked to obesity, family syndromes, such as hyperinsulinism, and the genetic influence on energy expenditure and eating behaviors (Bradford, 2009). Biologic factors can include endocrine disorders such as hypothyroidism, medications, and medical treatments. Although there are many associations between obesity and psychological diagnoses, the causal relationships are unclear. Environmental factors include parental obesity, sedentary lifestyles, eating habits, and sleep deprivation. Because of the relatively short time period in which this increase in obesity has occurred, it cannot be explained solely by genetic factors (Ferreira et al., 2006). It is more likely that behavioral and environmental factors play a greater role in the obesity epidemic.

One such behavioral factor is the recent increase in adolescent inactivity. Adolescents spent 75.5 % of their day inactive, with an average of 5.2 (SD = 1.8) hours spent engaging in television, computer, and homework activities (Strauss, Rodzilsky, Burack, & Colin, 2001). Only 1.4 % of an adolescent's day is spent engaging in vigorous activity (Strauss et al., 2001). This amounts to 10 hours of sedentary behavior per day with only 12–13 minutes of physical activity per day. Strauss and colleagues' findings are in sharp contrast with the international guidelines for physical activity that recommend engaging in at least an hour of physical activity on a daily basis (Biddle, Sallis, & Cavill, 1998). These activities should occur in the context of family, school, and community activities and should be enjoyable, engage a variety of muscle groups, and include weight-bearing activities (Sallis & Patrick, 1994). The Youth Risk Behavior Surveillance System estimated that 45.6 % of boys and 27.7 % of girls are meeting these guidelines (Camacho-Minano, LaVoi, & Barr-Anderson, 2011).

Benefits of Physical Activity Among Adolescents

Aside from managing overweight and obesity, there are many other physical, psychological, and social benefits of physical activity for adolescents. There is a consistent positive relationship between physical activity and overall mental well-being (Hallal, Victora, Azevado, & Wells, 2006; Mutrie & Parfitt, 1998). Psychological benefits of physical activity for adolescents include reduction of tension and anxiety, reduction in feelings of depression, strengthening of stress coping skills, improvement in concentration and memory, improvement in positive self-image and self-confidence, and improvement in sleeping patterns (Heaven, 1996, p. 153). A recent review found that adolescent exercise resulted in positive effects on self-esteem (Hallal et al., 2006). It was also found that exercise reduced need for thinness, changes in body composition, and frequency of bingeing, purging, and laxative abuse among bulimic adolescent and young adult females (Hallal et al., 2006).

Physical activity also has positive impacts on adolescent social health. Social advantages of physical activity include games and organized sports that provide opportunities to work with others on a team, interact with others, and develop social skills (Heaven, 1996, p. 153). Participating in school and community activities is associated with short- and long-term indicators of positive development (Barber, Stone, & Eccles, 2005). Furthermore, it has been found that athletic youth are more likely to have opportunities to play sports, make friendships, and be part of an in-group (Pender & Stein, 2002). These athletic activities provide a space for social development (Barber et al., 2005). Physical activities can serve to structure an adolescent's peer group: adolescents involved in extracurricular activities tend to have more academic friends and fewer friends who skip school and use drugs (Barber et al., 2005). Finally, in a study, participation in team sports was found to be linked to better academic outcomes as well as adult educational attainment, occupation, and income (Barber et al., 2005).

The research on the physiological benefits of physical activity has primarily focused on cardiovascular disease, skeletal health, and lung capacity. Because of the relatively low prevalence of morbidity and mortality related to cardiovascular disease in the adolescent population, most research investigating the relationship between physical activity and cardiovascular disease among adolescents has focused on cardiovascular risk factors (Twisk, 2001). Physical activity has been found to have a beneficial effect on high-density lipoprotein (HDL) cholesterol, body fatness, and cardiopulmonary fitness (Twisk, 2001) as well as aid in a range of factors associated with metabolic syndromes overall (hypertension, obesity, insulin resistance, impaired lipid and lipoprotein profile) (Hayman, 2002).

Knowledge regarding the long-term effects of exercise on skeletal health is incomplete; however, research suggests that vigorous physical activity may help to enhance bone mineral density in children. Furthermore, immobility and inactivity are associated with negative effects on skeletal health. Overall, it appears that low-impact activity, even without vigorous physical activity, is associated with better skeletal health (Riddoch, 1998). In a review by Hallal et al. (2006), the positive skeletal and bone density effects attained via adolescent physical activity were found to have a long-term protective effect on skeletal health in adulthood. There also appeared to be long-term positive effects for preventing breast cancer. Physical activity has also been found to significantly increase lung functioning among cystic fibrosis patients and certain types of physical exercise (e.g., swimming) in adolescence have been found to reduce the severity of asthma symptoms (Hallal et al., 2006).

Several large-scale studies have shown that physical inactivity in adolescence results in cardiovascular disease indirectly via the mechanisms that relate to beneficial effects of physical activities on blood pressure and serum lipoprotein profiles (Berlin & Colditz, 1990; Powell et al., 1987). Physical inactivity is a direct and indirect risk factor for adult diseases including cardiovascular diseases, cancer, and other chronic diseases. Atherosclerotic processes begin early in life, and it is possible that a sufficient amount and intensity of exercise during adolescence could decelerate this process. In a prospective study, it was found that being overweight during adolescence predicted a broad range of adverse health problems in adulthood independent of being overweight in adulthood (Riddoch, 1998). Obesity, cardiovascular problems, osteoporosis, and some kinds of cancer which are related to sedentariness in adults have also been found to originate in childhood (De Bourdeaudhuij, 1998).

Health behavior patterns established during adolescence affect the quality of life during adolescence and serve as the foundation for health-related lifestyles in adulthood (Pender & Stein, 2002). The specific goal of exercise promotion among children is to establish healthy exercise habits that will continue throughout life and subsequently improve current and future health outcomes (Riddoch, 1998).

Caveats When Considering Physical Activity in Adolescence

Although research has not found direct negative effects of physical activity on mental health, there is some concern that involvement in certain sports may increase the risk of some girls developing eating disorders. This is highlighted by the finding that 20 % of female athletes in Norway were defined as at risk of an eating disorder (Mutrie & Parfitt, 1998). Although it is unclear how being involved in athletics may be linked to eating disordered behavior, it is interesting that such a significant percentage of females with eating disorders are involved in athletics. There is some evidence that physical activity can have adverse effects on adolescent physical health. Epidemiological data has revealed that sports injury is the leading cause of physical injury among adolescents (Emery, 2003). Strenuous physical activity has been found to adversely affect the female reproductive system resulting in athletic amenorrhea and weight lifting during adolescence could lead to musculoskeletal injuries and interrupt growth (Hallal et al., 2006). It is possible that growing trends toward sports-related injuries among adolescents are associated with increased intensity of training, competition, skill, and duration of sports at increasingly younger ages (Emery, 2003).

Adolescents may be at risk for sports-related injuries due to improper technique, ill-fitting protective equipment, training errors, muscle weakness, and imbalance (Cassas & Cassettari-Wayhs, 2006). In a review by Emery (2005), the author revealed a number of non-modifiable and potentially modifiable risk factors that were found to be correlated with increased rates of injury. These risk factors included previous injury, older age, male gender, higher contact sports, higher level of skill, position played, weather, fitness level, training, flexibility, strength, joint stability, balance and proprioception, and psychological or social factors (Emery, 2005).

It is likely that knowledge regarding these risk factors will aid in efforts to prevent adolescent injury. In a review by Abernethy and Bleakley (2007), the authors found mixed results for protective equipment as a means of preventing sports-related injury. It appears that the use of headgear is related to an increased rate of head injury with little evidence supporting the use of mouth guards as a protective strategy. The authors also found little evidence supporting bracing methods with an increased rate of injury associated with the use of protective external bracing. They did find some evidence for the use of knee pads in reducing lower limb injury. Finally, the authors did find support for conditioning programs that included strength, flexibility, and technique training programs occurring both preseason and during the sport-specific season. The authors note that there was no evidence for programs that focused on stretching alone.

Although most adolescent injuries occur in sports contexts, there appears to be less support for adolescent injuries incurred in supervised physical education and after-school environments. In a review by Strong et al. (2005), the rate of injury in both settings was nearly zero. Overall, it appears that although there is some risk of injury when adolescents are involved in competitive sports, it appears that these risks are outweighed by the potential benefits of physical activity.

Recommendations for Adolescent Physical Activity

It is clear that there are many benefits of engaging in physical activity (Biddle et al., 1998; Hayman, 2002; Hallal et al., 2006; Mutrie & Parfitt, 1998; Twisk, 2001). For these reasons, guidelines have been established regarding optimal levels of adolescent physical exercise. The International Consensus Conference on Physical Activity Guidelines for Adolescents was convened in the 1990s and recommended that all adolescents should engage in physical activity daily or nearly every day, and adolescents should engage in moderate to vigorous levels of physical activity at least three times a week for at least 20 minutes (Sallis & Patrick, 1994).

In 1998, an international Health Education Symposium "Young and Active" modified the guidelines set forth by the International Consensus Conference on Physical Activity Guidelines for Adolescents and recommended that adolescents engage in at least 1 hour of moderate or greater intensity physical activity on a daily basis (Biddle et al., 1998). For adolescents who are not currently physically active, it was recommended that they should participate in at least half an hour of moderate or greater intensity exercise on a daily basis. Secondary recommendations included that at least twice a week, some of the aforementioned activities should help to enhance and maintain muscular strength, flexibility, and bone health. These secondary recommendations were based on the positive associations between strength and weight-bearing activities with bone mineral density. These activities are believed to reduce long-term risk of osteoporosis. Such activities include climbing, skipping, jumping, body conditioning, resistance exercises, gymnastics, aerobics, and most sports.

At a national level, the United States proposed Healthy People 2010 to increase adolescent physical activity (Office of Disease Prevention and Health Promotion, 2010). This initiative recommended vigorous physical activity that enhances cardiorespiratory fitness for at least 20 minutes at a time on at least 3 days a week. Although these guidelines and initiatives are in place at both international and national levels, adolescents continue to lead sedentary lives (Strauss et al., 2001).

Barriers to Physical Activity

There are several environmental, cognitive, and behavioral factors that appear to interfere with adolescent engagement in physical activity. These barriers to physical activity include not enough time, feeling too tired, feeling self-conscious when exercising, lack of motivation, lack of interest, and competition (Clemmens & Hayman, 2004; Park & Kim, 2008). It was also found that these perceived barriers mediated the relationship between perceived self-efficacy and physical activity. In another review by Sallis, Prochaska, and Taylor (2000), lack of perceived activity competence, lack of intent, depression, and low sensation seeking were found to be potential barriers to physical activity.

Past physical activity has been found to predict future physical activity (Park & Kim, 2008; Sallis, Prochaska et al., 2000); therefore if a child does not have a history of being physically active then it is not likely that he or she will be physically active in adolescence or adulthood. Also, sedentary family lifestyles on the weekends and after school have been found to be potential barriers to physical activity (Sallis, Prochaska et al., 2000).

While the above findings pertain to individual barriers that can interfere with adolescent physical activity, there are a number of social and environmental factors that can serve as impediments as well. Because adolescence tends to be a time of increased social activity, it is no surprise that a lack of social support (e.g., support from peers, parents, and others) can serve as a barrier to engaging in physical activity (Park & Kim, 2008). Other environmental barriers to physical activity are largely related to access. In Park and Kim's review (2008), the authors found that adolescents who were classified as low socioeconomic status emphasized proximity, cost, access, and safety of facilities as potential barriers to physical activity. The authors found mixed results regarding associations between physical activity and where adolescents lived. They found that among urban school students, the commute to school greatly affected any engagement in physical activity, with adolescents experiencing a longer commute being less physically active. Among rural school students, access was also a barrier to engaging in physical activity, and the addition of school physical education classes appeared to be an effective means of overcoming this barrier. Ferreira et al. (2006) found that attendance in vocational schools and living in a neighborhood with a high crime incidence were found to be negatively associated with physical activity, and therefore may serve as barriers to engaging in physical activity as well. It is possible that offering daily physical education programming in the school context as well as the availability of community sports and community recreation centers are effective means of counteracting access barriers, and these options will be further explored in later sections (Park & Kim, 2008; Sallis, Prochaska et al., 2000).

There are a number of demographic factors that appear to be negatively correlated with physical activity. Gender and age have consistently played a role in physical activity, with boys being more active than girls (Park & Kim, 2008; Sallis, Prochaska et al., 2000), and younger adolescents engaging in more physical activity than older adolescents (Park & Kim, 2008; Sallis, Prochaska et al., 2000). Also, minority status (i.e., nonwhite ethnicity) appears to be consistently associated with decreased physical activity when compared to other ethnicities (Sallis, Prochaska et al., 2000). High family income is associated with greater physical activity (Park & Kim, 2008; Sallis, Prochaska et al., 2000) as is high parental education with mother's education level being particularly positively correlated with physical activity (Ferreira et al., 2006; Park & Kim, 2008). Although these factors may not be altered via interventions, interventions can be informed by these factors and be designed to better accommodate these factors.

Interventions to Increase Physical Activity Among Adolescents

In order for interventions to effectively promote health behavior change, they must be developmentally appropriate, based on health behavior theory, systematic, and comprehensive (Sallis, Patrick et al., 2000). There are many avenues for intervention among adolescents (e.g., family, health care provider, school, and community), and these avenues are reviewed below. Ultimately, interventions that include multiple modalities will likely be more successful at increasing physical activity among adolescents.

Family-Based Interventions

Even during adolescence, an age where teens are experimenting with increased autonomy, parents can execute a great deal of control over the home environment, including their teen's diet and physical activity (Sallis, Patrick et al., 2000). Furthermore, parental, peer, siblings, and others' support have consistently been found to be positively associated with adolescent physical activity (Ferreira et al., 2006; Park & Kim, 2008; Sallis, Prochaska et al., 2000). In these studies, parental support has been described as both directly helping adolescents exercise as well as giving advice, role modeling, and engaging parents' own physical activity behaviors (Park & Kim, 2008; Sallis, Prochaska et al., 2000). These finding underscores the importance of interventions aimed at increasing physical activity and physical activity awareness within the family unit as a whole.

In a review of reviews by van Sluijs, Kriemler, and McMinn (2011), the authors found a generally positive impact of family-based interventions on adolescent physical activity, with half of family-based interventions having a positive impact on adolescent physical activity. The authors found no theoretical, methodological, or population differences identified between the effective and ineffective interventions. Many family-based interventions are aimed at altering the behaviors of the individuals within that particular family environment. Such individually based strategies can include activities such as screening, behavioral counseling and/or classes, and tracking of health behaviors (Pate et al., 2000).

Health Care Provider-Based Interventions

Health care providers are typically seen as being highly credible, and for a majority of adolescents, they are the first point of contact when there is a weight concern (Baranowski et al., 2000; Lobstein et al., 2004). These contacts can occur at private offices, community clinics, hospitals, schools, and other settings. The majority of adolescents visit a health care provider once a year (Ozer et al., 2005). Consequently, the main challenge to the success of interventions by health care providers is lack of contact between adolescents and health care providers (Sallis, Patrick et al., 2000). Providers may be resistant to intervening if they lack incentive to do so, do not have sufficient knowledge and skills, or lack evidenced-based interventions (Sallis, Patrick et al. 2000). In order for interventions involving health care providers to be successful, it is likely that the frequency, duration, and intensity of visits with health care providers will need to be increased (Sallis, Patrick et al. 2000). These could be increased by offering classes, groups, or workshops, referrals to other professionals, or communication via phone, mail, or Internet. Health care providers could also act as an additional stimulus to engage in home, school, and/or community-based interventions by recommending these programs during contact with their patients (Sallis, Patrick et al. 2000).

Although individual strategies can be effective at altering behavior, environmental strategies have the ability to reach larger audiences, and therefore have the potential to be less costly and more efficient (Wechsler, Devereaux, Davis, & Collins, 2000). These environmental strategies work to change physical structures and social norms to be more conducive to increasing physical activity (Wechsler et al., 2000). One type intervention that typically employs environmental strategies is school-based interventions.

School-Based Interventions

Nearly all children and adolescents spend the majority of their days at school (Kriemler et al., 2011). The school environment also provides many opportunities of physical activity including physical education classes, recess periods, extracurricular activities, and access to school facilities including gymnasiums, athletic fields, and playground equipment (Wechsler et al., 2000). School can also serve as an environment with trained professionals who could potentially implement theoretically driven interventions to promote physical activity among adolescents (Wechsler et al., 2000).

For these reasons, the CDC established guidelines for school and community programs to promote physical activity among children and adolescents (CDC, 1997). These guidelines included (1) establishing policies that would encourage enjoyable and lifelong physical activity; (2) providing physical structures and social environments that will support safe and enjoyable physical activity; (3) implementing physical education classes that stress enjoyable participation in physical activity as well as knowledge, attitudes, confidence, and skills to adopt and maintain physically active lifestyles; (4) implementing health education classes to aid in the development of knowledge, attitudes, confidence, and skills to adopt and maintain physically active lifestyles; (5) providing extracurricular programs that promote physical activity and are interesting and meet the needs of students; (6) involving parents and guardians in physical activity instruction and extracurricular and community programs and encouraging their support in their children's participation in physical activity; (7) providing personnel training for physical and health education, coaching, recreation, and health-care that is enjoyable and promotes lifelong physical activity; (8) assessing physical activity patterns among children and adolescents, counseling services around physical activity, and appropriate referrals to programs and interventions; (9) providing developmentally appropriate community sports and recreation programs that are appealing to children and adolescents; and (10) evaluating school and community physical activity instruction, programs, and facilities on a regular basis (CDC, 1997).

In a review of reviews by Kriemler et al. (2011), they found that school-based physical activity programs generally had positive effects on duration of physical activity and aerobic fitness, but found mixed results for how much school-based programs affected amount of physical activity engaged in outside of the school context. They also found that successful interventions tended to intervene for a longer period of time and applied multicomponent approaches (e.g., including family-, health care provider-, or community-based interventions).

Community-Based Interventions

Although community-based interventions can include strategies aimed at the individual level (e.g., screening, behavioral counseling, and tracking), these interventions have the capacity to alter the physical and social environment as well (Pate et al., 2000). Because adolescence is a time when teens become particularly aware of and influenced by their peer group (Bandura, 1969), this ability to potentially manipulate community and social norms around physical activity makes community-based interventions particularly interesting to explore within the adolescent population. In a study of social norms and diet and exercise by Baker, Little, and Brownell (2003), they found that adolescents' decisions to engage in physical activity were influenced by their perceptions of social norms around physical activity.

Because adolescents typically spend a substantial amount of time in community settings outside of school (Baranowski et al., 2000), community-based interventions are potentially powerful influencers of adolescent physical activity. These community-based interventions could take place at settings such as community organizations, religious institutions, businesses, and government agencies. Community-based interventions have the ability to involve other sources of influence and/or role models including parents and family, schools, and health care providers (Pate et al., 2000). In a review by Pate et al. (2000), the authors found that community-based interventions should be intense, long in duration, and involve as many different aspects of the community as possible. Although the rationale for community-based interventions appears to be strong, there appears to be a paucity of data to corroborate this rationale. In a recent review, van Sluijs et al. (2011) found only one out of four community-based interventions to have a significant positive impact on adolescent physical activity. This intervention was also the one intervention that was environmentally based and specifically targeted physical activity. It appears that, ideally, interventions will consist of a combination of individual- and environmentally based behavior change strategies.

Conclusion

Adolescence is a time of physical, psychosocial, cognitive, and emotional development that occurs amidst a backdrop of varied sociocultural contexts (Clemmens & Hayman, 2004). Each of these developmental changes affect and are affected by participation in physical activity (Sallis, Prochaska et al., 2000). Because of the dramatic increase in adolescent obesity as well as the short- and long-term physical, psychological, and social consequences associated with obesity, it is imperative that this obesity epidemic is addressed.

Although the increased prevalence of obesity is a persuasive argument for increasing adolescent physical activity, the physical, psychological, and social benefits of physical activity are also compelling. These benefits include physical benefits of decreasing cholesterol and fat, improving skeletal health, and increasing cardiopulmonary fitness; psychological benefits of decreasing tension, anxiety, and depression, increasing coping skills and self-confidence, and improving concentration, memory, and sleep; and social benefits of increasing teamwork and social skills, and increasing the likelihood of making academically oriented friends. It appears that although engaging in sports does convey some risk for injury, these injuries appear to be prevented by increased supervision and training. Overall, increasing adolescent physical activity is not only an appropriate strategy for managing overweight and obesity, but it also appears to be associated with significant physical, psychological, and social benefits.

A number of demographic, psychological, social, and environmental barriers have been identified. In order for interventions aimed at increasing physical activity to be effective, these barriers must be addressed as a part of the intervention. It appears that different types of interventions may be more effective at addressing certain barriers than others. For example, individual-based interventions such as family- or health care provider-based interventions may be more able to be tailored to individual characteristics of gender, age, and ethnicity, whereas environmentally based interventions such as school- or community-based interventions may be more effective at reducing social barriers. Furthermore, access to interventions should be considered as adolescents may not be able to obtain transportation; in this case family- or school-based approaches may be most effective. In sum, in order to be maximally effective, interventions should apply multicomponent approaches that include both individually and environmentally based strategies to increase physical activity to promote physical and emotional well-being during adolescence.

References

Abernethy, L., & Bleakley, C. (2007). Strategies to prevent injury in adolescent sport: A systematic review. *British Journal of Sports Medicine, 41*, 627–638.

Baker, C. W., Little, T. D., & Brownell, K. D. (2003). Predicting adolescent eating and activity behaviors: The role of social norms and personal agency. *Health Psychology, 22*, 189–198.

Bandura, A. (1969). *Principles of behavior modification*. Oxford, England: Holt, Rinehart, & Winston.

Baranowski, T., Mendlein, J., Resnicow, K., Frank, E., Cullen, K. W., & Baranowski, J. (2000). Physical activity and nutrition in children and youth: An overview of obesity prevention. *Preventive Medicine, 31*, S1–S10.

Barber, B. L., Stone, M. R., & Eccles, J. S. (2005). Adolescent participation in organized activities. In K. Moore (Ed.), *Conceptualizing and measuring indicators of positive development: What do children need to flourish?* (pp. 133–146). New York: Springer.

Berlin, J. A., & Colditz, G. A. (1990). A meta-analysis of physical activity in the prevention of coronary heart disease. *American Journal of Epidemiology, 132*, 612–628.

Biddle, S., Sallis, J., & Cavill, N. (1998). Policy framework for young people and health enhancing physical activity. In S. Biddle, J. Sallis, & N. Cavill (Eds.), *Young and Active? Young people and health-enhancing physical activity: Evidence and implications* (pp. 3–16). London: Health Education Authority.

Bradford, N. F. (2009). Overweight and obesity in children and adolescents. *Primary Care, 36*, 319–339.

Camacho-Minano, M. J., LaVoi, N. M., & Barr-Anderson, D. J. (2011). Interventions to promote physical activity among young and adolescent girls: A systematic review. *Health Education Research, 26*(6), 1025–1049.

Cassas, K. J., & Cassettari-Wayhs, A. (2006). Childhood and adolescent sports-related overuse injuries. *American Family Physician, 73*, 1014–1022.

Centers for Disease Control and Prevention. (1997). Guidelines for school and community programs to promote lifelong physical activity among young people. *Morbidity and Mortality Weekly Report, 46*, 1–36.

Centers for Disease Control and Prevention. (2004). *Prevalence of overweight among children and adolescents: United States, 2003–2004*. National Center for Health Statistics, CDC website. Retrieved August 21, 2011, from www.cdc.gov/nchs/products/pubs/pubd/hestats/overweight/overwght_chld_03.htm

Clemmens, D., & Hayman, L. L. (2004). Increasing activity to reduce obesity in adolescent girls: A research review. *Journal of Obstetric, Gynecologic, and Neonatal Nursing, 33*, 801–808.

De Bourdeaudhuij, I. (1998). Behavioural factors associated with physical activity in young people. In S. Biddle, J. F. Sallis, & N. Cavill (Eds.), Young and active? Young people and health-enhanced physical *activity: Evidence and implications* (pp. 17–48). London, UK: Health Education Authority.

Emery, C. (2003). Risk factors for injury in child and adolescent sport: A systematic review of the literature. *Clinical Journal of Sport Medicine, 13*, 256–268.

Emery, C. (2005). Injury prevention and future research. In N. Maffuli & D. J. Caine (Eds.), *Epidemiology of pediatric sports injuries: Team sports*. (Vol. 49, pp. 170–191). Basel: Karger. Med Sport Science.

Ferreira, I., van der Horst, K., Wendel-Vos, W., Kremers, S., van Lenthe, F. J., & Brug, J. (2006). Environmental correlates of physical activity in youth—a review and update. *Obesity Reviews, 8*, 129–154.

Hallal, P. C., Victora, C. G., Azevado, M. R., & Wells, J. C. K. (2006). Adolescent physical activity and health. *Sports Medicine, 36*, 1019–1030.

Hayman, L. L. (2002). Obesity: Nongenetic influences in childhood and adolescence. In L. L. Hayman, M. M. Mahon, & J. R. Turner (Eds.), *Health and behavior in childhood and adolescence* (pp. 213–232). New York: Springer.

Heaven, P. C. L. (1996). *Adolescent health: The role of individual differences*. London: Routledge.

Kemper, H. C. G. (2002). The importance of physical activity in childhood and adolescence. In L. L. Hayman, M. M. Mahon, & J. R. Turner (Eds.), *Health and behavior in childhood and adolescence* (pp. 105–144). New York: Springer.

Kriemler, S., Meyer, U., Martin, E., van Sluijs, E. M. F., Andersen, L. B., & Martin, B. W. (2011). Effect of school-based interventions on physical activity and fitness in children and adolescents: A review of reviews and systematic update. *British Journal of Sports Medicine, 45*, 923–930.

Lobstein, T., Baur, L., & Uauy, R. (2004). Obesity in children and young people: A crisis in Public health. *Obesity Reviews, 5*, 4–85.

Mutrie, N., & Parfitt, G. (1998). Physical activity and its link with mental, social and moral health in young people. In S. Biddle, J. Sallis, & N. Cavill (Eds.), *Young and active? Young people and health-enhancing physical activity: Evidence and implications* (pp. 3–16). London: Health Education Authority Office of Disease Prevention and Health Promotion, US Department of Health and Human Services. Healthy People 2010. Retrieved August 21, 2011, from www.healthypeople.gov

Ozer, E. M., Adams, S. H., Lustig, J. L., Gee, S., Garber, A. K., Gardner, L. R., et al. (2005). Increasing the screening and counseling of adolescents for risky health behaviors: A primary care intervention. *Pediatrics, 115*, 960–968.

Park, H., & Kim, N. (2008). Predicting factors of physical activity in adolescents: A systematic review. *Asian Nursing Research, 2*, 113–128.

Pate, R. R., Trost, S. G., Mullis, R., Sallis, J. F., Wechsler, H., & Brown, D. R. (2000). Community interventions to promote proper nutrition and physical activity among youth. *Preventive Medicine, 31*, S138–149.

Pender, N. J., & Stein, K. F. (2002). Social support, the self system and adolescent health and health behaviors. In L. L. Hayman, M. M. Mahon, & J. R. Turner (Eds.), *Health behavior in childhood and adolescence* (pp. 37–66). New York: Springer.

Powell, K. E., Thompson, P. D., Caspersen, C. J., & Kendrick, J. S. (1987). Physical activity and the incidence of coronary heart disease. *American Rev. Public Health, 8*, 253–287.

Riddoch, C. (1998). Relationships between physical activity and health in young people. In S. Biddle, J. F. Sallis, & N. Cavill (Eds.), *Young and active? Young people and health-enhanced physical activity: Evidence and implications* (pp. 17–48). London, UK: Health Education Authority.

Sallis, J. F., Prochaska, J. J., & Taylor, W. C. (2000). A review of correlates of physical activity of children and adolescents. *Medical Science Sports Excer, 32*, 963–975.

Sallis, J. F., & Patrick, K. (1994). Physical activity guidelines for adolescents: Consensus statement. *Pediatric Exercise Science, 6*, 302–314.

Sallis, J. F., Patrick, K., Frank, E., Pratt, M., Wechsler, H., & Galuska, D. A. (2000). Interventions in health care settings to promote healthful eating and physical activity in children and adolescents. *Preventive Medicine, 31*, S112–S120.

Strauss, R., & Pollack, H. (2001). Epidemic increase in childhood overweight, 1996–1998. *Journal of the American Medical Association, 286*, 2845–2848.

Strauss, R. S., Rodzilsky, D., Burack, G., & Colin, M. (2001). Psychosocial correlates of physical activity in healthy children. *Archives of Pediatric Adolescent Medicine, 155*, 897–902.

Strong, W. B., Malina, R. M., Blimkie, C. J. R., Daniels, S. R., Dishman, R. K., Gutn, B., et al. (2005). Evidence based physical activity for school age youth. *Journal of Pediatrics, 146*, 732–737.

Styne, D. M. (2001). Childhood and adolescent obesity. Prevalence and significance. *Pediatric Clinics of North America, 48*, 823–254.

Twisk, J. W. R. (2001). Physical activity guidelines for children and adolescents: A critical review. *Sports Medicine, 31*, 617–627.

van Sluijs, E. M., Kriemler, S., & McMinn, A. M. (2011). The effect of community and family interventions on young people's physical activity levels: A review of reviews and updated systematic review. *British Journal of Sports Medicine, 45*, 914–922.

Wechsler, H., Devereaux, R. S., Davis, M., & Collins, J. (2000). Using the school environment to promote physical activity and healthy eating. *Preventive Medicine, 31*, S121–S137.

Zametkin, A. J., Zoon, C. K., Klein, H. W., & Munson, S. (2003). Psychiatric aspects of child and adolescent obesity: A review of the past 10 years. *Journal of the American Academy of Child and Adolescent Psychiatry, 43*, 134–150.

Adolescent Sexual Assault: Prevalence, Risk Associates, Outcomes, and Intervention

Jenna L. McCauley, Kristyn Zajac, and Angela M. Begle

Introduction

Sexual assault is an unfortunate and all too common experience for adolescents in the USA. Although the majority of youth who experience sexual assault are resilient, these experiences can have both acute and chronic effects on adolescent development and adjustment in a substantial number of cases. The preponderance of the literature regarding sexual assault focuses on either the experiences of children (i.e., child sexual abuse) or adults, specifically adult women; however, attention to sexual assault experiences during adolescence is warranted, given that it is a particularly high-risk developmental period with respect to sexual assault. This chapter provides a brief introduction to the literature regarding adolescent sexual assault. Specifically, it discusses the scope of the problem among adolescents, factors potentiating risk for sexual assault, physical and mental health outcomes, as well as intervention and treatment relevant to sexual assault.

Terminology

Several terms are frequently used in the adolescent sexual assault literature. Gaining familiarity with these terms and their applications can be helpful in understanding the implications and limitations of the research discussed throughout this chapter.

Sexual abuse is a term broadly defined by Webster's New World Law Dictionary as meaning "unlawful sexual activity or contact with a person without his/her consent." Specific nonconsensual sexual acts constituting sexual abuse include (a) oral, anal, or genital penetration; (b) anal or genital digital or other penetration; (c) genital contact with no intrusion; (d) fondling of breasts or buttocks; (e) indecent exposure; (f) inadequate or inappropriate supervision of a child's voluntary sexual activities; and (g) use of a child in prostitution, pornography, Internet crimes, or other sexually exploitative activities (Goldman, Salus, Wolcott, & Kennedy, 2003). However, *sexual abuse* is most frequently used to address childhood sexual violence that is chronic or ongoing in nature. In this context, child sexual abuse may include acts such as incest (sexual contact among family members) or sexual contact between a child and an older child or adult. An important consideration in the determination of child sexual abuse is the age of

J.L. McCauley, Ph.D. (✉) • A.M. Begle, Ph.D.
Clinical Neuroscience Division,
Department of Psychiatry and Behavioral Sciences,
Medical University of South Carolina,
67 President Street, Charleston, SC 29425, USA
e-mail: mccaule@musc.edu; begle@musc.edu

K. Zajac, Ph.D.
Family Services Research Center, Department of Psychiatry and Behavioral Sciences, Medical University of South Carolina, 326 Calhoun Street, Charleston, SC 29425, USA
e-mail: zajac@musc.edu

W.T. O'Donohue et al. (eds.), *Handbook of Adolescent Health Psychology*,
DOI 10.1007/978-1-4614-6633-8_13,

legal consent—that is, the age at which a person can legally consent to sexual activity. The age of legal consent and specific definitions concerning child sexual abuse/assault are largely dictated by state legislation that vary from state to state; however, the Federal Child Abuse Prevention and Treatment Act (CAPTA; 42 U.S.C.A. §5,106 g) broadly addresses child sexual abuse. CAPTA defines the *minimum standards* of child abuse and neglect as "any recent act or failure to act on the part of the parent or caretaker, which results in the death, serious physical or emotional harm, sexual abuse or exploitation, or an act or failure to act which presents an imminent risk of serious harm."

As children enter adolescence, the risk of experiencing sexual violence is heightened. Terminology (and research) on peer-perpetrated and/or acute sexual violence often refers to these acts as sexual assault. *Sexual assault victimization* encompasses any form of unwanted sexual contact obtained through violent or nonviolent means (United States Department of Justice, 2008). Sexual assault victimization most often refers to acute victimization, rather than the more protracted or chronic victimization often referenced by the term *sexual abuse*. Sexual assault victimization includes the more distinctly defined acts of *rape* and *attempted rape*, as well as unwanted touching and/or fondling of breasts or genitalia. *Rape* is a form of sexual assault that involves some type of unwanted penetration of the victim's vagina, mouth, or anus. Rape may be perpetrated through several non-mutually exclusive tactics: (a) *forcible rape*, or the use of force or threat of other harm to the victim; (b) *drug- or alcohol-facilitated rape*, deliberately giving the victim alcohol or drugs with the intent of incapacitating the victim to the point at which they can no longer control their behavior, protect themselves, or consent; and (c) *incapacitated rape*, or when a perpetrator takes advantage of a victim who is passed out or too drunk or high from voluntary alcohol or drug use to consent or control their behaviors. *Attempted rape* is a type of sexual assault that involves attempted, but non-completed unwanted sexual penetration as defined above. *Statutory rape* occurs when a perpetrator has sexual penetration with someone who is defined by law as too young to be capable of giving consent. Again, age of consent varies from state to state, with most states setting the age between 16 and 18 years of age.

As discussed with child sexual abuse, there is also existing Federal legislation addressing the acts of rape and attempted rape. Although the Federal Criminal Code of 1986 (Title 18, Chapter 109A, Sections 2241–2233) does not explicitly use the term "rape," *aggravated sexual abuse* is referenced, including aggravated sexual abuse by force or threat of force and aggravated sexual abuse by other means. *Aggravated sexual abuse by force or threat of force* is defined within the code as follows: when a person knowingly causes another person to engage in a sexual act, or attempts to do so, by using force against that person, or by threatening or placing that person in fear of death, serious bodily injury, or kidnapping. *Aggravated sexual abuse by other means* is defined as follows: when a person knowingly renders another person unconscious and thereby engages in a sexual act with that other person or administers to another person by force or threat of force without the knowledge or permission of that person a drug, intoxicant, or similar substance and thereby, (a) substantially impairs the ability of that person to appraise or control conduct and (b) engages in a sexual act with that person. This definition has several important implications for what should be included in the assessment of rape. First, this definition includes more than just unwanted penile penetration of the vagina, and references other forms of penetration, such as oral and/or anal penetration. Second, the definition recognizes that not all perpetrators are male, and not all victims are female. Third, the definition acknowledges that unwanted sexual penetration should be recognized in both the instance of being obtained by force/threat of force and the instance of drug-alcohol facilitation/incapacitation. Fourth, the definition highlights that statutory rape (i.e., any type of non-forcible sexual penetration with a child) is a serious federal offense and should be measured in national surveys in order to capture the full scope of the problem of rape.

This basic review of terminology provides a foundation for the most common types of experiences being assessed in adolescent sexual assault research. Next, we will discuss several of the most prominent methodological issues implicit in the measurement and assessment of adolescent sexual assault.

Issues Related to the Estimation of Adolescent Sexual Assault Prevalence

Our best national estimates of the prevalence and scope of adolescent sexual assault are likely underestimates of the problem at hand. Several issues contribute to this likely underestimation. These include but are not limited to unacknowledged victims, low rates of disclosure and reporting, and methodological shortcomings of national prevalence surveys.

Acknowledgement and Disclosure

There is evidence that many victims of experiences meeting the legal definitions of rape or sexual assault do not perceive or acknowledge their experience as a rape or sexual assault (Kilpatrick, Resnick, Ruggiero, Conoscenti, & McCauley, 2007). These victims are often referred to as "unacknowledged victims" and are unlikely to report their cases to police, seek services from rape crisis centers or other service agencies, or participate in research projects that are recruiting for "sexual assault or rape victims," because they do not necessarily consider their experience to be rape and do not see themselves as "rape victims." Further, even if an adolescent acknowledges that what has happened to them is rape, the vast majority of rape victims do not report (or disclose) the assault to police or other authorities, especially if drugs or alcohol are involved. As an example of this phenomenon, a recent study recruiting a national sample of 2,000 women enrolled in US colleges and universities found that 11.5 % of women reported a lifetime history of forcible, incapacitated, or drug- and alcohol-facilitated rape (Kilpatrick et al., 2007). However, only about one out of six (16 %) of the women endorsing a history of *forcible rape* reported the incident to police or other authorities. An even smaller percentage (7 %; or about one out of fourteen) of those that experienced a drug- or alcohol-facilitated or incapacitated rape reported the incident to the authorities. These data indicate that most rape victims do not report their experiences to police or other authorities. More specific to adolescents, *only about one-half to one-third of adolescent victims tell anyone about their assault*, and even fewer—*one out of sixteen* (6 %)—report the incident to authorities (Broman-Fulks et al., 2007; Koss & Gidycz, 1985). Although it cannot be definitively stated that rates of sexual assault among adolescents are sixteen times those reported by annually released national sources like the National Crime Victimization Survey, it is clear that national prevalence estimates based solely on sexual assaults reported to authorities result in a gross underestimation of the scope of sexual assault among US adolescents.

Assessment Methodology

Getting an accurate picture of the scope of sexual assault is also made difficult by several notable measurement issues. The accuracy of the measurement is largely dependent on the sensitivity of assessment and methodology. Stronger, more comprehensive assessments utilize behaviorally specific questions, as opposed to relying on labels such as "sexual assault," and include the range of experiences described by state and federal definitions of sexual assault. An example of one such behaviorally specific question appears on the Sexual Experiences Survey (a standard assessment in sexual assault research; Koss & Gidycz, 1985): *Have you had sexual intercourse when you didn't want to because a man gave you alcohol or drugs to prevent you from resisting?* Comprehensive assessments also include specific language describing experiences where the victim was too intoxicated or high to provide consent, as well as statutory rape experiences, in addition to the more commonly assessed forcible and coerced assaults.

Method of assessment is also an important consideration in reviewing sexual assault research. Most nationally representative victimization surveys discussed in this chapter employed random-digit-dial methods to select their sample and interviewed their participants via telephone. Random-digit-dial methods generate telephone numbers at random giving it the advantage of sampling from residences with both listed and unlisted telephone numbers. Whereas this form of telephone assessment is relatively cost-effective, it also limits the data available to those who are contactable by phone (e.g., not institutionalized, residing in a home, having a home phone line) and willing to participate in a research survey, thus limiting the generalizability of findings. Additionally, all self-report methods are subject to recall bias and participants' willingness to disclose personal information. The assessment of experiences within the time frame of "lifetime" may be more susceptible to recall bias, particularly when adults are asked to recall sexual assault experiences that may have occurred many years prior to the conduct of the survey. Therefore, studies that survey adolescents directly and ask about shorter time frames (like the past year) tend to reduce the length of time that respondents are asked to recall and may increase accuracy in reporting.

Unfortunately, the perfect study on adolescent sexual assault does not exist. Each study aims to maximize the reliability, representativeness, validity, and accuracy of its findings within its given constraints (both time and cost). The subsequent sections of this chapter will review research findings from studies that employ rigorous methodology, utilize behaviorally specific assessment measures, and draw conclusions within the framework of the study's limitations. When this caliber of research is not available, we will briefly address the limitations of the literature in that area.

Prevalence of Adolescent Sexual Assault

Adolescence is a notable period of risk for sexual assault experience. More than half of all rape victims experience their first rape before the age of 18 (Kilpatrick, Edmunds, & Seymour, 1992; Tjaden & Thoennes, 2000). Moreover, national data indicate that adolescents and young adults experience the *highest rates* of rape and other sexual assault of all age groups, with approximately one-third of all lifetime forcible rapes occurring between the ages of 11 and 17 years (Kilpatrick et al., 1992; Rennison, 2002). Although there are numerous studies that produce prevalence estimates among nonrepresentative adolescent samples (e.g., clinical, regional, school-specific samples), we will focus only on national estimates, as they maintain the broadest degree of generalizability.

Two main general statistics are provided by national data on sexual assault: prevalence and incidence. *Prevalence* is the proportion or percent of the population that has been sexually assaulted at least once in a specific period of time, such as "lifetime" or "past-year." The Centers for Disease Control and Prevention monitors a compendium of health-risk behaviors among male and female youth enrolled in grades 9 through 12 and annually compiles their data in a report entitled Youth Risk Behavior Surveillance System (YRBSS; Centers for Disease Control and Prevention, 2007). Although the YRBSS uses a crude assessment of rape (asking only, "Have you ever been physically forced to have sexual intercourse when you didn't want to?"), the 2007 YRBSS report estimated the prevalence of rape among adolescents to be 7.8 % (11.3 % of females and 4.5 % of males). A more thorough, although less recent, assessment of the prevalence of sexual assault experiences among US adolescents was provided by the National Survey of Adolescents (NSA; Hanson et al., 2003; Kilpatrick et al., 2003a). Conducted in 1995, the NSA included a nationally representative sample of 4,023 adolescents (ages 12–17) and used validated epidemiological methods of assessment. According to the NSA, 3.4 % of male and 13 % of female adolescents endorsed a lifetime history of forced sexual assault.

Nationally representative studies have also produced recent estimates of the prevalence of adolescents' experience of dating violence and drug-facilitated/incapacitated assault.

Wolitzky-Taylor et al. (2009) estimated the overall prevalence of adolescent dating violence, defined as peer-to-peer sexual assault, physical assault, and drug-alcohol-facilitated sexual assault. Among teens ages 12–17, 1.6 % reported experiencing dating violence, equating to a population estimate of 400,000 US adolescents. Prevalence of dating violence increases by age, with estimates of 14 % and 22 % among 16- and 17-year-olds, respectively. Drug-facilitated and incapacitated sexual assaults appear to be even more prevalent among adolescents, with 2.1 % of adolescent girls reporting at least one such experience in their lifetime (McCauley et al., 2009). Similar to dating violence, incapacitated and drug- or alcohol-facilitated sexual assaults were notably more prevalent among older adolescents. This elevated risk for peer-to-peer or acquaintance-perpetrated assault continues into young-adulthood, with this time frame being second only to adolescence with respect to risk for sexual assault. Several large, nationally representative studies have focused exclusively on the impact of sexual assault among college women. These studies, the National College Women's Sexual Victimization Survey (NCWSV; Fisher, Cullen, & Turner, 2000) and the National Women's Study—Replication (NWS-R; Kilpatrick et al., 2007), estimated a 3 % annual prevalence rate for completed forcible rape, 2.1 % for incapacitated rape, and 1.5 % for drug-alcohol-facilitated rape. In total, over 300,000 college women in the USA (5.2 %) reported a rape experience in the year prior to this 2006 study.

Incidence refers to the number of new cases of sexual assault that occur in a specified period of time. Incidence is most often expressed as a victimization rate, or number of incidents per given number of people. Because incidence rates are case-based statistics, it is also important to note that there is a distinction between *sexual assault cases* and *sexual assault victims*, such that a single victim may have experienced more than one sexual assault case. The US Department of Justice National Crime Victimization Survey (2009) reports the recent annual incidence rates (per 1,000 persons) of sexual assault reported to authorities to be 0.9 for adolescents aged 12–15 years and 0.6 for adolescents aged 16–19 years. Note that these rates reflect cases of sexual assault or rape that were reported to authorities and, as previously discussed, are likely significant underestimates of the actual annual incidence.

Taken together, prevalence data indicate that adolescence is a very high-risk time period for sexual assault. When extrapolated into population estimates, the cost to society posed by adolescent sexual assault becomes glaring. It is not surprising that identification of individual, ecological, and sociocultural risk and protective factors has high public health relevance. Next, we will discuss and summarize what is known with regard to risk and protective factors for adolescent sexual assault, as well as provide an overview of the health and mental health outcomes associated with adolescent sexual assault experiences.

Risk Factors

While a well-established literature has identified that sexual assault can affect adolescents of a variety of ages, socioeconomic backgrounds, ethnic/racial groups, and familial backgrounds, several specific risk factors for sexual assault have been identified among this group, including demographic, individual characteristics, and behavioral factors (Finkelhor, Ormrod, Turner, & Hamby, 2005; Franklin, 2010; Kilpatrick, Saunders, & Smith, 2003b; Putnam, 2003). These categories of risk factors are addressed below.

Demographic factors conferring risk for adolescent sexual assault include gender, age, and family characteristics. When examining prevalence rates of sexual assault across gender, researchers have consistently found that a disproportionate number of adolescent girls report exposure to sexual assault (Bailey & McCloskey, 2005; Finkelhor, Turner, Ormrod, Hamby, & Kracke, 2009; Foster, Kuperminc, & Price, 2004; Hamburger, Leeb, & Swahn, 2008; Kilpatrick et al., 2003b; Tjaden & Thoennes, 2000). For example, results from a nationally representative sample of 12–17-year-olds indicated that 13.2 % of girls reported a lifetime prevalence of sexual assault, compared to 3.5 % of boys (Hanson et al., 2008). Similarly, a separate nationally representative study indicated that sexual assault prevalence among adolescent girls was 7.9 % over the past year and 18.7 % over the lifetime (Finkelhor et al., 2009). Again, these prevalence estimates likely underestimate actual prevalence among adolescents, and this may be especially true among adolescent boys; however, significant gender differences in prevalence are a consistent finding among nationally representative studies and indicate that female gender serves as an important risk factor for sexual assault in adolescence.

Adolescence represents the highest risk-period for sexual assault (U.S. Department of Health and Human Services [U.S. DHHS], 1998). Specifically, research indicates that, of people under age 18 reporting sexual assault, approximately 10 % were 0–3-year-olds, 28.4 % were between ages 4 and 7, 25.5 % were between ages 8 and 10, and 35.9 % were ages 12–17 (U.S. DHHS, 1998). Further, researchers have noted an interaction between age and gender, as age is a more significant risk factor for girls than boys (Bailey & McCloskey, 2005). Statistics from the Bureau of Justice indicated that women between age 16 and 24 have the highest risk of sexual assault (Hart, 2003), with reports of sexual assault from women in this age group consistently being four times higher than the overall sexual assault prevalence for women (Humphrey & Kahn, 2000). Socioeconomic status and ethnic/racial background are identified as risk factors for other forms of child and adolescent mistreatment (i.e., physical abuse, neglect); however, these factors have not been identified as risk factors for sexual assault.

In addition to demographic characteristics, personal and familial characteristics can confer increased risk for sexual assault. Presence of a disability, such as blindness, deafness, and mental retardation, increases the likelihood of sexual assault throughout development (Westcott & Jones, 1999). Findings have indicated that boys with disabilities display higher risk for sexual assault than either girls with disabilities or boys without disabilities (Sobsey, Randall, & Parrila, 1997). Further, a multitude of family characteristics increase the incidence of sexual abuse among adolescents (Putnam, 2003). Specifically, these familial factors include parental physical or mental disability, parental substance use and neglect, marital conflict or domestic violence, social isolation, and coercive or physically abusive parenting (Fergusson, Lynskey, & Horwood, 1996; Nelson et al., 2002). Finally, many studies have documented that prior incidences of sexual assault significantly increase risk for revictimization during adolescence (Krebs, Lindquist, Warner, Fisher, & Martin, 2009; Miller, Markman, & Handley, 2007; Stevens, Ruggiero, Kilpatrick, Resnick, & Saunders, 2005).

Commonly identified sexual assault risk factors also encompass the domain of high-risk behaviors, such as substance abuse. A study examining the trajectories of sexual assault and substance use demonstrated that early initiation of substance use leads to increased risk for sexual assault, presumably due to poor decision-making during intoxication (Kingston & Raghavan, 2009). In fact, it is estimated that alcohol is involved in approximately 50 % of sexual assaults perpetrated by a date or acquaintance during adolescence (Abbey, McAuslan, & Ross, 1998). Thus, early initiation of substance use may increase the risk for sexual assault exposure through several mechanisms, including impaired decision-making skills, impaired judgment while intoxicated, increased engagement in risk-taking behaviors, association with delinquent peers, greater exposure to potentially dangerous situations, and decreased ability to physically defend oneself in threatening situations (Danielson et al., 2006; Davis, George, & Norris, 2004; Kingston & Raghavan, 2009; Klaczynski, 2001; Koenen et al., 2005). In addition to substance use, other risk-taking behaviors have been associated with sexual assault among adolescents, including risky dating and sexual practices, such as unprotected sex and indiscriminate sexual contact (Combs-Lane & Smith, 2002). Other potential risk factors include decreased danger cue recognition and prior victimization. Specifically, frequent misperception of danger cues among adolescents may increase the likelihood of sexual assault, due to increased vulnerability and inability to accurately assess threat of personal danger, thus resulting in a slower response rate during potentially dangerous situations (Franklin, 2010).

Physical Health and Mental Health Consequences of Sexual Assault

The consequences of sexual assault experiences can be diverse and long-lasting. Researchers have identified a range of physical and mental health consequences faced by adolescents who have experienced a sexual assault. Some are evident immediately after the abuse and require acute care, whereas others represent risk for longer term health consequences that may not be apparent until later adolescence or adulthood.

The healthcare needs of adolescents immediately following a sexual assault vary depending on the characteristics of the sexual assault and length of time between assault and disclosure, but can include both treatment of physical needs and collection of evidence for forensic and legal purposes. In terms of medical needs, the most common problems faced by adolescent sexual assault victims are physical injuries and sexually transmitted infections (STIs). Though the estimates vary depending on the definition of injury, one study found that 64 % of female adolescents presenting for an acute sexual assault examination had some degree of genital or anal injury (Adams, Girardin, & Faugno, 2001). In a larger study of women ages 15 and older using a more stringent definition of injury, only 20 % of the sample presented with genital-anal trauma; however, adolescent victims were twice as likely as older women to present with these types of injuries, and an additional 52 % of the overall sample showed signs of general bodily injuries (Sugar, Fine, & Eckert, 2004). It should be noted that the majority of genital injuries, unless severe in nature, tend to heal quickly without intervention, such that victims presenting for treatment even within days or weeks after an assault may show no physical signs (McCann, Miyamoto, Boyle, & Rogers, 2007).

Another potential risk to adolescent sexual assault victims is the contraction of STIs. Studies show rates of STIs are low but significant in this population. Reports vary depending on referral source and data collection methods, but generally indicate higher rates for female adolescents (compared to male) and for adolescents who were sexually active prior to the assault (compared to sexually abstinent). For example, one study reported an overall rate for STIs (gonorrhea, chlamydia, syphilis, trichomonas, or HIV) of 14.6 % in pubertal girls during examinations for suspected sexual assault (Siegel, Schubert, Myers, & Shapiro, 1995), whereas a more recent study reported a rate of 24 % for girls who were not sexually active prior to the assault and 39 % for those who reported pre-assault sexual activity (Kawsar, Anfield, Walters, McCabe, & Forster, 2004). It should be noted that these are likely to be overestimates of prevalence rates due to research procedures restricting STI testing to a subsample of adolescents at the highest risk for testing positive (e.g., those who reported attempted or completed penetration, those with suspected symptoms of STIs). In studies where a majority of the adolescents were tested for STIs, rates are much lower (e.g., 5.6 % of victims testing positive for an STI; Kelly & Koh, 2006).

Medical assessments during adolescence are unlikely to detect the overall physical health problems that have been linked to sexual assault. However, sexual assault during childhood or adolescence is a risk factor for longer term health problems that manifest during later adolescence or adulthood. Generally, adult victims of adolescent sexual assault have higher rates of health care utilization and report significantly more health complaints compared to adults without such a history (Arnow, 2004; Golding, Cooper, & George, 1997; Thompson, Arias, Basile, & Desai, 2002). This finding is consistent for both self-reported doctor's visits and objective examination of medical records (Newman et al., 2000). Data from the National Comorbidity Survey, a large nationwide epidemiological study, indicate that adults with a history of sexual assault are more likely to have a serious medical problem including arthritis, asthma, diabetes, cancer, heart problems, stroke, hernia, hypertension, and multiple other problems compared to adults without such a history (Sachs-Ericsson, Blazer, Plant, & Arnow, 2005). This result is especially compelling because the association remained significant even when taking into account other adverse childhood events including physical abuse, family conflict, poverty, and separation from parents.

In addition to these global health concerns, studies have focused on more specific health problems among adults with a history of sexual assault. Researchers are unable to test whether the assault plays a causal role in these disorders, but rather examine prevalence rates of sexual assault history among groups of patients presenting with such health concerns. In studies of this type, prevalence rates of sexual assault history have been found to be elevated among patients who have chronic pelvic pain with or without a known medical cause, fibromyalgia, severe premenstrual syndrome, chronic headaches, irritable bowel syndrome, obesity, non-epileptic seizures, and a wide range of reproductive and sexual health complaints, including excessive bleeding, amenorrhea, pain during intercourse, lack of sexual pleasure, and menstrual irregularity (Ehlert, Heim, & Hellhammer, 1999; Fuemmeler, Dedert, McClernon, & Beckham, 2009; Golding, 1996; Golding, Taylor, Menard, & King, 2000; Peterlin, Ward, Lidicker, & Levin, 2007; Rohde et al., 2008; Ross, 2005; Sharpe & Faye, 2006; Walker et al., 1997). Though many of these health problems are potentially psychosomatic in nature, they represent a burden both to the sexual assault victim and the healthcare system.

Similar to physical health consequences, sexual assault has also been repeatedly linked to deleterious outcomes in both short- and long-term mental health functioning. Adolescents who have experienced sexual assault are at significantly increased risk for post-traumatic stress disorder (PTSD) and other anxiety symptoms, depression, suicide attempts, substance abuse, and delinquency (Fergusson, Boden, & Horwood, 2008; Kilpatrick et al., 2003a, 2003b; McLeer et al., 1998; Turner, Finkelhor, & Ormrod, 2006; Waldrop et al., 2007). These emotional and behavioral difficulties can lead to significant disruptions in normal adolescent development and interfere with their ability to meet important expectations and milestones, including school success, healthy peer and dating relationships, and the transition to adulthood. Further, sexual assault-related mental health problems often follow a chronic course, leading to mental health problems well into adulthood (Banyard, Williams, & Siegel, 2001; Dube et al., 2005; Young, Harford, Kinder, & Savell, 2007). Specifically, a large nationally representative study found that, among adults reporting a history of sexual assault during childhood or adolescence, 39.1 % of women and 29.1 % of men had a lifetime diagnosis of PTSD, 33.9 % of women and 37 % of men had a lifetime alcohol problem, and 39.3 % of women and 30.3 % of men had a lifetime diagnosis of depression (Molnar, Buka, & Kessler, 2001). Finally, physical and mental health consequences are likely to co-occur. For example, symptoms of PTSD have been found to at least partially account for the increased levels of certain physical health problems in victims of sexual assault (Eadie, Runtz, & Spencer-Rodgers, 2008).

Associated High-Risk Behaviors

In addition to the magnitude of mental and physical health consequences, adolescent sexual assault experiences have also been associated with elevated prevalence of subsequent risk behaviors including increased rates of substance use, disruptive behavior and impulsivity, delinquency, teen pregnancy, and HIV/AIDS/STI infection via adolescent risky sexual behavior (Bailey & McCloskey, 2005; Cuevas, Finkelhor, Turner, & Ormrod, 2007; Deas-Nesmith, Brady, White, & Campbell, 1999; Ford et al., 2000; Hamburger et al., 2008; Males & Chew, 1996; Noll, Shenk, & Putnam, 2009; Siegel & Williams, 2003).

Regarding elevated prevalence rates of substance use, data from the NSA indicated that adolescent victims of sexual assault were 2.4 times more likely to experience problems with alcohol use and/or dependence than non-victims, after controlling for age of onset of substance use and familial substance use problems (Kilpatrick et al., 2000). This study also found that age of onset for nonexperimental drug use (i.e., five or more drinks of alcohol on a given day; use of marijuana at least four times; or use of cocaine, heroin, inhalants, LSD, or prescription drugs non-medically, on at least four or more occasions) was 14.4 years for victims of sexual assault, compared to 15.1 years for adolescents without sexual assault experiences. Nationally representative prevalence estimates indicate that approximately 25.2 % of adolescents met criteria for past-year alcohol abuse, 11.2 % for drug abuse, and 7.4 % for abuse of both alcohol and drugs (Danielson et al., 2009). This elevated prevalence rate of substance use problems persists into adulthood, with 40.5 % of female adults with a history of adolescent sexual assault reporting substance use problems (compared to 14 % of the general population) and 65 % of males with adolescent sexual assault experiences reporting adult substance use problems (compared to 25 % in the general population; Simpson & Miller, 2002).

In addition to substance use, adolescents with a history of sexual assault display heightened levels of inattention and impulsivity compared to their non-victimized peers. Specifically, among a sample of school-age children diagnosed with clinically significant levels of inattention or impulsivity (attention-deficit/hyperactivity disorder, ADHD) and aggression (oppositional defiant disorder, ODD), approximately 31 % reported a history of sexual assault (Ford et al., 2000). Importantly, findings from this study indicated that exposure to sexual assault and PTSD may exacerbate the current symptoms of inattention, impulsivity, or aggression that are already present in children with ADHD or ODD (Ford et al., 2000). While these findings are relevant, causality cannot be inferred due to the cross-sectional nature of the data. Researchers have begun to examine trajectories of adolescent sexual assault, along with inattention, impulsivity, and aggression, and identified detrimental consequences such as delinquency that tend to develop as children become older (Stewart, Livingston, & Dennison, 2008; Thornberry, Ireland, & Smith, 2001; Widom & Maxfield, 2001). An examination of delinquency rates among adolescent sexual assault victims found that approximately 13.6 % had been arrested for a violent offense compared to 6.3 % of non-victims; victims were 1.35 times more likely to commit a property offense (9.2 % vs. 6.3 %), 17.67 times more likely to run away from home (5.3 % vs. 0.3 %), and 2.65 times more likely to be involved in a dependency hearing (18 % vs. 6.8 %; Cuevas et al., 2007). Further, researchers have found that 25 % of adolescents residing in a juvenile assessment center after arrest had been victims of sexual assault (Dembo, Schmeidler, & Childs, 2007). These delinquent acts are persistent, as adult victims of adolescent sexual assault are almost twice as likely to be arrested for a violent offense (20.4 % vs. 10.7 %) and 2.11 times more likely to be arrested for a property offense (9.3 % and 4.4 %; Siegel et al., 2003).

Teenage pregnancy has also been identified as a significant risk following sexual assault. Specifically, a meta-analysis of 21 studies showed that approximately 45 % of pregnant teenagers report a history of sexual assault, with adolescent sexual assault victims 2.21 times more likely to become mothers in their teenage years when compared to non-victimized adolescents (Noll et al., 2009). Similarly, another study indicated that 44 % of a sample of girls who became pregnant during adolescence reported a history of rape, with 4.8 % of these adolescents reporting pregnancy as a direct result of the sexual assault (Boyer & Fine, 1992). Also related to risky sexual behavior, adolescents exposed to sexual assault are at high risk for HIV/AIDS infection, based upon the well-documented link between adolescent risky sexual behavior and substance use—both of which are related to HIV/AIDS infection (Deas-Nesmith et al., 1999).

Finally, adolescents who experience sexual assault are at notably greater risk for subsequent victimization in adulthood (Hines, 2007; Humphrey & White, 2000). For example, in studies of college women, those with a history of adolescent rape are at 2–4.5 times greater risk for adult victimization than women without a rape history (Calhoun & Gidycz, 2002; Gidycz, Hanson, & Layman, 1995). Several mechanisms have been posited through which prior victimization may confer risk for subsequent victimization, many of which have associations with aforementioned risk factors and outcomes associated with assault (Breitenbecher, 2001; Macy, 2007). Impaired risk perception, emotion dysregulation and psychopathology, self-medication via substance abuse, and engagement in high-risk behaviors are among the factors hypothesized to potentiate revictimization risk (Cougle, Resnick, & Kilpatrick, 2009; Fargo, 2009; Gidycz, McNamara, & Edwards, 2006; Hedtke et al., 2008; Testa, Hoffman, & Livingston, 2010).

Intervention and Treatment

Whereas a complete review of this programming is beyond the scope of this chapter, primary and secondary prevention of sexual assault among adolescents has received increasing attention in the past decade (Schewe, 2007). A significant portion of intervention programming has been aimed specifically at older adolescents (i.e., college students), with representation of a wide range of target populations and varied outcomes. Programming targeting male perpetration has been developed, evaluated, and found to reduce rape myth acceptance, increase bystander intervention efficacy, and produce some sustainable behavior change (Garrity, 2011). Programming targeting college women typically focuses on risk reduction, and, overall, these interventions have evidenced limited success, with few being effective at reducing revictimization risk (Breitenbecher & Gidycz, 1998; Gidycz, Rich, & Marioni, 2002; Hanson & Broom, 2005; Hanson & Gidycz, 1993; Sochting, Fairbrother, & Kocj, 2004). Among younger adolescents, the majority of sexual assault risk reduction education occurs within school-based dating violence prevention programs; is presented to a range of audience compositions (all girls, all boys, co-ed); targets changes in knowledge, attitudes, and behaviors related to sexual assault; and generally produces small to moderate effects (Fay & Medway, 2006; Foshee et al., 1998; Jaycox et al., 2006; Wekerle & Wolfe, 1999; Wolfe, 2006). Future programming would likely benefit from employing ecological approaches to prevention and risk reduction that capitalize on changing peer- and community-level factors influencing sexual assault risk (Casey & Lindhorst, 2009).

Recent research has also focused on standards of care for adolescents after a sexual assault has occurred. When intervening with adolescent victims in the acute aftermath of a sexual assault, caring for any physical injuries and ensuring that basic needs are being met are the primary objectives. Treatment at a Child Advocacy Center (CAC), where both healthcare and forensic concerns can be addressed by specialists in this field, is considered best practice for child and adolescent victims (Cross et al., 2008). Studies have shown that adolescents receiving care at a CAC following a sexual assault are more likely to receive a physical exam, a genital exam when indicated, and a referral to counseling, compared with those receiving care at other community centers (Edinburgh, Saewyc, & Levitt, 2008). Although there were no differences between CAC and other community providers in forensic outcomes in this particular study (i.e., decisions to prosecute, convictions, or sentence length), another study found that CAC cases were more likely to have law enforcement involvement and case substantiation compared to those not receiving CAC services (Smith, Witte, & Fricker-Elhai, 2006). Thus, use of CACs for treatment of acute adolescent sexual assault should be facilitated whenever possible.

In addition to acute care, adolescent sexual assault victims often present for mental health problems in the months and years following the trauma. It should be noted that many sexual assault victims will not suffer long-term mental health consequences, with a significant minority of victims requiring formal interventions. A recent review of the effectiveness of treatments for children and adolescents with trauma-related mental health symptoms provided support for the efficacy of cognitive-behavioral treatments (CBT) provided in either individual or group formats, but concluded that there was not enough evidence to determine the effectiveness of other treatments, including play and art therapies, psychodynamic approaches, and psychological debriefing (Wethington et al., 2008). The CBT approach with the most empirical support in treating mental health symptoms resulting from adolescent sexual assault is trauma-focused cognitive behavioral therapy (TF-CBT), which is a manualized, components-based intervention targeting children ages 3–17. Specifically, TF-CBT addresses symptoms associated with trauma exposure, including PTSD, depression, and other significant emotional and behavioral techniques (Cohen, Mannarino, & Deblinger, 2006). The treatment utilizes components of multiple conceptual treatment modalities, including cognitive-behavioral, attachment, humanistic, empowerment, and family therapy techniques, and can be effectively used with a wide range of youth from multiple cultural backgrounds or with youth who have been multiply traumatized (Cohen, Deblinger, Mannarino, & Steer, 2004). The core components of TF-CBT are arranged according to the acronym, PRACTICE: (P)sychoeducation and (P)arenting skills, (R)elaxation, (A)ffective expression and modulation, (C)ognitive coping and processing, (T)rauma narrative, (I)n vivo exposure, (C)onjoint sessions, and (E)nhancing future safety and development, with each component directly targeting symptoms related to the traumatic experience (Cohen, Kelleher, & Mannarino, 2008). While each of these components are implemented for all children and adolescents throughout TF-CBT, the clinician has some discretion regarding the most appropriate way to incorporate the concepts into child and parent sessions, as trauma-related symptoms can present differently in children of different developmental or cognitive levels. See Cohen et al. (2006) for a more detailed description of the TF-CBT components.

Additional approaches that deserve attention include other individual CBT approaches and pharmacotherapy. For example, a developmentally adapted protocol of prolonged exposure (PE) therapy, a well-validated and widely used treatment for adult PTSD, has recently been tested on an adolescent population (Gilboa-Schetctman et al., 2010). Though this was a pilot study and thus requires replication, results were promising, with adolescents who received PE for adolescents showing greater decreases in PTSD and depression at treatment end and 17-month follow-up compared to an active treatment control group. Studies of the use of psychiatric treatments for adolescent PTSD show that a wide range of psychotropic medications, including selective serotonin reuptake inhibitors (SSRIs), alpha- and beta-adrenergic blocking agents, anxiolytic, tricyclic antidepressants, anticonvulsants, and antipsychotic medications are widely prescribed for this population (Cohen, Mannarino, & Rogal, 2001). Despite this clinical reality, there are very few studies that support the use of psychopharmacological approaches for adolescent PTSD. Among the two rigorously designed clinical trials, one found that sertraline performed no better than placebo in treating PTSD symptoms among a sample of children and adolescents (Robb, Cueva, Sporn, Yang, & Vanderberg, 2008). The second, a study comparing TF-CBT plus sertraline to TF-CBT alone, found no clear additive benefit for the medication among a group of sexually abused 10- to 17-year-olds (Cohen, Mannarino, Perel, & Staron, 2007). It should be noted that these studies were small, and further research is needed to understand that potential role of medications in the treatment of adolescent PTSD. Further, there have been few rigorously designed studies of medications other than SSRIs for this population.

Overall, there are effective treatment options available for adolescents who experience mental health difficulties following a sexual assault. The first-line treatment should be cognitive behavioral treatment provided by a mental health professional proficient in this approach. Currently, psychotropic medications have shown limited efficacy for this population, but additional studies are needed to understand the potential of those medications being prescribed in practice to treat symptoms following sexual assault. Unfortunately, less is known about preventing sexual assault among adolescents; thus, this is an area where program development and rigorous evaluation is sorely needed.

Conclusion

In sum, sexual assault is an unfortunate and all too common experience among US adolescents. Whereas various demographic, environmental, and personal characteristics have been identified as risk factors for sexual assault, few compelling options exist for primary and secondary prevention intervention programming. Whereas experience of sexual assault in adolescence is associated with elevated risk for numerous deleterious physical and mental health outcomes, a majority of teens experiencing sexual assault will display a high degree of resilience. However, for the significant minority of teens who display posttraumatic sequelae, effective treatment options are available.

References

Abbey, A., McAuslan, P., & Ross, L. T. (1998). Sexual assault perpetrated by college men: The role of alcohol, misperception of sexual intent, and sexual beliefs and experiences. *Psychology of Women Quarterly, 20*, 147–169.

Adams, J. A., Girardin, B., & Faugno, D. (2001). Adolescent sexual assault: Documentation of acute injuries using photo-colposcopy. *Journal of Pediatric and Adolescent Gynecology, 14*, 175–180.

Arnow, B. A. (2004). Relationships between childhood maltreatment, adult health and psychiatric outcomes, and medical utilization. *Journal of Clinical Psychiatry, 65*(Suppl 12), 10–15.

Bailey, J. A., & McCloskey, L. A. (2005). Pathways to adolescent substance use among sexually abused girls. *Journal of Abnormal Child Psychology, 33*(1), 39–53.

Banyard, V. L., Williams, L. M., & Siegel, J. A. (2001). The long-term mental health consequences of child sexual abuse: An exploratory study of the impact of multiple traumas in a sample of women. *Journal of Traumatic Stress, 14*, 697–715.

Boyer, D. & Fine, D. (1992). Sexual abuse as a factor in adolescent pregnancy and child maltreatment. *Family Planning Perspectives, 24*(1), 4–11.

Breitenbecher, K. H. (2001). Sexual revictimization among women: A review of the literature focusing on empirical investigations. *Aggression and Violent Behavior, 6*, 415–432.

Breitenbecher, K. H., & Gidycz, C. A. (1998). An empirical evaluation of a program designed to reduce the risk of multiple sexual victimization. *Journal of Interpersonal Violence, 13*, 472–488.

Broman-Fulks, J. J., Ruggiero, K. J., Hanson, R. F., Smith, D. W., Resnick, H. S., Kilpatrick, D. G., et al. (2007). Sexual assault disclosure in relation to adolescent mental health: Results from the National Survey of Adolescents. *Journal of Clinical Child an Adolescent Psychology, 36*(2), 260–266.

Bureau of Justice Statistics. (2009). *National Crime Victimization Survey 2009*. U.S. Department of Justice, Office of Justice Programs. Retrieved from http://www.ojp.usdoj.gov/bjs/cvict.htm#ncvs.

Calhoun, K. S. & Gidycz, C. A. (2002, November). Self-efficacy as a predictor of revictimization. Presentation at the annual meeting of the Association for the Advancement of Behavior Therapy, Reno, NV.

Casey, E. A., & Lindhorst, T. P. (2009). Toward a multi-level, ecological approach to primary prevention of sexual assault: Prevention in peer and community contexts. *Trauma, Violence, and Abuse, 10*(2), 91–114.

Centers for Disease Control and Prevention (2007). *Youth Risk Behavior Surveillance System 2007*. National Center for Chronic Disease Prevention and Health Promotion, Centers for Disease Control and Prevention. Retrieved from http://www.cdc.gov/HealthyYouth/yrbs/index.htm.

Cohen, J. A., Deblinger, E., Mannarino, A. P., & Steer, R. (2004). A multi-site, randomized controlled trial for children with abuse-related PTSD symptoms. *Journal of the American Academy of Adolescent Psychiatry, 43*(4), 393–402.

Cohen, J. A., Kelleher, K. J., & Mannarino, A. P. (2008). Identifying, treating, and referring traumatized children. *Archives of Pediatrics and Adolescent Medicine, 162*(5), 447–452.

Cohen, J., Mannarino, A. P., & Deblinger, E. (2006). *Treating trauma and traumatic grief in children and adolescents*. New York, NY: Guilford Publications.

Cohen, J. A., Mannarino, A. P., Perel, J. M., & Staron, V. (2007). A pilot randomized trial of combined trauma-focused CBT and sertraline for childhood PTSD symptoms. *Journal of the American Academy of Child and Adolescent Psychiatry, 46*, 811–819.

Cohen, J. A., Mannarino, A. P., & Rogal, S. (2001). Treatment practices for childhood posttraumatic stress disorder. *Child Abuse and Neglect, 25*, 123–135.

Combs-Lane, A. M., & Smith, D. W. (2002). Risk of sexual victimization in college women: The role of behavioral intentions and risk-taking behaviors. *Journal of Interpersonal Violence, 17*, 165–183.

Cougle, J. R., Resnick, H. S., & Kilpatrick, D. G. (2009). A prospective examination of PTSD symptoms as risk factors for subsequent exposure to potentially traumatic events among women. *Journal of Abnormal Psychology, 118*, 405–411.

Cross, T. P., Jones, L. M., Walsh, W. A., Simone, M., Kolko, D. J., Szczepanski, J., et al. (2008). Evaluating children's advocacy centers' response to child sexual abuse. *Office of Juvenile Justice and Delinquency Prevention: Juvenile Justice Bulletin*. Retrieved August 15, 2011, from www.ojp.usdoj.gov.

Cuevas, C. A., Finkelhor, D., Turner, H. A., & Ormrod, R. K. (2007). Juvenile delinquency and victimization: A theoretical typology. *Journal of Interpersonal Violence, 22*(12), 1581–1602.

Danielson, C. K., Amstadter, A. B., et al. (2009). Trauma-related risk factors for substance use among male versus female young adults. *Addictive Behaviors, 34*(4), 395–399.

Danielson, C. K., de Arellano, M. A., Ehrenreich, J. T., et al. (2006). Identification of high-risk behaviors among victimized adolescents and implications for empirically supported psychosocial treatment. *Journal of Psychiatric Practice, 12*, 364–383.

Davis, K. C., George, W. H., & Norris, J. (2004). Women's responses to unwanted sexual advances: The role of alcohol and inhibition confliect. *Psychology of Women Quarterly, 28*, 333–343.

Davis, T. C., Peck, G. Q., & Storment, J. M. (1993). Acquaintance rape in the high school student. *The Journal of Adolescent Health, 14*, 220–224.

Deas-Nesmith, D., Brady, K. T., White, R., & Campbell, S. (1999). HIV-risk behaviors in adolescent substance users. *Journal of Substance Abuse Treatment, 16*(2), 169–172.

Dembo, R., Schmeidler, J., & Childs, K. (2007). Correlates of male and female juvenile offender abuse experiences. *Journal of Child Sexual Abuse, 16*(3), 75–94.

Dube, S. A., Anda, R. F., Whitfield, C. L., Brown, D. W., Felitti, D. J., Dong, M., et al. (2005). Long-term consequences of childhood sexual abuse by gender of the victim. *American Journal of Preventive Medicine, 28*, 430–437.

Eadie, E. M., Runtz, M. G., & Spencer-Rodgers, J. (2008). Posttraumatic stress symptoms as a mediator between sexual assault and adverse health outcomes in undergraduate women. *Journal of Traumatic Stress, 21*, 540–547.

Edinburgh, L., Saewyc, E., & Levitt, C. (2008). Caring for young adolescent sexual abuse victims in a hospital-based children's advocacy center. *Child Abuse and Neglect, 32*, 1119–1126.

Ehlert, U., Heim, C., & Hellhammer, D. H. (1999). Chronic pelvic pain as a somatoform disorder. *Psychotherapy and Psychomatics, 68*, 87–94.

Fargo, J. D. (2009). Pathways to adult sexual revictimization: Direct and indirect behavioral risk factors across the lifespan. *Journal of Interpersonal Violence, 24*, 1771–1791.

Fay, K. E., & Medway, F. J. (2006). An acquaintance rape education program for students transitioning to high school. *Sex Education, 6*, 223–236.

Fergusson, D. M., Boden, J. M., & Horwood, L. J. (2008). The developmental antecedents of illicit drug use: Evidence from a 25-year longitudinal study. *Drug and Alcohol Dependence, 96*, 165–177.

Fergusson, D., Lynskey, M., & Horwood, L. (1996). Childhood sexual abuse and psychiatric disorder in young adulthood, I: Prevalence of sexual abuse and factors associated with sexual abuse. *Journal of the American Academy of Child and Adolescent Psychiatry, 35*, 1355–1364.

Finkelhor, D., Ormrod, R., Turner, H., & Hamby, S. L. (2005). The victimization of children and youth: A comprehensive, national survey. *Child Maltreatment, 10*, 5–25.

Finkelhor, D., Turner, J., Ormrod, R., Hamby, S., & Kracke, K. (2009, October). Children's exposure to violence: A comprehensive national survey (NCJ 227744). Accessed at: www.ncjrs.gov/pdffiles1/ojjdp/227744.pdf.

Fisher, B. S., Cullen, F. T., & Turner, M. G. (2000). *The sexual victimization of women*. NCJ 182369. Washington, DC: U.S. Department of Justice, National Institute of Justice.

Ford, J. D., Racusin, R., Ellis, C. G., Davis, W. B., Reiser, J., Fleischer, A., et al. (2000). Child maltreatment, other trauma exposure, and posttraumatic symptomatology among children with oppositional defiant and attention deficit-hyperactivity disorders. *Child Maltreatment, 5*, 205–217.

Foshee, V. A., Bauman, K. E., Arriaga, X. B., Helms, R. W., Koch, G. G., & Linder, G. F. (1998). An evaluation of safe dates, an adolescent dating violence prevention program. *American Journal of Public Health, 88*, 45–50.

Foster, J. D., Kuperminc, G. P., & Price, A. W. (2004). Gender differences in posttraumatic stress and related symptoms among inner-city minority youth exposed to community violence. *Journal of Youth and Adolescence, 33*(1), 59–69.

Franklin, C. A. (2010). Physically forced, alcohol-induced, and verbally coerced sexual victimization: Assessing risk factors among university women. *Journal of Criminal Justice, 38*, 149–159.

Fuemmeler, B. F., Dedert, E., McClernon, F. J., & Beckham, J. C. (2009). Adverse childhood events are associated with obesity and disordered eating: Results from a U.S. population-based survey of young adults. *Journal of Traumatic Stress, 22*, 329–333.

Garrity, S. E. (2011). Sexual assault prevention programs for college-aged me: A critical evaluation. *Journal of Forensic Nursing, 7*(1), 40–48.

Gidycz, C. A., Hanson, K., & Layman, M. (1995). A prospective analysis of the relationships among sexual assault experiences: An extension of previous findings. *Psychology of Women Quarterly, 19*, 5–29.

Gidycz, C. A., McNamara, J. R., & Edwards, K. M. (2006). Women's risk perception and sexual victimization: A review of the literature. *Aggression and Violent Behavior, 11*, 441–456.

Gidycz, C. A., Rich, C. L., & Marioni, N. L. (2002). Interventions to prevent rape and sexual assault. In J. Petrak & B. Hedge (Eds.), *The trauma of adult sexual assault: Treatment, prevention, and policy* (pp. 235–260). New York: Wiley.

Gilboa-Schetctman, E., Foa, E. B., Shafran, N., Aderka, I. M., Powers, M. B., Rachamim, L., et al. (2010). Prolonged exposure versus dynamic therapy for adolescent PTSD: A pilot randomized controlled trial. *Journal of the American Academy of Child and Adolescent Psychiatry, 49*, 1034–1042.

Golding, J. M. (1996). Sexual assault history and women's reproductive and sexual health. *Psychology of Women Quarterly, 20*, 101–121.

Golding, J. M., Cooper, M. L., & George, L. K. (1997). Sexual assault history and health perceptions: Seven general population studies. *Health Psychology, 16*, 417–425.

Golding, J. M., Taylor, D. L., Menard, L., & King, M. J. (2000). Prevalence of sexual abuse history in a sample of women seeking treatment for premenstrual syndrome. *Journal of Psychosomatic Obstetrics and Gynecology, 21*, 69–80.

Goldman, J., Salus, M. K., Wolcott, D., & Kennedy, K. Y. (2003). A coordinated response to child abuse and neglect: The foundation for practice. *United States Department of Health and Human Services, Administration for Children and Families*. Washington, DC: U.S. Retrieved November, 2010, from http://www.childwelfare.gov/pubs/usermanuals/foundation/foundationo.cfm.

Hamburger, M. E., Leeb, R. T., & Swahn, M. H. (2008). Child maltreatment and early alcohol use among high-risk adolescents. *Journal of Studies on Alcohol and Drugs, 69*, 291–295.

Hanson, R. F., Bontrager, C., Self-Brown, S., et al. (2008). Relations among gender, violence exposure, and mental health: The National Survey of Adolescents. *American Journal of Orthopsychiatry, 78*, 313–321.

Hanson, R. K., & Broom, I. (2005). The utility of cumulative meta-analysis: Application to programs for reducing sexual violence. *Sexual Abuse: A Journal of Research and Treatment, 17*(4), 357–373.

Hanson, K. A., & Gidycz, C. A. (1993). Evaluation of a sexual assault prevention program. *Journal of Consulting and Clinical Psychology, 61*(6), 1046–1052.

Hanson, R., Kievit, L., Saunders, B., Smith, D., Kilpatrick, D., Resnick, H., et al. (2003). Correlates of adolescent reports of sexual assault: Findings from the National Survey of Adolescents. *Child Maltreatment, 8*(4), 261–272.

Hart, T. C. (2003). *National Crime Victimization Survey, 1995–2000: Violent victimization of college students*. Washington, DC: US Department of Justice, Bureau of Justice Statistics.

Hedtke, K. A., Ruggiero, K. J., Fitzgerald, M. M., Zinzow, H. M., Saunders, B. E., Resnick, H. S., et al. (2008). A longitudinal investigation of interpersonal violence in relation to mental health and substance use. *Journal of Consulting and Clinical Psychology, 76*, 633–647.

Hines, D. A. (2007). Predictors of sexual coercion against women and men: A multilevel, multi-national study of university students. *Archives of Sexual Behavior, 36*, 403–422.

Humphrey, S. E., & Kahn, A. S. (2000). Fraternities, athletic teams, and rape: Importance of identification with a risky group. *Journal of Interpersonal Violence, 15*, 1313–1322.

Humphrey, J. A., & White, J. W. (2000). Women's vulnerability to sexual assault from adolescence to young adulthood. *Journal of Adolescent Health, 27*, 419–424.

Jaycox, L., McCaffrey, D., Eiseman, B., Aronoff, J., Shelley, G., Collins, R., et al. (2006). Impact of a school-based dating violence prevention program among Latino teens: Randomized controlled effectiveness trial. *Journal of Adolescent Health, 39*, 694–704.

Kawsar, M., Anfield, A., Walters, E., McCabe, S., & Forster, G. E. (2004). Prevalence of sexually transmitted infections and mental health needs of female child and adolescent survivors of rape and sexual assault attending a specialist clinic. *Sexually Transmitted Diseases, 80*, 138–141.

Kelly, P., & Koh, J. (2006). Sexually transmitted infections in alleged sexual abuse of children and adolescents. *Journal of Paediatrics and Child Health, 42*, 434–440.

Kilpatrick, K., Acierno, R., Saunders, B., Resnick, H., Best, C., & Schnurr, P. (2000). Risk factors for adolescent substance abuse and dependence: Data from a national sample. *Journal of Consulting and Clinical Psychology, 68*, 19–30.

Kilpatrick, D. G., Edmunds, C. N., & Seymour, A. K. (1992). *Rape in America: A report to the nation*. Arlington, VA: National Victim Center and Medical University of South Carolina.

Kilpatrick, D. G., Resnick, H. S., Ruggiero, K. J., Conoscenti, L. M., & McCauley, J. L. (2007, July). Drug-facilitated, incapacitated, and forcible rape: A National Study. Report to National Institute of Justice. Accessed at www.ncjrs.gov/pdffiles1/nij/grants/219181/pdf.

Kilpatrick, D. G., Ruggiero, K. J., Acierno, R., Saunders, B. E., Resnick, H. S., & Best, C. L. (2003a). Violence and risk of PTSD, major depression, substance abuse/dependence, and comorbidity: Results from the National Survey of Adolescents. *Journal of Consulting and Clinical Psychology, 71*(4), 692–700.

Kilpatrick, D., Saunders, B., & Smith, D. (2003b). *Youth victimization: Prevalence and implications*. (NIJ Research in Brief). Washington, DC: U.S. Department of Justice, National Institute of Justice.

Kingston, S., & Raghavan, C. (2009). The relationship of sexual abuse, early initiation of substance use, and adolescent trauma to PTSD. *Journal of Traumatic Stress, 22*(1), 65–68.

Klaczynski, P. A. (2001). Analytic and heuristic processing influences on adolescent reasoning and decision making. *Child Development, 72*, 844–861.

Koenen, K. C., Fu, Q. J., Lyons, M. J., Toomey, R., Goldberg, J., Eisen, S. A., et al. (2005). Juvenile conduct disorder as a risk factor for trauma exposure and posttraumatic stress disorder. *Journal of Traumatic Stress, 18*, 23–32.

Koss, M. P., & Gidycz, C. A. (1985). Sexual experiences survey: Reliability and validity. *Journal of Consulting and Clinical Psychology, 53*, 422–423.

Krebs, C. P., Lindquist, C. H., Warner, T. D., Fisher, B. S., & Martin, S. L. (2009). The differential risk factors of physically forced and alcohol- or other drug-enabled sexual assault among university women. *Violence and Victims, 24*, 302–321.

Macy, R. J. (2007). A coping theory framework toward preventing sexual revictimization. *Aggression and Violent Behavior, 12*, 177–192.

Males, M., & Chew, K. S. Y. (1996). The ages of fathers in California adolescent births, 1993. *American Journal of Public Health, 86*, 565–568.

McCann, J., Miyamoto, S., Boyle, C., & Rogers, K. (2007). Healing of hymenal injuries in prepubertal and adolescent girls: A descriptive study. *Pediatrics, 119*, 1094–1106.

McCauley, J. L., Conoscenti, L. M., Ruggiero, K. J., Resnick, H. S., Saunders, B. E., & Kilpatrick, D. G. (2009). Prevalence and correlates of drug/alcohol-facilitated and incapacitated sexual assault in a nationally representative sample of adolescent girls. *Journal of Clinical Child and Adolescent Psychology, 38*, 295–300.

McLeer, S. V., Dixon, J. F., Henry, D., Ruggiero, K., Escovitz, K., Niedda, T., et al. (1998). Psychopathology in non-clinically referred sexually abused children. *Journal of the American Academy of Child and Adolescent Psychiatry, 37*, 1326–1333.

Miller, A. K., Markman, K. D., & Handley, I. M. (2007). Self-blame among sexual assault victims prospectively predicts revictimization: A perceived sociolegal context model of risk. *Basic and Applied Social Psychology, 29*, 129–136.

Molnar, B. E., Buka, S. L., & Kessler, R. C. (2001). Child sexual abuse and subsequent psychopathology: Results from the National Comorbidity Survey. *American Journal of Public Health, 91*, 753–760.

Nelson, E., Heath, A., Madden, P., et al. (2002). Association between self-reported childhood sexual abuse and adverse psychosocial outcomes: Results from a twin study. *Archives of General Psychiatry, 59*, 139–146.

Newman, M. G., Clayton, L., Zuellig, A., Cashman, L., Arnow, B., Dea, R., et al. (2000). The relationship of childhood sexual abuse and depression with somatic symptoms and medical utilization. *Psychological Medicine, 30*, 1063–1077.

Noll, J. G., Shenk, C. E., & Putnam, K. T. (2009). Childhood sexual abuse and adolescent pregnancy: A meta-analytic update. *Journal of Pediatric Psychology, 34*, 366–378.

Peterlin, B. L., Ward, T., Lidicker, J., & Levin, M. (2007). A retrospective, comparative study on the frequency of abuse in migraine and chronic daily headache. *Headache, 47*, 397–401.

Putnam, F. W. (2003). Ten-year research update review: Child sexual abuse. *Journal of the American Acedemy of Child and Adolescent Psychiatry, 42*(3), 269–278.

Rennison, C. M. (2002). *Rape and sexual assault: Reporting to police and medical attention, 1992–2000. Bureau of Justice Report, NCJ 194530*. Washington, DC: Bureau of Justice Statistics, Office of Justice Programs, U.S. Department of Justice.

Resnick, H. S., Holmes, M. M., Kilpatrick, D. G., Clum, G., Acierno, R., Best, C. L., et al. (2000). Predictors of post-rape medical care in a national sample of women. *American Journal of Preventive Medicine, 19*, 214–219.

Robb, A. S., Cueva, J. E., Sporn, J., Yang, R., & Vanderberg, D. G. (2008). Sertraline treatment of children and adolescents with posttraumatic stress disorder: A double-blind placebo-controlled trial. *Journal of Child and Adolescent Psychopharmacology, 20*, 463–471.

Rohde, P., Ichikawa, L., Simon, G. E., Ludman, E. J., Linde, J. A., Jeffery, R. W., et al. (2008). Associations of child sexual and physical abuse with obesity and depression in middle-aged women. *Child Abuse and Neglect, 32*, 878–887.

Ross, C. (2005). Childhood sexual abuse and psychosomatic symptoms in irritable bowel syndrome. *Journal of Childhood Sexual Abuse, 14*, 27–38.

Sachs-Ericsson, N., Blazer, D., Plant, E. A., & Arnow, B. (2005). Childhood sexual and physical abuse and 1-year prevalence of medical problems in the National Comorbidity Survey. *Health Psychology, 24*, 32–40.

Schewe, P. A. (2007). Interventions to prevent sexual violence. In L. S. Doll, S. E. Bonzo, J. A. Mercy, & D. A. Sleet (Eds.), *Handbook of injury and violence prevention* (pp. 223–240). New York: Springer Science.

Sexual abuse. (2006). In Webster's New World Law Dictionary. Hoboken, NJ: Wiley.

Sharpe, D., & Faye, C. (2006). Non-epileptic seizures and child sexual abuse: A critical review of the literature. *Clinical Psychology Review, 26*, 1020–1040.

Siegel, R. M., Schubert, C. J., Myers, P. A., & Shapiro, R. A. (1995). The prevalence of sexually transmitted diseases in children and adolescents evaluated for sexual abuse in Cincinnati: Rationale for limited STD testing in prepubertal girls. *Pediatrics, 96*, 1090–1094.

Siegel, J. A., & Williams, L. M. (2003). The relationship between child sexual abuse and female delinquency and crime: A prospective study. *Journal of Research in Crime and Delinquency, 40*(1), 71–94.

Siegel, L. J., Welsh, B., & Senna, J. J. (2003). Juvenile delinquency: Theory, practice, and law. Belmont, CA: Thompson/Wadsworth.

Simpson, T. L., & Miller, W. R. (2002). Concomitance between child sexual and physical abuse and substance use problems: A review. *Clinical Psychology Review, 22*, 27–77.

Smith, D. W., Witte, T. H., & Fricker-Elhai, A. E. (2006). Service outcomes in physical and sexual abuse cases: A comparison of Child Advocacy Center-based and standard services. *Child Maltreatment, 11*, 354–360.

Sobsey, D., Randall, W., & Parrila, R. (1997). Gender differences in abused children whose experiences were documented by videotape. *Child Abuse and Neglect, 21*, 707–720.

Sochting, I., Fairbrother, N., & Kocj, W. J. (2004). Sexual assault of women: Prevention efforts and risk factors. *Violence Against Women, 10*(1), 73–93.

Stevens, T. N., Ruggiero, K. J., Kilpatrick, D. G., Resnick, H. S., & Saunders, B. E. (2005). Variables differentiating singly and multiply victimized youth: Results from the National Survey of Adolescents and implications for secondary prevention. *Child Maltreatment, 10*, 211–223.

Stewart, A., Livingston, M., & Dennison, S. (2008). Transitions and turning points: Examining the links between child maltreatment and juvenile offending. *Child Abuse and Neglect, 32*, 51–66.

Sugar, N. F., Fine, D. N., & Eckert, L. O. (2004). Physical injury after sexual assault: Findings of a large case series. *American Journal of Obstetrics and Gynecology, 190*, 71–76.

Testa, M., Hoffman, J. H., & Livingston, J. A. (2010). Alcohol and sexual risk behaviors as mediators of the sexual victimization-revictimization relationship. *Journal of Consulting and Clinical Psychology, 78*, 249–259.

Thompson, M. P., Arias, I., Basile, K. C., & Desai, S. (2002). The association between childhood physical and sexual victimization and health problems in adulthood in a nationally representative sample of women. *Journal of Interpersonal Violence, 17*, 1115–1129.

Thornberry, T., Ireland, T., & Smith, C. (2001). The importance of timing: The varying impact of childhood and adolescent maltreatment on multiple problem outcomes. *Development and Psychopathology, 13*(4), 957–979.

Tjaden, P., & Thoennes, N. (2000). *Full report of the prevalence, incidence, and consequences of violence against women: Findings from the National Violence Against Women Survey*. Washington, DC: National Institute of Justice, Office of Justice Programs, U.S. Department of Justice and Centers for Disease Control and Prevention, NCJ183781.

Turner, H. A., Finkelhor, D., & Ormrod, R. (2006). The effect of lifetime victimization on the mental health of children and adolescents. *Social Science and Medicine, 62*, 13–27.

U.S. Department of Health and Human Services. (1998). *Child Maltreatment 1996: Reports from the States to the National Child Abuse and Neglect Data System*. Washington, DC: US Government Printing Office.

United States Department of Justice. (2008). Criminal victimization in the United States, 2006 statistical tables. *National crime victimization survey*. Washington, DC, USA.

Waldrop, A. E., Hanson, R. F., Resnick, H. S., Kilpatrick, D. G., Naugle, A. E., & Saunders, B. E. (2007). Risk factors for suicidal behavior among a National sample of adolescents: Implications for prevention. *Journal of Traumatic Stress, 20*, 869–879.

Walker, E. A., Keegan, D., Gardner, G., Sullivan, M., Bernstein, D., & Katon, W. J. (1997). Psychosocial factors in fibromyalgia compared with rheumatoid arthritis: II. Sexual, physical, and emotional abuse and neglect. *Psychosomatic Medicine, 59*, 572–577.

Wekerle, C., & Wolfe, D. A. (1999). Dating violence in mid-adolescence: Theory, significance, and emerging prevention initiatives. *Clinical Psychology Review, 19*(4), 435–456.

Westcott, H., & Jones, D. (1999). Annotation: The abuse of disabled children. *Journal of Child and Adolescent Psychiatry, 40*, 497–506.

Wethington, H. R., Hahn, R. A., Fuqua-Whitley, D. S., Sipe, T. A., Crosby, A. E., Johnson, R. L., et al. (2008). The effectiveness of interventions to reduce psychological harm from traumatic events among children and adolescents: A systematic review. *American Journal of Preventive Medicine, 35*, 287–313.

Widom, C. S., & Maxfield, M. G. (2001). *An update on the "cycle of violence"*. Washington, DC: U.S. Department of Justice. National Institute of Justice.

Wolfe, D. (2006). Preventing violence in relationships: Psychological science addressing complex social issues. *Canadian Psychology, 47*, 44–50.

Wolitzky-Taylor, K. B., Ruggiero, K. J., Danielson, C. K., Resnick, H. S., Hanson, R. F., Smith, D. W., et al. (2009). Prevalence and correlates of dating violence in a National sample of adolescents. *Journal of the American Academy of Child and Adolescent Psychiatry, 47*(7), 755–762.

Young, M. S., Harford, K., Kinder, B., & Savell, J. K. (2007). The relationship between childhood sexual abuse and adult mental health among undergraduates: Victim gender doesn't matter. *Journal of Interpersonal Violence, 22*, 1315–1331.

Intimate Partner Violence in Adolescent Romantic Relationships

Ann T. Chu, Jane M. Sundermann, and Anne P. DePrince

Intimate partner violence (IPV) in adolescent romantic relationships is a serious public health problem. First, such violence is all too common, affecting a significant number of youth. In grades 9–12, approximately 10 % of male and female students report being physically hurt by a dating partner in the past 12 months (Centers for Disease Control and Prevention, 2011). Rates of exposure are even higher among certain populations: for example, an estimated 25–50 % of adolescent females in foster care report violence in dating relationships (Jonson-Reid & Bivens, 1999). Second, IPV in adolescent romantic relationships is linked to a range of serious negative health consequences, particularly maladaptive mental health outcomes (e.g., Banyard & Cross, 2008; Teten, Ball, Valle, Noonan, & Rosenbluth, 2009). Compared to male victims of adolescent IPV, some of these adverse health outcomes are uniquely elevated for female victims, including the physical and mental stress associated with higher rates of unwanted pregnancies among female IPV victims (versus non-victims; Silverman, Raj, Mucci, Lorelei, & Hathaway, 2001). Serious physical injury is also more likely to occur for female (versus male) victims of adolescent IPV (Coker et al., 2000).

A.T. Chu, Ph.D. (✉) • J.M. Sundermann
A.P. DePrince, Ph.D.
Department of Psychology, University of Denver, 2155 South Race Street, Denver, CO 80208, USA
e-mail: ann.chu@du.edu; Jane.Sundermann@du.edu; anne.deprince@du.edu

In addition to effects on health broadly, IPV victimization during adolescence contributes to IPV risk in adulthood, particularly for females. Both prospective and retrospective studies point to the critical role that IPV in adolescence plays in understanding lifetime risk for IPV among girls and women (Arata, 2002; Gidycz, Hanson, & Layman, 1995; Smith, White, & Holland, 2003). For instance, females who experienced childhood abuse were found to be at risk for dating violence as adults *only* when they experienced dating violence during adolescence (Smith et al., 2003). Humphrey and White (2000) documented that college women who had been sexually assaulted during adolescence were 4.6 times more likely than their peers to report sexual victimization in young adulthood. Women's revictimization in adolescence and adulthood, in turn, is linked to greater physical and psychological health costs than single victimizations (DePrince, 2005; Kimerling, Alvarez, Pavao, Kaminski, & Baumrind, 2007; Polusny, Rosenthal, Aban, & Follette, 2004). While some studies suggest that adolescent girls and boys do engage in mutually aggressive relationships (Foshee, Reyes, & Ennett, 2010; Teten et al., 2009), the safety and health trajectories for girls and women exposed to IPV in dating relationships differ significantly than those for boys. This current chapter focuses on understanding the risks and consequences of IPV victimization for girls and women.

Because one of the potential consequences of adolescent IPV is adult IPV, we distinguish adolescent IPV through use of the term teen dating

W.T. O'Donohue et al. (eds.), *Handbook of Adolescent Health Psychology*,
DOI 10.1007/978-1-4614-6633-8_14, © Springer Science+Business Media New York 2013

violence (TDV). TDV definitions have historically focused on physical violence, such as "the use or threat of physical force or restraint carried out with the intent of causing pain or injury to another" (Sugarman & Hotaling, 1989, p. 5). In more recent years, though, definitions of TDV have expanded to recognize a range of behaviors exerted in romantic relationships to "control or dominate another person physically, sexually, or psychologically *causing some level of harm*" (Wekerle & Wolfe, 1999, p. 436; italics ours). Unless otherwise noted, we use the term TDV to refer broadly to all three forms of aggression (physical, sexual, and psychological) that cause harm to either partner within adolescent romantic relationships.

Research on TDV has advanced rapidly in recent decades to include more sophisticated analyses and rigorous study designs. These advances, though, have revealed how complex studying TDV can be. While earlier epidemiological studies focused on establishing prevalence rates of TDV, recent studies take a more nuanced look at differences in prevalence rates among subgroups of adolescents (e.g., Jonson-Reid, Scott, McMillen, & Edmond, 2007). Advocates of ecological models (e.g., Connolly, Friedlander, Pepler, Craig, & Laporte, 2010; White, 2009) also recognize that violence and subsequent sequelae do not exist in a vacuum; rather, many factors at multiple levels interact to influence exposure and response to violence, including TDV. Each level of risk must be well understood in order to develop a valid ecological model that can be used to inform prevention/intervention efforts. Along with a review of TDV prevalence and health consequences, the current chapter uses an ecological model framework to organize existing research on risk factors for TDV victimization. We rely on an ecological model comprised of three levels of risk: individual, relationship, and societal. At each level we identify risk factors that have garnered consistent support across studies. We then review the empirical evidence for efficacious prevention programs. Throughout the chapter, we highlight unanswered questions and suggest areas for continued investigation.

Prevalence

Estimates of TDV prevalence vary greatly, likely due to methodological differences across studies. Research drawing on nationally representative samples tends to report lower prevalence rates of IPV victimization, ranging from 3 to 32 % (Halpern, Oslak, Young, Martin, & Kupper, 2001; Wolitzky-Taylor et al., 2008), while research using more extensive and in-depth questionnaires documents higher rates with studies reporting up to 80 % in school-based and inpatient samples (e.g., Hickman, Jaycox, & Aronoff, 2004; Rizzo, Esposito-Smythers, Spirito, & Thompson, 2010; Smith et al., 2003). The epidemiological surveys may provide more conservative estimates of TDV prevalence because questions regarding violence are typically limited to a few concrete and specific behaviors. For example, the Youth Risk Behavior Survey (YRBS), a biannual school-based survey by the Centers for Disease Control and Prevention (CDC), asks only one "Yes or No" question regarding dating violence (i.e., "During the past 12 months, did your boyfriend or girlfriend ever hit, slap, or physically hurt you on purpose?") and one "Yes or No" question regarding forced sexual intercourse (i.e., "Have you ever been physically forced to have sexual intercourse when you did not want to?"; CDC, 2011).

Prevalence estimates are also affected by varying operationalization and measurement of adolescent romantic relationships and TDV across studies. Despite the observation that teens have multiple dating partners across adolescence (e.g., Halpern et al., 2001), many TDV studies rely on cross-sectional approaches focused on a specific relationship, thereby precluding researchers' ability to examine individual differences in and across romantic relationships (e.g., Banyard & Cross, 2008; Coker et al., 2000; Noonan & Charles, 2009; Rizzo et al., 2010). Studies also include a range of TDV experiences, from victimization in the context of casual one-time dating to serious long-term relationships. Further, studies vary in the time frames used to assess violence in relationships; some questionnaires ask about relationships in a specific time frame (e.g., Conflict in Adolescent Dating Relationships Inventory (CADRI; Wolfe et al., 2001), across the lifespan (e.g., Youth Risk Behavior Survey; CDC, 2011), or violent experiences within the last relationship (e.g., Revised Conflict Tactics Scales (CTS-2); Straus, Hamby, Boney-McCoy, & Sugarman, 1996). Violence can vary from relatively benign (e.g., "He insulted me with put downs" from the CADRI; Wolfe et al., 2001) to serious abuse that affects psychological and physical health (e.g., "He threw something at me," "I touched him/her sexually when he/she didn't want me to" from the CADRI; Wolfe et al., 2001; Rizzo et al., 2010). In general, the field lacks systematic assessment for different types of romantic involvements and dating violence; methodological differences also present challenges to making comparisons across studies.

To date, knowledge on TDV from epidemiological and empirical studies primarily comes from school settings with adolescents who are or had been involved in heterosexual romantic relationships. To our knowledge, there have been no studies on TDV in same-sex romantic relationships in adolescence specifically; and few studies have recruited from nonschool settings. Additionally, most empirical studies have traditionally utilized samples that comprise primarily Caucasian adolescents. Although findings from school-based samples of primarily Caucasian adolescents in heterosexual relationships have established an important foundation from which to expand, focusing solely on such sampling methods ignores a large portion of US youth and likely limits our understanding of the heterogeneity of TDV experiences. Demonstrating the importance of expanding sampling methods, one study of TDV with an urban sample of homeless youth found higher prevalence rates among those youth involved with the child welfare system as compared to their peers without child welfare involvement (Goldstein, Leslie, Wekerle, Leung, & Erickson, 2010).

Prevalence and Gender

Some adolescent research suggests that females engage in as much psychological and/or physical aggression as males (e.g., Halpern et al., 2001), while other studies suggest that females engage in greater physical and/or psychological aggression than males (see Foshee & Matthew, 2007; Wolfe et al., 2003). Despite the fact that females may engage in physical and psychological aggression at approximately equal (or greater) rates to males, feminist theorists point to important characteristics of TDV to demonstrate that TDV remains a gendered phenomenon influenced by principles of social learning theory and sociocultural values (White, 2009). A review by Saunders (2002) indicated that female victims of male-perpetrated TDV suffer more serious negative consequences, particularly health outcomes, compared to male victims of female-perpetrated TDV. Straus' (1995) landmark finding that women needed medical attention seven times as often as husbands after a physically violent conflict in the relationship is echoed in studies with youth. For instance, Muñoz-Rivas, Graña, O'Leary, and González (2007) found that female TDV victims were more likely to receive injuries and need medical attention/hospitalization for injuries than male TDV victims. This disparity in consequences may be due to the fact that males engage in violence that is more severe and more often involves lethal weapons compared to females who engage in lower level violence such as kicking, slapping, or shoving (Schwartz, Magee, Griffin, & Dupuis, 2004).

Unlike psychological and physical aggression, researchers have documented that males are more likely to perpetrate sexual violence than females (Basile, Chen, Lynberg, & Saltzman, 2007; USDJ, 2008, National Crime Victimization Survey). Interestingly, Spitzberg (1999) conducted a review of 120 studies of sexual violence, 90 of which used adolescent or college samples. This review demonstrated that, when sexual violence was assessed at a broad level, males and females did not report significantly different perpetration rates; however, when more specific forms of sexual violence were assessed, such as rape, males were four times more likely than females to identify as perpetrators while females were four times more likely than males to identify as victims. Sexual violence in adolescence is particularly important to consider because statistics from nationally representative samples demonstrate that adolescents and young adults are disproportionately victims of sexual assault: the 2008 National Crime Victimization Survey found that half of all rape/sexual assault victims were aged 12–24 (USDJ, 2008).

Emerging qualitative studies examining motivations or reasons for perpetrating aggressive behaviors may be important to understanding gender differences in prevalence rates. Adolescent females appear to use physical violence as a means of self-defense or due to other situational factors whereas male teens use physical violence as a means to control their partners (Foshee, Bauman, Linder, Rice, & Wilcher, 2007; O'Keeffe, 1997). Further, rigid gender roles may result in inequities in power between male and female partners as well as expectancies that relationships involve harm to women (Wolfe et al., 2003). Supporting the latter argument, DePrince, Combs, and Shanahan (2009) documented expectances that relationships involve harm among college women who had been revictimized, compared to women who had not.

Prevalence and Race/Ethnicity

Several studies, including the CDC national survey, have found that adolescents from racial and ethnic minority groups report higher rates of dating violence compared to non-Hispanic Caucasian adolescents (e.g., CDC, 2011; Chapple, 2003; Connolly et al., 2010; Foshee et al., 2010). Specifically, the highest prevalence rates were found among Black adolescents, followed by Hispanic and Caucasian adolescents, and then Asian adolescents, even after controlling for socioeconomic status (SES). However, two separate reviews on risk factors for TDV also identified a number of studies that found either lower rates of dating violence in teens from racial/ethnic minority groups or no link at all between race/ethnicity and TDV (Lewis & Fremouw, 2001; Vézina & Hébert, 2007). The authors of the reviews suggest methodological variation and potential third variables as explanations for this discrepancy. For example, many studies do not distinguish between immigrants versus US-born racial/ethnic minority teens. This distinction may be important because racial/ethnic identity, involvement with culture of origin, and lower levels of acculturation have been found to be buffers against TDV for some racial/ethnic groups (for a review, see Smokowski, David-Ferdon, & Stroupe, 2009). Additionally, many general racial categories (e.g., Latino, Asian) are differentiated by specific subgroups (e.g., Cuban versus Mexican, Chinese versus Japanese), with great heterogeneity across the subgroups. Yet the variability between ethnic groups often gets washed out by comparisons of only the larger racial categories.

Recommendations

The differences in prevalence rates between genders and racial/ethnic groups highlight the importance of moving beyond documenting broad group differences (e.g., victimized youth versus non-victimized youth) to identifying the mechanisms and processes that lead to these disparities (e.g., relationship dynamics, acculturation). To date, however, TDV research has largely involved single informants in the context of heterosexual romantic relationships. Research involving both partners as well as same-gendered romantic relationships may help to clarify the impact of gender role expectations and gender differences in relationship dynamics on TDV. While studies are starting to pay more attention to cross-cultural and gender issues, these areas remain important topics for future research to fully examine.

Health Consequences of TDV

TDV is associated with a diverse array of maladaptive health-related outcomes measured proximally in adolescence as well as more distally in adulthood. Examples of maladaptive outcomes for health among victims include significantly higher levels of mental health symptomatology such as depression (Banyard & Cross, 2008; Yen et al., 2010). In a longitudinal survey of approximately 2,000 female high school students, Silverman et al. (2001) found that female teens reporting physical or sexual dating violence victimization also reported higher levels of substance use, unhealthy weight control behaviors, sexual risk behaviors, pregnancy, and suicidality as compared to their non-victimized peers. These associations held above and beyond the effects of potentially confounding demographics and other risk behaviors.

Few studies have examined differential health outcomes based on the distinctions between pure perpetrators, pure victims, or teens who are both perpetrators and victims. One of the few studies that examined these subtypes found a higher percentage of teens reporting as being both the offender and victim versus offender or victim only (Gray & Foshee, 1997). Furthermore, teens who identified as being both perpetrator and victim endorsed perpetrating more severe levels of violence and sustaining more injuries as compared to individuals who were victims only. Yen et al. (2010) also conducted a study that asked teens to make the distinction between being a perpetrator only, victim only, or both. Teens across all three groups had higher rates of depression, insomnia, suicidality, and alcohol abuse compared to teens with no experience of TDV as perpetrator or victim. However, teens reporting both victimization and perpetration experiences had significantly higher levels of alcohol abuse than pure victims and significantly higher rates of externalizing behaviors (i.e., truancy and theft) than pure perpetrators. These two studies point to important characteristic differences in teens who engage in mutually aggressive relationship as compared to teens who are perpetrators or victims only, though research to date has not focused a great deal of attention to this subgroup of teens.

Some studies have also suggested that rape has unique and severe health consequences relative to other types of violence. A study by Coker et al. (2000) revealed that forced-sex victimization was associated with suicidal ideation and attempts among both female and male high school students. Because suicidal ideation and attempts are clearly one of the most severe (i.e., by definition, life-threatening) mental health symptoms and female teens suffer much more from rape victimization than male teens, these findings provide yet further evidence for gender differences in the severity of TDV's consequences for victims, namely, that female teen victims, on average, suffer more severe consequences than male teen victims.

Recommendations

Existing research demonstrates a robust relationship between TDV and maladaptive health outcomes. However, identifying potential moderators and mediators linking TDV and deleterious consequences are sorely needed. For example, studies are starting to examine race and/or ethnicity as a moderator of health consequences in *adult* IPV; existing data suggest that racial/ethnic minority IPV victims suffer more severe consequences relative to Caucasian victims (Stark, 1990). However, researchers in the adult IPV field have yet to identify the mechanisms that drive these group differences. Importantly, researchers have also yet to examine race/ethnicity and/or associated variables as moderators of outcomes in the TDV literature. Understanding moderators could provide policy makers and practitioners insight into how to direct services in the context of limited resources.

Despite the heterogeneous nature of TDV, most studies examine broad-level differences (e.g., TDV versus no TDV) rather than identifying specific subgroup profiles of adolescents with different experiences of TDV (e.g., victim only versus perpetrator-victim; subtypes of violence); therefore, studies may inadvertently overlook important individual differences that lead to varied outcomes. Recently, researchers in the adult IPV literature have called for and started to adopt person-centered analyses to better understand the full variability of victimization experiences and responses that may be lost in group comparisons (see Macy, 2008). Given that not all adolescents who experience TDV report similar health problems as sequelae, adopting a person-centered approach in the field of TDV may help target subpopulations to more effectively ameliorate specific deleterious outcomes.

Risk Factors for TDV Victimization: Applying an Ecological Model

The ecological model, first proposed by Bronfenbrenner (1979), comprises multiple embedded levels (e.g., individual, family, societal) that work together to influence individual experiences. Ecological models have been applied to different aspects of violence exposure (for a discussion on the application to childhood maltreatment, see Chu, Pineda, DePrince, & Freyd, 2011). Using an ecological model to organize our review, we turn now to identifying risk factors for TDV at individual (e.g., internalizing/externalizing problems, age), relationship (e.g., peer, family), and societal (e.g., attitudes, affiliations, acculturation, neighborhood) levels. We focus on risk factors that have been replicated across studies.

Individual

At the individual level, researchers have identified both internalizing and externalizing problems as risk factors for TDV. For example, internalizing problems such as depressive symptoms have been consistently linked to TDV, according to a review of 61 studies conducted by Vézina and Hébert (2007). Though depression is a common consequence of violence, several longitudinal studies found that depression may also be an antecedent to TDV (see Vézina & Hébert, 2007). Depression might increase risk for TDV by decreasing female adolescents' perceptions of self-efficacy in relationships and potentially violent situations, by increasing tolerance of abusive behaviors from dating partners in order to maintain intimacy and to avoid feelings of isolation, or by increasing high-risk behaviors as a coping strategy against feelings of depression (see Vézina & Hébert, 2007). However, these explanations have yet to be supported consistently by empirical data. A few studies have also documented the finding that suicidal attempts increase risk for TDV in addition to being a consequence of violence (Vézina & Hébert, 2007). Again, the pathway by which suicidal attempts increase risk for TDV remains unexplored.

Externalizing problems such as substance abuse as well as risky/disruptive behaviors also appear to put teens at higher risk for experiencing TDV (Vézina & Hébert, 2007). Researchers have assumed that substance use makes youth vulnerable to high-risk situations that they would otherwise avoid or be able to protect themselves; however, we are aware of no empirical data that exist to support that link. Thus, the process by which substance use leads to dating violence remains unclear. As mentioned previously, substance use as well as other internalizing and externalizing problems could be either risk factors for and/or consequences of TDV. Only with more longitudinal research will researchers be able to tease out important causal/transactional processes related to TDV.

Age also appears to be linked to TDV risk. In the handful of TDV longitudinal studies available, researchers have documented a curvilinear relationship such that aggressive behaviors increase from early adolescence to a peak point around mid-adolescence, and then decline by the end of adolescence, though the exact age at which aggressive behaviors peaked differed across studies (see Foshee et al., 2009). Additionally, Wolfe and colleagues (2003) found that though girls reported engaging in higher rates of physical dating aggression than boys, this difference decreased over time such that by ages 16–18 there were no significant gender differences in aggression rates. Thus, the gender difference between rates of aggression may also vary as a function of age.

Relationships

Adolescents are embedded in multiple, complex relational systems that are linked to risk for TDV. For example, adolescents are just starting to form and explore their self-identities and sexuality (Erikson, 1968) while also experiencing considerable need to conform and be accepted in peer relationships. Though positive peer norms may provide a buffer against many negative experiences, negative peer influences may represent a risk factor. Drawing on the social learning framework, one well-established finding is that violent behavior appears in part to be learned through associations with peer reference groups (see Elliot & Menard, 1996). Indeed, Arriaga and Foshee (2004) found that having friends who experienced violence in their romantic relationships predicted teen girls' victimization 6 months later. Having peers who experience dating violence predicted victimization above the contribution of inter-parental violence. This pattern has been replicated in several other studies (for a review, see Vézina & Hébert, 2007).

Theories and emerging empirical findings suggest that gender differences in peer interactions may also impact romantic relationships and the experience of dating violence. For example, gender socialization in childhood of girls and boys may lead to different expectations for how males and females "should" behave in adolescence (see Maccoby, 1998). Male and female adolescents then come together in heterosexual romantic relationships within two different "cultures." The female culture emphasizes intimate relationships, self-disclosure, and emotional expression while the male culture focuses on activities, multiple superficial relationships, minimal disclosure, and anger expression. Data from one longitudinal study provide some preliminary evidence to support this theory (Underwood & Rosen, 2009). The authors found that girls' relational interactions and boy's aggression in same-gender peer relationships may relate to having emotionally intense arguments when they come together in romantic relationships in early adolescence.

Adolescent relationships within families can also increase TDV risk. For example, teens who live in single-parent households and/or who have inadequate parental supervision are at elevated risk of experiencing TDV (Vézina & Hébert, 2007). Findings also consistently show that childhood abuse and witnessing violence in the home increases risk for being a victim of TDV (see Vézina & Hébert, 2007). Reitzel-Jaffe and Wolfe (2001) postulate that living with aggressive parents leads to the development of aggressive social-cognitive information processing, which is then carried over to teens' abilities to form healthy relationships as well as their interpersonal interactions within romantic relationships. While these findings are starting to provide more comprehensive knowledge on the impact of relationships on the risk for TDV, the underlying mechanisms again remain theoretical. Empirical support is sorely needed to better understand the processes that drive these associations.

Societal

In studying interpersonal violence, it is difficult to measure environmental factors separate from the individual; however, the environmental context, with its affiliated attitudes, beliefs, and practices, may increase risk for or protect youth from TDV. For example, beliefs that violence is acceptable are linked to increases in TDV risk (Vézina & Hébert, 2007) while cultural affiliation appears to buffer against TDV risk (see Smokowski et al., 2009). Importantly, though, societal factors such as cultural affiliation may interact with individual- and relationship-level factors to influence risk for TDV in complex ways. For example, family violence exposure predicted the initiation of dating violence among Black, but not White, adolescents for reasons that are yet unclear (Foshee, Ennett, Bauman, Benefield, & Suchindran, 2005). The processes by which particular attitudes or cultural affiliations translate into TDV risk remain unclear across studies. Perhaps highly culturally affiliated teens with high values of collectivism tend to report dating violence less than their peers, or strong cultural affiliation may contribute to better social support as well as more prosocial peer and/or partner involvement. For example, being less involved in religious activities has been shown to be a risk factor (for a review, see Vézina & Hébert, 2007).

Other factors in adolescents' living contexts may also affect TDV risk. For example, the few available studies that involve youth from rural settings suggest that those teens are at higher risk for TDV relative to teens in more urban environments (see Spencer & Bryant, 2000; Vézina & Hébert, 2007). Unfortunately, researchers have been unable to identify the mechanisms by which living in a rural environment increases risk for TDV. It may be that the driving force behind the difference between rural and urban environments is the level of involvement in prosocial and supportive networks (Vézina & Hébert, 2007). The mechanisms for these contextual societal risk factors need to be further examined.

Recommendations

Research in the TDV field began by documenting broad group differences (e.g., gender, culture/ethnicity) and correlations (e.g., previous violence exposure, substance use) associated with TDV. As many researchers (e.g., Coulton, Crampton, Irwin, Spilsbury, & *Korbin*, 2007; White, 2009) have suggested, we must now employ an ecological perspective that includes all levels of analysis in order to fully understand the context within which TDV happens. Such studies may clarify nonlinear processes of risk and protective factors of TDV, which in turn can further inform risk for further victimization.

Increasingly, studies have started to examine interactions between and across levels of analyses. For example, Foshee et al. (2010) found that depression, marijuana use, and aggression against peers predicted perpetration of dating violence by girls but not by boys. Anxiety predicted dating violence perpetration by Caucasian adolescents, while anger predicted perpetration by African-American adolescents (Foshee et al., 2005). Reyes, Foshee, Bauer, and Ennett (2011) also found that the positive association between heavy alcohol use and dating violence perpetration increased as family violence severity and level of friend involvement in dating violence increased. This pattern was present in teens from grades 8 through 12. These research examining interactions across multiple ecological levels while using more complex analyses and multiple methods is sorely needed. Such research will have important implications for clinical practice with teens experiencing TDV (both as perpetrators and as victims) as it helps build an empirical base of knowledge to identify resources for preventions and interventions.

There also needs to be further systematic research on whether specific risk factors in certain subgroups of teens are particularly influential in predicting dating violence. For example, Wekerle and colleagues (2001) recruited two samples of female adolescents: one school-based group and one comprised of teens involved with the child welfare system. They found that different risk factors predicted victimization in romantic relationships. In the high school group, post-traumatic stress disorder (PTSD) symptoms completely mediated the relationship between childhood abuse and TDV. In the child welfare group, PTSD symptoms only partially mediated this relationship. Smokowski et al. (2009) also found that the buffer effects of low levels of acculturation, ethnic identity, and culture-of-origin involvement were particularly strong for female minority teens compared to male minority teens.

Whether risk factors vary according to the type of violence remains another question to be answered. In Vézina and Hébert's review (2007), only 5 out of 61 studies examined risk factors by specific types of dating violence. Findings from those five studies provide initial evidence that some risk factors may differentially impact TDV depending on type. However, additional studies need to be conducted to confirm these patterns.

Notably, the way that variables affect adolescents' risk for TDV may be different from the effects of variables on adult IPV. For example, SES is a risk factor for adult IPV (Field & Caetano, 2004; Riggs, Caulfield, & Street, 2000); however, two separate reviews failed to find consistent links between SES and TDV (Foshee & Matthew, 2007; Vézina & Hébert, 2007). Vézina and Hébert (2007) postulated that parents with higher SES may hold more prestigious occupations that lead to more hours of work; in turn, more time away from home may lead to lower levels of parental involvement and monitoring, which increases risk for TDV. This example illustrates the importance of testing (and not assuming) whether risk factors identified in the adult literature translate to youth.

Prevention

Whitaker and colleagues (2006) conducted a systematic review of 11 studies examining the efficacy of TDV prevention programs designed for middle- and high-school students. Though the reviewed efficacy studies were mostly randomized control trials (RCT), Whitaker et al. (2006) noted a lack of evidence for the efficacy of prevention programs in general. However, evidence did converge in support of two specific prevention programs: Safe Dates (Foshee et al., 1998, 2004) and Youth Relationships Project (Wolfe et al., 2003; Wolfe, Crooks, Chiodo, & Jaffe, 2009).

Safe Dates has both a school and community component and includes activities aimed at changing norms of dating violence and improving prosocial skills. Foshee et al. (1998, 2004) evaluated the efficacy of Safe Dates via a RCT design where the control group received exposure to general community activities. At a 1-year follow-up, Safe Dates students reported lower perceived acceptability of dating violence compared to control group students. At a 4-year follow-up, students who received Safe Dates (versus control) reported less physical and sexual TDV perpetration and victimization.

Whereas Safe Dates is a school-based prevention program that targets a broad group of adolescents, the Youth Relationships Project took place at community agencies and targeted high-risk adolescents who were identified through the child protective service (CPS) system. Wolfe et al. (2009, 2003) evaluated the Youth Relationships Project via a RCT design where the control group received standard CPS services. At a 16-month follow-up, adolescents who received the Youth Relationships Project intervention (versus control) reported less physical abuse perpetration and victimization.

Recommendations

With the exceptions of Safe Dates and the Youth Relationships Project, most prevention programs of TDV have not yet demonstrated a sufficient level of evidence for their efficacy. In order to increase the efficacy of TDV prevention programs, we make several recommendations. RCTs that compare adolescents who receive intervention versus an active control treatment should be the gold standard for evidence of efficacy. Whenever possible, studies should employ additional research methodologies to complement the RCT design. For instance, studies should utilize a multi-rater (i.e., parents, teachers, etc.) and multimethod (i.e., self-report, behavioral) approach to examining program efficacy. Behavioral measures of change and long-term follow-up assessments are crucial to sufficiently document the impact of the intervention.

As risk factors for TDV become more well-known, programs should specifically target teens with those specific risk factors. Such targeted interventions could provide more specific information regarding mediating variables between early risk factors like maltreatment and outcomes like TDV, as well as highlight the nuanced "active ingredients" of prevention programs. Programs should also continue to explore ways to enhance cultural-sensitivity to targeted populations of adolescents and to recruit adolescents from more diverse settings beyond schools. Though program recruitment through school-settings is an efficient way to reach large numbers of adolescents, adolescents who are at the highest risk for TDV may be the adolescents who are truant or simply not very engaged in school-related activities. Thus, the combination of school- and community-based approaches, as demonstrated by Safe Dates, appears critical for reaching both large numbers of teens as well as high-risk teens. More targeted prevention programs for high-risk youth certainly come with additional challenges. Rizzo et al. (2010) noted that at-risk teens may also have significant difficulties with affect regulation which in turn prevents them from responding appropriately when overwhelmed in various social situations. When working with such a population on reducing TDV, then, prevention/intervention components would also need to address broader affect regulation skills prior to addressing knowledge and attitudes about dating violence.

With the preponderance of universal prevention programs implemented in schools, Wolfe and colleagues (2009) argue for addressing well-being and enhancing resilience as a way to reduce TDV as well as to help adolescents develop adaptive skills more generally. In fact, Foshee and colleagues (1998) found that after completing an educational program teaching appropriate positive behaviors and adaptive socioemotional skills, adolescent participants reported perpetrating 25 % fewer psychological abuse, 60 % fewer physical abuse, and 60 % fewer sexual abuse at the 1-year follow-up. However, notably throughout this current chapter and the larger literature, information on protective factors and resilience is absent (with the exception of acculturation as buffer). All too often, studies that examine violence view protective factors as simply the flip side of vulnerability. That is, if female gender is a risk factor, then male gender is protective. Therefore, we know little about protective factors independent of risk. In order for prevention programs to enhance resilience, more research is needed to identify protective factors.

Future Directions

In addition to the specific recommendations we provided at the close of the major sections in this chapter, we turn now to highlighting additional recommendations for future research directions that are critical to improving TDV-related policy and practice.

Single Victimization Versus Repeat Victimization

Many studies on current adult symptomatology or level of functioning ask participants to retrospectively recount their experiences of childhood victimization, often defined as before age 18 (e.g., Masho & Ahmed, 2007). Studies also often define revictimization as at least one incident of childhood abuse (before age 18) and at least one incident of victimization in adulthood (after age 18; e.g., Kimerling et al., 2007). Both of these approaches completely exclude adolescence as a distinct category. This perspective continues even as recent findings suggest that victimization in adolescence is the crucial link between childhood victimization and increased risk for adulthood victimization (Arata, 2002; Gidycz et al., 1995; Smith et al., 2003). Victimization in early adolescence has also been shown to place individuals at increased risk for additional victimizations at a later time (e.g., Humphrey & White, 2000; Smith et al., 2003). To date, we know little about specific aspects of revictimization in adolescence.

Similarly, much of the past research has focused on identifying risk factors for experiencing victimization broadly defined. Many researchers on TDV do not measure or distinguish between singly victimization and multiple victimization. One of the few exceptions is a study conducted by Young and Furman (2008). They found that more sexual experience and higher levels of demonstrated sensitivity to rejection were risk factors for both single and repeat victimizations. To date, we are aware of no studies that have identified risk factors for single versus multiple victimizations in adolescence.

Part of the reason for the paucity of research on this topic may be due to the fact that we do not clearly understand whether revictimization represents a distinct phenomenon. In other words, are there different characteristics or risk factors for individuals who experience a single victimization versus individuals who experience multiple victimizations? Understanding the trajectory of dating violence throughout childhood and adolescence as well as any distinctions between single versus multiple victimizations may be crucial steps in preventing additional victimizations.

TDV Versus IPV in Adulthood

Given the persistence of dating violence exposure from adolescence to adulthood, more efforts should be made to design studies that are methodologically similar in adolescent and adulthood samples so that findings within these age groups can be more readily compared. This is especially important in the absence of longitudinal studies that can follow individuals over long periods of time, such as from adolescence to adulthood. Currently, several differences in the research design and methodologies stand out when comparing adolescent studies of dating violence and adulthood studies of dating violence. One difference is that adolescent studies often utilize schools as a source of recruitment while this source of recruitment is clearly not utilized in adult samples. Thus, adolescents who are assessed may not fully represent the population, but rather encompass a much narrower portion of the population that might not readily translate to findings on IPV in adulthood. Another important difference between studies in adolescence versus adulthood is that studies with adolescents have rarely included data from both partners in the relationship but have instead relied on the report of individuals. Thus, within the adolescent literature, important information related to the prevalence of mutual aggression or reporting biases from one partner versus another (i.e., victims versus perpetrators) are sometimes very difficult, if not impossible, to estimate. Such estimates in adolescence should be viewed as critical given that some level of mutual aggression often characterizes relationships and has important outcomes for both victims and perpetrators as demonstrated in adulthood. Even within a given adolescent community like a school, rates of perpetration and victimization do not as easily "match up" as they might in adulthood studies where relationships might be defined by households, living arrangements, or other indicators, like marriage or engagement, that are more present in adult relationships.

Health-related consequences of TDV may also differ in important ways from health-related consequences of adult IPV. A large scale study by Masho and Ahmed (2007) found that victimization by TDV was associated with worse mental health outcomes than adult IPV. Specifically, women who reported sexual assault in their adolescent years also reported higher levels of PTSD than women who reported sexual assault only in their adulthood years. Masho and Ahmed (2007) did not control for subsequent victimizations in adulthood, so the individuals who reported sexual assault in adolescence may be at higher risk for PTSD because that earlier victimization led to many other subsequent victimizations, not necessarily because it occurred in the context of adolescence. Given the paucity of longitudinal research or research that specifically compares adolescent versus adult victims, these findings need to be interpreted with caution until further replicated. Masho and Ahmed's (2007) study does demonstrate, though, that researchers should systematically present what the results may look like when controlling for earlier or subsequent victimizations.

Summary and Conclusion

Based on the research to date, TDV poses a serious public health issue. TDV affects a large number of adolescents. Though males and females endorse similar rates of TDV when defined broadly, female victims report more severe levels of TDV and suffer more serious consequences. The existing body of research on TDV clearly illustrates that TDV cannot be reduced to a single-risk model. Instead, risk factors need to be viewed through an ecological model at the individual, relationship, and societal levels; factors across and within levels influence each other in additive and interactive ways to increase or ameliorate risk for TDV. Importantly, even while we continue to gain a better understanding of the interaction between risk factors, many of the mechanisms that underlie these interactions remain poorly understood (see DePrince et al., 2009 for related discussions). With the important advances in research design and statistical tools, we need to continue asking more nuanced research questions. A better understanding of gender and racial/ethnic differences along with identifying subgroups of adolescents who may be particularly vulnerable to TDV will help to address some of the unanswered questions. In turn, researchers, clinicians, and policy makers must work together to provide comprehensive and collaborative services in both the prevention and treatment of TDV.

References

Arata, C. M. (2002). Child sexual abuse and sexual revictimization. *Clinical Psychology: Science and Practice, 9*, 135–164.

Arriaga, X. B., & Foshee, V. A. (2004). Adolescent dating violence: Do adolescents follow in their friends', or their parents', footsteps? *Journal of Interpersonal Violence, 19*, 162–184.

Banyard, V. L., & Cross, C. (2008). Consequences of teen dating violence: Understanding intervening variables in ecological context. *Violence and Victims, 14*, 998–1013.

Basile, K. C., Chen, J., Lynberg, M. C., & Saltzman, L. E. (2007). Prevalence and characteristics of sexual violence victimization among U.S. adults, 2001–2003. *Violence and Victims, 22*, 437–448.

Bronfenbrenner, U. (1979). Contexts of child rearing: problems and prospects. *American Psychologist, 34*(10), 844–850. doi:10.1037/0003-066X.34.10.844.

Centers for Disease Control and Prevention. (2011). *Youth Risk Behavior Survey.* Retrieved from Centers for Disease Control and Prevention website: http://www.cdc.gov/healthyyouth/yrbs/questionnaire_rationale.htm

Chapple, C. L. (2003). Examining intergenerational violence: Violent role modeling or weak parental controls? *Violence and Victims, 18*, 143–162.

Chu, A. T., Pineda, A. S., DePrince, A. P., & Freyd, J. J. (2011). Vulnerability and protective factors for child abuse and maltreatment. In J. W. White, M. P. Koss, & A. E. Kazdin (Eds.), *Violence against women and children* (Mapping the terrain, Vol. 1, pp. 55–75). Washington, DC: American Psychological Association.

Coker, A. L., McKeon, R. E., Sanderson, M., Davis, K. E., Values, R. F., & Huber, E. S. (2000). Severe dating violence and quality of life among South Carolina high school students. *American Journal of Preventive Medicine, 19*, 220–227.

Connolly, J., Friedlander, L., Pepler, D., Craig, W., & Laporte, L. (2010). The ecology of adolescent dating aggression: Attitudes, relationships, media use, and socio-demographic risk factors. *Journal of Aggression, Maltreatment and Trauma, 19*, 469–491.

Coulton, C. J., Crampton, D. S., Irwin, M., Spilsbury, J. C., & Korbin, J. E. (2007). How neighborhoods influence child maltreatment: A review of the literature and alternative pathways. *Child Abuse & Neglect, 31*, 1117–1142.

DePrince, A. P. (2005). Social cognition and revictimization risk. *Journal of Trauma & Dissociation, 6*, 125–141.

DePrince, A. P., Combs, M. D., & Shanahan, M. (2009). Automatic relationship-harm associations and interpersonal trauma involving close others. *Psychology of Women Quarterly, 33*, 163–171.

Elliot, D. S., & Menard, S. (1996). Delinquent friends and delinquent behavior: Temporal and developmental patterns. In J. D. Hawkins (Ed.), *Delinquency and crime: Current theories* (pp. 28–67). New York: Cambridge University Press.

Erikson, E. H. (1968). *Identity: Youth and crisis.* New York: Norton.

Field, C. A., & Caetano, R. (2004). Ethnic differences in intimate partner violence in the U.S. general population: The role of alcohol use and socioeconomic status. *Trauma, Violence & Abuse, 5*(4), 303–317.

Foshee, V. A., Bauman, K. E., Arriaga, X. B., Helms, R. W., Koch, G. G., & Linder, G. (1998). An evaluation of safe dates, an adolescent dating violence prevention program. *American Journal of Public Health, 88*, 45–50.

Foshee, V. A., Bauman, K. E., Ennett, S. T., Linder, G., Benefield, T., & Suchindran, C. (2004). Assessing the long-term effects of the safe dates program and a booster in preventing and reducing adolescent dating violence victimization and perpetration. *American Journal of Public Health, 94*, 619–624.

Foshee, V. A., Bauman, K. E., Linder, F., Rice, J., & Wilcher, R. (2007). Typologies of adolescent dating violence: Identifying typologies of adolescent dating violence perpetration. *Journal of Interpersonal Violence, 22*(5), 498–519. doi:10.1177/08862605 06298829.

Foshee, V. A., Benefield, T., Suchindran, C., Ennett, S. T., Bauman, K. E., Karriker-Jaffe, K. J., et al. (2009). The development of four types of adolescent dating abuse and selected demographic correlates. *Journal of Research on Adolescence, 19*, 380–400.

Foshee, V. A., Ennett, S. T., Bauman, K. E., Benefield, T., & Suchindran, C. (2005). The association between family violence and adolescent dating violence onset: Does it vary by race, socioeconomic status, and family structure? *The Journal of Early Adolescence, 25*, 317–344.

Foshee, V. A., & Matthew, R. A. (2007). Adolescent dating abuse perpetration: A review of findings, methodological limitations, and suggestions for future research. In D. J. Flannery, A. T. Vazsonyi, & I. D. Waldman (Eds.), *The Cambridge handbook of violent behavior and aggression* (pp. 431–449). New York: Cambridge University Press.

Foshee, V. A., Reyes, H. L. M., & Ennett, S. T. (2010). Examination of sex and race differences in longitudinal predictors of the initiation of adolescent dating violence perpetration. *Journal of Aggression, Maltreatment and Trauma, 19*, 492–516.

Gidycz, C. A., Hanson, K., & Layman, M. J. (1995). A prospective analysis of the relationships among sexual assault experiences. *Psychology of Women Quarterly, 19*, 5–29.

Goldstein, A. L., Leslie, B., Wekerle, C., Leung, E., & Erickson, P. (2010). A comparison of young women involved with child welfare and those utilizing street youth services: Implications for the transition from care. *Social Development Issues: Alternative Approaches to Global Human Needs, 32*(3), 16–34.

Gray, H. M., & Foshee, V. (1997). Adolescent dating violence: Differences between one-sided and mutually violent profiles. *Journal of Interpersonal Violence, 12*, 126–141.

Halpern, C. T., Oslak, S. G., Young, M. L., Martin, S. L., & Kupper, L. L. (2001). Partner violence among adolescents in opposite-sex romantic relationships: Findings from the National Longitudinal Study of Adolescent Health. *American Journal of Public Health, 91*, 1679–1685.

Hickman, L. J., Jaycox, L. H., & Aronoff, J. (2004). Dating violence among adolescents: Prevalence, gender distribution, and prevention program effectiveness. *Trauma, Violence & Abuse, 5*, 123–142.

Humphrey, J. A., & White, J. W. (2000). Women's vulnerability to sexual assault from adolescence to young adulthood. *Journal of Adolescent Health, 27*, 419–424.

Jonson-Reid, M., & Bivens, L. (1999). Foster youth and dating violence. *Journal of Interpersonal Violence, 14*, 1249–1262.

Jonson-Reid, M., Scott, L. D., McMillen, J. C., & Edmond, T. (2007). Dating violence among emancipating foster youth. *Children and Youth Services Review, 29*, 557–571.

Kimerling, R., Alvarez, J., Pavao, J., Kaminski, A., & Baumrind, N. (2007). Epidemiology and consequences of women's revictimization. *Women's Health Issues, 17*, 101–106.

Lewis, S. F., & Fremouw, W. (2001). Dating violence: A critical review of the literature. *Clinical Psychology Review, 21*, 105–127.

Maccoby, E. E. (1998). *The two sexes: Growing up apart, coming together*. Cambridge, MA: Belknap Press/Harvard University Press.

Macy, R. J. (2008). A research agenda for sexual revictimization: Priority areas and innovative statistical methods. *Violence Against Women, 14*(10), 1128–1147. doi:10.1177/1077801208322701.

Masho, S. W., & Ahmed, G. A. (2007). Age at sexual assault and post- traumatic stress disorder among women: Prevalence, correlates, and implications for prevention. *Journal of Women's Health, 16*, 262–271.

Muñoz-Rivas, M. J., Graña, J. L., O'Leary, K. D., & González, M. P. (2007). Aggression in adolescent dating relationships: Prevalence, justification, and health consequences. *Journal of Adolescent Health, 40*(4), 298–304.

Noonan, R. K., & Charles, D. (2009). Developing teen dating violence prevention strategies: Formative research with middle school youth. *Violence Against Women, 15*, 1087–1105.

O'Keeffe, M. (1997). Predictors of dating violence among high school students. *Journal of Interpersonal Violence, 12*, 546–568.

Polusny, M. A., Rosenthal, M., Aban, I., & Follette, V. M. (2004). Experiential avoidance as a mediator of the effects of adolescent sexual victimization on negative adult outcomes. *Violence And Victims, 19*(1), 109–120.

Reitzel-Jaffe, D., & Wolfe, D. A. (2001). Predictors of relationship abuse among young men. *Journal of Interpersonal Violence, 16*, 99–115.

Reyes, H. L. M., Foshee, V. A., Bauer, D. J., & Ennett, S. T. (2011). Heavy alcohol use and dating violence perpetration during adolescence: Family, peer, and neighborhood violence as moderators. *Prevention Science: The official Journal of the Society for Prevention Research.* doi:10.1007/s11121-011-0215-8. Advance online publication.

Riggs, D. S., Caulfield, M. B., & Street, A. E. (2000). Risk for domestic violence: Factors associated with perpetration and victimization. *Journal of Clinical Psychology, 56*, 1289–1316.

Rizzo, C. J., Esposito-Smythers, C., Spirito, A., & Thompson, A. (2010). Psychiatric and cognitive functioning in adolescent inpatients with histories of dating violence victimization. *Journal of Aggression, Maltreatment and Trauma, 19*, 565–583.

Saunders, D. G. (2002). Are physical assaults by wives and girlfriends a major social problem? A review of the literature. *Violence Against Women, 8*, 1424–1448.

Schwartz, J. P., Magee, M. M., Griffin, L. D., & Dupuis, C. W. (2004). Effects of a group preventive intervention on risk and protective factors related to dating violence. *Group Dynamics: Theory, Research, and Practice, 8*(3), 221–231.

Silverman, J. G., Raj, A., Mucci, L., Lorelei, A., & Hathaway, J. E. (2001). Dating violence against adolescent girls and associated substance use, unhealthy weight control, sexual risk behavior, pregnancy, and suicidality. *Journal of the American Medical Association, 286*, 572–579.

Smith, P. H., White, J. W., & Holland, L. J. (2003). A longitudinal perspective on dating violence among adolescent and college age women. *American Journal of Public Health, 93*, 1104–1109.

Smokowski, P. R., David-Ferdon, C., & Stroupe, N. (2009). Acculturation and violence in minority adolescents: A review of the empirical literature. *Journal of Primary Prevention, 30*, 215–263.

Spencer, G. A., & Bryant, S. A. (2000). Dating violence: A comparison of rural, suburban, and urban teens. *Journal of Adolescent Health, 27*, 302–305.

Spitzberg, B. H. (1999). An analysis of empirical estimates of sexual aggression victimization and perpetration. *Violence and Victims, 14*, 241–260.

Stark, E. (1990). Rethinking homicide: Violence, race, and the politics of gender. *International Journal of Health Services, 20*, 3–26.

Straus, M. A. (1995). Trends in cultural norms and rates of partner violence: An update to 1992. In S. M. Stich & M. A. Straus (Eds.), *Understanding partner violence: Prevalence, causes, consequences, and solutions* (pp. 30–33). Minneapolis, MN: National Council on Family Relations.

Straus, M. A., Hamby, S. L., Boney-McCoy, S., & Sugarman, D. B. (1996). The Revised Conflict Tactics Scales (CTS2): Development and preliminary psychometric data. *Journal of Family Issues, 17*, 283–316.

Sugarman, D. B., & Hotaling, G. T. (1989). Dating violence: Prevalence, context, and risk markers. In M. A. Pirog-Good & J. E. Stets (Eds.), *Violence in dating relationships: Emerging social issues* (pp. 3–32). New York: Praeger Publishers.

Teten, A. L., Ball, B., Valle, L. A., Noonan, R., & Rosenbluth, B. (2009). Considerations for the definition, measurement, consequences, and prevention of dating violence victimization among adolescent girls. *Journal of Women's Health, 18*, 923–927.

U.S. Department of Justice, Bureau of Justice Statistics. (2008). *National Crime Victimization Survey*. Washington, DC: Author. Retrieved August 9, 2011, from http://bjs.ojp.usdoj.gov/index.cfm?ty=dcdetail&iid=245#Questionnaires

Underwood, M. K., & Rosen, L. H. (2009). Gender, peer relations, and challenges for girlfriends and boyfriends coming together in adolescence. *Psychology of Women Quarterly, 33*, 16–20.

Vézina, J., & Hébert, M. (2007). Risk factors for victimization in romantic relationships of young women: A review of empirical studies and implications for prevention. *Trauma, Violence & Abuse, 8*, 33–66.

Wekerle, C., & Wolfe, D. A. (1999). Dating violence in mid-adolescence: Theory, significance, and emerging prevention initiatives. *Clinical Psychology Review, 19*, 435–456.

Wekerle, C., Wolfe, D. A., Hawkins, D., Pittman, A., Glickman, A., & Lovald, B. E. (2001). Childhood maltreatment, posttraumatic stress symptomatology, and adolescent dating violence: Considering the value of adolescent perceptions of abuse and a trauma mediational model. *Development and Psychopathology, 13*, 847–871.

Whitaker, D. J., Morrison, S., Lindquist, C., Hawkins, S. R., O'Neil, J. A., Nesius, A. M., et al. (2006). A critical review of interventions for the primary prevention of perpetration of partner violence. *Aggression and Violent Behavior, 11*, 151–166.

White, J. W. (2009). A gendered approach to adolescent dating violence: Conceptual and methodological issues. *Psychology of Women Quarterly, 33*, 1–15.

Wolfe, D. A., Crooks, C. C., Chiodo, D., & Jaffe, P. (2009). Child maltreatment, bullying, gender-based harassment, and adolescent dating violence: Making the connections. *Psychology of Women Quarterly, 33*, 21–24.

Wolfe, D. A., Scott, K., Reitzel-Jaffe, D., Wekerle, C., Grasley, C., & Straatman, A. L. (2001). Development and validation of the conflict in adolescent dating relationships inventory. *Psychological Assessment, 13*, 277–293.

Wolfe, D. A., Wekerle, C., Scott, K., Straatman, A., Grasley, C., & Reitzel-Jaffe, D. (2003). Dating violence prevention with at-risk youth: A controlled outcome evaluation. *Journal of Consulting and Clinical Psychology, 71*, 279–291.

Wolitzky-Taylor, K. B., Ruggiero, K. J., Danielson, C., Resnick, H. S., Hanson, R. F., Smith, D. W., et al. (2008). Prevalence and correlates of dating violence in a national sample of adolescents. *Journal of the American Academy of Child and Adolescent Psychiatry, 47*, 755–762.

Yen, C., Ko, C., Yen, J., Tang, T., Chang, Y., & Cheng, C. (2010). Internalizing and externalizing problems in adolescent aggression perpetrators, victims, and perpetrator-victims. *Comprehensive Psychiatry, 51*, 42–48.

Young, B. J., & Furman, W. (2008). Interpersonal factors in the risk for sexual victimization and its recurrence during adolescence. *Journal of Youth and Adolescence, 37*, 297–309.

Part II

Developmental Issues in Adolescent Health Psychology

Continuity of Behavior and Parenting from Childhood Through Adolescence

Carol R. Freedman-Doan and Amanda G. Ellis

Pediatricians see a wide range of behaviors in children as they present themselves for their annual appointments, from shy and fearful to unruly and willful. As these children approach adolescence, many pediatricians may be asked if these behaviors predict involvement with drugs, delinquent behaviors, poor school performance, depression, and/or anxiety disorders. When healthcare providers are asked for advice about how to parent through these difficult adolescent years, they are often at a loss to know what advice to give and how to best structure the discussion with parents. This is notable in light of the results of a recent study that looked at the identification of psychosocial problems in youth during pediatric visits and found that 75 % of pediatric visits included discussion about at least one psychosocial topic with 56.8 % discussing child behavior, 55.1 % child mood, and 65.6 % school problems (Brown, Riley, & Wissow, 2007). This chapter will present a longitudinal study spanning 9 years of data collection that we have conducted looking at how early childhood characteristics and early parenting practices, as well as current relationships and practices impact adolescents' behaviors. From this work, we will highlight what healthcare providers might say to parents who are struggling with their adolescents and turn to them for advice.

The adolescent behaviors we examine here include both internalizing and externalizing behaviors. We are interested in delinquent behaviors (cutting school, destroying property, getting in fights, etc.) and substance abuse, as well as depression, anxiety, and self-esteem problems. We focus on these behaviors because they are the ones that most concern parents and do affect a worrisome number of adolescents. However, in highlighting these behaviors, it is important to recognize that these behaviors do not affect the vast majority of adolescents and that occasional experimentation with alcohol or self-doubt about one's future capabilities do not portend a life of crime and misery. Rather, the majority of adolescents emerge from this period of adjustment relatively unscathed, ready to take on the challenges of work, family, and social relationships. We also want to impress the fact that when problems do arise in adolescents, they generally do not emerge as a result of adolescence per se, but rather are more often a continuation of problems evident during the early childhood years. In a study of 95 parent–child dyads during a routine pediatric visit, more than twice as many parents raised concerns about their child's behavior as had children with actual significant problem behaviors (as measured on a child behavior inventory) (Glascoe, MacLean, & Stone, 1991). Thus, pediatricians are cautioned that parents may report a variety of problem behaviors, but the severity of those problems and the likelihood that those problems will continue into adolescence are often minimal.

C.R. Freedman-Doan (✉) • A.G. Ellis
Department of Psychology, Eastern Michigan University, 341 Science Complex, Ypsilanti, MI 48197, USA
e-mail: cfreedman@emich.edu; afezzey@emich.edu

W.T. O'Donohue et al. (eds.), *Handbook of Adolescent Health Psychology*,
DOI 10.1007/978-1-4614-6633-8_15,

For parenting behaviors, we have examined several key areas that have been correlated, or thought to correlate, with later adolescent outcomes. These include harsh and gentle discipline strategies during childhood, how worried parents are about their children and the level of conflict between them prior to entering adolescence, the quality of the parent–child relationship during adolescence, parents' attempts to monitor their adolescents' behaviors, and parents' actual knowledge about their children's behaviors during adolescence as reported by the adolescents. We, therefore, want to examine how specific parenting behaviors both in childhood and in adolescence influence adolescent outcomes. We are interested in the continuity of these behaviors and relationships across time, as well as their interactions with each other. Where possible, we examine both mothers' and fathers' behaviors, as gender may play a role in how children respond to parenting practices. Similarly, we look at differences in boys' and girls' behaviors on the outcome behaviors because there is consistent evidence that there are significant differences between boys and girls in terms of delinquent behavior, depression, anxiety, and self-esteem.

The Sample

The research presented here utilizes data collected as part of a longitudinal investigation conducted by Eccles and her colleagues (Eccles, Blumenfeld, Harold, & Wigfield, 1990; Eccles, Wigfield, & Blumenfeld, 1984) from 1986 to 1996 called the Childhood and Beyond (CAB) study. The original sample was recruited through ten elementary schools in four school districts in Southeast Michigan. This population was chosen in order to examine the socialization and development of self-perceptions, activity choices, and task values in children in the absence of economic or neighborhood risk. Three cohorts of children, their parents, and teachers were identified and agreed to participate for 4 years in the original research study (Waves 1–4). These children were in kindergarten, first, and third grades at the beginning of the study. After a 4-year hiatus, funding was again secured to continue data collection for 5 more years, beginning when the children were in seventh, eighth, and tenth grades and continuing until each cohort was out of high school (Waves 5–9). Seventy-nine percent of the sample of over 1,100 children who were initially approached about the study agreed to participate ($N=875$) and obtained parental consent to participate in the study when it began in 1986. The sample consisted of 51 % girls and 49 % boys and was 92.2 % Caucasian. Of the parents surveyed in the sample, 91.9 % of the mothers and 97.6 % of the fathers in the sample were married. In addition, 36.9 % of mothers and 49.7% of fathers had attained a level of education at or above a college degree; and 52.5 % of the household in the study had an annual income greater than or equal to $50,000.

The CAB study began with 875 children, their parents, and teachers. A unique feature of this longitudinal study was the inclusion of both mother and father questionnaires in the initial 4 years of data collection (approximately 188 mothers of girls, 183 mothers of boys, 126 fathers of girls, and 125 fathers of boys filled out at least one parent survey at some point during the study). When data collection was resumed in 1994, 63 % of the original sample ($N=511$) agreed to participate. In general, throughout the years of data collection, students filled out surveys in classrooms. Parents were mailed questionnaires and given return envelopes.

The Outcome Measures

The adolescent outcomes were measured when all the subjects were in high school (grades 9, 10, and 12; Wave 7). The outcomes reported here are outlined on Table 1. The means, standard deviations, and reliabilities for the scales used are also reported. Because age is a factor for many of these behaviors [e.g., on average, 12th graders engage in more alcohol use than do 9th and 10th graders (Johnston, O'Malley, Bachman, & Schulenberg, 2011)], we controlled for age in all our analyses. We also report gender differences on these outcome measures and discuss possible explanations for these differences in each section.

Table 1 Descriptives of outcome variables and gender differences

	Mean (SD)	Range	Number of items	Reliability α	f	Significance of age as covariate	Gender main effects	Mean by gender	
								Female	Male
Community problem behavior	2.12 (1.02)	1–7	6	0.82	4.64* (548)	ns	8.52*	2.00 (0.06)	2.26 (0.06)
Alcohol use	2.49 (1.65)	1–7	3	0.81	4.73** (548)	5.86*	3.84ᵗ	2.61 (0.94)	2.34 (0.10)
School problem behavior	1.35 (0.68)	1–7	3	0.74	10.65** (548)	ns	21.28**	1.29 (0.04)	1.49 (0.04)
High-risk problem behavior	2.51 (2.56)	0–12	12	0.75	6.62** (548)	ns	12.62**	2.16 (0.15)	2.93 (0.16)
Sad depression	2.46 (1.20)	1–7	6	0.87	14.39** (547)	ns	28.59**	2.71 (0.07)	2.17 (0.07)
Angry depression	2.68 (1.40)	1–7	3	0.81	0.24^{NS} (548)	ns	ns	2.65 (0.08)	2.73 (0.09)
Anxiety	3.01 (1.09)	1–7	5	0.68	2.44^{NS} (545)	ns	4.54*	3.10 (0.06)	2.90 (0.07)
Self-esteem problems	3.12 (0.51)	1–7	7	0.81	3.67* (543)	ns	6.15*	3.17 (0.03)	3.06 (0.03)

Notes: ns not significant

$^{t}p \leq 0.10$; $*p \leq 0.05$ level; $**p \leq 0.01$

To create the externalizing behavior scales (community problem behavior, school problem behavior, and substance use), a factor analysis was conducted on the 12 items that were created to assess the level that adolescents in the study engaged in problem behaviors (Note: Factor analyses will not be reported here to save space; these analyses can be obtained from the authors). The items asked adolescents to indicate how often in the past 6 months they had engaged in a variety of illegal and risky behaviors. Responses were given on an 8-point Likert-type scale (1 = *never*, 2 = *once*, 3 = *2 to 3 times*, 4 = *4 to 6 times*, 5 = *7 to 10 times*, 6 = *11 to 20 times*, 7 = *21 to 30 times*, and 8 = *31 or more times*). Community problem behavior consisted of the items related to engaging in risky behavior, doing something dangerous for the thrill of it, disobeying parents, damaging property, lying to parents, and having contact with the police. These items involve problem behaviors that adolescents engage in at home and in the community. The alcohol use scale consisted of the items related to getting drunk, drinking alcohol, and skipping school, all items involving alcohol use and behaviors associated with the use of substances (i.e., skipping school in order to use substances). School problem behavior consisted of items related to being suspended from school, fist fighting, and being sent to the principal's office. As can be seen on Table 1, these behaviors were relatively infrequent for this, and there are some gender and age differences in frequency of behavior. Because of the low frequency of these behaviors across the sample, we created a high-risk problem behavior variable that consisted of the number of times an adolescent gave a response on a problem behavior item that fell in the upper quartile for the sample. This item yielded responses from 0 to 12 and further descriptive characteristics for this variable can be found in Table 1.

We also ran a factor analysis on the 9-item depression scale on which adolescents provided responses on a 7-point Likert scale with options ranging from 1 = *almost never* to 7 = *almost always* (derived from the Symptoms Checklist-90; SCL-90-R; Derogatis, Rickesl, & Rock, 1976) and created two subscales: angry depression and sad depression. Angry depression included the items related to feeling so angry that you wanted to smash or break something, feeling like you couldn't control your temper, and feeling as if you wanted to hit or hurt someone, while sad depression included items related to feeling hopeless, not caring anymore, feeling very sad, having thoughts of ending your life, and feeling unhappy. Again, as can be seen on Table 1, there were gender differences in sad, but not angry, depression, and no age differences.

The anxiety scale was comprised of six items that assessed social (e.g., How much do you worry that boys/girls don't like you?) and academic (e.g., How much do you worry about doing badly on tests? How fast does your heart beat when you take a test?) anxiety with responses given on the same 7-point Likert scale used for the depression scale. There were no age but significant gender differences in anxiety symptoms across the sample, with girls reporting higher levels of anxiety than did boys.

Self-esteem was measured using seven items from the Harter self-worth scale (Harter, 1982). This scale consists of seven forced-choice items that range from 1 (very much not like me) to 4 (very much like me). Items assess children's general self-evaluations of the way they do things, feel about themselves, act, and whether they feel like a good person. Higher scores reflect more self-esteem problems. Analyses revealed gender but not age differences on this measure as reported on Table 1.

Continuity of Behaviors from Childhood to Adolescence

Our first question was whether or not there is continuity of behavior patterns from childhood to adolescence. Is that shy child more likely than the more outgoing child to become anxious or depressed in adolescence? Does that difficult, impulsive, aggressive kid end up delinquent or abusing substances in adolescence?

Table 2 Correlations of parents' ratings of childhood behavior with adolescent outcomes

	Externalizing behavior problems in elementary school	Internalizing behavior problems in elementary school	Prosocial behaviors in elementary school
Community problem behavior	ns ns	ns ns	ns ns
Alcohol use	ns 0.23*	ns 0.23*	ns 0.20*
School problem behavior	ns ns	ns ns	ns ns
High-risk problem behavior	ns ns	ns −0.17*	ns ns
Sad depression	ns ns	ns ns	ns ns
Angry depression	ns 0.38***	ns ns	ns ns
Anxiety	ns 0.32**	ns ns	ns ns
Self-esteem problems	ns 0.38***	ns 0.20*	ns −0.33***

Notes: Correlations for girls are on top of each cell; correlations for boys are on the bottom. *ns* not significant
'*$p \leq 0.05$; **$p \leq 0.01$; ***$p \leq 0.001$

To begin to look at this question, we examined the relation between parents' ratings of their child's personality and temperament when they were in elementary school and the adolescent outcomes. The parents of the children in our sample rated their children on 44 personality/temperament items when the sample was in 3rd, 4th, and 6th grades. We combined mothers' and fathers' ratings when available, or used either mother or father ratings if the other were not available. A factor analysis of the 44 items was conducted that yielded seven factors, accounting for about 60 % of the variance: difficult personality (noisy, impulsive, and physically aggressive), prosocial (leader, assertive, outgoing, athletic, competitive), sensitive (shy, nervous), intellectual (persistent, intelligent), artistic (imaginative, creative, curious), caring (affectionate, caring), and relaxed (flexible, laid back). We then constrained the model to three factors: externalizing (difficult), internalizing (sensitive, artistic, caring, and relaxed), and prosocial (prosocial and intellectual). The following table contains the correlations of these three child personality/temperament constructs as reported by parents with the adolescent outcomes (Table 2).

As can be seen, none of the behaviors rated by parents of girls were related to later adolescent behaviors. In contrast, parents who rated their sons as more externalizing (i.e., being more difficult, aggressive, noisy) during childhood as compared to sons who were rated lower on these items had adolescents who indicated they used alcohol more, had more angry depression, had higher levels of anxiety, and had more self-esteem problems. Boys rated as having more internalizing problems (e.g., sensitive, artistic, shy) by their parents were more likely to have fewer high-risk problem behaviors but more self-esteem problems as compared to boys rated with fewer internalizing problems. Finally, boys who were identified as presenting several prosocial behaviors, including being a leader, athletic, and outgoing, were more likely to use alcohol, and have fewer self-esteem problems in adolescence than were boys with fewer prosocial behaviors.

So, when pediatricians experience children in their waiting rooms who are difficult or fearful or outgoing, how these behaviors manifest themselves in adolescence depends on the gender of the child and the kind of problem they are exhibiting. Boys who exhibit more externalizing behaviors may be most vulnerable to problems in adolescence, especially mood problems and alcohol use. Our findings are consistent with others who have found that difficult child temperament measured even as early as six months of age predicted later externalizing behavior problems at age 17 (Olson, Bates, Sandy, & Lanthier, 2000). Although no one has looked at gender differences in continuity of behavior over time, Schonberg and Shaw (2007) looked at the relationship between early temperament (measured at age 2) and later conduct problems (measured at ages 5 and 12) in a group of low-income boys. The researchers found a significant relationship between the measures at age 5, but not age 12. It is interesting to note that boys rated high on externalizing behaviors in childhood reported more internalizing behaviors (depression, anxiety, self-esteem problems) in adolescence. It may be that the externalizing behaviors were a reflection of the boys' negative emotions during childhood, or that the boys developed these internalizing problems in adolescence in response to parental interventions throughout their childhood. This is an area that needs further exploration.

Parenting Practices and Beliefs in Childhood

Does parenting matter? In her second edition 2009 book, *The Nurture Assumption*, Judith Rich Harris challenges the assumption that parenting matters in how a child turns out. Her view is that the countless studies that have demonstrated how various parenting practices and behaviors are correlated with a variety of child outcomes fail to control for genetic influences. Many healthcare providers familiar with Harris' work may counsel parents to not worry so much about what they do as parents and instead watch the child's peer group, which she claims is the most important shaper of the child's behavior. Nevertheless, many researchers have questioned Harris' analyses and find that parent behaviors and practices have a profound impact on children's academic outcomes (Bronstein et al., 1996; Steinberg, Lamborn, Dornbusch, & Darling, 1992), their mental health (Aseltine, Gore, & Colten, 1994; Lewinsohn, Gotlib, & Seeley, 1997; Steinberg, Lamborn, Darling, Mounts, Dornbusch, 1994), and their involvement with delinquency and alcohol use (Barnes, Farrell, & Banerjee, 1994; Baumrind, 1991). In addition, during regular pediatric checkups, parents often report to healthcare providers that they and their child have a lot of conflict and that they are worried about their child's behavior. How realistic are these conflicts and fears? Do they foreshadow some problematic behavior in the future, or should healthcare providers not be concerned?

In our work, we examined parenting strategies from early childhood when the children were in kindergarten, first, and third grades and two groups of strategies emerged: harsh and gentle discipline. Harsh discipline included items that assessed parents' use of threats, criticism/anger, showing disappointment, withdrawal of affection, guilt, and physical punishment to control child behavior. The second factor, labeled gentle discipline, consisted of the items related to the use of explanation/reasoning, praise/affection/kindness, and tangible rewards to control child behavior. Because this construct did not map onto any of the outcomes of interest, we only looked at the harsh parenting strategies. We looked at the correlation of these practices for mothers and fathers with both behaviors reported 3 years later (prosocial, externalizing, internalizing) and the adolescent outcomes for boys and girls separately. As can be seen on Table 3, not surprisingly the harsh parenting practices were more strongly related to childhood temperament than to later adolescent behaviors. Mothers' harsh parenting was related to both boys' and girls' prosocial (negatively related), externalizing, and internalizing problems. Fathers' harsh parenting was related to girls' prosocial and internalizing behaviors and boys' externalizing behaviors. The stronger relationships between mothers' parenting practices and the behaviors may reflect the fact that the mothers in this sample reported being the primary caretakers and disciplinarians of their

Table 3 Correlations of parental practices and beliefs in childhood and adolescent outcomes

	Harsh discipline moms (Wave 1–2)	Harsh discipline dads (Wave 1–2)	Maternal conflicted relationship with child (Wave 4)	Paternal conflicted relationship with child (Wave 4)	Maternal worry about child (Wave 4)	Paternal worry about child (Wave 4)
	($N_{girls} \approx 192$)	($N_{girls} \approx 145$)	($N_{girls} \approx 155$)	($N_{girls} \approx 98$)	($N_{girls} \approx 155$)	($N_{girls} \approx 98$)
	($N_{boys} \approx 157$)	($N_{boys} \approx 127$)	($N_{boys} \approx 144$)	($N_{boys} \approx 102$)	($N_{boys} \approx 144$)	($N_{boys} \approx 102$)
Childhood personality/temperament (Waves 1 and 2)						
Prosocial	−0.19** −0.16**	−0.14* ns	−0.27*** ns	ns −0.22*	−0.30*** −0.21**	−0.23* −0.28**
Externalizing	0.27*** 0.24***	ns 0.18*	0.38*** 0.38***	ns 0.31**	0.48*** 0.39***	0.34** 0.44***
Internalizing	0.21*** 0.19***	0.16* ns	0.23** ns	ns 0.22*	0.21** ns	ns ns
Adolescent behaviors						
Community	ns	ns	ns	ns	0.23**	ns
Problem behavior	ns	0.16'	ns	ns	ns	ns
Alcohol use	ns ns	ns ns	0.20* ns	ns ns	0.24** ns	ns ns
School problem	ns	ns	ns	ns	0.34***	0.22*
Behavior	ns	0.18*	ns	ns	0.18*	0.26**
High risk	ns	ns	ns	ns	0.27***	ns
Problem behavior	ns	ns	ns	ns	ns	ns
Sad depression	ns ns	ns ns	ns ns	ns ns	ns ns	ns ns
Angry depression	ns ns	ns ns	ns 0.17*	0.18* ns	ns 0.18*	0.21* ns
Anxiety	0.1' ns	ns ns	ns ns	ns ns	ns ns	ns ns
Self-esteem	ns	ns	ns	ns	ns	ns
Problems	ns	ns	ns	ns	ns	ns
Grade point	ns	ns	ns	ns	ns	−0.36***
Average	ns	ns	0.18*	ns	ns	−0.29**

Notes: Correlations for girls are on top of each cell; correlations for boys are on the bottom; *ns* not significant
'$p \leq 0.10$; *$p \leq 0.05$ level; **$p \leq 0.01$; ***$p \leq 0.001$

children. Interestingly, although the harsh discipline strategies were related to childhood behaviors, they were related to only a few adolescent problem behaviors. Most notably, fathers' harsh discipline strategies were related to boys' community and school problems in adolescence.

We also examined some negative aspects of the parent–child relationship (worried about child and conflicted relationship). There is some evidence that the history of family conflicts prior to the transition to adolescence is critical in predicting parent–adolescent conflicts (see Collins, 1990; Montemayor, 1986; Paikoff & Brooks-Gunn, 1991). Families that encounter the most problems during the child's adolescence are those that have had the most conflicts prior to the transition period. It was expected, then, that parents' perceptions of conflict with and their degree of concern about their children would relate to adolescent outcomes. As can be seen on Table 3, there are only a few significant relations for conflict and later adolescent outcomes; most notably, conflict between mothers and sons and fathers and daughters during childhood appears to be related to increased levels of angry depression in adolescence. However, parental worry about the child (worried that the child is up to something, worried about the kinds of friends this child has, worried that this child will get into trouble in the coming year, worried that I sometimes don't know where this child is or who he/she is with) is related to a number of outcomes 6 years later. Girls whose mothers reported high levels of worry about them in childhood also reported a number of externalizing problem behaviors in adolescence, including community problems, alcohol use, school behavior problems, and high-risk problem behaviors. Similarly, girls whose fathers worried about them in childhood reported more school behavior problems, and more angry depression than did girls whose fathers were less worried.

Putting together early parenting practices and child behavior, we begin to see a pattern in which harsh parenting practices appear to be related positively to internalizing and externalizing behaviors, and negatively to prosocial behaviors. Four years later, these same behaviors appear to be related to parents' conflicts with their child and their worries (or lack of them) about their behavior. This is especially true of externalizing and prosocial behaviors. Most surprisingly is that to some extent the level of these conflicts and to a greater extent the level of worry parents had when the child was in elementary school were related to several self-reported adolescent behaviors 6 years later, especially the externalizing behaviors for girls (community problem behavior, alcohol use, school problem behavior, and high-risk group), and angry depression.

Pediatricians are often the first health professional parents turn to when concerned about their child's behavior, with over one third of parents raising concerns about the conduct of their child (Glascoe et al., 1991). Nevertheless, in a random sample ($N=719$) of well-child visits, behavioral health issues (i.e., social or learning problems) were discussed 38 % of the time, while mood problems were discussed <1 % of the time (Williams, Burwell, Foy, & Foy, 2006). Given the data presented here, pediatricians are advised to listen to parents' concerns and develop a method of assessing the severity of the problems parents report. More will be said about this later in this chapter.

Parenting in Adolescence

We next looked at the relations of the adolescent outcomes with adolescents' reports of their parents' knowledge and monitoring of their behavior, as well as their relationship with their parents. Parental monitoring was assessed by asking adolescents how often their parents try to find out where they go at night, what they are doing on their free time, and where they are after school (1 = never, 5 = always). The second construct, knowledge, was assessed by asking adolescents how often their parents *actually* know about these three issues (1 = never, 5 = always). Although these two constructs are moderately correlated with each other ($r=0.45$), they each make an independent contribution to the adolescent outcomes.

Table 4 Correlations of parental practices and relationship in adolescence and adolescent outcomes

	Parental monitoring of adolescent behavior (Wave 6) ($N_{girls} \approx 284$) ($N_{boys} \approx 232$)	Parental knowledge of adolescent behavior (Wave 6) ($N_{girls} \approx 242$) ($N_{boys} \approx 175$)	Adolescent–mother relationship (Wave 6) ($N_{girls} \approx 269$) ($N_{boys} \approx 226$)	Adolescent–father relationship (Wave 6) ($N_{girls} \approx 268$) ($N_{boys} \approx 221$)
Community problem behavior	−0.26*** −0.17**	−0.37*** −0.15*	−0.22*** −0.22***	−0.31*** ns
Alcohol use	−0.30*** −0.23***	−0.33*** −0.17*	−0.15* −0.18**	−0.22*** −0.13ᵗ
School problem behavior	−0.23*** ns	−0.27*** −0.12ᵗ	−0.18** −0.15*	−0.18** ns
High-risk problem behavior	−0.31*** −0.19**	−0.34*** −0.19*	−0.22*** −0.22***	−0.27*** ns
Sad depression	−0.19** ns	−0.23** −0.15*	−0.31*** −0.20**	−0.21*** ns
Angry depression	−0.18** ns	−0.21** ns	−0.23*** −0.22***	−0.20*** −0.15*
Anxiety	ns ns	0.11ᵗ ns	ns ns	ns ns
Self-esteem problems	−0.13* −0.16*	−0.24*** −0.32***	−0.18** ns	−0.16** −0.26***

Notes: Correlations for girls are on top of each cell; correlations for boys are on the bottom; *ns* not significant
ᵗ$p \leq 0.10$; *$p \leq 0.05$ level; **$p \leq 0.01$; ***$p \leq 0.001$

As can be seen on Table 4, for girls, perceived parental monitoring was negatively related to all of the externalizing behaviors, along with lower levels of both sad and angry depression, and fewer self-esteem problems. For boys, parental monitoring was related to most of the externalizing behaviors and fewer self-esteem problems. Similarly, actual knowledge of behavior is related to all the relevant outcomes, including reported anxiety for girls. For boys, knowledge is related to all of the externalizing behaviors to some extent, but less so to depression and anxiety. Nevertheless, knowledge is significantly related to fewer self-esteem problems for boys. It may be that monitoring one's adolescent certainly curtails a variety of externalizing behaviors, and it reassures the adolescent that their parents are concerned about and protective of their well-being.

We next focused our attention on the quality of the relationship between the parent and child during adolescence. We asked adolescents how much they want to be like their moms/dads, how much they like being with their mom/dad, how much they respect their mom/dad, and how close they feel towards their mom/dad. As can be seen on Table 4, for girls, the quality of their relationship with their parents appears to be an important factor related to their behavior. Girls who report close, positive relationships with their mothers and fathers also report lower levels of externalizing problem behavior, lower levels of both sad and angry depression, and fewer self-esteem problems as compared to girls who report less positive relationships. For boys, the picture is a bit more complex. Their relationship with their mothers appears related to all the externalizing behaviors and angry and sad depression, but not to self-esteem. Boys' relationships with their fathers are related to more angry depression and self-esteem problems.

Putting the Data Together

What, then, can we say about how much parenting behaviors and the parent–adolescent relationship have on adolescent outcomes? Kerr, Stattin, Biesecher, and Ferrer-Wreder (2003) suggest that the typical unidirectional view of parenting behaviors affecting adolescent outcomes should be replaced with a bidirectional model in which child characteristics and experiences of the parents prompt certain parenting behaviors. They also propose that attachment theory provides a better model for understanding the effectiveness of parental rules and expectations on adolescent outcomes than does looking at specific parenting behaviors. Specifically, Kerr et al. suggest that parental warmth and closeness (attachment) create positive feelings in the children. These feelings, in turn, make children more likely to disclose information about themselves and their behaviors, leading to increased parental knowledge and trust. Monitoring the adolescent's behavior, then, becomes an interactive process built on a foundation of mutual warmth, affection, and trust. Stattin and Kerr (2000) found that reduced adolescent problem behavior was not due to parents' efforts to monitor their child's behavior, but rather because they were highly knowledgeable about their children's activities. Parents become knowledgeable through soliciting information from the children themselves or others in the environment, controlling their adolescent's behavior by requiring permission before going out, and through adolescent spontaneous disclosure.

Does this mean parents' attempts to control and/or monitor their children are unnecessary in preventing them from getting involved in risky behavior, as long as the parent–child relationship is warm and close? Not really, say Fletcher, Steinberg, and Williams-Wheeler (2004). Although parental warmth and child disclosure are highly correlated (Trost, 2000), parental warmth and parental monitoring and knowledge are only moderately correlated, and each make a unique contribution to both internalizing and externalizing behaviors. In addition, Fletcher et al. (2004) found that although the effects of warmth are mediated by parental knowledge in predicting both substance use and delinquency (Stattin and Kerr hypothesis), parental control and to some extent parental monitoring have both direct and indirect effects on these outcomes.

Mediation Effects

In our own research, we looked at both the mediating and moderating effects of parenting behaviors on the adolescent outcomes for mothers and fathers and boys and girls separately. In terms of mediation, first it should be noted that we did find significant modest relationships between parental monitoring and knowledge and both maternal and paternal/adolescent affective relationships (correlations between 0.25 and 0.29). Thus, we were able to conduct the regression analyses entering the maternal or paternal affective relationship first, followed by the parenting behaviors knowledge and monitoring (two regressions for each outcome). We found that parental monitoring for both parents, and also parental knowledge for mothers, mediated the relation between the parent–adolescent relationship and all four externalizing behaviors (community problems, alcohol use, school behavior problems, high-risk group). That is, the parent–child relationship was only indirectly related to the externalizing behaviors as it relates to parental monitoring and to some extent knowledge. Warmer mothers, it seems, tend to monitor their children's behaviors more, and are more knowledgeable (actually know) about their children's whereabouts. This monitoring, in turn, tends to lower rates of problem behavior. A model for these relationships is illustrated below (Fig. 1).

For the internalizing behaviors, specifically sad and angry depression and self-esteem problems, the relation between parental knowledge and monitoring and these outcome variables was mediated by the parent–adolescent affective relationship (see Fig. 2). Thus, it appears that an increase in parental monitoring of the adolescent's behavior and knowledge about his/her whereabouts increases the warmth the child feels towards his/her parent that then, in turn, leads to lower levels of depression and higher self-esteem. It may be that adolescents who are monitored feel that their parents are concerned about them and, therefore, they feel better about themselves and feel less depressed. It should be noted that these relations are stronger for girls, but that, in

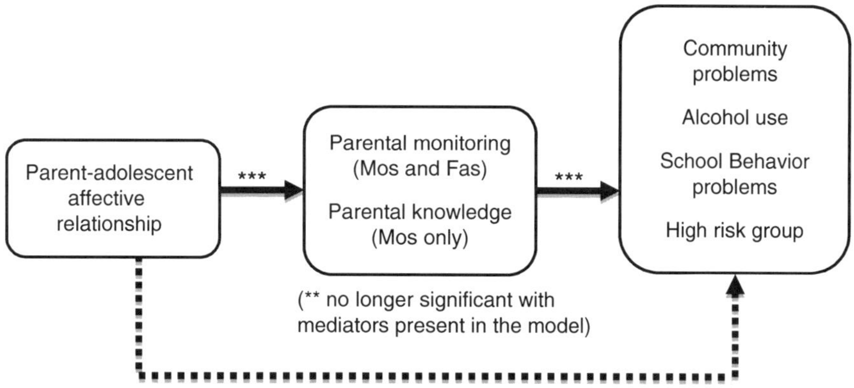

Fig. 1 Relation of parent–adolescent relationship, parental knowledge, and parental monitoring and externalizing adolescent outcomes

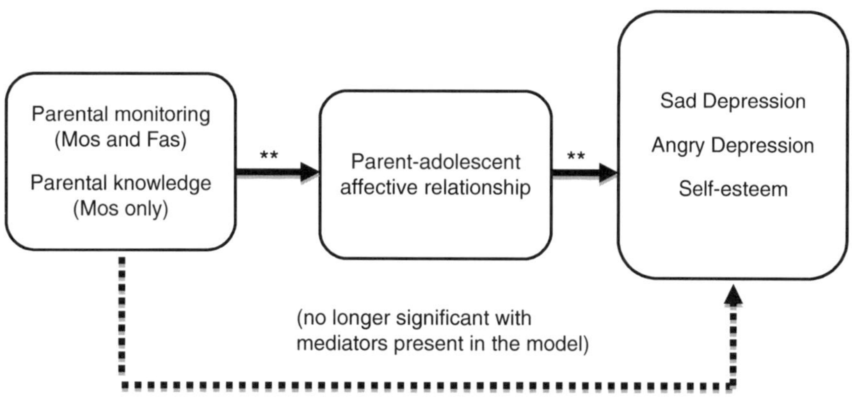

Fig. 2 Relation of parent–adolescent relationship, parental knowledge, and parental monitoring and internalizing adolescent outcomes

general, the amount of variance accounted for in predicting these outcomes is considerably less (range of adjusted R^2 for three internalizing outcomes = 0.03–0.13) as compared to the outcomes for the externalizing behaviors (range of adjusted R^2 for four externalizing outcomes = 0.13–0.23). It may be that parenting behaviors and the affective relationship only have a marginal effect on internalizing behaviors. Certainly it is the case that parenting behaviors and the affective relationship have little impact on adolescents' reported anxiety, as none of the predictors had a significant relation with this outcome.

Moderation Effects

To look at moderation, we first centered the parenting variables (parental monitoring and parental knowledge), as well as the two relationship variables (maternal–adolescent relationship and paternal–adolescent relationship), and computed

Table 5 Moderation effects of parental monitoring and knowledge with parent–adolescent relationship for GIRLS on adolescent outcomes

	Adjusted R squared (significance of change with interaction term)	Standardized beta coefficients
Community problem behavior	0.09*	
Parental monitoring		−0.19**
Maternal relationship		−0.19**
Monitoring × relationship		0.14*
School problem behavior	0.09**	
Parental monitoring		−0.18**
Maternal relationship		−0.16*
Monitoring × relationship		0.18**
High-risk group	0.12*	
Parental monitoring		−0.24***
Maternal relationship		−0.18**
Monitoring × relationship		0.14*
Anxiety	0.01*	
Parental monitoring		0.05^{ns}
Maternal relationship		-0.02^{ns}
Monitoring × relationship		−0.14*
Community problem behavior		
Parental knowledge	0.24***	−0.27***
Paternal relationship		−0.28***
Knowledge × relationship		0.23***
Alcohol use	0.13*	
Parental knowledge		−0.26***
Paternal relationship		−0.17*
Knowledge × relationship		0.13*
High-risk group	0.19**	
Parental knowledge		−0.26***
Paternal relationship		−0.25***
Knowledge × relationship		0.18**

*$p \leq 0.05$ level; **$p \leq 0.01$; ***$p \leq 0.001$

the interaction terms (as outlined by Holmbeck, 2002). We then looked at which interaction terms were related to the outcome variables for boys and girls separately. For the girls, the interaction of monitoring and the mother–daughter relationship was positively related to community problem behavior, school problem behavior, and high risk, and negatively related to anxiety. For dads of girls, although the interaction of parental monitoring and the father–daughter relationship was not related to any outcomes, the interaction of parental knowledge and the paternal–adolescent relationship was significantly related positively to community problem behaviors, alcohol use, and high risk. For boys, the only significant interaction was parental monitoring and the maternal–adolescent relationship negatively predicting anxiety. Following the procedures outlined by Holmbeck (2002), we next entered all centered main effects and interaction terms into simple regression equations for all the significant correlations of the interaction terms. Table 5 provides the adjusted R squares for these regression models, as well as the beta weights for the main and interaction effects.

To understand these interaction effects better, we have created figures to represent some of the stronger relationships using the methods outlined

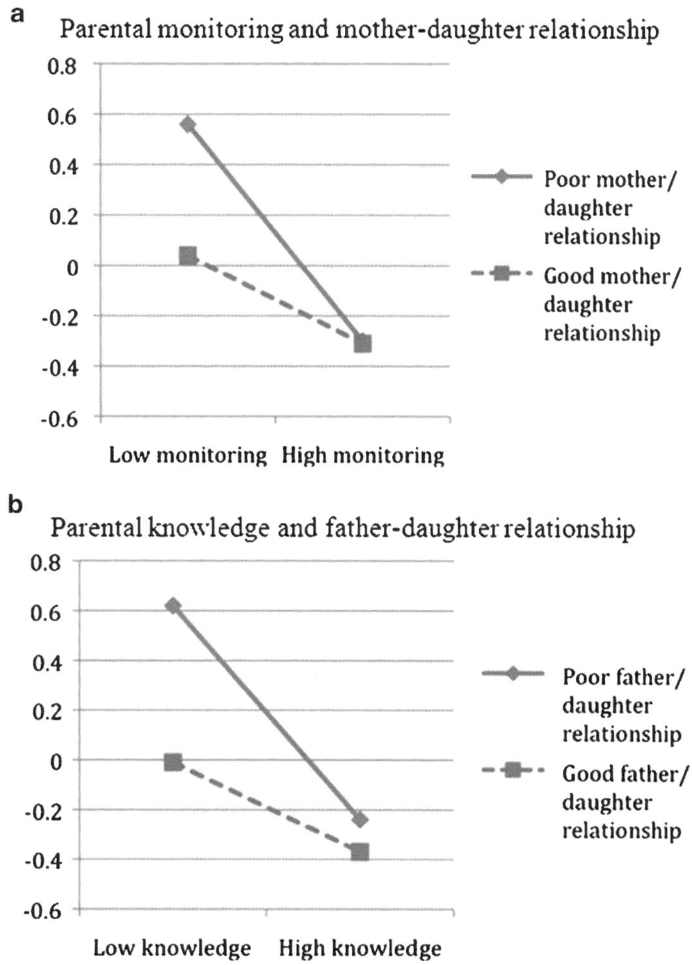

Fig. 3 Interaction effects of parental relationship on parental behavior in predicting. *High-risk problem behavior* for GIRLS (two examples). (**a**) Parental monitoring and mother–daughter relationship. (**b**) Parental knowledge and father–daughter relationship

by Holmbeck (2002) in which we looked at the regression lines for the interaction effects for values 1 standard deviation above and below the mean of each centered variable. The first figure (Fig. 3a) shows the interaction effect of the mother–daughter relationship on parental monitoring in predicting high-risk behavior problems. This is the number of times an adolescent gave a response on a problem behavior item that fell in the upper quartile for the sample. As can be seen, having a positive and warm mother–daughter relationship appears to keep high-risk problem behaviors relatively low. However, when the mother–daughter relationship is problematic, monitoring becomes crucial in keeping daughters safe from risky behaviors, lying, and involvement with the police. A similar pattern is seen for fathers (Fig. 3b), with the father–daughter relationship important in its interaction with parental knowledge in predicting high-risk behaviors. Why the interaction of monitoring and the parent–daughter relationship is important for mothers and knowledge and parent–daughter relationship is important for fathers is not clear. It may be that mothers do the bulk of the monitoring of girls' behaviors—who they are with, when they will be home, etc.—and so their efforts are modified through their relationship with their daughters. Fathers, in contrast, who are less involved with the details of their daughters' comings and goings, must rely on the strength of their relationship with their daughters to actually know what they are doing and whom they are with. This is in keeping with the Kerr and Stattin model

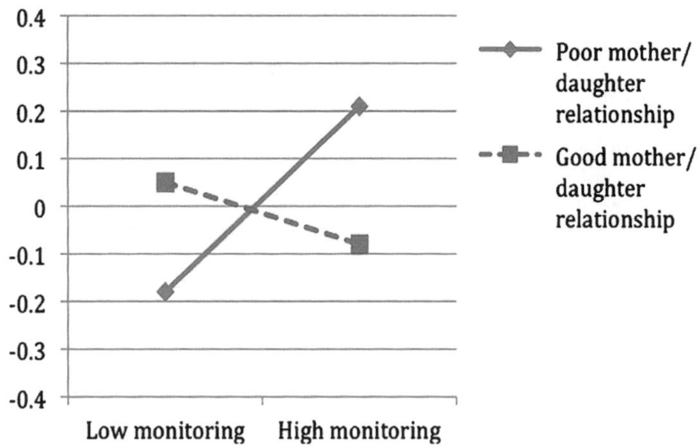

Fig. 4 Interaction effect of parental monitoring and mother–daughter relationship in predicting. *Anxiety* for GIRLS

presented above, in which there is an interactive process between the relationship and parental attempts to monitor behavior.

One other interaction is interesting to note. For mothers of girls, there was a significant positive interaction for monitoring and mother–daughter relationship in anxiety. The figure below illustrates this relationship. As can be seen, monitoring has little effect on girls' anxiety when the mother–daughter relationship is good. However, when the relationship is poor, low monitoring has a negative impact on their anxiety (lower anxiety), while high monitoring has a positive impact (higher anxiety). It should be noted that this model had a small effect size (see Table 5), but the interaction is interesting in that it demonstrates how the quality of the parent–child relationship might influence internalizing problems. It may be that adolescent girls interpret high monitoring as a sign of distrust or that the world is an unsafe place when the mother–daughter relationship is poor, but not when there is a good relationship (Fig. 4).

Parenting Advice from the Pediatrician

The data here present a complex picture of how childhood behaviors and parenting practices both in childhood and in adolescence influence adolescent outcomes. There is some continuity in behaviors over time, especially for boys. There is also some continuity in the impact of parenting practices and beliefs during childhood on childhood temperament and adolescent behaviors. Certainly the effects of conflict between parents and children, as well as parents' concerns about their children's behaviors, foreshadow a host of problematic behaviors. And, certainly, parenting behaviors during adolescence itself have an impact on adolescent behaviors, though how those behaviors work together differs depending on the gender of the child, the gender of the parent, and the particular behavior. Of note is the fact that the parent–adolescent relationship and the parenting practices (monitoring and knowledge) work in concert, sometimes mediating and sometimes moderating each other, in affecting adolescent behaviors.

What, then, can pediatricians do or say to parents concerned about what their preteen might be like in adolescence or how to parent their child now that they are an adolescent? Pediatricians have an advantage over mental healthcare providers who are often called into a problematic situation long after a pattern of difficult temperament interacting with harsh parenting and conflict have formed into problematic child behavior. These doctors are able to see problem behaviors—both in the child and in the parent—take shape early in the child's life. They can assess, advise, refer, and reassure as the situation warrants. Integrated primary care combines medical and behavioral health services to address the full spectrum of problems individuals bring to their medical providers (Blount, 1998). Such services offer pediatricians a means of assessing problematic behavior in their patients and then referring them to appropriate psychological treatment, if applicable. Blount (1998) suggests that pediatricians should not be expected to bear the responsibility of their patients' psychological problems alone and recommends that pediatricians use an integrated primary care framework which would include in-house behavioral health services.

The issue then becomes the following—how can pediatricians and other healthcare providers accurately screen for psychological problems in their patients? This can present a problem for many healthcare providers and questions can arise about the utility of psychological screening tools and how they can be used in their practice. Brown and Wissow (2010) took on the task of demonstrating the utility of the Strengths and Difficulties Questionnaire (a parent-report questionnaire designed for parents to report on their child's mental health symptoms and impairment) in identifying mental health problems in a sample of 767 child patients ages 5–16 above and beyond the assessment of a primary care provider (PCP). They had each child's parent fill out the screening questionnaire and then had each child's PCP identify whether or not they believed the child demonstrated symptoms of a mental health problem. Results indicated that the screening instrument identified 28 % more patients with high symptoms and twice as many patients with moderate symptoms, compared to PCP ratings. This work supports the routine use of a child mental health screening instrument at the child's primary care appointments in order to increase the identification of mental health problems and to aid healthcare providers in knowing when to make a behavioral referral. Given the results of our research, such mental health screening tools are likely to be helpful across the span of childhood and adolescents.

Besides screening for psychological problems, healthcare providers can be important informants for mental health workers about the parenting practices and behaviors they observe over the years. Do the parents appear appropriately warm and responsive to their child's behaviors? Are aggressive, acting out behaviors dealt with effectively without resorting to harsh parenting tactics? Do parents monitor their adolescent's behaviors—who they are with, where they go, etc.? Asking parents about how they get along with their child, what concerns they have about their child's behaviors, and what strategies they use to get their child/adolescent to comply with their expectations should be part of the routine pediatric visit. Detecting problems early and providing parents with resources to learn more effective parenting strategies can lead to positive adolescent outcomes. Through awareness of the parenting behaviors that lead to problematic adolescent behavior and partnering with mental health providers in primary care settings, pediatricians can be active participants in helping prevent problems during the adolescent years.

References

Aseltine, R., Gore, S., & Colten, M. (1994). Depression and the social developmental context of adolescence. *Journal of Personality and Social Psychology, 67*, 252–263.

Bandura, A. (1977). *Social learning theory*. Englewood Cliffs, NJ: Prentice-Hall.

Barnes, G., Farrell, M., & Banerjee, S. (1994). Family influences on alcohol abuse and other problem behaviors among black and white adolescents in a general population sample. *Journal of Research on Adolescence, 4*, 183–201.

Baumrind, D. (1991). The influence of parenting style on adolescent competence and substance use. *Journal of Early Adolescence, 11*, 56–95.

Blount, A. (Ed.). (1998). *Integrated primary care: The future of medical and mental health collaboration*. New York: W.W. Norton.

Bronstein, P., Duncan, P., D'Ari, A., Pieniadz, J., Fitzgerald, M., Abrams, C., et al. (1996). Family and parenting behaviors predicting middle school adjustment: A longitudinal study. *Family Relations, 45*, 415–426.

Brown, J. D., Riley, A. W., & Wissow, L. S. (2007). Identification of youth psychosocial problems during pediatric primary care visits. *Administration and Policy in Mental Health and Mental Health Services Research, 34*(3), 269–281.

Brown, J. D., & Wissow, L. S. (2010). Screening to identify mental health problems in pediatric primary care: Considerations for practice. *International Journal of Psychiatry in Medicine, 40*, 1–19.

Collins, W. A. (1990). Parent–child relationships I the transition to adolescence: Continuity and change in interaction, affect, and cognition. In R. Montemayor, G. Adams, & T. Gullotta (Eds.), *Advances in adolescent development: From childhood to adolescence: A transitional period?* (Vol. 2, pp. 85–106). Newbury Park, CA: Sage.

Derogatis, L. R., Rickesl, K., & Rock, A. F. (1976). The SCL-90 and the MMPI: A step in the validation of a new self-report scale. *The British Journal of Psychiatry, 128*, 280–289.

Eccles, J., Blumenfeld, P., Harold, R., & Wigfield, A. (1990). Ontogeny of self and task concepts and activity choice. (Grant No. RO1 HD17553-06). Bethesda, MD: National Institute of Child Health and Human Development.

Eccles, J. S., Wigfield, A. L., & Blumenfeld, P. C. (1984). Psychological predictors of competence development. (Grant No. 2 RO1 HD17553-01). Bethesda, MD: National Institute of Child Health and Human Development.

Fletcher, A. C., Steinberg, L., & Williams-Wheeler, M. (2004). Parental influences on adolescent problem behavior: Revisiting Stattin and Kerr. *Child Development, 75*, 781–796.

Freedman-Doan, C. R., Arbreton, A. J., Harold, R. D., & Eccles, J. S. (1993). Looking forward to adolescence: Mothers' and fathers' expectations for affective and behavioral change. *Journal of Early Adolescence, 13*(4), 472–502.

Glascoe, F. P., MacLean, W. E., & Stone, W. L. (1991). The importance of parents' concerns about their child's behavior. *Clinical Pediatrics, 30*, 8–11.

Harris, J. (2009). *The nurture assumption: Why children turn out the way they do*. New York: Free Press.

Harter, S. (1982). The perceived competence scale for children. *Child Development, 53*, 87–97.

Holmbeck, G. N. (2002). Post-hoc probing of significant moderational and meditational effects in studies of pediatric populations. *Journal of Pediatric Psychology, 27*, 87–96.

Johnston, L. D., O'Malley, P. M., Bachman, J. G., & Schulenberg, J. E. (2011). *Monitoring the future national results on adolescent drug use: Overview of key findings, 2010*. Ann Arbor: Institute for Social Research, The University of Michigan.

Kerr, M., Stattin, H., Biesecher, G., & Ferrer-Wreder, L. (2003). Relationships with parents and peers in adolescence. In R. M. Lerner, M. A. Easterbrooks, & J. Mistry (Eds.), *Handbook of psychology: Developmental psychology* (Vol. 6, pp. 395–419). Hoboken, NJ: Wiley.

Lewinsohn, P., Gotlib, I., & Seeley, J. (1997). Depression-related psychosocial variables: Are they specific to depression in adolescents? *Journal of Abnormal Psychology, 106*, 365–375.

Montemayor, R. (1986). Family variation in parent-adolescent storm and stress. *Journal of Adolescent Research, 1*, 15–31.

Olson, S. L., Bates, J. E., Sandy, J. M., & Lanthier, R. (2000). Early developmental precursors of externalizing behavior in middle childhood and adolescence. *Journal of Abnormal Child Psychology, 28*(2), 119–133.

Paikoff, R., & Brooks-Gunn, J. (1991). Do parent–child relationships change during puberty? *Psychological Bulletin, 110*, 47–66.

Schonberg, M. A., & Shaw, D. S. (2007). Risk factors for boys' conduct problems in poor and lower-middle-class neighborhoods. *Journal of Abnormal Child Psychology: An Official Publication of the International Society for Research in Child and Adolescent Psychopathology, 35*(5), 759–772.

Stattin, H., & Kerr, M. (2000). Parental monitoring: A reinterpretations. *Child Development, 71*, 1072–1085.

Steinberg, L., Lamborn, S. D., Darling, N., Mounts, N. S., & Dornbusch, S. M. (1994). Over-time changes in adjustment and competence among adolescents from authoritative, authoritarian, indulgent, and neglectful families. *Child Development, 65*(3), 754–770.

Steinberg, L., Lamborn, S. D., Dornbusch, S. M., & Darling, N. (1992). Impact of parenting practices on adolescent achievement: Authoritative parenting, school involvement, and encouragement to succeed. *Child Development, 63*(5), 1266–1281.

Trost, K. (2000, April). *Parental trust: A neglected concept in parenting research*. Paper presented at the meeting of the Society for Research on Adolescence, Chicago, IL, USA.

Williams, J., Burwell, S., Foy, C. G., & Foy, J. M. (2006). Addressing behavioral health issues during well child visits by pediatric residents. *Clinical Pediatrics, 45*, 734–740.

School Performance in Adolescence

Steven G. Little, Angeleque Akin-Little, and Keryn Lloyd

Adolescence is a time of transition that often involves decreases in academic achievement or perceptions of academic competence (Fredricks & Eccles, 2002; Ryan & Patrick, 2001). For example, Fredricks and Eccles studied beliefs of competence in math and found consistent declines in math ability perceptions across the school years. They speculate that this may be due to young children tending to be overly optimistic with regard to their competence and having less comparative standards with which to judge their competence than adolescents. It is entirely possible that adolescents are more accurate and critical in their assessment of their abilities than are younger children. They also note that elementary school teachers are more likely to use criterion-referenced testing while middle and high school students are faced with a greater range of norm-referenced assessment measures which allows them to become better judges of their ability relative to their peers. Is such a perception accurate however?

If one listened only to public media outlets, one may get the conclusion that the American public education system is broken, students are not learning much, and high school graduates are attaining less than those attending school in previous years. The data do not support that conclusion, however. The National Assessment of Educational Progress (NAEP) is a continuing and nationally representative measure of achievement in various subjects over time (U.S. Department of Education, 2008a). The trends in NEAP performance over the past four decades indicate a steady increasing trend in math performance for 9- and 13-year-olds and a consistent performance across time for 17-year-olds (U.S. Department of Education, 2008b). Results in reading performance were similar with an increasing trend noted for 9-year-olds and consistent performance for 13- and 17-year-olds. It should be noted, however, that the average score for the 2008 sample of students was higher for both reading and math at each age level than in the initial year of data collection (1971 for Reading, 1973 for Math).

School Attendance

To paraphrase Yogi Berra, school success is "90 percent showing up; the other half is mental" (Reeve, 2008, p. 90). In spite of the attempted humor of the remark, there is no question that a lack of consistent school attendance is a serious concern. Lack of consistent attendance in school is a major barrier to academic achievement which can lead to poor mental health (Goldstein, Little, & Akin-Little, 2003;

S.G. Little, Ph.D., B.C.B.A.-D. (✉) • K. Lloyd, B.A.
School of Education, Massey University,
Private Bag 102904, North Shore City, Auckland
0745, New Zealand
e-mail: s.little@massey.ac.nz

A. Akin-Little, Ph.D., B.C.B.A.-D.
68 Nautilus Drive, Gulf Harbour, Auckland
0930, New Zealand
e-mail: aakinlittle@gmail.com

W.T. O'Donohue et al. (eds.), *Handbook of Adolescent Health Psychology*,
DOI 10.1007/978-1-4614-6633-8_16,

Gottfried, 2010). Overall, American students with higher rates of attendance perform better on standardized achievement tests and have lower rates of dropping out of school, are less likely to engage in delinquent or destructive behaviors (Sheldon, 2007), and are more likely to graduate from high school (Gewertz, 2007). To that end, the *No Child Left Behind* legislation (NCLB, 2002) included attendance as one of the criteria in a school's evaluation for adequate yearly progress.

High School Graduation

Maintaining a high percentage of high school graduates is an important part of a nation's economy (Goldstein et al., 2003). Individuals who fail to graduate from high school can have an enduring effect on the economy because they are more likely to be unqualified to perform duties in an increasing technical and service-related economy. Graduation from high school is accomplished by successfully passing specific classes and, in most states, a state exit exam. Nationally, only 78 % of white students, 56 % of African American students, and 52 % of Hispanic students graduate from high school 4 years after they enter 9th grade (Greene, 2009). The states with the worst high school graduation rates are Georgia, which graduated only 54 % of its students in 4 years, Nevada (58 %), and Florida, Arizona, and the District of Columbia (all 59 %) (Greene). Additionally, students in predominantly African American and Latino schools are less likely to earn a high school diploma or equivalent (Goldsmith, 2009). Attendance is a major factor in high school graduation success (Pinkus, 2009) because when children and youth are in school, they have the opportunity to succeed academically, an opportunity not afforded to them when not in attendance. A study by the Consortium on Chicago School Research indicated that 9th-grade grades and attendance are two of the most important indicators of high school graduation (Gewertz, 2007).

Individuals with Disabilities

School performance can be impacted by several factors, including disabilities. Federal legislation has, since the early 1970s, guaranteed the rights of all children and youth in the United States to a "Free Appropriate Public Education" regardless of the presence of any disability. Prior to this time, many children and youth were denied access to education simply because they had a disability. For example, in 1970, US schools educated only one in five children with disabilities, and many states had laws excluding certain students, including children who were deaf, blind, emotionally disturbed, or mentally retarded (U.S. Department of Education, 2007). Current legislation (e.g., IDEA), however, mandates that schools provide appropriate educational opportunities for these children.

The first legislation addressing the rights of the disabled was Section 504 of the Rehabilitation Act of 1973. This law stated that recipients of federal assistance could not discriminate on the basis of a handicap. As all public schools receive federal assistance, the tenets of this law apply to schools. One specific part of Section 504 mandates a "Free Appropriate Public Education" to qualified people with a disability, regardless of the nature or severity of the disability. This was the first use of this term in federal legislation. This law was expanded in 1990 with the passage of the Americans with Disabilities Act (ADA).

Congress enacted the landmark *Education for All Handicapped Children Act* (Public Law 94-142), in 1975. This legislation insured the right to public education for all persons, including the disabled. It included four major provisions: (1) that all children and youth have available to them a free appropriate public education which emphasizes special education and related services designed to meet their unique needs, (2) that the rights of children and youth with disabilities and their parents are protected, (3) that the federal government will assist states and localities to provide for the education of all children and youth with disabilities, and (4) to assess and assure the effectiveness of efforts to educate all children with disabilities.

This law was amended in 1986 (PL 99-457) at which time early intervention services were authorized. At the time of the 1990 reauthorization, the name of the act was changed to the Individuals with Disabilities Education Act (IDEA). Further reauthorizations with modifications occurred in 1997 and 2005. There are 13 disability categories specified in IDEA. They are:

- *Autism*: A developmental disability significantly affecting verbal and nonverbal communication and social interaction, generally evident before age 3
- *Deafness*: A hearing impairment that is so severe that the student is impaired in processing linguistic information through hearing, with or without amplification
- *Deaf-blindness*: Simultaneous hearing and visual impairments
- *Emotional disturbance*: A disability whereby a student of typical intelligence has difficulty, over time and to a marked degree, building satisfactory interpersonal relationships; responds inappropriately behaviorally or emotionally under normal circumstances; demonstrates a pervasive mood of unhappiness; or has a tendency to develop physical symptoms or fears
- *Hearing impairment*: An impairment in hearing, whether permanent or fluctuating, that is not included under deafness
- *Mental retardation*: Significant subaverage general intellectual functioning existing concurrently with deficits in adaptive behavior and manifested during the developmental period
- *Multiple disabilities*: The manifestation of two or more disabilities (e.g., mental retardation-blindness), the combination of which requires special accommodation for maximal learning
- *Orthopedic impairment*: Physical disabilities, including congenital impairments (e.g., club foot), impairments caused by disease (e.g., poliomyelitis), and impairments from other causes (e.g., cerebral palsy)
- *Other health impairment*: Having limited strength, vitality, or alertness due to chronic or acute health problems (e.g., asthma, heart condition, attention-deficit/hyperactivity disorder)
- *Specific learning disability*: A disorder in one or more of the basic psychological processes involved in understanding or in using language, spoken or written, which may manifest itself in an imperfect ability to listen, think, speak, read, write, spell, or do mathematical calculations
- *Speech or language impairment*: A communication disorder such as stuttering, impaired articulation, a language impairment, or a voice impairment
- *Traumatic brain injury*: An acquired injury to the brain caused by an external physical force or by a certain medical condition (e.g., brain tumor) resulting in total or partial functional disability or psychosocial impairment, or both
- *Visual impairment*: A visual difficulty (including both partial sight and blindness) that, even with correction, adversely affects a student's educational performance

Factors Related to School Performance in Adolescence

Self-Regulation

Self-regulation has been defined as an individual's ability to control and regulate his/her own actions, cognitions, and emotions as well as the ability to begin and end activities based on situational demands, and to modulate their behavior in social and educational settings (Bronson, 2000). Self-regulation is believed to develop during adolescence and by the age of 13 or 14, adolescents generally develop the ability to be planful with regard to their short- and long-term goals and thus able to regulate their behavior to increase the likelihood that these goals will be attained (Demetriou, 2000). Research suggests that students who engage in self-regulatory behavior do better in school (Pintrich, 2000) and that students who observe and evaluate their performance accurately can react appropriately by keeping or changing their study strategies to achieve optimal results (Hartman, 2001). Bakracevic Vukman and Licardo (2010) examined the relationship between self-regulation and school achievement. Results indicated that metacognitive self-regulation was found to be an important predictor of school achievement in both primary and secondary school students, with self-regulation explaining 21 % of the variance of school performance their secondary school sample.

The process of self-regulation includes three subprocesses: self-monitoring, self-evaluation, and behavioral adjustment (Singer & Bashir, 1999). The question then arises: can self-regulation skills be improved via directed interventions? Research has consistently demonstrated that direct instruction, modeling, and practice and feedback have all been found effective in teaching students self-monitoring and self-regulation procedures which have subsequently been found to improve both academic performance and classroom behavior (Coleman & Webber, 2002; Zimmerman, 1996).

Social and Emotional Functioning: Depression and Conduct Disorder

Two psychological disorders which can have a major impact on both academic achievement and graduation are depression and conduct disorder. An increase in adjustment problems, such as depression, is not uncommon during adolescent development (Graber, 2004). The rate of depression increases throughout the adolescent years, with a rate of 3.9 % for 12-year-olds, 11.6 % for 16-year-olds, and 10.6 % for 17-year-olds with the rate among girls being three times that for boys (National Institute for Mental Health, 2010). By later adolescence, the prevalence of major depression is very similar to prevalence for adults (Hankin, 2006) with 18–24-years-olds having the highest rate of overall depression of any age group (Centers for Disease Control and Prevention, 2011).

Depression in adolescence has been found to be related to academic performance and high school graduation (Humensky et al., 2010). For example, Wilcox-Gok, Marcotte, Farahati, and Borkoski (2004) found that men who retrospectively recalled onset of depression prior to age 16 were less likely to graduate from high school. Similarly, Fletcher (2008) found that adolescent girls diagnosed with depression were less likely to graduate from high school or enroll in college. In addition, Ding, Lehrer, Rosenquist, and Audrain-McGovern (2009) found that female adolescents with depression had greater decreases in school performance than males.

Humensky and colleagues (2010) examined school performance among adolescents at risk for major depression. Results indicated that the relationship between depressive symptoms and actual school performance was not statistically significant; however, adolescent perception of functioning and school performance was related to depressive symptoms. They found that depressive symptoms affected adolescents' perception of their ability to perform in school, do their homework, concentrate, and engage in other adaptive academic behaviors.

Fröjda et al. (2008) found, in a large sample of Finnish 7th through 9th graders, that when participants reported a lower GPA or when their academic performance had decreased from the previous term, they were more likely to self-report depressive symptoms at a level consistent with moderate to severe depression. A relationship was also found between depression and other factors such as concentration and social relationships. The study concluded that the lower a student's GPA, the higher the likelihood of them being depressed.

Conduct-disordered (CD) youth are at an even greater risk of failure to achieve academically. That is because, by definition, children and adolescents diagnosed with CD are likely to eventually come into contact with the criminal justice system. Virtually every one of the 15 criteria listed in the *DSM-IV* for CD involves a behavior that, if manifested to a sufficient magnitude and chronicity, will eventually lead to arrest and possible incarceration. This generally necessitates dismissal from school or low attendance which can negatively affect both grades and graduation rate. Grisso (1998) reviewed the epidemiological research with regard to the prevalence of childhood mental disorders in delinquent populations and found that CD is the most prevalent diagnosis with a rate probably about 50–60 %.

In terms of prevalence, conduct disorder is diagnosed more frequently in males than females. A study by Keenan, Wroblewski, Hipwell, Loeber, and Stouthamer-Loeber (2010) indicated 2–16 % of boys and 1–9 % of girls may be diagnosed. Age of onset is an additional important consideration. However, presently, data are somewhat sparse regarding developmental patterns particularly for females. Some authors have suggested a need to consider differing criteria for girls in terms of overt versus covert aggression in the diagnosis of CD (Delligatti, Akin-Little, & Little, 2003).

Kazdin (1998) and Sholevar and Sholevar (1995) both discuss the correlation between school-related factors and CD. These factors include attending school where little emphases is placed on academic work, the poor physical condition of the school building(s), infrequent use of teacher praise, low teacher expectancy, and teacher unavailability to deal with students' problems. Given the lack of promise to both scholastic achievement and graduation for students diagnosed with CD (Boden, Fergusson, & Horwood, 2010), all studies emphasize the critical nature of early, wraparound (i.e., inclusion of school and familial environment), efficacious intervention (e.g., Murray & Farrington, 2010).

Finally, Crick and Dodge (1994) present a reformulated social information-processing (SIP) model that can help explain the development of aggressive and antisocial behavior in school-age children. They proposed that children process social information in six steps: (1) encoding cues, (2) interpreting cues, (3) clarifying goals, (4) accessing or constructing responses, (5) deciding on responses, and (6) enacting behaviors. Research has consistently supported links between this model and overt aggressive behavior, particularly in boys (Crick & Dodge, 1996; Dodge et al., 2003). In addition, social rejection, as predicted from this model, has been found to reduce inhibit classroom participation (Ladd, 2008) and increase antisocial behavior (Martens & Witt, 2004).

Obesity

Obesity is usually defined as having a body mass index (BMI) of 30 or greater (Centers for Disease Control and Prevention, 2010). Further the CDC has identified obesity rates in the United States ranging from a low of 18.6 % of the population in Colorado to a high of 34.4 % of the population in Mississippi with African Americans and Hispanics both having a higher rate of obesity than Whites (51 % and 21 % higher, respectively) with similar patterns found in children and adolescents (Ogden, Carroll, Curtin, Lamb, & Flegal, 2010). Sabia (2007) found a consistent negative relationship between BMI and grade point average (GPA) for white adolescent females. In a review of research on the association between obesity and academic performance in school-age children, Taras and Potts-Datema (2005) concluded being overweight or obese was associated with lower academic achievement; however, the directionality of this relationship is not clear.

Studies have shown that there is also a relationship between obesity and low self-esteem and mental health conditions such as anxiety and depression (Zametkin, Zoon, Klein, & Munson, 2004). It is entirely possible that it is these conditions that predispose children and adolescents to both obesity and poor school performance (Datar, Sturm, & Magnabosso, 2004). However, in a study of Korean adolescents, Cho, Lambert, Kim, and Kim (2009) concluded from their data that obesity and poor academic performance are simultaneously determined.

Chronic Illness

Chronic medical conditions are defined as those having debilitating symptoms or which last for more than 3 months a year (Thompson & Gustafson, 1996) and include developmental illnesses (e.g., cerebral palsy) and chronic diseases (e.g., diabetes, epilepsy). About 10.3 million children and adolescents in the United States have chronic medical conditions or illnesses, which involve limitations in cognitive, physical, or psychosocial development (Algozzine & Ysseldyke, 2006; Valletutti, 2004; Walsh & Murphy, 2003). In addition, about 4.4 million children with chronic conditions face problems hindering their participation in school (Kaffenberger, 2006; Thies & McAllister, 2001) which may interfere with their school performance (Nabors, Little, Akin-Little, & Iobst, 2008).

It is not uncommon for factors related to the chronic illness and not the illness itself to contribute to poor academic performance. Smith, Taylor, Newbould, and Keady (2008) suggested that the adverse effects of medication may be related to school performance. Calsbeek, Rijken, Bekkers, Dekker, and van Berge Henegouwen (2006) examined adolescents and young adults with chronic digestive disorders and found a relationship between the disease and academic performance. Their conclusions, however, was that it was depression associated with the disease that led to the academic difficulties and not the disease itself. McNelis, Johnson, Huberty, and Austin (2005) examined the relationship between chronic epilepsy and academic performance. While their results indicated that most students with chronic seizures perform in the average range, teachers rate 25 % as at or below one standard deviation of the mean. Similarly, Nabors and colleagues' (2008) results indicated that relatively few teachers in their survey indicated having high knowledge of chronic illnesses or confidence in working with students with all but the most common chronic illnesses (e.g., asthma). Spilkin and Ballantyne (2007) found that while children with cystinosis, a genetic disorder characterized by the abnormal accumulation of the amino acid cystine, may have real academic limitations related to their disease, teachers do not always recognize this and misattribute it to laziness. Finally, in discussing children with cancer and academic performance, Armstrong and Horn (1995) noted that school performance may be affected by the cancer but the type and severity of the performance deficit is dependent on the type and location of the tumor. Further, cancer treatments (e.g., radiation, chemotherapy) may interfere with a child or adolescent's ability to attend school or result in long-term cognitive deficits (e.g., processing speed) which may affect school performance.

Pregnancy

Approximately 750,000 girls and women age 15–19 become pregnant each year in the United States, with 59 % of these pregnancies resulting in birth (Guttmacher Institute, 2010), a rate nearly twice that of Canada (McKay & Barrett, 2010). Teenage childbearing has been found to have unfavorable outcomes for both mother and child (Meade, Kershaw, & Ickovics, 2008), including lower educational attainment (Coley & Chase-Lansdale, 1998). For example, Jones, Astone, Keyl, Kim, and Alexander (1999) found that teen childbearing reduces the probability of completing high school by 8–10 %.

Trauma

Unfortunately, it is not uncommon for adolescents to be exposed to traumatic events (Little, Akin-Little & Somerville, in press). Children and adolescents may experience a number of different types of trauma. These can include abuse (e.g., sexual, physical), grief, exposure to domestic and community violence, natural disasters, or a combination of the above (Little, Akin-Little, & Gutierrez, 2009). Felitti and colleagues (1998) conducted a retrospective study of over 17,000 adults and found that more than one half of their sample reported experiencing at least one adverse event in childhood with approximately one quarter reporting having experienced two or more.

While not every child exposed to a traumatic event experiences negative outcomes, trauma symptoms are not uncommon and have been categorized into four domains: affective, behavioral, cognitive, and physical (Cohen, Mannarino, &

Deblinger, 2006). Common affective symptoms include fear, depression, anger, and frequent mood changes; behavioral symptoms usually center on avoiding reminders of the trauma; cognitive symptoms usually involve distorted cognitions about themselves, others, the event, or the world (e.g., "the event is my fault"); and physical symptoms include stress related responses such as elevated heart rates and blood pressure, increased muscle tension, and hypervigilance. It has also been found that prolonged exposure to trauma and maltreatment can decrease brain size and functioning (De Bellis et al., 1999). With regard to school performance, few studies exist that directly relate trauma exposure to decreases in school performance. The trauma symptoms described by Cohen and colleagues above all are likely to have an impact on school performance however. In one of the few empirical studies comparing trauma exposure to a no trauma control group, Green et al. (2001) found that a traumatic loss group had higher rates of impaired school performance compared to the no trauma control group. Similarly, in a more recent study from the UK, Abdelnoor and Hollins (2004) found significant underachievement in secondary school performance for adolescents who lost a parent to death.

Bullying

Studies have recognized the relationship between substance use, poor academic achievement, mental health problems, and bullying (Gini & Pozzoli, 2009; Nansel et al., 2001). Bullying can take the form of overt or covert behaviors intended to physically harm or ostracize a particular student (Little, Akin-Little, & Medley, 2011). While fewer schools reported weekly occurrences of student bullying in 2005 than in 2000 (24.5 % and 29.3 %, respectively), in 2005 28 % of students reported having been bullied during the last 6 months (Dinkes, Cataldi, & Lin-Kelly, 2007). Additionally, the last 3–4 years have seen an increase in the occurrence of cyber-bullying. There are reports of 20–40 % of middle and high school students being bullied at least one time online (Stover, 2006). A recent study in Massachusetts indicated that 26.8 % of middle school students and 15.6 % of high school students were categorized as victims of bullying (McKenna, Hawk, Mullen, & Hertz, 2011). While our schools may be relatively safer in terms of the threat of physical harm than public perception, the rate of bullying remains disturbingly high.

Increases in loneliness, lower self-esteem, psychosomatic complaints, depression, suicidal ideations, and suicide have all been reported as characteristic of victims of bullying (Cook, Williams, Guerra, Kim, & Sadek, 2010). In addition, fear of being bullied increases the likelihood of victims dropping out of school (Sharp, 1995). A recent meta-analysis of 33 studies concluded that bullied students are more likely to earn lower grades and score lower on standardized achievement tests than nonbullied students (Nakamoto & Schwartz, 2010). In an even more recent study, Juvonen, Wang, and Espinoza (2011) found robust associations between bully victimization and compromised academic achievement in a longitudinal study of 2,300 middle school students. This effect was noted with both GPA and teacher-rated academic engagement. It appears clear that being the victim of bullying can negatively impact school performance in both children and adolescents.

Schools and Intervention

Schools are the only single location where the educational, emotional, and behavioral needs of children and youth can all be addressed (Adelman & Taylor, 2010; Burns et al., 1995; Paternite, 2005). Schools are located in every community in the United States, and school attendance is mandatory up to the age of 16–18 depending on the state (U.S. Department of Education, 2009). In addition, schools are convenient for families and provide an environment ideally suited for the implementation of a variety of different treatment modalities. Willie Sutton, a bank robber in the 1930s through 1950s, allegedly replied to a reporter's inquiry as to why he robbed banks by saying "because that's where the money is."

This idea has led medical schools to teach their students "Sutton's law" which suggests that when diagnosing illness, physicians should first consider the obvious. "Sutton's law" also applies to meeting the physical and mental health needs of children and adolescents. It is just obvious because "that's where the children are."

In an extensive review of the literature on school-based mental health services for children, Hoagwood and Erwin (1997) found empirical support for three types of interventions: cognitive-behavioral therapy, social skills training, and teacher consultation. Similarly, Durlak and Wells (1997) conducted a meta-analysis of 177 programs designed to prevent behavioral and social problems in children and adolescents. Results indicated that programs involving modifications in the school environment, individual mental health promotion efforts, and providing children help in negotiating stressful transitions produced significant effect sizes ranging from 0.24 to 0.93. They noted that most programs had positive effects in both reducing problem behavior and increasing student social competence.

Anglin, Naylor, and Kaplan (1996) concluded that adolescents with mental health symptoms who were referred to school-based clinics were more likely to receive treatment than students who were referred for services in other settings. Bruns and colleagues (1999) found that personnel in schools with expanded school mental health (ESMH) programs were more likely to refer students with suspected emotional and behavioral problems for services than were individuals in non-ESMH schools (52 % vs. 28 %). Not only do children who receive metal health services in schools show improvements in behavior (e.g., Hall, 2000) and emotional functioning (e.g., Nabors & Reynolds, 2000), they also have shown improvements in academic outcomes (e.g., Jennings, Pearson, & Harris, 2000; Kalafat, Illback, & Sanders, 1997). It is clear then that school-based provision of mental health services is beneficial and not only makes the provision of mental health services more efficient, it makes it more likely that students in these schools will receive the services they need. Clinical, health, and counseling psychologists, in addition to school psychologists, need to recognize the potential of schools in meeting the mental and physical health needs of children and youth including primary, secondary, and tertiary prevention efforts.

Summary

Schools are the one location where virtually all children and youth are present. High school graduation, the culmination of an individual's high school education, is important with regard to the individual's future earnings and the economy of the entire country. School performance (grades) and attendance are the two most critical variables affecting high school graduation. In spite of that, multiple factors can influence school performance in adolescence. These include disability, self-regulation, social and emotional functioning, chronic illness, exposure to trauma, and factors such as obesity, pregnancy, bullying, or a combination of these. This chapter reviewed each of these with respect to their influence on school performance.

The United States Congress recognized the importance of school performance in passing the No Child Left Behind Act of 2001 (2002) (NCLB). This act is based on the belief that setting high standards and establishing measurable goals can improve individual outcomes in education. NCLB increased federal funding for education but in doing so required schools to increase accountability. While parts of NCLB have been controversial (e.g., increased use of norm-referenced assessment of basic skills), some data suggest that reading and math scores are improving (U.S. Department of Education, 2008a, 2008b). It is too early to determine, however, if these improvements are a direct result of NCLB. More recently, the Obama Administration has proposed revisions to NCLB which are designed to (1) improve teacher and principal effectiveness, (2) provide information to families to help them evaluate and improve their children's schools, (3) implement college- and career-ready standards, and (4) improve student learning and achievement in America's lowest-performing schools by providing intensive support and effective interventions (U.S. Department of Education, 2010).

It is clear that school performance is an important variable in the future success of students. Psychologists and other mental health professionals can play a vital and important role in maximizing the potential for all students to succeed in the classroom, graduate from high school, and go on to a productive life.

References

Abdelnoor, A., & Hollins, S. (2004). The effect of childhood bereavement on secondary school performance. *Educational Psychology in Practice, 20*, 43–54. doi: 10.1080/0266736042000180401.

Adelman, H. S., & Taylor, L. (2010). *Mental health in schools: Engaging learners, preventing problems, and improving schools*. Thousand Oaks, CA: Corwin.

Algozzine, B., & Ysseldyke, J. (2006). *Teaching students with medical, physical, and multiple disabilities: A practical guide for every teacher*. Thousand Oaks, CA: Corwin.

Anglin, T. M., Naylor, K. E., & Kaplan, D. W. (1996). Comprehensive school based health care: High school students' use of medical, mental health, and substance services. *Pediatrics, 97*, 318–330.

Armstrong, F. D., & Horn, M. (1995). Educational issues in childhood cancer. *School Psychology Quarterly, 10*, 292–304. doi:10.1037/h0088313.

Bakracevic Vukman, K., & Likardo, M. (2010). How cognitive, metacognitive, motivational, and emotional self-regulation influence school performance in adolescence and early adulthood. *Educational Studies, 36*, 259–268. doi:10.1080/03055690903180376.

Boden, J. M., Fergusson, D. M., & Horwood, L. J. (2010). Risk factors for conduct disorder and oppositional/defiant disorder: Evidence from a New Zealand birth cohort. *Journal of the American Academy of Child & Adolescent Psychiatry, 49*(11), 1125–1133.

Bronson, M. B. (2000). Recognizing and supporting the development of self-regulation in young children. *Young Children, 55*, 32–37.

Bruns, E., Walrath, C., Glass-Siegel, M., Acosta, O., Anderson, K., & Weist, M. (1999). *Outcomes associated with expanded school mental health in Baltimore: The school mental health climate survey*. Baltimore, MD: Baltimore Mental Health Systems, Inc.

Burns, B. J., Costello, E. J., Angold, A., Tweed, D., Stangl, D., Farmer, E. M., et al. (1995). Children's mental health use across service sectors. *Health Affairs, 14*, 411–488.

Calsbeek, H., Rijken, M., Bekkers, M. J. T. M., Dekker, J., & van Berge Henegouwen, G. P. (2006). School and leisure activities in adolescents and young adults with chronic digestive disorders: Impact of burden of disease. *International Journal of Behavioral Medicine, 13*, 121–130. doi:10.1207/s15327558ijbm1302_3.

Centers for Disease Control and Prevention. (2010). State specific obesity prevalence among adults—United States, 2009. *Morbidity and Mortality Weekly Report, 59*(30), 951–955.

Centers for Disease Control and Prevention. (2011). *Current depression among adults in the United States, 2006 and 2008*. Retrieved from Revised_Table_Estimates_for_Depression_MMWR_Erratum_Feb %202011[1].pdf.

Cho, S. H., Lambert, D. M., Kim, H. J., & Kim, S. G. (2009). Overweight Korean adolescents and academic achievement. *Journal of Family and Economic Issues, 30*, 126–136. doi:10.1007/s10834-009-9147-x.

Cohen, J. A., Mannarino, A. P., & Deblinger, E. (2006). *Treating trauma and traumatic grief in children and adolescents*. New York: The Guilford Press.

Coleman, M. C., & Webber, J. (2002). *Emotional and behavioral disorders*. Boston: Pearson.

Coley, R. L., & Chase-Lansdale, P. L. (1998). Adolescent pregnancy and parenthood: Recent evidence and future directions. *American Psychologist, 53*, 152–166. doi:10.1037/0003-066X.53.2.152.

Cook, C. R., Williams, K. R., Guerra, N. G., Kim, T. E., & Sadek, S. (2010). Predictors of bullying and victimization in childhood and adolescence: A meta-analytic investigation. *School Psychology Quarterly, 25*, 65–83. doi:10.1037/a0020149.

Crick, N. R., & Dodge, K. A. (1994). A review and reformulation of social information-processing mechanisms in children's social adjustment. *Psychological Bulletin, 115*, 74–101. doi:10.1037/0033-2909.115.1.74.

Crick, N. R., & Dodge, K. A. (1996). Social information processing mechanisms in reactive and proactive aggression. Child Development 67, 993–1002.

Datar, A., Sturm, R., & Magnabosso, J. L. (2004). Childhood overweight and academic performance: National study of kindergarteners and first-graders. *Obesity Research, 12*, 58–68. doi:10.1038/oby.2004.9.

De Bellis, M. D., Keshavan, M. S., Clark, D. B., Casey, B. J., Giedd, J. N., Boring, A. M., et al. (1999). Developmental traumatology: II. Brain development. *Biological Psychiatry, 45*, 1271–1284.

Delligatti, N., Akin-Little, K. A., & Little, S. G. (2003). Conduct disorder in girls: Diagnostic and intervention issues. *Psychology in the Schools, 40*, 183–192.

Demetriou, A. (2000). Organization and development of self-understanding and self-regulation: Toward a general theory. In M. Boekaerts, P. R. Pintrich, & M. Zeidner (Eds.), *Handbook of self-regulation* (pp. 209–251). New York: Academic.

Ding, W., Lehrer, S., Rosenquist, J. N., & Audrain-McGovern, J. (2009). The impact of poor health on academic performance: New evidence using genetic markers. *Journal of Health Economics, 28*, 578–597. doi:10.1016/j.jhealeco.2008.11.006.

Dinkes, R., Cataldi, E. F., & Lin-Kelly, W. (2007). *Indicators of school crime and safety: 2007* (NCES 2008-021/NCJ 219553). National Center for Education Statistics, Institute of Education Sciences, U.S. Department of Education, and Bureau of Justice. Statistics, Office of Justice Programs, U.S. Department of Justice: Washington, DC.

Dodge, K. A., Lansford, J. E., Burks, V. S., Bates, J. E., Pettit, G. S., Fontaine, R., et al. (2003). Peer rejection and social information-processing factors in the development of aggressive behavior problems in children. *Child Development, 74*, 374–393. doi:10.1111/1467-8624.7402004.

Durlak, J. A., & Wells, A. M. (1997). Primary prevention mental health programs for children and adolescents: A meta-analytic review. *American Journal of Community Psychology, 25*, 115–152. doi:10.1023/A:1024654026646.

Felitti, V. J., Anda, R. F., Nordenberg, D., Williamson, D. F., Spitz, A. M., Edwards, V., et al. (1998). Relationship of childhood abuse and household dysfunction to many of the leading causes of death in adults. The Adverse Childhood Experiences (ACE) Study. *American Journal of Preventive Medicine, 14*, 245–258. doi:10.1016/S0749-3797(98)00017-8.

Fletcher, J. (2008). Adolescent depression: Diagnosis, treatment, and educational attainment. *Health Economics, 17*, 1215–1235. doi:10.1002/hec.1319.

Fredricks, J. A., & Eccles, J. S. (2002). Children's competence and value beliefs from childhood through adolescence. *Developmental Psychology, 38*, 519–533. doi:10.1037/0012-1649.38.4.519.

Fröjda, S. A., Nissinena, E. S., Pelkonenb, M. U. I., Marttunenb, M. J., Koivistoa, A. M., & Kaltiala-Heinoa, R. (2008). Depression and school performance in middle adolescent boys and girls. *Journal of Adolescence, 31*, 485–498. doi:10.1016/j.adolescence.2007.08.006.

Gewertz, C. (2007). Graduation predictors. *Education Week, 27*(1), 5.

Gini, G., & Pozzoli, T. (2009). Association between bullying and psychosomatic problems: A meta-analysis. *Pediatrics, 123*, 1059–1065. doi:10.1542/peds.2008-1215.

Goldsmith, P. (2009). Schools or neighborhoods or both? Race and ethnic segregation and educational attainment. *Social Forces, 87*, 1913–1941.

Goldstein, J. S., Little, S. G., & Akin-Little, K. A. (2003). Increasing attendance in the public schools: A review of most effective techniques. *The California School Psychologist, 8*, 127–139.

Gottfried, M. A. (2010). Evaluating the relationship between school attendance and achievement in urban elementary and middle schools: An instrumental variables approach. *American Educational Research Journal, 47*, 434–465. doi:10.3102/0002831209350494.

Graber, J. A. (2004). Internalizing problems during adolescence. In R. M. Lerner & L. Steinberg (Eds.), *Handbook of adolescent psychology* (2nd ed., pp. 587–626). Hoboken, NJ: Wiley.

Green, B. L., Krupnick, J. L., Stockton, P., Goodman, L., Corcoran, C., & Petty, R. (2001). Psychological outcomes associated with traumatic loss in a sample of young women. *American Behavioral Scientist, 44*, 817–837. doi:10.1177/00027640121956511.

Greene, J. P. (2009). *High school graduation rates in the United States*. New York: Manhattan Institute for Policy Research, Inc. Retrieved from http://www.manhattan-institute.org/html/cr_baeo.htm.

Grisso, T. (1998). *Forensic evaluation of juveniles*. Sarasota, FL: Professional Resource Press.

Guttmacher Institute. (2010). *U.S. teenage pregnancies, births and abortions: National and state trends and trends by race and ethnicity*. Retrieved from http://www.guttmacher.org/pubs/USTPtrends.pdf.

Hall, S. (2000). *Final report: Youth and family centers program: 1999–2000*. Dallas, TX: Dallas Public Schools Division of Evaluation, Accountability, and Information Systems.

Hankin, B. L. (2006). Adolescent depression: Description, causes and interventions. *Epilepsy & Behavior, 8*, 102–114. doi:10.1016/j.yebeh.2005.10.012.

Hartman, H. J. (2001). Developing students' metacognitive knowledge and skills. In H. J. Hartman (Ed.), *Metacognition in learning and instruction* (pp. 33–67). New York: Springer.

Hoagwood, K., & Erwin, H. D. (1997). Effectiveness of school-based mental health services for children: A 10-year research review. *Journal of Child and Family Studies, 6*, 435–451. doi:10.1023/A:1025045412689.

Humensky, J., Kuwabara, S. A., Fogel, J., Wells, C., Goodwin, B., & Van Voorhees, B. W. (2010). Adolescents with depressive symptoms and their challenges with learning in school. *The Journal of School Nursing, 26*, 377–392. doi:10.1177/1059840510376515.

Jennings, J., Pearson, G., & Harris, M. (2000). Implementing and maintaining school-based mental health services in a large, urban school district. *Journal of School Health, 70*, 201–206. doi:10.1111/j.1746-1561.2000.tb06473.x.

Jones, A. S., Astone, N. M., Keyl, P. M., Kim, Y. J., & Alexander, C. S. (1999). Teen childbearing and educational attainment: A comparison of methods. *Journal of Family and Economic Issues, 20*, 387–418. doi:10.1023/A:1022932305898.

Juvonen, J., Wang, Y., & Espinoza, G. (2011). Bullying experiences and compromised academic performance across middle school grades. *The Journal of Early Adolescence, 31*, 152–173. doi:10.1177/0272431610379415.

Kaffenberger, C. J. (2006). School reentry for students with a chronic illness: A role for professional school counselors. *Professional School Counseling, 9*, 223–230.

Kalafat, J., Illback, R., & Sanders, D. (1997). Implementation and outcome evaluation of statewide school-based family/youth services. In C. Liberton, K. Kutash, & R. Friedman (Eds.), *The 10th annual research conference proceedings: A system of care for children's mental health: Expanding the research base* (pp. 163–168). Tampa, FL: Research & Training Center for Children's Mental Health.

Kazdin, A. E. (1998). Conduct disorders. In R. J. Morris & T. R. Kratochwill (Eds.), *The practice of child therapy* (3rd ed., pp. 199–230). Boston: Allyn and Bacon.

Keenan, K., Wroblewski, K., Hipwell, A., Loeber, R., & Stouthamer-Loeber, M. (2010). Age of onset, system threshold, and expansion of the nosology of conduct disorder for girls. *Journal of Abnormal Psychology, 119*, 689–698.

Ladd, G. W. (2008). Does chronic classroom peer rejection predict the development of children's classroom participation during the grade school years? *Child Development, 79*, 1001–1015. doi:10.1111/j.1467-8624.2008.01172.x.

Little, S. G., Akin-Little, A., & Gutierrez, G. (2009). Children and traumatic events: Therapeutic techniques for psychologists working in the schools. *Psychology in the Schools, 46*, 199–205. doi:10.1002/pits.20364.

Little, S. G., Akin-Little, A., & Medley, N. (2011). Interventions to address school crises and violence. In T. Kehle & M. Bray (Eds.), *The oxford encyclopedia of school psychology* (pp. 483–503). New York: Oxford University Press.

Little, S. G., Akin-Little, A., & Somerville, M. (in press). Response to trauma in children: An examination of effective intervention and post-traumatic growth. *School Psychology International*.

Martens, B. K., & Witt, J. C. (2004). Competence, persistence, and success: The positive psychology of behavioral skill instruction. *Psychology in the Schools, 41*, 19–30. doi:10.1002/pits.10135.

McKay, A., & Barrett, M. (2010). Trends in teen pregnancy rates from 1996–2006: A comparison of Canada, Sweden, U.S.A., and England/Wales. *The Canadian Journal of Human Sexuality, 19*, 43–52.

McKenna, M., Hawk, E., Mullen, J., & Hertz, M. (2011). Bullying among middle school and high school students—Massachusetts, 2009. *Morbidity and Mortality Weekly Report, 60*, 465–471.

McNelis, A. M., Johnson, C. S., Huberty, T. J., & Austin, J. K. (2005). Factors associated with academic achievement in children with recent-onset seizures. *Seizure, 14*, 331–339. doi:10.1016/j.seizure.2005.04.005.

Meade, C. S., Kershaw, T. S., & Ickovics, J. R. (2008). The intergenerational cycle of teenage motherhood: An ecological approach. *Health Psychology, 27*, 419–429. doi:10.1037/0278-6133.27.4.419.

Murray, J., & Farrington, D. P. (2010). Risk factors for conduct disorder and delinquency: Key findings from longitudinal studies. *Canadian Journal of Psychiatry, 55*, 633–642.

Nabors, L. A., Little, S. G., Akin-Little, A., & Iobst, E. A. (2008). Teacher knowledge of and confidence in meeting the needs of children with chronic medical conditions: Pediatric psychology's contribution to education. *Psychology in the Schools, 45*, 217–226. doi:10.1002/pits.20292.

Nabors, L., & Reynolds, M. (2000). Program evaluation activities: Outcomes related to treatment for adolescents receiving school-based mental health services. *Children's Services: Social Policy, Research, and Practice, 3*, 175–189. doi:10.1207/S15326918CS0303_4.

Nakamoto, J., & Schwartz, D. (2010). Is peer victimization associated with academic achievement? A meta-analytic review. *Social Development, 19*, 221–242. doi:10.1111/j.1467-9507.2009.00539.x.

Nansel, T. R., Overpeck, M., Pilla, R. S., Ruan, W. J., Simons-Morton, B., & Scheidt, P. (2001). Bullying behaviors among US youth: Prevalence and association with psychosocial adjustment. *Journal of the American Medical Association, 285*, 2094–3100. doi:10.1001/jama.285.16.2094.

National Institute for Mental Health. (2010). *Major depressive disorder in children*. Retrieved from http://www.nimh.nih.gov/statistics/1MDD_CHILD.shtml.

No Child Left Behind Act of 2001 (2002). Pub. L. No. 107–110, 115 Stat. 1425.

Ogden, C. L., Carroll, M. D., Curtin, L. R., Lamb, M. M., & Flegal, K. M. (2010). Prevalence of high body mass index in US children and adolescents, 2007–2008. *Journal of the American Medical Association, 303*, 242–249. doi:10.1001/jama.2009.2012.

Paternite, C. E. (2005). School-based mental health programs and services: Overview and introduction to the special issue. *Journal of Abnormal Child Psychology, 33*, 657–663. doi:10.1007/s10802-005-7645-3.

Pinkus, L. M. (2009). *Action required: Addressing the nation's lowest-performing high schools. Policy brief*. Washington, DC: Alliance for excellent education. Retrieved from www.all4ed.org/files/ActionRequired.pdf.

Pintrich, P. R. (2000). The role of goal orientation in self-regulated learning. In M. Boekaerts, P. R. Pintrich, & M. Zeidner (Eds.), *Handbook of self-regulation* (pp. 451–502). New York: Academic.

Reeve, D. B. (2008). Improving school attendance. *Educational Leadership, 65*(8), 90–91.

Ryan, A. M., & Patrick, H. (2001). The classroom social environment and changes in adolescents' motivation and engagement during middle school. *American Educational Research Journal, 38*, 437–460. doi:10.3102/00028312038002437.

Sabia, J. J. (2007). The effect of body weight on adolescent academic performance. *Southern Economic Journal, 73*, 871–900.

Sharp, S. (1995). How much does bullying hurt? The effects of bullying on the personal well-being and educational progress of secondary-aged students. *Educational and Child Psychology, 12*, 81–88.

Sheldon, S. B. (2007). Improving student attendance with school, family and community partnerships. *The Journal of Educational Research, 100*, 267–275.

Sholevar, G. P., & Sholevar, E. H. (1995). Overview. In G. P. Sholevar (Ed.), *Conduct disorders in children and adolescents* (pp. 3–26). Washington, DC: American Psychiatric Press.

Singer, B. D., & Bashir, A. S. (1999). What are executive functions and self-regulation and what do they have to do with language-learning disorders? *Language, Speech, and Hearing Services in Schools, 30*, 265–273.

Smith, F. J., Taylor, K. M. G., Newbould, J., & Keady, S. (2008). Medicines for chronic illness at school: Experiences and concerns of young people and their parents. *Journal of Clinical Pharmacy and Therapeutics, 33*, 537–544. doi:10.1111/j.1365-2710.2008.00944.x.

Spilkin, A., & Ballantyne, A. (2007). Behavior in children with a chronic illness: A descriptive study of child characteristics, family adjustment, and school issues in children with cystinosis. *Families, Systems & Health, 25*, 68–84. doi:10.1037/1091-7527.25.2.161.

Stover, D. (2006). Treating cyberbullying as a school violence issue. *Education Digest, 72*, 40–42.

Taras, H., & Potts-Datema, W. (2005). Obesity and student performance at school. *Journal of School Health, 75*, 291–295. doi:10.1111/j.1746-1561.2005.00040.x.

Thies, K. M., & McAllister, J. W. (2001). The Health Education Leadership Project: A school initiative for children and adolescents with chronic health conditions. *Journal of School Health, 71*, 167–172. doi:10.1111/j.1746-1561.2001.tb07309.x.

Thompson, R. J., & Gustafson, K. E. (1996). *Adaptation to chronic childhood illness*. Washington, DC: American Psychological Association.

U. S. Department of Education. (2010). *A blueprint for reform: The reauthorization of the Elementary and Secondary Education Act*. Retrieved from http://www2.ed.gov/policy/elsec/leg/blueprint/publicationtoc.html.

U.S. Department of Education (2007). *History: Twenty-five years of progress in educating children with disabilities through DEA*. Retrieved from http://www2.ed.gov/policy/speced/leg/idea/history.html.

U.S. Department of Education (2008a). *About the Nation's Report Card*. Retrieved from http://nationsreportcard.gov/about_nrc.asp.

U.S. Department of Education. (2008b). *NAEP 2008: Trends in academic progress*. Jessup, MD: Author.

U.S. Department of Education, National Center for Education Statistics. (2009). *Age range for compulsory school attendance and special education services, and policies on year-round schools and kindergarten programs, by state: Selected years, 1997 through 2008*. Retrieved from http://nces.ed.gov/programs/digest/d09/tables/dt09_166.asp.

Valletutti, P. J. (2004). The crucial role of the teacher. In H. A. Haslam & P. J. Valletutti (Eds.), *Medical problems in the classroom: The teacher's role in diagnosis and management* (4th ed., pp. 1–28). Austin, TX: Pro-Ed.

Walsh, M. E., & Murphy, J. A. (2003). Children, health, and learning: A guide to the issues. In R. M. Lerner (Series Ed.), *Contemporary youth issues*. Westport, CT: Praeger.

Wilcox-Gok, V., Marcotte, D. E., Farahati, F., & Borkoski, C. (2004). Early onset depression and high school dropout. In D. E. Marcotte & V. Wilcox-Gok (Eds.), *The economics of gender and mental illness*. Amsterdam: Elsevier.

Zametkin, A. J., Zoon, C. K., Klein, H. W., & Munson, S. (2004). Psychiatric aspects of child and adolescent obesity: A review of the past 10 years. *Journal of the American Academy of Child and Adolescent Psychiatry, 43*, 134–150. doi:10.1097/00004583-200402000-00008.

Zimmerman, B. J. (1996). Enhancing student's academic and health functioning: A self-regulatory perspective. *School Psychology Quarterly, 11*, 47–66. doi:10.1037/h0088920.

Brain Development and Health Implications in Adolescents

Brian D. Leany

Introduction

The development of the human brain during adolescence is not insignificant. In fact, as a result of the developmental theories of Erickson and Piaget as well as our own anecdotal experiences, most of us are aware of the behavioral changes exhibited in adolescence. Given these obvious behavioral milestones, it would stand to reason that there are neurodevelopment and thus cognitive changes that underlie these behaviors. Understanding the normal genesis of development, as well as potential risk factors and limitations, is critical to helping us better understand the adolescent. An example of this is the relative paradox pointed out by Dahl and Spears (2004). This review identifies our knowledge of neurocognitive superiority of the adolescent in contrast to the seemingly unintelligent choices that result contemporaneously (e.g., high number of accidents occurring at a time of optimal reaction time and cognitive processing).

The consideration then for this chapter is, given what we know about adolescent brain development, what can we do to promote healthy behavior in exchange for preventing or limiting unhealthy behaviors. While we may not necessarily find definitive guidelines or protocols for such a goal, we can make some observations that help explain the resulting behaviors, both troubling and reassuring, with a biological explanation as an underpinning. Covered in this chapter is an explanation for the perplexing risk-taking behaviors of adolescents, the differences between males and females in neural and sociocognitive developmental trajectory as well as sex-specific risk and protective factors.

Neurological Changes

Neurological changes can be thought of in terms of being both structural and functional. Structurally we want to consider the aspects of white matter (association between cortices) myelination and growth, as well as the growth of gray matter areas, which can be thought of as the individual processing centers. To describe the process as one of growth might be a misnomer. In fact, much research has shown that the real change is not purely one of volume (which is to be expected in a maturing organism), but rather a change of function and efficiency of the brain. The adolescent growth spurt is much more a reorganization marked by shrinkage and recession in some areas co-occurring with growth in other areas. Thus it has been posited that this is a secondary process of synaptic pruning and dendritic expansion or reorganization not unlike the one seen in infancy, perhaps in preparation for new roles and expectations (e.g., preparation for

B.D. Leany, Ph.D. (✉)
State of California Department of Corrections and Rehabilitation, California Correctional Health Care System, Susanville, CA 96127-0750, USA
e-mail: leanyb@gmail.com

W.T. O'Donohue et al. (eds.), *Handbook of Adolescent Health Psychology*,
DOI 10.1007/978-1-4614-6633-8_17, © Springer Science+Business Media New York 2013

relationships and work roles; Blakemore & Choudhury, 2006).

The white matter of the cortex is responsible for associations between cortical areas, and thus expansion in this area is what we deem responsible for the speed of processing between say the visual cortex responsible for perceiving information and the motor cortex responsible for the resulting behavioral response to the perceived stimuli. It has been largely shown that this myelination process may reach its peak at adolescence, and in fact much of the current fMRI research supports that this is the case (Giedd et al., 1999).

Gray matter on the other hand is responsible for the density of neural cells which process information. The growth pattern throughout the life span is one in which growth occurs from the top down, and the center out. Neurological development occurs in a pattern that develops from the brain stem forward, with the frontal cortex being the last to develop. Given that the frontal lobe has been considered largely responsible for impulse control, coordination (or executive processing), and higher-order thinking/abstract reasoning, it is no wonder that much of the importance of our focus on adolescent brain development focuses on the development of this area.

In general, while past research has suggested that there is an increase in white matter, while gray matter decreases, recent research has shown this to be untrue. In particular the areas of the prefrontal cortex as well as the temporal, parietal, and occipital lobes all show changes during the preadolescent, adolescent, and postadolescent stages. Further, these stages are not considered to be proportional. That is, the growth of the parietal lobe, for example, is not equivalent to that of the occipital or prefrontal cortices. This suggests that the maturation may be specific to a genetic "readiness," and potentially indicates a critical stage of development in which environmental factors could influence the developmental trajectory and ultimately the functional outcome (Giedd et al., 1999; Perrin et al., 2008; Thompson, 2006).

Given that there are physical differences between genders it would stand to reason that we should explore potential differences in neurological development between the genders and as extension behavioral differences. There is no one-to-one correspondence however in these comparisons. For example while the female brain is, on average, smaller than that of her male counterpart, there is no corresponding difference in intellectual functioning or capacity. However, there are distinct hormonal differences, which we would expect are uniquely different (and research has shown are different in adults) throughout the developmental process.

While there has been much debate recently regarding the exact parameters of adolescence (largely due to the earlier onset of menarche for girls and some later prolonged puberty for males), the most traditional marking of adolescence has been from puberty to legal adulthood, and this would be the most reasonable parameters to consider when discussing neurological development. Additionally, we need to consider the function of the various lobes that demonstrate change in adolescence.

Parietal Lobe

The parietal is responsible for visuospatial processing and integration with the motor cortex. Thus, changes in this area would be relative to visuospatial acuity and resulting motor response. It is in fact during adolescence when most states allow for driving privileges in the form of temporary learning permits or restricted licenses. In fact, many states have recently considered and even passed legislation for graduated licenses related to the discordance between capacity and ability, which was all to evident in the disproportionate number of accidents for this age group, which should theoretically have the greatest ability to avoid them.

Temporal Lobe

The most prominent function of the temporal is language production, reception, and integration. It is no wonder that we begin to see this rapid acquisition of language capabilities not since seen in the childhood language explosion described by various developmental psychologists. This change in language abilities suggests that when we interact with adolescents, we can use a more sophisticated manner of communication than we would with children. However, it also means that we must assess who we are communicating to (an individual patient, a group of teens, or a broad-based preventative health campaign), in order to maximize the effectiveness of that communication.

Occipital Lobe

The occipital lobe is the only one whose growth pattern is linear in nature. That is, we see none of the spurts and stops observed in the other cortical regions previously discussed. Thus, while the implications for this nonlinear growth are not fully understood, one could posit that this is more of a normal developmental trajectory consistent with the overall growth of the human organism.

Prefrontal Cortex

The greatest area of interest for this discussion would be the development and functional processes associated with the prefrontal cortex. It is in this cortical region where we believe the true higher order functioning of human reason occurs. Here we believe the ability to control impulses and integrate various sensory information and the corresponding outputs of behavior occurs. An important aspect of this system is the dopamine feedback system. This system has been labeled as our basic reinforcement feedback loop and is responsible for those thoughts and behaviors we deem to be intrinsically motivating. Dysfunction in this area has been associated with several mental and physical health concerns such as schizophrenia, Parkinson's, Alzheimer's, and drug addiction. In fact, research (Iacono & McGue, 2006) has shown that it may be a decrease in activation of this area during adolescence that predicts externalized psychopathology (e.g., substance use disorders, risky sexual behaviors, and antisocial personality features).

The prefrontal cortex is also the area we associate with inhibition for socially inappropriate behavior as well as the basic constitution of our personality. We have some prominent examples of the role of the frontal cortex come from case studies of cortical injury such as that of Phineas Gage (Chap. 6 in Macmillan, 2000) where the loss of frontal cortical gray matter resulted in lasting personality changes and socially inappropriate disinhibition in individuals previously described as mild mannered and polite. Conversely, the decades of 1940s saw a period in the USA where intentional ablation of this area was utilized to reduce inappropriate behavior and deviance (Swayze, 1995).

Not all changes in the cortex can easily be seen as a result of pure structural change. In fact some of the more interesting research has discussed a differential pattern of activation for emotional discrimination and processing of such responses as fear and anger (Monk et al., 2003). Additionally and seemingly of critical importance are the changes seen in the reward system of our brain. This system is the dopaminergic system and is located here in the prefrontal cortex. Research has shown that adolescence is an extremely sensitive period for human development of sensation seeking and a period where we may attribute greater value to potentially rewarding behavior (Ernst & Spear, 2009). This inflation of rewarding value may explain the development of both adaptive and maladaptive patterns of behavior as well as addictions.

It is the development of the prefrontal cortex, which gives most who work with adolescents the most frustration. This area is the fastest and largest region of brain development in adolescence, and is responsible for rational thinking and impulse control, yet adolescents are often (and rightly so) portrayed as impulsive, irrational, and labile. In a review Schwartz (2008) discusses how the paradox is really not a paradox at all, but in fact just another misunderstood process of development. The review provides support for a rapidly developing yet immature prefrontal cortex. Thus, it is akin to gangly first steps we take as toddlers, where we have these rapidly growing and refining synaptic connections for bipedal locomotion, yet we stumble and fall with varying rates in development of true coordination. An additional caveat for this paradox suggests that it is a developmentally necessary process that actually guides the synaptic pruning process (Bessant, 2008). Thus suggesting that it is the experience of bad decisions and judgment which prevents us from making more serious errors in the future, and becoming more efficient at this improved (and informed) decision-making process.

Females

Gray matter in the parietal and frontal lobes peaks nearly a year earlier in females than in males. This peak corresponds to physiological developmental processes in puberty and thus may indicate differential periods of readiness to learn as well as corresponding behavioral patterns that would impact health and wellness.

Given that the parietal lobe is responsible for visuospatial acuity and the temporal lobe allows for more abstract and what we consider adult-type thinking, we could expect adolescent females to be more mature with better reaction times and coordination, as well as a greater level of insight and impulse control than their male counterparts. Thus, they may be more receptive to adult-like treatment paradigms and preventative interventions.

Males

In adolescence, males show a sharp increase in white matter as compared to females. To reiterate, white matter consists of the axons or communication pathways of the neurons within and between brain regions. It has been reported that this increase is mediated by an increase in the production of testosterone and number of androgen receptors (Perrin et al., 2008). This research goes on to suggest that interruptions or alterations (e.g., the use of androgen-based steroids) in testosterone production and androgen receptors could be implicated in adolescent and adult male depression.

In addition to volume of white and gray matter, we can also see a differentiation in activation. For males, one particular area of interest is the amygdala. Here research has shown a change in patterns of activation between males and females exposed to emotion-laden (read angry) faces, with males showing greater activation of the right hemisphere (and almost exclusive for the particular paradigm) of the amygdala than females (Schneider et al., 2011). This research goes on to suggest that given the greater prevalence rates for males of mental disorders related to emotional processing (e.g., conduct disorder, antisocial PD, schizophrenia), this may be an area of dysfunction and potential intervention/ assessment. The problem currently lies in the inability to detect whether the dysfunction is a result of hyper- or hypoactivation of the amygdala or yet some other unexplained mechanism.

Resulting Behaviors

The benefits of adolescent brain development are many, the most obvious being largely due to the increased myelination and resulting increase in processing speed, as well as more efficient communication between cortices due to white matter association cortices that are expanded and pruned for maximum efficiency. This improvement is not limited to processing speed however, and multiple domains are impacted. This can be seen through observable changes in a broad range of behaviors.

Emotional Development

Probably the most salient for many of us, and especially for those who work with or have adolescents of their own, is the emotional development that occurs during puberty. This development is multimodal, in that it is not wholly isolated to the expression of emotion we so readily attribute to the tumult and turmoil of teenage years, but also includes changes in the way that adolescents perceive the emotion of others.

Much of what we know about adolescent emotional development can be found in the literature of emotional intelligence. As suggested at the onset of this chapter, this is not wholly a result of pure structural growth or transformation (that we have been able to see anyway), but rather a change in the pattern of activation. This change has been shown to differ between the sexes. Research has shown that during adolescence, females (and emotionally receptive or intuitive males) show a pattern of activation that shifts emotional processing from the amygdala to the prefrontal and parietal cortices (Whittle et al., 2008). Given that the amygdala is what we would consider a primitive system (similar to the medulla, which is responsible for basic survival functions of breathing and the beating of the heart), this shift suggests a movement from visceral responses to emotional stimuli to responses we would consider more thoughtful and evolved. Conversely, this same research shows males who persist in more aggressive behaviors also have correspondingly larger amygdala volume and smaller association cortices in the prefrontal cortex (which does not exist in female adolescents).

This more sophisticated processing of human interactions is an important change for the adolescent. No longer might they be concerned about positive health practices to avoid immediate consequences or for instant gratification. They now have the capability of foresight and planning to maintain health for the benefit of others and future prevention (e.g., exercise to avoid diabetes or high blood pressure).

Communication

Similar to the other changes discussed, we can identify a direct correlation between brain development and resulting changes in communication related behavior. Just as we see in the parietal lobe, the development trajectory in the temporal lobe has readily identifiable behavioral correlates. For our developing adolescents, we often see a much more sophisticated level of conversation, which more closely resembles that of adults. In conjunction with the developing executive processes and improved abstract reasoning, the adolescent not only has a larger repertoire of vocabulary but also has an additional way to represent old words in and concepts in a new manner (e.g., through metaphorical and abstract relation of words to ideas and exemplars), which was not previously available. In fact it has been suggested that this social isolation may lead to actual neurotropic atrophy, in areas that suggest potential causes for depression (Meng, Li, Han, & Wang, 2011).

Changes (Perhaps Lapses) in Judgment

Given the changes seen in emotional responsiveness and communication we naturally want to consider the aspect of adolescent social interactions. Adolescent development is typically marked by the onset of puberty. We thus have a dramatic shift in hormones. These hormones naturally impact (and often signal) changes in the brain. A major shift in adolescence is the significant shift in the adolescent social system. It is in adolescence (citation) that teens shift their social alliances to their peers, away from their parents and family. It has been suggested that there is an interplay between the developing brain regions, associative cortices, and the hormonal feedback loop in the brain that helps signify desire, arousal, and satiation (the limbic system). This review of the literature identified changes in brain activity, relative to maturational development and hormonal influence (Eric, Ellen, Erin, & Daniel, 2005), and correlates them with resulting changes in social perception and value. The research indicates that these hormonal changes in effect change how we value social interactions, and suggests that this change is responsible for the increased value placed on opinions of potential romantic partners and peers. The research also suggests that this process creates a sensitive period for psychopathology for anxiety and depression, as a result of perceived rejection or failed social interactions. This same hormonal process also influences adolescent sexual behavior.

Research has worked to examine the influence of hormones on adolescent male and female sexual interest and involvement. Here we see gender differences with males being largely driven by physiological changes (e.g., puberty and increases in testosterone), whereas females are driven by both the biological changes resulting from increased estrogen and androgens as well as their peers. More precisely, males who are more adult like in their development are more likely to be interested and engaged in sexual behavior, whereas females can be influenced by their peers' sexual interest and behavior. However, this peer influence is only seen in those females who are further along (or near the end) of the pubescent maturational period (Smith, Udry, & Morris, 1985).

Impact of Teratogens

While there is a great deal of plasticity in the adolescent brain due to the processes that underlie organization, there is also the risk that this is a developmentally sensitive period where environmental factors can influence later functioning. Because there is increased impulsivity and risk-taking behavior that occurs in adolescence, and in light of this sensitive period, we must examine the potential impact of drug and alcohol use.

One important thing to consider in this discussion of teratogenic influences on brain development is research which shows that not all teratogenic effects or risk factors occur during the adolescent period itself. In fact, research has shown that exposure to drugs and alcohol most typically occurs during infancy, but has lasting compounding effects into adolescence and adulthood.

The effects of alcohol in infancy have obvious lasting effects that are not abated by the neurological changes seen in adolescence. In fact, many aspects of socially problematic behavior considered normal in adolescence are exacerbated. In particular the problem of increased impulsivity appears to be exponentially magnified in adolescents with fetal alcohol effects (FAE) or fetal alcohol syndrome (FAS).

In adolescents, it appears to be the differences in white matter development that impacts teratogenic outcomes. Researchers (Thatcher, Pajtek, Chung, Terwilliger, & Clark, 2010) have shown that there is a differential susceptibility to white matter insult that occurs in adolescence. In fact, white matter growth (the communication pathways) can be stunted by substance use during this critical period, with females being more susceptible than males.

Research has also suggested that tobacco exposure can also have an impact on brain development (Jacobsen, Slotkin, Mencl, Frost, & Pugh, 2007). While the exact neural mechanism was not studied in adolescence, the current research was an extension of a prenatal study on the cholinergic impact of nicotine and tobacco exposure during the prenatal period. The current research demonstrated a decrease in auditory and visual attention, which was greater for males than females who are exposed to tobacco (nicotine) at either the prenatal or the adolescent period, with the greatest impact for males seen as for those who used tobacco during adolescence only.

Physical Health Risks

The previously mentioned risk-taking behavior is of greatest concern to the physical health of our adolescents. While they seemingly have the capacity to be more thoughtful, and efficient judges of risk, statistics show us that they are either not fully capable of or not willing to take advantage of these new resources. Thus, adolescents are at a great risk for injury due to risk taking or lapses in judgment. These risks include choices regarding substance use, sex, driving behaviors, and decisions regarding everyday activities where teens actually seek out risk. The organic reasons for why they engage in risk have already been discussed. The additional concern is the potential long-term cerebral consequences when they make poor choices.

The repeated use of substances can lead to long-term changes in organization and functioning of the brain that will extend into adulthood for many of these teens. The immediate consequence of alcohol (and other substance use for that matter) is acutely impaired judgment and decision-making that can lead to other physical and punitive consequences. Chronic alcohol use can lead to long-term organic problems such as Korsakoff's syndrome, which looks very much like dementia or psychosis, leading to an early need for long-term care and death. With amphetamines and stimulants, there are cardiac consequences that impact the brain through vascular changes, but also the long-term effects of stimulants that appear to alter the ability of individuals to utilize foresight and planning, as well as the adolescents developing ability to process human communication in a more sophisticated manner. This occurs through the deterioration of the frontal lobe, its association cortices for executive functioning and impulse control, as well as the amygdala.

Poor decisions related to sex can have obvious physiological consequences (e.g., pregnancy). However, sexually transmitted infections (STI) are a growing concern among teens. The largest concern related to cerebral health is diseases like hepatitis C, HIV/AIDS, and syphilis.

While the quality of life and overall longevity for individuals with HIV and AIDS is increasing, there are new consequences that result. At later stages, individuals infected with HIV are likely to develop an AIDS related dementia, which impairs one's ability to engage in activities of daily living (ADLs). Thus, they may no longer be able to engage in the day-to-day activities of self-care and advocacy (like taking a shower and bathing, or even knowing that they are ill). Similar to HIV/AIDS, hepatitis C has shown an expansion in treatment and longevity, but is still incurable.

There is no associated dementia, but there are vascular changes due to impaired functioning of the liver, as well mental illness complications related to treatment. Some of the most effective treatments for hepatitis C also cause mood dysregulation, which can lead to depression and suicidal ideation.

Syphilis is concerning at any age, but more so in adolescence. Syphilis is a disease that has only visible symptoms in males, and these symptoms last only a couple of weeks. In females, symptoms may go completely undetected due to the fact that they are largely internal. For males, the symptoms are obvious but only for a couple weeks. Given that adolescents are reluctant to seek medical care for sex-related symptoms, they may just wait for the symptoms to "clear up." The problem with syphilis is that visible symptoms will abate within a couple of weeks. However, the internal process will continue. An infection can lie dormant, and not become detectable again, until the disease reaches the brain and develops into incurable encephalitis. The impact of such a disease is extremely debilitating and often incurably fatal.

Finally, the day-to-day risks that adolescents engage in can lead to death or serious head injuries. The impact of a traumatic brain injury (TBI) is dependent on many variables. These variables include the location (e.g., an injury to the frontal lobe could lead to impairments in planning and impulse control, while a temporal lobe injury could present as problems in language), severity, as well as type of injury (open or closed). More severe deficits tend to occur with closed head injuries due to the displacement of brain tissue by bleeding and swelling, whereas open head injuries would reduce this displacement, but make the brain more susceptible to infection.

While adolescents are at a greater risk for TBI, they do have some protective factors going for them. Because the adolescent brain is not fully formed, and there is a great deal of reorganization occurring, there is also a good deal of plasticity. This means that while there could be a great deal of injury to a particular brain region, the brain is capable of repairing and, if necessary, reorganizing some processes to compensate for the insult. A good indicator of prognosis for TBI is the adolescent's premorbid level of functioning. This means that those with a higher level of functioning prior to injury are likely to have a better outcome than those with lower levels of premorbid functioning.

Mental Health Awareness

As the frontal lobe develops in conjunction with white matter track myelination, there are unique mental health concerns that arise. While the myelination is an important and critical aspect of becoming a more thoughtful adult, this same process is the time period where we begin to see early signs of mental illness such as schizophrenia (Mana, Martinot, & Martinot, 2010) as well as precursors to personality disorders. Symptom awareness is critical, at this period, because the best prognosis for serious mental disorders, and in fact for many personality disorders, the only efficacious intervention, occurs during adolescence at the onset of these disorders. Point prevalence rates indicate that 20–25 % of all adolescents may be at risk for a major mental illness, such as substance abuse, mood disorders, or self-injurious behavior (Patel, Flisher, Hetrick, & McGorry, 2007).

One common disorder seen in adolescents, attention-deficit/hyperactivity disorder (ADHD), illustrates the problematic nature of adolescent mental illness. While ADHD is a disorder that must be evidenced by age 7, it is often not detected until comorbid disorders of mood and substance use/dependence arise. While the prevalence rate is greater for males, this may be a protective factor for them, as clinicians, teachers, and parents may be more open or alert for this disorder in males. It has been suggested that in fact females may go undetected or misattributed to the more frequent mood, anxiety, and substance use disorders that we see in adolescent females (Quinn, 2005).

Preventative Steps

Much of the preventative steps that can be taken are simply based in knowledge, communication, and a clinical awareness of current research related specifically to adolescence. For example, research conducted by Spano (2003) suggests that the behavior of a teen (e.g., the choice to use drugs or not or engaging in activities that promote engaging adolescents in cognitive exercises) can influence the pattern of neurodevelopment. Thus a physician could encourage adolescents and their parents to "exercise" their brains, much like teachers or coaches encourage homework and training.

Knowledge is something that is becoming easier to obtain. With the proliferation of technology, we not only have better studies; with higher resolution, we have access. The key is to find reliable and current sources of information, specific to adolescent health. For clinicians, health care providers, and educators, this technology also allows us greater access to continuing education related to our specific demographic. In many of my own institutions we had a clinical reference guide of best-practices, specific to current journals throughout the developmental lifespan. If one does not exist in your own setting, you may want to develop this resource and share it with others.

Communication of our knowledge is just as important. For adolescents, we not only have to provide them information in a manner that reaches them; we often must also help parents find a way to help their adolescent at a period when they may be less than receptive. Additionally, communication is a two-way street. We are the experts, but we cannot get information from our clients, patients, or students without really listening. We need to occasionally slow down and really pay attention to what is being said. Is she talking about being depressed, or is this more the dysphoria that we see in adolescent, female ADHD?

Our clinical awareness is a combination of knowledge and communication. We need to stay current in the research to identify new findings, diagnostic and treatment tools, as well as new or changing interventions.

Conclusion

Adolescence has always been considered a period of change and passage. The development of the brain does not necessarily provide us with any unique solutions to the difficulty adolescents (and thus their parents, teachers, and clinicians) encounter in this time period, nor does it allow us to elucidate a specific algorithm for the exploitation of the newly acquired or developing abilities of the adolescent. However, a better understanding of the neuro-developmental process does allow us to have a better understanding of the limitations, as well as the potential pitfalls of adolescent abilities, thus providing us a more informed foundation upon which to base our interventions.

In understanding these abilities and limitations, it is the hope that we may better address related health care education and interventions for greater efficiency and efficacy. One final note relates to policy. In a letter to the editor, Steinberg (2009) discusses the history of neuroscience research and public policy. Here he provides support for the use of neuroscientific evidence in developing policy (relating it to the largely successful of head start and early childhood education), yet also recommends a balanced approach to evaluating the evidence in order to avoid the undue influence that neuroscience research tends to hold on the general public. For example, Males (2009) points out that while we know that there are significant changes in brain areas that have the potential to influence risk-taking behavior, it is not the "teenage brain" that is the best predictor of risky behavior, but rather the socioeconomic status of the adolescent that presents the greatest risk (e.g., poverty and exposure to violent crimes). Thus, while we can use this information to inform our approach to adolescent health, we should maintain a perspective on what is in the best interest of the individual adolescent.

References

Bessant, J. (2008). Hard wired for risk: Neurological science, 'the adolescent brain' and developmental theory. *Journal of Youth Studies, 11*(3), 347–360.

Blakemore, S., & Choudhury, S. (2006). Development of the adolescent brain: Implications for executive function and social cognition. *Journal of Child Psychology and Psychiatry, 47*(3/4), 296–312.

Dahl, R. E., & Spear, L. P. (2004). *Adolescent brain development: Vulnerabilities and opportunities*. New York: Academy of Sciences.

Eric, E. N., Ellen, L., Erin, B. M., & Daniel, S. P. (2005). The social re-orientation of adolescence: A neuroscience perspective on the process and its relation to psychopathology. *Psychological Medicine, 35*(2), 163–174.

Ernst, M., & Spear, L. (2009). Reward systems. In M. de Haan & M. Gunnar (Eds.), *Handbook of developmental social neuroscience* (pp. 324–341). New York: Guilford Press.

Giedd, J., Blumenthal, J., Jeffries, N., Castellanos, F., Liu, H., Zijdenbos, A., et al. (1999). Brain development during childhood and adolescence: A longitudinal MRI study. *Nature Neuroscience, 2*(10), 861–863.

Iacono, W. G., & McGue, M. (2006). Association between P3 event-related brain potential amplitude and adolescent problem behavior. *Psychophysiology, 43*(5), 465–469. doi:10.1111/j.1469-8986.2006.00422.x.

Jacobsen, L. K., Slotkin, T. A., Mencl, W., Frost, S. J., & Pugh, K. R. (2007). Gender-specific effects of prenatal and adolescent exposure to tobacco smoke on auditory and visual attention. *Neuropsychopharmacology, 32*(12), 2453–2464. doi:10.1038/sj.npp. 1301398.

Macmillan, M. (2000). *The damage to gage's psyche.* MIT Press. Cambridge, MA.

Males, M. (2009). Does the adolescent brain make risk taking inevitable? *Journal of Adolescent Research, 24*(1), 3–20.

Mana, S., Martinot, M., & Martinot, J. (2010). Brain imaging findings in children and adolescents with mental disorders: A cross-sectional review. *European Psychiatry, 25*, 345–354.

Meng, Q., Li, N., Han, X., & Wang, W. (2011). Effects of adolescent social isolation on the expression of brain-derived neurotrophic factors in the forebrain. *European Journal of Pharmacology, 650*, 229–232.

Monk, C., McClure, E., Nelson, E., Zarahn, E., Bilder, R., Leibenluft, E., et al. (2003). Adolescent immaturity in attention-related brain engagement to emotional facial expressions. *NeuroImage, 20*, 420–428.

Patel, V., Flisher, A. J., Hetrick, S., & McGorry, P. (2007). Mental health of young people: A global public health challenge. *The Lancet, 369*, 13402–13413.

Perrin, J. S., Hervé, P., Leonard, G., Perron, M., Pike, G., Pitiot, A., et al. (2008). Growth of white matter in the adolescent brain: Role of testosterone and androgen receptor. *Journal of Neuroscience, 28*(38), 9519–9524. doi:10.1523/JNEUROSCI.1212-08.2008.

Quinn, P. O. (2005). Treating adolescent girls and women with ADHD: Gender-specific issues. *Journal of Clinical Psychology, 61*(5), 579–587. doi:10.1002/jclp. 20121.

Schneider, S. S., Peters, J. J., Bromberg, U. U., Brassen, S. S., Menz, M. M., Miedl, S. F., et al. (2011). Boys do it the right way: Sex-dependent amygdala lateralization during face processing in adolescents. *NeuroImage, 56*(3), 1847–1853. doi:10.1016/j.neuroimage.2011.02.019.

Schwartz, K. (2008). Adolescent brain development: An oxymoron no longer. *The Journal of Youth Ministry, 6*(2), 85–93.

Smith, E. A., Udry, J., & Morris, N. M. (1985). Pubertal development and friends: A biosocial explanation of adolescent sexual behavior. *Journal of Health and Social Behavior, 26*(3), 183–192.

Spano, S. (2003). Adolescent brain. *Youth Studies of Australia, 22*(1), 36–38.

Steinberg, L. (2009). Should the science of adolescent brain development inform public policy? *American Psychologist, 64*(8), 739–750.

Swayze, V. W. (1995). Frontal leukotomy and related psychosurgical procedures in the era before antipsychotics (1935–1954): A historical overview. *The American Journal of Psychiatry, 152*(4), 505–515.
Thatcher, D. L., Pajtek, S., Chung, T., Terwilliger, R. A., & Clark, D. B. (2010). Gender differences in the relationship between white matter organization and adolescent substance use disorders. *Drug and Alcohol Dependence, 110*(1–2), 55–61. doi:10.1016/j.drugalcdep. 2010.02.004.
Thompson, P. (2006). Time-lapse imaging tracks brain maturation from ages 5 to 20, National Institutes of Mental Health, and the University of California Los Angeles, May 2004; also, author interview with Robin Jenkins, Ph.D., June 2006.
Whittle, S., Yap, M., Yucel, M., Fornito, A., Simmons, J., Barrett, A., et al. (2008). Prefrontal and amygdala volumes are related to adolescents' affective behaviors during parent–adolescent interactions. *PNAS, 105*(9), 3652–3657.

Puberty: Its Role in Adolescent Maturation

John S. Fuqua and Alan D. Rogol

Introduction

The objective of this chapter is to describe the pubertal process in boys and girls, especially to note its great physiological variability in both timing and *tempo*. Later in the chapter, we shall describe some effects on those parameters by pathophysiological processes—diseases, therapeutic agents, and the environment—in greater depth.

Normal Growth

Growth can occur in at least three complementary categories: incremental (height), hypertrophic (body composition), and reparative (from physical work or training or recovery from injury). Although all forms are important to those who exercise, the third component is often subsumed under the second.

J.S. Fuqua, M.D. (✉)
Section of Pediatric Endocrinology and Diabetology, Indiana University School of Medicine, Riley Hospital for Children, Room 5960, 705 Riley Hospital Drive, Indianapolis, IN 46202, USA
e-mail: jsfuqua@iupui.edu

A.D. Rogol, M.D., Ph.D.
Division of Pediatric Endocrinology and Diabetes, University of Virginia School of Medicine, Charlottesville, VA, USA
e-mail: adrogol@comcast.net

A normal pattern of linear growth is generally accepted as strong evidence that the general health of a child or adolescent is good. However, acute, subacute, and chronic illnesses or stressors may perturb this physiological pattern. Linear growth is often partitioned into three phases: infantile, childhood, and pubertal (Karlberg, 1989). The *infantile phase* is characterized by rapid but decelerating growth during the first 2 years of life, and lengths/heights may cross several growth percentile lines as children grow toward their genetic potential and gradually move from the excesses or constraints of the intrauterine environment.

The *childhood phase* is characterized by a relatively constant growth rate of 5–7 cm/year and growth along or parallel to one of the percentile lines on the standard (distance) growth chart. The *pubertal phase* is characterized by a growth spurt of 8–14 cm/year and is the most variable in terms of its timing, tempo, and duration. This is the phase that may be vulnerable to variation in energy balance (nutrition and energy expenditure) and other potential environmental stressors. Factors affecting the processes of physiological growth and maturation include genetic and epigenetic background, the intrauterine environment, general state of health, living conditions and home environment, and at least the hormones GH/IGF-I, sex steroids, thyroid, and adrenal, with modulation by an ever increasing host of others, including insulin, leptin and other adipokines, and cytokines.

W.T. O'Donohue et al. (eds.), *Handbook of Adolescent Health Psychology*,
DOI 10.1007/978-1-4614-6633-8_18, © Springer Science+Business Media New York 2013

Puberty (L. *pubertas*, from *pubes*, *puber* of ripe age, adult) is the state of *physical* maturation at which persons are first able to bear children. However, it is really a *process* beginning many years before the first outward signs (testicular enlargement in boys and breast maturation in girls). This process begins as the prepubertal neuroendocrine hiatus ("juvenile pause") between fetal life/early infancy and adolescence comes to a close, with increasing secretion of gonadotropins and gonadal steroid hormones in both sexes and diminishing strength of the gonadal steroid feedback inhibition on the entire system that regulates gonadotropin-releasing hormone (GnRH)-mediated gonadotropin release (see below). Collectively this is noted as gonadarche—the onset of significant gonadal function.

Puberty is an important process to understand because its evolution often forms an integral part of the evaluation and treatment of endocrine disorders in children and adolescents. Its disorders herald effects with lifelong consequences. These include adult height and body composition, especially bone mineralization, and effects on the regional distribution of body fat and its cardiovascular consequences.

Thelarche refers to the development of breast tissue due to circulating estradiol derived from the ovaries after gonadarche in girls. Pubarche is the development of pubic hair and often axillary hair and axillary odor. It is due to the onset of adrenal androgen secretion (adrenarche) and usually occurs 6–12 months after gonadarche. Thelarche usually occurs 6–12 months before pubarche, and as noted, the two are due to quite different mechanisms. The sequence is reversed in perhaps 10 % of children and has a racial/ethnic imbalance in that premature pubarche is more common in African American and Hispanic children.

Assessment of Sexual Maturity Stages

Accurate staging of the physical alterations of sexual maturation provides an important framework for the diagnosis and management of disorders of growth and maturation. The process of "Tanner staging" is a now nearly universal system of sexual maturity rating based on the work of Marshall and Tanner for girls (Marshall & Tanner, 1969) and boys (Marshall & Tanner, 1970).

Girls

The original five stages for breast maturation were derived from photographs rather than palpation; however, especially with the increasing prevalence of obesity, it may be difficult to detect whether breast stage 2 (Table 1 and Fig. 1) is actual breast tissue or adipomastia (adipose tissue *without* any glandular breast tissue). The latter is not indicative of pubertal maturation. Similarly, pubic hair is divided into five stages (Table 2 and Fig. 1) from stage 1 (none) to stage 5 where there is dark hair of adult type (coarse and curled) and distributed in an inverted triangle. Menarche is a late development in the progression of biological maturation but may occur several years before full sexual maturation and many years before the attainment of adult body composition and the regional distribution of body fat.

Marshall and Tanner (1969, 1970) have noted the mean ages and variability of reaching the individual stages of sexual maturation (Table 3) for girls and boys. They have also shown the mean duration to pass through some significant maturational stages (Table 3) and the mean age for menarche. Although present data may indicate an earlier beginning of the stages of pubertal maturation and menarche (Rosenfield, Lipton, & Drum, 2009),

Table 1 Breast maturation in females

Stage	Physical characteristics
1	Prepubertal
2	Breast budding, elevation of both breast and nipple as a small mound
3	Continued enlargement of both breast and areola without separation of their contours
4	The areola and nipple form a secondary mound projecting above the contour of the breast
5	Adult shape, areola and nipple recessed to the contour of the breast

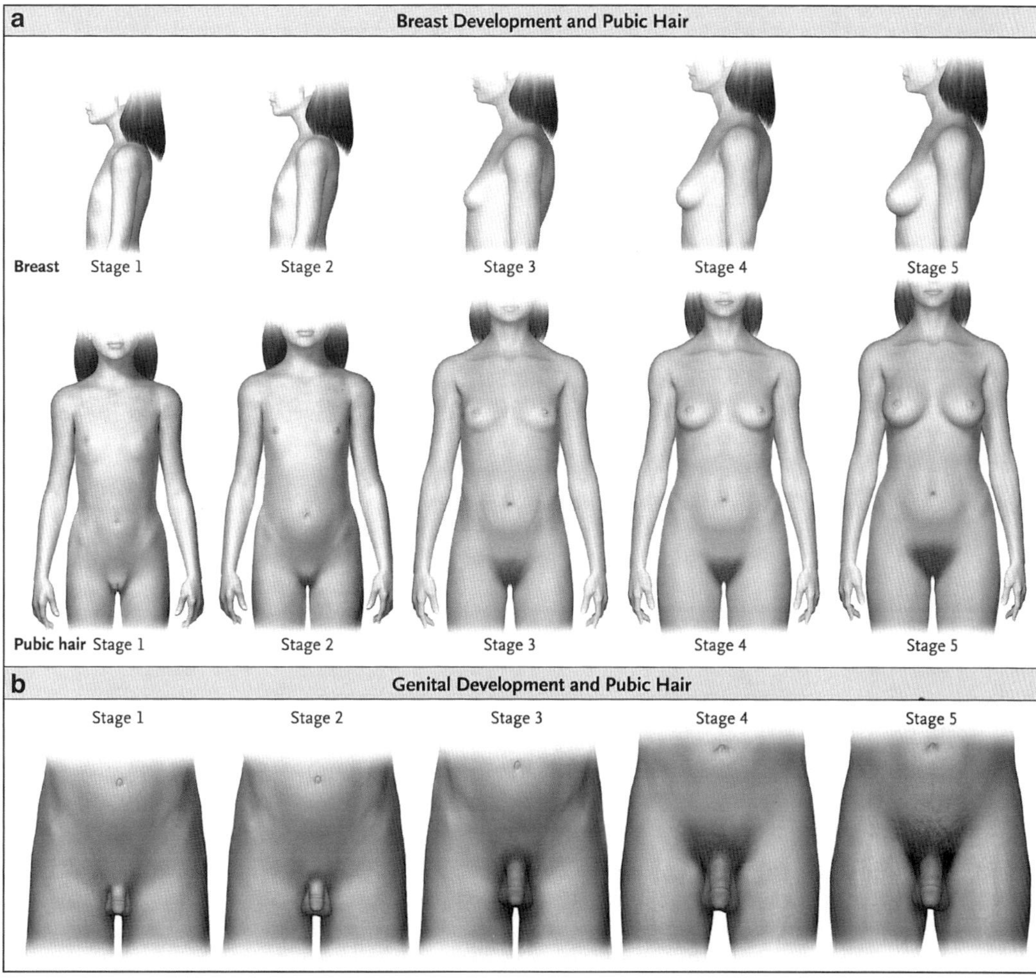

Fig. 1 Stages of sexual maturation according to Tanner. The *top two rows* illustrate stages of breast and pubic hair maturation in girls. The *bottom row* illustrates stages of genital and pubic hair maturation in boys. See Tables 1, 2, and 4 for additional details. Used with permission from Carel JC, Leger J. (2008). Precocious puberty. *N Engl J Med*, 358:2366–77. Copyright Massachusetts Medical Society

Table 2 Pubic hair maturation in males and females

Stage	Physical characteristics
1	Prepubertal
2	Sparse growth of long, lightly pigmented hairs at the base of the penis in males or the mons veneris/labia majora in females
3	Additional darkening and coarsening of hair, spreading over the pubic symphysis
4	Adult in character but has not spread to the lower abdomen in males or to the medial surface of the thighs in males and females
5	Adult in distribution, extension to the lower abdomen in males and/or the medial surface of the thighs in males and females

the process remains similar in terms of time between these various stages. The exception occurs in the very youngest of girls (Rosenfield et al., 2009), in whom the time from breast Tanner stage 2 to menarche is prolonged, so that although starting breast maturation considerably early, menarche is but several months earlier than previous data indicate.

There is also great variability in the timing of peak height velocity (PHV), which is an excellent biological anchor of pubertal maturation, in terms of stages of breast or genital maturation or in terms of the progression of pubic

Table 3 Mean ages at entry into pubertal stages for boys and girls from NHANES III (Anderson & Must, 2005; Chumlea et al., 2003; Herman-Giddens et al., 2001; Sun et al., 2002)

Boys			Girls		
	Mean	95% CI		Mean	95% CI
G 2	10.1[a]	9.6–10.6	B 2	10.4	10.1–10.7
G 3	12.4	12.0–12.7	B 3	11.8	11.5–12.0
G 4	13.5	13.2–13.8	B 4	13.3	13.0–15.9
G 5	15.9	15.3–16.4	B 5	15.5	15.0–15.9
PH 2	12.0	11.7–12.3	PH 2	10.6	10.3–10.9
PH 3	12.6	12.3–13.0	PH 3	11.8	11.5–12.1
PH 4	13.5	13.2–13.8	PH 4	13.0	12.7–13.3
PH 5	15.7	15.3–16.0	PH 5	16.3	15.9–16.9
G 2–G 5	5–6		B 2–B 5	5	
			Menarche	12.55	12.31–12.79

[a]All values in terms of years

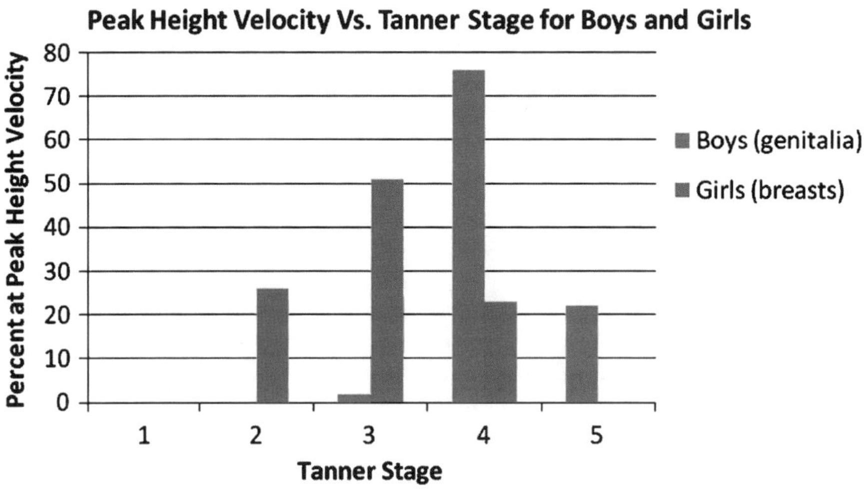

Fig. 2 Relationship between peak height velocity and breast and genital maturation in boys and girls, respectively. In girls, peak height velocity occurs at a median Tanner stage of 3, whereas in boys it occurs later, at a median Tanner stage of 4. Data are from Tanner, Whitehouse, Marubini, and Resele (1976)

hair (Figs. 2 and 3). Thus, the mid-pubertal growth spurt may occur at virtually any of the mid-pubertal breast or genital stages or pubic hair stages. Similarly, there is variability in the timing of pubic hair maturation in all of the stages of genital or breast maturation (Fig. 4).

Boys

Similarly, genital maturation in boys is divided into five stages from stage 1 (prepubertal) in which the penis, testes, and scrotum are about the same size and proportions as in early childhood to stage 5 (fully mature, see Table 4 and Fig. 1). In a manner similar to that in girls, pubic hair is divided into stages 1 (none) to 5 (dark, coarse mainly in the triangular distribution but may spread to the medial thighs or vertically). Adolescent boys may attain adult height and mature sexual maturation years before acquiring their adult body composition.

Testicular maturation (size) is conveniently measured by comparison to a Prader orchidometer, which is a set of ellipsoids roughly of the

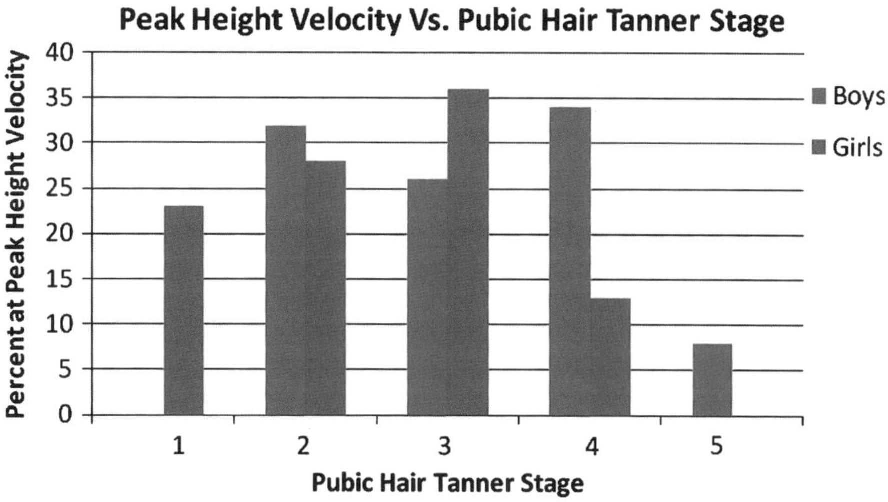

Fig. 3 Relationship between peak height velocity and pubic hair maturation in boys and girls. Unlike breast and genital maturation, there is a wide variation in the degree of pubic hair maturation at the time of peak height velocity, although boys tend to be further advanced than girls. Data are from Tanner et al. (1976)

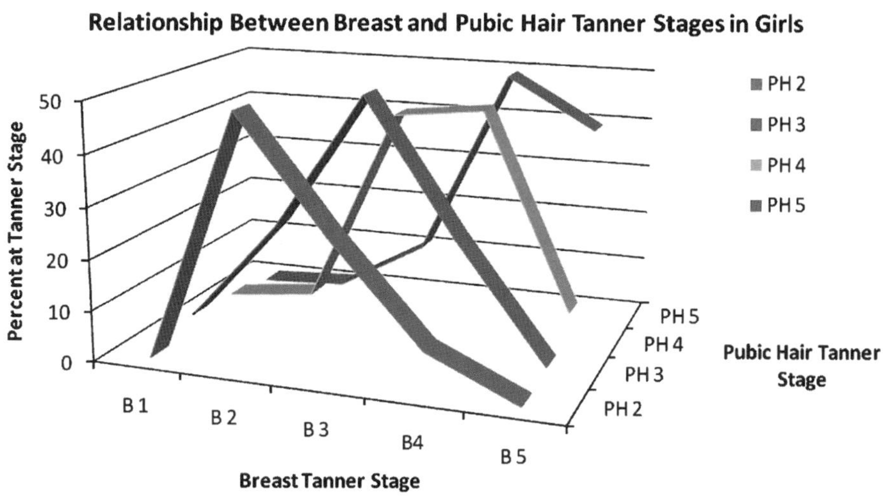

Fig. 4 Relationship between breast and pubic hair maturation in girls. Although there is a general concordance between breast and pubic hair maturation, significant variability exists. Data are from Tanner et al. (1976)

Table 4 Genital maturation in males

Stage	Physical characteristics
1	Prepubertal
2	Enlargement of the testes and scrotum, thinning and reddening of the scrotal skin, penis remains prepubertal
3	Further growth of testes and scrotum, enlargement of the penis in length and width
4	Further growth of testes and scrotum with pigmentation of the scrotal skin, further enlargement of the penis with maturation of the glans
5	Testes, scrotum, and penis are adult in size and shape

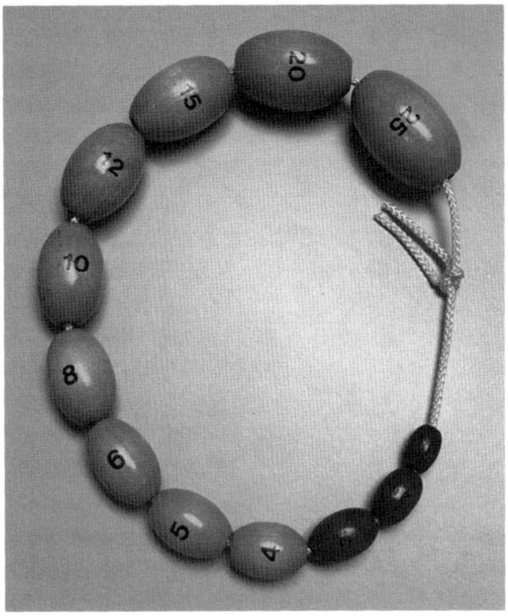

Fig. 5 The Prader orchidometer is a series of calibrated ellipsoid beads ranging from 1 mL to 25 mL in volume. Testicular volumes up to 3 mL (blue beads) are considered prepubertal. Normal adult testicular volume is 15–25 mL

size and shape of testes from prepubertal to fully adult (Fig. 5). Other available methods include rulers (semimajor and semiminor axes), calipers, and ultrasound. The normal prepubertal testis is 1–2 mL and the fully mature one 15–25 mL. One considers puberty to have begun when the testes are >3 mL. There is a rough correlation between testicular size and the Tanner stages for genital and pubic hair maturation. The common practice is to denote each parameter individually.

Pubertal Growth Spurt

The pubertal growth spurt can be divided into three stages: the stage of minimal growth velocity just before the spurt (takeoff velocity), the stage of most rapid growth or peak height velocity (PHV), and the stage of decreased velocity and cessation of growth at epiphyseal fusion. Boys reach PHV approximately 2 years later than girls and are taller at takeoff; PHV occurs at stages 3 to 4 of puberty in most boys and is completed by stage 5 in more than 95 % of boys (Largo, Gasser, Prader, Stuetzle, & Huber, 1978; Tanner, Whitehouse, Marubini, & Resele, 1976). The mean takeoff age is 11 years, and the PHV occurs at a mean age of 13.5 years in boys. The total height gain in boys between takeoff and cessation of growth is approximately of 31 cm (Abbassi, 1998). The mean height difference (boys taller than girls) between adult height men and women is 12.5 cm.

Hypothalamic-Pituitary-Gonadal Axis

In physiologically mature individuals, the secretion of gonadal steroids (testosterone in boys and estradiol in girls) is controlled by the gonadotropic hormones, luteinizing hormone (LH), and follicle-stimulating hormone (FSH), secreted by the pituitary gland. LH and FSH secretion are themselves regulated by gonadotropin-releasing hormone (GnRH) which is produced in the hypothalamus. In the adult, GnRH is secreted in tightly regulated bursts (pulses) every 60–120 min throughout the day (Knobil, 1980). This pulsatility is required for normal gonadotropin secretion and gonadal steroid production. In the circulation, estradiol and testosterone travel not only to target organs but also to the CNS, where they act to suppress production of GnRH, LH, and FSH, thus establishing a negative feedback loop.

Maturation of the HGP Axis

In the prepubertal child, the situation differs markedly from the adolescent and adult. During early infancy, the HPG axis is active, but it then becomes suppressed until the approach of puberty. This suppression is known as the juvenile pause. During this stage, GnRH and gonadotropin secretion are highly suppressed by the low concentrations of circulating gonadal steroids (Sisk & Foster, 2004). With currently available assays, the serum concentrations of testosterone and estradiol are usually unmeasurable, but they circulate at levels below those necessary for the physical changes of puberty. However, estradiol levels are sufficient to add to the growing difference in fat mass in boys and girls between the ages of approximately 6 years and the onset of the external signs of pubertal maturation. The heightened negative feedback keeps sex hormone concentrations low and prevents pubertal maturation, although GnRH continues to be produced in small, irregular, and widely spaced pulses (Sisk & Foster, 2004). Gonadotropins are also secreted, again at very low rates that may be difficult to detect in routine clinical laboratory assays.

In late childhood, before any physical evidence of puberty is present, the intensity of the negative feedback diminishes. Although the mechanism for this process is poorly understood, GnRH pulse amplitude and frequency both increase as the sensitivity to sex steroids decreases (Dunkel, Alfthan, Stenman, Tapanainen, & Perheentupa, 1990). The increased GnRH pulsatility first occurs primarily at night, with resulting diurnal variation in gonadotropin secretion and waxing and waning levels of sex hormones over the course of the day (Fig. 6). The increasing circulating sex-steroid levels directly lead to the physical and behavioral alterations noted during pubertal maturation. As puberty progresses, GnRH pulses become more consistent throughout the day, and the troughs and peaks in sex hormone concentrations tend to even out somewhat. However, the diurnal testosterone variation in boys persists into adulthood, although with a smaller day/night difference (Manasco et al., 1995). For this reason, measurement of testosterone in adolescent and young adult males is best performed in the AM, when levels tend to be at their highest. In girls, serum estradiol concentrations increase from <5 pg/mL (~18 pmol/L) before puberty up to >100 pg/mL (~370 pmol/L) in a post-menarchal girl, varying greatly over the menstrual cycle. Testosterone concentrations in prepubertal males generally are below 10 ng/dL, (~0.3 nM) and in young adults they are above 300 ng/dL (~10 nM).

Establishment of the Menstrual Cycle

During the prepubertal years, the ovaries gradually increase in size, and the number of small follicles increases (Bridges, Cooke, Healy, Hindmarsh, & Brook, 1993; Peters, Byskov, & Grinsted, 1978). In response to increased GnRH pulses primarily during the nighttime, gonadotropin secretion increases, particularly FSH. The increased serum concentration of FSH leads to increased follicular recruitment. Acting via its receptor, LH promotes androgen production, primarily androstenedione, from the ovarian thecal cells. FSH stimulates aromatase activity in the granulosa cells and leads to estradiol production. Before menarche, estradiol levels peak approximately 12 h after the diurnal peaks in gonadotropin secretion (Norjavaara, Ankarberg, & Albertsson-Wikland, 1996).

As puberty progresses, a cyclic pattern emerges in estradiol secretion (Rosenfield, Cooke, & Radovick, 2008). In this setting, estradiol comes from the small antral follicles developing midway through pubertal maturation. As estradiol concentrations increase and promote endometrial proliferation, anovulatory bleeding may occur following cyclic declines in estradiol. True ovulatory cycles do not begin until after the HPG axis matures to the point at which the mid-cycle LH surge takes place.

Endocrine Regulation of the Menstrual Cycle

Before ovulation (the follicular phase), gradually increasing FSH and LH production prompt the recruitment of small follicles, which begin to secrete estradiol. With increasing stimulation, the follicle with the greatest FSH sensitivity becomes dominant and begins to produce progesterone as well as additional estradiol. Estradiol causes proliferation of the endometrial lining of the uterus. Although in boys, sex steroids consistently have a suppressive effect on GnRH and gonadotropin secretion, such is not the case for girls. In the mid-part of the menstrual cycle, increasing serum concentrations of estradiol, acting synergistically with progesterone, cause a dramatic increase in LH secretion, with levels approaching 60 IU/L. In the dominant (ovulatory) follicle, alterations in gene transcription in response to the LH surge result in the formation of inflammatory mediators and disruption of cellular integrity, causing rupture of the follicle and ovulation (Russell & Robker, 2007). After ovulation (the luteal phase), estradiol concentrations initially decline, but as the

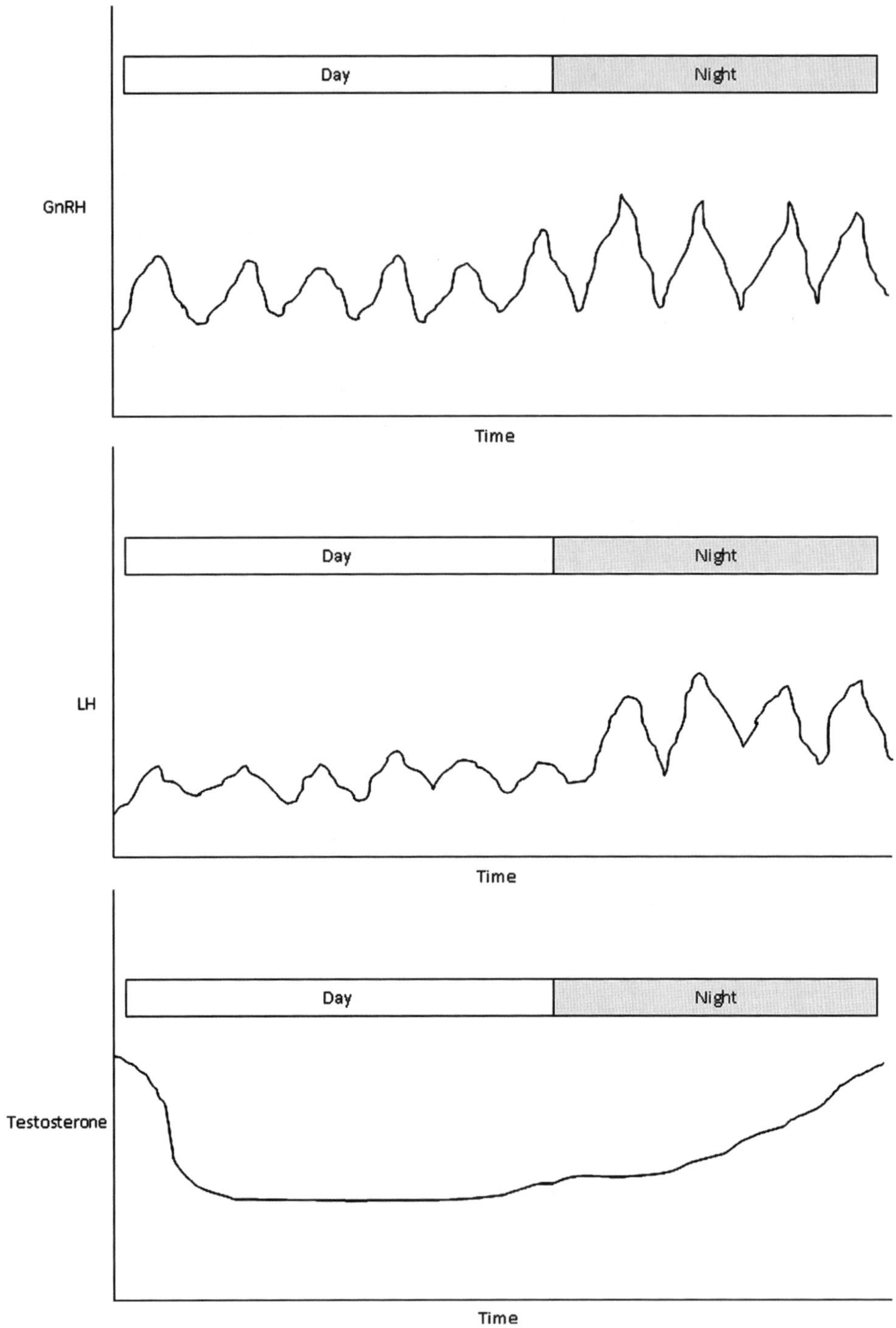

Fig. 6 GnRH, LH, and testosterone secretion in the early to mid-pubertal adolescent boy. GnRH is secreted in a pulsatile manner, with parallel pulses of LH release. The pulse amplitudes of both GnRH and LH increase at night, resulting in a gradual rise in serum testosterone concentrations as the night progresses. Testosterone peaks in the morning, and levels decline during the day

corpus luteum forms, both estradiol and progesterone levels increase, resulting in endometrial maturation. In the absence of embryonal hCG, however, the corpus luteum has a limited lifespan, and hormone production declines. With falling estradiol and progesterone levels, the endometrium becomes ischemic and sloughs off, resulting in menstrual bleeding. The high FSH levels observed during the follicular phase and at the end of the luteal phase cause the initial recruitment of another wave of small follicles, one of which will become the dominant follicle 2½ cycles later (Gougeon, 1996).

Regulation of Pubertal Timing

The timing of puberty is a complex trait, and in the general population, it has a Gaussian distribution. There are many influences on the regulation of pubertal timing, including nutritional factors, environmental influences, and genetic input. Complex traits often demonstrate a high degree of genetic regulation, and it is estimated that between 50 and 80 % of the variance of normal pubertal timing is explained by genetic factors (Palmert & Boepple, 2001). Efforts to understand the genetics of pubertal timing have led to the discovery of many genes that are clearly necessary for pubertal maturation. Many of these, when mutated, cause specific syndromes of delayed or absent puberty. However, it is not clear that these genes individually or as a group explain much of the variability of the onset of *normal* puberty.

In 2003, the kisspeptin/GPR54 system was discovered. It is a key regulatory system in the initiation of increased GnRH pulsatility at the onset of puberty (Seminara et al., 2003). Kisspeptin is produced by hypothalamic neurons and interacts with its receptor, GPR54, on GnRH-secreting neurons. In humans, inactivating mutations are associated with pubertal delay, and an activating mutation has led to precocious puberty (Teles et al., 2008). Exogenous administration of kisspeptin increases the pulse amplitude of GnRH. Short-term administration of kisspeptin to healthy male and female volunteers increases gonadotropin concentrations, although chronic dosing appears to induce tachyphylaxis (Dhillo et al., 2005, 2007; Jayasena et al., 2009). The kisspeptin/GPR54 system may also be involved in the negative and positive feedback effects of sex steroids on GnRH secretion. Although it is clear that kisspeptin plays a role upstream of GnRH, the factors regulating its release are not presently fully understood (Kauffman, Clifton, & Steiner, 2007).

Both inhibitory and stimulatory factors in the central nervous system are involved in the initiation of puberty. Gamma-aminobutyric acid (GABA)-secreting neurons play an inhibitory role and may be involved in the temporary suppression of the HPG axis during childhood. Suppression of GABAergic neuronal input may lead to the initiation of puberty (Terasawa & Fernandez, 2001). Additional factors may include increased glutamate stimulation of *N*-methyl-D-aspartate (NMDA) receptors, which are stimulatory to GnRH release, and neuropeptide Y-expressing neuron activity (Gamba & Pralong, 2006). Leptin, acting through its receptor, links nutritional status to puberty, and sufficient levels of leptin are thought to be required to initiate puberty (Farooqi et al., 2002).

Role of Energy Balance in Pubertal Maturation and the Menstrual Cycle

One must have sufficient energy to support body growth and to store energy, predominantly as fat, for longer-term energy requirements such as the menstrual cycle, pregnancy, and lactation (Loucks, 2007). Thus, energy availability is one of the factors that contribute to the regulation of timing of puberty and the menstrual cycle. Energy availability is defined as the difference between energy intake and energy expenditure, and it may be decreased by either lowering food intake or increasing caloric expenditure through exercise. Loss of energy availability leads to alterations in puberty and the menstrual cycle by decreasing the frequency of GnRH pulses, thus lowering mean serum levels of gonadotropins, decreasing ovarian follicle formation, and decreasing estradiol secretion (Gordon, 2010). This phenomenon may be mediated by loss of body fat and decreases in circulating leptin, considered permissive for normal hypothalamic-pituitary-ovarian activity. Younger women and adolescents are particularly prone to hypothalamic amenorrhea as a result of decreased energy availability. Loss of energy availability is reflected clinically by decreases in percent body fat and, to a lesser extent, body weight and BMI. In athletes, weight and BMI may not accurately reflect body fat stores due to the higher density of muscle. Restoration of energy availability results in increased body weight. Return of body weight to >90 % of ideal usually, but not always, results in resumption of menses in amenorrheic patients (Golden et al., 1997). Whether weight loss occurs from excessive exercise or by severe caloric restriction, as seen in starvation and anorexia nervosa, the hypothalamic effects appear the same.

Hypothalamic-Pituitary Axis for Growth Hormone/IGF-1

Growth hormone release is intermittent ("burst-like" or pulsatile) at all ages and is magnified in low energy states, such as malnutrition (Soliman et al., 1986) and anorexia nervosa (Argente et al., 1997; Scacchi et al., 1997). Once a regular day/night cycle is established, there is a major burst of GH release 45–90 min following the onset of deep sleep (Martha, Gorman, Blizzard, Rogol, & Veldhuis, 1992). Generally, more than 75 % of the total daily production of GH accompanies sleep during the nighttime hours. However, this amount is dampened to a variable degree by the amount of body fat and its distribution in the subcutaneous vs. abdominal/visceral regions. There are significant increases in GH release during the newborn period, possibly related to a state of transient nutritional insufficiency (see Anorexia Nervosa, below) (Wright, Northington, Miller, Veldhuis, & Rogol, 1992) and more marked increases during adolescence (see below) (Martha et al., 1992).

Changes in GH release during pubertal maturation are large. There is an approximately threefold increase in the amount of GH released, which translates into a similar increase in serum IGF-I concentrations (Martha et al., 1992; Martha, Rogol, Veldhuis, & Blizzard, 1996; Roemmich et al., 1998). These increases are tied to the rising levels of sex steroids, but toward the end of pubertal maturation the GH secretory alterations return virtually to the prepubertal state (Kerrigan & Rogol, 1992). Variation in body composition and the regional distribution of fatness also influence GH release during puberty and into adulthood (Roemmich et al., 1998; Roemmich & Rogol, 1999; Veldhuis et al., 2005; Veldhuis, Roemmich, & Rogol, 2000).

Hypogonadism and Delayed Puberty

Constitutional Delay of Growth and Puberty

Constitutional delay of growth and puberty is a very frequent variant of normal pubertal maturation. Pubertal maturation is pathological if it has not started by 14 or 15 years of age (Styne & Grumbach, 2008). However, it is unlikely that the boy or his family would wait until that time for evaluation. When a boy presents for evaluation of delayed puberty it is more likely due to perceived psychosocial issues than those of growth or sexual maturation. Therefore, the precise incidence is undefined, perhaps because a majority of the boys do not come to medical evaluation. It is likely that only a minority are referred to an endocrinologist.

Constitutional delay of growth and puberty is characterized by a slowing of the growth rate (preadolescent dip), as well as by a delay in the timing and, perhaps, *tempo* of pubertal maturation. The patients are typically boys who seek medical evaluation in their early teenage years as they become aware of the discrepancy in linear growth and adolescent maturation compared with their age peers. Clinically, these boys have a height age (the age at which the patient's height would be at the 50th centile) that is delayed but often concordant with the bone age, meaning that the height potential is normal. Sexual maturation lags behind that of the peers, and there is likely to be a family history of other "late bloomers."

The suppressed HPG axis in children with CDGP represents an extension of the physiological hypogonadotropic hypogonadism present since infancy. Without intervention, most will undergo normal pubertal maturation spontaneously and most, but not all, will nearly reach their genetically determined mid-parental height (Crowne, Shalet, Wallace, Eminson, & Price, 1990). Pubertal maturation is likely to occur several years later than that of their peers. Many adolescents suffer significant emotional distress because they differ in their appearance from their peers during these years. Androgen therapy was initially proposed for boys with CDGP to alleviate their psychological discomfort, in addition to the beneficial effects on bone mineral accrual, lean body mass, protein metabolism, and the regional distribution of body fat.

Psychological benefits of treatment were examined in the Oakland Growth Study (Gross & Duke, 1980), in which 16 early- and 16 late-maturing boys were followed from age 11 years until adulthood. Multiple behavioral and social characteristics were assessed by peer ratings, adult perceptions, and psychological projective tests. The late-maturing boys were characterized as less mature, less attractive, and more talkative than young boys. As adolescents, the late-maturing boys expressed more feelings of inadequacy and rejection, and needed more social acceptance. Many of these traits persisted into adulthood. The National Health Examinations Survey found that pubertally delayed boys had lower teacher ratings of intellectual ability, lower intellectual test scores, and lower parental expectations for educational achievement than normally maturing boys in all age groups from 13 to 17 years (Duke et al., 1982). This makes a strong case for aggressive therapy in boys with CDGP, especially older ones. Other studies have shown no significant residual effects of delayed puberty; however, retrospectively, many of those not treated wished that they had received treatment. Despite these conflicting studies, the authors recognize that the majority of boys are anxious to begin androgen therapy and are generally pleased with the results, albeit subtle, even after 3 months of therapy with 50–75 mg long-acting testosterone esters per month. Their reasons to begin therapy fall into the appearance (too young), social (not considered a peer), and athletic (cannot compete because of size and lack of strength) spheres.

Pathologic Causes of Hypogonadism (Table 5)

Central Hypogonadism

Traumatic Brain Injury

Traumatic brain injury (TBI) affects a growing number of children and adolescents, with an incidence of at least 180–250 per 100,000 children each year and with infants/toddlers and adolescents being the most commonly affected (Bruns & Hauser, 2003; Langlois, Rutland-Brown, & Thomas, 2005). Disordered pituitary function, especially for the GH and HPG axes, is prevalent in adult survivors of TBI (Agha et al., 2004; Agha, Sherlock, Phillips, Tormey, & Thompson, 2005; Aimaretti et al., 2004, 2005; Leal-Cerro et al., 2005), but has only recently been reported in children and adolescents in case-reports and case-series (Einaudi et al., 2006; Niederland et al., 2007; Poomthavorn, Maixner, & Zacharin, 2008).

Among abnormalities in pituitary function after TBI in children, growth hormone deficiency (GHD) appears the most common (Einaudi et al., 2006; Niederland et al., 2007; Poomthavorn et al., 2008). GHD not only may affect linear growth but also has been implicated in lipid abnormalities and body composition alterations in children and adolescents (Boot, Engels, Boerma, Krenning, & De Muinck Keizer-Schrama, 1997; Gleeson et al., 2007; Hulthen et al., 2001; Roemmich, Huerta, Sundaresan, & Rogol, 2001) and associated with cognitive impairments and poor recovery from TBI (Bavisetty et al., 2008; Behan, Phillips, Thompson, & Agha, 2008; Bondanelli et al., 2007; Kelly et al., 2006; Popovic et al., 2004). Knowledge of the associated features of GHD after TBI in children and adolescents may improve the ability of treating physicians to recognize and refer patients suspected of having pituitary abnormalities, especially GHD, for appropriate diagnostic evaluation and treatment.

Table 5 Pathologic causes of hypogonadism

Hypogonadotropic hypogonadism
Traumatic brain injury
Hyperprolactinemia
Exercising adolescent and adult women (female athlete triad)
Anorexia nervosa
Infiltrative and inflammatory diseases of the hypothalamus and pituitary
Pituitary
Granulomatous
Sarcoidosis
Histiocytosis
Metastasis (rare in adolescence)
Breast
Lung
Gastrointestinal tract
Hypophysitis
Lymphocytic (especially postpartum)
Xanthomatous
Lipid-laden macrophages
Hypothalamus
Histiocytosis
Sarcoidosis
Infectious (multiple pathogens)
Combined pituitary hormone deficiencies (with gonadotropin deficiency)
Multiple causes
Isolated hormone abnormalities
Kallmann syndrome and normosmic idiopathic hypogonadotropic hypogonadism
KAL1 mutation
GPR54/kisspeptin mutation
Fibroblast growth factor receptor 1 mutation
GnRH mutation
GnRHR mutation
Hypergonadotropic hypogonadism
Congenital hypergonadotropic hypogonadism
Disorders of sex chromosome number
47,XXY (Klinefelter syndrome) and its variants
45,X (Turner syndrome) and its variants
47,XXX
XY and XX gonadal dysgenesis
Complete androgen insensitivity syndrome
Galactosemia
Resistance to gonadotropins
Acquired hypergonadotropic hypogonadism
Radiation exposure
Chemotherapy
Trauma
Infection
Autoimmune oophoritis

To date, there have been few prospective studies that assess for GHD in children and adolescents who have sustained a TBI (Einaudi et al., 2006; Kaulfers et al., 2010). The former was only partially prospective and showed a much lower incidence of hypopituitarism (~30 %) than some of the retrospective studies. The latter showed a varying incidence, 15 % at 1 month, 75 % at 6 months, but 29 % at 1 year. After 12 months only 5 % had GH deficiency. Our preliminary data indicate that GH deficiency is found in ~16 % of children and adolescents who sustained moderate-to-severe head trauma (Norwood et al., 2010). Those with GH deficiency exhibited more rapid weight gain following injury than those with a normal GH/IGF-I axis (~25 kg/year vs. ~0 kg/year).

Prolactin

Abnormalities of prolactin (PRL) secretion are well-known causes of disordered puberty and reproductive function. PRL is produced in the anterior pituitary gland. It is unique among the pituitary hormones in that it is secreted tonically and undergoes inhibition by hypothalamic dopamine release, rather than being secreted only after stimulation by a trophic hormone as are most anterior pituitary hormones. Additional physiologic factors influencing PRL secretion include estradiol and thyrotropin-releasing hormone.

At physiologic concentrations, PRL acts to increase milk production in lactating women and also stimulates mammary gland development during puberty; however, PRL does not appear to influence normal breast maturation during puberty. Pathologically elevated PRL concentrations have a suppressive effect on GnRH secretion, thus decreasing LH and FSH levels and leading to insufficient production of estradiol in females and testosterone in males. In adolescents, these endocrine changes manifest as delayed or arrested pubertal maturation or primary or secondary amenorrhea in females. Males may have additional evidence of decreased testosterone, including decreased libido, erectile dysfunction, or infertility. Hyperprolactinemia is associated with gynecomastia in males, not as a result of direct stimulation of breast growth but due to hypogonadism and a decrease in the androgen/

estrogen ratio. Galactorrhea, or milky breast discharge, may occur as a symptom or sign of hyperprolactinemia. This finding occurs in about 50 % of female patients and 35 % of males (Melmed & Kleinberg, 2008).

Hyperprolactinemia may be detected in a variety of conditions. Most commonly, it is a result of treatment with one of many medications. These include agents used to treat neurologic or psychiatric conditions, including anticonvulsants (phenytoin), selective serotonin reuptake inhibitors (fluoxetine), tricyclic antidepressants (amitriptyline), opiates (methadone), phenothiazines (chlorpromazine), and other medications known to decrease the actions of dopamine and serotonin (olanzapine, risperidone). Hyperprolactinemia may also occur in association with polycystic ovary syndrome, hypothyroidism, and renal failure. Central nervous system causes include conditions that prevent normal dopamine inhibition of PRL secretion, such as traumatic, neoplastic, or inflammatory injury of the pituitary stalk. Pituitary tumors may cause hyperprolactinemia, either from direct secretion of PRL from the tumor (prolactinoma) or from compression of the surrounding gland from a non-PRL-secreting pituitary adenoma.

Prolactinomas are the most commonly identified functional pituitary tumors, with an annual incidence of 6/100,000 and a prevalence of 10 per 100,000 in the general population (Colao & Lombardi, 1998). In the pediatric and adolescent age group, prolactinomas make up about 50 % of all pituitary adenomas (Colao, 2009). They occur far more commonly in females, especially during adolescence. Prolactinomas are divided into two classes: microprolactinomas, measuring ≤10 mm diameter, and macroprolactinomas, measuring >10 mm. Macroprolactinomas typically secrete more PRL, and serum concentrations typically are >200 ng/mL. Patients with microprolactinomas usually have PRL levels between 50 and 200 ng/mL. Serum PRL concentrations <100 ng/mL typically occur with non-tumoral causes of hyperprolactinemia, but may occasionally occur in association with small microprolactinomas.

Measurement of a serum PRL level is a standard part of the evaluation of delayed puberty, amenorrhea, or oligomenorrhea. If elevated, magnetic resonance imaging of the head should be the next step, particularly if the concentration is high or if there is no other explanation. Treatment of hyperprolactinemia is indicated if sexual or reproductive function is impaired or if galactorrhea is problematic. Treatment involves removal of the offending agent if possible. Prolactinomas are usually treated with dopamine agonists, such as bromocriptine or cabergoline. Surgical therapy is rarely indicated.

Female Athlete Triad

Adolescent girls and young women who participate in physical activities and sports, especially those that emphasize a lean physique, may be prone to disordered eating, primary or secondary amenorrhea, and low bone mineral density (osteopenia or frank osteoporosis), denoted collectively as the female athlete triad. Although core functions are maintained until the lowest levels of energy availability, some of the less immediately necessary processes, e.g., growth and reproductive function, are diminished. Thus, some aspects of the body's adaptation to low energy availability tend to restore energy balance and promote survival but impair health.

The evidence for this disorder comes from a number of studies in young adult women (see ACSM statement for review, Nattiv et al., 2007) but clearly is relevant to the maturing adolescent, for whom there is strong evidence that the hypothalamic-pituitary-end organ axes are more susceptible to perturbation by a low energy balance, than in the more mature young woman. (Loucks, 2006) An elegant series of experiments done by Dr. Anne Loucks and her associates has likely determined the pathophysiologic basis for at least the disordered HPG axis physiology in women with the female athlete triad and also perhaps the underlying heightened susceptibility in the adolescent athlete (Loucks, 2006; Loucks & Thuma, 2003). If the energy availability is insufficient to support physiologic processes after the energy expenditure of athletic training, then there is less energy available for cellular maintenance, thermoregulation, growth, and reproduction (Wade, Schneider, & Li, 1996).

The health-related consequences of a deficit of energy output compared to intake are poten-

Table 6 Guidelines for assuring safe and healthy sports participation for children and adolescents

Dietary practices; exercise intensity, duration, and frequency; and menstrual history should be reviewed during evaluations that precede participation in sports
Amenorrhea should not be considered a normal response to exercise. That is, the underlying cause should be sought before denoting it as "athletic amenorrhea" in these gynecologically young women
Disordered eating should be considered in adolescents with amenorrhea
Education and counseling should be provided to athletes, parents, and coaches regarding disordered eating, menstrual dysfunction, decreased bone mineralization, and adequate energy and nutrient intake to meet energy expenditure and maintain normal growth and development
An adolescent with menstrual dysfunction attributed to exercise should be encouraged to increase energy intake and to modify excessive exercise activity to return to energy balance
Estrogen-progesterone supplementation may be considered in mature amenorrheic (late adolescent) athletes
Measurement of bone mineral density and level of 25-hydroxyvitamin D should be considered tools to help make treatment decisions. The adolescent athlete is unlikely to have reached peak bone mass, and thus, it is appropriate to use age-adjusted Z-scores rather than T-scores

Modified in part from the American Academy of Pediatrics, Committee on Sports Medicine and Fitness, 1999–2000, with relevance to the female athlete triad

tially irreversible and the operative imperative is to prevent the consequences by early diagnosis and appropriate treatment. Except for stress fractures, the consequences are most often delayed in time, and are mediated by failure to accrue an appropriate peak bone mass, causing osteoporosis of greater severity and at younger ages than in the general population. The likely pathogenesis is that low energy availability directly impairs bone health and maturation by suppressing the hormones that promote bone formation. Indirectly, low energy availability leads to primary or secondary amenorrhea, removing estrogen's restraint on bone resorption. Bone mineral accrual is diminished for a long enough interval to develop wide-ranging deficits in bone mineral content.

Similarly, there is significant variability in the sensitivity of the hypothalamic-pituitary-gonadal axis suppression by energy deficits, thus failing to preserve body growth and energy storage for longer-term energy requirements such as the menstrual cycle, pregnancy, and lactation (Nattiv et al., 2007). In addition, the hypothalamic-pituitary-thyroid axis is altered to preserve energy (Nattiv et al., 2007).

Treatment of the female athlete triad is often difficult. The most direct approaches are to prescribe greater caloric intake or to decrease exercise energy expenditure. These are difficult for a highly competitive athlete, likely a gymnast, dancer, or long-distance runner. The American Academy of Pediatrics Committee of Sports Medicine and Fitness, 1999–2000, has presented a series of recommendations. Those relevant to the female athlete triad are shown in Table 6.

Table 7 Diagnostic criteria for anorexia nervosa

Refusal to maintain weight within a normal range for height and age (<85% of ideal body weight)
Intense *fear of becoming fat* or gaining weight, even though underweight
Severe body disturbance—weight or shape impacts greatly sense of self-worth with denial of the seriousness of the illness
Amenorrhea (either primary or secondary) with the absence of at least three consecutive menstrual cycles due to lack of estrogen

Diagnostic and statistical manual of mental disorders, 4th edition. (DSM-IV). Washington, DC. American Psychiatric Association 1994:544–545

Anorexia Nervosa

In western cultures anorexia nervosa affects approximately 0.6 % of adolescent girls (Stice, Marti, Shaw, & Jaconis, 2009). The DSM-IV cri-

Table 8 Systemic abnormalities related to the endocrine system in subjects with anorexia nervosa

Delayed puberty
Oligo/amenorrhea
Hypothyroidism
Hypercortisolism
Impaired growth
Polyuria
Defective thermogenesis with sensitivity to cold temperatures
Electrolyte abnormalities Hypokalemia Hypophosphatemia Hypomagnesemia
Osteopenia/osteoporosis
Decreased metabolic rate
Decreased fat mass
Alterations in appetite-regulating factors Leptin NPY PYY Melanocortins CRH

Table 9 Circulating levels of some hormones in subjects with anorexia nervosa

Endocrine axis	Hormone abnormalities
Hypothalamic-pituitary-gonadal axis	↓ or inappropriately low gonadotropins ↓ sex steroids
GH/IGF-I axis	↑ GH ↓ IGF-I Consistent with GH resistance
Hypothalamic-pituitary-adrenal axis	↑ CRH ↑ ACTH ↑cortisol Consistent with "stress response," diurnal variation preserved
Hypothalamic-pituitary-thyroid axis	↓ T_3 ↓ or normal T_4 Normal TSH Consistent with the low T_3 syndrome and preferential deiodination of T_4 to rT_3
Vasopressin system	↓ secretion of vasopressin Consistent with partial diabetes insipidus

teria for the diagnosis are listed in Table 7. Systemic abnormalities and endocrinopathies related to the endocrine system in patients with anorexia nervosa are shown in Tables 8 and 9.

Other Causes of Central Hypogonadism

Central hypogonadism may be due to one of a rapidly expanding group of genetic conditions affecting development of the HPG axis. The prototypic genetic condition causing abnormal pubertal maturation is Kallmann syndrome (KS). This is an association between anosmia or hyposmia and central hypogonadism. The first gene identified to cause KS was the KAL1 gene, located on the X chromosome. The KAL1 gene encodes a neural cell adhesion molecule required for the migration of both olfactory and GnRH neurons (Legouis et al., 1991). Affected individuals classically have a lifelong impairment of their sense of smell, but usually come to medical attention when they fail to enter puberty. Questioning patients with pubertal delay about their ability to smell may establish the diagnosis clinically. Since the identification of the KAL1 gene, mutations in other genes have been identified in patients with Kallmann syndrome (Bianco & Kaiser, 2009) .

Interestingly, affected KS patients may have family members with central hypogonadism but a normal sense of smell, termed normosmic isolated hypogonadotropic hypogonadism (nIHH). The variable presence of anosmia/hyposmia may also be seen in other genetic defects leading to KS and/or nIHH, including abnormalities of FGFR1, PROK2, and PROK2R (Bianco & Kaiser, 2009).

Several genetic conditions cause nIHH alone, including defects of kisspeptin and its receptor, GPR54; GnRH and its receptor; and leptin and its receptor. Defects of the genes for neurokinin B and its receptor also lead to nIHH. Affected patients with abnormalities of these genes (TAC3 and TAC3R) have occasionally experienced partial or complete recovery of endocrine function during their adult years when observed following sex-steroid treatment. Defective TAC3/TAC3R genes may comprise up to 5 % of subjects with nIHH (Gianetti et al., 2010).

Primary Hypogonadism

Primary hypogonadism refers to a group of conditions in which the hypothalamus and pituitary are intact but there is a defect in the testis or ovary that leads to inadequate gonadal function. This may be difficult to distinguish clinically from central hypogonadism, as patients with either condition have low circulating levels of testosterone or estradiol. Low testosterone secretion in pubertal boys causes poor genital growth, lack of progression of pubic hair growth, and decreased muscle development and linear growth. In older adolescent males who have already progressed through puberty, hypogonadism of any cause may lead to loss of libido, gynecomastia, erectile dysfunction, and decreased body hair. In girls with hypogonadism, breast maturation may be absent or nonprogressive, linear growth may be slow, and primary amenorrhea may be present. Girls with isolated hypogonadism typically have normal pubic and axillary hair, as these occur under the influence of adrenal androgens. Older adolescents with newly developed hypogonadism may experience oligo- or amenorrhea, hot flashes, and reduction of breast volume. Primary hypogonadism is easily distinguished from central hypogonadism in the laboratory, however. Causes of primary hypogonadism lead to elevations of one or both gonadotropins, while these are typically low or normal in cases of central hypogonadism.

Causes of Primary Hypogonadism

Radiation Exposure

Both testicular and ovarian tissues are highly radiosensitive, and gonadal failure is a frequent long-term sequela of cancer treatment. However, because of the differing physiology, the effects of exposure to low doses of radiation differ in boys and girls. Within both testes and ovaries, germ cells are more sensitive to radiation effects than stromal cells. At low radiation doses in boys, germ cell loss occurs, but Leydig cell function may be maintained. Because Leydig cells are the source of testosterone, radiation doses under 20–30 Gy may cause infertility in boys but preserved sex hormone production. The prepubertal testis may be more radioresistant than adult testes (Shalet, Tsatsoulis, Whitehead, & Read, 1989). Higher radiation doses damage Leydig cells and lead to both reproductive and endocrine dysfunction.

In contrast, low-dose radiation exposure in girls is more likely to cause both infertility and estrogen deficiency. This is because estradiol production is intimately linked to follicle formation around germ cells, and loss of these germ cells prevents normal estrogen secretion. Girls are born with a limited number of germ cells that declines throughout the lifespan. Hence, younger prepubertal girls have a higher stockpile of oocytes, and a given amount of radiation exposure does not deplete them as much as radiation exposure in an adolescent or adult. Radiation exposure in doses above 18 Gy in a 5-year-old prepubertal girl uniformly leads to sterility, while doses above 15 Gy consistently lead to sterility in 20-year-olds (Wallace, Thomson, Saran, & Kelsey, 2005).

Chemotherapy

Chemotherapy is associated with decreased fertility in both sexes. Alkylating agents are associated with the highest rates of gonadal injury (Howell & Shalet, 1998). Examples of this class of chemotherapy include cyclophosphamide, ifosfamide, procarbazine, chlorambucil, and busulfan. Because these agents damage germ cells, females are more likely to develop sex hormone deficiency than males, as germ cells are required for estrogen synthesis in girls but not for testosterone synthesis in boys. Higher dose protocols are more likely to cause gonadal injury than lower dose regimens.

In pubertal children undergoing cancer treatment, fertility preservation should be considered. In pubertal boys, this usually requires collection and freezing of semen. Preservation of fertility in girls is more problematic. While embryo freezing is commonly practiced, this is not typically feasible in adolescent girls. Both cryopreservation of ovarian tissue and collection and freezing of oocytes after ovarian stimulation are clinically available in some areas and should be discussed with the adolescent and her family.

Other Causes of Primary Hypogonadism

In addition to radiation exposure and chemotherapy, causes of acquired hypogonadism include trauma or vascular compromise of testes and less commonly ovaries; autoimmune oophoritis, either isolated or as part of type I autoimmune polyglandular syndrome; galactosemia in females; and rarely viral infections. Many genetic etiologies of congenital primary hypogonadism exist, often related to disorders of sex chromosome number or function. In boys, these include Klinefelter syndrome (47,XXY and variants), and in girls Turner syndrome (45,X and variants), deletion of Xq, 47,XXX syndrome, XX and XY complete gonadal dysgenesis, and complete androgen insensitivity syndrome.

Distinguishing Between Delayed and Absent Puberty in Boys and Girls

Although signs of puberty usually become apparent before age 14 years in boys and 13 years in girls, delays are common but are usually not medically significant. Particularly in boys, constitutional delay of growth and puberty is very prevalent, especially when the family history is positive. A challenge arises, however, when spontaneous puberty does not occur after a reasonable period of time. It is difficult to distinguish the "physiologic hypogonadism" of constitutional delay from pathologic causes of central hypogonadism. Anosmia or hyposmia points to Kallmann syndrome, and a history of CNS disease will suggest a permanent impairment of the HPG axis. In the otherwise healthy adolescent, however, nIHH often presents as constitutional delay. Laboratory and radiographic findings may be helpful but not diagnostic. Testosterone levels that are low for the stage of puberty or do not increase over time suggest central hypogonadism, as do concentrations of LH in the adult range with relatively low testosterone production. Teens with constitutional delay usually have delayed bone maturation as assessed by a bone age radiograph, and a normal bone age in the setting of delayed puberty suggests a pathologic diagnosis. Advanced laboratory testing, including measurement of ultrasensitive LH (Sequera et al., 2002), morning testosterone concentrations, administration of GnRH or GnRH agonists (Street et al., 2002), or human chorionic gonadotropin administration (Degros, Cortet-Rudelli, Soudan, & Dewailly, 2003) have all been evaluated, but none offers high degrees of sensitivity or specificity and a conveniently performed study. More recently, a combination approach has been effective, but the high cost and testing burden make this unfeasible (Segal, Mehta, Anazodo, Hindmarsh, & Dattani, 2009).

Treatment of Delayed and Absent Puberty in Boys and Girls

A detailed discussion of the hormonal induction of puberty is beyond the scope of this text. Boys, and rarely girls, with presumed constitutional delay of growth and puberty often receive courses of low-dose sex steroids in an attempt to promote the early stages of puberty and possibly accelerate the onset of endogenous sex hormone production. If low doses are used, this is unlikely to suppress endogenous puberty or accelerate skeletal maturation.

If central hypogonadism is suspected in either sex, estrogen or testosterone administration as appropriate begins at relatively low doses, with gradual increases over the span of several years, the goal being to attain adult serum concentrations at an appropriate age. Testosterone is typically initiated using depot injectable preparations, the doses of which can be customized for adolescents. Although oral, buccal, and transdermal preparations are available, these are usually formulated for adult replacement and are not suitable for pubertal induction.

In girls, estrogen may be administered in the form of oral micronized estradiol, estradiol esters, or conjugated estrogens. Transdermal preparations have become more widely used in recent years with the availability of low-dose patches that generate physiologic estradiol concentrations, avoid hepatic first pass effects, and may reduce some of the long-term risks of estrogen replacement therapy.

Outcomes of Children with Delayed Puberty

Boys and girls with delayed puberty are short relative to their peers due to the absence of a sex-steroid-mediated growth spurt, thus appearing younger than their classmates. Additionally, they appear much younger due to the lack of pubertal maturation. After entering spontaneous or induced puberty, however, affected individuals are not distinguishable from their peers in terms of their sexual maturation. Long-term studies of boys and girls with delayed puberty have shown that their adult heights typically reach the levels predicted during adolescence. However, these adult heights are usually less than expected based on their family backgrounds (Crowne, Shalet, Wallace, Eminson, & Price, 1991; Poyrazoglu et al., 2005). The lower adult height is due to a combination of factors, including short stature at the onset of puberty, a relatively small amount of height gained during the pubertal growth spurt, and a relatively small amount of spinal growth (Poyrazoglu).

Long-term studies of adult men with constitutional delay of puberty demonstrate decreased bone mineral density at the wrist and spine (Finkelstein, Neer, Biller, Crawford, & Klibanski, 1992). Similar findings have been noted in women with delayed menarche and hypothalamic amenorrhea, even in the presence of exercise (Warren et al., 2002). Children with other causes of hypogonadism in adolescence also have decreases in bone density (Galli-Tsinopoulou, Nousia-Arvanitakis, Mitsiakos, Karamouzis, & Dimitriadis, 2000; Petraroli et al., 2007). These findings make earlier treatment with sex steroids an important clinical consideration.

Children with delayed puberty often experience emotional difficulty, presumably related to the difference in their physical appearance compared to peers (Mazur & Clopper, 1991; Mobbs, 2005). Psychological effects of delayed puberty are more marked in adolescence and tend to diminish as the individuals enter adulthood (Crowne et al., 1991), although some problems may persist (Mazur & Clopper, 1991). Treatment with sex steroids improves some of the psychological abnormalities in girls and boys, with minimal effects on mood and behavior problems (Schwab et al., 2001; Susman et al., 1998).

Precocious Puberty

Definition

Precocious puberty may be defined as pubertal changes occurring before the age of 8 years in girls and before 9 years in boys. Many studies over the last 10 years, however, suggest that girls may be experiencing the earliest changes of puberty at younger ages than previously (Freedman et al., 2002; Herman-Giddens et al., 1997; Wattigney, Srinivasan, Chen, Greenlund, & Berenson, 1999). The reason for this is unclear, but may be related to the increasing prevalence of obesity in children (Kaplowitz, Slora, Wasserman, Pedlow, & Herman-Giddens, 2001; Wattigney et al., 1999). Additionally, there are clear differences in the timing of puberty among certain racial and ethnic groups. Previous studies typically cited in support of the lower limit of normal for puberty being 8 years included homogenous populations of middle class white girls, while more recent studies included African American and Hispanic girls, who often demonstrate signs of puberty at earlier ages than white girls, irrespective of body weight (Rosenfield et al., 2009). While there is some evidence that boys also may be entering puberty at younger ages (Herman-Giddens, Wang, & Koch, 2001; Juul, Magnusdottir, Scheike, Prytz, & Skakkebaek,

2007), the lower limit of 9 years continues to be generally accepted.

Precocious puberty is much more common in girls than boys. The first symptoms typically mirror those of normal pubertal maturation. Hence, in girls the first evidence of precocious puberty is usually breast maturation, which may be slowly or rapidly progressive. In boys, testicular enlargement is usually the first sign of pubertal maturation. Pubic hair growth typically follows in both sexes, although there are exceptions. Affected children usually have rapid height gain due to a pubertal growth spurt. In addition to pubic hair, boys and girls may have other signs of androgen production, such as facial acne, axillary hair, and adult body odor. In advanced cases, girls may develop a physiologic vaginal discharge or may have vaginal bleeding. Alternatively, some children may have variant forms of precocious puberty featuring isolated and nonprogressive breast or pubic hair growth as discussed below.

Etiologies of Precocious Puberty

The etiologies of precocious puberty may be separated into two categories based on how sex hormone secretion is regulated. The term "central precocious puberty" (CPP) refers to puberty that is regulated by the hypothalamus and pituitary, analogous to normally timed pubertal maturation that occurs under the influence of GnRH. "Peripheral precocious puberty," or GnRH-independent precocious puberty, refers to conditions in which sex-steroid secretion occurs from the gonad or adrenal gland in the absence of CNS control. Causes of GnRH-dependent and -independent precocious puberty are listed in Table 10.

Table 10 Etiologies of precocious puberty

GnRH-dependent (central precocious puberty)
Idiopathic (95% of girls)
Hypothalamic hamartoma
CNS tumor
Germinoma
Hypothalamic astrocytoma
Pinealoma
Traumatic brain injury
Cerebral palsy
Hydrocephalus
Encephalitis
CNS radiation (low dose)
Neurofibromatosis, type 1
Activating mutation of Kisspeptin/GPR54 system
GnRH-independent (peripheral precocious puberty)
Adrenal tumor (androgen or estrogen secreting)
McCune-Albright syndrome
Severe primary hypothyroidism (Van Wyk-Grumbach syndrome)
Exposure to exogenous sex steroids
Males only
Familial male-limited precocious puberty
Congenital adrenal hyperplasia
Human chorionic gonadotropin (hCG)-secreting tumor
Females only
Ovarian cysts
Estrogen-secreting ovarian tumor
Variations of normal puberty
Premature adrenarche (males and females)
Premature thelarche (females)

The majority of cases of CPP are of indeterminate cause, or "idiopathic." Approximately 90 % of girls and 50 % of boys with CPP have no definable etiology. Of the remainder, most will have an identifiable disorder of the CNS. Commonly encountered abnormalities include cerebral palsy or developmental delay related to birth injury, head trauma, post-infectious damage, or metabolic abnormalities. Tumors of the CNS may also cause CPP, including gliomas, astrocytomas, and germinomas. Hypothalamic hamartomas are found most commonly in young children with CPP and do not require surgical therapy.

Premature adrenarche and premature thelarche are non- or slowly progressive conditions in which androgen or estrogen production occurs as an isolated finding. Premature thelarche classically occurs in toddler or preschool aged girls and presents as bilateral or unilateral breast enlargement without other findings of puberty. This usually regresses spontaneously, although a few will develop CPP. Premature adrenarche refers to the onset of adrenal androgen secretion before the age of 8–9 years and is manifested by pubic or axillary hair growth in boys or girls. Adult body odor and occasionally mild facial acne may be present, but there is no testicular enlargement in boys. Other signs of puberty are absent, and the hair growth is usually very gradual. The onset of other findings of puberty occurs at a normal age. Girls with a history of premature adrenarche have an increased risk of polycystic ovary syndrome, hyperinsulinism, and metabolic syndrome in adolescence and adulthood, particularly if born small for gestational age (Ibanez et al., 1993).

Diagnosis of Precocious Puberty

Precocious puberty may be diagnosed on the basis of early pubertal maturation before a defined age (see above). In girls, the presence of both breast maturation and pubic hair usually signal a progressive process, as does testicular maturation in boys. Determination of the etiology of precocious puberty usually first requires the establishment of GnRH dependence or independence. Measurement of casual LH and FSH levels is often not helpful, as there is a significant overlap in the ranges observed in the early stages of puberty with those of normal prepubertal children. However, administration of GnRH or a GnRH analog such as leuprolide to a child with CPP causes a dramatic increase in serum LH concentrations. This is in contrast to the findings in a child with GnRH-independent precocious puberty, whose LH levels are low at baseline and do not increase following GnRH administration.

Children with CPP, particularly boys and younger girls, require CNS imaging studies to exclude the presence of a tumor or other pathologic process. Children with peripheral causes of precocious puberty should have an investigation for the etiology, which may be pathology of the gonads or adrenal glands.

Treatment of Precocious Puberty

CPP is effectively treated with delayed-release GnRH analogs. Commonly used forms include intramuscular depot preparations of leuprolide and subdermal implants of histrelin. Treatment of GnRH-independent precocious puberty is based on the underlying pathologic process.

Outcomes of Precocious Puberty

Growth

Treatment of children with CPP leads to increases in adult height (Brito et al., 2008). This is because sex steroids cause advancement of skeletal maturation leading to early cessation of growth, despite relatively tall stature in childhood. Compared to pretreatment predictions of adult height, therapy with GnRH agonists increased measured adult height by an average of 4.8 cm in one study (Carel et al., 1999). The mean height standard deviation score at adulthood was zero, indicating that patients' average height was equivalent to the population average. Other studies have confirmed the magnitude of this height increase (Cacciari et al., 1994; Neely et al., 1992). The success of treatment in terms of height varies inversely with the age of the child, and treatment does not increase the height of children with borderline early puberty (Couto-Silva, Adan, Trivin, & Brauner, 2002). In selected situations, the addition of growth hormone or oxandrolone, a non-aromatizable androgen, may be beneficial (Pucarelli et al., 2000; Vottero et al., 2006).

Reproductive Function

Several long-term studies of women who were treated for CPP with GnRH agonists have been published. Cessation of therapy usually occurs between 10 and 11 years of age, and menarche follows on average about 1 year later. Menses are regular in the vast majority of patients, and the rate of oligomenorrhea is similar to that of controls (Cassio et al., 2006; Heger et al., 2006; Pasquino et al., 2008). Evaluation has indicated normal endocrine function. Fertility has been assessed in several of these long-term studies, and no abnormalities have been noted (Heger et al., 2006; Pasquino et al., 2008). Although not a consistent finding, ovarian volume is increased relative to age-matched controls in some studies, and there have been concerns for an increased incidence of polycystic ovary syndrome (Heger et al., 2006).

Body mass index is commonly elevated in girls with CPP before treatment. In most studies, however, there is no change in BMI SD scores over the course of treatment and long-term follow-up (Cassio et al., 2006; Heger et al., 2006; Pasquino et al., 2008). There are very few long-term data for adult men who were treated for CPP.

Psychological Problems

Several studies of psychological functioning in girls with CPP have been reported (Dorn, 2007). Although some did not demonstrate behavioral abnormalities (Mul et al., 2001), others show increased internalizing scores on the Child Behavior Checklist, including withdrawal and anxiety/depression as well as increased somatic complaints (Xhrouet-Heinrichs et al., 1997). Externalizing scores are increased compared to controls (Sonis et al., 1985). Although there is some evidence that treatment with GnRH analogs may improve the psychological functioning of girls with CPP (Xhrouet-Heinrichs et al., 1997), additional longitudinal studies are clearly required. One study of girls with premature adrenarche has shown a higher incidence of oppositional defiant disorder and more anxiety, mood, or disruptive behavior disorders (Dorn et al., 2008).

In contrast to girls with true precocious puberty, there are many studies that have assessed outcomes of girls with early but normal puberty. Adolescent girls who have menarche before age 11 years have earlier sexual debuts and more sex partners than girls with later menarche, as well as more delinquent behaviors (Johansson & Ritzen, 2005). However, these differences were not apparent when the same subjects were examined as adults or even in later adolescence (Lien, Haavet, & Dalgard, 2010). Similar problems have been noted in early maturing boys (Michaud, Suris, & Deppen, 2006).

It is not known if children with true precocious puberty, who may demonstrate problems with psychological functioning, are also at increased risk for the problems detected in early normal maturing adolescents. Additionally, the efficacy of treatment of patients with CPP in prevention of long-term emotional or behavioral dysfunction remains a matter for debate, although this is commonly used as a justification for treatment. Additional long-term well-designed clinical studies are required.

Conclusion

Puberty is a critical time in the life of a child as he or she transitions into adolescence and young adulthood. In addition to the many psychological changes, dramatic physical changes also occur, not only the development of secondary sexual characteristics but also the alteration of body size, shape, and composition. A complex neuroendocrine system initiates and coordinates these changes, and while the process usually proceeds normally, variations in timing and duration are common. Many pathological conditions may cause delayed or incomplete pubertal maturation and may require short- or long-term sex hormone administration. Alternatively, puberty may begin abnormally early and require suppression of sex hormone secretion. Referral to a pediatric endocrinologist is appropriate when puberty is not following the normal course.

References

Abbassi, V. (1998). Growth and normal puberty. *Pediatrics, 102*(2 Pt 3), 507–511.

Agha, A., Rogers, B., Sherlock, M., O'Kelly, P., Tormey, W., Phillips, J., et al. (2004). Anterior pituitary dysfunction in survivors of traumatic brain injury. *The Journal of Clinical Endocrinology and Metabolism, 89*(10), 4929–4936.

Agha, A., Sherlock, M., Phillips, J., Tormey, W., & Thompson, C. J. (2005). The natural history of post-traumatic neurohypophysial dysfunction. *European Journal of Endocrinology, 152*(3), 371–377.

Aimaretti, G., Ambrosio, M. R., Di Somma, C., Fusco, A., Cannavo, S., Gasperi, M., et al. (2004). Traumatic brain injury and subarachnoid haemorrhage are conditions at high risk for hypopituitarism: Screening study at 3 months after the brain injury. *Clinical Endocrinology (Oxford), 61*(3), 320–326.

Aimaretti, G., Ambrosio, M. R., Di Somma, C., Gasperi, M., Cannavo, S., Scaroni, C., et al. (2005). Residual pituitary function after brain injury-induced hypopituitarism: A prospective 12-month study. *The Journal of*

Clinical Endocrinology and Metabolism, 90(11), 6085–6092.

Anderson, S. E., & Must, A. (2005). Interpreting the continued decline in the average age at menarche: Results from two nationally representative surveys of US girls studied 10 years apart. *The Journal of Pediatrics, 147*(6), 753–760.

Argente, J., Caballo, N., Barrios, V., Munoz, M. T., Pozo, J., Chowen, J. A., et al. (1997). Multiple endocrine abnormalities of the growth hormone and insulin-like growth factor axis in patients with anorexia nervosa: Effect of short- and long-term weight recuperation. *The Journal of Clinical Endocrinology and Metabolism, 82*(7), 2084–2092.

Bavisetty, S., McArthur, D. L., Dusick, J. R., Wang, C., Cohan, P., Boscardin, W. J., et al. (2008). Chronic hypopituitarism after traumatic brain injury: Risk assessment and relationship to outcome. *Neurosurgery, 62*(5), 1080–1093.

Behan, L. A., Phillips, J., Thompson, C. J., & Agha, A. (2008). Neuroendocrine disorders after traumatic brain injury. *Journal of neurology, neurosurgery, and psychiatry, 79*(7), 753–759.

Bianco, S. D., & Kaiser, U. B. (2009). The genetic and molecular basis of idiopathic hypogonadotropic hypogonadism. *Nature Reviews. Endocrinology, 5*(10), 569–576.

Bondanelli, M., Ambrosio, M. R., Cavazzini, L., Bertocchi, A., Zatelli, M. C., Carli, A., et al. (2007). Anterior pituitary function may predict functional and cognitive outcome in patients with traumatic brain injury undergoing rehabilitation. *Journal of Neurotrauma, 24*(11), 1687–1697.

Boot, A. M., Engels, M. A., Boerma, G. J., Krenning, E. P., & De Muinck Keizer-Schrama, S. M. (1997). Changes in bone mineral density, body composition, and lipid metabolism during growth hormone (GH) treatment in children with GH deficiency. *The Journal of Clinical Endocrinology and Metabolism, 82*(8), 2423–2428.

Bridges, N. A., Cooke, A., Healy, M. J., Hindmarsh, P. C., & Brook, C. G. (1993). Standards for ovarian volume in childhood and puberty. *Fertility and Sterility, 60*(3), 456–460.

Brito, V. N., Latronico, A. C., Cukier, P., Teles, M. G., Silveira, L. F., Arnhold, I. J., et al. (2008). Factors determining normal adult height in girls with gonadotropin-dependent precocious puberty treated with depot gonadotropin-releasing hormone analogs. *The Journal of Clinical Endocrinology and Metabolism, 93*(7), 2662–2669.

Bruns, J., Jr., & Hauser, W. A. (2003). The epidemiology of traumatic brain injury: A review. *Epilepsia, 44*(Suppl 10), 2–10.

Cacciari, E., Cassio, A., Balsamo, A., Colli, C., Cicognani, A., Pirazzoli, P., et al. (1994). Long-term follow-up and final height in girls with central precocious puberty treated with luteinizing hormone-releasing hormone analogue nasal spray. *Archives of Pediatrics & Adolescent Medicine, 148*(11), 1194–1199.

Carel, J. C., Roger, M., Ispas, S., Tondu, F., Lahlou, N., Blumberg, J., et al. (1999). Final height after long-term treatment with triptorelin slow release for central precocious puberty: Importance of statural growth after interruption of treatment. French study group of Decapeptyl in Precocious Puberty. *The Journal of Clinical Endocrinology and Metabolism, 84*(6), 1973–1978.

Cassio, A., Bal, M. O., Orsini, L. F., Balsamo, A., Sansavini, S., Gennari, M., et al. (2006). Reproductive outcome in patients treated and not treated for idiopathic early puberty: Long-term results of a randomized trial in adults. *The Journal of Pediatrics, 149*(4), 532–536.

Chumlea, W. C., Schubert, C. M., Roche, A. F., Kulin, H. E., Lee, P. A., Himes, J. H., et al. (2003). Age at menarche and racial comparisons in US girls. *Pediatrics, 111*(1), 110–113.

Colao, A. (2009). Pituitary tumours: The prolactinoma. *Best Practice & Research. Clinical Endocrinology & Metabolism, 23*(5), 575–596.

Colao, A., & Lombardi, G. (1998). Growth-hormone and prolactin excess. *The Lancet, 352*(9138), 1455–1461.

Couto-Silva, A. C., Adan, L., Trivin, C., & Brauner, R. (2002). Adult height in advanced puberty with or without gonadotropin hormone releasing hormone analog treatment. *Journal of Pediatric Endocrinology & Metabolism, 15*(3), 297–305.

Crowne, E. C., Shalet, S. M., Wallace, W. H., Eminson, D. M., & Price, D. A. (1990). Final height in boys with untreated constitutional delay in growth and puberty. *Archives of Disease in Childhood, 65*(10), 1109–1112.

Crowne, E. C., Shalet, S. M., Wallace, W. H., Eminson, D. M., & Price, D. A. (1991). Final height in girls with untreated constitutional delay in growth and puberty. *European Journal of Pediatrics, 150*(10), 708–712.

Degros, V., Cortet-Rudelli, C., Soudan, B., & Dewailly, D. (2003). The human chorionic gonadotropin test is more powerful than the gonadotropin-releasing hormone agonist test to discriminate male isolated hypogonadotropic hypogonadism from constitutional delayed puberty. *European Journal of Endocrinology, 149*(1), 23–29.

Dhillo, W. S., Chaudhri, O. B., Patterson, M., Thompson, E. L., Murphy, K. G., Badman, M. K., et al. (2005). Kisspeptin-54 stimulates the hypothalamic-pituitary gonadal axis in human males. *The Journal of Clinical Endocrinology and Metabolism, 90*(12), 6609–6615.

Dhillo, W. S., Chaudhri, O. B., Thompson, E. L., Murphy, K. G., Patterson, M., Ramachandran, R., et al. (2007). Kisspeptin-54 stimulates gonadotropin release most potently during the preovulatory phase of the menstrual cycle in women. *The Journal of Clinical Endocrinology and Metabolism, 92*(10), 3958–3966.

Dorn, L. (2007). Psychological and social problems in children with premature adrenarche and precocious puberty. In O. Pescovitz & E. Walvoord (Eds.), *When puberty is precocious: Scientific and clinical aspects* (pp. 309–330). Totowa, NJ: Humana.

Dorn, L. D., Rose, S. R., Rotenstein, D., Susman, E. J., Huang, B., Loucks, T. L., et al. (2008). Differences in endocrine parameters and psychopathology in girls with premature adrenarche versus on-time adrenarche. *Journal of Pediatric Endocrinology & Metabolism, 21*(5), 439–448.

Duke, P. M., Carlsmith, J. M., Jennings, D., Martin, J. A., Dornbusch, S. M., Gross, R. T., et al. (1982). Educational correlates of early and late sexual maturation in adolescence. *The Journal of Pediatrics, 100*(4), 633–637.

Dunkel, L., Alfthan, H., Stenman, U. H., Tapanainen, P., & Perheentupa, J. (1990). Pulsatile secretion of LH and FSH in prepubertal and early pubertal boys revealed by ultrasensitive time-resolved immunofluorometric assays. *Pediatric Research, 27*(3), 215–219.

Einaudi, S., Matarazzo, P., Peretta, P., Grossetti, R., Giordano, F., Altare, F., et al. (2006). Hypothalamo-hypophysial dysfunction after traumatic brain injury in children and adolescents: A preliminary retrospective and prospective study. *Journal of Pediatric Endocrinology & Metabolism, 19*(5), 691–703.

Farooqi, I. S., Matarese, G., Lord, G. M., Keogh, J. M., Lawrence, E., Agwu, C., et al. (2002). Beneficial effects of leptin on obesity, T cell hyporesponsiveness, and neuroendocrine/metabolic dysfunction of human congenital leptin deficiency. *The Journal of Clinical Investigation, 110*(8), 1093–1103.

Finkelstein, J. S., Neer, R. M., Biller, B. M., Crawford, J. D., & Klibanski, A. (1992). Osteopenia in men with a history of delayed puberty. *The New England Journal of Medicine, 326*(9), 600–604.

Freedman, D. S., Khan, L. K., Serdula, M. K., Dietz, W. H., Srinivasan, S. R., & Berenson, G. S. (2002). Relation of age at menarche to race, time period, and anthropometric dimensions: The Bogalusa Heart Study. *Pediatrics, 110*(4), e43.

Galli-Tsinopoulou, A., Nousia-Arvanitakis, S., Mitsiakos, G., Karamouzis, M., & Dimitriadis, A. (2000). Osteopenia in children and adolescents with hyperprolactinemia. *Journal of Pediatric Endocrinology & Metabolism, 13*(4), 439–441.

Gamba, M., & Pralong, F. P. (2006). Control of GnRH neuronal activity by metabolic factors: The role of leptin and insulin. *Molecular and Cellular Endocrinology, 254–255*, 133–139.

Gianetti, E., Tusset, C., Noel, S. D., Au, M. G., Dwyer, A. A., Hughes, V. A., et al. (2010). TAC3/TACR3 mutations reveal preferential activation of gonadotropin-releasing hormone release by neurokinin B in neonatal life followed by reversal in adulthood. *The Journal of Clinical Endocrinology and Metabolism, 95*(6), 2857–2867.

Gleeson, H., Barreto, E. S., Salvatori, R., Costa, L., Oliveira, C. R., Pereira, R. M., et al. (2007). Metabolic effects of growth hormone (GH) replacement in children and adolescents with severe isolated GH deficiency due to a GHRH receptor mutation. *Clinical Endocrinology, 66*(4), 466–474.

Golden, N. H., Jacobson, M. S., Schebendach, J., Solanto, M. V., Hertz, S. M., & Shenker, I. R. (1997). Resumption of menses in anorexia nervosa. *Archives of Pediatrics & Adolescent Medicine, 151*(1), 16–21.

Gordon, C. M. (2010). Clinical practice. Functional hypothalamic amenorrhea. *The New England Journal of Medicine, 363*(4), 365–371.

Gougeon, A. (1996). Regulation of ovarian follicular development in primates: Facts and hypotheses. *Endocrine Reviews, 17*(2), 121–155.

Gross, R. T., & Duke, P. M. (1980). The effect of early versus late physical maturation on adolescent behavior. *Pediatric Clinics of North America, 27*(1), 71–77.

Heger, S., Muller, M., Ranke, M., Schwarz, H. P., Waldhauser, F., Partsch, C. J., et al. (2006). Long-term GnRH agonist treatment for female central precocious puberty does not impair reproductive function. *Molecular and Cellular Endocrinology, 254–255*, 217–220.

Herman-Giddens, M. E., Slora, E. J., Wasserman, R. C., Bourdony, C. J., Bhapkar, M. V., Koch, G. G., et al. (1997). Secondary sexual characteristics and menses in young girls seen in office practice: A study from the Pediatric Research in Office Settings network. *Pediatrics, 99*(4), 505–512.

Herman-Giddens, M. E., Wang, L., & Koch, G. (2001). Secondary sexual characteristics in boys: Estimates from the national health and nutrition examination survey III, 1988–1994. *Archives of Pediatrics & Adolescent Medicine, 155*(9), 1022–1028.

Howell, S., & Shalet, S. (1998). Gonadal damage from chemotherapy and radiotherapy. *Endocrinology and Metabolism Clinics of North America, 27*(4), 927–943.

Hulthen, L., Bengtsson, B. A., Sunnerhagen, K. S., Hallberg, L., Grimby, G., & Johannsson, G. (2001). GH is needed for the maturation of muscle mass and strength in adolescents. *The Journal of Clinical Endocrinology and Metabolism, 86*(10), 4765–4770.

Ibanez, L., Potau, N., Virdis, R., Zampolli, M., Terzi, C., Gussinye, M., et al. (1993). Postpubertal outcome in girls diagnosed of premature pubarche during childhood: Increased frequency of functional ovarian hyperandrogenism. *The Journal of Clinical Endocrinology and Metabolism, 76*(6), 1599–1603.

Jayasena, C. N., Nijher, G. M., Chaudhri, O. B., Murphy, K. G., Ranger, A., Lim, A., et al. (2009). Subcutaneous injection of kisspeptin-54 acutely stimulates gonadotropin secretion in women with hypothalamic amenorrhea, but chronic administration causes tachyphylaxis. *The Journal of Clinical Endocrinology and Metabolism, 94*(11), 4315–4323.

Johansson, T., & Ritzen, E. M. (2005). Very long-term follow-up of girls with early and late menarche. *Endocrine Development, 8*, 126–136.

Juul, A., Magnusdottir, S., Scheike, T., Prytz, S., & Skakkebaek, N. E. (2007). Age at voice break in Danish boys: Effects of pre-pubertal body mass index and secular trend. *International Journal of Andrology, 30*(6), 537–542.

Kaplowitz, P. B., Slora, E. J., Wasserman, R. C., Pedlow, S. E., & Herman-Giddens, M. E. (2001). Earlier onset

of puberty in girls: Relation to increased body mass index and race. *Pediatrics, 108*(2), 347–353.
Karlberg, J. (1989). A biologically-oriented mathematical model (ICP) for human growth. *Acta Paediatrica Scandinavica. Supplement, 350*, 70–94.
Kauffman, A. S., Clifton, D. K., & Steiner, R. A. (2007). Emerging ideas about kisspeptin- GPR54 signaling in the neuroendocrine regulation of reproduction. *Trends in Neurosciences, 30*(10), 504–511.
Kaulfers, A. M., Backeljauw, P. F., Reifschneider, K., Blum, S., Michaud, L., Weiss, M., et al. (2010). Endocrine dysfunction following traumatic brain injury in children. *The Journal of Pediatrics, 157*(6), 894–899.
Kelly, D. F., McArthur, D. L., Levin, H., Swimmer, S., Dusick, J. R., Cohan, P., et al. (2006). Neurobehavioral and quality of life changes associated with growth hormone insufficiency after complicated mild, moderate, or severe traumatic brain injury. *Journal of Neurotrauma, 23*(6), 928–942.
Kerrigan, J. R., & Rogol, A. D. (1992). The impact of gonadal steroid hormone action on growth hormone secretion during childhood and adolescence. *Endocrine Reviews, 13*(2), 281–298.
Knobil, E. (1980). The neuroendocrine control of the menstrual cycle. *Recent Progress in Hormone Research, 36*, 53–88.
Langlois, J. A., Rutland-Brown, W., & Thomas, K. E. (2005). The incidence of traumatic brain injury among children in the United States: Differences by race. *The Journal of Head Trauma Rehabilitation, 20*(3), 229–238.
Largo, R. H., Gasser, T., Prader, A., Stuetzle, W., & Huber, P. J. (1978). Analysis of the adolescent growth spurt using smoothing spline functions. *Annals of Human Biology, 5*(5), 421–434.
Leal-Cerro, A., Flores, J. M., Rincon, M., Murillo, F., Pujol, M., Garcia-Pesquera, F., et al. (2005). Prevalence of hypopituitarism and growth hormone deficiency in adults long-term after severe traumatic brain injury. *Clinical Endocrinology, 62*(5), 525–532.
Legouis, R., Hardelin, J. P., Levilliers, J., Claverie, J. M., Compain, S., Wunderle, V., et al. (1991). The candidate gene for the X-linked Kallmann syndrome encodes a protein related to adhesion molecules. *Cell, 67*(2), 423–435.
Lien, L., Haavet, O. R., & Dalgard, F. (2010). Do mental health and behavioural problems of early menarche persist into late adolescence? A three year follow-up study among adolescent girls in Oslo, Norway. *Social Science & Medicine (1982), 71*(3), 529–533.
Loucks, A. B. (2006). The response of luteinizing hormone pulsatility to 5 days of low energy availability disappears by 14 years of gynecological age. *The Journal of Clinical Endocrinology and Metabolism, 91*(8), 3158–3164.
Loucks, A. B. (2007). Energy availability and infertility. *Current Opinion in Endocrinology, Diabetes, and Obesity, 14*(6), 470–474.
Loucks, A. B., & Thuma, J. R. (2003). Luteinizing hormone pulsatility is disrupted at a threshold of energy availability in regularly menstruating women. *The Journal of Clinical Endocrinology and Metabolism, 88*(1), 297–311.
Manasco, P. K., Umbach, D. M., Muly, S. M., Godwin, D. C., Negro-Vilar, A., Culler, M. D., et al. (1995). Ontogeny of gonadotropin, testosterone, and inhibin secretion in normal boys through puberty based on overnight serial sampling. *The Journal of Clinical Endocrinology and Metabolism, 80*(7), 2046–2052.
Marshall, W. A., & Tanner, J. M. (1969). Variations in pattern of pubertal changes in girls. *Archives of Disease in Childhood, 44*(235), 291–303.
Marshall, W. A., & Tanner, J. M. (1970). Variations in the pattern of pubertal changes in boys. *Archives of Disease in Childhood, 45*(239), 13–23.
Martha, P. M., Jr., Gorman, K. M., Blizzard, R. M., Rogol, A. D., & Veldhuis, J. D. (1992). Endogenous growth hormone secretion and clearance rates in normal boys, as determined by deconvolution analysis: Relationship to age, pubertal status, and body mass. *The Journal of Clinical Endocrinology and Metabolism, 74*(2), 336–344.
Martha, P. M., Jr., Rogol, A. D., Veldhuis, J. D., & Blizzard, R. M. (1996). A longitudinal assessment of hormonal and physical alterations during normal puberty in boys. III. The neuroendocrine growth hormone axis during late prepuberty. *The Journal of Clinical Endocrinology and Metabolism, 81*(11), 4068–4074.
Mazur, T., & Clopper, R. R. (1991). Pubertal disorders. Psychology and clinical management. *Endocrinology and Metabolism Clinics of North America, 20*(1), 211–230.
Melmed, S., & Kleinberg, D. (2008). Anterior pituitary. In H. Kronenberg, S. Melmed, K. Polonsky, & P. Larsen (Eds.), *Williams textbook of endocrinology* (11th ed., pp. 155–261). Philadelphia: Saunders Elsevier.
Michaud, P. A., Suris, J. C., & Deppen, A. (2006). Gender-related psychological and behavioural correlates of pubertal timing in a national sample of Swiss adolescents. *Molecular and Cellular Endocrinology, 254–255*, 172–178.
Mobbs, E. J. (2005). The psychological outcome of constitutional delay of growth and puberty. *Hormone Research, 63*(Suppl 1), 1–66.
Mul, D., Versluis-den Bieman, H. J., Slijper, F. M., Oostdijk, W., Waelkens, J. J., & Drop, S. L. (2001). Psychological assessments before and after treatment of early puberty in adopted children. *Acta Paediatrica, 90*(9), 965–971.
Nattiv, A., Loucks, A. B., Manore, M. M., Sanborn, C. F., Sundgot-Borgen, J., & Warren, M. P. (2007). American College of Sports Medicine position stand. The female athlete triad. *Medicine and Science in Sports and Exercise, 39*(10), 1867–1882.
Neely, E. K., Hintz, R. L., Parker, B., Bachrach, L. K., Cohen, P., Olney, R., et al. (1992). Two-year results of treatment with depot leuprolide acetate for central precocious puberty. *The Journal of Pediatrics, 121*(4), 634–640.

Niederland, T., Makovi, H., Gal, V., Andreka, B., Abraham, C. S., & Kovacs, J. (2007). Abnormalities of pituitary function after traumatic brain injury in children. *Journal of Neurotrauma, 24*(1), 119–127.

Norjavaara, E., Ankarberg, C., & Albertsson-Wikland, K. (1996). Diurnal rhythm of 17 beta-estradiol secretion throughout pubertal development in healthy girls: Evaluation by a sensitive radioimmunoassay. *The Journal of Clinical Endocrinology and Metabolism, 81*(11), 4095–4102.

Norwood, K. W., Deboer, M. D., Gurka, M. J., Kuperminc, M. N., Rogol, A. D., Blackman, J. A., et al. (2010). Traumatic brain injury in children and adolescents: Surveillance for pituitary dysfunction. *Clinical Pediatrics, 49*(11), 1044–1049.

Palmert, M. R., & Boepple, P. A. (2001). Variation in the timing of puberty: Clinical spectrum and genetic investigation. *The Journal of Clinical Endocrinology and Metabolism, 86*(6), 2364–2368.

Pasquino, A. M., Pucarelli, I., Accardo, F., Demiraj, V., Segni, M., & Di Nardo, R. (2008). Long-term observation of 87 girls with idiopathic central precocious puberty treated with gonadotropin-releasing hormone analogs: Impact on adult height, body mass index, bone mineral content, and reproductive function. *The Journal of Clinical Endocrinology and Metabolism, 93*(1), 190–195.

Peters, H., Byskov, A. G., & Grinsted, J. (1978). Follicular growth in fetal and prepubertal ovaries of humans and other primates. *Clinics in Endocrinology and Metabolism, 7*(3), 469–485.

Petraroli, M., D'Alessio, E., Ausili, E., Barini, A., Caradonna, P., Riccardi, R., et al. (2007). Bone mineral density in survivors of childhood brain tumours. *Child's Nervous System, 23*(1), 59–65.

Poomthavorn, P., Maixner, W., & Zacharin, M. (2008). Pituitary function in paediatric survivors of severe traumatic brain injury. *Archives of Disease in Childhood, 93*(2), 133–137.

Popovic, V., Pekic, S., Pavlovic, D., Maric, N., Jasovic-Gasic, M., Djurovic, B., et al. (2004). Hypopituitarism as a consequence of traumatic brain injury (TBI) and its possible relation with cognitive disabilities and mental distress. *Journal of Endocrinological Investigation, 27*(11), 1048–1054.

Poyrazoglu, S., Gunoz, H., Darendeliler, F., Saka, N., Bundak, R., & Bas, F. (2005). Constitutional delay of growth and puberty: From presentation to final height. *Journal of Pediatric Endocrinology & Metabolism, 18*(2), 171–179.

Pucarelli, I., Segni, M., Ortore, M., Moretti, A., Iannaccone, R., & Pasquino, A. M. (2000). Combined therapy with GnRH analog plus growth hormone in central precocious puberty. *Journal of Pediatric Endocrinology & Metabolism, 13*(Suppl 1), 811–820.

Roemmich, J. N., Clark, P. A., Mai, V., Berr, S. S., Weltman, A., Veldhuis, J. D., et al. (1998). Alterations in growth and body composition during puberty: III. Influence of maturation, gender, body composition, fat distribution, aerobic fitness, and energy expenditure on nocturnal growth hormone release. *The Journal of Clinical Endocrinology and Metabolism, 83*(5), 1440–1447.

Roemmich, J. N., Huerta, M. G., Sundaresan, S. M., & Rogol, A. D. (2001). Alterations in body composition and fat distribution in growth hormone-deficient prepubertal children during growth hormone therapy. *Metabolism, 50*(5), 537–547.

Roemmich, J. N., & Rogol, A. D. (1999). Hormonal changes during puberty and their relationship to fat distribution. *American Journal of Human Biology, 11*(2), 209–224.

Rosenfield, R., Cooke, D., & Radovick, S. (2008). Puberty and its disorders in the female. In M. Sperling (Ed.), *Pediatric endocrinology* (3rd ed., pp. 530–609). Philadelphia: Saunders Elsevier.

Rosenfield, R. L., Lipton, R. B., & Drum, M. L. (2009). Thelarche, pubarche, and menarche attainment in children with normal and elevated body mass index. *Pediatrics, 123*(1), 84–88.

Russell, D. L., & Robker, R. L. (2007). Molecular mechanisms of ovulation: Co-ordination through the cumulus complex. *Human Reproduction Update, 13*(3), 289–312.

Scacchi, M., Pincelli, A. I., Caumo, A., Tomasi, P., Delitala, G., Baldi, G., et al. (1997). Spontaneous nocturnal growth hormone secretion in anorexia nervosa. *The Journal of Clinical Endocrinology and Metabolism, 82*(10), 3225–3229.

Schwab, J., Kulin, H. E., Susman, E. J., Finkelstein, J. W., Chinchilli, V. M., Kunselman, S. J., et al. (2001). The role of sex hormone replacement therapy on self-perceived competence in adolescents with delayed puberty. *Child Development, 72*(5), 1439–1450.

Segal, T. Y., Mehta, A., Anazodo, A., Hindmarsh, P. C., & Dattani, M. T. (2009). Role of gonadotropin-releasing hormone and human chorionic gonadotropin stimulation tests in differentiating patients with hypogonadotropic hypogonadism from those with constitutional delay of growth and puberty. *The Journal of Clinical Endocrinology and Metabolism, 94*(3), 780–785.

Seminara, S. B., Messager, S., Chatzidaki, E. E., Thresher, R. R., Acierno, J. S., Jr., Shagoury, J. K., et al. (2003). The GPR54 gene as a regulator of puberty. *The New England Journal of Medicine, 349*(17), 1614–1627.

Sequera, A. M., Fideleff, H. L., Boquete, H. R., Pujol, A. B., Suarez, M. G., & Ruibal, G. F. (2002). Basal ultrasensitive LH assay: A useful tool in the early diagnosis of male pubertal delay? *Journal of Pediatric Endocrinology & Metabolism, 15*(5), 589–596.

Shalet, S. M., Tsatsoulis, A., Whitehead, E., & Read, G. (1989). Vulnerability of the human Leydig cell to radiation damage is dependent upon age. *The Journal of Endocrinology, 120*(1), 161–165.

Sisk, C. L., & Foster, D. L. (2004). The neural basis of puberty and adolescence. *Nature Neuroscience, 7*(10), 1040–1047.

Soliman, A. T., Hassan, A. E., Aref, M. K., Hintz, R. L., Rosenfeld, R. G., & Rogol, A. D. (1986). Serum insulin-like growth factors I and II concentrations and growth hormone and insulin responses to arginine infusion in children with protein-energy malnutrition before and after nutritional rehabilitation. *Pediatric Research, 20*(11), 1122–1130.

Sonis, W. A., Comite, F., Blue, J., Pescovitz, O. H., Rahn, C. W., Hench, K. D., et al. (1985). Behavior problems and social competence in girls with true precocious puberty. *The Journal of Pediatrics, 106*(1), 156–160.

Stice, E., Marti, C. N., Shaw, H., & Jaconis, M. (2009). An 8-year longitudinal study of the natural history of threshold, subthreshold, and partial eating disorders from a community sample of adolescents. *Journal of Abnormal Psychology, 118*(3), 587–597.

Street, M. E., Bandello, M. A., Terzi, C., Ibanez, L., Ghizzoni, L., Volta, C., et al. (2002). Leuteinizing hormone responses to leuprolide acetate discriminate between hypogonadotropic hypogonadism and constitutional delay of puberty. *Fertility and Sterility, 77*(3), 555–560.

Styne, D., & Grumbach, M. (2008). Puberty: Ontogeny, neuroendocrinology, physiology, and disorders. In H. Kronenberg, S. Melmed, K. Polonsky, & P. Larsen (Eds.), *Williams textbook of endocrinology* (11th ed., pp. 969–1166). Philadelphia: Saunders Elsevier.

Sun, S. S., Schubert, C. M., Chumlea, W. C., Roche, A. F., Kulin, H. E., Lee, P. A., et al. (2002). National estimates of the timing of sexual maturation and racial differences among US children. *Pediatrics, 110*(5), 911–919.

Susman, E. J., Finkelstein, J. W., Chinchilli, V. M., Schwab, J., Liben, L. S., D'Arcangelo, M. R., et al. (1998). The effect of sex hormone replacement therapy on behavior problems and moods in adolescents with delayed puberty. *The Journal of Pediatrics, 133*(4), 521–525.

Tanner, J. M., Whitehouse, R. H., Marubini, E., & Resele, L. F. (1976). The adolescent growth spurt of boys and girls of the Harpenden growth study. *Annals of Human Biology, 3*(2), 109–126.

Teles, M. G., Bianco, S. D., Brito, V. N., Trarbach, E. B., Kuohung, W., Xu, S., et al. (2008). A GPR54-activating mutation in a patient with central precocious puberty. *The New England Journal of Medicine, 358*(7), 709–715.

Terasawa, E., & Fernandez, D. L. (2001). Neurobiological mechanisms of the onset of puberty in primates. *Endocrine Reviews, 22*(1), 111–151.

Veldhuis, J. D., Roemmich, J. N., Richmond, E. J., Rogol, A. D., Lovejoy, J. C., Sheffield-Moore, M., et al. (2005). Endocrine control of body composition in infancy, childhood, and puberty. *Endocrine Reviews, 26*(1), 114–146.

Veldhuis, J. D., Roemmich, J. N., & Rogol, A. D. (2000). Gender and sexual maturation-dependent contrasts in the neuroregulation of growth hormone secretion in prepubertal and late adolescent males and females–a general clinical research center-based study. *The Journal of Clinical Endocrinology and Metabolism, 85*(7), 2385–2394.

Vottero, A., Pedori, S., Verna, M., Pagano, B., Cappa, M., Loche, S., et al. (2006). Final height in girls with central idiopathic precocious puberty treated with gonadotropin-releasing hormone analog and oxandrolone. *The Journal of Clinical Endocrinology and Metabolism, 91*(4), 1284–1287.

Wade, G. N., Schneider, J. E., & Li, H. Y. (1996). Control of fertility by metabolic cues. *The American Journal of Physiology, 270*(1 Pt 1), E1–E19.

Wallace, W. H. B., Thomson, A. B., Saran, F., & Kelsey, T. W. (2005). Predicting age of ovarian failure after radiation to a field that includes the ovaries. *International Journal of Radiation Oncology, Biology, Physics, 62*(3), 738–744.

Warren, M. P., Brooks-Gunn, J., Fox, R. P., Holderness, C. C., Hyle, E. P., & Hamilton, W. G. (2002). Osteopenia in exercise-associated amenorrhea using ballet dancers as a model: A longitudinal study. *The Journal of Clinical Endocrinology and Metabolism, 87*(7), 3162–3168.

Wattigney, W. A., Srinivasan, S. R., Chen, W., Greenlund, K. J., & Berenson, G. S. (1999). Secular trend of earlier onset of menarche with increasing obesity in black and white girls: The Bogalusa Heart Study. *Ethnicity & Disease, 9*(2), 181–189.

Wright, N. M., Northington, F. J., Miller, J. D., Veldhuis, J. D., & Rogol, A. D. (1992). Elevated growth hormone secretory rate in premature infants: Deconvolution analysis of pulsatile growth hormone secretion in the neonate. *Pediatric Research, 32*(3), 286–290.

Xhrouet-Heinrichs, D., Lagrou, K., Heinrichs, C., Craen, M., Dooms, L., Malvaux, P., et al. (1997). Longitudinal study of behavioral and affective patterns in girls with central precocious puberty during long-acting triptorelin therapy. *Acta Paediatrica, 86*(8), 808–815.

Adolescent Sexuality and Sexual Behavior

Candace Best and J. Dennis Fortenberry

This chapter presents a theoretical framework that incorporates eight significant factors that have been associated with adolescent sexuality and sexual behaviors. Specifically, we discuss genetics, antenatal experiences, gender, parents, siblings, peers, partners, and neighborhood and cultural influences. Next, we provide an overview of the developmental trajectory of sexual behavior during adolescence. We also highlight the role of media in influencing adolescent sexual behavior. We then review psychosexual development and four dimensions of adolescent sexual self-concept (i.e., sexual self-esteem, sexual openness, sexual ambivalence, sexual anxiety). Finally, our chapter concludes with a discussion of adolescent sexual health and the limits of our current sexual health curriculum.

Adolescent Sexuality and Sexual Behavior

Adolescence represents a sociosexual developmental period through which sexuality and sexual behavior initiates, develops, and matures. Adolescence is closely tied to the hormonal and physical changes of puberty (Graber, Nichols, & Brooks-Gunn, 2010) in the context of ongoing neuropsychological brain development, achievement of adult body habitus, and an emerging autonomy from parents. Through use of a developmental approach, we present an overview of seven multifaceted factors that have been demonstrated to influence adolescent sexuality to varying degrees. These factors include genetic, antenatal, family, peer, partner, gender, and cultural influences. This chapter also highlights the relative impact of these factors on sexual behaviors, psychosexual development, sexual self-concept, and sexual health during adolescence.

A Theoretical Framework for Understanding Sexuality and Sexual Behavior in Adolescence

Our general theoretical perspective is that adolescent sexual behaviors are microsocial events organized as subjective and situational experiences. These events occur within the context of specific interpersonal relationships and are represented by fixed psychological and social features related to developmental life-stage, gender, sexuality, and interpersonal relationships. Because sexual behavior is a repetitively enacted experience, variations in motivation, context, affect, and outcomes may occur from event to event. Features of situations interact with cognitive, affective, and/or behavioral mediating elements, which create a typical response pattern. These features encompass the

C. Best, Ph.D. (✉) • J.D. Fortenberry, M.D., M.S.
Department of Pediatrics, Indiana University School of Medicine, 410 W. St, HITS 1001, Indianapolis, IN 46202, USA
e-mail: cabest@iu.edu; jfortenb@iu.edu

W.T. O'Donohue et al. (eds.), *Handbook of Adolescent Health Psychology*,
DOI 10.1007/978-1-4614-6633-8_19, © Springer Science+Business Media New York 2013

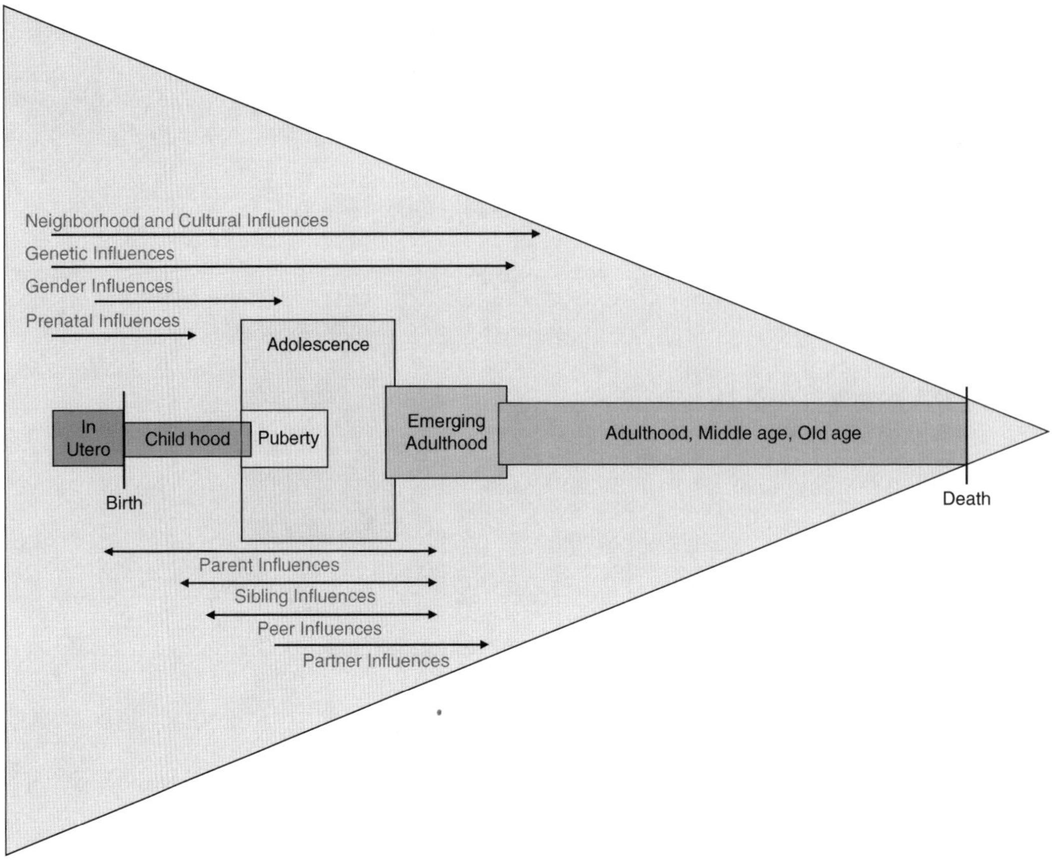

Fig. 1 Theoretical factors influencing adolescent development

social and interpersonal situation (i.e., a potential sexual event) as well as more variable circumstances such as mood and the everyday stream of experience and feeling. Sexual situations are rarely, if ever, entirely defined by sexual exchanges conducted without regard to cultural, social, or personal contexts. The affective and behavioral phenomena associated with dyad interactions and sexual situations thus do not occur randomly. Rather, meanings develop from social interactions with significant others and are modified through reflection and interpretation, which ultimately influences subsequent interactions. Simply stated, the combination of accrued learning, development of sexual expectations, and improved sexual skills throughout adolescence is the basis of adult sexuality (Fig. 1).

Genetic Influences

Genes influence various adolescent sexual behaviors including sexual abstinence, sexual initiation, and number of sexual partners. These influences also appear to be more significant for males (Mustanski, Viken, Kaprio, Winter, & Rose, 2007). For instance, Verweij and colleagues (2009) examined current risky sexual behaviors in adults and retrospective misconduct during adolescence and discovered that genetics accounted for approximately one-third of the variance in understanding risky sexual behaviors among late adolescent and adult twins. In addition, gender trends were observed such that shared environmental factors seemed to be more significant in the relationship between adolescent misconduct and risky sexual behaviors for females, while genetic influences were more significant for males (Verweij, Zietsch, Bailey, & Martin, 2009). In another study, researchers discovered a much closer relationship in the timing of sex among identical twins as compared to fraternal twins. For example, the probability of first sex was approximately 30 % greater when an identical twin had initiated sex as compared to the twin being a virgin. This relationship was not observed among same-sex fraternal twins. Also, Asian American, European American, and Hispanic American adolescents who possessed a 3R allele of the dopamine receptor DRD4 gene were significantly more likely to have engaged in first sex. This relationship was not found among African American adolescents (Guo & Tong, 2006).

Gender nonconformity also seems to have a heritable quality for both males and females (Bailey, Dunne, & Martin, 2000). In fact, genes have been implicated in gender atypical behavior during childhood and later sexual orientation. Again, the relationship between genes and behavior appears stronger for males (Alanko et al., 2010). Significant skewing of X-chromosome inactivation has also been associated in mothers with gay sons. This relationship appears to be stronger among mothers with more than one son who identifies as homosexual (Bocklandt, Horvath, Vilain, & Hamer, 2006). Similarly, having more female relatives, such as aunts, is more prevalent in female-to-male transsexuals. This relationship has not yet been established in male-to-female transsexuals (Green & Keverne, 2000).

These studies suggest that genes are involved in adolescent sexual behaviors with early displays of genetic influences observed in gender atypical behavior during childhood. Variations in genetic influences have been observed among different ethnic groups and among males. Moreover, genes appear to be implicated in the development of sexual orientation to some degree. All the same, it is likely that a combination of genetic and non-shared environmental factors influence adolescent sexual behaviors.

Antenatal Influences

Variation in adolescent development of sexual identity and sexual behaviors has been consistently highlighted within research investigating congenital adrenal hyperplasia (CAH). In fact, substantial understanding of the influence of congenital hormone anomalies on gender identity, sexual orientation, and sexual interest has emerged during the past 30 years. In attempting to understand variation in adolescent development of sexual identity and sexual behaviors, examining research of CAH is particularly illustrative. CAH occurs as a result of a variety of intra-uterine sex hormone exposure, via fetal or maternal sources. Specifically, key enzymes involved in the synthesis of adrenal glucocorticoid hormones become mutated. These mutations render the enzyme partially or completely ineffective, leading to an excess of hormone intermediaries. These intermediaries may have potent effects on expressions of sexuality during adolescence or on genitals themselves (girls with CAH are born with an XX chromosome pattern but may be substantially virilized). The majority of women with CAH report different-sex (i.e., heterosexual) sexual orientation, although women with CAH are much more likely than unaffected women to express same-sex fantasies and behaviors (Cohen-Bendahan, van de Beek, & Berenbaum, 2005). Some studies show that young women with CAH do not differ from other women in terms of age at menarche, age of initiation of masturbation, age at first partnered sex, and age of first orgasm (Meyer-Bahlburg, Dolezal, Baker, & New, 2008). However, other studies suggest that women with CAH may be delayed in terms of onset of partnered sexual activity (Dittmann, Kappes, & Kappes, 1992).

Another illustration of potential antenatal influences on sexual orientation relates to the ratio of the lengths of the second and fourth fingers (2D:4D). Males typically develop a smaller 2D:4D ratio, presumably as an effect of intrauterine androgen exposure (Rahman & Wilson, 2003). This gender dimorphism becomes especially apparent during puberty

(Friedman & Downey, 2008). A substantial body of research has addressed 2D:4D ratio as a marker for sexual orientation. A recent meta-analysis of these studies confirmed the markedly lower 2D:4D ratio in males with different-sex orientation compared to females with different-sex orientation. Women with same-sex orientation have smaller (i.e., more masculine) 2D:4D ratios compared to women with different-sex orientations. However, no differences were noted in men with same- and different-sex orientations (Grimbos, Dawood, Burriss, Zucker, & Puts, 2010).

Overall, understanding potential antenatal influences on other characteristics of adolescent sexuality and sexual behavior, such as age at first coitus or preferred number of sexual partners, remains quite meager. Data are emerging to provide a more detailed understanding of antenatal hormonal effects on characteristics such as sexual orientation, but some of these data remain controversial. Additionally, very few studies have gathered prospective data from adolescents themselves. Thus, we still know little about the developmental experience of sexuality and sexual behaviors of various potential antenatal exposures as they unfold during adolescence.

Gender Influences

Gender differences in sexuality are often noticeable early in development and include behaviors such as preferences for sex-typed toys among boys and girls (Hassett, Siebert, & Wallen, 2008). It has been argued that these types of preferences occur at their earliest stages because young girls are programmed to seek objects that imply nurturance, while young boys are interested in objects that suggest movement or excitement (Alexander & Hines, 2002). However, these differences are also likely to occur within an environment that reinforces or punishes such behaviors. From early age, young boys and girls are treated differently by parents and peers for engaging in play behaviors that are deemed appropriate for their gender. Fathers tend to display more positive reactions to daughters and provide more negative feedback to boys playing with cross-gendered toys. On the other hand, mothers and peers exhibit more rewards for play with gendered toys and mothers tend to be more positive overall about their children's play (Langlois & Downs, 1980). Play preferences are a significant part of sexuality development, as it has been linked with later homosexual orientation (Alanko et al., 2010). Even when play behavior decreases, other gender differences still persist throughout adolescence.

In a study of middle and late adolescent women, researchers examined two qualities, relationship authenticity and body objectification, associated with feminist ideology. They discovered that young women who were less authentic in friendships and those who felt more negative about their body demonstrated less sexual self-efficacy or feelings of being in sexual control within their sexual relationship. Lower sexual self-efficacy was also predictive of less hormonal contraceptive use and greater use of condoms during first sex. Similarly, negative feelings about one's body were related to lower rates of condom use. The authors argued that being less authentic and feeling less positive about one's body may be associated with traditional feminine ideology and less perceived sexual control. Ironically, young women also tended to view aggression as a desirable quality in a potential partner (Impett, Schooler, & Tolman, 2006). This relationship might be due to the association that young men who display aggressive qualities may appear older or more distinctive (Bukowski, Sippola, & Newcomb, 2000).

Pleck and others (1993) examined the masculine ideology of middle and late adolescent men and discovered that young men who held more traditional views of romantic relationships viewed heterosexual relationships as more oppositional, believed that it was their partner's responsibility to prevent pregnancy, believed that getting a relationship partner pregnant is a vital part to being a man, endorsed more overall sexual partners, demonstrated a negative view of condoms, and used condoms less regularly (Pleck, Sonenstein, & Ku, 1993). In a more recent study, Giordano and colleagues (2006) found disparate results which indicated that young men expressed greater feelings of awkwardness when communicating with a dating partner. Young men were also less confident within romantic relationships, although young men who engaged in sexual activity with their romantic partner felt more confident within their relationship. Participants also endorsed greater levels of attempted interpersonal influence and this influence increased throughout the length of the relationship. However, young men were less likely to view themselves positively with regard to having power within their relationship, as they endorsed actual influence deriving from their relationship partner (Giordano, Longmore, & Manning, 2006).

In a retrospective account of gender differences within partnered relationships, Morgan and Zurbriggen (2007) found that sexual gender roles are very prevalent among adolescents engaging in sexual intercourse. When recounting their first sexual experience during adolescence, adult women reported feeling pressured to engage in sex. Adult women also had beliefs that their male sexual partner ascribed to masculine values. Adult men recounted that their first female sexual partner wanted to set sexual boundaries. However, both men and women highlighted the significance of sexual negotiations within their first sexual encounter. This suggests that sexual negotiating is an important part of developing one's sexual identity and communicating within an adolescent sexual relationship.

Gender influences likely occur through a system of reinforcement and punishment from parents, family members, and peers. Adolescents appear to ascribe to specific gendered roles which are quite different for young men and young women. Young women in particular tend to report feeling pressured to engage in sex. Nonetheless, our understanding of these experiences appears to be more complex then early research in this area has suggested. That is, young men may be more aware of and in touch with the emotional component of sexuality than previous research has asserted. Young women may also be making partnering decisions with the intent of locating a more distinctive, aggressive partner, but may, in actuality, be increasing their probability of lowered sexual self-efficacy. Overall, adolescent pathways of gender development may be more similar than divergent for young men and young women. It is probable that both young men and young women have similar sexuality experiences, but they may experience very different reinforcement strategies from parents and peers. Accordingly, they may encounter a host of punishing behaviors if they do not display their sexual emotions and behaviors in a gendered-specific manner.

Parent Influences

Throughout childhood, parents play an increasing role in their children's lives. From managing their basic survival necessities, they also present morals, values, and messages regarding acceptable and appropriate sexual behavior. Parents who engage in open and responsive communication, tend to have adolescents with intentions to delay sexual activity for at least 1 year (Fasula & Miller, 2006). Whitaker and Miller (2000) also discovered that adolescents who had discussion with their parents about sex tended to initiate sex later and have fewer sexual partners. Additionally, parents who discussed condom use were more likely to have adolescents who had ever used condoms, had used condoms at their most recent sexual event, and who used condoms more consistently overall. Moreover, they found that adolescents who communicated with their parents about sex and condom use were less influenced by peers and more likely to report that their parents provided more accurate information about sex as compared to adolescents who had not engaged in such conversations.

Another way that parents have been shown to be a significant influence on adolescent sexual behavior is through parental monitoring. Adolescents with lower levels of parental monitoring tend to engage in sexual intercourse at a younger age. This relationship is especially significant among young women who have more sexual partners and are less likely to use any form of contraceptives during sex intercourse (Wight, Williamson, & Henderson, 2006). Researchers have also found that parental monitoring techniques and its effects vary across ethnic groups. For example, Pearson and colleagues (2006) examined the specific aspects of parental involvement that influence initiation of sexual activity among European American, African American, and Latino American adolescents. Results from this study indicated that adolescents living with two biological parents were less likely to engage in sexual behaviors as compared to adolescents with other family formations. However, African American adolescents residing with step-parents were no more likely than those residing with biological parents to initiate sex. In addition, shared dinnertime, parent-adolescent communication about sex, shared parent-adolescent activities, and having a close parent-adolescent relationship was related to European American adolescents being less likely to ever initiating sex. However, with regard to sexual initiation, engaging in shared activities was the only significant parent-adolescent factor for African American adolescents and communicating about sex was the only significant parental monitoring technique among Latino American adolescents (Pearson, Muller, & Frisco, 2006). Although it is likely that other parental factors do in fact influence feelings of social support and sexual behaviors among African American and Latino American adolescents, it is possible that cultural differences within parent–adolescent relationships may not have been captured by the instruments utilized in this study.

Taken together, parents play a vital role in the engagement of their adolescent's sexual behaviors. Both parental communication and parental monitoring have significant influences on not only adolescent beliefs but also the behaviors with which they engage. These techniques appear to delay intent to engage in sexual intercourse, an increase in parental status regarding sexual information, and reduced sexual risk-taking through increased condom use and fewer sexual partners. Parents are strongly encouraged develop an open dialogue with their adolescents about sexuality, sexual behaviors, contraceptive use and parental values of preferred adolescent behavior. Preferably, these conversations would occur during preadolescence. This would promote an open dialogue for adolescents to seek out additional information from their parents, clarify inconsistencies in sexual knowledge, and problem-solve sexual conflicts.

Sibling Influences

Similar to parents, siblings also provide a significant model with regard to sexual behavior. These effects tend to be more influential when siblings are older and more alike. For example, adolescents with older siblings are more likely to have engaged in sexual behaviors. This effect appears to be most significant for adolescent with siblings who are 4 or more years older than themselves. In addition, research demonstrates a subthreshold trend that young women with an older sibling tend to be less likely to use contraception during their first sexual intercourse encounter (Argys, Rees, Averett, & Witoonchart, 2006).

Having a good relationship with a sibling or having a sibling who is more genetically similar has also been linked to risky sexual behaviors. Also, stronger attitudes about becoming pregnant have also been associated among siblings who are more biologically similar (McHale, Bissell, & Kim, 2009). For instance, young women who report higher levels of companionship with their older sister are more likely to become pregnant. Likewise, young women have a greater probability of becoming pregnant if their older sister has experienced a pregnancy or if both their older sister and mother have experienced a teenage pregnancy. However, when teenage pregnancies of mothers and older siblings are compared, young women have a greater chance of becoming pregnant if their older sister experienced a pregnancy as compared to their mother having experienced a pregnancy when she was a teenager (East, Reyes, & Horn, 2007).

Overall, having an older sexually active sibling shapes adolescent sexuality and sexual behaviors. Adolescents with older siblings have the opportunity to learn from their sibling's experience, be more encouraged to participate in sexual activity, or be less inclined to follow in their sibling's footsteps. These relationships appear to be stronger when adolescents are more biologically similar to their siblings or share a closer relationship to their sibling. However, much of the research conducted to date has investigated sibling relationships among young women. Although it is likely that older male siblings also influence sexual behaviors among young men, additional research is needed to examine these relationships.

Peer Influences

The impact of peers on adolescent sexual behaviors is notable, complex, and strengthens across time. Not surprisingly, peers often set norms for sexual behaviors (Kinsman, Romer, Furstenberg, & Schwarz, 1998) and these norms are likely established both overtly (e.g., increased social status) or subtly (e.g., encouraging the perception of participation in sexual behaviors). Although the differences in sexual behavior as a result of either norm has yet to be clearly established, perception of peer engagement of sexual activity has been associated with having more sexually experienced friends, perceiving more respect from friends, being more involved with friends (Sieving, Eisenberg, Pettingell, & Skay, 2006), and initiating sexual activity (Zimmer-Gembeck & Helfand, 2008). The literature has also highlighted that adolescents who are not themselves engaging in sexual behaviors may feel hindered by their limited ability to contribute to conversations with peers (Skinner, Smith, Fenwick, Fyfe, & Hendriks, 2008). This suggests that adolescents may perceive the peer norm to participate in discussions about sexual behaviors through sharing relevant and personal experience.

Peer influences also vary across sexual behaviors. One such example is that peers influence oral sex behaviors more readily than vaginal intercourse behaviors. Prinstein and colleagues (2003) found a relationship between the reported numbers of oral sex partners among adolescents and their perceived number of oral sex partners for their best friends. Adolescents who endorsed engaging in more oral sex were considered to be more popular but less friendly. The researchers also found that peers shape sexual intercourse behaviors, especially if adolescents perceive that their peers engaged in sexual intercourse at a younger age, were currently engaging in sexual intercourse, or that social status would be gained as a result of sexual intercourse (Prinstein, Meade, & Cohen, 2003). Ironically, in the same way that peer influence may be negative through increased pressure to initiate sexual activity, peer pressure may also be protective with regard to contraceptive use. In another study, it was found that having the belief that peers are more likely to use condoms during sexual activity was linked to a greater desire to use condoms at first sex and an increased use of some form of contraception during sexual intercourse, especially among young men (Potard, Courtois, & Rusch, 2008).

Some have even suggested that the media may represent a "super peer" by influencing early adolescents' interest in advanced sexual behaviors (Brown, Halpern, & L'Engle, 2005). This hypothesis was demonstrated by a study that investigated adolescent sexual behavior and the media domain of music, adolescents who listened to greater amounts of sexually degrading music lyrics were more likely to engage in sexual intercourse and other sexual behaviors (i.e., masturbation). Notably, music with strong sexual themes without degrading lyrics was not related to adolescent sexual behaviors (Martino et al., 2006). This implies that sexual themes alone do not promote sexual behavior. Rather, the addition of degrading lyrics appears to be the key feature in encouraging adolescents to participate in sexual behavior. Another media study examined the relationship between sexual content from four media domains (i.e., television, movies, music, and magazines) among African American and European American adolescents across time. Researchers discovered that adolescents aged 12–14 with the highest media exposure to sexual content were more likely to have engaged in sexual intercourse 2 years later. However, this trend was more widely observed among European American adolescents (Brown et al., 2006). It is possible that the association between the media was not as prevalent for African American adolescents because much of the content within these domains did not reflect basic demographic characteristics of these adolescents (i.e., skin color). Thus, the likely reduced salience across media domains may have led to reduced media comparisons, resulting in less media influence among African American adolescents.

By and large, peers have a substantive influence on perception of sexual activity, contraception, and various sexual behaviors. The influence of peers may be more subtle, such as making adolescents feel bad if they cannot contribute to a conversation about sexual activity or more overt such as improved social status through engaging in various sexual behaviors. Paradoxically, the media which is operated and controlled by adults also functions as a peer by providing explicit cues about appropriate sexual activity, although the influence of these effects may be more relevant across groups of adolescents. Nevertheless, peers influence is most apparent among adolescents who lack adequate communication with their parents about sexual behaviors and using condoms (Whitaker & Miller, 2000).

Partner Influences

As the common saying goes, "it takes two to tango," most sexual behaviors involve a sexual partner. Sexual partnerships often play an increasing role as individuals shift from middle to late adolescence and early adulthood. These relationships encompass a wide variety of dynamics including age of first partnership, age differentials between partners, emotional connectedness, sexual power, sexual gender roles, and sexual negotiation. While many of these variables may be involved in adolescent sexual relationships to some degree, the literature is clear that the outcomes of these variables may differ among young men and young women.

In a longitudinal study investigating relationship experiences between adolescent men and women, researchers discovered interesting gender similarities and differences. Both young men and young women who participated in a relationship in the seventh grade demonstrated a greater probability of being sexual active by the ninth grade. However, young women who had older boyfriends in the seventh grade were even more likely to have engaged in sexual activity in ninth grade. This relationship was not found among young men. In addition, when young women were compared to each other, those who experienced menarche in sixth grade were more likely to be in relationships with young men who were at least 2 years older than themselves (Marín, Kirby, Hudes, Coyle, & Gómez, 2006). Another study found that approximately one-third of adolescents engage in sexual partnerships with older individuals. Characteristics associated with these adolescents include having an older peer group, attending a school with a wider grade span, being younger, using substances, endorsing higher levels of communication with their parents, having less educated parents, or being foreign born (Manlove, Ryan, & Franzetta, 2007).

Other partner characteristics such as feeling emotionally close to a romantic partner or perceiving that a romantic partner has more power has been demonstrated to influence adolescent sexual behaviors. For example, when adolescent participants were asked who they perceived to have more power within romantic relationships, both young men and young women agreed that they perceived young women to have more power within romantic relationships. However, young men were found to have more actual power in adolescent relationships (Giordano, Manning, & Longmore, 2010). Power differentials are important as risky sexual behaviors have been observed among adolescents who want to please their partner because they perceive their partner as having more relationship control (Marston & King, 2006). For instance, young women have reported that despite not feeling ready to initiate sexual intercourse, they have done so out of fear of losing a relationship partner or due to concern that their relationship partner may feel unsatisfied (Skinner et al., 2008). Moreover, Blythe and colleagues (2006) found that within a 3-month span, approximately 40 % of young adolescent women reported experiencing unwanted sexual intercourse at least once and over one-third of young women reported engaging in unwanted sexual intercourse out of concern that their partner would become angry if they refused (Blythe, Fortenberry, Temkit, Tu, & Orr, 2006).

These studies reveal that sexual partners play a very significant role in influencing adolescent sexual behaviors. Early experiences with a romantic partner are related to the increased probability that adolescent young women will become sexual active. In addition, perception of relationship power and actual relationship power has been demonstrated to be important components of adolescent relationships. This may be especially relevant among young women who may feel pressured to engage in unwanted sexual behaviors because they perceive that their sexual partners have more relationship power or that their partner may become angry and/or decide to leave the relationship. Also, young women who participate in romantic partnerships with older young men may experience an even greater power dynamics within their relationship. Of note, a lack of parental involvement and monitoring was implicated as a risk factor for young women participating in relationships with older partners. This again highlights the role that parents play in mitigating the effects of undesirable partner influences. Moreover, additional partner research that is squarely focused on young men would be valuable to better understanding this area.

Neighborhood and Cultural Influences

Social environments have also been shown to influence adolescent sexuality and sexual behaviors. Previous research has demonstrated distinct differences in the sexual behaviors of adolescents who reside in communities that are poor, structurally disadvantaged, lack supervision, experience greater incidents of crime, and/or have fewer available community resources (Cubbin, Santelli, Brindis, & Braveman, 2005; DiClemente et al., 2008; Sampson, Morenoff, & Gannon-Rowley, 2002). Accordingly, it is no surprise that adolescents who spend more time at home alone are more likely to engage in sexual behaviors (Buhi & Goodson, 2007).

Neighborhood influences on sexual behaviors have also been observed in a study by Browning and colleagues (2008). The investigators examined how immigrant populations, neighborhood level covariates and collective efficacy or the combined effects of parental and adult supervision of adolescents within one's neighborhood predicted adolescents engaging in multiple sexual partnerships across time. Using data derived from the Project on Human Development in Chicago Neighborhoods and 1990 Census data, the researchers discovered that adolescents were more likely to report ever having a sexual partner if they were older, male, in the latter stages of puberty, living in concentrate poverty and/or if they had ever experienced past problem behaviors. Adolescents who reported higher levels of parental attachment and those who were first or second generation immigrants and lived in neighborhoods with low levels of immigrant populations were less likely to ever report having a sexual partner. Having ever had more than one sexual partner was related to being older, male and African American. Adolescents who endorsed greater collective efficacy were less likely to have ever experienced more than one sexual partner (Browning, Burrington, Leventhal, & Brooks-Gunn, 2008).

Perhaps one of the most frequently considered cultural aspects of adolescent sexuality and sexual behavior is religiosity. Religiosity has been associated with reduced risk-taking behaviors such as delinquency (Armour & Haynie, 2007) and delay of initiation of first sex among early, middle, and late adolescents (Zimmer-Gembeck & Helfand, 2008). In a recent study, adolescent young women who were affiliated with a religious organization during childhood were less likely to have ever engaged in oral sex or vaginal sex. Also, young men who consistently endorsed attending religious services during their childhood were more likely to be virgins and never have engaged in oral sex (Brewster & Tillman, 2008).

Norms and limits established within one's culture and neighborhood likely serves as an example of appropriate adolescent sexual behavior. This is possibly why significant differences in sexual behaviors have been observed among adolescents residing in disadvantaged communities. Adolescents in these communities may have reduced opportunities and less parental monitoring experiences, thus increasing the influence of peers, relationship partners or perhaps other individuals in their community. Similarly, religiosity also models acceptable sexual behaviors as adolescents who ascribe to a particular religion delay initiating in sexual behaviors. These studies emphasize that adolescent sexual behaviors cannot be viewed in isolation. That is, consideration must be given to the context of one's environment and relevant cultural factors.

Sexual Behavior During Adolescence

Adolescents engage in a variety of sexual behaviors, with vaginal sex representing one of many forms of sexual expression. Accordingly, the variety and prevalence of sexual behaviors with which adolescents engage is central to understanding adolescent sexuality. For example, masturbation is a very common form of sexual expression throughout one's life course. In studies of older adolescents and adults, masturbation is nearly universal among men and reported by a majority of women (Gerressu, Mercer, Graham, Wellings, & Johnson, 2008; Kinsey, Pomery, & Martin, 1948; Kinsey, Pomeroy, Martin, & Gebhard, 1953; Laumann, Gagnon, Michael, & Michaels, 2000; Pinkerton, Bogart, Cecil, & Abramson, 2003). In a recent national sample of sexual behaviors in the USA (see Table 1), masturbation was more common than any partnered sexual behavior among 14–17-year-old adolescents (Herbenick et al., 2010). In addition, masturbation onset has been shown to occur by early adolescence (between the ages of 11 and 13) in 53 % of males and 25 % of females (Janus & Janus, 1993).

Despite the prevalence of masturbation, it remains an extremely sensitive topic, and accordingly is often underreported adolescents, even with the use of confidential reporting techniques (Halpern, Udry, Suchindran, & Campbell, 2000). This is likely due to themes of guilt, shame, and indulgence often being associated with this behavior (Bullough, 1995; Patton, 1986). Perhaps this is the rationale behind omitting masturbation from sexuality education, (Moore & Rienzo, 2000), even in the context of abstinence-only education (Fine & McClelland, 2006). Moreover, many parents omit discussions of masturbation in hopes that children will view masturbation unfavorably (Friedrich et al., 1991; Gagnon, 1985; Leung & Robson, 1993). Few data directly explore associations of adolescent masturbation and other sexual behaviors, although a recent paper shows that masturbation in the past year was associated with partnered sexual behaviors among young men and young women (Robbins et al., 2011).

Noncoital sexual behaviors such as kissing, nongenital touching, and genital touching are also common adolescent sexual behaviors that often precede first sexual intercourse (O'Sullivan, Cheng, Harris, & Brooks-Gunn, 2007). The prevalence of oral sex has also become more common in recent years, perhaps in response to a greater emphasis on the value of virginity and media popularized "risks" associated with sexual intercourse. Oral sex, in particular, also allows for sexual learning that emphasizes exchange, physical intimacy, and pleasure as well as "safer" sexual behaviors (Halpern-Felsher et al., 2005). To the extent that noncoital sexual behaviors provide opportunity to experience partnered arousal, sexual agency, and sexual control, oral sex is likely an important part of the development of healthy sexuality during adolescence and young adulthood (Horne & Zimmer-Gembeck, 2005). Frequencies by age of giving and receiving oral sex with same- and different-sex partners are summarized in Table 1.

Vaginal sex is often viewed in both popular and professional dialogue as the *sine qua non* of sexual development. Many societies develop separate language and social status for adolescents before and after an initial vaginal sexual experience (Fasula & Miller, 2006). However, the range and meanings of sexual behaviors available to adolescents suggest the need for a more nuanced perspective. For example, a recent daily diary study showed no difference in daily mood on days before and after first coitus (Tanner et al., 2010). Recent data from the National Survey of Sexual Health and Behavior (NSSHB) provided age-specific rates of a range of sexual behaviors of

Table 1 Sexual behavior during adolescence

	Adolescent males (N=482)			Adolescent females (N=450)		
	14–15 (n=191)	16–17 (n=219)	18–19 (n=72)	14–15 (n=188)	16–17 (n=212)	18–19 (n=50)
Masturbated alone						
Past month (%)	42.9	58.0	61.1	24.1	25.5	26.0
Past year (%)	62.1	74.8	80.6	40.4	44.8	60.0
Lifetime (%)	67.5	78.9	86.1	43.3	52.4	66.0
Masturbated with partner						
Past month (%)	3.6	7.1	14.5	4.3	11.2	18.4
Past year (%)	5.2	16.0	42.0	7.5	18.9	36.0
Lifetime (%)	5.7	20.3	49.3	9.0	19.7	38.8
Received oral from female						
Past month (%)	7.8	17.5	22.9	0	2.3	0
Past year (%)	11.9	30.9	53.6	1.1	4.7	3.9
Lifetime (%)	13.0	34.4	59.4	3.8	6.6	8.0
Received oral from male						
Past month (%)	0.5	1.4	1.5	3.7	16.4	32.0
Past year (%)	0.5	2.8	5.9	10.0	23.5	58.0
Lifetime (%)	1.6	3.2	8.8	10.1	25.8	62.0
Gave oral to female						
Past month (%)	2.6	13.8	20.3	0.5	4.2	2.0
Past year (%)	7.8	18.3	50.7	1.6	7.1	2.0
Lifetime (%)	8.3	20.2	60.9	5.4	9.0	8.2
Gave oral to male						
Past month (%)	1.0	0.9	1.4	8.0	14.6	34.7
Past year (%)	1.0	2.3	4.3	11.8	22.4	58.5
Lifetime (%)	1.6	2.8	10.1	12.8	29.1	61.2
Vaginal intercourse						
Past month (%)	7.9	16.1	31.0	5.9	20.8	43.1
Past year (%)	8.9	30.3	52.8	10.7	29.7	62.0
Lifetime (%)	9.9	30.3	62.5	12.4	31.6	64.0
Receptive anal sex						
Past month (%)	1.0	0.9	1.4	3.2	0.5	8.0
Past year (%)	1.0	0.9	4.2	3.7	4.7	18.0
Lifetime (%)	1.0	0.9	4.3	4.3	6.6	20.0
Insertive anal sex						
Past month (%)	0.5	1.4	0	–	–	–
Past year (%)	3.1	5.5	5.6			
Lifetime (%)	3.7	6.0	9.7			

Herbenick et al. (2010)

adolescents aged 14–19 years. Vaginal intercourse was a rare event for the majority of 14–15-year-olds with 90 % of males and 88 % of females never having engaged in sex. Among 16–17-year-olds, vaginal sex occurred more frequently. However, only approximately one-third of males and females in this age group reported ever having vaginal sex. Among 18–19-year-olds, 63 % of males and 64 % of females reported experiencing vaginal sex at least once during their lifetime. Anal sex, and especially receptive anal sex, was a low occurring behavior among most adolescents. For instance, among 18–19-year-old males, lifetime prevalence rates of receptive anal sex was 4 %, while 10 % of males in this age group reported ever engaging in insertive anal sex.

Among adolescent women, anal sex was also a very low occurring event and was endorsed at a rate of 4 % among 14–15-year-olds and 7 % among 16–17-year-olds. Higher rates of anal sex were reported among 18–19-year-old adolescent females with over 20 % having experienced anal sex once during their lifetime (Table 1; Herbenick et al., 2010).

Sexual Behavior and Sexually Explicit Media

One aspect of adolescent sexual behavior that is gaining increasing attention is adolescent access to sexually explicit media through use of the internet, cell phones, television, and movies. Whether such material is obtained intentionally or unintentionally, it appears to be linked to pubertal development (Peter & Valkenburg, 2006) with approximately 90 % of adolescents who view it being age 14 or older (Ybarra & Mitchell, 2005). It is also becoming apparent that exposure to such material influences adolescent sexual behaviors (Cooper, McLoughlin, & Campbell, 2000; Štulhofer, Buško, & Landripet, 2010). For example, accessing sexually explicit material has been associated with male gender, a higher level of sensation seeking, a reduced odds of condom use during last sex (Luder et al., 2011), more lifetime sexual partners, having multiple sexual partners in the last 3 months, and having used alcohol or substances during a last sexual encounter (Braun-Courville & Rojas, 2009). Greater levels of sexually explicit material also have been linked to lower socioeconomic status, having less educated parents, being older, being African American, being more likely to have engaged in some form of sexual harassment, and having less developed gender role beliefs (Brown & L'Engle, 2009). Adolescents who view sexually explicit material also are more likely to endorse that it depicts sexually realistic behaviors and that sex is more of a physical rather than a relational activity (Peter & Valkenburg, 2010).

Sexting, or the transmission of sexual text, seminude, or nude photographs via cell phone use is a contemporary form of sexually explicit media. Despite considerable attention of this topic, very little scientific research has been conducted in this area (Weiss & Samenow, 2010). This is significant in that sexting is a unique form of sexually explicit media. Some jurisdictions view sexting within the framework of child pornography laws (Ostrager, 2010) and multiple adolescents have been prosecuted for self-produced child pornography (Arcabascio, 2010).

Sexting appears to be a somewhat frequent behavior. According to a recent survey of adolescents and young adults, approximately 22 % of adolescent young women and 18 % of adolescent young men report having sent or received sexting picture messages, with the vast majority of these messages being sent to a relationship partner. With regard to sexting text messages, 37 % of adolescent young women and 40 % of adolescent young men have sent or posted such messages. Of note, approximately 59 % of young adults (aged 20–26) have sent or posted sexting text messages (The National Campaign to Prevent Teen and Unplanned Pregnancy & Cosmo Girl.com, 2008). This suggests that despite the focus of adolescent sexting, late adolescents and young adults are regularly engaging in sexing behaviors.

Notwithstanding the novelty of many new forms of sexually explicit media, glaring behavioral differences between adolescents and adults has yet to be found. Any pattern differences suggest that adults utilize sexually explicit media much more frequently than adolescents, with adult males endorsing the highest rates (Peter & Valkenburg, 2011). By and large, additional research is needed in this area to examine longitudinal trends of sexually explicit media among adolescents. Likewise, more consistent definitions are necessary so that generalized findings can be made across studies (Short, Black, Smith, Wetterneck, & Wells, 2011).

Psychosexual Development

Normal prepubertal children display a range of sexual behaviors, including masturbation, interest in sexual topics, revealing genitals to adults or children, and efforts to observe the genitals of others (Friedrich et al., 1991; Thigpen, 2009). Many children demonstrate knowledge of sexual

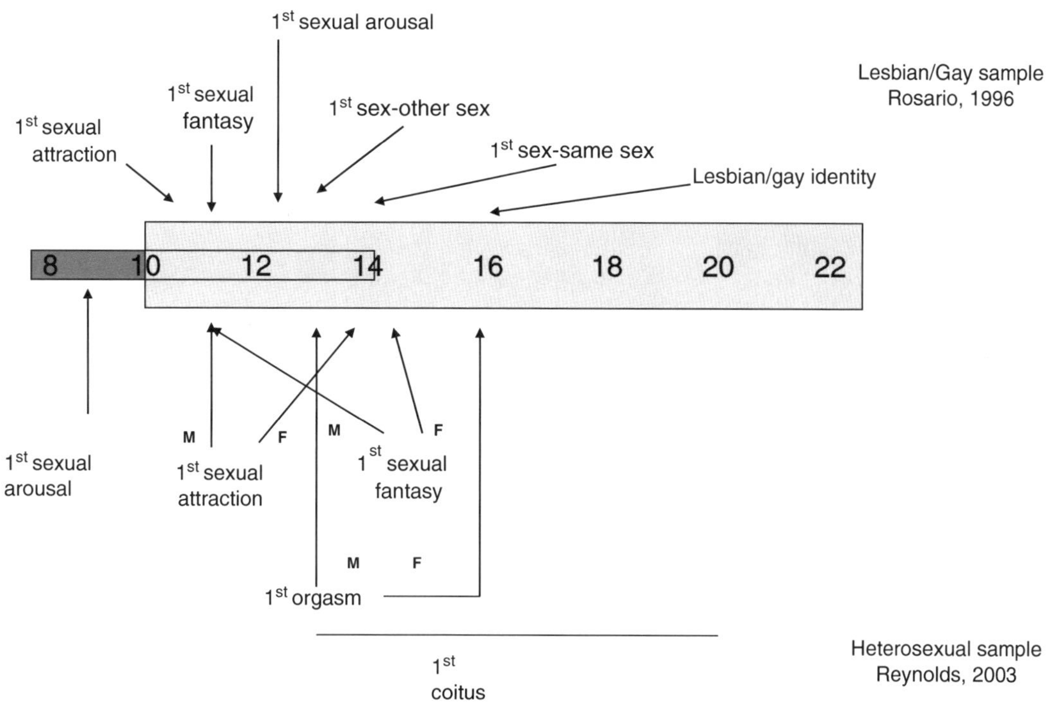

Fig. 2 Milestones in adolescent psychosexual development

body parts, the functions of those parts, and other aspects of sexuality (Grocke et al., 1995) and engage in both same-gender and cross-gender sexual play (Okami et al., 1997). Familial attitudes, familial and environmental stressors and responses to manifestations of sexuality in a child, likely influence subsequent psychosexual development (Thigpen & Fortenberry, 2009). However, there is no evidence that children have a self-awareness of themselves as *sexual*, and some authors argue for a clear conceptual distinction between children's and adolescents' sexuality (Rademakers, Laan, & Straver, 2003).

The developmental connections of childhood and adolescent sexuality and sexual behavior are not clearly specified. Figure 2 depicts a general timeline. Although linear growth and breast and genital development (gonadarche) during puberty are generally identified as the starting place for adolescent sexuality, first sexual attractions (to same or different sex persons) are reported around age 10 (Herdt & McClintock, 2000). This age roughly corresponds to the process of adrenarche and it is associated with increases in levels of two androgenic steroid hormones dehydroepiandrosterone (DHEA) and dehydroepiandrosterone sulfate (DHEAS) (Campbell, 2006). This suggests that the developmental origins of adolescent sexuality precede puberty (Herdt & McClintock, 2000).

Sexual Self-Concept

Sexual self-concept is a multidimensional construct encompassing an individual's positive and negative perceptions of themselves as a sexual person (Rostosky et al., 2008). These perceptions are developed from identities, self-evaluations, attitudes, beliefs, values, and desires of one's sexual self. Accordingly, the sexual self encompasses feelings to help interpret sexual experiences and provides both structure and motivation for sexual behavior in different sexual scenarios (Birnbaum et al., 2006).

Some elements of sexual self-concept are apparent in early adolescence, often months or years before any physical sexual contact (Butler, Miller, Holtgrave, Forehand, & Long, 2006; Ott,

Pfeiffer, & Fortenberry, 2006). However, as sexual self-concept develops, new behaviors reshape existing generalizations about the sexual self. This process, in turn, influences the choice of future sexual behaviors (Houlihan et al., 2008; O'Sullivan & Brooks-Gunn, 2005). Previous research has varied in its operationalization of sexual self-concept, with some using uni-dimensional definitions (e.g., Breakwell & Millward, 1997) and more recent studies postulating multiple domains of sexual self-concept (e.g., O'Sullivan et al., 2006). Four domains of sexual self-concept (i.e., sexual openness, sexual self-esteem, sexual ambivalence, and sexual anxiety) are considered in more detail.

Sexual Self-Esteem

Sexual self-esteem includes one's affective reactions and appraisals of their sexual thoughts, feelings, and behaviors as well as perceptions of their body in a sexual context (Horne & Zimmer-Gembeck, 2006). Australian adolescents who classified themselves as sexually "competent," "adventurous," or "driven" reported a more positive view of their sexual activity, perceived themselves as more sexually attractive, felt more assured in sexual situations, and were more satisfied with their bodies as compared to those who reported themselves as less sexually experienced (Buzwell & Rosenthal, 1996). Higher sexual self-esteem has also been linked with more sexual experience and higher sexual satisfaction, but not with earlier onset of intercourse or with increased number of partner changes (Hensel, Fortenberry, O'Sullivan, & Orr, 2011; Impett et al., 2006). It is possible that adolescents with higher sexual self-esteem place more value on their sexuality and sexual experiences, and by extension are willing to engage sexual partner discussions related to sexual satisfaction, emotions, and openness to participate in risk (Oattes & Offman, 2007).

Sexual Openness

Sexual openness refers to recognition of sexual pleasure or sexual arousal, as well as deriving a sense of well-being from understanding one's entitlement to experience and express sexual desire (Horne & Zimmer-Gembeck, 2006). In general, greater sexual openness is associated with greater desire to explore (or not explore) new sexual behaviors, greater use of condoms and contraception, lower pregnancy rates, and later onset of sexual intercourse (O'Sullivan et al., 2006). Sexual openness increases with age among young women, with higher levels of sexual openness being associated with a greater frequency of oral and vaginal sex (Hensel et al., 2011).

Sexual Ambivalence

Sexual ambivalence has been defined as two processes including individuals wanting to engage in sex but not consenting to it (nonconsensual wanted sex) or individuals not desiring sex but deciding to consent to it (unwanted consensual sex) (Muehlenhard & Peterson, 2005). Sexual ambivalence is a common, normal developmental process during adolescence, with higher levels associated with younger adolescents, less body satisfaction, pressure to engage in first sex, a stronger desire to be in a relationship prior to engaging in first sex, being on an educational track intended for college, or delaying first sex (Pinquart, 2010). Greater levels of sexual ambivalence have also been linked to a reduced ability to predict engaging in sexual behavior and decreased use of condoms (MacDonald & Hynie, 2008).

Sexual Anxiety

Negative emotions associated with sexuality (e.g., anxiety and guilt) can serve as a deterrent to sexual behavior or contribute to sexual dysfunction. Sexual anxiety, for example, has been associated with more abstinence beliefs, lower perceived likelihood of intercourse in the near future, fewer reports of having a partner, having been in love, or having engaged in kissing, fondling, or vaginal sex. Also, older adolescents had lower negative sexual affect as compared to younger adolescents (O'Sullivan et al., 2006). This reveals that reduced negativity regarding sexual topics appears to align with increasing sexual experience, perhaps as an anticipatory effect (O'Sullivan & Brooks-Gunn, 2005).

Sexual Health

Sexual health has gained prominence in recent years as a guiding concept for understanding STIs and for the organization of testing, treatment, and prevention services. Sexual health is likely more explicitly linked to developmental change than at any other point during the sexual life span, with the possible exception of menopause. The approximately one decade span from age 10–20 encompasses the physical, psychological, social, and relational changes that become critical parameters of sexual health in the decades after adolescence (Bolton & MacEachron, 1988; Christopher & Cate, 1988; Dornbusch et al., 1981; Ehrhardt, 1996; Furman & Wehner, 1997; Gfellner, 1986; Halpern, 2010; Miller & Benson, 1999; O'Sullivan, Cheng, Harris, & Brooks-Gunn, 2007; Ott, Pfeiffer, & Fortenberry, 2006; Rosenthal, Cohen, & Biro, 1996). The World Health Organization (WHO) provides the following definition of sexual health.

> Sexual health is a state of physical, emotional, mental and social well-being related to sexuality; it is not merely the absence of disease, dysfunction or infirmity. Sexual health requires a positive and respectful approach to sexuality and sexual responses, as well as the possibility of having pleasurable and safe sexual experiences, free of coercion, discrimination and violence. For sexual health to be attained and maintained, the sexual rights of all persons must be respected, protected and fulfilled (Koyama, Corliss, & Santelli, 2009).

A somewhat different definition of adolescent sexual health was proposed in the Consensus Statement of the National Commission on Adolescent Sexual Health and endorsed by more than 50 national medical and policy organizations. They stated that

> Sexual health encompasses sexual development and reproductive health, as well as such characteristics as the ability to develop and maintain meaningful interpersonal relationships; appreciate one's own body; interact with both genders in respectful and appropriate ways; and express affection, love, and intimacy in ways consistent with one's own values (Bacon, 1999).

The Consensus Statement additionally notes that "responsible adolescent intimate relationships" should be "consensual, nonexploitative, honest, pleasurable, and protected against unintended pregnancy and STD's if any type of intercourse occurs."

The WHO and the National Consensus statement raise some additional issues to consider in thinking about the sexual health of adolescents. First, adolescents' sexual behavior is substantially limited by legal proscriptions. Most states have specific age thresholds to distinguish illegal and legal sexual activity (English, 2002; Findholt & Robrecht, 2002). For example, in the state of Indiana, partnered sexual activity before age 14 is defined as child abuse. Whether or not the sexual activity is consensual is not considered by these laws. Other states have established different age thresholds, up to age 18 years, meaning that the precept of individual sexual autonomy implicit in the WHO definition is legally restricted. We do not argue for or against the appropriateness of this restriction. Rather, it is important to note that adolescents do not have full sexual autonomy in most jurisdictions.

One additional difficulty in applying sexual health concepts to adolescents is the relative lack of data regarding sexual functioning and the subjective experience of sex among adolescents. Approximately, two-thirds of young men and just under half of young women reported orgasm associated with a sexual event, proportions similar to those reported by 16–19-year-olds in Australia: 84 % and 52 % for young men and young women, respectively (Richters, Visser, Rissel, & Smith, 2006). Orgasm is strongly associated with vaginal intercourse for both young men and young women and with oral sex for young men. Relationship status has also been associated with orgasm, consistent with a two-dimensional model of orgasm, reflecting both physical and emotional aspects, demonstrated among adults (Mah & Binik, 2002, 2005). Research also suggests that orgasm among adolescents is affected by factors such as cognitive distractions due to body image issues or performance anxieties (Meana & Nunnink, 2006). Pain is another relevant factor during adolescence and it is especially common among young women as one-third to half of young women report at least some pain with sexual intercourse (Landry & Bergeron, 2011).

Sexual Health Curricula

The limitations of the educational system in addressing sexual health have been noted for years (Fine, 1988). Access by adolescents to sexual health information is often restricted by local governmental or school board policy, as well as by state and national statutes. The content of sex education curricula is often skewed toward abstinence, pregnancy, and STI, with little or no mention of masturbation, sexual pleasure or orgasm (Koyama et al., 2009; Santelli, 2008). Similarly, the educational system has failed to attend to other pertinent adolescent sexuality issues such as sexual desire and it frequently stigmatizes youth who differ from mainstream society (Fine & McClelland, 2006). Adolescents who feel ashamed may instead turn to the internet for sexual health information. Even so, inaccuracies persist in large amounts online, even among websites touted as reputable (Yen, 2010). Additionally, much of the sexual health information portrayed in other aspects of the media tends to be incorrect, vague and vastly undervalue conscientious sexual behavior through use of humor. In a study examining four types of media content (i.e., movies, television, music, and magazines) less than half of 1 % of all media domains were represented by sexual health information. Furthermore, the sexual health information was organized around three key themes: (1) sexual health is awkward and comical, (2) young men are consumed by thoughts of sex and their sexual ability, and (3) young women are responsible for all prevention (e.g., contraceptives) and potential negative outcomes (e.g., pregnancy, STIs) of sexual behavior (Hust, Brown, & L'Engle, 2008).

Curriculum designed to teach sexual health is extremely important as adolescents are one of the most vulnerable populations to contract STI infections (Bearinger, Sieving, Ferguson, & Sharma, 2007) and large knowledge deficits regarding STIs and HIV continually persist, especially among some of the most vulnerable adolescent groups (Swenson et al., 2010). For example, one study found that approximately 14 % of adolescents believed that it was not possible to acquire an STI or HIV during oral sex. Oral sex was also viewed as less risky and less compromising (Halpern-Felsher, Cornell, Kropp, & Tschann, 2005). However, research has demonstrated negative emotional outcomes for adolescents who engage in only oral sex. These adolescents tend to feel guiltier and are less likely to experience the positive sexual feelings endorsed by peers who have participated in vaginal intercourse. Negative emotional outcomes are also markedly salient for young women participating in any sex, as they tend to be approximately three times more likely to endorse "feeling used" and twice as likely to have negative feelings about themselves after engaging in either vaginal or oral sex (Brady & Halpern-Felsher, 2007).

Adolescents require access to clinical health services and accurate information regarding sexual behaviors, negative outcomes of sex, and sexual decision-making. These programs appear to be most effective when implemented in both school and community settings. In addition, providing accurate sexual information and engaging adolescents to become advocates for themselves are also very important (Bearinger et al., 2007), as adolescents tend to be more proactive about their sexual health when provided with sexual health services (Maticka-Tyndale, 2008). Potential programs may include a combination of focus groups and a peer-socialization framework, as both appear to be useful in facilitating conversations about sex (Campbell & MacPhail, 2002; Hyde, Howlett, Brady, & Drennan, 2005). Regardless of the precise composition of these programs, much work is needed to begin implementing these changes into the existing adolescent sexual health curriculum. We suspect that few persons within the public health arena would endorse purposeful under-education as a national health strategy, but that persists as the de facto approach in much of the USA.

Conclusion

Overall, adolescence represents a period of trial and error. Entering and navigating through the world of sexual exploration, sexual initiation, and sexual maturity is certainly complex. Additional research is needed to understand the various sexual behaviors with which adolescents at different developmental stages engage. Furthermore, as the vast majority of early and middle adolescents have never participated in vaginal intercourse, polling only for this form of sexual behavior truncates our knowledge of sexuality and sexual behavior during adolescence. Supplementary work is needed to explicate the nuances of these relationships, and especially prospective research on young men. These literary pieces would be useful to help expand our understanding of adolescent sexual development and provide additional information to develop and refine sexual health venues that provide adolescents with skills to make informed decisions about their sexual health.

References

Alanko, K., Santtila, P., Harlaar, N., Witting, K., Varjonen, M., Jern, P., et al. (2010). Common genetic effects of gender atypical behavior in childhood and sexual orientation in adulthood: A study of Finnish twins. *Archives of Sexual Behavior, 39*, 81–92.

Alexander, G. M., & Hines, M. (2002). Sex differences in response to children's toys in nonhuman primates (Cercopithecus aethiops sabaeus). *Evolution and Human Behavior, 23*, 467–479.

Arcabascio, C. (2010). Sexting and teenagers: OMG RU Going 2 Jail???, XVI Rich. *JL & Tech, 10*.

Argys, L. M., Rees, D. I., Averett, S. L., & Witoonchart, B. (2006). Birth order and risky adolescent behavior. *Economic Inquiry, 44*, 215–233.

Armour, S., & Haynie, D. (2007). Adolescent sexual debut and later delinquency. *Journal of Youth and Adolescence, 36*, 141–152.

Bacon, J. L. (1999). Adolescent sexuality and teen pregnancy prevention. *Journal of Pediatric and Adolescent Gynecology, 12*, 185–193.

Bailey, J. M., Dunne, M. P., & Martin, N. G. (2000). Genetic and environmental influences on sexual orientation and its correlates in an Australian twin sample. *Journal of Personality and Social Psychology, 78*, 524–536.

Bearinger, L. H., Sieving, R. E., Ferguson, J., & Sharma, V. (2007). Adolescent health 2: Global perspectives on the sexual and reproductive health of adolescents: Patterns, prevention, and potential. *The Lancet, 369*, 1220–1231.

Birnbaum, G. E., Reis, H. T., Mikulincer, M., Gillath, O., & Orpaz, A. (2006). When sex is more than just sex: Attachment orientations, sexual experience, and relationship quality. *Journal of Personality and Social Psychology, 91*, 929.

Blythe, M. J. M. D., Fortenberry, J. D. M. D. M. S., Temkit, M. H. M. S., Tu, W. P., & Orr, D. P. M. D. (2006). Incidence and correlates of unwanted sex in relationships of middle and late adolescent women. *Archives of Pediatrics & Adolescent Medicine, 160*, 591–595.

Bocklandt, S., Horvath, S., Vilain, E., & Hamer, D. (2006). Extreme skewing of X chromosome inactivation in mothers of homosexual men. *Human Genetics, 118*, 691–694.

Bolton, F. G., Jr., & MacEachron, A. E. (1988). Adolescent male sexuality: A developmental perspective. *Journal of Adolescent Research, 3*, 259–273.

Brady, S. S., & Halpern-Felsher, B. L. (2007). Adolescents' reported consequences of having oral sex versus vaginal sex. *Pediatrics, 119*, 229–236.

Braun-Courville, D. K., & Rojas, M. (2009). Exposure to sexually explicit web sites and adolescent sexual attitudes and behaviors. *The Journal of Adolescent Health, 45*, 156–162.

Breakwell, G. M., & Millward, L. J. (1997). Sexual self-concept and sexual risk-taking. *Journal of Adolescence, 20*, 29–41.

Brewster, K. L., & Tillman, K. H. (2008). Who's doing it? Patterns and predictors of youths' oral sexual experiences. *The Journal of Adolescent Health, 42*, 73–80.

Brown, J. D., Halpern, C. T., & L'Engle, K. L. (2005). Mass media as a sexual super peer for early maturing girls. *The Journal of Adolescent Health, 36*, 420–427.

Brown, J. D., & L'Engle, K. L. (2009). X-rated. *Communication Research, 36*, 129–151.

Brown, J. D., L'Engle, K. L., Pardun, C. J., Guo, G., Kenneavy, K., & Jackson, C. (2006). Sexy media matter: Exposure to sexual content in music, movies, television, and magazines predicts black and white adolescents' sexual behavior. *Pediatrics, 117*, 1018–1027.

Browning, C. R., Burrington, L. A., Leventhal, T., & Brooks-Gunn, J. (2008). Neighborhood structural inequality, collective efficacy, and sexual risk behavior among urban youth. *Journal of Health and Social Behavior, 49*, 269–285.

Buhi, E. R., & Goodson, P. (2007). Predictors of adolescent sexual behavior and intention: A theory-guided systematic review. *The Journal of Adolescent Health, 40*, 4–21.

Bukowski, W. M., Sippola, L. K., & Newcomb, A. F. (2000). Variations in patterns of attraction of same- and other-sex peers during early adolescence. *Developmental Psychology, 36*, 147–154.

Bullough, V. L. (1995). Sexuality and religion. In L. Diamant & R. D. McAnulty (Eds.), *The pscyhology of sexual orientation, behavior, and identity: A handbook*. Westport, CT: Greenwood.

Butler, T. H., Miller, K. S., Holtgrave, D. R., Forehand, R., & Long, N. (2006). Stages of sexual readiness and six-month stage progression among African American pre-teens. *Journal of Sex Research, 43*, 378–386.

Buzwell, S., & Rosenthal, D. (1996). Constructing a sexual self: Adolescents' sexual self-perceptions and sexual risk-taking. *Journal of Research on Adolescence, 6*, 489–513.

Campbell, C., & MacPhail, C. (2002). Peer education, gender and the development of critical consciousness: Participatory HIV prevention by South African youth. *Social Science & Medicine, 55*, 331–345.

Campbell, B. (2006). Adrenarche and the evolution of human life history. *American Journal of Human Biology, 18*, 569–589.

Christopher, F. S., & Cate, R. M. (1988). Premarital sexual involvement: A developmental investigation of relational correlates. *Adolescence, 23*, 793–803.

Cohen-Bendahan, C. C. C., van de Beek, C., & Berenbaum, S. A. (2005). Prenatal sex hormone effects on child and adult sex-typed behavior: Methods and findings. *Neuroscience and Biobehavioral Reviews, 29*, 353–384.

Cooper, A., McLoughlin, I. P., & Campbell, K. M. (2000). Sexuality in cyberspace: Update for the 21st century. *Cyberpsychology & Behavior, 3*, 521–536.

Cubbin, C., Santelli, J., Brindis, C., & Braveman, P. (2005). Neighborhood context and sexual behaviors among adolescents: Findings from the national longitudinal study of adolescent health. *Perspectives on Sexual and Reproductive Health, 37*, 125–134.

DiClemente, R. J., Crittenden, C. P., Rose, E., Sales, J. M., Wingood, G. M., Crosby, R. A., et al. (2008). Psychosocial predictors of HIV-associated sexual behaviors and the efficacy of prevention interventions in adolescents at-risk for HIV infection: What works and what doesn't work? *Psychosomatic Medicine, 70*, 598–605.

Dittmann, R. W., Kappes, M. E., & Kappes, M. H. (1992). Sexual behavior in adolescent and adult females with congenital adrenal hyperplasia. *Psychoneuroendocrinology, 17*, 153–170.

Dornbusch, S. M., Carlsmith, J. M., Gross, R. T., Martin, J. A., Jennings, D., Rosenberg, A., et al. (1981). Sexual development, age, and dating: A comparison of biological and social influences upon one set of behaviors. *Child Development, 52*, 179–185.

East, P. L., Reyes, B. T., & Horn, E. J. (2007). Association between adolescent pregnancy and a family history of teenage births. *Perspectives on Sexual and Reproductive Health, 39*, 108–115.

Ehrhardt, A. A. (1996). Our view of adolescent sexuality—A focus on risk behavior without the developmental context. *American Journal of Public Health, 86*, 1523–1525.

English, A. (2002). The health of adolescent girls: Does the law support it? *Current Women's Health Reports, 2*, 442–449.

Fasula, A. M., & Miller, K. S. (2006). African-American and Hispanic adolescents' intentions to delay first intercourse: Parental communication as a buffer for sexually active peers. *The Journal of Adolescent Health, 38*, 193–200.

Findholt, N., & Robrecht, L. C. (2002). Legal and ethical considerations in research with sexually active adolescents: The requirement to report statutory rape. *Perspectives on Sexual and Reproductive Health, 34*, 259–264.

Fine, M. (1988). Sexuality, schooling, and adolescent females: The missing discourse of desire. *Harvard Educational Review, 58*, 29–51.

Fine, M., & McClelland, S. I. (2006). Sexuality education and desire: Still missing after all these years. *Harvard Educational Review, 76*, 297–338.

Friedman, R. C., & Downey, J. I. (2008). Sexual differentiation of behavior: The foundation of a developmental model of psychosexuality. *Journal of the American Psychoanalytic Association, 56*, 147–175.

Friedrich, W. N., Grambsch, P., Broughton, D., Kuiper, J., & Beilke, R. L. (1991). Normative sexual behavior in children. *Pediatrics, 88*, 456–464.

Furman, W., & Wehner, E. A. (1997). Adolescent romantic relationships: A developmental perspective. *New Directions for Child Development, 78*, 21–36.

Gagnon, J. H. (1985). Attitudes and responses of parents to pre-adolescent masturbation. *Archives of Sexual Behavior, 14*, 451–466.

Gerressu, M., Mercer, C. H., Graham, C. A., Wellings, K., & Johnson, A. M. (2008). Prevalence of masturbation and associated factors in a British national probability survey. *Archives of Sexual Behavior, 37*, 266–278.

Gfellner, B. M. (1986). Concepts of sexual behavior: Construction and validation of a developmental model. *Journal of Adolescent Research, 1*, 327–347.

Giordano, P. C., Longmore, M. A., & Manning, W. D. (2006). Gender and the meanings of adolescent romantic relationships: A focus on boys. *American Sociological Review, 71*, 260–287.

Giordano, P. C., Manning, W. D., & Longmore, M. A. (2010). Affairs of the heart: Qualities of adolescent romantic relationships and sexual behavior. *Journal of Research on Adolescence, 20*, 983–1013.

Graber, J. A., Nichols, T. R., & Brooks-Gunn, J. (2010). Putting pubertal timing in developmental context: Implications for prevention. *Developmental Psychobiology, 52*, 254–262.

Green, R., & Keverne, E. B. (2000). The disparate maternal aunt-uncle ratio in male transsexuals: An explanation invoking genomic imprinting. *Journal of Theoretical Biology, 202*, 55–63.

Grimbos, T., Dawood, K., Burriss, R. P., Zucker, K. J., & Puts, D. A. (2010). Sexual orientation and the second to fourth finger length ratio: A meta-analysis in men and women. *Behavioral Neuroscience, 124*, 278–287.

Grocke, M., Smith, M., & Graham, P. (1995). Sexually abused and nonabused mothers' discussions about sex and their children's sexual knowledge. *Child Abuse & Neglect, 19*, 985–996.

Guo, G., & Tong, Y. (2006). Age at first sexual intercourse, genes, and social context: Evidence from twins and the dopamine D4 receptor gene. *Demography, 43*, 747–769.

Halpern, C. T. (2010). Reframing research on adolescent sexuality: Healthy sexual development as part of the life course. *Perspectives on Sexual and Reproductive Health, 42*, 6–7.

Halpern, C. J. T., Udry, J. R., Suchindran, C., & Campbell, B. (2000). Adolescent males' willingness to report masturbation. *Journal of Sex Research, 37*, 327–332.

Halpern-Felsher, B. L., Cornell, J. L., Kropp, R. Y., & Tschann, J. M. (2005). Oral versus vaginal sex among adolescents: Perceptions, attitudes, and behavior. *Pediatrics, 115*, 845–851.

Hassett, J. M., Siebert, E. R., & Wallen, K. (2008). Sex differences in rhesus monkey toy preferences parallel those of children. *Hormones and Behavior, 54*, 359–364.

Hensel, D. J., Fortenberry, J. D., O'Sullivan, L., & Orr, D. P. (2011). The developmental association of sexual self-concept with sexual behavior among adolescent women. *Journal of Adolescence, 34*, 675–684.

Herbenick, D., Reece, M., Schick, V., Sanders, S. A., Dodge, B., & Fortenberry, J. D. (2010). Sexual behavior in the United States: Results from a national probability sample of men and women ages 14–94. *The Journal of Sexual Medicine, 7*, 255–265.

Herdt, G., & McClintock, M. (2000). The magical age of 10. *Archives of Sexual Behavior, 29*, 587–606.

Horne, S., & Zimmer-Gembeck, M. J. (2005). Female sexual subjectivity and well-being: Comparing late adolescents with different sexual experiences. *Sexuality Research and Social Policy, 2*, 25–40.

Horne, S., & Zimmer Gembeck, M. J. (2006). The female sexual subjectivity inventory: Development and validation of a multidimensional inventory for late adolescents and emerging adults. *Psychology of Women Quarterly, 30*, 125–138.

Houlihan, A. E., Gibbons, F. X., Gerrard, M., Yeh, H. C., Reimer, R. A., & Murry, V. M. (2008). Sex and the self the impact of early sexual onset on the self-concept and subsequent risky behavior of african american adolescents. *The Journal of Early Adolescence, 28*, 70–91.

Hust, S. J. T., Brown, J. D., & L'Engle, K. L. (2008). Boys will be boys and girls better be prepared: An analysis of the rare sexual health messages in young adolescents' media. *Mass Communication and Society, 11*, 3–23.

Hyde, A., Howlett, E., Brady, D., & Drennan, J. (2005). The focus group method: Insights from focus group interviews on sexual health with adolescents. *Social Science & Medicine, 61*, 2588–2599.

Impett, E., Schooler, D., & Tolman, D. (2006). To be seen and not heard: Femininity ideology and adolescent girls' sexual health. *Archives of Sexual Behavior, 35*, 129–142.

Janus, S. S., & Janus, C. L. (1993). *The Janus report on sexual behavior*. New York: Wiley.

Kinsey, A. C., Pomeroy, W. B., Martin, C. E., & Gebhard, P. (1953). *Sexual behavior in the human female*. Philadelphia: Saunders.

Kinsey, A. C., Pomery, W. B., & Martin, C. E. (1948). *Sexual behavior in the human male*. Philadelphia: Saunders.

Kinsman, S. B., Romer, D., Furstenberg, F. F., & Schwarz, D. F. (1998). Early sexual initiation: The role of peer norms. *Pediatrics, 102*, 1185–1192.

Koyama, A., Corliss, H. L., & Santelli, J. S. (2009). Global lessons on healthy adolescent sexual development. *Current Opinion in Pediatrics, 21*, 444–449.

Landry, T., & Bergeron, S. (2011). Biopsychosocial factors associated with dyspareunia in a community sample of adolescent girls. *Archives of Sexual Behavior, 40*, 877–889.

Langlois, J. H., & Downs, A. C. (1980). Mothers, fathers, and peers as socialization agents of sex-typed play behaviors in young children. *Child Development, 51*, 1237–1247.

Laumann, E., Gagnon, J., Michael, R., & Michaels, S. (2000). *The social organization of sexuality: Sexual practices in the United States*. Chicago: University of Chicago Press.

Leung, A. K. C., & Robson, W. L. M. (1993). Childhood masturbation. *Clinical Pediatrics, 32*, 238–241.

Luder, M.-T., Pittet, I., Berchtold, A., Akré, C., Michaud, P.-A., & Surís, J. C. (2011). Associations between online pornography and sexual behavior among adolescents: Myth or reality? *Archives of Sexual Behavior, 40*, 1027–1035.

MacDonald, T. K., & Hynie, M. (2008). Ambivalence and unprotected sex: Failure to predict sexual activity and decreased condom use. *Journal of Applied Social Psychology, 38*, 1092–1107.

Mah, K., & Binik, Y. M. (2002). Do all orgasms feel alike? Evaluating a two-dimensional model of the orgasm experience across gender and sexual context. *Journal of Sex Research, 39*, 104–113.

Mah, K., & Binik, Y. M. (2005). Are orgasms in the mind or the body? Psychosocial versus physiological correlates of orgasmic pleasure and satisfaction. *Journal of Sex & Marital Therapy, 31*, 187–200.

Manlove, J. S., Ryan, S., & Franzetta, K. (2007). Risk and protective factors associated with the transition to a first sexual relationship with an older partner. *The Journal of Adolescent Health, 40*, 135–143.

Marín, B. V., Kirby, D. B., Hudes, E. S., Coyle, K. K., & Gómez, C. A. (2006). Boyfriends, girlfriends and teenagers' risk of sexual involvement. *Perspectives on Sexual and Reproductive Health, 38*, 76–83.

Marston, C., & King, E. (2006). Factors that shape young people's sexual behaviour: A systematic review. *The Lancet, 368*, 1581–1586.

Martino, S. C., Collins, R. L., Elliott, M. N., Strachman, A., Kanouse, D. E., & Berry, S. H. (2006). Exposure to degrading versus nondegrading music lyrics and sexual behavior among youth. *Pediatrics, 118*, e430–e441.

Maticka-Tyndale, E. (2008). Sexuality and sexual health of Canadian adolescents: Yesterday, today and tomorrow. *The Canadian Journal of Human Sexuality, 17*, 85–95.

McHale, S. M., Bissell, J., & Kim, J.-Y. (2009). Sibling relationship, family, and genetic factors in sibling similarity in sexual risk. *Journal of Family Psychology, 23*, 562–572.

Meana, M., & Nunnink, S. E. (2006). Gender differences in the content of cognitive distraction during sex. *Journal of Sex Research, 43*, 59–67.

Meyer-Bahlburg, H., Dolezal, C., Baker, S., & New, M. (2008). Sexual orientation in women with classical or non-classical congenital adrenal hyperplasia as a function of degree of prenatal androgen excess. *Archives of Sexual Behavior, 37*, 85–99.

Miller, B. C., & Benson, B. (1999). Romantic and sexual relationship development during adolescence. In W. Furman, B. B. Brown, & C. Feiring (Eds.), *The development of romantic relationships in adolescence* (pp. 99–121). New York: Cambridge University Press.

Moore, M. J., & Rienzo, B. A. (2000). Utilizing the SIECUS guidelines to asses sexuality education in one state: Content scope and importance. *The Journal of School Health, 70*, 56–60.

Morgan, E. M., & Zurbriggen, E. L. (2007). Wanting sex and wanting to wait: Young adults' accounts of sexual messages from first significant dating partners. *Feminism & Psychology, 17*, 515–541.

Muehlenhard, C. L., & Peterson, Z. D. (2005). Wanting and not wanting sex: The missing discourse of ambivalence. *Feminism & Psychology, 15*, 15–20.

Mustanski, B., Viken, R. J., Kaprio, J., Winter, T., & Rose, R. J. (2007). Sexual behavior in young adulthood: A population-based twin study. *Health Psychology, 26*, 610–617.

National Campaign to Prevent Teen and Unplanned Pregnancy & CosmoGirl.com. (2008). Sex and tech: Results from a survey of teens and young adults. Retrieved from http://www.thenationalcampaign.org/sextech/pdf/sextech_summary.pdf.

Oattes, M. & Offman, A. (2007). Global self-esteem and sexual esteem as predictors of sexual communication in intimate relationships. *Canadian Journal of Human Sexuality, 16*, 89–100.

Okami, P., Olmstead, R., & Abramson, P. R. (1997). Sexual experiences in early childhood: 18-year longitudinal data from the UCLA family lifestyles project. *Journal of Sex Research, 34*, 339–347.

Ostrager, B. (2010). SMS. OMG! LOL! TTYL: Translating the law to accommodate today's teens and the evolution from texting to sexting. *Family Court Review, 48*, 712–726.

O'Sullivan, L. F., & Brooks-Gunn, J. (2005). The timing of changes in girls' sexual cognitions and behaviors in early adolescence: A prospective, cohort study. *Journal of Adolescent Health, 37*, 211–219.

O'Sullivan, L. F., Meyer-Bahlburg, H. F. L., & McKeague, I. W. (2006). The development of the sexual self-concept inventory for early adolescent girls. *Psychology of Women Quarterly, 30*, 139–149.

O'Sullivan, L. F., Cheng, M. M., Harris, K. M., & Brooks-Gunn, J. (2007). I wanna hold your hand: The progression of social, romantic and sexual events in adolescent relationships. *Perspectives on Sexual and Reproductive Health, 39*, 100–107.

Ott, M. A., Pfeiffer, E. J., & Fortenberry, J. D. (2006). Perceptions of sexual abstinence among high-risk early and middle adolescents. *The Journal of Adolescent Health, 39*, 192–198.

Patton, M. (1986). Twentieth-century attitudes toward masturbation. *Journal of Religion and Health, 25*, 291–302.

Pearson, J., Muller, C., & Frisco, M. L. (2006). Parental involvement, family structure, and adolescent sexual decision making. *Sociological Perspectives, 49*, 67–90.

Peter, J., & Valkenburg, P. M. (2006). Adolescents' exposure to sexually explicit material on the internet. *Communication Research, 33*, 178–204.

Peter, J., & Valkenburg, P. M. (2010). Processes underlying the effects of adolescents' use of sexually explicit internet material: The role of perceived realism. *Communication Research, 37*, 375–399.

Peter, J., & Valkenburg, P. (2011). The use of sexually explicit internet material and its antecedents: A longitudinal comparison of adolescents and adults. *Archives of Sexual Behavior, 40*, 1015–1025.

Pinkerton, S., Bogart, L., Cecil, H., & Abramson, P. (2003). Factors associated with masturbation in a collegiate sample. *Journal of Psychology and Human Sexuality, 14*, 103–121.

Pinquart, M. (2010). Ambivalence in adolescents' decisions about having their first sexual intercourse. *Journal of Sex Research, 47*, 440–450.

Pleck, J. H., Sonenstein, F. L., & Ku, L. C. (1993). Masculinity ideology: Its impact on adolescent males' heterosexual relationships. *Journal of Social Issues, 49*, 11–29.

Potard, C., Courtois, R., & Rusch, E. (2008). The influence of peers on risky sexual behaviour during adolescence. *The European Journal of Contraception & Reproductive Health Care, 13*, 264–270.

Prinstein, M. J., Meade, C. S., & Cohen, G. L. (2003). Adolescent oral sex, peer popularity, and perceptions of best friends' sexual behavior. *Journal of Pediatric Psychology, 28*, 243–249.

Rademakers, J., Laan, M., & Straver, C. J. (2003). Body awareness and physical intimacy: An exploratory study. In J. Bancroft (Ed.), *Sexual development in childhood* (pp. 121–125). Bloomington, IN: Indiana University Press.

Rahman, Q., & Wilson, G. D. (2003). Sexual orientation and the 2nd to 4th finger length ratio: Evidence for organising effects of sex hormones or developmental instability? *Psychoneuroendocrinology, 28*, 288–303.

Richters, J., Visser, R., Rissel, C., & Smith, A. (2006). Sexual practices at last heterosexual encounter and occurrence of orgasm in a national survey. *Journal of Sex Research, 43*, 217–226.

Robbins, C. L., Schick, V., Reece, M., Herbenick, D., Sanders, S. A., Dodge, B., et al. (2011). Prevalence, frequency, and associations of masturbation with partnered sexual behaviors among US adolescents. *Archives of Pediatrics & Adolescent Medicine, Published online*. doi:10.1001/archpediatrics. 2011.142.

Rosenthal, S. L., Cohen, S. S., & Biro, F. M. (1996). Developmental sophistication among adolescents of negotiation strategies for condom use. *Developmental and Behavioral Pediatrics, 17*, 94–97.

Rostosky, S. S., Dekhtyar, O., Cupp, P. K., & Anderman, E. M. (2008). Sexual self-concept and sexual self-efficacy in adolescents: A possible clue to promoting sexual health? *Journal of Sex Research, 45*, 277–286.

Sampson, R. J., Morenoff, J. D., & Gannon-Rowley, T. (2002). Assessing "neighborhood effects": Social processes and new directions in research. *Annual Review of Sociology, 28*, 443–478.

Santelli, J. S. (2008). Medical accuracy in sexuality education: Ideology and the scientific process. *American Journal of Public Health, 98*, 1786–1792.

Short, M. B., Black, L., Smith, A. H., Wetterneck, C. T., & Wells, D. E. (2011). A review of internet pornography use research: Methodology and content from the past 10 years. *Cyberpsychology, Behavior and Social Networking, 15*(1), 13–23. doi:10.1089/cyber.2010.0477.

Sieving, R. E., Eisenberg, M. E., Pettingell, S., & Skay, C. (2006). Friends' influence on adolescents' first sexual intercourse. *Perspectives on Sexual and Reproductive Health, 38*, 13–19.

Skinner, S. R., Smith, J., Fenwick, J., Fyfe, S., & Hendriks, J. (2008). Perceptions and experiences of first sexual intercourse in Australian adolescent females. *The Journal of Adolescent Health, 43*, 593–599.

Štulhofer, A., Buško, V., & Landripet, I. (2010). Pornography, sexual socialization, and satisfaction among young men. *Archives of Sexual Behavior, 39*, 168–178.

Swenson, R. R., Rizzo, C. J., Brown, L. K., Vanable, P. A., Carey, M. P., Valois, R. F., et al. (2010). HIV knowledge and its contribution to sexual health behaviors of low-income African American adolescents. *Journal of the National Medical Association, 102*, 1173–1182.

Tanner, A. E., Fortenberry, J. D., Zimet, G. D., Reece, M., Graham, C. A., & Murray, M. (2010). Young women's use of a microbicide surrogate: The complex influence of relationship characteristics and perceived male partners' evaluations. *Archives of Sexual Behavior, 39*, 735–747.

Thigpen, J. W. (2009). Early sexual behavior in a sample of low-income, African American children. *Journal of Sex Research, 46*, 67–79.

Thigpen, J. W., & Fortenberry, J. D. (2009). Understanding variation in normative childhood sexual behavior: The significance of family context. *Social Service Review, 83*, 611–631.

Verweij, K. J. H., Zietsch, B. P., Bailey, J. M., & Martin, N. G. (2009). Shared aetiology of risky sexual behaviour and adolescent misconduct: Genetic and environmental influences. *Genes, Brain, and Behavior, 8*, 107–113.

Weiss, R., & Samenow, C. P. (2010). Smart phones, social networking, sexting and problematic sexual behaviors—A call for research. *Sexual Addiction & Compulsivity, 17*, 241–246.

Whitaker, D. J., & Miller, K. S. (2000). Parent-adolescent discussions about sex and condoms. *Journal of Adolescent Research, 15*, 251–273.

Wight, D., Williamson, L., & Henderson, M. (2006). Parental influences on young people's sexual behaviour: A longitudinal analysis. *Journal of Adolescence, 29*, 473–494.

Ybarra, M. L., & Mitchell, K. J. (2005). Exposure to internet pornography among children and adolescents: A national survey. *Cyberpsychology & Behavior, 8*, 473–486.

Yen, S. (2010). Reputable but inaccurate: Reproductive health information for adolescents on the web. *Knowledge Quest, 38*, 62–65.

Zimmer-Gembeck, M. J., & Helfand, M. (2008). Ten years of longitudinal research on U.S. adolescent sexual behavior: Developmental correlates of sexual intercourse, and the importance of age, gender and ethnic background. *Developmental Review, 28*, 153–224.

Part III

Treatment and Training in Adolescent Health Psychology

Intervention Effectiveness Research in Adolescent Health Psychology: Methodological Issues and Strategies

Norman A. Constantine

Interventions to promote adolescent health have been widely implemented with a variety of goals, settings, populations, and approaches. Many of these interventions focus on preventing risky behaviors, promoting healthy behaviors, or more broadly promoting healthy development—all within the province of adolescent health psychology. Research evidence regarding effectiveness has been accumulating for some intervention approaches, yet the validity and integrity of this evidence and the way in which it is used require careful scrutiny. The issues and challenges in conducting, interpreting, appraising, and synthesizing this type of research are substantial.

This chapter examines the nature of intervention effectiveness evidence, together with the scientific foundations for effectiveness research and its use. The fundamental strategy of identifying and addressing plausible alternative explanations for research findings is emphasized, together with the importance of qualitative reasoning and well-justified argument. The essential roles of theory and demonstrated mechanisms of change, converging evidence, and research critique are discussed. Common threats to validity are reviewed, as are threats to research integrity potentially fueled by largely unintentional conflicts of interest and motivated reasoning. A case example critiquing research syntheses on the effectiveness of interventions to reduce adolescent sexual risk behaviors is used to illustrate frequently encountered issues and challenges.

Interventions in Adolescent Health Psychology

> Health is a state of complete physical, mental and social well-being, and not merely the absence of disease or infirmity.
>
> (World Health Organization, 1946)

In the context of adolescent health psychology, an intervention is a systematic effort to promote the physical, mental, and social well-being of adolescents. Interventions are typically intended to work at one or more of the levels of individuals, families, systems, and communities. Interventions can involve population-based efforts such as outreach, social marketing, community organizing, and policy advocacy, or person-based efforts such as health education, case management, mentoring, consultation, and counseling. Because a majority of adolescents attend school, schools are common settings for adolescent health interventions, but interventions for adolescents also take place in community-based organizations, religious institutions, and in the broader community.

N.A. Constantine, Ph.D. (✉)
Center for Research on Adolescent Health and Development, Public Health Institute, 555 12th Street, Oakland, CA 94607, USA

School of Public Health, University of California, Berkeley, CA 94720, USA
e-mail: nconstantine@berkeley.edu

W.T. O'Donohue et al. (eds.), *Handbook of Adolescent Health Psychology*,
DOI 10.1007/978-1-4614-6633-8_20, © Springer Science+Business Media New York 2013

Interventions are sometimes classified within a disease-prevention framework comprising primary, secondary, and tertiary prevention (Williams, Holmbeck, & Greenley, 2002). Primary prevention interventions focus on avoiding the development of new health problems. In adolescent health psychology, this generally involves attempts to prevent or reduce health risk behaviors, for example, tobacco use, unsafe sex, or sedentariness. Positive health promotion and healthy development interventions also are considered primary interventions. Secondary prevention interventions provide early identification and treatment of existing health problems or established harmful health behaviors. Tertiary prevention interventions focus on the management and treatment of chronic diseases and conditions and of diseases with long-lasting consequences. This chapter focuses on methodological issues and strategies relevant to research on primary prevention and health promotion interventions, with most examples drawn from school-based risk behavior prevention interventions. The issues and strategies addressed, however, generally apply across other types of adolescent health psychology interventions as well.

Intervention Effectiveness

Increasingly, interventions are expected to be backed by evidence of effectiveness, and many funding sources formally require interventions to be "science-based" or "evidence-based." Intuitively this makes sense, especially in times of decreasing funds and increasing need. But it also raises potentially perplexing questions and opportunities for misunderstanding about the nature of effectiveness evidence and about standards of scientific evidence.

The concept of effectiveness might appear simple and straightforward—does an intervention accomplish what it was designed for? But answering this question requires complex judgments and tradeoffs. Part of the complexity involves specifying what is meant by effectiveness. In its broadest sense, effectiveness refers to meeting one or more intervention goals.[1] Most interventions have multiple goals, and the question of relative priority among goals is important. In appraising effectiveness, it is generally advisable to specify just one or a small number of primary-intended outcomes tied to the intervention's primary goal. Yet, it is possible that an intervention might not achieve its primary goal but still achieve one or more secondary goals. And by specifying a large enough number of secondary goals and outcomes, most interventions can be expected to statistically demonstrate success on at least one or a few of these just by chance alone, leaving the overall question of effectiveness debatable.

A related issue is that of socio-demographic and other moderators. Moderators are factors that affect the relationship between an intervention and its intended outcomes, leading to differential effectiveness in different subpopulations (also referred to as interactions). So another important question that must be addressed asks for which subpopulations is the intervention effective? What if an intervention appears to achieve its primary goal for girls but not boys? And what if this same intervention does not achieve its primary goal in a combined sample of girls and boys? What if it achieves its goal for Latina girls but not for non-Latina girls or for boys of any ethnicity? This subgroup division process could be further continued, increasing the likelihood that through chance differences alone a finding of effectiveness would emerge for some demographic or other subgroup level, again leaving the overall question of effectiveness debatable. And even if a purported effect of the intervention limited to a

[1] A separate question related to the meaning of effectiveness is how it differs from the concept of efficacy. Efficacy is used to refer to an intervention's success under ideal and highly controlled conditions, whereas effectiveness refers to an intervention's success under more typical real world conditions. Especially in medical research, efficacy studies are often conducted prior to effectiveness studies. While the focus of this chapter is on intervention effectiveness research, much of the discussion applies to efficacy studies as well.

specific subgroup is real, rather than due to chance, does it make sense to label an intervention as effective when it might only be so for a subgroup that represents a small proportion of the population for which the intervention was developed, and for which it is being promoted?

Evidence of Effectiveness

Evidence provides the grounds for a belief or judgment. It is "the raw material from which judgments, both of probability and of fact, are made" (Shafer & Tversky, 1985, p. 337). Evidence of effectiveness in regard to interventions in adolescent health psychology usually refers to research evidence, with special credibility given to research evidence that is believed to be scientific. For example, The National Campaign to Prevent Teen and Unplanned Pregnancy (Suellentrop, 2010) publishes a series of research briefs on the effectiveness of teen-pregnancy-prevention interventions titled *Science Says*, and Advocates for Youth (2008) publishes a similar series titled *Science and Success*. This focus on purported science is reinforced by a front page headline in a recent issue of the American Public Health Association membership newspaper: "Ineffective abstinence-only lessons being replaced with science: Teen pregnancy prevention focusing on evidence" (Krisberg, 2010). To be clear, this last example is not about replacing abstinence-only lessons with lessons on biology or chemistry. Instead, the use of the word science is intended to convey some ultimate credibility for the particular evidence that is the focus of the headline.

It is hard to argue with the desire for scientific evidence in evaluating intervention effectiveness and informing intervention adoption and funding decisions that follow. But to use evidence appropriately and responsibly requires that some critical questions are first addressed. For example, what counts as evidence, and when is evidence compelling? What counts as science, and what makes evidence scientific? Are some methods of developing evidence fundamentally better than others? What role do values, biases, and potential conflicts of interest play in selecting and appraising evidence? These and other related questions about the nature and use of evidence in science are sometimes minimalized or overlooked. A publication by the Centers for Disease Control and Prevention (2008) illustrates this tendency, defining a "science-based" teen pregnancy prevention program merely as "a program that research has shown to be effective in changing at least one (specified behavior)" (p. 24).

When these types of questions about scientific evidence and its use are addressed, intense disagreement among experts can result. Consider, for example, a debate within the American Evaluation Association (AEA) over the US Department of Education's priority statement on "scientifically based evaluation methods." The heart of the issue was the Department's statement, with substantial implications for funding eligibility, that "evaluation methods using [a randomized] experimental design are best for determining project effectiveness" (Scientifically Based Evaluation Methods, 2003, p. 62446). AEA submitted a board-approved position statement to the Department, objecting to the blanket nature of this conclusion and discussing other options and contextual considerations to inform the selection of the best methods. Shortly thereafter, a group of prominent evaluation theorists and methodologists, including several former AEA presidents, submitted a competing statement endorsing the Department's priority and its conclusions regarding the superiority of randomized experiments. One of the consequences of this debate was the resignation from the organization of a prominent former president and leading evaluation textbook author, who publicly stated his view that "AEA now has the same relationship to the field of evaluation as the Flat Earth Society has to the field of geology" (Lipsey, 2004, p. 9). When it comes to standards of scientific evidence, reasonable minds can differ, sometimes strongly.

Principles of Scientific Inquiry

A common belief among some researchers, many policy influentials and practitioners, and much of the general public is that science is defined by its use of the "scientific method." In the general sense, this is supposed to consist of a series of steps beginning with observation and progressing to prediction, hypothesis, experimentation, and finally conclusion. More specifically, in intervention research the methods often equated to science are the randomized experiment (involving random assignment of units, for example, persons, schools, clinics, or communities, to intervention versus no-intervention control conditions) and the meta-analysis of randomized experiments (involving statistical cumulation of measures of effects across multiple studies). But science in the real world tends to be quite a bit more complicated and less orderly and defies any simple definition or defining characteristic. Many methods are used in science, and decisions about appropriate methods depend first and foremost on the particular research question to be addressed. Yet, even when a research method is well matched to the research question at hand, the science is only beginning. Methods are a means for obtaining evidence, but evidence rarely speaks for itself. And making good sense of evidence can be quite challenging.

Philosopher of science Susan Haack (2003) described scientific evidence as "complex and ramifying, structured more like a crossword puzzle than a mathematical proof. A tightly interlocking mesh of reasons well-anchored in experience" (p. 58). Campbell (2009) similarly spoke of the extended networks of implications within which scientific evidence must be presented and evaluated, and he emphasized the essential roles of plausible rival hypotheses and critical examination of their ramifications (i.e., implications):

> The core of the scientific method is not experimentation per se but rather the strategy connoted by the phrase "plausible rival hypotheses."… This strategy includes making explicit other implications of the hypothesis for other available data and reporting how these fit. It also includes seeking out rival explanations of the focal evidence and examining their plausibility. The plausibility of these rivals is usually reduced by ramification extinction, that is, by looking at their other implications on other data sets and seeing how well these fit. (p. 7)

Weiss (1980) concluded that "researchers bring not so much discrete findings as their whole theoretical, conceptual, and empirical fund of knowledge into the decision making process" (p. 12). From her cognitive-developmental psychology work on scientific reasoning and evidence appraisal, Koslowski similarly emphasized the importance of one's network of evidentially relevant collateral information to thinking in general and to scientific explanation in particular (Koslowski, 1996; Koslowski & Thompson, 2002). A common theme across these and other analyses (e.g., Chinn & Brewer, 2001; Evans, 1989; Gigerenzer, 2009) of the nature of scientific research evidence and its use is that "neither theory nor data alone is sufficient to achieve scientific success; each must be evaluated in the context of, and constrained by, the other" (Koslowski, 1996, p. 252).

These views of the inherent complexity of scientific evidence and the essential role of theory are at odds with the apparent beliefs of many adolescent health promotion researchers and research users, as well as evidence-based policy and practice proponents more generally. As currently understood and widely implemented, evidence-based policy and practice involve the assumption that scientific research evidence can be validly classified into hierarchical levels of quality according to the type of research methods employed to generate the evidence. And when theory is invoked it is often in name only, or in the form of what Gigerenzer (1998, 2009) has called *theoretical minimalism*—the application of surrogate theories such as one-word explanations, circular restatements, lists of vague dichotomies, and data fitting:

> The problem is not that a majority of researchers would say that theory is irrelevant; the problem is that almost anything passes as a theory…What distinguishes these surrogates from genuine theory is that they are vague, imprecise, and/or practically unfalsifiable. (Gigerenzer, 1998, p. 195)

In spite of an understandable desire for simplicity among consumers of research on intervention effectiveness, adequate appraisal of this evidence requires more than consulting a hierarchy of design and analysis methods or a checklist of basic research quality criteria. Most fundamentally, scientific research interpretation and appraisal requires scrupulous attention to theory-informed plausible rival hypotheses or plausible alternative explanations and their implications, by scientists as well as by research consumers. Doing this well calls for deep substantive knowledge of the subject matter and context, strong theoretical grounding, and rigorous critical thinking and reasoning (Abelson, 1995; Campbell, 1982; Freedman, 2010; Levy, 2010).

National Research Council Report

To help mediate the debate regarding the appropriate role of randomized experiments in educational research, the National Research Council (NRC) Committee on Scientific Principles for Educational Research (2002) discussed science as "competent inquiry that produces warranted assertions, and ultimately develops theory that is supported by pertinent evidence" (p. 54). Consistent with modern views of scientific evidence such as those discussed above as espoused by Haack (2003), Campbell (2009), Weiss (1980), and Gigerenzer (1998), six guiding principles for scientific research emerged from the committee's work (see Table 1). These principles "provide a framework for how valid inferences are supported, characterize the grounds on which scientists criticize one another's work, and with hindsight, describe what scientists do" (p. 54). Although developed in the context of educational research, they provide a solid frame of reference for intervention effectiveness research in adolescent health psychology (and many other fields) as well. The committee emphasized the following:

> Scientific research, whether in education, physics, anthropology, molecular biology, or economics, is a continual process of rigorous reasoning supported by a dynamic interplay among methods, theories, and findings. It builds understandings in the form of models or theories that can be tested. Advances in scientific knowledge are achieved by the self-regulating norms of the scientific community over time, not, as sometimes believed, by the mechanistic application of a particular scientific method to a static set of questions. (p. 2)

In discussing these principles, committee members made clear that they were specifically focusing on scientific research, yet not intending to minimize the importance of other types of scholarship such as humanistic, historic, and philosophical approaches (Feuer, Towne, & Shavelson, 2002; NRC Committee on Scientific Principles for Educational Research, 2002). A key point made throughout the committee's report and supporting materials was that particular research methods or designs do not make a study or program of research scientific:

> Judgments about scientific merit of a particular method can only be accomplished with respect to its ability to address a particular question at hand....No method is good, bad, scientific, or unscientific in itself: Rather, it is the appropriate application of method to a particular problem that enables judgments about scientific quality. (Feuer et al., 2002, pp. 7–8)

The committee distinguished between three interrelated types of research questions: *description* (What's happening?), *cause* (Is there a systematic effect?), and *process or mechanism* (Why or how is this happening?). It discussed a variety of methods that have been successfully applied to each type of question, and it emphasized the importance of addressing all three types of questions in a program of research, together with the concurrent need for multiple methods (NRC Committee on Scientific Principles for Educational Research, 2002; Shavelson & Towne, 2004).

The committee's report was generally well received as articulating a responsible middle ground between the simplistic and extremist view that only randomized experiments can provide credible scientific evidence, and the equally simplistic and extremist view that science is hopelessly flawed and all research standards are arbitrary. For example, Berliner (2002) supported the committee's recommendations and commended its strong emphasis on science beyond randomized experiments. At the same time, he criticized the report for insufficiently addressing the unique complexity of educational research as compared with other fields of scientific research,

Table 1 Guiding principles of scientific research

Scientific principle 1 *Pose significant questions that can be investigated empirically* Moving from hunch to conceptualizing and specifying a worthwhile question is essential to scientific research. The questions, and the designs developed to address them, must reflect a solid understanding of the relevant theoretical, methodological, and empirical work that has come before.
Scientific principle 2 *Link research to relevant theory* It is the long-term goal of much of science to generate theories that can offer stable explanations for phenomena that generalize beyond the particular. Science generates cumulative knowledge by building on, refining, and occasionally replacing, theoretical understanding.
Scientific principle 3 *Use methods that permit direct investigation of the question* Methods can only be judged in terms of their appropriateness and effectiveness in addressing a particular research question. Moreover, scientific claims are significantly strengthened when they are subject to testing by multiple methods.
Scientific principle 4 *Provide a coherent and explicit chain of reasoning* Making scientific inferences is not accomplished by merely applying an algorithm for using accepted techniques in correct ways. Rather, it requires the development of a logical chain of reasoning from evidence to theory and back again that is coherent, shareable, and persuasive to the skeptical reader.
Scientific principle 5 *Replicate and generalize across studies* Scientific inquiry emphasizes checking and validating individual findings and results. Ultimately, scientific knowledge advances when findings are reproduced in a range of times and places and when findings are integrated and synthesized.
Scientific principle 6 *Disclose research to encourage professional scrutiny and critique* Scientific studies do not contribute to a larger body of knowledge until they are widely disseminated and subjected to professional scrutiny by peers. Indeed, the objectivity of science derives from publicly enforced norms of the professional community of scientists, rather than from the character traits of any individual person or design features of any study.

NRC Committee on Scientific Principles for Educational Research (2002, *pp. 3–5*)

especially in regard to the importance of personal, cultural, and educational contexts and to the ubiquity of interactions (differential effects in different subpopulations) in education research. Maxwell (2004) went further in his critique, arguing that the report inadequately addressed the importance of process, mechanism, and context in establishing and understanding intervention effects and other types of causation, and that it misrepresented the nature and potential value of qualitative research. According to Maxwell, qualitative methods should not be relegated to just descriptive and exploratory research questions but are important components of fully addressing questions of causation and mechanism as well. Despite these and other criticisms, the committee's report was a remarkable accomplishment and its primary messages still stand well. Its six principles of scientific inquiry provide a sound framework for designing, interpreting, and critically appraising intervention effectiveness research in adolescent health psychology.

Validity: How Might Research Conclusions Be Wrong?

Validity refers to the correctness of an inference or conclusion. "Validity is a property of inferences. It is not a property of designs or methods, as the same design may contribute to more or less valid inferences under different circumstances" (Shadish, Cook, & Campbell, 2002, p. 35). Validity is important to all types of scientific research. One of the best summaries of validity has been provided by a qualitative researcher:

> Validity is a goal rather than a product. It is never something that can be proven or taken for granted. Validity is also relative. It has to be assessed in relationship to the purposes and circumstances of the research, rather than being a context independent property of methods or conclusions. Validity threats are made implausible by evidence, not methods, methods are only a way of getting evidence that can help you rule out these threats. (Maxwell, 2005, p. 105)

A distinction between two primary types of validity that are especially relevant to quantitative research on intervention effectiveness was first articulated by Campbell (1953, 1957) and further developed by Campbell and Stanley (1963). *Internal validity* is the basic minimum for interpretation of an intervention study's findings, and it relates to the fundamental question of causation: Did the intervention contribute causally to a change in the outcome? *External validity* is concerned with generalizability: To which populations, settings, times, treatments, and outcomes can results be generalized? Subsequently (Cook & Campbell, 1979; Shadish et al., 2002), two additional types of validity were spun off from these original two and further developed. *Statistical conclusion validity* is a basic component of internal validity, regarding the magnitude of the association between an intervention and an outcome and the possibility that it might be due to chance, regardless of the question of causality. *Construct validity* like external validity involves questions of generalizability, but specifically in reference to the link between abstract constructs and operationalization of these constructs in the research: did we implement the intervention we intended to implement and did we measure the outcome we intended to measure?

Common Threats to Validity

The foundation of building a case for the validity of research inferences involves identifying and ruling out plausible rival hypotheses, or plausible alternative explanations, for research findings. For example, if adolescents who voluntarily sign a virginity pledge are found more likely to remain virgins, is this difference between pledgers and nonpledgers due to the pledging itself, or might it be due to a preexisting inclination to abstain from sex among those adolescents who voluntarily sign the pledge? Such plausible alternative explanations are also referred to as threats to validity. Campbell and Stanley (1963) originally discussed eight threats to internal validity and four threats to external validity in the context of intervention effectiveness research. These lists of threats have grown over time and with the further development of the validity typology. Shadish et al. (2002) discussed 36 specific threats, together with additional threats due to combinations of or interactions between the basic threats. Each of these threats represents a potential alternative explanation for a particular research finding that can challenge the conclusions and interpretations drawn by researchers and research users.

Threats to internal validity have received the most attention, and seven of the most prominent of these threats are listed in Table 2. Among these, selection threats can be especially daunting and often are insufficiently addressed in intervention research (Larzelere, Kuhn, & Johnson, 2004). Although selection threats can involve preexisting group differences from any nonrandomized selection mechanism, such as natural, administrative, and convenience selection, the most dangerous type of selection threat arises from motivated self-selection of individuals into intervention versus control conditions.

Threats to external validity involve the potential for unwarranted generalizations of intervention effectiveness inferences, including any interactions of the intervention's potential effectiveness with settings, populations, or outcomes. Threats to statistical conclusion validity include low statistical power due to small sample sizes or unreliable measures, as well as inflated probability of finding significant intervention effects due solely to chance (i.e., Type I error) through inappropriate use of statistical analysis methods. Two common practices that can substantially increase the probability of a Type I error are the conduct of large numbers significance tests without statistical adjustment for this multiple testing, and failure to adjust for the statistical clustering that results from assigning groups rather than individuals to

Table 2 Threats to internal validity

Selection. Preexisting differences between intervention and control groups, which can be especially serious when these differences are due to individuals' motivated self-selection
History. Extraneous events occurring during the intervention that could affect the outcome
Maturation. Naturally occurring changes in participants over time
Regression. Natural movement on subsequent measurements toward the overall group average—especially for groups composed on the basis of extreme scores
Attrition. Differential loss of participants between groups
Testing. Practice effects or other factors based on repeated exposure to the assessment instrument
Instrumentation. Changes in the function or meaning of the measures used over time or between groups

intervention and control conditions. Construct validity threats include inadequate implementation of an intervention (Dane & Schneider, 1998) and inadequate development of construct definitions and operationalizations, as well as situations in which program administrators or staff provide unplanned compensatory services to those not receiving the intervention (compensatory equalization) or when those not receiving the intervention are so resentful that they respond more negatively than they otherwise would have (resentful demoralization). Other threats to validity and in-depth discussions and examples of these threats can be found in Shadish et al. (2002).

Trochim and Donnelly (2007) discussed five general approaches to addressing threats to validity in quantitative research. First, a well-reasoned *argument* that explains why a potential threat is not likely can sometimes suffice. Second, systematic *measurement or observation* of plausible alternative explanations can provide evidence on whether a potential threat is occurring. Third, *research design* is commonly used to rule out alternative explanations through strategies such as employing control groups that do not receive the intervention, or incorporating multiple waves of measurement to obtain data on existing trends in outcomes independent of the intervention. Fourth, *statistical analysis* can be used to test for suspected threats, such as differential attrition between the intervention and control groups, and under some special circumstances and strong assumptions, to reduce these threats through statistical adjustment. Finally, anticipated threats can sometimes be eliminated through *preventive action*, such as use of sample incentives to reduce attrition, or quality control procedures to identify and remediate data errors. These five approaches are not mutually exclusive, and in general it is preferable to use multiple methods to minimize threats to validity. In particular, argument development is always part of making a case for the validity of inferences or conclusions (Maxwell, 2005; Victora, Habicht, & Bryce, 2004).

Maxwell (2005) discussed validity issues in qualitative research from a similar perspective of identifying plausible alterative explanations and threats to the valid interpretation and understanding of research findings. These included biased selection or interpretation of data by the researcher (researcher bias) and any influence of the researcher on the setting or individuals studied (reactivity and reflexivity). These two threats can be relevant to quantitative research as well.

Research Designs

Research designs provide the blueprints from which research studies are built, and play a central role in addressing threats to validity, especially internal validity. Many threats to internal validity can be minimized or eliminated through the careful use of an appropriate randomized experimental or quasi-experimental design. Nonexperimental observational designs also can be used to address threats to validity, but generally on a more limited basis. Finally, qualitative designs have a unique and complementary role to play in addressing validity threats and enhancing intervention effectiveness research.

Randomized Experiments and Quasi-Experiments

Randomized experiments (sometimes referred to as randomized controlled trials [RCTs] or randomized field trials) involve the random assignment of units such as persons, schools, clinics, or communities to intervention versus nonintervention control conditions. This is done to control or minimize potential threats to internal validity and can be especially powerful in reducing or eliminating selection effects. The putative power of randomization is its potential "to control an infinite number of rival hypotheses without specifying what any of them are" (Campbell, 2009, p. viii). Scriven (2008) cautioned, however, that most randomized experiments as actually implemented do not eliminate all plausible alternative explanations for purported effects, and that "the RCT banner in applied human sciences is in fact being flown over pseudo-RCT's" (p. 13).

This criticism derives from the understanding that randomization alone does not yield an RCT—other essential aspects of an RCT include, for example, a focus on a single or very few primary outcome measures that are specified prior to the start of data collection, and double-blinding of treatment and control group conditions so that neither the investigators nor the participants know the participants' treatment assignments (Meinert, 1986). These conditions are rarely met in field-based intervention research, and in fact, the ideal of double-blinding is commonly not met even in clinical research (Abel & Koch, 1999; Meinert, 1986).

Additional criticisms related to internal validity threats are based on other fundamental assumptions of an RCT. One of the most important of these assumptions is that participants accept and maintain their intervention assignments and that any refusal to participate (selection), loss of participants (attrition), or differential levels of participation that occur during the course of a study are not related to group assignment (West, 2009). RCTs have also been criticized for threats to external validity and construct validity (e.g., differences between the study protocol and routine practice) that are widely believed to be greater in randomized designs than in other types of designs (Rothwell, 2005). Cook (2002) provided a comprehensive review of criticisms of randomized experiments in school-based research. Although still supporting random assignment as the best and most credible mechanism for justifying causal conclusions about intervention effectiveness, he acknowledged that

> random assignment cannot be considered the "gold standard" for justifying causal inferences in school-based research. It creates only a probabilistic equivalence between the groups being contrasted, and then only at pretest. Moreover, treatment-correlated attrition is likely when treatments differ in intrinsic desirability. Also, treatments are not always independent of each other in practice like they are supposed to be in theory, and many of the ways used to increase internal validity can also reduce external validity. (p. 195)

None of these criticisms negate the potential power of a properly designed, implemented, maintained, and interpreted randomized experiment to yield strong evidence with regard to intervention effectiveness. Instead, they are reminders that randomization in itself does not necessarily eliminate important threats to validity (Abel & Koch, 1999; Scriven, 2008).

Quasi-experiments do not involve random assignment to intervention and control conditions but instead employ some combination of other design features to help rule out alternative explanations of observed effects. The quasi-experimental label is often applied to weak designs based on comparisons of preexisting groups composed of members who have self-selected into intervention and control conditions, and characterized by just one or two waves of data collection. Yet much more powerful and sophisticated quasi-experimental designs can be developed through the use of strategies such as matching or stratifying participants into intervention and control conditions, scheduling of multiple preintervention and postintervention measurements and time points, employing multiple treatment and comparison groups, and manipulating intervention timing. A variety of quasi-experimental designs involving these strategies has evolved over time (Campbell & Stanley, 1963; Cook & Campbell, 1979), and these designs have been discussed in depth by Shadish et al. (2002).

Both randomized experiments and quasi-experiments offer the potential to reduce the likelihood of plausible alternative explanations for a purported effect. To be realized, this potential requires skillful application under the right circumstances and conditions. It is the researcher's responsibility to argue and sufficiently document the case that an appropriate design has been developed and skillfully applied to the research questions addressed.

Nonexperimental Observational Studies

Observational studies employ quantitative research methods to make inferences about causal risk factors or intervention effects in the absence of researcher control over most threats to internal validity. Intervention and control groups are based on existing memberships or conditions, and no controlled manipulation of intervention exposure occurs. These groups may or may not be based on self-selection, for example, an adolescent voluntarily choosing to make a virginity pledge. Observational studies often involve secondary analysis of existing population-based data sets. The National Longitudinal Study of Adolescent Health (Add Health) and the National Survey of Family Growth (NSFG) are two large national survey databases sometimes used in observational studies in adolescent health psychology. With observational studies that involve comparisons of respondents who experienced some type of intervention with those who did not, statistical analyses are commonly used to try to remove (i.e., statistically adjust or control for) preintervention group differences that could be the cause of group outcome differences. For example, using the Add Health dataset, Bearman and Bruckner (2001) attempted to show that virginity pledging delays initiation of sexual intercourse. Because pledgers and nonpledgers differed on many background variables (such as religiosity) that were associated with making the decision to pledge, the researchers statistically adjusted their data in an attempt to remove these prepledge differences. In this situation, however, it is hard to imagine how preexisting motivational inclinations among voluntary (self-selected) pledgers to abstain from sex could be meaningfully removed by statistical methods. As Anderson (1963) complained nearly a half century ago, in situations like this, "One may well wonder what exactly it means to ask what the data would look like were they not what they are" (p. 170). Along the same lines, Lord (1967) cautioned:

> With the data usually available for such studies, there is simply no logical or statistical procedure that can be counted on to make proper allowances for uncontrolled preexisting differences between groups. The researcher wants to know how the groups would have compared if there had not been preexisting uncontrolled differences. The usual research study of this type is attempting to answer a question that simply cannot be answered in any rigorous way on the basis of the available data. (p. 305)

Further critique and discussion of the virginity pledge example is provided in Constantine and Braverman (2004).

Modern statistical analysis methods provide an abundance of complex methodologies intended to better achieve the types of statistical adjustments that so perplexed Anderson and Lord. Yet, in most real world situations, these new methods are plainly unable to meet their hypothetical potential. Light, Singer, and Willett's (1990) admonition that "you can't fix by analysis what you bungled in design" (p. v) remains relevant. A lament by the editors of the International Journal of Epidemiology reinforces this point:

> Observational studies revealed strong apparently protective effects of beta-carotene, but long term RCTs found that, if anything, beta-carotene increased cardiovascular disease risk. There are now a series of similar examples: hormone replacement therapy, vitamin E and vitamin C intake in relation to cardiovascular disease, or fiber intake in relation to colon cancer among them. What these examples have in common is that the groups of people who were apparently receiving protection from these substances in the observational studies were very different from the groups not using them, on a whole host of characteristics of their lives. Belief that these differences could be summed up in measures of a few "potential confounders" and adequately adjusted for in statistical analyses, fails to recognize the complexity of the reasons why people differ with regard to particular and general characteristics of their lives. (Davey Smith & Ebrahim, 2001, p. 5)

Observational studies can provide evidence relevant to the understanding of the effectiveness of an adolescent health intervention. This generally occurs not through automatic use of complex statistics, but instead through a careful analysis and understanding of potential alternative explanations and threats to validity (Constantine, 2012). Evidence from the best of these observational studies can then be used for two primary purposes. First, this evidence can help justify the need for more controlled and expensive randomized or quasi-experimental studies. Second, as one component of a comprehensive evidence review to be combined with evidence from other studies, observational study results can be part of a critical review of the convergence of evidence across studies that experience different threats to validity and have complementary strengths and weaknesses.

For example, Kohler, Manhart, and Lafferty (2008) employed 2002 NSFG data to evaluate the effectiveness of sex education programs at the United States population level. They found that adolescents who received comprehensive sex education were significantly less likely to report teen pregnancies than were those who received either no sex education or abstinence-only sex education. These findings resulted from a strong design and analysis that statistically controlled for plausible alternative explanations based on preexisting group differences. The main reason that this was possible is that type of sex education received is much less likely due to purposeful self-selection than are such conditions as virginity pledging or dietary habits. Absent purposeful self-selection, preexisting group differences (e.g., family income) that might influence both sex education received and sexual behavior outcomes can be more amenable to meaningful statistical adjustment. Nevertheless, cautious interpretation and further study is warranted. One of the strengths of the findings from this study is that it provided convergent validity when combined with other types of available research evidence on the relative effectiveness of comprehensive versus abstinence-only sex education (Constantine, 2008a).

Qualitative Research

Unlike randomized experiments, quasi-experiments, and observational studies, all of which primarily employ the analysis of quantitative data, qualitative research involves the analysis of unstructured data such as interview transcripts, open-ended survey responses, behavior observations, and text materials. Typically, qualitative research focuses more on the why and how of behavior and other phenomena, whereas quantitative research focuses more on the what, whether, where, when, and how much.

Qualitative research is commonly regarded as a useful adjunct (or precursor) to experimental or quasi-experimental designs. Yet, Maxwell (2004) took issue with this hierarchical characterization, arguing that valid causal inference requires that qualitative research be given an equal place at the table. While acknowledging the important and more typically recognized exploratory value of qualitative research for hypothesis and theory development and its explanatory value in helping to elucidate quantitative findings, Maxwell saw a more fundamental role for qualitative research in supporting causal inferences about intervention effectiveness, arguing that the qualitative study of causal processes is indispensable for most causal inferences. This argument was supported by Freedman (2008): "Scientific inquiry is a long and tortuous process, with many false starts and blind alleys. Combining qualitative insights and quantitative analysis—and a healthy dose of skepticism—may provide the most secure results" (p. 313). Freedman (2008) further explicated the role of qualitative causal process observations in 10 of the major scientific discoveries from the histories of medicine and public health, such as the discovery of penicillin and the development of the smallpox vaccine, illustrating how

> progress depends on refuting conventional ideas if they are wrong, developing new ideas that are better, and testing the new ideas as well as the old ones. The examples show that qualitative methods can play a key role in all three tasks. (p. 312)

Several qualitative research frameworks for rigorous causal analysis have been developed, including Maxwell's (2005) interactive approach,

Miles and Huberman's (1994) cross-case analysis approach, and Yin's (2008) multiple case study approach. As with all types of methods and designs used in intervention effectiveness research, these approaches require diligence in recognizing and minimizing threats to validity and are best used as part of a well-integrated combination of complementary methods within a study or across a program of research.

Research Integrity: How Might Research Conclusions Be Biased?

> Bias is not a crime, is not necessarily intentional, and is not a sign of lack of [personal] integrity; rather, it is a natural human phenomenon . . . everyone is likely capable of rationalizing beliefs and denying influences that bias them.
>
> (Cain & Detsky, 2008)

Research integrity involves a commitment to intellectual honesty and to a range of practices that characterize responsible research conduct (National Research Council [NRC] Committee on Assessing Integrity in Research Environments, 2002). Although practices related to human subject protection, accurate representation of authorship roles, and research management are important aspects of research integrity, this section focuses specifically on those related to intellectual honesty in performing, interpreting, and using research. These issues apply not only to research scientists and their institutions, but also to advocates, journalists, bureaucrats, and other policy shapers who are part of the chain of research creation, communication, and use.

Conflicts of Interest and Motivated Reasoning

Issues in research integrity are often based in conflicts of interest, which occur when individuals' personal interests are in conflict with their professional judgment and obligations (Gorman & Conde, 2007; Kumar, 2008; Young, 2009). These competing personal interests can be directly or indirectly financial, or more broadly related to the goals of the individuals or their organization (Bachrach & Newcomer, 2002; Ioannidis, 2011; Smith, Feachem, Feachem, Koehlmoos, & Kinlaw, 2009; Young, 2009). MacCoun (2005) has placed conflicts of interest in public policy research "on a continuum from blatant pecuniary bias to more subtle ideological bias" (p. 233), whereas Chugh, Bazerman, and Banaji (2005) have distinguished among three types of conflicts of interest: the plainly visible, the visible yet dismissed through disclosure or denial, and the invisible.

For any type of conflict of interest, *bounded ethicality* can make it difficult to overcome or even to recognize one's own conflicts and biases. Bounded ethicality involves ethically limited judgment and decision making due to largely unconscious biases and ego protective mechanisms. This is enabled by "an ethical blind spot [that] emerges as decision makers view themselves as moral, competent, and deserving, and thus assume that conflicts of interest are non-issues" (Chugh et al., 2005, p. 80). Bounded ethicality has been well documented in studies of the psychological aspects of conflicts of interest and implausible denials in the field of financial auditing (Chugh, et al., 2005; Moore, Lowenstein, Tanlu, & Bazerman, 2003).

Feinstein (1988) discussed several types of biases in the quest for scientific truth, especially distinguishing between deliberately planned fraud and inadvertent deception. Inadvertent deception was further divided into one-time distortions of evidence versus more robust delusions: "A distortion is usually produced by failure to recognize important distinctions in the complexity of nature, [whereas] a delusion usually arises from excessive zeal in the expectations, beliefs, or behavior of the investigators" (pp. 475–476). Each of these can contribute to deluded consensus among experts, or the *consensus syndrome*, which Feinstein argued is particularly detrimental to scientific progress. MacCoun (1998) similarly concluded that "under a wide variety of circumstances, collective decision making will significantly amplify individual bias, rather than attenuate it" (p. 278). Both Feinstein and MacCoun emphasized the importance and prevalence of bias and deception that occur outside of the realm of deliberately planned fraud. Cain and Detsky (2008) concurred:

> Conflicts of interest are problematic not only because they are widespread but also because most people incorrectly think that succumbing to them is due to intentional corruption, a problem for only a few bad apples. . . . (S)uccumbing to a conflict of interest is more likely to result from unintentional bias, something common in everyone. (p. 2893)

Much conflict of interest involves *motivated reasoning*, the unintentionally biased appraisal of evidence to support one's goals through a set of preconscious cognitive processes. These processes include biased selection of evidence, biased access to background beliefs, and biased selection of statistical reasoning heuristics (Dawson, Gilovich, & Regan, 2002; Evans, 1989; Kunda, 1990). Heuristics are simple rules of thumb that are generally true in many but not all situations. For example, a common statistical reasoning heuristic is the belief that larger sample sizes lead to more reliable and valid results. Statistical reasoning heuristics are often applied differentially to research evidence that supports or challenges one's motivated beliefs:

> Heuristics that have judgmental implications congenial to perceivers' existing beliefs are especially likely to be used, whereas incongenial heuristics may be ignored or disparaged. . . . Information that is congruent with one's existing beliefs, such as research supporting one's position on abortion, will be judged more favorably than incongruent information . . . [while] incongruent information may be scrutinized in an effort to derogate its validity. (Chen & Chaiken, 1999, p. 45)

Level of motivation and type of motivation are both important determinants of the nature of biased cognitive processing that occurs (Chen & Chaiken, 1999). Motivated reasoning and its biases can affect research design and implementation, research interpretation, and research appraisal and synthesis.

In adolescent health psychology, common situations that might lead to real or apparent conflicts of interest, bounded ethicality, and motivated reasoning include effectiveness research conducted by intervention program developers or publishers, and research reviews or syntheses conducted by researchers involved in some of the reviewed research. Moskowitz (1993) argued that "much of the drug abuse (prevention) research conducted to date suffers from real or apparent conflicts of interest" (p. 7), and discussed a variety of motivations and pressures for these conflicts, primarily arising from investigators evaluating programs that they or their institutions developed. Weiss and colleagues (Gandhi, Murphy-Graham, Petrosino, Chrismer, & Weiss, 2007; Weiss, Murphy-Graham, Petrosino, & Gandhi, 2008) raised similar concerns regarding conflict of interest in drug prevention intervention research and research use. Gorman and Conde (2007) quantified this phenomenon in a study of the 34 model school-based interventions for drug and violence prevention in the Substance Abuse and Mental Health Services Administration National Registry of Effective Programs. Of the 246 published evaluation reports located for these interventions, 78 % included the intervention developer as an author of the evaluation report, and for another 11 %, the developer had some other association such as working in the same organization as one of the evaluation report authors. Only 11 % showed no identifiable association between the evaluation authors and the program developer.

Threats to Research Integrity

Threats to validity have been well studied and publicized, and a variety of strategies for dealing with these threats has been developed. Threats to research integrity can be just as damaging or even more so. Growing bodies of research on unconscious conflicts of interest, bounded rationality, unintentional biases, and motivated reasoning in evidence selection and appraisal help explain the etiology of these threats and some of the cognitive and affective mechanisms behind them. It is also useful to consider the common methodological mechanisms that comprise these threats.

1. *Multiple significance testing* (*fishing for significance, data dredging*). Sometimes referred to as simply as *multiplicity*, this involves testing large numbers of potential

outcomes for statistical significance, and capitalizing on the increased likelihood of finding spurious effects due to chance as more outcomes are tested (Feinstein, 1988; Howel & Bhopal, 1994; Mills, 1993).

2. *Within-study selective reporting* (*data suppression, cherry picking*). This type of threat builds on multiple significance testing but goes a step further, involving the selective reporting or combining of results across multiple outcomes, subgroup analyses, and other multiplicities, such that results that support the researcher's hypotheses are more likely to be reported than are those that do not (Chan, Hrobjartsson, Haahr, Gotzsche, & Altman, 2004; Dwan et al., 2008; Hahn, Williamson, & Hutton, 2002; Ioannidis, 2005; Kumar, 2008; Mills, 1993; Simmons, Nelson, & Simonsohn, 2011).
3. *Exploiting ambiguities* (*researcher degrees of freedom*). Simmons and colleagues (2011) discussed a variety of ambiguities that researchers commonly exploit to increase the likelihood of a positive result. In addition to multiple significance testing, these include decisions about deleting outliers (suspicious extreme values in the data), choosing sample size, using covariates, and reporting subsets of treatment conditions. Testing several of these through computer simulations of experimental data, they reported a 61 % false positive rate, i.e., "A researcher is more likely than not to falsely detect a significant effect by using these four common researcher degrees of freedom." (p. 1361).
4. *Biased misreporting of statistical results.* Errors in reporting of statistical results have been found widely prevalent in peer reviewed articles published in natural science and medicine (Garcia-Berthou & Alcarz, 2004), psychiatry (Berle & Starcevic, 2007), and psychology (Bakker & Wicherts, 2011). Bakker and Wicherts found in their sample of articles that these errors fell overwhelmingly (92 % for congruence errors and 100 % for rounding errors) in the direction to lend support for the researcher's hypotheses and expectations. Friedlander (1964) commented nearly a half century ago on this particular mechanism of Type I bias, which he attributed to the natural tendency of researchers, himself included, to more readily investigate and verify results that do not support their expectations.
5. *Hypothesizing after the results are known* (*HARKing, data-driven hypothesizing*). HARKing involves presenting a post hoc hypothesis developed from a study's results as if it were an a priori hypothesis confirmed by these results (Kerr, 1998; Kumar, 2008).
6. *Methodological impenetrability* (*statisticization*). This involves the use of unnecessarily complex analysis methods and impenetrable descriptions of these methods to discourage critical appraisal by others. "If the assumptions and strength of a simpler method are reasonable for your data and research problem, use it. Occam's razor applies to methods as well as to theories." (Wilkinson & APA Task Force on Statistical Inference, 1999).
7. *Selective publication* (*publication bias*). Selective publication of manuscripts based on the direction and magnitude of results has been well documented. See especially a systematic review of eleven studies investigating publication bias in health-care intervention research by Dwan and colleagues (2008). In particular, research with statistically significant positive results is more likely to be submitted for publication, to be published, and to be published more quickly than research with negative or null results (Constantine, 2008c; Dwan et al., 2008).
8. *Redundant publication*. This involves publication of the same results multiple times as if they were independent replications (Constantine, 2008c; Huston & Moher, 1996; Kassirer & Angell, 1995; Rennie, 1999). In addition, *data augmentation* occurs when after publishing results, additional data are collected and combined with the originally published data and then published as a new study (Kumar, 2008).
9. *Biased peer-review*. The influence of a reviewer's personal biases on the results and recommendations of their peer reviews has

been widely demonstrated (Altman, 2002; Ioannidis, Tatsioni, & Karassa, 2010; Mahoney, 1977; Shatz, 2001; Young, Ioannidis, & Al-Ubaydi, 2009). *Confirmation bias* in peer review involves the general tendency to less critically evaluate evidence that is consistent with one's existing beliefs. *Ideological bias* occurs when a reviewer's values-based views for or against an author's position unduly influence a review. *Ad hominem* and *affiliation biases* are found when a review is influenced by knowledge of the author's identity or affiliation (Constantine, 2008b).

10. *Postpublication peer review limitations.* Postpublication peer review includes letters to the editor as well as full articles critiquing a published work. As Altman (2002) cautioned, "many readers seem to assume that articles published in peer-reviewed journals are scientifically sound, despite much evidence to the contrary. It is important, therefore, that misleading work be identified after publication" (p. 2766). Authors sometimes choose to ignore a published critique or respond minimally to peripheral issues in place of the specific criticisms made. Even when serious errors are detailed in a critique, retractions or corrections are the exception. PsycINFO and other databases rarely link postpublication critiques to the original article, and narrative reviews and other research syntheses that cite a criticized work frequently ignore the critique (Altman, 2002; Rennie, 1998). Another aspect of this threat is *selective data sharing*—researchers' reluctance to share raw data for reanalysis and external verification (Wolins, 1962; Wicherts, Borsboom, Kats, & Molenaar, 2006), and the inverse relationship between this reluctance and strength of evidence and reporting quality (Wicherts, Bakker, & Molenaar, 2011).
11. *Motivated communication of results.* This involves selective emphasis of a study's supportive versus limiting conclusions by researchers, funders, media, or advocates (Constantine & Braverman, 2004; Scher, Lin, & Constantine, 2009), and more generally, the minimization of study limitations by researchers, reviewers, and research users (Ioannidis, 2007). Cronbach's (1982, p. 108) caution that "validity depends not only on data collection and analysis but also on the way a conclusion is stated and communicated," applies to research integrity as well as research validity.
12. *Biased research synthesis.* As with individual studies, research syntheses can be affected by selective inclusion of studies or outcomes based on the direction of their results (Dwan et al., 2008; Hahn, Williamson, Hutton, Garner, & Flynn, 2000; Ioannidis & Karassa, 2010). In addition, biases in the included individual studies can carry over to the research synthesis, especially when these threats appear in multiple studies.

Issues in Consolidating Research Evidence

Rarely is a research question settled by a single study. To better address questions of intervention effectiveness, research evidence from multiple sources must be located, appraised, and consolidated. This activity is referred to as research synthesis, comprising a set of processes through which multiple research studies are reviewed and assessed with the objective of summarizing the evidence relating to a particular question. The most common types of research synthesis in adolescent health psychology are narrative reviews, programs-that-work lists, and systematic reviews and meta-analyses.

Narrative Reviews

The *narrative review* designation is used in a variety of ways, sometimes to indicate a review that does not meet standards of rigor expected of a systematic review. It also is sometimes used synonymously with the term literature review. Narrative reviews range from primarily descriptive to primarily critical. A *descriptive narrative review* attempts to summarize research results relating to a particular question, whereas a *critical narrative review*, sometimes referred to as an integrative literature review, "presents a logically argued case founded on a comprehensive understanding of the current state of knowledge about a topic of study" (Machi & McEvoy, 2009, p. 4).

Descriptive narrative reviews frequently include a *box score* presentation of empirical results. This takes the form of a table of intervention studies and outcomes tested, with check marks or other indicators to denote whether the study reported a statistically significant result in the expected direction on each tested outcome. Descriptive narrative reviews have been widely criticized as especially susceptible to reviewer bias and publication bias due to insufficiently objective and transparent criteria for selection of studies and appraisal of results. And the use of box score approaches in narrative reviews has been criticized as an inappropriate overuse of statistical significance tests without regard for magnitudes of the reported effects (Egger & Davey Smith, 1997; Shadish et al., 2002; Slavin, 1995).

Whereas descriptive narrative reviews tend to focus on empirical evidence alone, critical narrative reviews generally make more extensive use of theory to integrate empirical evidence. The latter consider both supportive and challenging evidence, with special attention to plausible alternative explanations and their implications. Good examples of a theory-focused critical narrative reviews can be found in such journals as *Psychological Bulletin*, *Perspectives on Psychological Science*, and *School Psychology Review*. Compared with other forms of research synthesis, critical narrative reviews tend to involve more complex forms of argumentation and justification, and more nuanced answers to research questions. Accordingly, they can be more difficult to develop, and more difficult to translate into black and white research-based policy and practice decisions. This might explain why they have not been more commonly used in synthesizing intervention research.

Programs-That-Work Lists

Programs-that-work lists are a second type of research synthesis, comprising lists of interventions that meet prespecified criteria of effectiveness findings. They are sometimes referred to as evidence-based or science-based program lists, or best practice lists. Lists of this nature are often used to determine program eligibility for federal or other types of funding, and they have been prevalent at least since the introduction in 1992 of the Centers for Disease Control and Prevention now-defunct lists of effective health education programs (Collins et al., 2002). There is now a proliferation of lists in many areas of adolescent health psychology.

Although they vary widely in the criteria used, most programs-that-work lists allow the inclusion of a program based on just one study with one statistically significant result, regardless of the number of outcomes tested within a study or the number of studies conducted on the same intervention. In other words, an intervention program for which just 1 of 20 relevant tested outcomes is found to be statistically significant could earn a place on a programs-that-work list as an evidence-based program. In fact, exactly this did happen with the Second Step violence prevention curriculum—this intervention received an "exemplary program" certification by a U.S. Department of Education Safe, Disciplined, and Drug-Free Schools Expert Panel based on a randomized study yielding just 1 statistically significant outcome out of 20 relevant tests conducted (Grossman et al., 1997; critiqued in Constantine & Braverman, 2004 and Gorman, 2002). Although this example exhibits statistical irony in its precise details (1 in 20 statistically significant outcome tests is exactly what is expected by chance when an intervention has no effect and the tests are conducted with the usual significance level criterion of 0.05), the problem reflected is not at all unique.

Weiss and colleagues (Gandhi et al., 2007; Petrosino, 2003; Weiss et al., 2008) investigated seven prominent programs-that-work lists of school-based drug prevention interventions and the five programs appearing most frequently across the seven lists, concluding that "when we look at all of the evaluations cited across the lists, we are disturbed by the frailty of evidence for some of the 'proven' programs" (Gandhi et al., 2007, p. 65). Several factors were identified to explain how so many questionably effective programs were ending up on these lists. These included the following: (a) the insufficient standard of requiring just one or two evaluations to designate a program as effective, (b) the common practice of conducting multiple significance tests of outcomes (with an example provided of a program that was listed based on two statistically significant outcomes out of 100 tests conducted), (c) the failure to adjust for clustering when interventions were assigned to groups rather than individual persons, and (d) the potential for conflicts of interest and biases due to the common practice of program developers' evaluating their own programs (Gandhi et al., 2007). This last point was extended to the review process itself: "The [program review] procedures used, even by a prestigious group of outside experts, seem to reflect a degree of bias and favoritism. Experts, it seems, may be as subject to human frailties as the rest of us" (Weiss et al., 2008, p. 43). A similar set of issues has been raised by Gorman (2002; Gorman & Conde, 2007), who concluded that "with regard to the entry criterion of one effect from one evaluation, this is far too low a standard by which to designate Exemplary status" (Gorman, 2002, p. 301).

An unusually rigorous programs-that-work system is the What Works Clearinghouse (2008), which is focused on educational programs and strategies. Among other evidence standards employed, What Works Clearinghouse requires that study results be adjusted for biases that arise from assigning interventions at the group (e.g., school or classroom) level rather than at the individual student level, and for biases due to conducting multiple significance tests. Studies that have been published without properly adjusting for these biases are retroactively adjusted as part of the review and synthesis process. This system also goes further than most programs-that-work lists in attempting to consider the full body of relevant program effectiveness study results in supporting a judgment of positive effects. Yet it still suffers from one of the fundamental validity and integrity threats that all such systems experience—the ease with which a program can meet the stated criteria of having positive effects based on chance findings alone. For example, consider a program that had been evaluated ten times with each evaluation testing ten outcomes, for a total of 100 tests of statistical significance. According to the What Works Clearinghouse rules, this program could qualify as a positive effects program (the systems highest rating) if just one outcome in each of two studies, one of which was judged to have a strong design, were found to be statistically significant—even with all other 98 tested outcomes not yielding statistically significant results (What Works Clearinghouse, p. 22).

Systematic Reviews and Meta-Analyses

The *systematic review* label is generally used to describe a quantitative review based on a standardized protocol intended to protect the process from bias. A *meta-analysis* is a type of systematic review employing quantitative procedures for averaging effect sizes across multiple studies. In meta-analyses of intervention studies, one commonly used effect size is the standardized mean difference between intervention and control groups (McCartney & Rosenthal, 2000). Systemic reviews are generally found in the same journals that publish critical narrative reviews, such as *Psychological Bulletin*, *Perspectives on Psychological Science*, and *School Psychology Review*. In addition, two international organizations sponsor, monitor, and maintain systematic reviews and meta-analyses of interventions in different areas—the Cochrane Collaboration for health-care interventions and the Campbell Collaboration for social interventions. Both collaborations include reviews related to adolescent health psychology interventions.

Quantitative systematic reviews of multiple randomized controlled trials are generally considered to occupy the top rung of the hierarchy of sources of effectiveness evidence. Yet, just as with individual research studies, inferences resulting from systematic reviews and meta-analyses are subject to a variety of validity and integrity threats. Any of the threats experienced by individual studies, such as selection or attrition threats to internal validity, can be carried over to the systematic review. Additional threats are related to the nature of the research syntheses itself. These include publication bias and biased sampling of studies, biased selection of outcomes, lack of statistical independence among multiple effect sizes used, study rater biases and rating instability, and many others (Dwan et al., 2008; Hahn et al., 2000; Ioannidis & Karassa, 2010; Matt & Cook, 2009; Shadish et al., 2002). Briggs (2005) has gone so far as to argue that "researcher subjectivity is no less problematic in the context of a meta-analysis than in a narrative review" (p. 87).

Case Example: Interventions to Reduce Adolescent Sexual Risk Behaviors

An extensive body of research and research syntheses on the effectiveness of interventions to reduce adolescent sexual risk behavior provides for a compelling case example. Hundreds of individual studies exist, along with numerous narrative reviews, programs-that-work lists, and meta-analyses. This case example involves a brief methodological critique focusing on the most influential research syntheses in this area.

Scher, Maynard, and Stagner (2006) identified 14 descriptive narrative reviews of effectiveness studies of sexual risk behavior interventions for adolescents. Now in its third incarnation, *Emerging Answers* (Kirby, 2007) is the most extensive and influential of such reviews. One of its main components is a descriptive summary of risk and protective factors that purportedly affect teens' sexual behavior. The author concluded that more than 500 specific factors affect one or more adolescent sexual risk behaviors and their outcomes. A box score table was provided for the 71 factors deemed most important, based on a large collection of primarily observational studies reviewed, and employing statistical criteria such as three or more studies reporting statistically significant associations for the specific risk or protective factor (pp. 54–61). A fundamental limitation in this review was not sufficiently distinguishing between factors that are merely associated with and occur before the sexual behaviors (*risk or protective markers*) and those for which evidence of causality has been found, for example when a manipulation of the factor has been shown to contribute to a change in the outcome (*causal risk or protective factors*). Causal claims were made repeatedly, as in referring to this group of factors as "affecting teen sexual behavior and its outcomes" (p. 54) and "influential on teen's sexual behavior" (p. 63), and in arguing that each factor "exerted an effect," (p. 54). Yet evidence of causality over and above mere association was weak or completely absent for many or most of the factors listed, for example, hours of paid work and peer substance use (risk markers), and taking a virginity pledge and peer condom-use support (protective markers). This not uncommon failure to adequately distinguish between association and causation, referred to by Rosenthal (1994) as the problem of *causism*, has important negative implications for the development and evaluation of interventions. Kraemer and colleagues (Kraemer et al., 1997; Kraemer, Lowe, & Kupfer, 2005) provide in-depth discussions on the differentiation between risk markers and causal risk factors and the fundamental importance of recognizing these distinctions.

The primary focus of *Emerging Answers* was a review of the evidence of effectiveness across a large number of adolescent sexual behavior and other related outcomes for sexual risk behavior prevention interventions. Studies were selected for review based on criteria such as program goals and measured outcomes, and having follow-up data collected at least 3 months after intervention completion, as well as several vague methodological criteria:

> Include a reasonably strong experimental or quasi-experimental design, have reasonably well matched intervention and comparison groups, collect data both before and after implementation of the program, have a sample size of at least 100 persons [and] employ appropriate statistical analyses. (Kirby, 2007, p. 83)

No further specification was provided of the criteria used to identify studies that met the inclusion standards of "a reasonably strong" design or "appropriate statistical analysis." While several issues of design and statistical analysis were discussed, these were not used as a basis for exclusion of weaker studies. For example, the author disclosed that "almost one-third of the studies in this review are biased in favor of more significant results because they did not adjust statistically for clustering" (p. 93), and that "99 of the 115 studies conducted multiple tests of significance, but only seven studies adjusted for them" (p. 96), yet no remedial adjustments were made for these biases as part of this synthesis.

Emerging Answers concluded with a programs-that-work list of 15 programs characterized as having "strong evidence of positive impact on sexual behavior or pregnancy or STD rates" (Kirby, 2007, pp. 190–191). This list included seven curriculum-based interventions, four of which are published by the author's employer, ETR Associates. Many of the 15 listed programs are characterized by questionable evidence of effectiveness, involving such issues as unadjusted multiple significance testing, selective reporting, differential attrition, and failure to adjust for clustering (for example, see Constantine and Braverman's (2004) critique of the effectiveness evidence and its use for ETR Associate's *Reducing the Risk* curriculum). In addition, programs for which the preponderance of reported outcomes showed no statistically significant effects were nevertheless included on the list. In fact, of the seven curriculum-based interventions listed in *Emerging Answers* as having strong evidence of effectiveness, six were subsequently judged by the Coalition for Evidence-Based Policy (2010) as not having strong evidence of effectiveness for pregnancy or STD prevention (the seventh was not addressed by the Coalition).

Various other programs-that-work lists have been developed and promoted for adolescent sexual risk behavior interventions. Most recently, the federal Personal Responsibility Education Program requests for applications required that grantees "replicate evidence-based effective program models or substantially incorporate elements of effective programs that have been proven on the basis of rigorous scientific research to change [sexual] behavior" (US Department of Health and Human Services, Office of Adolescent Health, 2010). Partly but incompletely modeled after What Works Clearinghouse (2008) principles, this list of programs eligible for funding is more rigorous than the lists in this area typically developed by advocates and publishers. Nevertheless, it suffers from many of the same validity problems. For example, no adjustments were made by the reviewers for biases due to clustering or multiple significance testing in studies that had neglected to do so. Programs designated as evidence-based were initially classified into eight levels of evidence strength, but ultimately all were collapsed into one list of "evidence-based programs" preapproved for federal funding eligibility. Upon release of the request for applications employing this list, the independent Coalition for Evidence-Based Policy (2010) commented that "HHS's evidence-based teen pregnancy prevention program is an excellent first step, but only 2 of 28 approved models have strong evidence of effectiveness" (p. 1).

Systematic reviews and meta-analyses in this area have been almost as prolific as narrative reviews and programs-that-work lists. In their Campbell Collaboration review of interventions intended to reduce pregnancy-related outcomes among adolescents, Scher and colleagues (2006) identified six previously published meta-analyses on adolescent sexual risk behavior interventions. Subsequently, Oringanje et al. (2010) published a Cochrane Collaboration review on interventions for preventing unintended pregnancies among adolescents, and Johnson, Scott-Sheldon, Huedo-Medina, and Carey (2011) updated their original 2003 meta-analysis on adolescent HIV prevention interventions. These reviews vary in program type, intervention focus, eligible research designs, outcomes considered, and number of studies analyzed and in patterns of strengths and weaknesses exhibited. They also vary in findings and conclusions. Four of these reviews that are arguably the most influential, either because of their Cochrane Collaboration or Campbell Collaboration sponsorship or as evidenced by a relatively large number of citations are worth considering.

Oringanje et al.'s (2010) Cochrane Collaboration systematic review was based on analyses of 15 of 41 eligible randomized studies for which appropriate data were available. It reported no significant effects for any type of intervention on any type of sexual behavior or pregnancy-related outcome based on full sample analyses. Among the many subgroup analyses included, one significant effect was reported for "gender mixed or not specified" (p. 65) subgroups' initiation of sexual intercourse in interventions that combine education with contraception promotion. Inexplicably, one nonsignificant result that "approached significance" (p. 14) and was based on just two studies led the authors to erroneously conclude in their abstract, without qualification, that this type of combined education with contraception promotion "lowered the rate of unintended pregnancy among adolescents" (p. 2).

Scher and colleagues (2006), in their Campbell Collaboration review, analyzed 19 studies of school-based sex education programs. These were selected based on explicit criteria, such as employing a randomized design, reporting at least one of three prespecified outcomes (sexual experience, unprotected sexual activity, and pregnancy rates), and meeting defined sample retention standards. For sex education programs with an abstinence focus, the authors found "limited evidence" of a negative effect involving *higher* pregnancy rates among intervention groups (p. 3). For sex education programs with a comprehensive focus "no consistent evidence" was found that these programs "altered the likelihood that youth would initiate sex, would risk pregnancy, or would become [or get someone] pregnant" (p. 3). "Promising results" based on six randomized studies were reported for intensive multicomponent youth development programs serving higher risk adolescents (p. 3). The authors noted that these results did not show the programs to be ineffective, but rather, were most likely a reflection of the dearth of high quality research evidence available in this field.

In one highly cited systematic review, DiCenso, Guyatt, Willan, and Griffith (2002) analyzed 26 randomized studies of interventions developed to reduce unintended adolescent pregnancies and found no effects on initiation of sexual intercourse, use of birth control, or number of pregnancies. Methodological quality scores were calculated for each included study but used only descriptively to illustrate the poor methodological quality of most of the studies analyzed. Most recently, Johnson et al. (2011) updated their highly cited 2003 review, analyzing 67 adolescent HIV prevention intervention studies selected based on criteria that included a single methodological standard, "use [of] a randomized trial or a quasi-experimental design with rigorous controls" (p. 78), without further elaboration on how rigor was evaluated. Again, methodological quality scores were computed, but this was done subsequent to study inclusion and they were used only descriptively. In this review, intervention effects in the desired directions were found across the 67 studies for condom use, incidence of sexually transmitted infections, reducing or delaying sex, and negotiation skills.

Although hundreds of individual studies have been conducted, many of the synthesis authors have commented on the dearth of high quality studies. The largest and most rigorous individual study in this area to date was a 5-year randomized trial of the U.S. Title V, Section 510 Abstinence Education Program, which tested four of the most promising abstinence-only interventions. The results indicated no significant differences between individually randomized trial participants and control students on any of the primary outcomes (Trenholm et al., 2007, 2008). This study provides compelling evidence for the limited potential of abstinence-only education approaches, especially when considered in light of converging evidence derived from other studies based on complementary research designs, such as the previously discussed Kohler and colleagues' (2008) NSFG observational study. Yet, no study of the scope and rigor of this Trenholm and colleagues trial has ever been conducted of abstinence-plus interventions. Together with differences in the criteria used to select research studies for inclusion in a synthesis, this dearth of high quality research might help explain the wide disparity of conclusions across the many narrative reviews, programs-that-work lists, and meta-analyses.

At the same time, these research syntheses as a group are characterized by neglect of some of the most serious and common threats to validity and integrity found in the individual studies analyzed, such as failure to adjust for clustering bias when intervention assignments are made at the group rather than individual level and failure to account for multiple significance testing biases. Additional threats introduced at the research-synthesis level in some reviews include the potential for conflict of interest due to close reviewer connections to the programs and studies reviewed, and insufficiently systematic and transparent criteria for study selection. And for the narrative reviews and programs-that-work lists, the same one study/one outcome criterion for effectiveness that has been widely criticized in other areas of intervention research continues to be perhaps the most serious threat of all.

A further weakness in this and many other areas of research synthesis and evidence-based policy has been insufficient attention to additional relevant and important sources of evidence, especially evidence from basic science research (Hirsch, 2002; Lochman, 2000; Westen & Bradley, 2005). This includes evidence from established and emerging programs of research in social, cognitive, developmental, and educational psychology and neuropsychology. For example, programs and curricula focused on prevention of adolescent sexual risk behaviors tend to view adolescents as rational, deliberative decision makers motivated to maximize positive outcomes. Yet basic research in developmental, cognitive, and social psychology has for some time demonstrated how judgment and decision making are much more complex in general (Gigerenzer & Selten, 2002; Schneider & Shanteau, 2003), and specifically regarding health behavior (Wiers, et al., 2010), adolescents (Jacobs & Klaczynski, 2005; Moshman, 2011; Reyna & Rivers, 2008), and adolescent sexual health behavior (Goldfarb & Constantine, 2011). Evidence from this type of basic science research is essential to appraising and understanding intervention effectiveness and its contexts and practices, yet it is routinely ignored.

This brief methodological critique of research syntheses on the effectiveness of interventions to reduce adolescent sexual risk behaviors illustrates several of the commonly encountered validity and integrity threats discussed in the chapter. It demonstrates how the etiological roots of some of the most insidious threats can be found in the quest for black and white answers within an area characterized by varied shades of gray. These roots are nurtured by the abundance of poor quality research in the field.

In spite of these weaknesses, several broad conclusions are supported by the full body of evidence in this area:

(a) Abstinence-only interventions as typically conceived and implemented have limited potential.
(b) Abstinence-plus interventions that directly focus on promoting behavioral change and include instruction on condoms and contraception methods have better potential, and evidence is accumulating of some modest positive effects overall.
(c) With few exceptions, the effectiveness of specific individual abstinence-plus interventions, programs, or curricula is not well supported by the available evidence. This does not necessarily mean that these programs are ineffective, just that the nature and quality of the available research is woefully inadequate to answering questions at this level.
(d) The full potential to enhance adolescents' sexual health and development through primary prevention and health promotion interventions is not being realized by the currently popular abstinence-only and abstinence-plus intervention models.

Concluding Comments and Recommendations

> Failed certainties in social science litter the landscape like so many elephant bones bleaching in the African sun. Honest hard scientists never claim final answers; good social science shouldn't either.
>
> (Carter, 2004)

> In considering the ways in which research data are typically interpreted, I became convinced that there is a strong cult of naive and overconfident empiricism in psychology and the social sciences with an excessive faith in data as the direct source of scientific truth and an inadequate appreciation of how misleading data can be. I concluded that the commonly held belief that research progress requires only that we "let the data speak" is sadly erroneous. If data are allowed to speak for themselves, they will typically lie to you.
>
> (Schmidt, 2010)

There exists an important need for interventions based in adolescent health psychology to reduce adolescent risk behaviors and to promote adolescent health and development more broadly. Appropriately, questions of intervention effectiveness have been and are continuing to receive steadfast attention. Funders, policy shapers, practitioners, and other stakeholders understandably seek direct and straightforward answers, especially to the one deceptively decisive question of highest perceived importance—does an intervention achieve its intended effect, yes or no? But reality rarely yields to such desired simplicity, nor does principled scientific inquiry enable it. Oversimplification of research, its appraisal, and its use in the service of this single yes or no question opens the door to unchecked threats to research validity and research integrity, neglect of valuable types of relevant evidence, and ultimately to misleading research conclusions, misinformed policy and funding decisions, and unfulfilled potential.

Consistent with the National Research Council (2002) principles of scientific inquiry and other modern views on the nature of science, there are a number of ways in which intervention effectiveness research and its use in adolescent health psychology could be improved to better support the development, evaluation, and dissemination of effective interventions. A good start would be to move beyond the widely embraced myth that method determines validity and its corollary fiction that methodological hierarchies and methodological quality checklists can substitute for genuine critical appraisal. This would be supported by a better understanding and acceptance of the need for and importance of qualitative reasoning (Brady & Collier, 2010; Freedman, 2008; Maxwell, 2005) and carefully reasoned argument (Abelson, 1995; Campbell, 1982; Victora, Habicht, & Bryce, 2004) in all types of research. As Abelson has noted, "the purpose of statistics is to organize a useful argument from quantitative evidence, using a form of principled rhetoric" (1995, p. xiii). And Lancet editor Richard Horton's (1998) advice to physicians should resonate with adolescent health psychology researchers and practitioners as well: "The argument is the fundamental unit of all medical thought" (p. 249).

A principal tool for putting this into practice would be the critical narrative review, characterized by deeper and more meaningful attention to theory and mechanisms. This would embrace basic research evidence from relevant fields such as social, cognitive, developmental, and educational psychology and neuropsychology. It would focus on cumulative evidence and theoretical replications, together with theoretically expected convergence of evidence across multiple studies, research groups, methods, and contexts. And its essence would involve the spirited consideration of plausible alternative explanations for all results and potential conclusions, with attention to the implications of competing explanations on multiple data sets and to the fit between these implications and actual data (Campbell, 2009).

At a more fundamental level, research programs based on theory-driven model-building approaches have the potential to strengthen intervention development and evaluation. A model-building approach has been described as "iterative within a program of research, cycling though the following phases: theory, field observations, construct definition, measurement development, construct analysis, model testing, experimental field trials, and model revision" (Dishion & Patterson, 1999). Such an approach includes the probing of theory-based moderators and mediators to increase the understanding of relevant processes and mechanisms of change (Cook, 2002; Hinshaw, 2002; Kazdin, 1997; Kotchick, Shaffer, & Forehand, 2001; Lochman, 2006; Weersing & Weisz, 2002), consistent with the understanding that

> The "gold standard" studies in intervention research are those that not only demonstrate efficacy but also demonstrate that the postulated change mechanisms . . . do indeed carry the weight of improvement on (intervention) outcomes. (Hughes, 2000, p. 307)

Although programs-that-work lists have been characterized by what might appear to be insurmountable problems, the quest for such straightforward direction by funders and program administrators is not surprising, and these types of lists are unlikely to disappear anytime soon. One strategy to address this challenge would be the development of a new generation of evidence-based program lists that are grounded upon more genuinely scientific criteria of effectiveness. In place of the currently popular practice of trolling through individual research studies for any possible signs of effectiveness, this would involve critically appraising intervention content, approach, and intended populations for consistency with more inclusive theory-grounded evidence and principles derived from comprehensive and integrative critical narrative reviews. This process would not be easy, but like principled scientific inquiry more generally, principled scientific research synthesis rarely is easy.

Finally, recognizing that biases associated with conflict of interests are pervasive and generally not intentional or even within one's conscious awareness, a greater separation among program developers, researchers, and research reviewers is needed.

> We must move beyond mere disclosure of conflicts of interest toward developing additional regulatory mechanisms aimed at minimizing their pervasive influence. Like George Washington admitting that he chopped down his father's cherry tree, our willingness to disclose conflicts of interest does not absolve us of further responsibility. (Abi-Jaoude & Gorman, 2010, p. 1546)

The issues and strategies discussed in this chapter are intended to address the need for fundamental improvements in the conduct and use of research and research synthesis on intervention effectiveness in adolescent health psychology. Through better understanding and application of principled scientific inquiry, better attention to common threats to research validity and research integrity, and better use of theory, evidence, and reasoned argument, the field of adolescent health psychology should be able to make further progress toward reaching its full potential.

Acknowledgments The author thanks Eva Goldfarb, Petra Jerman, Wendy Constantine, and Jessica Lin for critical review and suggestions. Preparation of this chapter was facilitated by grants from the Ford Foundation and the William and Flora Hewlett Foundation.

References

Abel, U., & Koch, A. (1999). The role of randomization in clinical studies: Myths and beliefs. *Journal of Clinical Epidemiology, 52*, 487–497. doi:10.1016/S0895-4356(99)00041-4.

Abelson, R. (1995). *Statistics as principled argument*. Hillsdale, NJ: Erlbaum.

Abi-Jaoude, E., & Gorman, D. A. (2010). Disclosure: Only a first step. *Canadian Medical Association Journal, 182*, 1546. doi:10.1503/cmaj.110-2109.

Advocates for Youth. (2008). *Science and success: Sex education and other programs that work to prevent teen pregnancy, HIV & sexually transmitted infections* (2nd ed.). Retrieved June 6, 2011, from http://www.advocatesforyouth.org/storage/advfy/documents/sciencesuccess.pdf.

Altman, D. G. (2002). Poor quality medical research: What can journals do? *Journal of the American Medical Association, 287*, 2765–2767. doi:10.1001/jama.287.21.2765.

Anderson, N. H. (1963). Comparison of different populations: Resistance to extinction and transfer. *Psychological Review, 70*, 162–179. doi:10.1037/h0044858.

Bachrach, C., & Newcomer, S. F. (2002). Addressing bias in intervention research: Summary of a workshop. *Journal of Adolescent Health, 31*, 311–321. doi:10.1016/S1054-139X(02)00395-6.

Bakker, M., & Wicherts, J. M. (2011). The (mis)reporting of statistical results in psychology. *Behavior Research Methods, 43*, 666–678. doi:10.3758/s13428-011-0089-5.

Bearman, P. S., & Bruckner, H. (2001). Promising the future: Virginity pledges and first intercourse. *American Journal of Sociology, 106*, 859–912. doi:10.1086/320295.

Berle, D., & Starcevic, V. (2007). Inconsistencies between reported test statistics and p-values in two psychiatry journals. *International Journal of Methods in Psychiatric Research, 16*, 202–207. doi:10.1002/mpr.225.

Berliner, D. (2002). Comment: Educational research: The hardest science of all. *Educational Researcher, 31*(8), 18–20. doi:10.3102/0013189X031008018.

Brady, H. E., & Collier, D. (Eds.). (2010). *Rethinking social inquiry: Diverse tools, shared standards* (2nd ed.). Lanham, MD: Rowman and Littlefield.

Briggs, D. C. (2005). Meta-analysis: A case study. *Evaluation Review, 29*, 87–127. doi:10.1177/0193841X04272555.

Cain, D. M., & Detsky, A. S. (2008). Everyone's a little bit biased (even physicians). *Journal of the American Medical Association, 299*, 2893–2895. doi:10.1001/jama.299.24.2893.

Campbell, D. T. (1953). *Designs for social science experiments*. Evanston, IL: Northwestern University.

Campbell, D. T. (1957). Factors relevant to the validity of experiments in social settings. *Psychological Bulletin, 54*, 297–312. doi:10.1037/h0040950.

Campbell, D. T. (1982). Experiments as arguments. In E. R. House, S. Mathison, J. A. Pearsol, & H. Preskill (Eds.), *Evaluation studies review annual* (Vol. 7, pp. 117–127). Beverly Hills, CA: Sage.

Campbell, D. T. (2009). Forward. In R. K. Yin (Ed.), *Case study research: Design and methods* (4th ed., pp. vii–viii). Thousand Oaks, CA: Sage.

Campbell, D. T., & Stanley, J. C. (1963). *Experimental and quasi-experimental designs for research*. Boston: Houghton-Mifflin.

Carter, H. (2004). Presidential perspective. In M. T. Braverman, N. A. Constantine, & J. K. Slater (Eds.), *Foundations and evaluation: Contexts and practices for effective philanthropy*. San Francisco: Jossey-Bass.

Centers for Disease Control and Prevention. (2008). *10 steps to promoting science-based approaches to teen pregnancy prevention using Getting To Outcomes: A summary*. Retrieved from http://www.cdc.gov/reproductivehealth/adolescentreprohealth/PDF/LittlePSBA-GTO.pdf.

Chan, A. W., Hrobjartsson, A., Haahr, M. T., Gotzsche, P. C., & Altman, D. G. (2004). Empirical evidence for selective reporting of outcomes in randomized trials: Comparison of protocols to published articles. *Journal of the American Medical Association, 291*, 2457–2465. doi:10.1001/jama.291.20.2457.

Chen, S., & Chaiken, S. (1999). The heuristic-systematic model in its broader context. In S. Chaiken & Y. Trope (Eds.), *Dual-process theories in social psychology* (pp. 73–96). New York: Guilford.

Chinn, C. A., & Brewer, W. F. (2001). Models of data: A theory of how people evaluate data. *Cognition and Instruction, 19*, 323–393. Retrieved from http://www.jstor.org/stable/3233918.

Chugh, D., Banaji, M., & Bazerman, M. (2005). Bounded ethicality as a psychological barrier to recognizing conflicts of interest. In D. Moore, D. Cain, G. Loewenstein, & M. Bazerman (Eds.), *Conflicts of interest: Challenges and solutions in business, law, medicine, and public policy*. New York: Cambridge University Press.

Coalition for Evidence-Based Policy. (2010). *HHS's evidence-based teen pregnancy prevention program*. Retrieved June 6, 2011, from http://coalition4evidence.org/wordpress/wp-content/uploads/Coalition-comments-HHS-Teen-Pregnancy-Prevention-May-2010.pdf.

Collins, J., Robin, L., Wooley, S., Fenley, D., Hunt, P., Taylor, J., et al. (2002). Programs-that-work: CDC's guide to effective programs that reduce health-risk behavior of youth. *Journal of School Health, 72*, 93–99. doi:10.1111/j.1746-1561.2002.tb06523.x.

Constantine, N. A. (2008a). Converging evidence leaves policy behind: Effectiveness of and support for school-based sex education programs [Editorial]. *Journal of Adolescent Health, 42*, 324–326. doi:10.1016/j.jadohealth.2008.01.004.

Constantine, N. A. (2008b). The peer review process. In S. Boslaugh (Ed.), *Encyclopedia of epidemiology* (Vol. 1, pp. 794–796). Thousand Oaks, CA: Sage.

Constantine, N. A. (2008c). Publication bias. In S. Boslaugh (Ed.), *Encyclopedia of epidemiology* (Vol. 1, pp. 853–854). Thousand Oaks, CA: Sage.

Constantine, N. A. (2012). Regression analysis and causal inference: Cause for concern? *Perspectives on Sexual and Reproductive Health, 44*, 134–137. doi:10.1363/4413412.

Constantine, N. A., & Braverman, M. T. (2004). Appraising evidence on program effectiveness. In M. T. Braverman, N. A. Constantine, & J. K. Slater (Eds.), *Foundations and evaluation: Contexts and practices for effective philanthropy* (pp. 236–258). San Francisco: Jossey-Bass.

Cook, T. D. (2002). Randomized experiments in educational policy research: A critical examination of the reasons the educational evaluation community has offered for not doing them. *Educational Evaluation and Policy Analysis, 24*, 175–199. doi:10.3102/01623737024003175.

Cook, T. D., & Campbell, D. T. (1979). *Quasi-experimentation: Design and analysis issues for field settings*. Chicago: Rand-McNally.

Cronbach, L. J. (1982). *Designing evaluations of educational and social programs*. San Francisco: Jossey-Bass.

Dane, A. U., & Schneider, B. H. (1998). Program integrity in primary and early secondary prevention: Are implementation effects out of control? *Clinical Psychology Review, 18*, 23–45. doi:10.1016/S0272-7358(97)00043-3.

Davey Smith, G., & Ebrahim, S. (2001). Epidemiology—is it time to call it a day? *International Journal of Epidemiology, 30*, 1–11. doi:10.1093/ije/30.1.1.

Dawson, E., Gilovich, T., & Regan, D. T. (2002). Motivated reasoning and performance on the Wason Selection Task. *Personality and Social Psychology Bulletin, 28*, 1379–1387. doi:10.1177/014616702236869.

DiCenso, A., Guyatt, G., Willan, A., & Griffith, L. (2002). Interventions to reduce unintended pregnancies among adolescents: Systematic review of randomized controlled trials. *British Medical Journal, 324*, 1426–1434. doi:10.1136/bmj.324.7351.1426.

Dishion, T. J., & Patterson, G. R. (1999). Model building in developmental psychopathology: A pragmatic approach to understanding and intervention. *Journal of Clinical Child Psychology, 28*, 502–512. doi:10.1207/S15374424JCCP2804_10.

Dwan, K., Altman, D. G., Arnaiz, J. A., Bloom, J., Chan, A.-W., Cronin, E., et al. (2008). Systematic review of the empirical evidence of study publication bias and outcome reporting bias. *Public Library of Science (PLoS) ONE, 3*, e3081. doi:10.1371/journal.pone.0003081.

Egger, M., & Davey Smith, G. (1997). Meta-analysis: Potentials and promise. *British Medical Journal, 315*, 1371–1374.

Evans, J. (1989). *Bias in human reasoning: Causes and consequences*. London: Erlbaum.

Feinstein, A. R. (1988). Fraud, distortion, delusion, and consensus: The problems of human and natural deception in epidemiologic science. *American Journal of Medicine, 84*(3, Pt. 1), 475–478. doi:10.1016/0002-9343(88)90268-9.

Feuer, M. J., Towne, L., & Shavelson, R. J. (2002). Scientific culture and educational research. *Educational Researcher, 31*(8), 4–14. doi:10.3102/0013189X031008004.

Freedman, D. A. (2008). On types of scientific inquiry: The role of qualitative reasoning. In J. M. Box-Steffensmeier, H. E. Brady, & D. Collier (Eds.), *The Oxford handbook of political methodology* (pp. 300–318). New York: Oxford University Press.

Freedman, D. A. (2010). *Statistical models and causal inference: A dialogue with the social sciences*. Cambridge, UK: Cambridge University Press.

Friedlander, F. (1964). Type I and Type II bias. *American Psychologist, 19*, 198–199. doi:10.1037/h0038977.

Gandhi, A. G., Murphy-Graham, E., Petrosino, A., Chrismer, S. S., & Weiss, C. H. (2007). The devil is in the details: Examining the evidence for "proven" school-based drug abuse prevention programs. *Evaluation Review, 31*, 43–74. doi:10.1177/0193841X06287188.

Garcia-Berthou, E., & Alcaraz, C. (2004). Incongruence between test statistics and P values in medical papers. *BMC Medical Research Methodology, 4*, 13. doi:10.1186/1471-2288-4-13.

Gigerenzer, G. (1998). Surrogates for theories. *Theories & Psychology, 8*, 195–204. doi: 10.1177/0959354398082006.

Gigerenzer, G. (2009). Surrogates for theory. *Association for Psychological Science Observer, 22*, 21–23.

Gigerenzer, G., & Selten, R. (Eds.). (2002). *Bounded rationality: The adaptive toolbox*. Cambridge, MA: The MIT Press.

Goldfarb, E. S., & Constantine, N. A. (2011). Sexuality education. In B. B. Brown & M. Prinstein (Eds.), *Encyclopedia of adolescence*. New York: Academic.

Gorman, D. M. (2002). Defining and operationalizing 'research-based' prevention: A critique (with case studies) of the US Department of Education's Safe, Disciplined and Drug-Free Schools exemplary programs. *Evaluation and Program Planning, 25*, 295–302.

Gorman, D. M., & Conde, E. (2007). Conflict of interest in the evaluation and dissemination of "model" school-based drug and violence prevention programs. *Evaluation and Program Planning, 30*, 422–429. doi:10.1016/j.evalprogplan.2007.06.004.

Grossman, D. C., Neckerman, H. J., Koespell, T. D., Liu, P. Y., Asher, K. N., Beland, K., et al. (1997). Effectiveness of a violence prevention curriculum among children in elementary school: A randomized controlled trial. *Journal of the American Medical Association, 277*, 1605–1611. doi:10.1001/jama.1997.03540440039030.

Haack, S. (2003). *Defending science—within reason: Between scientism and cynicism*. New York: Prometheus.

Hahn, S., Williamson, P. R., & Hutton, J. L. (2002). Investigation of within-study selective reporting in clinical research: Follow-up of applications submitted to a local research ethics committee. *Journal of Evaluation in Clinical Practice, 8*, 353–359. doi:10.1046/j.1365-2753.2002.00314.x.

Hahn, S., Williamson, P. R., Hutton, J. L., Garner, P., & Flynn, V. (2000). Assessing the potential for bias in meta-analysis due to selective reporting of subgroup analyses within studies. *Statistics in Medicine, 19*, 3325–3336. doi:10.1002/1097-0258(20001230)19:24<3325::AID-SIM827>3.0.CO;2-D.

Hinshaw, S. P. (2002). Intervention research, theoretical mechanisms, and causal processes related to externalizing behavior patterns. *Development and Psychopathology, 14*, 789–818. doi:10.1017/S0954579402004078.

Hirsch, E. D. (2002). Classroom research and cargo cults. *Policy Review, 115*, 51–69.

Horton, R. (1998). The grammar of interpretive medicine. *Canadian Medical Association Journal, 159*, 245–249.

Howel, D., & Bhopal, R. (1994). Assessing cause and effect from trials: A cautionary note. *Controlled Clinical Trials, 15*, 331–334. doi:10.1016/0197-2456(94)90030-2.

Hughes, J. N. (2000). The essential role of theory in the science of treating children: Beyond empirically supported treatments. *Journal of School Psychology, 38*, 301–330. doi:10.1016/S0022-4405(00)00042-X.

Huston, P., & Moher, D. (1996). Redundancy, disaggregation, and the integrity of medical research. *The Lancet, 347*, 1024–1026. doi:10.1016/S0140-6736(96)90153-1.

Ioannidis, J. P. A. (2005). Why most published research findings are false. *Library of Science (PLoS) Medicine, 2*, 696–701. doi:10.1371/journal.pmed.0020124.

Ioannidis, J. P. A. (2007). Limitations are not properly acknowledged in the scientific literature. *Journal of Clinical Epidemiology, 60*, 324–329. doi:10.1016/j.jclinepi.2006.09.011.

Ioannidis, J. P. A. (2011). An epidemic of false claims: Competition and conflicts of interest distort too many medical findings. *Scientific American, 304*, 16.

Retrieved from http://www.scientificamerican.com/article.cfm?id=an-epidemic-of-false-claims.
Ioannidis, J. P. A., & Karassa, F. B. (2010). The need to consider the wider agenda in systematic reviews and meta-analyses: Breadth, timing, and depth of the evidence. *British Medical Journal, 341*, c4875. doi:10.1136/bmj.c4875.
Ioannidis, J. P. A., Tatsioni, A., & Karassa, F. B. (2010). Who is afraid of reviewers' comments? Or, why anything can be published and anything can be cited. *European Journal of Clinical Investigation, 40*, 285–287. doi:10.1111/j.1365-2362.2010.02272.x.
Jacobs, J. J., & Klaczynski, P. A. (2005). *The development of judgment and decision making in children and adolescents*. Mahwah, NJ: LEA.
Johnson, B. T., Scott-Sheldon, L. A. J., Huedo-Medina, T. B., & Carey, M. P. (2011). Interventions to reduce sexual risk for human immunodeficiency virus in adolescents: A meta-analysis of trials, 1985–2008. *Archives of Pediatrics & Adolescent Medicine, 165*, 77–84. doi:10.1001/archpediatrics.2010.251.
Kassirer, J. P., & Angell, M. (1995). Redundant publication: A reminder [Editorial]. *New England Journal of Medicine, 333*, 449–450. Retrieved from http://www.nejm.org/doi/pdf/10.1056/NEJM199508173330709.
Kazdin, A. E. (1997). A model for developing effective treatments: Progression and interplay of theory, research, and practice. *Journal of Clinical Child Psychology, 26*, 114–129.
Kerr, N. L. (1998). HARKing (hypothesizing after the results are known). *Personality and Social Psychology Review, 2*, 196–217. doi:10.1207/s15327957pspr0203_4.
Kirby, D. (2007). *Emerging answers 2007: Research findings on programs to reduce teen pregnancy and sexually transmitted diseases*. Washington, DC: National Campaign to Prevent Teen and Unplanned Pregnancy.
Kohler, P. K., Manhart, L. E., & Lafferty, W. E. (2008). Abstinence-only and comprehensive sex education and the initiation of sexual activity and teen pregnancy. *Journal of Adolescent Health, 42*, 344–351. doi:10.1016/j.jadohealth.2007.08.026.
Koslowski, B. (1996). *Theory and evidence: The development of scientific reasoning*. Cambridge, MA: MIT Press/Bradford Books.
Koslowski, B., & Thompson, S. (2002). Theorizing is important, and collateral information constrains how well it is done. In P. Carruthers, S. Stich, & M. Siegal (Eds.), *The cognitive basis of science* (pp. 171–192). Cambridge, UK: Cambridge University Press.
Kotchick, B. A., Shaffer, A., & Forehand, R. (2001). Adolescent sexual risk behavior: A multi-system perspective. *Clinical Psychology Review, 21*, 493–519. doi:10.1016/S0272-7358(99)00070-7.
Kraemer, H. C., Kazdin, A. E., Offord, D. R., Kessler, R. C., Jensen, P. S., & Kupfer, D. J. (1997). Coming to terms with the terms of risk. *Archives of General Psychiatry, 54*, 337–343.
Kraemer, H. C., Lowe, K. K., & Kupfer, D. J. (2005). *To your health: How to understand what research tells us about risk*. Oxford, UK: Oxford University Press.
Krisberg, K. (2010). Teen pregnancy prevention focusing on evidence: Ineffective abstinence-only lessons being replaced with science. *The Nation's Health, 40*, 1–14. Retrieved from http://thenationshealth.aphapublications.org/content/40/3/1.1.full.
Kumar, M. N. (2008). A review of the types of scientific misconduct in biomedical research. *Journal of Academic Ethics, 6*, 211–228. doi:10.1007/s10805-008-9068-6.
Kunda, Z. (1990). The case for motivated reasoning. *Psychological Bulletin, 108*, 480–498. doi:10.1037/0033-2909.108.3.480.
Larzelere, R. E., Kuhn, B. R., & Johnson, B. (2004). The intervention selection bias: An underrecognized confound in intervention research. *Psychological Bulletin, 130*, 289–303. doi:10.1037/0033-2909.130.2.289.
Levy, D. A. (2010). *Tools of critical thinking: Metathoughts for psychology* (2nd ed.). Long Grove, IL: Waveland.
Light, R. J., Singer, J. D., & Willett, J. B. (1990). *By design: Planning research on higher education*. Cambridge, MA: Harvard University Press.
Lipsey, M. W. (2004). *The 2004 Claremont debate: Lipsey vs. Scriven. Determining causality in program evaluation & applied research: Should experimental evidence be the gold standard?* Retrieved October 31, 2010, from http://www.cgu.edu/include/SBOS_2004_Debate.pdf.
Lochman, J. E. (2000). Theory and empiricism in intervention research: A dialectic to be avoided. *Journal of School Psychology, 38*, 359–338. doi:10.1016/S0022-4405(00)00038-8.
Lochman, J. E. (2006). Translation of research into interventions. *International Journal of Behavioral Development, 30*, 31–38. doi:10.1177/0165025406059971.
Lord, F. M. (1967). A paradox in the interpretation of group comparisons. *Psychological Bulletin, 68*, 304–305.
MacCoun, R. (1998). Biases in the interpretation and use of research results. *Annual Review of Psychology, 49*, 259–287. doi:10.1146/annurev.psych.49.1.259.
MacCoun, R. (2005). Conflicts of interest in public policy research. In D. A. Moore, D. M. Cain, G. Lowenstein, & M. H. Bazerman (Eds.), *Conflicts of interest: Challenges and solutions in business, law, medicine, and public policy* (pp. 233–262). Cambridge, UK: Cambridge University Press.
Machi, L. A., & McEvoy, B. T. (2009). *The literature review*. Thousand Oaks, CA: Corwin.
Mahoney, M. J. (1977). Publication prejudices: An experimental study of confirmatory bias in the peer-review system. *Cognitive Therapy and Research, 1*, 161–175. doi:10.1007/BF01173636.
Matt, G. E., & Cook, T. D. (2009). Threats to the validity of generalized inferences. In H. Cooper, L. V. Hedges, & J. C. Valentine (Eds.), *The handbook of research synthesis and meta-analysis* (2nd ed., pp. 537–556). New York: Russell Sage Foundation.
Maxwell, J. A. (2004). Causal explanation, qualitative research, and scientific inquiry in education. *Educational Researcher, 33*(2), 3–11. doi:10.3102/0013189X033002003.

Maxwell, J. A. (2005). *Qualitative research design: An interactive approach* (2nd ed.). Thousand Oaks, CA: Sage.

McCartney, K., & Rosenthal, R. (2000). Effect size, practical importance, and social policy for children. *Child Development, 71*, 173–180. doi:10.1111/1467-8624.00131.

Meinert, C. L. (1986). *Clinical trials: Design, conduct, and analysis*. Oxford, UK: Oxford University Press.

Miles, M. B., & Huberman, A. M. (1994). *Qualitative data analysis: An expanded sourcebook* (2nd ed.). Thousand Oaks, CA: Sage.

Mills, J. L. (1993). Data torturing. *New England Journal of Medicine, 329*, 1196–1199.

Moore, D. A., Loewenstein, G., Tanlu, L., & Bazerman, M. H. (2003). *Auditor independence, conflict of interest, and the unconscious intrusion of bias*. Harvard Business School Working Paper #03-116. Retrieved October 7, 2011, from http://citeseerx.ist.psu.edu/viewdoc/download?doi=10.1.1.9.2829&rep=rep1&type=pdf.

Moshman, D. (2011). *Adolescent rationality and development: Cognition, morality, and identity*. New York, NY: Psychology.

Moskowitz, J. M. (1993). Why reports of outcome evaluations are often biased or uninterpretable: Examples from evaluations of drug abuse prevention programs. *Evaluation and Program Planning, 16*, 1–9. doi:10.1016/0149-7189(93)90032-4.

National Research Council Committee on Assessing Integrity in Research Environments. (2002). *Integrity in scientific research: Creating an environment that promotes responsible conduct*. Washington, DC: National Academies Press.

National Research Council Committee on Scientific Principles for Educational Research. (2002). *Scientific research in education*. Washington, DC: National Academies Press.

Oringanje, C., Meremikwu, M. M., Eko, H., Esu, E., Meremikwu, A., & Ehiri, J. E. (2010). Interventions for preventing unintended pregnancies among adolescents. *Cochrane Database of Systematic Reviews, 4*. doi:10.1002/14651858.CD005215.pub2.

Petrosino, A. (2003). Standards for evidence and evidence for standards: The case of school-based drug prevention. *Annals of the American Academy of Political and Social Science, 587*, 180–207. doi:10.1177/0002716203251218.

Rennie, D. (1998). Freedom and responsibility in medical publication: Setting the balance right. *Journal of the American Medical Association, 280*, 300–302. doi:10.1001/jama.280.3.300.

Rennie, D. (1999). Fair conduct and fair reporting of clinical trials. *Journal of the American Medical Association, 282*, 1766–1768. doi:10.1001/jama.282.18.1766.

Reyna, V. F., & Rivers, S. E. (2008). Current theories of risk and rational decision making. *Developmental Review, 28*, 1–11. doi:10.1016/j.dr.2008.01.002.

Rosenthal, R. (1994). Science and ethics in conducting, analyzing, and reporting psychological research. *Psychological Science, 5*, 127–134. doi:10.1111/j.1467-9280.1994.tb00646.x.

Rothwell, P. M. (2005). External validity of randomised controlled trials: "To whom do the results of this trial apply?". *The Lancet, 365*, 82–93. doi:10.1016/S0140-6736(04)17670-8.

Scher, S., Lin, J., & Constantine, N. A. (2009). *Motivated translation of ambiguous scientific research findings: A case study from the sex education debates. Paper presented at the International Conference on Science in Society*. United Kingdom: University of Cambridge.

Scher, L. S., Maynard, R. A., & Stagner, M. (2006). Interventions intended to reduce pregnancy- related outcomes among adolescents. *Campbell Collaboration Systematic Reviews, 12*. Campbell Collaboration. doi: 10.4073/csr.2006.12.

Schmidt, F. (2010). Detecting and correcting the lies that data tell. *Perspectives on Psychological Science, 5*, 233–242. doi:10.1177/1745691610369339.

Schneider, S. L., & Shanteau, J. (2003). *Emerging perspectives on judgment and decision making*. Cambridge, UK: Cambridge University Press.

Scientifically Based Evaluation Methods, 68 Fed. Reg. 62,445 (October 29, 2003).

Scriven, M. (2008). A summative evaluation of RCT methodology and an alternative approach to causal research. *Journal of Multidisciplinary Evaluation, 5*, 11–24.

Shadish, W. R., Jr., Cook, T. D., & Campbell, D. T. (2002). *Experimental and quasi-experimental designs for generalized causal inference*. Boston: Houghton-Mifflin.

Shafer, G., & Tversky, A. (1985). Languages and designs for probability judgment. *Cognitive Science, 9*, 309–339. doi:10.1207/s15516709cog0903_2.

Shatz, D. (2001). *Peer review: A critical inquiry*. New York: Rowman and Littlefield.

Shavelson, R., & Towne, L. (2004). What drives scientific research in education? Questions, not methods, should drive the enterprise. *American Psychological Society Observer, 17*(4), 27–30. Retrieved from http://www.psychologicalscience.org/observer/getArticle.cfm?id=1557.

Simmons, J. P., Nelson, L. D., & Simonsohn, U. (2011). False-positive psychology: Undisclosed flexibility in data collection and analysis allows presenting anything as significant. *Psychological Science, 22*, 1359–1366. doi:10.1177/0956797611417632.

Slavin, R. E. (1995). Best evidence synthesis: An intelligent alternative to meta-analysis. *Journal of Clinical Epidemiology, 48*, 9–18. doi:10.1016/0895-4356(94)00097-A.

Smith, R., Feachem, R., Feachem, N. S., Koehlmoos, T. P., & Kinlaw, H. (2009). The fallacy of impartiality: Competing interest bias in academic publications. *Journal of the Royal Society of Medicine, 102*(2), 44–45. doi:10.1258/jrsm.2009.080400.

Suellentrop, K. (2010). *Effective and promising teen pregnancy prevention programs for Latino youth. Science Says, 43*. Retrieved June 6, 2011, from http://www.thenationalcampaign.org/resources/pdf/SS/SS43_TPPProgramsLatinos.pdf.

Trenholm, C., Devaney, B., Fortson, K., Clark, M., Quay, L., & Wheeler, J. (2008). Impacts of abstinence education on teen sexual activity, risk of pregnancy, and risk of sexually transmitted diseases. *Journal of Policy Analysis and Management, 27*, 255–276. doi:10.1002/pam.20324.

Trenholm, C., Devaney, B., Fortson, K., Quay, L., Wheeler, J., & Clark, M. (2007). *Impacts of four Title V Section 510 abstinence education programs: Final report.* Retrieved January 12, 2011, from http://www.mathematica-mpr.com/publications/pdfs/impactabstinence.pdf.

Trochim, M. K., & Donnelly, J. P. (2007). *The research methods knowledge base* (3rd ed.). Mason, OH: Thomson.

U.S. Department of Health and Human Services, Office of Adolescent Health. (2010). *Overview of the teen pregnancy prevention research evidence review.* Retrieved May 16, 2011, from http://www.hhs.gov/ash/oah/prevention/research/index.html.

Victora, C. G., Habicht, J., & Bryce, J. (2004). Evidence-based public health: Moving beyond randomized trials. *American Journal of Public Health, 94*, 400–405.

Weersing, V. R., & Weisz, J. R. (2002). Mechanisms of action in youth psychotherapy. *Journal of Child Psychology and Psychiatry, 43*, 3–29. doi:10.1111/1469-7610.00002.

Weiss, C. H. (1980). *Social science research and decision-making*. New York: Columbia University Press.

Weiss, C. H., Murphy-Graham, E., Petrosino, A., & Gandhi, A. G. (2008). The fairy godmother—and her warts: Making the dream of evidence-based policy come true. *American Journal of Evaluation, 29*, 29–47. doi:10.1177/1098214007313742.

West, S. G. (2009). Alternatives to randomized experiments. *Current Directions in Psychological Science, 18*, 299–304. doi:10.1111/j.1467-8721.2009.01656.x.

Westen, D., & Bradley, R. (2005). Empirically supported complexity: Rethinking evidence-based practice in psychotherapy. *Current Directions in Psychological Science, 14*, 266–271. doi:10.1111/j.0963-7214.2005.00378.x.

What Works Clearinghouse. (2008). *Procedures and standards handbook (Version 2.0).* Retrieved June 6, 2011, from http://ies.ed.gov/ncee/wwc/pdf/wwc_procedures_v2_standards_handbook.pdf.

Wicherts, J. M., Bakker, M., & Molenaar, D. (2011). Willingness to share research data is related to the strength of the evidence and the quality of reporting of statistical results. *Public Library of Science (PLoS) ONE, 6*, e26828. doi:10.1371/journal.pone.0026828.

Wicherts, J. M., Borsboom, D., Kats, J., & Molenaar, D. (2006). The poor availability of psychological research data for reanalysis. *American Psychologist, 61*, 726–728.

Wiers, R. W., Houben, K., Roefs, A., de Jong, P., Hofmann, W., & Stacy, A. W. (2010). Implicit cognition in health psychology: why common sense goes out of the window. In B. Gawronski & B. K. Payne (Eds.), *Handbook of implicit social cognition* (pp. 463–488). New York: Guilford.

Wilkinson, L., & APA Task Force on Statistical Inference. (1999). Statistical methods in psychology journals: Guidelines and explanations. *American Psychologist, 54*, 594–604. doi:10.1037/0003-066X.54.8.594.

Williams, P. G., Holmbeck, G. M., & Greenley, R. N. (2002). Adolescent health psychology. *Journal of Consulting and Clinical Psychology, 70*, 828–842. doi:10.1037/0022-006X.70.3.828.

Wolins, L. (1962). Responsibility for raw data. *American Psychologist, 17*, 657–658. doi:10.1037/h0038819.

World Health Organization. (1946). *Constitution of the World Health Organization*. Retrieved July 28, 2011, from http://apps.who.int/gb/bd/PDF/bd47/EN/constitution-en.pdf.

Yin, R. K. (2008). *Case study research: Design and methods* (4th ed.). Thousand Oaks, CA: Sage.

Young, S. N. (2009). Bias in the research literature and conflict of interest: An issue for publishers, editors, reviewers and authors, and it is not just about the money [Editorial]. *Journal of Psychiatry & Neuroscience, 34*, 412–417.

Young, N. S., Ioannidis, J. P. A., & Al-Ubaydi, O. (2009). Why current publication practices may distort science. *Public Library of Science (PLoS) Medicine, 5*, 1418–1422. doi:10.1371/journal.pmed.0050201.

Training Issues in Adolescent Health

Catherine Cook-Cottone, Stephanie Grella, and Amanda Sommers Smith

Introduction

> One of the most important commitments a country can make for future economic, social, and political progress and stability is to address the health and development needs of its adolescents.
>
> (World Health Organization, 1995, p. 3)

Appropriate and adequate training of medical, educational, and mental health professionals working with adolescents is essential for the improvement of physical and psychological health outcomes (Michaud, Stronski, Fonesca, & Macfarlane, 2004). Despite the substantial rigor across training programs, many professionals do not feel adequately prepared to address adolescent health psychology issues in their practice (Michaud et al., 2004; Williams, Klinepeter, Palmes, Pulley, & Meschan, 2004). Review of the literature indicates that despite adolescence being a period of relatively low disease risk, it is a pivotal developmental period in terms of engagement in behaviors that are potentially harmful to both short-term and long-term health outcomes (Skopelja, Whipple, & Richwine, 2008; Walker & Townsend, 1999). Specifically, reviews indicate risky behaviors in adolescence result in immediate health outcomes (i.e., accidental injury, suicide and self-injury, sexually transmitted diseases) as well as long-term health problems (e.g., increased risk of cancer and heart disease; Walker & Townsend, 1999).

Unique Features of Adolescence

The physical and mental health care needs of adolescence, the period between 10 and 19, are often compromised by three separate but intersecting issues: (a) adolescence is a time period that includes rapid and co-occurring cognitive, physiological, sexual, and behavioral change, (b) adolescents are likely to be exposed to adult issues that often require mature decision-making and self-regulatory skills (e.g., sexual behavioral, substance use, self-regulated eating and exercise, and driving), and (c) training programs are unable to adequately address the breadth and complexity of this period and associated interventions (Holmbeck, 2002; Mokdad, Marks, Stroup, Gerberding, 2004; Williams et al., 2002).

First, it is well known that adolescence is a distinct developmental period qualitatively different from childhood or adulthood (Holmbeck, 2002). Adolescence offers both opportunities and challenges for teenagers. Despite the increased risk for exposure, there are also opportunities to develop lifestyle choices that positively impact long-term health throughout adulthood. Empirical

C. Cook-Cottone, Ph.D. (✉) • S. Grella, M.A.
A.S. Smith, M.S.
Department of Counseling, School, and Educational Psychology, Graduate School of Education, University at Buffalo, State University of New York, 409 Baldy Hall, Buffalo, NY 14260, USA
e-mail: cpcook@buffalo.edu; slgrella@buffalo.edu; amssmith@buffalo.edu

W.T. O'Donohue et al. (eds.), *Handbook of Adolescent Health Psychology*,
DOI 10.1007/978-1-4614-6633-8_21, © Springer Science+Business Media New York 2013

evidence indicates that numerous biological, social, and psychological changes occur during this transitional time period that have the potential to shape long-term health trajectories positively or negatively (Holmbeck, 2002; Williams, Holmbeck, & Neff, 2002). During this time of tremendous physiological and cognitive changes, ecological factors may be especially important. For example, in a qualitative study of multidisciplinary adolescent health care providers, McManus, Shejavali, and Fox (2003) concluded that the physical and mental health of adolescents appears to be profoundly shaped by both family and social environment. Providers believed that the most common adolescent health conditions are not signs of inherent medical problems. Rather, they see these conditions as indicators of a considerable lack of parental involvement as well as the chaotic and disordered context in which many adolescents live.

Second, a range of physical and mental health-related conditions are known to begin during adolescence and continue to impact functioning and quality of life in later adulthood (Williams et al., 2002). This sector of life poses a window of time in which intervention is critical in order to prevent the development of unhealthy behaviors that compromise adolescents' immediate health and contribute to pathology and disease in adulthood. For example, Mokdad et al. (2004) found that approximately half of the mortality rates in adulthood are result of risky behaviors (e.g., tobacco use) developed in adolescence.

Third, the distinct nature of this developmental period warrants specialized training. Knowledge in pediatric or adult physical and mental health issues cannot be effectively applied to adolescence. It is important to note that the unique challenges related to this stage of development can be further exacerbated by poverty, racial and ethnic minority status, involvement in the juvenile justice system, homelessness, immigration status, and sexual orientation (lesbian, gay, bisexual, or transgender; Lawrence et al., 2009; McManus et al., 2003). Given these complexities, comprehensive care is required to address the various factors related to adolescent health. Although there are several initiatives designed to improve training (e.g., interdisciplinary training and policy initiatives), many health care, education, and mental health providers remain underprepared in the area of adolescent health (Michaud et al., 2004). Moreover, training across professional disciplines often fails to adequately meet the needs of this population (Lawrence et al., 2009). Therefore, as the gap between training programs and applied practice widens, many adolescents remain underserved.

Training Issues in Adolescent Health

The demand for professionals trained in adolescent health is high, yet the supply remains sparse. Although the American Academy of Pediatrics recommends one physician to every 6,000 adolescents, on average, there exists only one adolescent medical physician to 105,000 adolescents in the United States alone (Lawrence et al., 2009). The gap is huge and the need for competent, highly trained professions in the field of adolescent health is evident. As a result, the burden falls on training programs to adequately prepare providers to serve the needs of adolescents. Effective training must address the development of knowledge (e.g., developmental and contextual) and skills (e.g., assessment and communication) associated with adolescent physical and mental health service provision in order for professionals to provide efficient care and treatment (Astroth, Garza, & Taylor, 2004).

Training Programs in Adolescent Health

The utilization of a multidisciplinary approach to understanding and treating adolescents is the recommended gold standard for providing health care treatment (Lawrence et al., 2009). As such, training in adolescent health spans cross several disciplines including medicine, psychology, and education. Across disciplines, specifically focused programmatic curriculum, fellowship, continuing education, and/or self-study programs are needed.

Limitations of Training Programs

Across all levels of professional education, providers must be attuned to the nature of adolescents' health problems and demonstrate the skills necessary to provide effective risk assessment, disease prevention, treatment, and health promotion. Unfortunately, many practitioners do not possess unique training in order to effectively work with this population (Fox et al., 2008a). Evidence offered by provider self-report, as well as adolescent ratings of heath care, indicates disparities in providing a workforce suited to meet the unique needs of adolescents (Blum & Bearinger, 1990; Fox et al., 2008a). Self-assessments of competencies provided by various clinicians reveal inadequacies regarding their training as well as practices when working with adolescents. For example, Blum and Bearinger (1990) assessed the competencies across several disciplines and found physicians and nurses alike, perceived the greatest limitations in the areas of eating disorders, learning disabilities, chronic illness, and delinquent behavior in adolescents. Limitations reported by psychologists and social workers included sexual concerns, sexual orientation conflict, eating disorders, and chronic illness. Nearly half of all nutritionists surveyed acknowledged training deficits across all adolescent food-related issues. According to Fox and colleagues (2008a) medical pediatric residency programs are not designed to provide specialized training in adolescent health. Alarmingly, residency programs may require as little as 1 month training in adolescent medicine, although many extend over the course of several years. Therefore, it is not surprising that there is a consensus among fellowship and residency training directors, as well as adolescent medicine faculty to improve the training experiences provided to those in adolescent medicine programs (Fox et al., 2008a).

There are a variety of barriers that make it challenging to teach the necessary knowledge base and skills needed to work effectively with adolescents. Within many training programs, educators are faced with the lack of adolescent-specific training resources (curricular and financial; Fox et al., 2008b). To overcome these barriers, classroom textbooks and curricular plans should emphasize adolescent health content and not attempt to simply extend pediatric content upward and adult content downward.

Framework for Adolescent Health Training

As a field, adolescent health reflects a set of issues that are comparatively distinct to the physical and mental health of the developing adolescent. Therefore, programmatic, state/province, and federal training initiatives, guidelines, and policy should be based on empirically supported knowledge on the subject of the adolescent developmental period (see Fig. 1). In practice, training program curriculum, fellowship opportunities, continuing education offerings, and self-study programs should be grounded upon informed guidelines and policy.

Best-Practices

Training in adolescent health psychology should be grounded in empirical evidence and a solid theoretical foundation. Within the past several decades, knowledge about adolescent health psychology has grown substantially with both researchers and practitioners recognizing the pivotal nature of the adolescent developmental period in terms of immediate and long-term health and mental health outcomes (Michaud et al., 2004; Walker & Townsend, 1999). Accordingly, outcome-based education models evolved from this recognition. These models base specific learning objectives and curricular content on the particular needs delineated by researchers, professionals, and educators (Michaud et al., 2004).

Consistent with outcome-based models, policy and practice in training should integrate key content areas as indicated by the current empirical knowledge (i.e., epidemiological, group outcome, and case study designs), as well use empirically supported format and processes for training (Ford, 2008; Michaud et al., 2004). Key content areas include knowledge of adolescent-specific developmental characteris-

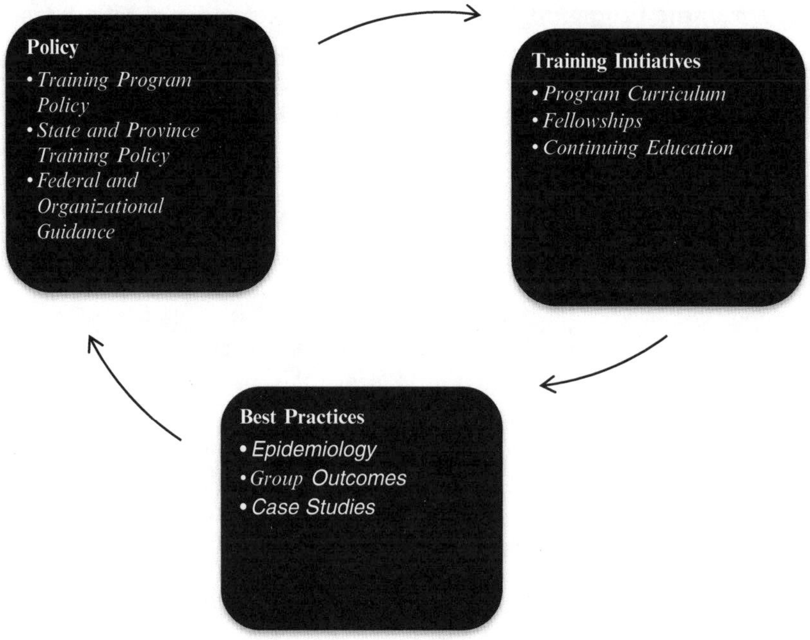

Fig. 1 Framework for training in adolescent health

tics, disorders, diseases, and psychosocial problems unique to this population (e.g., eating disorders, sexually transmitted disease, and teenage pregnancy), treatment needs (e.g., treatment compliance and adherence), and prevention and wellness issues (e.g., emotional regulation, physical activity, and nutrition; Ford, 2008; Michaud et al., 2004). According to researchers, educational strategies have proven effective for trainees and professions such as interactive lectures, role playing, and focus group and problem-based learning (Michaud et al., 2004).

Policy

Policy regarding training in adolescent health can be informed by national, organizational (e.g., American Pediatric Association, American Medical Association, and the American Psychological Association), and state/local agencies. Resources to construct such curricula include the *Guide to Clinical Preventive Services* which was developed by the US Preventive Services Task Force (1996); *Bright Futures: Guidelines for Health Supervision of Infants, Children and Adolescents* (Green, 1994), created by the Maternal and Child Health Bureau; the American Academy of Pediatrics *Health Supervision Guidelines* (Stein, 1997); *The Clinician's Handbook of Preventive Services* (US Department of Health and Human Services, 1994); *Improving the Health of Adolescents & Young Adults: A Guide for States and Communities* (National Adolescent Health Information Center, 2010); and the American Medical Association *Guidelines for Adolescent Preventive Services* (GAPS; Elster & Kuznets, 1994). Specifically, the GAPS provides recommendations pertinent to the delivery of health care services, including the promotion of health and well-being of adolescents, the necessity of screening tools relevant to specific conditions prevalent to adolescents, and the utilization of immunizations (Elster & Kuznets, 1994). Additionally, the National Adolescent Health Information Center (NAHIC, 2010) provides guidance, initiatives, and resources to communities and state agencies with the goal to enhance adolescent health and safety by addressing mortality, unintentional injury, violence, mental health and substance abuse, reproductive health, and chronic diseases. The development of standards or guidelines for the delivery of adolescent health services makes it possible to assess the gaps in the provision of such services and help guide appropriate corrective action.

Training Initiatives

Training is conceptualized broadly and is flexible in terms of delivery methods and format. The available training initiatives can be viewed in terms of levels that ultimately serve to prepare professionals for work with adolescents. Training in adolescent health involves traditional programmatic curriculum (level one) as well as specialized fellowships (level two) and a variety of continuing educational programs (level three).

Standards for Programmatic Curricula Training relevant to adolescent health psychology tends to occur at the graduate and specialist level. As such, training programs are specifically designed to prepare students for a particular profession and are often beholden to external training mandates. Specifically, programmatic curricula frequently adhere to the standards set by the program's corresponding professional organization (e.g., APA, AMA) as well as state licensure and certification requirements. The formulation of these guidelines and requirements is an ongoing and fluid process. Using an outcome-based approach, evolving guidelines ideally reflect the needs of key stakeholders (Michaud et al., 2004). Such stakeholders include individuals from a variety of settings: hospital physicians and practitioners, university staff and students, patients, researchers and epidemiologists, and leaders of patient groups (Michaud et al., 2004). This process involves identifying needs, translating needs into desired outcomes, and formulating desired outcomes into training objectives.

Likely related to the breadth of issues that are considered necessary to many training programs, the coverage of adolescent health issues is often deficient in many programs across disciplines. Those who desire in-depth training at this level must seek out programs dedicated to training in adolescent issues. For example, the Society of Adolescent Health and Medicine provides an updated listing of training opportunities in adolescent health medicine across five disciplines (i.e., medicine, nutrition, psychology, nursing, social work). However, the number of specific training programs varies, with 30 programs in adolescent medicine, ten in nutrition and psychology, nine in nursing, and eight in social work.

Educational Training Programs, Fellowships/Residency Programs, and Continuing Education. For those who do not receive training in adolescent health psychology as part of their graduate of specialist training curricula, or those who desire further specialization, there are additional opportunities at the next level of training. Currently, there are a variety of programs designed to provide multidisciplinary training. For example, to provide interdisciplinary training in adolescent health, The Leadership Education in Adolescent Health (LEAH) program was created to integrate the training of future physicians, psychologists, nurses, social workers, and nutritionists. Seven programs currently receive federal funding from the Maternal and Child Health Bureau, which include Baylor College of Medicine, Harvard Medical School (Children's Hospital Boston), Indiana University, Johns Hopkins School of Medicine, University of California at San Francisco, University of Minnesota, and the University at Rochester School of Medicine. These programs are designed with the purpose of preparing future leaders in adolescent health care and are the only multidisciplinary training programs specifically targeted toward adolescent health supported by federal funding. Since its inception in 1977, LEAH programs have trained more than 600 long-term professionals across all disciplines. Graduates of these programs are prepared as health professionals for leadership roles in clinical care, research, training, advocacy, and administrators. In addition to multidisciplinary training, within medicine, the Accreditation Council for Graduate Medical Education (ACGME) oversees accreditation of post medical training programs. To date, there are 26 accredited programs that provide fellowship training in adolescent medicine. Moreover, specialized postdoctoral fellowships exist in psychology.

Another layer of training initiatives is continuing education. Continuing education in adolescent health is critical to ensure appropriate professional development for health service providers already in the field. The Society of Adolescent Health and Medicine offers up-to-date information on presentations, workshops, and conferences related to adolescent health and medicine. The European Training Effective Adolescent Care and Health (EuTEACH) also offers opportunities for educating practicing health care professionals.

Curricular Development in Adolescent Health Training

Syllabi from graduate level courses in adolescent health, adolescent development, psychology of adolescence, and adolescent risk taking and health, as well as pertinent textbooks, and journal articles were obtained to review essential content areas relevant to adolescent health. Key areas of focus included graduate course work objectives and topics, frameworks used for training programs, curricular development, and training methodologies. Government agencies and professional organizations were also reviewed to provide national data on adolescent health care services and guidelines and recommendations for best practice.

In addition to syllabi reviewed, the Society for Adolescent Health and Medicine, EuTEACH, the material provided through the RESOURCE project, and the adolescent health curriculum outlined by Dr. Lawrence S. Neinstein at The University of Southern California were utilized to identify the key content areas. The EuTEACH has created a framework used in curricular development designed for adolescent health using a multidisciplinary model. Starting in 1999, a group of 16 physicians across various specialties met to develop a consensual curriculum that intended to cover essential learning objectives for training adolescent health and medicine. Since that time, the group has reconvened biannually to discuss the goals of the curriculum, instructional trategies, specific content areas and modules, evaluation, and refinement. The EuTEACH curriculum targets trainees in health care professions and aims to enhance training in adolescent health (Michaud et al., 2004). The main function of the program is to offer training curriculum to all health professionals involved in teaching adolescent medicine and health. The program provides (a) descriptions of the main teaching objects, (b) training methods, (c) practical examples, (d) evaluation procedures, and (e) references (Michaud et al., 2004). Prospective trainers can select from curriculum that is both broad and narrow in scope depending on the needs of the target audience. Further, each training module focuses on knowledge, studies, and skills providing the instructor with the following strategies and methodologies: teaching objectives, corresponding teaching methods, concrete examples (i.e., case-stories), issues to be debated in small groups, and themes for role playing (Michaud et al., 2004). Each objective is accompanied by suggested readings and suggestions for assessment.

Overview of Key Content Areas

A consistent finding across the literature and syllabi reviewed was the importance of understanding adolescent health utilizing developmental-contextual and biopsychosocial frameworks. Ideally adolescent health needs should be understood in terms of the biological, psychological, and social changes that take place during this vulnerable time (Holmbeck, 2002; Williams et al., 2002), as well as understood within relevant systems, familial and community contexts. The interrelatedness of family support, school connections, peer influences, work opportunities, community resources, and media influences all collectively impact adolescents' abilities to adapt successfully to these changes.

In nearly all graduate course syllabi, the key content area covered reflected variables and topics related to interpersonal, developmental, demographic, and intrapersonal variables. Particular content areas covered in courses included common mental health issues prevalent in adolescent populations, risky behaviors demonstrated during ado-

Table 1 Key content areas and suggested topics for training in adolescent health

1. Adolescent development and ecological context	
Understanding adolescent development	*Ecological factors*
Growth and puberty	Family influences and dynamic
Cognitive development	Socioeconomic status
Sexual identity and gender	Cultural and ethnic issues
Nutritional needs	Social context
Reproductive health	
Common medical conditions	
Variance in chronic conditions	
Variance in developmental disabilities	
2. Resiliency, specific disorders, exploratory and risky behaviors	
Risk and outcomes for specific disorders and problems	*Adolescent risk behavior*
Overweight and obesity	Resiliency in adolescents
Sexually transmitted diseases	Risky and exploratory behaviors
Mental illness (anxiety, depression, suicide)	Sexual behavior
Eating disorders	Mental health
Substance use and abuse	Smoking
Accidental injuries	Illegal drug use
Self-harm	Diet exercise
Abuse in relationships	
3. Adolescent characteristics, health education, and advocacy	
Adolescent characteristics, knowledge, and skills	*Health education and promotion*
Health literacy	Adolescent health literacy
Locus of control	Positive youth development
Health optimism	Personal advocacy
Self-efficacy	
Socio-environmental context	
4. Prevention, treatment, clinical skills, and multidisciplinary environments	
Prevention	*Clinical skills*
Screening	Setting
Assessment	Communication skills
Treatment	Process skills
	Multidisciplinary work
5. Confidentiality, privacy, treatment adherence, and access	
Confidentiality	*Treatment adherence*
Consent	Health decision-making
Privacy rights	Access/health care disparity

lescence (e.g., substance use, sexual behaviors, injury, and violence), ecological systems (e.g., family, school, community), interpersonal variables, and intrapersonal variables (e.g., identity development, gender, ethnicity) as well as current prevention and treatment programs. Additional content areas were reflective of unique issues related to adolescent health such as confidentiality, privacy, and treatment adherence. Research on adolescent development through the integration of a wide variety of disciplines and contexts was also an emphasis in various syllabi. Specifically, theoretical perspectives and content were incorporated from interdisciplinary fields including biology, education, sociology, and anthropology. Another goal of training courses included current assessment and treatment issues relevant to understanding adolescent psychopathology such as examining symptom characteristics, screening tools, assessment methods, treatment protocols, and research issues. Based on the information gathered, the table below was organized and depicts key content areas and suggested training topics in adolescent health (Table 1).

Key Concepts for Training Programs

The following five sections review key concepts to be covered in training programs relevant to the specific needs of the adolescent developmental period.

1. *Adolescent development and ecological context.* Adolescent development is an essential component to understanding and managing health-related issues during this period. Pertinent factors are related to biological, cognitive, psychological, and social influences. Specific issues include puberty, sexual identity, cognitive development, individuation, identity development, gender roles, unique nutritional needs, and medical conditions.

   Training should also encompass ecological factors such as family influences and dynamics (Michaud et al., 2004). Numerous factors impact teenager's adaptation, which can be organized and categorized within the following four realms: interpersonal, developmental, demographic, and intrapersonal. *Interpersonal* variables include family, peers, school, and work. *Developmental transformation* variables include biological, cognitive, and social changes. *Developmental outcome* factors include achievement, autonomy, identity, intimacy, psychosocial adjustment, and sexuality. *Intrapersonal* factors include family structure, ethnicity, race, gender, neighborhood, community, economic opportunities, and socio-economic status.
2. *Resiliency, specific disorders, and exploratory and risky behaviors.* The European Training in Effective Care and Health provides definitions detailing the concepts of exploratory and risky behavior, resilience, and protective factors related to adolescence from a bio-psychosocial context. Exploratory behaviors are considered highly related to this period of development, and are essentially integrated in teenagers' learning experiences. Risk behaviors are defined as variables that increase one's likelihood of experiencing negative outcomes. Some common exploratory and risky behaviors associated with adolescence include sexual behaviors, drug and alcohol experimentation, excessive dieting or exercise, inadequate physical activity, violence, and dangerous driving practices (US Department of Health & Human Services, 2008). Protective factors are related to the variables (individual competencies or external support) that shield a teen from negative outcomes. Resiliency is then the culmination of protective factors that allow an individual to successfully cope and manage stressors.

   This knowledge directly impacts adolescent heath training programs. It is vital for programs to adequately prepare future practitioners to assess, treat, and provide education to teens who engage in risky behaviors. Equally important, training programs should prepare future educators and researchers to develop and implement effective prevention and intervention programs designed to provide psycho-education and treatment.

   Mental health issues: Mental health issues are common in the adolescent population. Annual rates of mental health diagnoses are between 10 and 20 % (Kataoka, Zhang, & Wells, 2002), with depression, anxiety, attention-deficit/hyperactivity, and substance use the most commonly diagnosed (Knopf, Park, & Mulye, 2008). A recent study examining the lifetime prevalence data across a broad range of mental disorders in a nationally representative sample of 10,123 US adolescents (ages 13–18) revealed that approximately 1 out of 4 or 5 youth suffers from a mental illness (Merikangas et al., 2010). The survey demonstrated that approximately 32 % met the lifetime criteria for anxiety disorder, followed by behavioral disorders (19 %), mood disorders (14 %), and substance-related disorders (11 %). Due to the high prevalence rates of mental health problems in adolescence, health care providers must be able to recognize symptoms associated with disorders, understand the contextual and systemic factors contributing to the issue, and be able to provide the most effective treatment plan to address the problem.

   Further, there are health disparities regarding access to mental health treatment and lower quality of care based on socioeconomic, minority, or gender status. For instance, when compared to Caucasian clients, minority clients are less likely to obtain mental health services, receive poorer services, and are underrepresented in research (US Department of Health and Human Services 2001). Given that mental illness is significantly correlated with low socioeconomic status, being female, single, and being non-Hispanic black (Kessler et al., 2006), training programs must recognize these disparities and inadequacies of health care toward certain groups to ensure equality of treatment and unbiased mental health care.

Suicide: In a survey conducted in 2005, nearly 17 % of teenagers in the United States seriously considered attempting suicide; and approximately 8 % attempted suicide (Eaton et al., 2006). Thus, suicide risk assessment is an important goal for training, as suicidal ideation and attempts are more likely during this developmental time period.

Depression: Depression is a common psychiatric illness diagnosed in adolescence (APA, 2000), with prevalence rates at 8 % for a Major Depressive Episode (Erk, 2008; Substance Abuse and Mental Health Services Administration, SAMHSA, 2009).

Sleep disturbances: Sleep disturbances is an additional area that affects a large percentage of teenagers. According to Ohayon, Roberts, Zulley, Smirne, and Priest (2000) it is estimated that 25 % of adolescents report symptoms associated with sleep disturbances.

Disruptive behavior disorders: In 2005, approximately 9 % adolescents aged 12–17 had a lifetime diagnosis of attention-deficit/hyperactivity disorder (Pastor & Reuben, 2008). Estimates of oppositional defiant disorder prevalence rates have ranged from 1 to 6 %; the prevalence of conduct disorder in preadolescents and older teens (ages 9 to 17) varies from 1 to 4 % (Shaffer et al., 1996).

Eating disorders: Eating disorders are categorized into four diagnostic classifications including anorexia nervosa, bulimia nervosa, binge eating disorder, and eating disorder not otherwise specified (APA, 2000). Hoek and van Hoeken (2003) reviewed the prevalence rates of diagnosed eating disorders in females and found average prevalence rate for anorexia nervosa is 0.3 % (aged 11–36). The prevalence rates for bulimia nervosa were 1.0 % for women (aged 12–44) and 0.1 % for men of all ages. Adolescent females are more likely to exhibit eating disorder symptoms than males. To ensure that health care providers are able to identify, assess, and treat eating disorders, training programs should emphasize the range of adolescent body shape, social influences on body image, psychosocial factors contributing to symptoms, and treatment strategies targeted toward patients with specific types of eating disorders.

Disordered eating and obesity: An extraordinarily large number of young women exhibit subthreshold symptomology associated with disordered eating (i.e., excessive exercise, dieting pills, laxative use). Furthermore, 31 % of adolescents aged 12–19 were considered at risk of being overweight and overweight in 1999–2002 (Hedley et al., 2004). Specifically, obesity has become an increasing health concern faced by youth and can result in serious health consequences for adolescents, increasing the risk of high cholesterol, hypertension, diabetes, and the metabolic syndrome (Dietz, 1998).

Drugs and alcohol: The rate of illicit drug use among those ages 12–17 and 18–25 has increased from 9.3 to 10.0 and from19.6 to 21.2, respectively (SAMHSA, 2010). According to the 2009 survey, illicit drug use varied by educational attainment, employment status, and race/ethnicity. The engagement in these behaviors poses serious health risks both during adolescence and into adulthood. Specifically, use in adolescence greatly increases the risk for developing a clinical substance use disorder in adulthood.

Pregnancy and sexually transmitted disease: A qualitative study conducted by McManus and colleagues (2003) across four cities identified reproductive health issues as the second most pervasive category impacting adolescents. In addition to sexually transmitted diseases, teenage pregnancies are an additional reproductive health issue. A national survey conducted in 2006 revealed that 750,000 females aged 20 and younger became pregnant (Kost, Henshaw, & Carlin, 2010). More specially, among teens ages 15–19, the pregnancy rate was nearly 72 pregnancies per 1,000 (Kost, Henshaw, & Carlin, 2010).

Furthermore, according to the Youth Risk Behavior Surveillance System (YRBSS), 47 % of teens reported having sexual intercourse, and 37 % of sexually active students had not used a condom during their last sexual intercourse (Grunbaum et al., 2004). These risky sexual behaviors in adolescence contribute to high rates of sexually transmitted diseases (STDs). For example, according to the Center for Disease Control and Prevention (2006), 5,259 individuals ages 13–24 were diagnosed with HIV/AIDS, which accounted for 14 % of new cases that year. It is crucial for health care providers to be cognizant of the issues related to adolescent sexuality in order to help decrease risk of STDs, and provide appropriate counseling services and treatment for pregnant adolescent females.

Mortality rates: According to the US Department of Health and Human Services (2008), there were reportedly 13,703 deaths among adolescents aged 15–19 years in 2005. The leading cause of mortality among this age aggregate is unintentional injury (i.e., motor vehicle accidents), which accounts for nearly half (49 %) of deaths.

Chronic illnesses: According to the Society for Adolescent Health and Medicine, common medical problems in adolescence include abdominal pain, chest pain, headaches, orthopedic problems (i.e., scoliosis), dermatological problems (e.g., acne), and asthma. Physical health conditions identified as the most prevalent in adolescents include obesity and asthma, which are believed to be influenced by poor nutrition, lack of exercise, and sleep disturbances (McManus et al., 2003). On the EuTEACH website, there are specific training modules with training goals and objectives relevant to chronic medical conditions in adolescents. Goals outlined include communicating to the adolescent that his or her experiences are understood, understanding the illness within the bio-psychosocial framework, demonstrating competencies in creating and implementing an appropriate treatment plan, and communicating effectively with all stakeholders.

3. *Adolescent characteristics, health education, and advocacy.* As part of the unique and dynamic developmental changes, there are new challenges faced during adolescence that are related to increasing autonomy and individuation. Factors related to locus of control, health optimism, and self-efficacy differentiate this period from childhood. To address these characteristics and promote optimal heath, adolescents need to acquire new knowledge and skills, which can be accomplished through health literacy, promotion, and education.
4. *Prevention, treatment, clinical skills, and multidisciplinary environments.* Clinical skills refer to practice-oriented variables including setting, communication skills, clinical skills, and multidisciplinary work. In regard to setting variables, both inpatient and outpatient facilities should be targeted toward adolescent populations. Adolescent-friendly settings should offer an adequate waiting area, pertinent literature, and unique confidentiality practices for teenagers (World Health Organization, 2002). Effective communication skills are also important to effectively work with adolescents. Successful communication with adolescents is developed via the provider's trustworthiness, openness, honesty (Ehrman & Matson, 1998), and active listening (Coupey, 1997). The goal is to establish a partnership with the adolescent and parents to facilitate all stages of treatment. To establish this partnership, clinical skills need to be drawn upon to create a nonjudgmental atmosphere.

Training should include effective preventative techniques, tools for screening and assessment, and empirically supported treatment method for physical and mental health problems (Sieving & Shrier, 2009). Measurement modalities relevant to adolescents include self-report, observation, and biological measurement. Specifically, self-reported anthropometric measures pose problems as adolescents tend to inaccurately report their weight and height. The greatest discrepancies between actual and self-reported weight tend to be in adolescent females and youth who are overweight while older Caucasian youth tend to report their height as taller than measured height (Brener, McManus, Galuska, Lowry, & Wechsler, 2003). Underestimations of height are most often seen in overweight adolescents (Lee, Valeria, Kochman, & Lenders, 2006). Body mass index (BMI) calculated from self-reported weight and heights therefore maybe underestimated (Brener, McManus et al., 2003). Additionally, self-reported puberty stage in comparison to a clinician's examination have found similar discrepancies, indicating adolescents to be poor reporters of their pubertal stage (Bonat, Pathomvanich, Keil, Field, & Yanovski, 2002; Lee et al., 2006). Overall, self-reported information tends to be bias and maybe a better reflection of adolescents' misperceptions and/or distortions of information deemed as unacceptable (i.e., alcohol/drug use, sexual behavior).

Several screening procedures and interview techniques have been established to conduct culturally sensitive and developmentally appropriate interviews. One tool used is called HEEADSSS (home, education, eating, peer activities, drugs, sexuality, suicide/depression, and safety), which is a practical, complementary screening tool to build rapport with teenagers by moving from less threatening items to more intrusive questions. An additional method used is Motivational Interviewing, which is a client-centered, directive counseling technique that was developed out of the transtheoretical model of change literature which identifies five stages of change (i.e., precontemplation, contemplation, action, maintenance, relapse prevention; Prochaska & DiClemente, 1982). Each stage corresponds with a patient's readiness to change. Matching interventions with the patient's level of readiness increases the individual's chance of successful behavioral change. In order to explore ambivalence to change a stance is made that behavioral change is effected more substantially by internal motivation rather than imparting information. To assess participant's level of motivation, four basic principles are utilized that include the (a) expression of empathy, (b) development of discrepancies, and the (c) clinician's ability to manage resistance and (d) support the patient's self-efficacy (Miller & Rollnick, 2002; Rollnick, Miller, & Butler, 2007).

Lastly, in addition to setting, communication, and clinical factors, the utilization of an interdisciplinary approach is critical to provide adolescents with optimal care. Adolescent health care requires intervention and treatment by professionals across several fields. The success of a multidisciplinary approach depends on regular communication, continuous cooperation, and the coordination of service delivery, while simultaneously ensuring the patient is informed throughout the process.

5. *Confidentiality, privacy, treatment adherence, and access.* Confidentiality is an important issue in the treatment of adolescents. The Convention on the Rights of the Child provides a special status for adolescents. Specifically, adolescents are viewed as "active rights holders" which allows them to be recognized as having their own human rights (United Nations, 2003). As adolescents develop an emerging sense of independence to make choices about their health, their views are increasingly considered and valued. However, they are still vulnerable to making poor decisions. As such, the rights' of parents to provide guidance are also recognized. From a legal stand point, adolescents have the right to nondiscrimination, information, privacy, and confidentiality, along with the right to express their views freely, gain legal protections about health care, and remain protected from abuse, neglect, violence, and exploitation (United Nations, 2003).

Although adolescents' cognitive development is nearly complete, these teenagers possess the forthcoming legal status of adults, yet lack the life experience that allows adults to make informed decisions. This leads to a unique legal and ethical situation that is essentially different from that of younger children. The majority of health care disciplines acknowledge that adolescents ought to be provided confidential services (Morreale, Stinnett, & Dowling, 2005). Nonetheless, a balance must be maintained between protecting confidentiality and ensuring safety as adolescents often participate in harmful or unacceptable behavior and therefore, warranting parental involvement (English, Santelli, & Rogers, 2009). It is the professional's responsibility to establish the limits of confidentiality with both the parents and the adolescent, honoring adolescent's privacy unless there is a potential harm to self or others, including a duty to warn. In the instance that inappropriate or harmful information is shared, it is important to engage the patient in a collaborative process to disclose this information to the parents. To make unilateral contact between the provider and parent, excluding the adolescent, may turn the patient away from receiving health care services in the future (English, Santelli, & Rogers, 2009).

Treatment adherence: Adherence to prescribed medical treatment varies across the lifespan. However, difficulties with adherence appear to emerge around the age of 11 years old and peak in adolescence (Shaw, 2001). This change in treatment adherence is best explained by the developmental and psychopathological issues that are pertinent to adolescents. With chronically ill patients, dependency on medical advice is necessary. However, this dependency is incongruent with the desired autonomy and individualization sought in adolescence, and therefore may result in refusal to adhere (Shaw, 2001). Additionally, adolescents struggle to understand the long-term consequences that may result from not following medical advice. Thus, the inability to adequately assess the risks associated with noncompliance can contribute to a lack of treatment adherence. Lastly, acceptance in peer groups and pressure to conform may create resistance to follow through with medical procedures or treatment, particularly when there is a negative side effect. In order to increase treatment adherence in adolescents, Shaw (2001) recommends interventions should (a) emphasize educational approaches specifically targeted toward placing greater responsibility on the adolescent; (b) incorporate a feedback system such that the adolescent is seen more frequently by the physician, receives reminder phone calls or e-mails, or participates in self-monitoring; (c) utilize incentives for treatment adherence; and (d) increase peer and family support and involvement.

Adolescent health decision-making: For many years it has been understood that adolescents have a developmentally unique conceptualization of personal health risk (Walker & Townsend, 1999). Reviews of the literature indicate that although many adolescents have substantial knowledge about the health risk associated with particular behaviors, they do not use this knowledge when they are making behavioral choices (Walker & Townsend, 1999). The specific psychology of this phenomenon is not well understood and the basis of much research. Researchers have been exploring constructs such as locus of control, health optimism, self-efficacy, and socio-environmental context (Walker & Townsend, 1999) to determine the variables that contribute to the difficulties associated with adolescent health decision-making.

Access/health care disparities: There are numerous barriers impeding on adolescents' abilities to obtain proper health care. For instance, on average adolescents have a low rate of primary care use (Hing, Cherry, & Woodwell, 2006) and a high rate of being uninsured when compared to other age aggregates (Agency for Healthcare Research & Quality, 2006).

Likely contributing to lack of insurance, poverty is considered one of the most influential factors impacting adolescent health (Klein, Slap, Elster, & Schonberg, 1992). In addition, professional training and medical models remain focused on pediatric or child-age and adult populations. The current model inadequately addresses the needs of adolescents, which ultimately has a negative impact on their overall health-related well-being.

Teaching Methodologies

The EuTEACH website provides guidance to instructors and trainers on how best to educate learners studying adolescent health. An interactive teaching methodology is emphasized, as a didactic strategy alone is recognized as an insufficient teaching method. Three areas of competencies are recognized: (a) knowledge (the cognitive domain); (b) attitudes (the affective domain that encompasses values, beliefs, biases, emotions, and role expectations); and (c) skills (the ability to put knowledge into practice). Well-trained professionals in each of these areas result in competent health service providers for adolescents.

Instructors are also provided with guidelines on how to structure a course in adolescent health. Dr. Charles E. Irwin at the Policy Center located within the School of Medicine at the University of California, San Francisco, reports on the RESOURCE project aimed at providing educational materials and resources to enhance the training in adolescent health. Sample syllabi along with training tools, assignments, and case studies are presented (see the Resources for Training in Adolescent Health below for the website). Additionally, EuTEACH website recommends that course objectives should be defined, teaching methodologies selected, and evaluation of outcomes chosen. It is recommended that objectives are based on the areas of competencies (i.e., knowledge, attitudes, skills). According to Astroth et al. (2004) competencies are developed in training programs and in practice by (a) conceptualizing the scope of practice, (b) offering recommendations for curriculum, and (c) creating standards to measure knowledge and skills in both practitioners and educational training programs. Table 2 provides examples of broad objectives relevant to knowledge, attitudes, and skills. Health professionals working with adolescents should be competent in these areas in prior to entering the field.

In order to support the learning of each objective while also building knowledge, attitudes, and skills, the EuTEACH website provides teaching techniques that can be utilized (see Table 3). A brief description of each methodology is reviewed on the website (www.euteach.com) but is not presented here. Additionally, in-depth and specific teaching objectives and modules are presented for targeted content areas that include, but are not limited to, the bio-psychosocial development during adolescents, setting communication and clinical skills, confidentiality, chronic conditions, mental health, and eating disorders.

Future Recommendations

Regardless of the type of training program appropriate certification and licensure plays a part in ensuring that practitioners are adequately trained. In addition, accreditation boards impact training programs, curriculum content, and continuing education. Educational institutions must follow the goals and objectives set forth by the appropriate accreditation committees in order to prepare their students for specializing in adolescent health. Moreover, a consistent set of competencies established by the accrediting bodies targeted toward each discipline lead to uniformity of the training in adolescent health across the workforce of providers including the clinicians who provide direct care services, the educators who teach others, and the scholars who conduct research to inform best practice.

Challenges and Barriers in Teaching Adolescent Health

Areas of competency clearly vary according to discipline. Depending on the type of setting and type of provider, guidelines and recommendations

Table 2 Examples of adolescent health objectives[a]

Competencies		
1. Develop patient-centered treatment plans for adolescents based on comprehensive risk-based assessments that considers cultural, linguistic, and socioeconomic background 2. Optimize treatment plans based on knowledge of adolescent care resources that include local, state, and federal agencies 3. Coordinate ambulatory, inpatient, and institutional care across health care providers, institutions, and governmental agencies 4. Demonstrate the ability to communicate effectively with the adolescent and his or her family in order to establish and maintain therapeutic relationships 5. Demonstrate sensitivity to the patient's race, ethnicity, culture, language, gender, sexual orientation, gender identity, and disabilities		
Knowledge	Attitudes	Skills
Students should know: 1. The normal growth and development in the adolescent years that include physical, mental, emotional, and sexual milestones 2. Health risks and behaviors of adolescents and methods to address them 3. Strategies for providing preventive services, health promotion, and guidance 4. Challenges faced as they try to establish their identity and learn responsible behaviors, including self-care, attention to mental health, sexual health, and reproductive health 5. Core conditions that may affect the health of an adolescent, such as family problems, poverty, depression, school failure, obesity, eating disorders, violence, drug use, unintended pregnancy, and sexually transmitted infections	*Students should be able to*: 1. Recognize strengths, which serve as protective factors and support development 2. Connect parents, school, and community 3. Provide confidentiality of sensitive information and the encouragement of adolescents to communicate with his or her parents 4. Treat each encounter as an opportunity to act as a caring adult and to engage the adolescent in conversations about healthy living 5. Understand that adolescence is a time of experimenting, learning, and development. The goal of the provider is to offer guidance that encourages the healthiest behaviors and responsible decision-making	*Students should be able to*: 1. Establish clinical rapport based on respect, explain confidential services to teens and parents 2. Respond to parental questions and concerns; collect data and information regarding teen history, risk factors, and strengths 3. Use appropriate assessment tools 4. Assess for high-risk behaviors (i.e., tobacco, alcohol, or drug use, sexual behavior, eating disorders) 5. Assess well-being at home, in school, and in peer relationships 6. Express sensitivity toward topics that include sexual activity, sexual orientation, gender identification, and development of sexual identity and orientation 7. Discuss contraceptive use and options for counseling regarding unintended pregnancy; assess mental health status and exposure to violence 8. Conduct a suicide assessment

[a]Adapted from the American Academy of Family Physicians http://www.aafp.org/online/etc/medialib/aafp_org/documents/about/rap/curriculum/adolescent_health.Par.0001.File.tmp/Reprint278.pdf

of best practice may differ. Guidelines targeted toward generalists may require training in proper screening procedures assessing areas of maladaptive functioning common in adolescents; specialists would benefit from more targeted knowledge in specific treatment and intervention procedures for sub-aggregates of adolescents; educators should be encouraged to utilize current research in adolescent heath and provide trainees information on effective strategies, interventions, and assessments of key areas pertinent to adolescent health; and scholars need to address the inadequacies by researching needs and current practices in adolescent health care services, as well as provide recommendations for more optimal care. Overall, in order to address the gap in health care disparities and prepare future providers to effectively meet the needs of adolescents, consistency is needed in the dissemination of knowledge and skills related to adolescent health practices across all disciplines.

In addition to consistency, adequate financial resources are necessary in order to address the health care needs of adolescents, to implement prevention and intervention programs, to ensure that training programs have access to adequate

Table 3 Suggested teaching methodologies[a]

Methodology	Knowledge	Attitudes	Skills
Formal lecture	X		
Mini lecture	X		
Interactive lecture	X		
Reading	X		
Audio visual materials	X		
Case studies	X		
Individual research (databases, Cochrane review)	X		
Group discussion	X		
Field work	X	X	X
Group discussion	X	X	X
Exploration of personal attitudes		X	
Focus groups		X	
Exposure to views using real or simulated patients		X	
Promotion of attitudes of openness and introspection		X	
Simulations (artificial models, standardized patients)			X
Supervised clinical practice			X
Videotaping clinical practice			X
Guidelines for good practice (checklists, handouts)			X

[a]Adapted from www.euteach.com

resources, and to address the current state of treatment provided to this age group. Unfortunately, the resources allocated to adolescent health care issues are minimal. Currently, there is one federal agency in the United States that provides grants to enhance adolescent health practices (The Maternal and Child Health Bureau). The grant provides $2.6 million dollars in funds to seven multidisciplinary Leadership Education in Adolescent Health (LEAD) programs in seven universities. In comparison to other populations, including pediatric or geriatric, the funding invested is scarce, especially when examining the number of teenagers in the United States. There are nearly 42 million adolescents in this country, which means that only 6 cents is invested per adolescent, per year, across researchers, training programs, educators, and scholars (Lawrence et al., 2009). As such, in order to address the needs of adolescents, funds need to be made available so that training programs can more adequately prepare professionals to work in the field of adolescent health.

Resources for Training in Adolescent Health

Journal Articles

Anglin, T. M., Naylor, K. E., & Kaplan, D. W. (1996). Comprehensive school-based health care: High school students' use of medical, mental health, and substance abuse services. *Pediatrics, 97*(3), 318–330.

Bethell C., Klein, J., & Peck, C. (2001). Assessing health system provision of adolescent preventative services: The Young Adult Health Care Survey. *Medical Care, 39*(5), 478–490.

Bower, P., Garralda, E., Kramer, T., Harrington, R., & Sibbald, B. (2001). The treatment of child and adolescent mental health problems in primary care: a systematic review. *Family Practice, 18,* 373–82.

Brindis, C. D., Jr., Ozer, E. M., Handley, M., Knopf, D. K., Millstein, S. G. & Irwin, C.E. (1998). *Improving Adolescent Health: An Analysis and Synthesis of Health Policy Recommendations, Full Report.* San Francisco, CA: University of California, San Francisco. National Adolescent

Health Information Center. Retrieved from http://nahic.ucsf.edu//downloads/IAH_Full.pdf.

Garofalo, R., Katz, E. (2001). Health care issues of gay and lesbian youth. *Current Opinion in Pediatrics, 13*(4), 298–302.

Goldenting, J.M., Rosen, D.S. (2004). Getting into adolescent heads: an essential update. *Contemporary Pediatrics. 21*(1), 64–90.

Hampton, H.L. (2000). Examination of the adolescent patient. *Obstetrics and Gynecology Clinics of North America. 27*(1), 1–18.

Holmbeck, G. N. (2002). A developmental perspective on adolescent health and illness: An introduction to the special issues. *Journal of Pediatric Psychology, 27*, 409–416.

Kann L. (2001). The Youth Risk Behavior Surveillance System: Measuring health-risk behaviors. *American Journal of Health Behavior, 25*(3):272–277.

Kotchick, B. A., Shaffer, A., Forehand, R. (2001). Adolescent sexual risk behavior: A multi-system perspective. *Clinical Psychology Review, 21*(4), 493–519.

Michaud, P., Stronski, S., Fonesca, H., & Macfarlane, A., Members of the EuTEACH Working Group (2004). The development and pilot-testing of training curriculum in adolescent medicine and health. *Journal of Adolescent Health, 35,* 51–57.

Minehan, J. A., Newcomb, M. D., & Galaif, E. R. (2000). Predictors of adolescent drug use: Cognitive abilities, coping strategies, and purpose in life. *Journal of Child and Adolescent Substance Abuse, 10*(2), 33–52.

Walker, Z. A. K., Townsend, J. (1999). The role of general practice in promoting teenage health. A review of the literature. *Family Practice, 16,* 164–172.

Williams, P.G., Holmbeck, G.N., & Neff, R. (2002). Adolescent Health Psychology. *Journal of Consulting and Clinical Psychology, 70*, 828–842.

Wilson, K. M., Klein, J. D. (2000). Adolescents who use the emergency department as their usual source of care. *Archives of Pediatric and Adolescent Medicine, 154*(4), 361–365.

Webpages

www.euteach.com. The European Training in Effective Adolescent Care and Health (EuTEACH) website provides information on training professionals to provide effective adolescent health care, and permits access to curriculum and modules that can be utilized in the education of health care professionals.

www.usc.edu/adolhealth. This website was created by Professor Laurence Neinstein at University of Southern California. It was developed to provide educational materials used to improve the clinical care provided to adolescents. It is indicated that this material can be used in isolation or in conjunction with the EUTEACH curriculum. Specific material on core content areas is provided.

http://www.who.int/topics/adolescent_health. The World Health Organization's website on Adolescent Health provides information regarding statistics and fact sheets on health risks, prevention and promoting healthy development and publications on the topic of adolescent health. Additionally, information regarding adolescent health in various regions around the world is presented.

http://kidshealth.org/parent/kh_misc/classroom.html. The Kids Health in the Classroom website offers school personnel (i.e., teachers, school nurses, coaches, and guidance counselors) free health curriculum materials aligned to the national health education standards.

http://www.nlm.nih.gov/medlineplus/teenhealth.html. As a service of the US National Library of Medicine and National Institutes of Health, the MedlinePlus—Teen Health website provides resources and links to information targeted for the adolescent reader.

http://www.keepkidshealthy.com/adolescent/adolescent.html. Teen Health Center's website provides information regarding teen nutrition, growth and development, advice to caregivers about parenting their teen, safety and mental health concerns.

http://healthypeople.gov/2020/topicsobjectives2020/overview.aspx?topicid=2. The Healthy

People.gov website provides a page on Adolescent Health with the goal of improving the health, safety and wellbeing of adolescents. An overview of issues that plaque adolescent health, objectives to improving adolescent health in accordance with Health People 2020, interventions, and resources.

http://www.naswdc.org/pippah/home.asp?hp=yes. The Partnership in Program Planning for Adolescent Health website is provided through the National Association of Social Workers and outlines new perspectives and strategies in order to promote public health awareness and ensure concerns regarding adolescents are addressed.

http://hhd.org. The Health and Human Development website provides assessment tools, curricula, and resources to on various health topics across the lifespan and include adolescents.

http://www.hhs.gov/opa/familylife/. The US Department of Health and Human Services Adolescent Family Life (AFL) Demonstration and Research program supports the development and implementation of intervention programs to postpone sexual activity and educate adolescents on pregnancy and parenting.

http://www.hhs.gov/ash/oah/. The US Depart ment of Health and Human Services Office of Adolescent Health (OAH) provides programs and initiatives to help support and improve adolescent health. This organization also collects and distributes information pertinent to adolescents.

http://www.cdc.gov/HealthyYouth/az/index.htm. The Centers for Disease Control and Prevention provides information on Adolescent Health that includes alcohol and drug use, sexual behaviors, injuries, tobacco use, skin cancer, asthma, crisis preparedness and response, health tips, food safety, nutrition, physical activity, suicide, worker safety, and youth violence.

http://www.mchb.hrsa.gov/chusa08/hstat/hsa/pages/200hsa.html. Through the US Department of Health and Human Services the Health Resources and Services Administration webpage provides information regarding specific topics relevant to adolescents that include HIV/AIDS, physical activity, mental health, cigarette smoking, substance abuse, violence, adolescent mortality, adolescent childbearing, sexual activity, and sexually transmitted infections.

http://mchb.hrsa.gov/. The Maternal and Child Health Bureau provides funding and grant opportunities in order to improve the health of mothers, children, and families.

http://www.adolescenthealth.org. The Society for Adolescent Health and Medicine (SAHM) is a multidisciplinary organization that strives to enhance the physical and mental health, as well as well-being of adolescents. The website provides information and resources regarding advocacy, continuing education, research, and professional resources (including curriculum development).

http://policy.ucsf.edu/index.php/resources/. The Public Policy Analysis and Education Center for Middle Childhood, Adolescent, and Young Adult Health provides information on this website about the RESOURCE project. This project provides resources and materials to enhance training in adolescent health.

http://monitoringthefuture.org/. Monitoring the Future is a continuous study of the behaviors, attitudes, values, and viewpoints of adolescents in 8th–12th grade, as well as college students. Approximately 50,000 adolescents are surveyed annually.

Books

Committee on Adolescent Health Care Services and Models of Care for Treatment, Prevention, and Healthy Development, National Research Council (2009). *Adolescent Health Services: Missing Opportunities.* Washington, DC: The National Academies Press

Davis, B. J. & Voegtle, K. H. (1994). *Culturally competent health care for adolescents: A guide for primary care providers.* Chicago: American Medical Association.

DiClemente, R. J., Santelli, J. S., & Crosby, R. A. (2009). Adolescent Health: Understanding and

Preventing Risk Behaviors. San Francisco, CA: Jossey-Bass.

Igra V, Irwin CE, Jr. Theories of Adolescent Risk-Taking Behavior. (1996). In: DiClemente R, Hansen W, Ponton L, eds. *Handbook of Adolescent Health Risk Behavior*. New York: Plenum Press.

Kern, D., & Hopkins, J. (1998). Curriculum development for medical education: A six-step approach. Baltimore, MD: Johns Hopkins University Press.

Lerner, R. M., & Steinberg, L. (Eds.). (2004). *Handbook of Adolescent Psychology* (2nd ed). Hoboken, NJ: John Wiley and Sons, Inc.

Muuss, R. (1996). *Theories of Adolescence*, 6th Edition. New York: McGraw-Hill Publishers

Steinberg, L. Adolescence: Seventh Edition. McGraw-Hill: New York

Videos

http://www.euteach.com/euteach_home/euteach-resources-tools/euteach-summer-school-videos.htm

This section of the EuTEACH website includes videos on how interactively teach

http://video.google.com/videoplay?docid=-5939446517701113787&ei=9YI-SZnDHZOwrALVi9muCQ&q=national+academies,+adolescent+health#

This video was created in conjunction with the book: *Adolescent Health Services: Missing Opportunities* and illustrated the difficulties adolescents face in obtaining appropriate health care.

References

Agency for Healthcare Research and Quality. (2006). *Medical Expenditure Panel Survey: Table 1. Health insurance coverage of the civilian noninstitutionalized population: Percent by type of coverage and selected population characteristics, United States, first half of 2006*. Retrieved from http://www.meps.ahrq.gov/mepsweb/data_stats/quick_tables_results.jsp?component=1&subcomponent=0&year=2006&tableSeries=4&searchText=&searchMethod=1&Action=Search.

American Academy of Family Physicians. (2008). *Recommended curriculum guidelines for family medicine residents. Adolescent health*. AAFP Reprint No. 278. Retrieved December 16, 2010, from http://www.aafp.org/online/etc/medialib/aafp_org/documents/about/rap/curriculum/adolescent_health.Par.0001.File.tmp/Reprint278.pdf.

American Psychiatric Association. (2000). *Diagnostic and statistical manual of mental disorders-IV-TR*. Washington, DC: American Psychiatric Association.

Astroth, K. A., Garza, P., & Taylor, B. (2004). Getting down to business: Defining competencies for entry-level youth workers. *New Directions for Youth Development, 104*, 25–37.

Blum, R. W., & Bearinger, L. H. (1990). Knowledge and attitudes of health professionals toward adolescent health care. *Journal of Adolescent Health Care, 11*(4), 289–294.

Bonat, S. H., Pathomvanich, A., Keil, M. F., Field, A. E., & Yanovski, J. A. (2002). Self-assessment of pubertal maturation in overweight children. *Pediatrics, 110*(4), 743–747.

Brener, N. D., Billy, J. O. G., & Grady, W. R. (2003). Assessment of factors affecting the validity of self-reported health-risk behavior among adolescents: Evidence from the scientific literature. *Journal of Adolescent Health, 33*(6), 436–457.

Brener, N., McManus, T., Galuska, D., Lowry, R., & Wechsler, H. (2003). Reliability and validity of self-reported height and weight among high school students. *Journal of Adolescent Health, 32*(4), 281–287.

Brindis, C. D., Jr., Ozer, E. M., Handley, M., Knopf, D. K., Millstein, S. G., & Irwin, C. E., (1998). *Improving adolescent health: An analysis and synthesis of health policy recommendations, full report*. San Francisco, CA: University of California, San Francisco. National Adolescent Health Information Center. Retrieved from http://nahic.ucsf.edu//downloads/IAH_Full.pdf.

Centers for Disease Control and Prevention. (2006). *Sexually Transmitted Disease Surveillance, 2005*. Atlanta, GA: Division of Sexually Transmitted Disease Prevention.

Centers for Disease Control and Prevention. (2010). Positive youth development promoting adolescent sexual and reproductive health: A review of observational and intervention research. *Journal of Adolescent Health, 46*(3), S1–S6.

Coupey, S. M. (1997). Interviewing adolescents. *Pediatric Clinics of North America, 44*(6), 1349–1364.

DiClemente, C. C., & Prochaska, J. O. (1982). Self-Change and Therapy Change of Smoking Behavior: A Comparison of Processes of Change in Cessation and Maintenance. *Addictive Behaviors, 7*, 133–142.

Dietz, W. H. (1998). Health consequences of obesity in youth: Childhood predictors of adult disease. *Pediatrics, 101*(3), 518–525.

Eaton, D. K., Kann, L., Kinchen, S., Ross, J., Hawkins, J., Harris, W. A., et al. (2006). Youth risk behavior surveillance—United States, 2005. *MMWR, Surveillance Summaries, 55*(SS-5), 1–108. Retrieved December 12, 2010, from http://www.cdc.gov/mmwR/preview/mmwrhtml/ss5505a1.htm.

Ehrman, W. G., & Matson, S. C. (1998). Approach to assessing adolescents on serious or sensitive issues. *Pediatric Clinics of North America, 45*(1), 189–204.

Elster, A. B., & Kuznets, N. J. (1994). *Guidelines for adolescent preventive services (GAPS). Recommendations and rationale*. American Medical Association: Chicago.

English, A., Santelli, J. S., & Rogers, A. S. (2009). Legal and ethical issues in adolescent health care and research. In R. Crosby, R. DiClemente, & J. Santelli (Eds.), *Adolescent health: Understanding and preventing risk behaviors and adverse health outcomes*. San Francisco, CA: Jossey-Bass.

Erk, R. R. (2008). *Counseling treatment for children and adolescents with DSM-IV-TR Disorders*. Columbus, OH: Merrill Prentice Hall.

Ford, T. (2008). Practitioner review: How can epidemiology help us plan and deliver effective child and adolescent mental health services. *Journal of Child Psychology and Psychiatry, 49*, 900–914.

Fox, H. B., McManus, M. A., Diaz, A., Elster, A., Felice, M., Kaplan, D., et al. (2008). Advancing medical education training in adolescent health. *Pediatrics, 121*, 1043–1045.

Fox, H. B., McManus, M. A., Wilson, J., Diaz, A., Elster, A. B., Felice, M. E., et al. (2008). *Adolescent medicine at the crossroads: A review of fellowship training and recommendations for reform*. Washington, DC: Maternal and Child Health Policy Research Center.

Green, M. (Ed.). (1994). *Bright futures: Guidelines for health supervision of infants, children, and adolescents*. Arlington, VA: National Center for Education in Maternal and Child Health.

Grunbaum, J., Kann, L., Kinchen, S., Ross, J., Hawkins, J., Lowry, R., et al. (2004). Youth Risk Behavior Surveillance—United States, 2003. *Morbidity and Mortality Weekly Report, 53*(SS-2), 1–96.

Hedley, A. A., Ogden, C. L., Johnson, C. L., Carroll, M. D., Curtin, L. R., & Flegal, K. M. (2004). Prevalence of overweight and obesity among US children, adolescents, and adults, 1999-2002. *Journal of the American Medical Association, 291*(23), 2847–2850.

Higgins, J. W., Begoray, D., & MacDonald, M. (2009). A social ecological conceptual framework for understanding adolescent health literacy in the health education classroom. *American Journal of Community Psychology, 44*, 350–362.

Hing, E., Cherry, D. K., & Woodwell, D. A. (2006). National Ambulatory Medical Care Survey: 2004 summary. *Advance Data from Vital and Health Statistics, 374*, 1–36.

Hoek, H. W., & van Hoeken, D. (2003). Review of the prevalence and incidence of eating disorders. *International Journal of Eating Disorders, 34*(4), 383–396.

Holmbeck, G. N. (2002). A developmental perspective on adolescent health and illness: An introduction to the special issues. *Journal of Pediatric Psychology, 27*, 409–416.

Kataoka, S. H., Zhang, L., & Wells, K. B. (2002). Unmet need for mental health care among US children: Variation by ethnicity and insurance status. *The American Journal of Psychiatry, 159*(9), 1548–1555.

Kessler, R. C., Chiu, W. T., Colpe, L., Demler, O., Merikangas, K. R., Walters, E. E., et al. (2006). The prevalence and correlates of serious mental illness (SMI) in the National Comorbidity Survey Replication (NCS-R). In R. W. Manderscheid & J. T. Berry (Eds.), *Mental health, United Sates, 2004* (pp. 134–148). Center for Mental Health Services, Substance Abuse and Mental Health Services Administration. Retrieved December 12, 2010, from http://mentalhealth.samhsa.gov/publications/allpubs/SMA06-4195/Chapter15.asp.

Klein, J. D., Slap, G. B., Elster, A. B., & Schonberg, S. K. (1992). Access to health care for adolescents: A position paper of the Society for Adolescent Medicine. Journal of Adolescent Health, 13(2), 162–170.

Knopf, D., Park, M. J., & Paul Mulye, T. A. (2008). *Mental health profile of adolescents 2008 brief*. National Adolescent Health Information Center. Retrieved from http://nahic.ucsf.edu/downloads/MentalHealthBrief.pdf.

Kost, K., Henshaw, S., & Carlin, L. (2010). *US teenage pregnancies, births and abortions: National and state trends and trends by race and ethnicity.* Retrieved from http://www.guttmacher.org/pubs/USTPtrends.pdf.

Lawrence, R. S., Gootman, J. A., & Sim, L. J. (Eds.). (2009). *Adolescent health services: Missing opportunities*. Washington, DC: The National Academy of Sciences.

Lee, K., Valeria, B., Kochman, C., & Lenders, C. M. (2006). Self-assessment of height, weight, and sexual maturation: Validity in overweight children and adolescents. *Journal of Adolescent Health, 39*(3), 346–352.

McManus, M. A., Shejavali, K. I., & Fox, H. B. (2003). *Is the health care system working for adolescents?* Washington, DC: Maternal and Child Health Policy Research Center.

Substance Abuse and Mental Health Services Administration, Office of Applied Studies (2009). *The NSDUH Report: Major depressive episode and treatment among adolescents*. Rockville, MD. Retrieved December 5, 2010, from http://oas.samhsa.gov/2k9/youthDepression/MDEandTXTforADOL.pdf.

Merikangas, K. R., He, J. P., Brody, D., Fisher, P. W., Bourdon, K., & Koretz, D. S. (2010). Prevalence and treatment of mental disorders among US children in the 2001-2004 NHANES. *Pediatrics, 125*(1), 75–81.

Michaud, P., Stronski, S., Fonesca, H., Macfarlane, A., & Members of the EuTEACH Working Group. (2004). The development and pilot-testing of training curriculum in adolescent medicine and health. *Journal of Adolescent Health, 35*, 51–57.

Miller, W. R., & Rollnick, S. (2002). *Motivational interviewing: Preparing people for change*. New York, NY: Guilford Press.

Mokdad, A. H., Marks, J. S., Stroup, D. F., & Gerberding, J. L. (2004). Actual causes of death in the United States, 2000. *Journal of the American Medical Association, 291*(10), 1238–1245.

Morreale, M., Stinnett, A. J., & Dowling, E. C. (Eds.). (2005). *Policy Compendium on Confidential Health*

Services for Adolescents (2nd ed.). Chapel Hill, NC: Center of Adolescent & the Law.

National Adolescent Health Information Center (2010). Retrieved December 16, 2010, from http://nahic.ucsf.edu/index.php/about/index/.

Ohayon, M. M., Roberts, R. E., Zulley, J., Smirne, S., & Priest, R. G. (2000). Prevalence and patterns of problematic sleep among older adolescents. *Journal of the American Academy of Child and Adolescent Psychiatry, 39*, 1549–1556.

Pastor, P. N., & Reuben, C. A. (2008). Diagnosed attention deficit hyperactivity disorder and learning disability: United States, 2004–2006. National Center for Health Statistics. *Vital Health Statistics, 10*(237), 1–14.

Prochaska, J. O., & DiClemente, C. (1982). Transtherortical therapy. Toward a comprehensive model of change. *Psychotherapy Theory, Research Practice, 19*, 267–288.

Rollnick, S., Miller, W. R., & Butler, C. C. (2007). *Motivational interviewing in health care: Helping patients change*. New York, NY: Guilford Press.

Shaffer, D., Fisher, P., Dulcan, M. K., Davies, M., Piacentini, J., Schwab-Stone, M. E., et al. (1996). The NIMH Diagnostic Interview Schedule for Children Version 2.3 (DISC-2.3): Description, acceptability, prevalence rates, and performance in the MECA Study. Methods for the Epidemiology of Child and Adolescent Mental Disorders Study. *Journal of the American Academy of Child and Adolescent Psychiatry, 35*(7), 865–887.

Shaw, R. J. (2001). Treatment adherence in adolescents: Development and psychopathology. *Clinical Child Psychology and Psychiatry, 6*(1), 137–150.

Sieving, R. E., & Shrier, L. (2009). Measuring adolescent health behavior. In R. Crosby, R. DiClemente, & J. Santelli (Eds.), *Adolescent health: Understanding and preventing risk behaviors and adverse health outcomes*. San Francisco, CA: Jossey-Bass.

Skopelja, E. N., Whipple, E. C., & Richwine, P. (2008). Reaching and teaching teens: Adolescent health literacy and the internet. *Journal of consumer Health on the Internet, 12*, 105–118.

Stein, M. (Ed.). (1997). *Health supervision guidelines* (3rd ed.). Elk Grove Village, IL: American Academy of Pediatrics.

Substance Abuse and Mental Health Services Administration. (2010). *Results from the 2009 National Survey on Drug Use and Health: Volume I. Summary of National Findings* (Office of Applied Studies, NSDUH Series H-38A, HHS Publication No. SMA 10-4586Findings).Rockville, MD.

US Department of Health and Human Services, Health Resources and Services Administration, Maternal and Child Health Bureau. (2008). *Child Health USA 2007*. Rockville, Maryland: US Department of Health and Human Services.

US Preventive Services Task Force. (1996). *Guide to clinical preventive services* (2nd ed.). Baltimore, MD: Williams & Wilkins.

United Nations Convention on the Rights of the Child, G.A. Res. 44/25, U.N. GAOR, 44th Sess., at 3, U.N. Doc. A/RES/44/25 (1989, November 20). Retrieved December 16, 2010, from http://www.unicef.org/crc/.

Walker, Z. A. K., & Townsend, J. (1999). The role of general practice in promoting teenage health. A review of the literature. *Family Practice, 16*, 164–172.

Williams, P. G., Holmbeck, G. N., & Neff, R. (2002). Adolescent health psychology [Special Issue: Behavioral Medicine and Clinical Health Psychology]. *Journal of Consulting and Clinical Psychology, 70*, 828–842.

Williams, J., Klinepeter, K., Palmes, G., Pulley, A., & Meschan, J. (2004). Diagnosis and treatment of behavioral health disorders in pediatric practice. *Pediatrics, 114*, 601–606.

World Health Organization. (2002). *Adolescent friendly health services—An agenda for change*. WHO/FCH/CAH/02.12. WHO, 2002. Retrieved from http://www.who.int/reproductive-health/publications/cah_docs/cah_02_14.pdf.

Reforming the Behavioral Health Delivery System for Adolescents: Why Is It Needed and What Is Psychology's Role?

William T. O'Donohue, Clair Rummel, Alexandros Maragakis, and Cassandra Snipes

The United States health care system is in crisis. Spending on health care has grown at an unsustainable rate over the past 40 years. In 1960 the US health care spending accounted for approximately 5 % of the gross national income (GDP). By 2007 health care spending accounted for 16–17 % of the GDP, reaching $2.4 trillion or $7,290–$7,900 per person (Angrisano, Farrell, Kocher, Laboissiere, & Parker, 2007; Keehan et al., 2008; Organisation for Economic Co-Operation and Development, 2009). Recent projections show a continuation of this trend with spending reaching 25 % of the GDP in 2025 and close to 50 % in 2082 (Congressional Budget Office, 2008). This dramatic growth in health care costs affects both the public and private sectors. This dramatic growth in health-care costs affects both the public and private sectors. In 1966 Medicare and Medicaid costs were 1 % of the federal budget. Currently these entitlements, along with the children's health insurance program (CHIP), account for 21 % of the federal budget and are rising quickly (Center on Budget and Policy Priorites, 2012)—particularly when new benefits such as those delineated in the new health care reform bill are factored in. These costs drive the federal deficit (currently approximately $13 trillion or about $40,000 for every US citizen; interest on the national debt in 2009 was an additional $260 billion), and the rate of taxation. This is of concern as some have called the federal debt an intergenerational transfer of wealth (Labonte & Makinen, 2000), meaning a significant part of the current generation's health care bill is to be paid by future generations.

Due to what economists call opportunity costs, the more funds spent on one sector of the economy means by necessity fewer funds to be spent on other sectors, such as education, infrastructure, and poverty programs. To put these numbers in perspective, the United States now spends more money on health care than it does on food or automobiles, and more than the Chinese spend, per capita on everything (Angrisano et al., 2007; Lowenstein, 2009), yet millions of Americans fail to receive effective care (Institute of Medicine, 2001).

Another part of the health care crisis as President Obama points out is that these high costs reduce the competitiveness of American products in a global economy. General Motors, for example, until it terminated health insurance for its retirees this year, paid more for health care for its retirees ($3.6 billion) than for its current employees and health care costs added about $1,700 to the price of one of its cars (www.whcoa.gov/about/policy). General Motors, for example, spends roughly $5 billion on health-care expenses annually and claims that health care costs add between $1,500 and $2,000 to the price of each automobile produced (Johnson, 2010). At the most personal level, medical debt is also the principal cause of personal

W.T. O'Donohue, Ph.D. (✉) • C. Rummel • A. Maragakis
C. Snipes, B.A.
Department of Psychology: MS 0296 Reno, University of Nevada, Mail Stop 297, Reno, NV 89557, USA
e-mail: wto@unr.edu

W.T. O'Donohue et al. (eds.), *Handbook of Adolescent Health Psychology*,
DOI 10.1007/978-1-4614-6633-8_22, © Springer Science+Business Media New York 2013

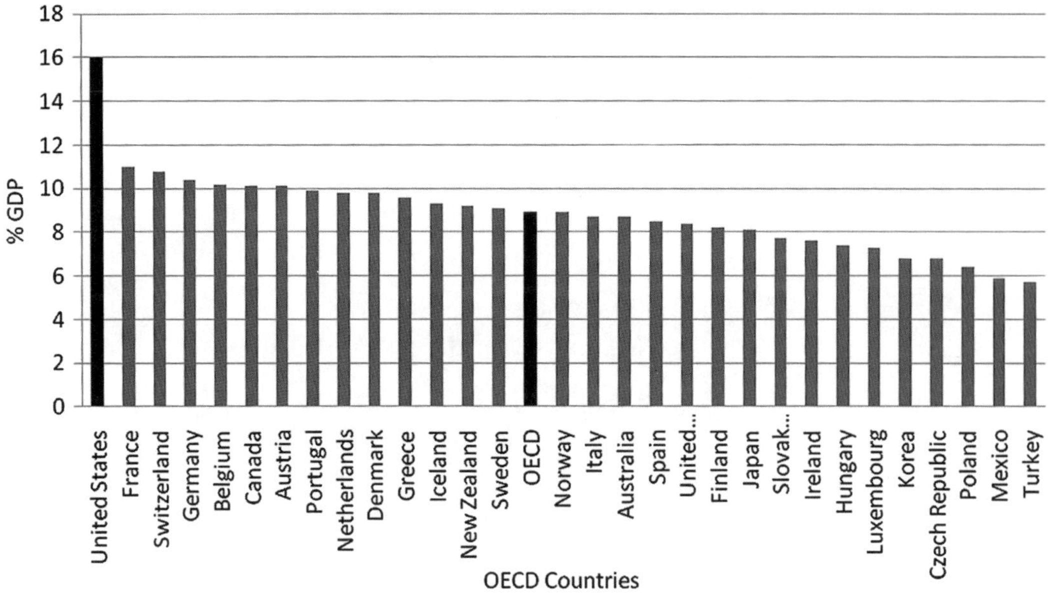

Fig. 1 Health expenditures as a share of GDP, 2007 (OECD, 2009)

bankruptcy in the USA (Himmelstein, Thorne, Warren, & Woolhandler, 2009). This chapter will discuss how we have arrived at the current health care crisis, the drivers of health care spending, the role of adolescent behaviors on current and future health care expenditures, and the role psychologists can play in cost-effective reforms.

How Does the United States Compare?

Health care expenditures in the United States far exceed money spent on health care in other developed nations, as a total or as a percentage of GDP. According to the Organization for Economic Co-Operation and Development (OECD, 2009), health care spending in the United States in 2007 accounted for 16 % of the GDP; more than seven percentage points higher than the average 8.9 % in OECD countries, yet the United States stands alone with Turkey and Mexico as the only OECD countries without universal health coverage (see Fig. 1 for a full list of OECD nations' health expenditures as a share of their GDP). Per person Americans spend more than any other nation on health care services, consuming $7,290 each in 2007, almost two and a half times more than the OECD average ($2,964) (OECD, 2009). The next closest country Norway spent $4,763 while relatively wealthy nations like France, Germany, and the United Kingdom spent less than half the US average.

Although there are concerns that one of the drivers of costs in the USA is that Americans are unhealthier (e.g., due to higher rates of obesity, diabetes, coronary problems) it is unclear what factors contribute how much to this. There is some evidence that there is a higher disease burden in the United States (Mackay & Mensah, 2004; World Health Organization, 2009), and that the medical system in the USA expends more on treatments for these diseases (Cutler, 2005). A key question is to what extent are these costs driven by higher incomes (wealthier individuals can afford more health care), higher disease burden, more expensive treatments and technology, inefficiencies such as administrative costs and defensive medicine, or to problematic incentives (called moral hazards by economists) producing overtreatment.

One cause of the high per capita costs is that the United States spends six times more per capita on the administration of the health care system than its peer Western European nations.

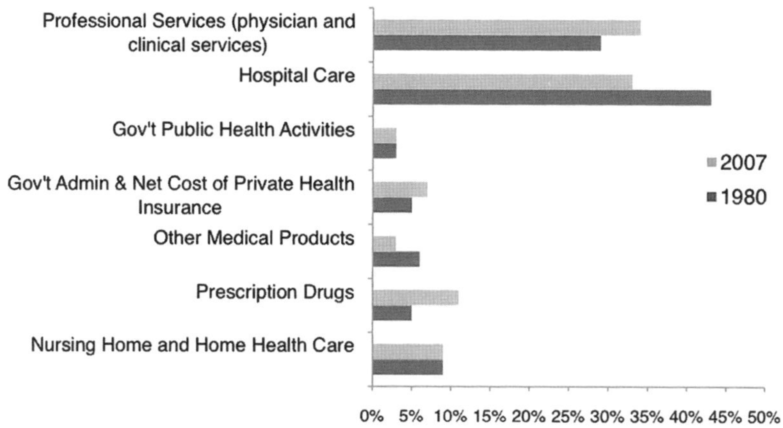

Fig. 2 National health expenditures as a percentage of total spending for 1980 and 2007 (CMS, 2009). Total health care expenditures in 1980 = \$253.4 billion, 2007 = \$2,241 billion

An analysis of how money is spent revealed that high costs are due to a "failure of the intermediation system to (a) provide sufficient incentives to patients and consumers to be value-conscious in their demand decisions, and (b) establish the necessary incentives or mandates to promote rational supply by providers and their suppliers" (Angrisano et al., 2007, p. 8). Findings point to an array of unnecessary costs specific to the United States due to its present structure. For example, Danzon and Furukawa (2008) found that foreign prices on pharmaceutical drugs are 20–40 % lower than manufacturer's prices in the USA and 10–30 % lower than public prices in the USA. However, some of this may be a segmenting marketing strategy by pharmaceutical companies to reclaim research and development costs in richer countries.

How Is Money Spent on Health Care in the United States?

According to the Centers for Medicare and Medicaid Services (2009), total health care expenditures jumped from 253.4 billion in 1980 to 2.2 trillion in 2007. A comparison of health expenditures for 1980 versus those for 2007 (Fig. 2) reveal several notable trends: (1) expenditures on prescription drugs saw the biggest increase over the time period as they increased from 5 % of total health care expenditures in 1980 to 11 % in 2007 and (2) a shift in spending away from hospital care towards professional services and prescription drugs. As services shifted to outpatient settings, expenditures on hospital care decreased significantly from 43 % of total expenditures in 1980 to 33 % in 2007.

Over the past 40 years a trend towards increased public spending and decreased private spending on health care expenditures has been observed (CMS, 2008). Government expenditures (paid through taxes and borrowing) accounted for close to 50 % of all health-care expenditures in 2006, up from 30.0 % in 1966 (CMS, 2008).

Behavioral Health Care Spending

Behavioral health care spending makes up a minority of total health care spending in the USA. According to the Substance Abuse and Mental Health Services Administration (Mark et al., 2007), national expenditures for the treatment of mental health (\$100 billion) and substance abuse (\$21 billion) amounted to \$121 billion in 2003 accounting for only 7.5 % of the total health care expenditures. Broken down further, mental health expenditures account for 6.2 % of total health care expenditures and substance abuse spending accounts for 1.3 %.

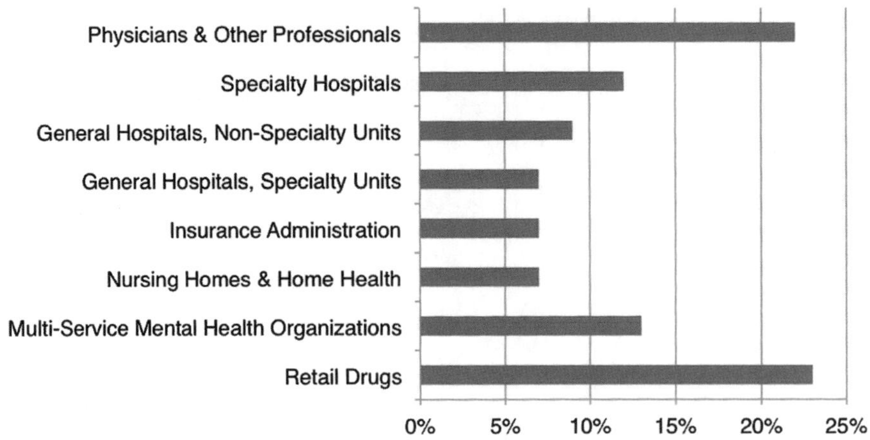

Fig. 3 Distribution of mental health expenditures by services, 2003 (Mark et al., 2007)

Trends in Direct Spending on Mental Health

The allocation of mental health spending has shifted over the last three decades. The trend of decreased inpatient services continued with inpatient expenditures dropping from 36 % of total mental health spending to only 24 % between 1993 and 2003 (Mark et al., 2007). The decrease in spending on inpatient services was picked up by prescription drug purchases, which increased from 8 % of total mental health spending to 23 % during the same time period (for a breakdown of mental health spending see Fig. 3). In 2003, close to 1 in 4 dollars spent on mental health services was spent on prescription medications (Mark et al., 2007). The rapid rise in the prescription of psychotropic medications has been well documented (Olfson, Marcus, Druss, & Pincus, 2002; Zuvekas, 2003). In an analysis of results from the Medical Expenditure Panel Survey, Zuvekas (2005) found that an increasing number of individuals take prescription medications without an accompanying visit to a mental health professional (40 % in 1996 and 45 % in 2001). The sharp increase in out-of-pocket spending on mental health seen between 1998 and 2003 may have largely been the result of increased spending on prescription medications. It is important for psychologist to realize that the major competitor in the marketplace—with an increasing share of the market—is the physician (most often a primary care doctor) with a prescription pad.

Individuals with mental health disorders rely on public sources of spending to a greater extent than people with other chronic diseases (Mark, et al., 2007). Public sources of funding account for 58 % of total mental health spending, while only 45 % of total health care spending comes from public sources. The largest portion of mental health expenditures is covered by state and local funding while private insurance accounts for only 4.0 %. The full economic costs of mental illness are not captured by the above breakdown of expenditures. Indirect costs such as reduced labor supply, public income support payments, high rates of homelessness among the seriously mentally ill (SMI), and incarceration often overshadow other indirect costs such as the high rates of medical complications, the high prevalence of pulmonary disease (individuals with mental illness smoke 44 % of all cigarettes in the USA), and early mortality (Colton & Manderscheid, 2006; Insel, 2008). While exact figures of indirect costs are difficult to quantify, a recent analysis by Kessler et al. (2008) estimated that serious mental illness is associated with an annual loss of earnings totaling $193.2 billion (Fig. 4).

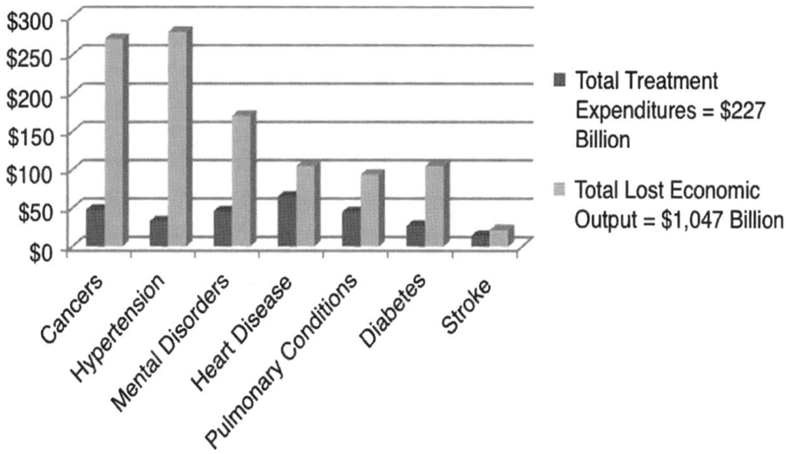

Fig. 4 Economic impact of chronic disease, 2003 (DeVol & Bedroussian, 2007)

The Major Drivers of Health Care Spending

Chronic Disease and Unhealthy Lifestyles

Advances in medical care and prevention efforts have resulted in an epidemiological shift in the leading cause of death from infectious disease and acute illness to chronic disease, defined by the Centers for Disease Control and Prevention as noncommunicable illnesses that are prolonged in duration, do not resolve spontaneously, and are rarely cured completely (2009; CDC, 2003). Currently, 7 of 10 deaths in the USA are caused by chronic disease (CDC, 2009). Nearly half of all Americans (133 million) suffer from one or more chronic disease and a quarter of those who do experience significant limitations in daily activities (CDC, 2009). The increase in the prevalence of chronic diseases has spread across the lifespan with chronic diseases affecting 1.8 % of children and adolescents in the 1960s to more than 7 % in 2004 (CDC, 2009). Recent analysis reveals that the seven most common chronic diseases (cancer, diabetes, hypertension, stroke, heart disease, pulmonary conditions, and mental disorders) cost the economy more than $1 trillion annually in 2003 (see Fig. 5, DeVol & Bedroussian, 2007). Currently, more than 75 % of health care costs are due to chronic conditions (CDC, 2009). Costs go beyond health care expenditures for each chronic disease and capture a host of indirect costs including sick days, low performance rates, output loss, and losses incurred by the caregiver, such as finances (DeVol & Bedroussian, 2007). The costs to the economy are projected to continue to grow and may reach close to $6 trillion by 2050 (DeVol & Bedroussian, 2007). An analysis of the modifiable behavioral risk factors that can lead to the nation's leading chronic diseases found that close to 35 % of US deaths in 2000 were due to tobacco use, poor diet, and physical inactivity (Mokdad, Marks, Stroup, & Gerberding, 2004). In an examination of the effects of obesity, smoking, and drinking on medical problems and costs, Strum (2002) found that obesity far outranks the negative effects of drinking and smoking. Obesity was associated with a 36 % increase in outpatient and inpatient spending and a 77 % increase in medications while current smokers were associated with a 21 % increase in inpatient and outpatient spending and a 28 % increase in medications and even smaller effects for problem drinkers (Strum, 2002). Obesity has become an epidemic among children and adolescents (O'Donohue, Moore, & Scott, 2009) (Fig. 6).

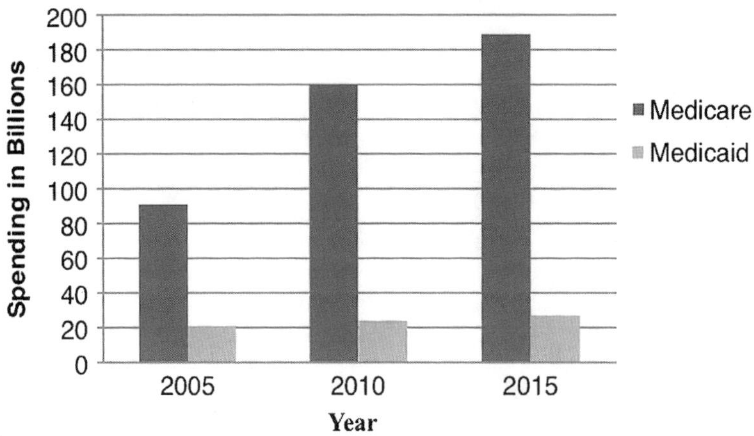

Fig. 5 Projected direct costs for Alzheimer's disease care (Alzheimer's Association, 2008)

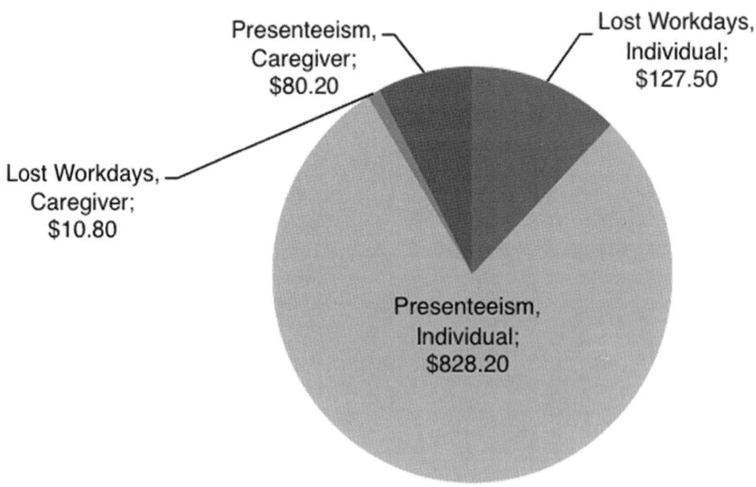

Fig. 6 Lost productivity in billions by source for 2003 (DeVol & Bedroussian, 2007)

Comorbid Conditions

A review of the literature reveals that individuals with mental illnesses tend to be high utilizers of medical care, as they routinely present to their primary care physicians with a high number of comorbid illnesses and incur longer hospital stays (Chiles, Lambert, & Hatch, 1999). Schizophrenia in particular is associated with substantial direct and indirect costs in excess of those incurred by matched controls (Wu et al., 2005). Wu et al. (2005) found that the overall cost of schizophrenia in the USA in 2002 was estimated to be $62.7 billion with $22.7 billion in direct health care costs. Treatment for comorbidity has been found to add 20–90 % to the annual spending among patients with schizophrenia (McDonald, Hertz, Lustik, & Unger, 2005).

Comorbid depression has been associated with higher health-care costs for patients with chronic medical disorders such as diabetes mellitus (Ciechanowski, Katon, & Russo, 2000; Gilmer et al., 2005) and congestive heart failure (Sullivan et al., 2005). In a population-based cross-sectional survey of 130,880 Canadians, Stein et al. (2006) found that the presence of comorbid major depressive disorder and a chronic physical illness was associated with approximately double the likelihood of health care utilization, increased functional disability, and work absence compared to a chronic physical illness without the comorbid depression. The increase in health care costs is particularly notable in older adults with comorbid depression (Himelhoch et al., 2004; Katon, 2003). In recent analysis of health care costs for close to 15,000 Medicare recipients with diabetes and/or congestive heart failure found that individuals with depression had significantly higher total health care costs over a 12-month period than those without depression ($20,046 vs. $11,956) (Unutzer et al., 2009). Interestingly, depressed individuals had higher health care costs across all cost categories except specialty mental health services, which accounted for less than 1 % of total costs.

A possible driver of increased costs for individuals with chronic disease and comorbid depression is the higher rates of adverse health-risk behaviors that depressed individuals have been shown to experience, such as smoking, maintaining a high-fat diet, sedentariness, drinking, and obesity (Goodman & Whitaker, 2002; Rosal et al., 2001). A meta-analysis of the effects of anxiety and depression on patient treatment adherence found that depressed individuals are three times more likely to be noncompliant with medical treatment recommendations than non-depressed patients (DiMatteo Lepper, & Croghan, 2000). The relationship between anxiety disorders and comorbid medical illnesses is less well studied, but Roy-Byrne et al. (2008) argue that anxiety and anxiety disorders may have as great a negative impact on physical illness as depression does. In a review of the literature, the authors found that anxiety disorders amplify symptoms of some medical illnesses and appear to worsen outcomes. Thus, it has increasingly become recognized that some of the key drivers of health care expenditures are behavioral: poor diet, insufficient exercise, smoking, poor treatment adherence, anxiety, and depression. These are factors that psychologists have something to offer.

The Importance of Adolescent Health Care Consumers

Adolescents are of particular importance when examining the current health care crisis in the United States. First, this population is a driver of high health care costs, at least in part due to the fact that adolescents underuse office visits and overuse emergency department care when compared with persons in other age groups (Newacheck, Wong, Galbraith, & Hung, 2003). Second, during the transition from childhood to adulthood, adolescents establish patterns of behavior and make lifestyle choices that affect both their current and future health (Centers for Disease Control and Prevention, 2011; O'Donohue & Tolle, 2009). Third, adolescence has been identified as a particularly important phase to address health behavior and it is a significant intervention point for behavior change (O'Donohue & Tolle, 2009). Adolescents are unique consumers of health care and must be considered when examining the current health care reform.

The financial burdens of preventable health problems in adolescence are large and include the long-term costs of chronic diseases that are a result of a pattern of behavior initiated during adolescence. Alarmingly, national surveys report that 70 % of adolescents engage in one or more health-risk behaviors (Klein & Matos Auerbach, 2002, as cited by Olson, Gaffney, Lee, & Starr, 2008). These behavioral problems are an important cause of adolescent morbidity and mortality (Catalano, et al., 2012). For example, the annual health-related financial burden of adult cigarette smoking, which usually starts by age 18, is $193 billion (Health People.gov, 2012). Unfortunately, adolescents have seemed to be neglected by health care providers and researchers, and as a result, adolescence health has improved far less than that of younger children over the past 50 years (Sawyer, et al., 2012). As the nation's spending in health care continually increases it is important to target adolescences in order to improve health behaviors early in life to prevent long-term problems, reduce health care costs, and most importantly, improve quality of life.

Adolescents engage in risk behaviors that may create problems both in the short and long term for not only the individual but also society as a whole. Adolescents engage in risky driving, dieting, substance use, and sexual activity. In 2005, teen birthrates went up for the first time since 1990 (Mulye et al., 2009). We see that teen pregnancy not only influences the quality of life of the teen, but that the health of the baby is usually compromised due to the higher likelihood of the mother engaging in unhealthy behaviors (Sawyer, et al., 2012). Obesity in adolescence is projected to increase coronary heart disease 5–16 % in adults by 2035 (Bibbins-Domingo, Coxson, Pletcher, Lightwood, & Goldman, 2007). To confound these behavioral problems, one in seven adolescents lacks full-year medical coverage, making access to care difficult if not financially impossible (Mulye et al., 2009).

Because adolescence is a developmental transition, teens are particularly sensitive to environmental (or contextual) influences such as family and societal cues (Health People.gov, 2012). Adolescence is a critical transitional period that includes the biological changes of puberty and the need to negotiate key developmental tasks, such as increasing independence and normative experimentation (Health People.gov, 2012). Specifically, adolescents begin to take more personal responsibility for managing their own health (O'Donohue & Tolle, 2009). Some adolescents struggle to adopt behaviors that could decrease their risk of developing chronic diseases in adulthood, such as eating nutritiously, engaging in physical activity, and choosing to not use tobacco (Centers for Disease Control and Prevention, 2011; National Institute of Child Health and Human Development, 2007). Fortunately, adolescences view health care providers as a credible source of information, and wish to discuss their issues with health-care providers (Klein, Graff, Santelli, Hedberg, Allan, Elster, 1999, as cited by Olson, Gaffney, Lee, & Starr, 2008). If adolescents can be influenced to visit health care providers, there is a good chance of guiding adolsence behavior towards positive outcomes.

Adolescence as the Origin of Chronic Disease and Unhealthy Lifestyles

As aforementioned, chronic disease is now the leading cause of death and the origin of lifestyle choices that increase the likelihood of developing chronic disease often begins in adolescence (O'Donohue & Tolle, 2009). Obesity, diabetes, and smoking are of particular concern during this developmental phase.

The incidence of youth obesity is rising sharply and has significant health implications. It is reported that 18 % of adolescents in the United States are overweight, a number that has more than tripled from 1980 to 2008 (Centers for Disease Control, 2011a, 2011b). Obesity at this age has both immediate and long-term health effects. Of those adolescents who were considered obese, 70 % had at least one risk factor for cardiovascular disease (Li, Ford, Zhao, & Mokdad, 2009, as cited by Centers for Disease Control, 2011a, 2011b). Obese adolescents are also more likely to suffer from prediabetes, bone and joint problems, and social and psychological problems (Li, Ford, Zhao, & Mokdad, 2009 as cited by Centers for Disease Control, 2011a, 2011b). Also, obese adolescents are more likely to be considered obese as adults, which is associated with health problems such as certain types of cancer, heart disease, diabetes, stroke, and osteoarthritis (Centers for Disease Control, 2011a, 2011b).

Related to the problem of obesity, the prevalence of type 2 diabetes has increased dramatically in the recent years and in most studies all youth diagnosed with type 2 diabetes were also obese (Delamater, Jacquez, & Patino-Fernandez, 2009). In the United States, approximately 176,500 individuals under the age of 20 years have diabetes (LaGreca & Mackey, 2009). Prior to the mid-1990s, only 1–2 % of children met the criteria for type 2 diabetes and in the recent years the incidence has increased to 8–45 % of youth. In addition, 1 out of every 400–600 children has type 1 diabetes. The annual cost for diabetes management is determined to be $174 billion (LaGreca & Mackey, 2009). Diabetes is a lifelong chronic illness that requires management across the lifespan and is often diagnosed in adolescence (O'Donohue & Tolle, 2009).

In 2009, 25.6 % of high school students and 9.5 % of middle school students reported using tobacco products (Centers for Disease Control, 2011a, 2011b). While these numbers are steadily declining (34.5 % of high school students and 15.1 % of middle school students reported using tobacco products in 2000), there are still many health implications associated with smoking. Those adolescents that do smoke are more likely to engage in high-risk sexual behavior and use alcohol and other illicit drugs (Centers for Disease Control 2012). Adolescents that begin smoking will likely continue to smoke regularly throughout their adulthood (WHO, 2012). Smoking is associated with short-term health consequences that include respiratory problems, decreased lung functioning, and addiction to nicotine. Long-term effects include increase risk of heart disease, stroke, and certain forms of cancer (WHO, 2012).

Comorbid Conditions

Individuals with mental illnesses tend to be high utilizers of medical care and comorbid conditions in adolescence, such as depression, can have lifelong health implications. In 2009, about 8 % of adolescents suffered at least one major depressive episode over the course of 1 year (Childstats.gov 2011). Rates of depressive disorders peak in mid-adolescence, particularly in females (Street & Garber, 2009). Of those adolescents that experienced a major depressive episode only 35 % received some kind of treatment, either talking to a medical or mental health professional about their problem and/or taking prescription medications (Childstats.gov 2011). Not only does depression affect school and social relationships, but it also exacerbates health conditions such as obesity, asthma, migraine headaches, and allergies (Street & Garber, 2009). Adolescences that experience depression are more likely to engage in alcohol and drug use and are more likely to smoke on a daily basis Childstats.gov 2011. Additionally, depressive symptoms in adolescence have been shown to predict not only the likelihood of recurrent depressive episodes in adult life but also the onset of subsequent clinical disorders (Street & Garber, 2009). Depression can also increase the risk for other medical problems through the occurrence of sleep problems, lack of exercise, and poor eating habits (Street & Garber, 2009).

The Problem of the Uninsured

Although the United States spends more on health care than other industrialized nations nearly 46 million individuals living in the USA do not have health insurance (Carey, Herring & Lenain, 2009). The number of uninsured individuals has increased significantly in the last decade, from 38 million (14 % of the population) in 2000 to 46 million (16 % of the population) in 2007 (Carey et al., 2009). The uninsured are a heterogeneous group, including about 10 million illegal immigrants (Gruber, 2008). The increase in the uninsured is due in part to a decline in the percent of employees with employer-sponsored insurance (80.4 % in 2000–2001 to 75.7 % in 2007 (Cunningham, Artiga, & Schwartz, 2008). The largest declines (53.0–40.8 %) have been seen among low-income employees, whose family incomes are less than 200 % of poverty. Employers, particularly small businesses, have struggled to provide health insurance as a benefit due to the increases in employers' health care costs (up to 7.3 % in 2009; Thomson Reuters, 2010).

The recently signed Patient Protection and Affordable Care Act (H.R. 3590) is focused on decreasing the number of uninsured by expanding coverage for 32 million Americans. The legislation will establish among other things a mandate for most Americans to obtain health insurance, significantly expand eligibility for Medicaid, set up insurance exchanges through which individuals can receive federal subsidies to reduce the cost of purchasing coverage, substantially reduce the growth of Medicare's payment rates for most services, and impose an excise tax on insurance plans with high premiums

(Congressional Budget Office, 2010). As detailed above, the health care reform legislature will increase the government's role in providing health to its citizens. An analysis of the bill by the Congressional Budget Office (2010) found that health care costs will be lowered over time although this point continues to be debated.

Due to the high rate of uninsured children and adolescence and the poor quality of care associated with being uninsured the Children's Health Insurance Program (CHIP) was enacted by Congress in 1997 to provide insurance for children and improve access to care for low-income families (Szilagyi, et al., 2004). Originally, Congress had set aside 40 billion dollars to provide states with grants to create and provide their own CHIP. However, due to budget cuts some of this original money was taken away, and in 2007, former President George W. Bush vetoed two bills to renew and expand CHIP. Due to these vetoes Congress passed a bill that extended the fund of CHIP until 2009, but fell far short of the original two bills to expand the program. In 2009, Congress passed another bill to renew and expand CHIP that was signed by President Barack Obama.

Though it has had a turbulent finically and political history, CHIP has proved to be beneficial for adolescents. One third of the individuals enrolled in CHIP are adolescences (Klein, Shone, Szilagyi, Bajorska, & Wilson, 2007). The program has been effective in reducing the amount of uninsured adolescents from 15.2 to 12.2 % since its inception (Newacheck, Park, Brindis, Biehl, & Irwin, 2004). Through CHIP, adolescences have improved access, continuity, and quality of care and this care is delivered within the usual primary care source (Szilagyi, et al., 2004). Those who have CHIP use more preventative care and have fewer unmet medical needs (Klein et al., 2007). Also, enrollment in CHIP also is associated with eliminating racial disparities in access to medical services (Klein et al., 2007).

While some improvements have been made through programs like CHIP, there is still much progress to be made. Adolescents' access to health care is among the worst of all age groups, and relatively few interventions have shown to be effective in improving their access to care (Klein et al., 2007, p. 891). Adolescents that would qualify for programs like CHIP make up for one third of the total adolescent population but account for two thirds of the uninsured population (Newacheck et al., 2004). Since health and health behaviors are of utmost importance for this age group, it is important that we continue to target and improve access to care for these individuals.

Cost vs. Value

Cutler (2005) makes the important point that examining increasing costs misses an important part of the issue, i.e., do these incremental costs bring increased value? Cutler answers that for the most part they do. He suggests, for example, that no one would want to revert to 1950s medicine with its lower costs but also with its decreased effectiveness. Thus, a significant part of the increased costs over time is driven by actual improvements in the technology of health care, e.g., cures for cancer, more surgical options (e.g., bypass surgery and hip replacements), additional prescriptions (e.g., HAART treatments for HIV), and improved imaging. Cutler examined in detail the technological improvements in care for low birth weight babies and argues that each additional \$1 spent produces \$5 of derived benefit. This raises an important point: we need to realize that often improvements in medical technology translate into increased costs. Part of the increased costs in the USA may be due to the increased technology developed and used in the USA. Some improvements are very cheap (e.g., aspirin to decrease heart attacks), but these tend to be the exception. Cutler suggests that the key is not finding a lower cost health care but a more *efficient* health care system. He suggests that too much emphasis has been placed on high-cost, high-tech, medicine and not enough on lower cost, lower technology medicine which can produce this higher value proposition. But still the question remains what expenditures in the current system fail to represent good value?

Focus on Understanding Incentives and Moral Hazards in Payment Systems

Health care economists examine how reimbursement systems (e.g., direct consumer payment vs. third-party payments, prepaid capitated payments vs. fee for service insurance, various managed care arrangements, pay for performance, etc.) affect the behavior—and hence the overall costs—of consumers, providers, and third-party reimbursers. The assumption is that none of these stakeholders should be expected to behave as "economic eunuchs" but rather respond to whatever incentives and disincentives—perverse or constructive—the system contains. The supply and demand of health care is determined by these incentives. For example, prepaid capitated plans provide disincentives for health care professionals to provide care: fee for service has the opposite effect—it provides incentives to provide more care.

Wennberg et al. (2002) found that, for Medicare spending there was a twofold variation among regions, and the variations persist even after differences in health are corrected for. The study found that "higher levels of Medicare spending are due largely to increased use of supply sensitive services—physician visits, specialist consultations, and hospitalizations, particularly for those with chronic illness or in their last 6 months of life (p. 11)." Specifically, he found that the difference between lifetime Medicare spending for a typical 65-year-old Medicare recipient in Miami vs. one in Minnesota was $50,000. One of the ways health care is somewhat unique is that the supply of health care has a major role in determining the demand for health care.

"Free" care—either because it is paid by the government or because the consumer directly pays nothing and a third-party insurer pays everything—provides a huge incentive (by removing the normal disincentive of direct consumer payment) for consumers to demand a lot of care; hence the demand created by free care is often rationed by policy or by lines. More expensive care generally reduces demand, if demand is not perfectly inelastic—a point professionals may not completely understand as they argue for higher fees.

Properly aligning the incentives on all stakeholders is perhaps the key and most difficult question in health-care reform. Goldhill (2009) states:

> …I suspect that our collective search for villains—for someone to blame—has distracted us and our political leaders from addressing the fundamental cause of our nation's health-care crisis. All of the actors in health care—from doctors to insurers to pharmaceutical companies—work in a heavily regulated, massively subsidized industry full of structural distortions. They all want to serve patients well. But they also all behave rationally in response to the economic incentives those distortions create. Accidentally, but relentlessly, America has built a health-care system with incentives that inexorably generate terrible and perverse results. Incentives that emphasize health *care* over any other aspect of health and well-being. That emphasize treatment over prevention. That disguise true costs. That favor complexity, and discourage transparent competition based on price or quality. That result in a generational pyramid scheme rather than sustainable financing. And that—most important—remove consumers from our irreplaceable role as the ultimate ensurer of value (p. 40).

A major part of properly aligning incentives in the health care system is to ask basic questions about the proper role of health care insurance. No one has asked more probing questions about this topic than the late Nobel laureate, Milton Friedman. First, Friedman (2001) suggested that the health care system is distorted by the fact that most individuals receive health-care insurance from their employers. Interestingly this happened due to a historical accident: During WWII there were federal wage and price controls so that employers could not attract employees by higher wages. However employers could offer benefit packages as the government did not prohibit this. So employers offered health insurance and the government decided not to tax this (this is often criticized as it is also regressive taxation—the relatively wealthier are more likely to have a job with health care benefits than the poor, and thus more of the relatively wealthy avoid taxes on this income, while the poor do not). Friedman pointed out that the employer paying for health care distorts usual market mechanisms as the employee is not shopping with their own dollars.

What health care expenses ought to be insured? According to Friedman (2001), part of the concern is that the current system is too insurance centric. Insurance is generally regarded as reasonable for expenditures that are rare but are not affordable (a $200,000 house burning down or tens or hundreds of thousands of dollars for some cancer treatments, for example). Friedman has long argued that we spend other people's money (i.e., the third-party insurer's) differently than we spend our own. Thus, third-party payments for expenses we can actually afford (but would like to not pay directly) are considered moral hazards as they distort normal consumer spending. As Goldhill (2009) has stated it, " we can't imagine paying for gas with our auto-insurance policy, or for our electric bills with our homeowners insurance, but we all assume that our regular checkups and dental cleanings will be covered at least partially by insurance" (p. 42). This gives rise to the saying, "If you are concerned with how much healthcare costs now, just wait until it is free." Price is a mechanism for rationing. Insurers in benefit design use co-pays and deductibles to disincent and incent consumer demand. Followers of Friedman's arguments argue for the use of medical savings accounts—tax free accounts that can only be used for medical expenses and that can roll over each year—so that consumers experience the normal disincentive of price for their first few thousand of their health care purchases.

Psychology's Role in Health Care Reform

The final section will discuss new opportunities for psychologists arising from the recent health care reform bill and ten suggested major reforms for the health care system. Psychology has the potential to be a major player in health care reform given the large and diverse roles that behavioral pathways play in medical presentations (Cucciare & O'Donohue, 2003). However, to take on this role, and not to be relegated to the sidelines, psychology needs to reform itself. It can no longer be business as usual.

The Patient Protection and Affordable Care Act: What Does It Mean for Psychology?

The American Psychological Association's Public Interest Government Relations Office (2010) reviewed the 2,400 pages of the Patient Protection and Affordable Care Act and found numerous legislative provisions that are favorable for the field of psychology. The provisions sited focused on increasing integrated health care and mental and behavioral health parity, enhancing prevention and wellness, developing the psychology workforce, elimination of health disparities support for psychological research, and increasing involvement with consumers, families, and caregivers (APA, 2010). Table 1 highlights several key provisions.

Ten Key Reforms

There are 10 key reforms (see Table 2); eight of these can be seen as nested under the first and most general reform: a systematic and thorough adoption of quality improvement philosophies and technology. These reforms will expand psychology's role in health care but should produce a more efficient overall health care system with reduced total costs.

Reform 1: A systematic adoption of quality improvement philosophy and technology

According to a 2001 report by the Institute of Medicine, Crossing the Quality Chasm, "health care today harms too frequently and routinely fails to deliver its potential benefits" (p.1). There is a significant amount of variance across practitioners and settings in diagnosis and treatment. The IOM report suggested that approximately 90,000 Americans die each year due to medical errors. As an example, it is now understood that "paper kills." Health records continue to be mostly handwritten, poorly organized, and difficult to retrieve making it challenging to manage multiple illnesses and treatments (IOM, 2001).

Table 1 Patient protection and affordable care act: key provisions for psychology

Integrated health care: • Grants to establish community-based integrated care to support primary care (members may include behavioral and mental health professionals) • Grants to colocate primary and specialty care • Grants to support community-based collaborative care networks
Mental and behavioral health care: • Mental health, substance abuse, and behavioral health treatment are included in the essential benefits package that plans must provide • Federal and mental health parity law shall apply to qualified health plans, health insurance issuers, and group health plans • Eligibility rules for group or individual health insurance coverage may not be based on any of the following: health status, medical condition (mental and physical), claims experience, receipt of health care, genetic information, evidence of insurability or disability
Prevention and wellness: • Provides a fund for an expanded and sustained national investment in prevention and public health programs • Grants for the implementation, evaluation, and dissemination of evidence-based community preventive health activities • Provides coverage for annual wellness visits that include a personalized prevention plan with a health risk assessment • Provides incentives for individuals participating in comprehensive, evidence-based programs focused on the prevention of chronic diseases through lifestyle changes. The program may also address co-morbidities such as depression • Grants for school-based health centers providing comprehensive primary health services including mental health services • Grants to establish national centers of excellence for depression and continue research on postpartum depression • Authorize a task force to review the scientific evidence related to the effectiveness, appropriateness, and cost-effectiveness of clinical and community preventive services • Authorizes a national strategy to improve the delivery of health care services, patient health outcomes and population health
Psychology workforce development: • Grants for mental and behavioral health education • Funding for geriatric education and training • Loan repayment program for qualified health professionals, including psychologists, providing pediatric care
Elimination of health disparities: • Mandates increased data collection and analysis of federally conducted or supported health care or public health program to increase understanding of health disparities
Support for psychological research • Authorizes the establishment of a private, nonprofit corporation to assist patients, clinicians, purchasers, and policy makers in making informed health decisions
Involvement with consumers, families, and caregivers: • Establishes a new national insurance program to increase community living assistance services and supports • Expands funding for state aging and disability resource centers • Provides incentives for states to offer home- and community-based services as long-term care alternatives to nursing homes

Quality improvement techniques can be a transformative technology: e.g., it transformed Japan from a producer of inferior goods to the second largest economy in the world. Computers, electronics, and retail shopping have been reformed to bring better value and exceed customer's expectations. QI is a meta-strategy that has the enormous potential to overcome long-standing and rather stale debates in our field, yet psychology has been slow to adopt QI (O'Donohue & Fisher, 2006). Continuously measuring outcomes such as consumer satisfaction would determine which therapies to practice. QI initiatives could resolve the debate over the generalizability and level of proof for efficacy and effectiveness studies through the

Table 2 Ten key reforms

1.	A systematic adoption of quality improvement philosophy and technology
2.	An increase in a consumer-centric orientation towards health care
3.	Increased development of a health system, not just a sickness system
4.	The adoption of evidence-based assessment and treatment
5.	An immediate adoption of key information technology such as electronic medical records, clinical decision tools, and e-health
6.	A systematic improvement in management and business education and practices
7.	An increased focus on the demonstration of integrated care delivery systems, including those that focus on the high medical utilizer
8.	An examination of the viability of alternative payment mechanisms which have fewer moral hazards and more rational incentives, including pay for performance
9.	Becoming developmentally aware, with a renewed focus on the health needs of adolescents and the elderly
10.	An increased focus on the sophistication of outcome studies of psychological interventions so that they show more relevant dimensions

use of continuous feedback on clinical outcomes and consumer satisfaction ratings. We need to understand how we can constantly increase our value proposition—e.g., making our services less expensive and more impactful. Look at the example of Moore's law in the computer industry where every 3 years computing power doubles and prices are halved.

The medical field is far ahead of behavioral health in the area of quality control (Pelonero & Johnson, 2007). Medicine is systematically embracing quality improvement philosophy and technology to reduce errors, create more efficient delivery systems, and increase consumer satisfaction. Psychology must reform itself by adopting the QI orientation of exceeding our customer's expectations. Psychology's motto should be similar to Honda's, "our customer's are satisfied because we never are." We suggest that the following seven reforms are highly related to quality improvement and can be seen as nested within this meta-strategy:

Reform 2: An increase in a consumer-centric orientation towards health care

As psychologists, we need to understand more clearly what our customers want—all our customers (i.e., employers, insurers, clients). A consumer-centric orientation to health care should be based, as the Institute of Medicine (2001) suggests, a continuous healing relationship where the care is customized to patient needs and values, and clinics cooperate to increase the quality and continuity of care. A system where consumers can take responsibility for their own health and health care is vital to this orientation, but for it to work knowledge and information needs to be easily accessible. We need to produce tools to increase consumer responsibility, such as transparent report cards that allow consumers to make intelligent choices between health-care alternatives.

Reform 3: Increased development of a health system, not just a sickness system

A priority should be to develop tools to keep individuals healthy instead of tools to help them restore health after they have been ill. There are basic questions about what is psychological health and what can be done to foster this. Positive psychology is a notable movement in this reform (Seligman, Steen, Park, & Peterson, 2005), but there is certainly room for the development and demonstration of other tools.

Psychologists are also in a position to address concerns beyond those of psychological health. As mentioned earlier in the chapter, chronic diseases account for 7 out of 10 deaths in the USA. Many of these chronic conditions are attributed to unhealthy behaviors such as smoking, lack of exercise, and improper diets. Despite public attempts to change these behaviors, 1 in 5 Americans still smokes, with lung cancer being the leading cause of cancer death, and 1 in 3 adults is obese, while 1 in 3 adults does not meet recommendations for aerobic physical activity (Centers for Disease Control and Prevention, 2010). To ensure the development of a health system would also entail developing tools that promote healthy behaviors (exercise, diet, smoking cessation), and developing contingencies would maintain these behaviors. Unfortunately, the broad attempts to prevent many of these behavioral issues have had mixed results due to the difficult nature of pinpointing the mechanism that causes these problems. Keeping in mind reform 2, psychologist, with the best interest of all customers, can be a driving force of developing a health system. We have seen for decades techniques such as self-rewarding along with tracking one's progress in regard to weight change not only leads to an immediate loss in weight, but individuals were more likely to maintain these loses at a 4-month follow-up (Mahoney, Moura, & Wade, 1973). A reduction of 5–15 % of an overweight or obese individual's weight can reduce the risk factors of many of the chronic diseases associated with being overweight (Zelman, 2011).

This being said, for these treatments to be effective, a change in the system as a whole is required as regards how one pays for service, incentives for remaining healthy on the clients part, and incentives for keeping clients healthy on the clinicians part.

Reform 4: The adoption of evidence-based assessment and treatment

Behavioral health fails to systematically apply evidence-based treatments and assess outcomes. Medicine is attempting multiple avenues to eliminate medical errors; while in psychology due to long-standing arguments about fundamentals it is difficult to define and identify psychological error (O'Donohue & Engle, in preparation). If no professional act is mistaken, what then is our expertise?

Psychotherapy has what economists call a "lemon problem": the lemons drive down the price of competent clinical services. Psychology has been slowly working towards creating formal treatment guidelines. The 1994 task force appointed by the Society for Clinical Psychology (Division 12) of the APA developed a set of criteria for empirically supported treatments (Chambless et al., 1996; Task Force, 1995). Unfortunately there is resistance towards adoption of ESTs at many levels, including the graduate training level (Horan & Blanchard, 2001; Weissman et al, 2006). Currently there is a widespread lack of incentives for mental health practitioners to align their practices with national quality improvement standards (see O'Donohue & Fisher, 2006 for a further discussion of these issues).

This movement is much less controversial in medicine. Evidence-based reforms have been shown to save millions of dollars, to increase customer satisfaction, and to decrease medical errors (James & Savitz, 2011). The success of these reforms in physical medicine has placed health care decision makers in a position to insist upon evidence-based practice.

It is important to note that even though the medical field has much better at implementing evidence-based care, it also has problems. As pointed out by the IOM (2001), it takes about 17 years for new knowledge from RCTs to be incorporated in general practice. Since the implementation of new and cutting-edge methods of delivering better care provides not only more effective but more efficient care ((James & Savitz, 2011), it is important that psychology quickly adapts its' practices on all levels, from graduate training to delivery of care. The persistence of psychologist to allow for assessments and therapies that are not based from empirical evidence will further marginalize psychology in the health care system.

Reform 5: An immediate adoption of key information technology

Currently, only around 2 % of the health care budget is consumed by information technology-related activities (Hauser & Johnston, 2008). The Institute of Medicine (2001) has called for the construction of an information infrastructure to support health care delivery, consumer health information, quality measurement and improvement, public accountability, clinical and health services research, and clinical education. A number of barriers stand in the way to this development but one place to start is with electronic medical records.

Medical records, which have historically been handwritten and hard to transport, need to be accessible and up to date in order to provide the best quality of care to all patients. Electronic medical records (EMRs) that are easily accessible, yet protect patients' health care confidentiality, would greatly decrease medical errors and health care professionals' time. Less than a quarter of physicians in the United States use any form of EMRs and the number is far lower for behavioral health providers (Hauser & Johnston, 2008). European countries are markedly ahead of the US system with some countries having 100 % use of electronic medical records.

The largest system in the United States is the one currently used throughout the Veterans Affairs System. In a recent analysis of the impact of implementing a comprehensive electronic health record system on ambulatory care use in the Kaiser Permanente health care delivery system (more than 225,000 members), Chen et al. (2009) found significant effects. The total office visit rate decreased 25.3 % and the specialty care office visit rate decreased by 21.5 %. Scheduled telephone calls and secure e-mail messaging increased eightfold and sixfold, respectively. The authors conclude that "introducing an electronic health record creates operational efficiencies by offering nontraditional, patient-centered ways of providing care" (p. 323).

A principle of quality improvement is that it is management's principal job to make sure that workers have the right tools to be most productive and to produce at the highest quality (Deming, 1986). We need to realize that incomplete written records impair productivity, that lack of decision support tools decreases quality, and that e-health options can provide lower cost treatment to those with access problems. Decision tools need to help make practice "knowledge intense," instead of knowledge disconnected.

Reform 6: A systematic improvement in management and business education and practices

There is a management crisis in behavioral health. As a profession, we do not have a traditionally educated management class as in most other fields. Managers are usually psychologists who have been there the longest or who for whatever reasons are attracted to the tasks. However, the dilettantish approach to management in our profession has produced a lack of real leadership and a lack of the ability to run a successful business (e.g., financial management), and generally hampered the progress of the application of psychology to applied problems. Health care has industrialized but we still take a "mom-and-pop" approach to our business. We need education and commitment to education and training in management, business, and entrepreneurship (see Cummings & O'Donohue, 2008).

While management course are not taught in other health care professions, such as medicine or dentistry, the model of service delivery is distinctly different from that of most mental health professionals. For example, when one goes to the dentist, they do not expect to get their teeth cleaned by the dentist themselves. Rather, the dentist comes in briefly to double-check the work, and finishes any work that may require their expertise, such as a filling. In the dentist example, they may have a client cancel their appointment, but are still being productive due to the other clients that are booked in the same hour. In the case of psychologist, if a client cancels a session shortly before the session occurs, that hour is completely lost in regard to productivity. Therefore, the notion of seeing one client for a 50-min session is not a sustainable course of action in improving mental health.

A very clear example of where psychologist have been able to make a profound impact by moving away from this 50-min session, once a week model has been with the treatment of autism. Autism costs society about $35 billion a year, with the average cost per individual being at about $3.2 million over their lifetime (Datz, 2006). However, providing intensive behavioral therapy at a very young age can usually help almost 50 % of those children succeed in regular education classrooms (Sallows & Graupner, 2005). To do this, it only takes one board-certified behavior analyst (B.C.B.A) and teams of "tutors" that consist of individuals with a wide range of education (high school students to graduate students). By engaging in this model, the professional in this case, the B.C.B.A, can provide useful, effective, and empirically supported treatment to many individuals at once and does not lose much productivity if one client cancels, and if a tutor cannot make a session for some reason, another can replace them. Until the whole of psychology adopts a model of treatment delivery similar to that of the dentist or the B.C.B.A, it is imperative that psychologist understand management practices that will make them more productive in providing services.

Reform 7: An increased focus on the demonstration of integrated care delivery systems

This reform is probably the one that has been best adopted to date as consumers seem to like "one-stop shopping." In a meta-analytic review of the impact of psychological interventions on medical cost offset, Chiles et al. (1999) found a significant broad cost-offset effect for individuals with a mental health diagnosis. The effect was greatest for behavioral medicine interventions to treat surgical inpatients and psychoeducation interventions. Results indicated that the average treatment group exhibited a reduction in utilization across all dependent variables by 15.7 %. This result is significant when compared to the 12.3 % increase in service utilization observed in the control group. It appeared as though the cost-offset was larger for older adult participants, although it was difficult to draw clear conclusions due to methodological issues. Katzelnick et al. (1997, 2000) found that an integrated approach to treating depression in medical "high utilizers" within primary care settings enhanced quality of life, work productivity, and improved depression symptoms as well as lowering health care expenditures. In a review of the cost-effectiveness of behavioral health services in medical settings, Blount et al. (2007) determined that the greatest opportunity for potential savings is through better identification and treatment of the behavioral health needs that patients bring to their primary care physicians via a multidisciplinary collaborative care. The examination of cost-offset in integrated systems has led to mixed results with some researchers finding that providing mental health treatment does not reduce medical costs (Bickman, 1996; Carbone et al., 2000). A closer examination of the effectiveness of the services provided would enhance the discussion and clarify the potential benefits of an integrated system.

There are literally billions of dollars in potential revenue for psychologists if medical cost-offset savings can be demonstrated. Cummings (1994) for example, in a randomly controlled study of high medical utilizers from a sample of 123,000 Medicaid recipients and federal workers on Oahu, reduced medical utilization 40 % within 18 months. Cummings found that the vast majority of the high medical utilizers suffered from chronic medical conditions, such as diabetes, asthma, COPD, and chronic pain, and provided individual and group treatment that focused on these patients' psychological issues such as lifestyle, treatment compliance, social support, stress, and depression. This kind of intervention should represent a new paradigm in psychological care. The disease management industry was created in the 1980s to address the problem of the high utilizer, but it is currently experiencing major problems because its actual outcomes have generally been disappointing. Part of the problem with the outcomes is that they have relied on less clinically intensive interventions than Cummings such as nurse telephonic outreach, pamphlets, and other less intensive and individualized interventions.

Reform 8: An examination of the viability of alternative payment mechanisms

The use of pay-for-performance health care programs has increased in the past decade with the primary goal of providing incentives to practitioners who deliver safe, effective, evidence-based health care. The medical field is far ahead of behavioral health, yet has had mixed results. A recent assessment of the California Integrated

Healthcare Association's pay-for-performance program found that after 3 years breakthrough quality improvements had not occurred (Damberg, Raube, Teleki, & dela Cruz, 2009).

On the behavioral health side, Anthem Blue Cross Blue Shield implemented a pay-for-performance program in 1999 with the goals of improving the quality of care, recognizing the practitioners who provide higher-quality care, demonstrating the value of behavior health services to providers, and helping providers align their practices with national standards (Pelonero & Johnson, 2007). Preliminary results have shown a higher quality of care. A future goal of the program is to provide consumers with data on provider quality to inform their treatment decisions. The authors described several challenges of implementing the pay-for-performance program in a behavioral health setting, including how to decide what outcome measures to use and how to avoid overly burdensome data collection.

Reform 9: Becoming developmentally aware, with a renewed focus on the health needs of adolescents and the elderly

It is imperative that the health care needs of specific age groups have a renewed focus. Specifically, prevention of disability and promotion of effective health behaviors must be targeted in adolescence in order to reduce health care spending as each cohort ages. Health care spending on the elderly is extremely costly (as specified below) and health behavior in adolescence can play a role in curtailing this spending.

The first baby boomer cohort turned 65 in the year 2011 and the last will turn 65 in 2029. During this time period the United States will be confronted with the greatest incidence of age-related health problems in history (APA, 2008). The cost of providing health care for an older American is three to five times greater than the cost for someone younger than 65. In recent decades, older adults' health care expenditures have outpaced the growth of the GDP by 3.5–4.0 % (Fuchs, 1998). Projections based on trends of the past two decades reveal that by the year 2020, older adults health care consumption will reach $25,000 annually, compared with $9,200 in 1995 (Fuchs, 1999). As a result, by 2030, the nation's health care spending is projected to increase by 25 % (CDC, 2009). Based on these projections, there is a strong economic incentive for action.

One large factor effecting health care costs is that individuals are living longer than ever. The average life expectancy at birth has increased from 70.2 years between 1960 and 1962 to an average of 77.7 years between 2003 and 2005 (OECD, 2009). The last two or three decades of life, although obviously a great boon, are very expensive medically. According to a study by Jacobzone (2000) the total number of disabled older people in the United States will increase by 15.4 % if past trends in disability continue and 38.3 % if age-specific rates of disability and institutionalization are held constant. One unintended consequence of universal health care is that it is regressive: i.e., it transfers money from the relatively healthy but poorer young to the relatively richer and less healthy elderly.

A vast strain on the health care system will be caused by the rapid increase in the number of individuals with Alzheimer's disease (AD) and other forms of dementia. According to a report by the Alzheimer's Association (2008), there are currently more than 5.2 million Americans with AD, and projections suggest that by the year 2050 the prevalence rate will increase to 11–16 million Americans. As the majority of individuals with AD are over the age of 65, Medicare picks up the bill for the high rates of hospital stays and other health care services associated with individuals with AD. Medicaid too is affected, due to the high costs of nursing home and long-term care services for older adults with low income. With the population aging, spending on care for individuals with AD will rapidly rise over the next decade (See Fig. 7).

Much of the health care increase that will occur in the next decade due to the increase in the elderly population is unavoidable. However, targeting adolescents may provide an avenue to not only reduce future health care cost in late life, but will also lead to improvement of overall quality of life across the lifespan.

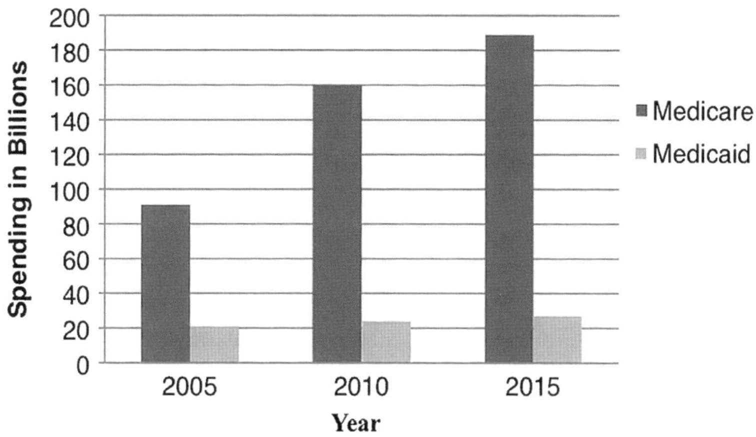

Fig. 7 Projected direct costs for Alzheimer's disease care (Alzheimer's Association, 2008)

As previously mentioned, the rates of disabled older adults are continuing to rise. Along with an increased lifespan, the final years of life may be hindered due to the disability. However, while the likelihood of disability increases with age, there is promising data in regard to decreasing the likelihood of this happening. Longitudinal studies that compare individuals who do or do not engage in healthy behaviors (i.e., daily exercise, nonsmokers, healthy diet) suggest that those who engage in healthy behaviors not only will have life longer than their counterparts but will spend less years of their lives suffering from a disability (Fries, Bruce, & Chakravarty, 2011).

Due to the fact that adolescence is a time where behavioral patterns are set that maintain throughout an individual's life, promotion of these healthy behaviors is imperative (O'Donohue & Tolle, 2009). Adolescence is also a time when an individual begins to take more responsibility for their health behaviors (as opposed to caregivers bearing the bulk of the responsibility) (O'Donohue & Tolle, 2009). The promotion of these behaviors does entail initial capital costs. Programs that promote and provide incentives to adolescents and their health care providers may increase health care costs initially, but if successful in reducing disability and morbidity it would greatly reduce costs in later life, reduce health care costs overall, and improve quality of life throughout one's lifetime.

Reform 10: An increased focus on the sophistication of outcome studies of psychological interventions so that these include measures of satisfaction, safety, efficiency, functioning, and medical cost offset

The standard efficacy or effectiveness study in psychotherapy typically contains several clinical outcome measures but few measures of cost, no measures of overall medical costs, and few measures of functional change. Employers, who pay about 50 % of all health care costs, care about functioning: is the employee absent less and when they come to work are they productive? Insurers care about overall medical cost reductions (found for example in the integrated care studies cited above) as well as efficient psychotherapy. In the future we suggest that psychotherapy outcome studies should include these measures so that the business case and the value proposition as well as the clinical efficacy of the intervention can be evaluated. Including these measures will go a long way to making the case for decision makers for the increased adoption of the therapy.

With the field of psychology beginning to emphasize mediating and moderating variables of psychopathology (Kazdin, 2007), researchers have a perfect opportunity to examine these proposed measures. While it has been stated that there is a "dodo bird" effect and all psychotherapies work equal well (Luborskey, et al., 2002), these studies have not looked at more sophisticated measures like the ones proposed here. It would provide a quite different picture for what kind of therapy one would engage in if two treatments are equally effective at reducing symptoms, but one helps the individual be more effective in areas such as work or their social domain.

References

Alzheimer's Association. (2008). Alzheimer's disease facts and figures. *Alzheimer's & Dementia, 4*(2), 1–41.

American Psychological Association. (2010). *Healthcare reform legislation: Key provisions of interest to psychology*. Retrieved from www.apa.org/health-reform/pdf/key-provisions.pdf.

American Psychological Association, Presidential Task Force on Integrated Health Care for an Aging Population. (2008). *Blueprint for change: Achieving integrated health care for an aging population*. Washington, DC: American Psychological Association.

Angrisano, C., Farrell, D., Kocher, B., Laboissiere, M., & Parker, S. (2007). *Accounting for the cost in the United States*. Retrieved April 13, 2009, from McKinsey & Company website: http://www.mckinsey.com/mgi/reports/pdfs/healthcare/MGI_US_HC_synthesis.pdf.

Bickman, L. (1996). A continuum of care: More is not always better. *American Psychologist, 51*, 689–701.

Bibbins-Domingo, K., Coxson, P., Pletcher, M. J., Lightwood, J., & Goldman, L. (2007). Adolescent overweight and future coronary heart disease. *The New England Journal of Medicine, 357*(23), 2371–2379.

Blount, A., Schoenbaum, R., Kathol, R., Rollman, B. L., Thomas, M., O'Donohue, W., et al. (2007). *Professional Psychology: Research and Practice, 38*, 290–297.

Carbone, L., Barsky, A., Orav, E., Fife, A., Fricchione, G., Minden, S., et al. (2000). Psychiatric symptoms and medical utilization in primary care patients. *Psychometrics, 41*, 512–518.

Carey, C., Herring, B., & Lenain, P. (2009). *Health care reform in the United States: Economics department working paper no. 665*. Retrieved May 10, 2009, from Organisation for Economic Co-Operation and Development website: http://www.olis.oecd.org.

Catalano, R. F., Fagan, A. A., Gavin, L. E., Greenberg, M. T., Irwin, C. T., Ross, D. A., et al. (2012). Worldwide application of prevention science in adolescent health. *Lancet, 379*(9826), 1653–1664.

Center on Budget and Policy Priorities. (2012). *Policy basics: Where do our federal tax dollars go?* Retrieved from http://www.cbpp.org/cms/index.cfm?fa=view&id=1258.

Centers for Disease Control and Prevention. (2003). Public health and aging: trends in aging—United States and worldwide. *Morbidity and Mortality Weekly Report, 52*(06), 101–106.

Centers for Disease Control. (2012, February 14). *Youth and tobacco use*. Retrieved from Smoking and Tobacco Use: http://www.cdc.gov/tobacco/data_statistics/fact_sheets/youth_data/tobacco_use/index.htm.

Center for Disease Control. (2009). *Chronic diseases: The power to prevent, the call to control: At a glance 2009*. Retrieved June 3, 2010, from http://www.cdc.gov/chronicdisease/resources/publications/AAG/chronic.htm.

Centers for Disease Control. (2011a, November 1). *Smoking and tobacco use*. Retrieved from Centers for Disease Control and Prevention: http://www.cdc.gov/tobacco/data_statistics/surveys/nyts/index.htm.

Centers for Disease Control. (2011b, September 15). *Adolescent and school health*. Retrieved from Centers for Disease Control and Prevention: http://www.cdc.gov/HealthyYouth/obesity/facts.htm

Childstats.gov. (2011). *Adolescent depression*. Retrieved from Childstats.gov: http://www.childstats.gov/americaschildren/health4.asp.

Centers for Disease Control and Prevention. (2010, July 7). *Chronic disease prevention and health promotion*. Retrieved April 2012, from Centers for Disease Control and Prevention: http://www.cdc.gov/chronicdisease/overview/index.htm.

Centers for Disease Control and Prevention. (2011). *Adolescent health*. Retrieved from Adolescent and School Health.

Centers for Medicare & Medicaid Services. (2008). *Historical data on national health expenditure data*. Retrieved from http://www.cms.gov/NationalHealthExpendData/02_NationalHealthAccountsHistorical.asp#TopOfPage.

Centers for Medicare & Medicaid Services. (2009). *National health expenditure data*. Retrieved April 12, 2009, from the Centers for Medicare & Medicaid Services website: http://www.cms.hhs.gov/NationalHealthExpendData/downloads/tables.pdf.

Chambless, D. L., Sanderson, W. C., Shoham, V., Johnson, S. B., Pope, K. S., Crits-Christoph, P., et al. (1996). An update on empirically validated therapies. *The Clinical Psychologist, 49*, 5–18.

Chen, C., Garrido, T., Chock, D., Okawa, G., & Liang, L. (2009). The Kaiser Permanente electronic health record: Transforming and streamlining modalities of care. *Health Affairs, 28*(2), 323–333.

Chiles, J. A., Lambert, M. J., & Hatch, A. L. (1999). The impact of psychological interventions on medical cost offset: A meta-analytic review. *Clinical Psychology: Science and Practice, 6*, 202–220.

Ciechanowski, P. S., Katon, W. J., & Russo, J. E. (2000). Depression and diabetes: Impact of depressive symptoms on adherence, function, and costs. *Archives of Internal Medicine, 160*, 3278–3285.

Colton, C. W., & Manderscheid, R. W. (2006). Congruencies in increased mortality rates, years of potential life lost, and causes of death among public mental health clients in eight states. *Preventing Chronic Disease, 3*, A42.

Congressional Budget Office. (2010). *Letter to the Honorable Harry Reid regarding the update estimate of budgetary impact of the Patient Protection and Affordable Care Act. (March 11, 2010).* Retrieved from http://www.cbo.gov/doc.cfm?index=11307&zzz=40511.

Congressional Budget Office. (2008). *Budget options volume I: Health care*. (Publication # 3185) Retrieved from http://www.cbo.gov/ftpdocs/99xx/doc9925/12-18-HealthOptions.pdf.

Cucciare, M. A., & O'Donohue, W. T. (2003). Integrated care and the high utilizer: An explication of medical usage patterns and the role in the healthcare crisis. In N. A. Cummings, W. T. O'Donohue, & K. E. Ferguson (Eds.), *Behavioral health as primary care: Beyond efficacy to effectiveness*. Reno, NV: Context Press.

Cummings, N. A. (1994). The successful application of a medical offset in program planning and delivery. *Managed Care Quarterly, 2*(2), 1–6.

Cummings, N. A., & O'Donohue, W. T. (2008). *Eleven blunders that cripple psychotherapy in America: A remedial unblundering*. New York: Routledge (Taylor and Francis Group).

Cunningham, P., Artiga, S., & Schwartz, K. (2008). *The fraying link between work and health insurance: Trends in employer-sponsored insurance for employees, 2000–2007*. (Report #7840). Retrieved from http://www.kff.org/uninsured/upload/7840.pdf.

Cutler, D. (2005). *Your money or your life: Strong medicine for America's healthcare system*. Oxford: Oxford University Press.

Damberg, C. L., Raube, K., Teleki, S. S., & dela Cruz, E. (2009). Taking stock of pay-for-performance: A candid assessment from the front lines. *Health Affairs, 28*(2), 517–527.

Danzon, P. M., & Furakawa, M. F. (2008). International prices and availability of pharmaceuticals in 2005. *Health Affairs, 27*(1), 221–233.

Datz, T. (2006). *Autism Has High Costs to US Society*. Cambridge: Harvard School of Public Health.

Delamater, A. M., Jacquez, F., & Patino-Fernandez, A. M. (2009). Type 2 diabetes in youth. In W. T. O'Donohue & L. W. Tolle (Eds.), *Behavioral approaches to chronic disease in adolescence: A guide to integrative care*. New York, NY: Springer.

Deming, W. E. (1986). *Out of Crisis*. Cambridge, MA: The W. Edwards Deming Institute.

DeVol, R., & Bedroussian, A. (2007). *An unhealthy America: The economic burden of chronic disease charting a new course to save lives and increase productivity and economic growth*. Retrieved April 1, 2009, from the Milken Institute website: http://www.milkeninstitute. org/pdf/chronic_disease_report.pdf.

DiMatteo, M. R., Lepper, H. S., & Croghan, T. W. (2000). Depression is a risk factor for noncompliance with medical treatment. *Archives of Internal Medicine, 160*, 2101–2108.

Friedman, M. (2001). *How to cure healthcare*. Retrieved December 9, 2009, from Hoover Digest website: http://www.hoover.org/publications/digest/3459466.html.

Fries, J. F., Bruce, B., Chakravarty, E. (2011). Compression of morbidity 1980–2011: A focused review of paradigms and process. *Journal of Aging Research 2011*, Article ID 261702.

Fuchs, V.R. (1998). Provide, provide: The economics of aging. *National Bureau of Economic Research*, Working Paper No. 6642.

Fuchs, V. R. (1999). Health care for the elderly: How much? Who will pay for it? *Health Affairs, 18*, 11–21.

Gilmer, T. P., O'Connor, P. J., Rush, W. A., Crain, A. L., Whitebird, R. R., Hanson, A. M., & Solberg, L. I. (2005). Predictors of health care costs in adults with diabetes. *Diabetes Care, 28*(1), 59–64.

Goldhill, D. (2009, September). How American health care killed my father. *Atlantic Monthly*.

Goodman, E., & Whitaker, R. (2002). A prospective study of the role of depression in the development and persistence of adolescent obesity. *Pediatrics, 109*, 497–506.

Gruber, J. (2008). *Covering the uninsured in the US Working Paper 13758*. Retrieved June 1, 2009, from the National Bureau of Economic Research website: http://www.nber.org/papers/w13758.

Health People.gov. (2012, February 8). *2020 topics & objectives*. Retrieved from Adolescent Health.

Hauser, S. L., & Johnston, S. C. (2008). Electronic medical records: Does it take a village of a thousand points of light? *Annals of Neurology, 63*(4), A13–A14.

Himelhoch, S., Weller, W. E., Wu, A. W., Anderson, G. F., & Cooper, L. A. (2004). Chronic medical illness, depression, and use of acute medical services among Medicare beneficiaries. *Medical care, 42*(6), 512–521.

Himmelstein, D. U., Thorne, D., Warren, E., & Woolhandler, S. (2009). Medical bankruptcy in the United States, 2007: Results of a national study. *American Journal of Medicine, 122*(8), 741–746.

Horan, W. P., & Blanchard, J. J. (2001). Training opportunities in empirically supported treatments and their relationship to intern recruitment and post-internship placement: A survey of directors of internship training. *Clinical Science*, 1–10.

Insel, T. (2008). Assessing the economic costs of serious mental illness. *The American Journal of Psychiatry, 165*(6), 663–665.

Institute of Medicine. (2001). *Crossing the quality chasm: A new health system for the 21st Century*. Washington, DC: National Academy Press.

James, B. C., & Savitz, L. A. (2011). How Intermountain trimmed health care costs through robust quality improvement efforts. *Health Affairs, 30*(6), 1185–1191.

Jacobzone, S. (2000). Coping with aging: International challenges. *Health Affairs, 19*(3), 213–225.

Johnson, T. (2010). *Healthcare costs and US competitiveness*. (Publication 13325). Retrieved from http://www.cfr.org/publication/13325/.

Katzelnick, D. J., Kobak, K. A., Greist, J. H., Jefferson, J. W., & Henk, H. J. (1997). Effect of primary care treatment of depression on service use by patients with high medical expenditures. *Psychiatric Services, 48*, 59–64.

Katzelnick, D. J., Simon, G. E., Pearson, S. D., Manning, W. G., Helstad, C. P., Henk, H. J., et al. (2000). Randomized trial of a depression management program in high utilizers of medical care. *Archives of Family Medicine, 9*, 345–351.

Katon, W. J. (2003). Clinical and health services relationships between major depression, depressive symptoms, and general medical illness. *Biological psychiatry, 54*(3), 216–226.

Kazdin, A. E. (2007). Mediators and mechanisms of change in psychotherapy research. *Annu. Rev. Clin. Psychol., 3,* 1–27.

Keehan, S., Sisko, A., Truffer, C., Smith, S., Cowan, C., Polsal, J., et al. (2008). Health spending projections through 2017. *Health Affairs Web Exclusive*, w145–w155.

Kessler, R. C., Heeringa, S., Lakoma, M. D., Petukhova, M., Rupp, A. E., Schoenbaum, M., ... & Zaslavsky, A. M. (2008). The individual-level and societal-level effects of mental disorders on earnings in the United States: Results from the National Comorbidity Survey Replication. *The American journal of psychiatry, 165*(6), 703.

Klein, J. D., Shone, L. P., Szilagyi, P. G., Bajorska, A., & Wilson, K. (2007). Impact of the State Children's Health Insurance Program on Adolescents in New York. *Pediatrics, 119*(4), 885–892.

Labonte, M., & Makinen, M. (2000). *Paying off the national debt: Some intergenerational consequences. CRS Report for congress.* Retrieved from the CRS Web, Order Number RS20654.

LaGreca, A. M., & Mackey, E. R. (2009). Type 1 diabetes mellitus. In W. T. O'Donohue & L. W. Tolle (Eds.), *Behavioral approaches to chronic disease in adolescence: A guide to integrative care*. New York, NY: Springer.

Lowenstein, R. (2009). *The quality cure? The New York Times Magazine*, March 13, 2005.

Luborskey, L., Rosenthal, R., Diguer, L., Andrusyna, T. P., Berman, J. S., Levitt, J. T., et al. (2002). The Dodo bird verdict is alive and well-mostly. *Clincal Psychology; Science and Practice, 9*(1), 2–12.

Mackay, J., & Mensah, G. (2004). *The atlas of heart disease and stroke*. Retrieved December 10, 2009, from the World Health Organization website: http://www.who.int/cardiovascular_diseases/resources/atlas/en.

Mahoney, M. J., Moura, N. G., & Wade, T. C. (1973). Relative efficacy of self-reward, self-punishment, and self-monitoring techniques for weight loss. *Journal of Consulting and Clinical Psychology, 40*(3), 404–407.

Mark, T., Levit, K., Coffey, R., McKusick, D., Harwood, H., King, E., et al. (2007). *National expenditures for mental health services and substance abuse treatment, 1999–2003*. Rockville, MD: Substance Abuse and Mental Health Services Administration.

McDonald, M., Hertz, R. P., Lustik, M. B., & Unger, A. N. (2005). Healthcare spending among community-dwelling adults with schizophrenia. *The American Journal of Managed Care, 11*(8), S242–S247.

Mokdad, A. H., Marks, J. S., Stroup, D. F., & Gerberding, J. L. (2004). Actual causes of death in the United States, 2000. *Journal of the American Medical Association, 291*(10), 1238–1245.

Mulye, T. P., Park, M. J., Nelson, C. D., Adams, S. H., Irwin, C. E., & Brindis, C. D. (2009). Trends in Adolescent and Young Adult Health in the United States. *Journal of Adolescent Health, 45*(1), 8–24.

National Institute of Child Health & Human Development. (2007, May 24). *Add Health Study*. Retrieved from National Institutes of Health.

Newacheck, P. W., Park, M. J., Brindis, C. D., Biehl, M., & Irwin, C. E. (2004). Trends in Private and Public Health Insurance for Adolescents. *Journal of the American Medical Association, 291*(10), 1231–1237.

Newacheck, P. W., Wong, S. T., Galbraith, A. A., & Hung, Y. (2003). Adolescent health care expenditures: a descriptive profile. *Journal of Adolescent Health, 32*(6), 3–11.

O'Donohue, W., & Fisher, J. (2006). The role of practice guidelines in systematic quality improvement. In J. Fisher & W. O'Donohue (Eds.), *Clinician's handbook of evidence based practice guidelines*. NY: Sage.

O'Donohue, W. & Engle, J. (In preparation). Errors in psychological practice: Devising a system to promote client well-being. Professional Psychology: Research and Practice.

O'Donohue, W. T., & Tolle, L. W. (2009). Introduction: Adolescents with chronic illnesses: Issue and answers. In W. T. O'Donohue & L. W. Tolle (Eds.), *Behavioral approaches to chronic disease in adolescence: A guide to integrative care*. New York, NY: Springer.

O'Donohue, W. T., Moore, B. A., & Scott, B. J. (Eds.). (2007). *Handbook of pediatric and adolescent obesity treatment*. Routledge.

Olfson, M., Marcus, S. C., Druss, B., & Pincus, H. A. (2002). National trends in the use of outpatient psychotherapy. *The American Journal of Psychiatry, 159*(11), 1914–1920.

Olson, A. L., Gaffney, C. A., Lee, P. W., & Starr, P. (2008). Changing Adolescent Helath Behaviors: The Healthy Teens Counseling Approach. *American Journal of Preventive Medicine, 35*(5S), 359–364.

Organisation for Economic Co-Operation and Development. (2009). *OECD health data 2009: How does the United States compare*. Retrieved May 27, 2010, from the Organization for Economic Co-Operation and Development website: http://www.oecd.org/dataoecd/46/2/38980580.pdf.

Pelonero, A., & Johnson, R. (2007). A pay-for-performance program for behavioral health care practicioners. *Psychiatric Services, 58*(4), 442–444.

Rosal, M., Ockene, J., Ma, Y., Herbert, J., Merriam, P., Matthews, C., et al. (2001). Behavioral risk factors among members of a health maintenance organization. *Preventive Medicine, 33*, 586–59.

Roy-Byrne, P., Davidson, K., Kessler, R., Asmundson, G., Goodwin, R., Kubzansky, L., et al. (2008). Anxiety disorders and comorbid medical illness. *General Hospital Psychiatry, 30*, 208–225.

Sallows, G. O., & Graupner, T. D. (2005). Intensive behavioral treatment for children with Autism: Four-year outcome and predictors. *American Journal of Mental Retardation, 110*(6), 417–438.

Sawyer, S. M., Afifi, R. A., Bearinger, L. H., Blakemore, S.-J., Dick, B., Ezeh, A. C., et al. (2012). Adolescence: A foundation for future health. *Lancet, 379*(9826), 1630–1640.

Seligman, M., Steen, T., Park, N., & Peterson, C. (2005). Positive psychology progress. *American Psychologist, 60*(5), 410–421.

Stein, M. B., Cox, B. J., Afifi, T. O., Belik, S., & Sareen, J. (2006). Does co-morbid depressive illness magnify the impact of chronic physical illness? A population-based perspective. *Psychological Medicine, 36*, 587–596.

Street, B. M., & Garber, J. (2009). Adolescent depression. In W. T. O'Donohue & L. W. Tolle (Eds.), *Behavioral approaches to chronic disease in adolescence: A guide to integrative care*. New York, NY: Springer.

Strum, R. (2002). The effects of obesity, smoking, and drinking on medical problems and costs. *Health Affairs, 21*(2), 245–253.

Sullivan, P. W., Morrato, E. H., Ghushchyan, V., Wyatt, H. R., & Hill, J. O. (2005). Obesity, inactivity, and the prevalence of diabetes and diabetes-related cardiovascular comorbidities in the US, 2000–2002. *Diabetes Care, 28*(7), 1599–1603.

Szilagyi, P. G., Dick, A. W., Klein, J. D., Shone, L. P., Zwanziger, J., & McInerny, T. (2004). Improved access and quality of care after enrollment in the New York state children's health insurance program. *Pediatrics, 113*(5), 395–404.

Task Force on Promotion and Dissemination of Psychological Procedures. (1995). Training in and dissemination of empirically validated psychological treatments. *The Clinical Psychologist, 48*(1), 3–23.

Thomson Rueters. (2010). *Healthcare costs rise more than 7 percent for US employers in 2009*. Retrieved from http://factsforhealthcare.com/management/Assets/EmployerNormsBook0210_2.pdf.

Unutzer, J., Schoenbaum, M., Katon, W., Fan, M., Pincus, H. A., Hogan, D., et al. (2009). Healthcare costs associated with depression in medically ill fee-for-service Medicare participants. *Journal of American Geriatrics Society, 57*, 506–510.

Weissman, M. N., Verdeli, H., Gameroff, M., Bledsoe, S., Betts, K., Mufson, L., et al. (2006). National survey of psychotherapy training in psychiatry, psychology and social work. *Archives of General Psychiatry, 63*, 925–934.

Wennberg, J. E., Fisher, E. S., & Skinner, J. S. (2002). Geography and the debate over Medicare reform. *Health Affairs: Supplement Web Exclusives*, W96–W114.

World Health Organization. (2009). *The WHO global infobase*. Retrieved December 12, 2009, from the World Health Organization website: https://apps.who.int/infobase/report.aspx.

World Health Organization. (2012). *Health effects of smoking among young people*. Retrieved from World Health Organization: http://www.who.int/tobacco/research/youth/health_effects/en/.

Wu, E. Q., Birnbaum, H. G., Shi, L., Ball, D. E., Kessler, R. C., Moulis, M., et al. (2005). The economic burden of schizophrenia in the United States in 2002. *The Journal of Clinical Psychiatry, 66*(9), 1122–1129.

Zelman, K. (2011, October 20). *Lose weight, gain tons of benefits*. Retrieved April 2012, from WebMD: http://www.webmd.com/diet/features/lose-weight-gain-tons-of-benefits?page=3.

Zuvekas, S. H. (2003). Trends in mental health service use and spending, 1987–1997. *Health Affairs, 20*(2), 214–224.

Zuvekas, S. H. (2005). Prescription drugs and the changing patterns of treatment for mental disorders, 1996–2001. *Health Affairs, 24*(1), 195–205.

Confidentiality and Care of the Adolescent Patient

Yolanda N. Evans and David J. Breland

Background

Providing care to adolescent patients has a unique set of challenges including, but not limited to, confidentiality, age of consent, and autonomy from parents and family. There is limited research on the topic of medical errors specifically in the care of adolescent patients. In this chapter we will discuss aspects of caring for the adolescent patient that may lead to errors. Aside from medical errors common in all disciplines of medicine (such as medication error), errors that occur in adolescent care may be more frequent in the outpatient setting (as opposed to the intensive care unit or medical ward) and will likely be the result of breaches in confidentiality, occur from the omission of behavioral health counseling and preventive options (such as immunizations), or errors in minor legal consent.

The American Academy of Pediatrics (AAP) produced a policy statement in 2011 about pediatric patient safety in order to raise awareness of patient safety risks. They describe a study on errors in pediatric ambulatory care that found 147 medical errors from 14 practices. Most errors were in the form of medical treatment (37 %), with 15 % being due to errors in preventive care, including immunizations. Among medical treatment errors, 85 % were due to medication errors with 55 % of those being related to medication ordering (Steering Committee on Quality Improvement and Management and Committee on Hospital Care 2011). These studies included young children and adolescents, so generalizability specifically to teens is limited; however it is our presumption that lack of anticipatory guidance and prevention, including discussing immunizations, alcohol and substance use, reproductive health, self-esteem and mood, as well as violence prevention, is likely often omitted during encounters with adolescent patients due to lack of time or possibly provider comfort in discussing these issues. There is evidence that providers list time constraints as a major barrier to providing confidential care (Helitzer, Sussman, Urquieta de Hernandez, & Kong, 2011; McKee, Rubin, Campos, & O'Sullivan, 2011) and the assurance of confidentiality is important to teens and their likelihood to disclose risky behaviors (Ford, Millstein, Halpern-Felsher, & Irwin, 1997).

Also included in the AAP statement is the concept that patient safety problems and solutions in children are multifactorial and the AAP references the definition of three key domains of these factors including physical characteristic, developmental issues, and minor legal status issues as described by Woods et al. (2005). In adolescent patients, developmentally, they may be less abstract thinkers and unable to fully grasp the consequences of actions,

Y.N. Evans, M.D., M.P.H. (✉)
D.J. Breland, M.D., M.P.H. (✉)
Division of Adolescent Medicine,
Department of Pediatrics, University of Washington,
4800 Sand Point Way NE Mailstop W-7831,
Seattle, WA 98105, USA
e-mail: yolanda.evans@seattlechildrens.org;
david.breland@seattlechildrens.org

W.T. O'Donohue et al. (eds.), *Handbook of Adolescent Health Psychology*,
DOI 10.1007/978-1-4614-6633-8_23, © Springer Science+Business Media New York 2013

yet mature enough to be decision makers regarding their own health. Minor status concerns around consent for care are a real dilemma. While all states and the District of Columbia have laws that allow minors to consent for their own care in certain situations, each has varying laws on the age of consent for adolescent health around the topics of mental health diagnosis and treatment, reproductive health, sexually transmitted infection and HIV screening and treatment, and substance abuse screening and treatment (Berlan & Bravender, 2009). These rules and regulations can be challenging for the medical provider to navigate, yet are extremely important to be aware of. Adolescents' concerns about confidentiality and privacy may keep them from seeking care (Klein, McNulty, & Flatau, 1998) and they may not correctly interpret the confidentiality assurances offered by the medical provider (Ford, Thomsen, & Compton, 2001). Providing confidential services may be the one factor that keeps an adolescent returning for ongoing care.

Due to the unique challenges of adolescent health care, the authors of this chapter thought it best to illustrate possible sources of medical error through the use of a case presentation of a typical adolescent patient followed by a discussion.

Case

A 17-year-old female, who we will call Sara, presents to her primary care provider's office for a yearly physical exam. She is accompanied by her mother who states her main concern today is about Sara's lack of sleep each night. She describes Sara as being a very good student who is on the honor society and involved in soccer. Sara admits that she often stays awake to study. You ask her mom to step out in order to speak with Sara alone.

After her mother leaves, you assure Sara the topics discussed will remain confidential unless she tells you she wants to harm herself, harm someone else, or someone is harming her. You define the term "confidential" as stating the conversation will not be shared with her mother unless she is agreeable to this, but you cannot assure her that her mother will not receive an insurance bill for any laboratory tests performed and that the general topics discussed will be a part of the visit summary in her medical records.

Sara tells you she lives at home with her mother and younger brother. Her parents divorced 2 years ago and she rarely sees her father. She is in 11th grade and finds the pressures to achieve high grades in school very stressful. In fact, she has been using her brother's ADHD stimulant medication to stay awake at night in order to study. She does not feel like this is a problem as other people in her school use medications and caffeine to stay awake. She denies other drug or alcohol use. She confides in you that her mood has been sadder lately and she often finds herself worried about how her teachers will react to her assignments. She stays up at night with racing thoughts as well. You ask her about her relationships and friendships and she responds that she has spent less time with friends lately because she is too busy. She is also on an advanced soccer team and is worried that her weight has been increasing so has started to restrict her food intake. She typically skips breakfast and lunch, eats a light dinner, and has increased her exercise. She is in a romantic relationship with a boy from her school. They became sexually active about 1 month ago and have used condoms on occasion. She tells you she plans to attend college and has no desire to become pregnant.

Discussion

This case has many features that are not uncommon to hear from a typical teen in the United States. It illustrates multiple areas of adolescent care where medical errors can occur. We will focus on the areas of confidentiality (which overlaps in all the areas discussed), sexual and reproductive health, mental health, and substance use.

Confidentiality

The Health Information Portability and Accountability Act of 1996 (HIPAA) is a federal privacy rule that allows for individuals to have access to their health information and for that information to be protected unless authorized. HIPAA does have provisions for adolescent care and any person who is age 18 or older and emancipated minors can utilize their individual rights for accessing their protected health information. For those adolescents under age 18 years who are not emancipated, their parents or legal guardians have the right to make health care decisions for them (English & Ford, 2004). There are three specific circumstances where parents may not be the personal representatives of their minor children. First, a minor can exercise their right as an individual under HIPAA when they have consented to the treatment of a sexually transmitted infection (STI) under a state minor consent law. Second, a minor may request or receive a court approval for an abortion without parent consent or notification. Many states require parent consent or notification to allow an abortion otherwise. Third, a minor has a right as an individual under HIPAA when the parent has assented to an agreement of confidentiality between the health care provider and the minor (English & Ford, 2004). For this final situation, providers who are unfamiliar with a family may be reluctant to offer to speak with a minor patient confidentially for fear of parent disapproval. Reluctance due to parental concerns may be unwarranted and can lead to errors in the omission of anticipatory guidance and behavioral health services. In a study of over 500 parents of teenagers, only 35 % disagreed or strongly disagreed that there were good reasons for a provider to speak with their child alone. All parents in the study received education on minor consent and confidentiality. After education, only 13.8 % of parents felt this way. The vast majority of parents agreed that there are good reasons to have their teen speak with a health care provider alone (Hutchinson & Stafford, 2005).

Sexual and Reproductive Health

As stated previously, all states and the District of Columbia have laws for the provision of STI diagnosis and treatment as well as reproductive health services, which are under federal legislation through Title X family planning programs (English & Ford, 2004). There is evidence that teens that do not have confidential care are less likely to disclose risky behaviors and may even forgo seeking health care (Ford et al., 1997; Thrall et al., 2000). In order for adolescents to feel comfortable bringing up the topics of reproductive health concerns, not only must confidentiality be assured, but the adolescent must perceive that the provider is comfortable and open to discussing these topics. The error of not discussing these topics can lead to delays in care. Lack of care can lead to a delay in the treatment of sexually transmitted infections, which could lead to serious complications including pelvic inflammatory disease and infertility. Delay in reproductive health care can lead to unintended pregnancy from lack of contraception. Due to these potential complications, access to reproductive care is extremely important for anyone seeking these services.

Mental Health

Medical errors in adolescent medicine can occur in other areas of the adolescent's life, such as mental health. Mental health problems can emerge or become more prevalent in adolescence. Eating disorders, depression, suicidal ideation, and substance use and/or abuse can cause significant morbidity and mortality in adolescence. Ensuring confidentiality, the assessment of competence, and gaining consent from adolescents are potential areas where errors can occur. In addition, disparity in insurance coverage and legal/societal and ethical issues can complicate early diagnosis and treatment of mental health disorders. Substance abuse may be missed if confidentiality is not assured or no questions regarding the use of substances are asked; thus confidentiality is essential in the health care of adolescents; without it, adolescents may refrain from seeking care and receiving treatment (Ford, English, & Sigman, 2004; Ford et al., 1997).

All states have a range of situations that allow for a minor to consent to their own health care.

Exceptions are provided to the rule of parental permission for certain health care conditions. Often the distinction between "mature minor" and "emancipated minor" can be quite ambiguous for clinicians. "Mature minor" relates to a situation or conditions in which the adolescent demonstrates the capacity to make a decision (Campbell, 2006). "Emancipated minor" relates to a serious of events viewed as conferring adult status, such as marriage (Campbell, 2006). These definitions can overlap and have the potential to lead to medical errors. For example, the adolescent's capacity to consent for treatment of clinical depression or substance abuse could be effected by the cognitive impairment that often accompanies depression or addiction to substances. Clinicians could consult legal counsel, but this is often impractical given the busy nature of a clinical setting. In general, most states encourage clinicians to promote shared or participatory decision-making behavior between the adolescent and parents (Campbell, 2006).

Mental health decision-making authority for adolescents, in many states, is often restricted to outpatient counseling only for a limited period (Campbell, 2006). However, along with the mature minor doctrine, adolescents can give consent in situations where the risk of not seeking care outweighs the risk of averting parental involvement. For instance, a clinician could decide to treat a homeless 17-year-old who is severely depressed with a tricyclic antidepressant and the teen could die from an overdose of this drug because of cardiac complications. This could be viewed as a medical error given the side effect profile of this medication. Many homeless youth often seek care in free clinics where medication choices may be limited due to funding. In this case, the clinician felt that the benefit of providing a tricyclic antidepressant for depression outweighed the risk of using this medication.

Another potential error that can occur relates to the ability to correctly diagnose mental health illnesses. Clinicians may misdiagnose maladaptive behaviors as "normal teen behaviors" and miss opportunities for counseling and treatment. For example, adolescent who is irritable and rebellious may state that they want to die after an argument with a parent. Is this teen exhibiting signs of depression or is this normal teen behavior? The ability to decipher between the two may be hard in a busy clinic. Therefore, clinicians must be aware screening questionnaires and/or have the ability to speak to the adolescent separately to facilitate a more comfortable environment for them.

Ethical perspectives must also be considered in regard to adolescent consent. Autonomy is the bioethical principle that plays an integral part in the capacity to give consent for mental health care during adolescence (Campbell, 2006). The adolescent needs to know the facts regarding treatment, and understand any risks, benefits, and treatment alternatives available. For mental health, maturity based on age cannot be assumed; the most important issue is whether the teen is competent to make a decision freely (Campbell, 2006).

Mental health is commonly connected to societal stigma, and often hinders help-seeking behaviors at any age (Ford et al., 1997, 2004; Klein et al., 1998). This can be especially true for adolescents who have concerns about discussing sensitive mental health issues with their health provider. The exceptions to minor consent laws were designed, in part, to enable adolescents to seek care for these sensitive issues. This can go against parental beliefs regarding their obligations to their children and the need for access to health care information. Parents often have the financial responsibility for health care for their children, and to deny access to medical/mental information could cause conflict. Clinicians must balance the pros and cons in allowing an adolescent to consent to care and obtain confidential care without involving parents or guardians. Lawsuits against clinicians have occurred because of completed suicides, with allegations of wrongful deaths secondary to previous threats (Campbell, 2006). Therefore, it is imperative that clinicians know the laws of the state in which they practice regarding confidentiality and consent for mental health care services by minors and use appropriate judgement of when to involve parents/guardians in health care decisions covered under minor consent laws.

Solutions to Errors and Challenges in Adolescent Health Care

The Institute of Medicine (IOM) acknowledges six core aims for improving care. These include care that is safe, effective and based on scientific knowledge, patient-centered, timely and avoids delays, efficient, and equitable (Institute of Medicine and Care, 2001). Adopting the IOM's recommendations for health care systems in the USA could potentially prevent medical errors and provide comprehensive care for adolescents. When caring for adolescent patients, providers should take care to remember these basic principles. In our current health care system, care is often fragmented between primary care, acute care, and specialty providers. Adolescents may see various providers in a given year who lack a consistent means for communicating patient information. Information, such as immunization status, may be unknown so vaccines are given multiple times or not at all. In addition, teens may not be given the opportunity to speak to providers alone, so information pertinent to safe and equitable care may never be disclosed. The IOM has ten rules for the redesign of the health care system that are applicable to adolescent health care as well. Care should be based on a continuous healing relationship and customized to the individual patient with the patient being the source of control. Medical knowledge should be shared and flow freely between provitders and patients. Transparency is necessary with safety being a system priority. This means that decisions are based on scientific evidence and needs of patients are anticipated. For all of these things to occur, the system should not waste resources and providers must cooperate with each other. In adolescent care, checklists or prompts in an electronic medical record system could be used for any patient encounter (including acute care, sports physicals, and yearly checkups) as a solution for remembering to ask about adolescent risky behaviors and anticipatory guidance. A local of national database for immunization documentation could be developed to ensure all teens receive the recommended vaccinations.

Summary

Adolescent health is unique in its range of services provided and that the nature of those services almost always involves provision of confidential care to minors. Though there is a lack of specific research on medical errors in adolescent health care, there is sufficient evidence of the importance of confidential services in ensuring that youth disclose risky behaviors. Lack of disclosure can lead to unintended pregnancy, untreated sexually transmitted infections, or undisclosed and untreated mental health conditions and/or substance abuse. More research is needed to determine exactly which medical errors may be occurring in adolescent health and how these errors impact teens.

References

Berlan, E., & Bravender, T. (2009). Confidentiality, consent, and caring for the adolescent patient. *Current Opinion in Pediatrics, 21*, 450–456.

Campbell, A. (2006). Consent, competence, and confidentiality related to psychiatric conditions in adolescent medicine practice. *Adolescent Medicine Clinics, 17*, 25–47.

English, A., & Ford, C. A. (2004). The HIPAA privacy rule and adolescents: Legal questions and clinical challenges. *Perspectives on Sexual and Reproductive Health, 36*(2), 80–86.

Ford, C., English, A., & Sigman, G. (2004). Confidential health care for adolescents: position paper for the Society for Adolescent Medicine. *Journal of Adolescent Health, 35*, 160–167.

Ford, C., Millstein, S., Halpern-Felsher, B., & Irwin, C. (1997). Influence of physician confidentiality assurances on adolescents' willingness to disclose information and seek future health care. A randomized controlled trial. *JAMA: The Journal of the American Medical Association, 278*, 1029–1034.

Ford, C., Thomsen, S., & Compton, B. (2001). Adolescents' interpretations of conditional confidentiality assurances. *Journal of Adolescent Health, 29*, 156–159.

Helitzer, D. L., Sussman, A. L., Urquieta de Hernandez, B., & Kong, A. S. (2011). The "ins" and "outs" of provider-parent communication: Perspectives from adolescent primary care providers on challenges to forging alliances to reduce adolescent risk. *Journal of Adolescent Health, 48*, 404–409.

Hutchinson, J. W., & Stafford, E. M. (2005). Changing parental opinion about teen privacy through education. *Pediatrics, 116*, 966–971.

Institute of Medicine and Care. (2001). *Crossing the quality chasm: A new health system for the 21st century.* Retrieved March 7, 2013, from http://iom.edu/~/media/Files/Report%20Files/2001/Crossing-the-Quality-Chasm/Quality%20Chasm%202001%20%20report%20brief.pdf.

Klein, J., McNulty, L., & Flatau, C. (1998). Teenager's self-reported use of services and perceived access to confidential care. *Archives of Pediatrics & Adolescent Medicine, 152*, 676–682.

McKee, D. M., Rubin, S. E., Campos, G., & O'Sullivan, L. F. (2011). Challenges of providing confidential care to adolescents in urban primary care: Clinician perspectives. *Annals of Family Medicine, 9*(1), 37–43.

Steering Committee on Quality Improvement and Management and Committee on Hospital Care. (2011). Principles of pediatric patient safety: Reducing harm due to medical care. *Pediatrics, 127*, 1199–1210.

Thrall, J., McCloskey, L., Ettner, S., Rothman, E., Tighe, J., & Emans, S. (2000). Confidentiality and adolescents' use of providers for health information and pelvic exams. *Archives of Pediatrics & Adolescent Medicine, 154*, 885–892.

Woods, D., Holl, J., Shonkoff, J., Mehra, M., Ogata, E., & Weiss, K. (2005). Child-specific risk factors and patient safety. *Journal of Patient Safety, 1*, 17–22.

Treatment Adherence in Adolescence

M. Robin DiMatteo and Tricia A. Miller

Treatment Adherence in Adolescence

Quality health care outcomes depend upon patients' adherence to a variety of treatments including medication, medical device use, and lifestyle management such as diet and exercise. Adherence refers to the degree to which an individual follows disease management activities as directed by their health professional. The empirical study of adherence now spans more than 50 years in the scientific literatures of psychology, medicine, and public health. Nonadherence has been found to be a pervasive threat to health and well-being and imposes an appreciable economic burden estimated at 290–300 billion dollars per year (DiMatteo, 2004a; New England Healthcare Institute, 2010). More than 240 million medical visits per year are wasted due to nonadherence (Haskard-Zolnierek & DiMatteo, 2009) and both providers and patients often remain unaware that a major cause of poor health outcomes is poor adherence (DiMatteo, Haskard-Zolnierek, & Martin, 2012).

While adherence behavior is not itself a health outcome, adherence is significantly related to both acute and chronic disease outcomes. Meta-analysis shows substantial and statistically significant outcome differences (26 %) between high and low adherence in all disease realms. Among pediatric (including adolescent) patients, adherence is significantly more strongly related to health outcomes than it is for adults. The difference in risk of a poor health outcome is 33 % greater with poor adherence than with good adherence in samples of children and adolescents; for adults, this risk difference is only 23 % ($z=2.64$, $p<0.01$) (DiMatteo, Giordani, Lepper, & Croghan, 2002).

Adolescent Nonadherence

The challenges of treatment adherence have been studied extensively in adult populations, but less so in child and adolescent care. In a meta-analysis of 569 empirical studies of adherence spanning the history of adherence research to that time, DiMatteo (2004a) found four times as many studies of adult populations (18 and older) as pediatric, and only a portion of the pediatric studies involved only adolescents. Since 2004, the corpus of studies of adolescent adherence has grown appreciably, however, with a recent search producing over 900 empirical research references, 162 of which were published in the year 2010 alone.

Adolescent nonadherence typically takes a number of forms. Although parents are likely to be in charge of filling/refilling medication prescriptions, scheduling medical appointments, and transporting the patient to treatment, adolescents themselves are likely to be expected to take

M.R. DiMatteo, Ph.D. (✉) • T.A. Miller, M.A.
Department of Psychology, University of California, 900 University Ave, Riverside, CA 92521, USA
e-mail: robin@ucr.edu; trishmiller122@gmail.com

W.T. O'Donohue et al. (eds.), *Handbook of Adolescent Health Psychology*,
DOI 10.1007/978-1-4614-6633-8_24, © Springer Science+Business Media New York 2013

responsibility for various health actions including testing blood sugar levels, taking insulin injections, following a prescribed diet or avoiding proscribed foods (e.g., those containing gluten), doing specific exercises for a sports injury, and following a daily asthma treatment regimen to avoid a breathing crisis.

The prevalence of nonadherence across a wide variety of diseases, regimens, and patient populations averages 25 %, although in some disease conditions such as the complex management of diabetes, nonadherence can be 50 % or more. In meta-analytic work with stable estimates, there is a significant trend for (401) studies of adults to yield higher adherence (76.8 %) than (116) studies of pediatric patients (70.6 %) ($t(515)=2.84$, $p=0.005$). Among adult patients, there is no relationship between age and adherence (83 studies, $r=0.01$, $d=0.02$), but among pediatric patients (41 studies, $r=-0.06$, $d=-0.12$) adherence is lower among adolescents than it is among children ($p<0.10$) (DiMatteo 2004a).

Treatment nonadherence in pediatric populations is estimated, in further studies, to be about 50–55 % (Rapoff, 1999); among children with asthma followed in a specialist clinic, medication adherence was about 70 % (Phelan, 1984). Based on structured interviews and daily phone diaries, more than 50 % of adolescents with cystic fibrosis reported doing less than their prescribed airway clearance regimen and 30 % indicated that they were not doing any of their prescribed regimens (DiGirolmo, Quittner, Ackerman, & Stevens, 1997). In a study of prescription medication adherence among adolescents, complete adherence to the prescription was only 36.2 % (Chappuy, Treluyer, Faesch, Giraud, & Cheron, 2009). Between 50 and 60 % of children and adolescents with adherence problems were found to underuse their prescribed medication (while less than 10 % overused it) (Chmelik & Doughty, 1994; Coutts, Gibson, & Paton, 1992). Among adolescent patients with adequate functional health literacy, 35.7 % were categorized as adherent, but only 23.5 % of those with marginal/inadequate health literacy were categorized as adherent (Murphy et al., 2010). Twenty-five percent of adolescents with type 1 diabetes reported mismanagement behaviors such as missing insulin shots (Kovacs, Goldston, Obrosky, & Iyengar, 1992; Weissberg-Benchell et al., 1995). In asthma treatment, the average overall adherence rate among African-American adolescents (measured as daily mean percent of prescribed inhaler puffs) was only 31.5 %. Adherence also decreased over time, from 42 % at the start of the study to only 20.2 % of prescribed puffs after a year on treatment (Rohan et al., 2010).

Simmons, Logan, Chastain, and Cerullo (2010) found variability in adherence as a function of the treatment regimen. Among adolescents who were recommended a medication change, 53.1 % were fully adherent; 87.5 % were fully adherent to obtaining additional recommended tests. Of participants prescribed physical therapy, 100 % were fully adherent to continuing if they had already started, but only 75 % began; 90.9 % were fully adherent to use of a TENS unit, but only 60 % were fully adherent to an independent exercise program. Adherence to psychological recommendations varied as well: 85.7 % of adolescents were fully adherent to continuing treatment with their current therapist; but only 46.7 % were fully adherent to beginning cognitive behavioral therapy (Simmons et al., 2010).

Understanding Treatment Adherence in Adolescent Patients

The empirical literature on treatment adherence in all age groups has documented a wide variety of factors that influence the degree to which patients follow medical recommendations. Researchers have offered empirical evidence for the contribution of dozens of intra- and interpersonal, environmental, disease-related, and regimen-related factors. Practical applications of this research are somewhat limited, however, because there are so many causes of nonadherence. It is critical to understand these causes in a workable conceptual framework in order to design successful programs to advance adherence among adolescents. DiMatteo et al. (2012) describe the Information, Motivation, Strategy (IMS) model which distills the findings of the complex literature into three main elements for understanding adherence. According to the IMS model, patients of all ages are non-adherent for three straightforward classes of reasons: (1) They do not understand what they are supposed to do (e.g., information transmittal and gathering are lacking; they have not participated in the decision-making process; their communication and rapport with their health professionals is limited), (2) they are not motivated to follow their treatment (e.g., they do not believe that the benefits outweigh the costs; their social network and/or cultural environment do not support the behavior), and (3) they do not have a workable strategy for following the treatment (e.g., they do not have help; practical barriers stand in the way). In the following section of this chapter, we examine the specific challenges in treatment of chronic illness among adolescents in the context of this model, attempting to understand three categories of factors related to adolescent nonadherence. We also examine the effectiveness of adherence-enhancing interventions in the context of this model.

Information

The communication of information between health professionals and their patients is a primary element essential for the achievement of treatment adherence; patients cannot follow treatments they do not fully understand. Communication is essential for a realistic assessment of patients' knowledge and understanding of their regimen, and communication is essential for building trust in the therapeutic relationship. In a recent meta-analysis, the relationship between physician–patient communication and treatment adherence was found to be higher (borderline significant) in pediatric practice (average $r=0.24$) than in the care of adult patients (average $r=0.18$) ($t(101)=1.75$, $p=0.08$). Further, training to improve physician communication showed significantly more improvement in patient adherence when pediatricians were trained (average effect size $r=0.27$) than when non-pediatricians were trained (average effect size $r=0.10$) ($t(19)=3.42$, $p=0.003$) (Haskard-Zolnierek & DiMatteo, 2009).

At the most basic level, recall of recommendations is essential, although studies have shown the majority of adults (e.g., Kravitz et al., 1993) as well as children and their parents (Ievers et al., 1999; Lewis, Pantell, & Sharp, 1991) fail to recall what they are told about disease management during their medical visits. Patients and caregivers need the opportunity to ask questions and have them answered, to clarify information they are given, and to "teach back" to their health professionals what they have learned. All patients, including adolescents, need the chance to participate in the decision process and to determine how they will follow their treatment (Golin, DiMatteo, & Gelberg, 1996). When patients and their doctors share similar beliefs about patient participation (that is, when patients are motivated to participate and their physicians allow them to do so), patient outcomes tend to be more positive and patients are more satisfied (Jahng, Martin, Golin, & DiMatteo, 2005). Patients are also more adherent to physicians who answer their questions (DiMatteo et al., 1993) and patients are typically willing to follow treatment recommendations only for health professionals they trust and who provide satisfactory interpersonal quality of care (Sherbourne, Hays, Ordway, DiMatteo, & Kravitz, 1992).

Whether patients understand and can follow their treatment is related strongly to their health literacy, which has been found to be a major factor among HIV-infected adolescents (of whom almost 15 % were found to have inadequate or marginal health literacy). Among the 85 % of participants with adequate functional health literacy, only 36 % were categorized as adherent, and among those with marginal or inadequate health literacy, only 23.5 % were categorized as adherent (Murphy et al., 2010). Adjusting for age and education level, viral load, and self-efficacy to adhere to medication regimens, however, adolescents' own health literacy was not significantly associated with their medication adherence (Murphy et al., 2010). But, as Janisse, Naar-King, and Ellis (2010) found among high-risk adolescents with IDDM, *parental* literacy/reading comprehension was significantly related to treatment adherence among adolescents on an intensive insulin regimen (Janisse et al., 2010). Parents with low health literacy struggled to help their children adhere to increasingly complex diabetes treatment regimens, leading the authors to suggest that families may benefit from more intensive diabetes education or different approaches to teaching diabetes management skills (Janisse et al., 2010).

Essential elements of improving communication involve strengthening physician–family interactions and the relationship between the adolescent and health professionals; the goal is to help understand the adolescent as well as the disease (Drotar, 2009; Simmons et al., 2010). Drotar (2009) studied both parents' and children's perceptions of their pediatricians' behavior in the management of pediatric chronic illness treatment management, and correlated the providers' communication behavior with treatment adherence. The findings showed that discrepancies between the needs of parents and their children, and inconsistencies in physicians' behavior while explaining treatment procedures, were related to limitations in the children's adherence to treatment. Further, understanding and implementing complex treatments, such as for diabetes, can be challenging to even the most motivated parents and their adolescents (Rudy, Murphy, Harris, Muenz, & Ellen, 2009).

Motivation

Probably more than in any other age group, adherence among adolescents is affected by issues of motivation. The motivations of the adolescents themselves as well as of their parents, siblings, and peers can have strong effects on commitment to a treatment regimen, and ultimately on its fulfillment (Wysocki, Greco, & Buckloh, 2003). Motivation for treatment adherence is built upon a number of factors (DiMatteo et al., 2012). These include the following: (1) belief in the treatment (the necessity of it, and its value), (2) the perceived costs of the treatment (particularly in terms of potential losses of social status, cultural norm maintenance, and peer acceptance), and (3) attitudes about the illness (i.e., its meaning) and treatment (i.e., expectations that the benefits outweigh any costs) and about the self in relation to disease management (self-efficacy). Beliefs, attitudes, motivations, and their resultant commitment to treatment may be particularly difficult to achieve for an adolescent patient, because he or she is embedded within a social system comprised of influential family members as well as peers who may not support the regimen (or with whom the adolescent is resistant to share the issues of care). Further, adult caregivers and parents may struggle to bridge the differences in attitudes and beliefs between the adolescent and all of the adults with whom they deal.

Models of health behavior and general behavior change (e.g., the Health Belief Model, the Theory of Planned Behavior) (Martin, Haskard-Zolnierek, & DiMatteo, 2010) posit beliefs and attitudes as the building blocks of commitment to action. Commitment requires belief in potentially negative and serious consequences of *not* acting, the expectation that the benefits of acting will outweigh the costs (broadly defined) of doing so, a synchrony between the beliefs and desires of the individual and his or her social (including cultural) environment, as well as the individual's belief in his or her own ability to act (i.e., self-efficacy). These models suggest that, clinically, it is vital to know the patient well, and to identify and manage realistic treatment goals and expectations for therapy. In the case of adolescent care, it is also vital to know the adult caregivers. Understanding what patients and their parents/guardians expect and believe, what they are influenced by, and what they can be inspired or prompted to do allows for health professionals to support adolescent motivation to adhere to treatment.

Chronic illness management can challenge the self-esteem of some adolescents (Friedman et al., 1986), who may become frustrated and view themselves as "defective" because of their illness; such feelings can potentially contribute to significant emotional distress (Rudy et al., 2009). Adolescents may view their illness and treatment regimens as forcing an unwanted dependence on their parents, guardians, and health professionals (Rudy et al., 2009). Sometimes, in an attempt to understand the full meaning and implications of their condition, adolescents might stop taking their medications as an experiment to determine the effect on their health or well-being. Not all medications produce immediate results, however, so their benefits may not be at all obvious; and the health consequences of not following treatment might also be delayed (e.g., celiac disease, cystic fibrosis). Some consequences might not be noticed at all, or might not be clearly connected to nonadherence. Distal future outcomes might be ignored completely, because adolescents are likely to have some difficulty with focused commitment to the future (Ingerski, Baldassano, Denson, & Hommel, 2010). The belief that treatment is not necessary to their current interests and goals may severely limit some adolescents' commitment to disease management (Ingerski et al., 2010).

For many adolescent patients, the perceived stigma of being ill is one of the major factors limiting active adherence to treatment (Wysocki et al., 2003). The developmental period of adolescence is one in which the struggle to "fit in" and to be accepted by peers is a primary concern. The everyday management of a chronic disease (such as with blood sugar testing and insulin injections by the diabetic, or the avoidance of popular foods such as pizza by the patient with celiac disease) can be a source of embarrassment and "differentness" leading the adolescent to avoid social stigma by avoiding the treatment regimen (Friedman et al., 1986; Salamon, Hains, Fleischman, Davies, & Kichler, 2010). Some adolescents may even have difficulty with management of their disease within certain social contexts because of *direct* peer pressure and actually being singled out for criticism because of their condition (Wysocki et al., 2003).

The sociocultural norms of adolescence (including expectations that adolescents have for each other regarding dress, activities, and behavior) may carry a great deal of weight in an adolescent patient's decisions about health action and treatment adherence (Hampson, Glasgow, & Toobert, 1990). These cultural norms can affect responses to treatment plans as well as perceptions of the meaning of illness and the sick role, and the acceptability of seeking and accepting advice from adult caregivers (Hampson et al., 1990; La Greca, Bearman, & Moore, 2002). For adolescents, friends and peer group members may be the strongest influences in their lives and in their commitment to care (La Greca et al., 2002). Thus, culture not only refers to racial and ethnic identification but extends to the broader adolescent culture, underscoring the need for health professionals who work with adolescent patients to fully understand adolescent culture (both broadly and regionally), perhaps working with psychologists who are experts in adolescent treatment (Christian & D'Auria, 1997). Providers should identify the important individuals and influences in the adolescent's life, and examine their understanding of, beliefs about, and influences on the patient's treatment and adherence (La Greca et al., 2002; Thomas, Peterson, & Goldstein, 1997). Concerns about norms and adolescent culture should be discussed with the patient and his or her caregivers in an effort to increase awareness of the factors that can affect the success of medical recommendations (Christian & D'Auria, 1997).

Adolescents with chronic disease can face daily challenges of social pressure, especially when their medical condition makes them appear different from their friends (Christian & D'Auria, 1997; La Greca & Hanna as cited in La Greca et al., 2002). For the diabetic, for example, the complexities of dietary adherence and invasive activities such as blood glucose testing and insulin injection are potentially significant issues that can derail adherence (Thomas et al., 1997). Promoting patient adherence requires health professionals to determine the degree to which their adolescent patients feel their disease affects their friendships, and to try to find ways to deal with these challenges (La Greca et al., 2002).

Although the findings are mixed, some research suggests that by being generally supportive (though not necessarily helping directly with treatment), peers can help to motivate adolescents to be adherent to chronic disease management. In a review by La Greca et al. (2002), data suggested that adolescents perceive the support of their friends to be more important in certain areas (e.g., meals and exercise) than in other areas of management (e.g., insulin injections and blood testing). Friends may also be helpful with emotional reactions. Bearman and La Greca (2002), however, did find that friend support, although not related to overall treatment adherence, was related to higher adherence for blood glucose testing. These findings argue for the importance of identifying the specific areas of disease management in which friends can be most supportive, and facilitating that support with education and encouragement. Providers should respectfully address patients' beliefs (including their concerns about the role of peers), and should serve as both partners and persuaders, working together with adolescent patients to arrive at mutually agreed-upon courses of action and using the strength of the therapeutic relationship to facilitate the adolescent's commitment to the treatment regimen. Identification of the "stage of change" at which the adolescent is approaching the treatment, and working with the patients' beliefs, attitudes, subjective norms, and cultural context, providers can help the patient to develop and maintain a commitment to long-term disease management (Prochaska, DiClemente, & Norcross, 1992).

Strategy

Even with a full understanding of the disease and treatment, strongly held commitment, the best of intentions, and supportive norms, individuals may still fail to adhere to necessary health behaviors because they encounter practical difficulties. Patients can only do what they are capable of doing within their resource limitations; those resources can range from affordable treatments to organized and supportive families to well-developed habits. Thus, the third element of achieving adherence involves identifying the barriers that adolescent patients face in following their treatment and assisting them to gain the necessary resources and supports to solve their strategic challenges.

Practical Barriers

Practical barriers can represent some of the most common challenges to patient adherence. At the simplest level, a medication's bad taste has been found to limit adherence among children and early adolescents (Ingerski et al., 2010). Economic challenges may limit the affordability of treatment (Rohan et al., 2010) and combined, with other pressures such as difficult parental work schedules, can result in parents' failures to obtain on-time refills of medications. In a study of adolescents with inflammatory bowel disease who were taking oral medications, the most commonly reported barriers included forgetting (87.8 %), being away from home (47.3 %), interference with an activity (44.6 %), refusal/defiance (17.6 %), not feeling well (16.2 %), and running out of the medication (16.2 %). Intensive treatments (such as for HIV, diabetes, CF) may be quite demanding and difficult for adolescents and families to manage (Ingerski et al., 2010). Orban et al. (2010) found that the most frequent stressors reported by adolescents receiving treatment for HIV were related to medication-taking (Orban et al., 2010), even despite the availability of clinic support services for adhering. These services, however, tended to focus more on tangible aspects of adherence such as medication reminders; in fact, some efforts such as passive coping strategies made youth feel helpless and frustrated, increasing depression and reducing adherence (Orban et al., 2010).

Treatments for chronic disease interfere with the lives of adolescents in major ways. Medication schedules can disrupt normal routines and both school and after-school schedules. Dosage frequency influences adherence to prescriptions, with more frequent dosing resulting in lower adherence; average adherence was 73 % for once daily regimens, 70 % for twice daily, 52 % for thrice daily, and 42 % for four times a day regimens (Chappuy et al., 2009). Researchers have found that adherence to complex and intrusive treatments such as dietary modification, glucose monitoring, and physical therapy is even lower than adherence to medical regimens in adolescents (Rapoff, 1999). Length of treatment also influences adherence. In one study with children treated for pneumococcal infection, adherence was significantly better for shorter therapy of 5 days than for the longer therapy of 10 days (Schrag et al., 2001). Of course, long-term chronic disease management is likely to produce even lower adherence (World Health Organization, 2003).

One of the most important factors in patients' ability to follow treatment involves the degree of practical support available to them to deal with the barriers encountered (Sherbourne et al., 1992). A meta-analytic review of the literature from 122 studies found a significant positive relationship of patients' adherence with the practical support available to them; adherence was 27 % higher when patients had practical social support (DiMatteo, 2004b). Social networks affect adherence. In a meta-analysis, DiMatteo (2004a, 2004b) assessed 40 studies of adult patients in which the average correlation between subjects' marital status and their adherence was only 0.05. However, among nine samples of pediatric patients, the average correlation between parents' marital status and children's treatment adherence was significant ($r=0.15$). The risk of nonadherence among children with unmarried parents was found to be 1.35 times higher (standardized relative risk from the binomial effect-size display) than the risk of nonadherence among children and adolescents with married parents (DiMatteo, 2004b). Furthermore, this meta-analysis showed a trend such that a greater number of people in the family was associated with lower adherence in the care of pediatric patients (median $r=-0.22$; mean $r=-0.17$). A likely explanation would involve greater competition for both physical and emotional resources including parental attention and energy in larger families.

Shorter duration of hospital stays and limits on physician time spent with patients have significantly shifted care to families and increased the need for family responsibility in treatment management for children and adolescents. For example, cancer medications that, in the past, were given to children in hospital may now be administered by parents at home. Certainly there are advantages to home care for pediatric patients, including the comfort and familiarity of setting and availability of relatives and friends. However, although some families are able to administer treatments effectively, not all are capable of taking on the organization and planning necessary to manage treatment responsibly (Riekert & Drotar, 1999). Some families may have difficulty independently caring for medical symptoms (such as of asthma) and instead rely on health care providers in clinic or emergency room visits (Rohan et al., 2010).

Emotional Distress and Family Conflict

Stress and emotional distress, in the patient and in the family, can be significant barriers to adherence (Cox & Gonder-Frederick, 1992). Depression and distress can be common in medical patients, and are associated with diminished health status (Sherbourne, Wells, Meredith, Jackson, & Camp, 1996) and increased health care utilization (Manning & Wells, 1992; Simon, Ormel, VonKorff, & Barlow, 1995). In a meta-analysis, the relationship between depression and nonadherence was substantial and significant (DiMatteo, Lepper, & Croghan, 2000). Compared with nondepressed patients, the odds were three times greater that depressed patients would be non-adherent, suggesting the importance of recognizing depression as a risk factor for poor outcomes among patients who might not be adhering to medical advice. In the Medical Outcomes Study, a longitudinal study of 1,198 patients with chronic medical diseases (hypertension, diabetes, heart disease), patients who were distressed about their health, used avoidant coping strategies, or reported worse physical and role functioning were less likely to adhere in general (Sherbourne et al., 1992). Blotcky, Cohen, Conaster, and Klopovich (1985) found that subjective distress was significantly related ($r=-0.48$) to refusal of treatment among children with cancer. Brownbridge and Fielding (1989) found adherence to be significantly lower in the care of children with end-stage renal disease when the main caregiver was depressed ($r=-0.45$).

There is a negative relationship between adherence and family conflict (including dysfunctional family interactions, the anger of a healthy sibling, and family pathology); an average r effect size of -0.21 indicated that poorer adherence was associated with greater family conflict and that the odds of nonadherence among patients in higher conflict families were 2.35 times higher than among those in families with lower levels of conflict (DiMatteo, 2004b). Effective communication about decision-making autonomy is also critical. Miller and Drotar (2003) documented the relationship between discrepancies in mother and adolescent perceptions of diabetes-related decision-making autonomy, diabetes-related conflict, and regimen adherence; discrepancies between mothers' and their adolescents' perceptions of decision-making autonomy were related to greater maternal report of diabetes-related conflict. In particular, mothers reported greater conflict with their adolescents when the adolescents reported that they were more in charge of decisions than their mothers believed that they were (Miller & Drotar, 2003).

In a meta-analysis, DiMatteo (2004b) found that the odds of adherence are three times higher if patients come from cohesive families than if they do not ($r=0.27$). Higher levels of mother-reported spousal support were associated with less conflict and with greater adherence to treatment (Lewandowski & Drotar, 2007). This latter study was important because it demonstrated that the spousal support mothers receive may play an important role in the health care behaviors of their adolescents (Lewandowski & Drotar, 2007). DeLambo, Ievers-Landis, Drotar, and Quittner (2008) examined associations between observations of the quality of family relationships and reported adherence to medical treatments for older children and adolescents with cystic fibrosis. Based on children's reports of treatment adherence, the positivity of the observed family relationship quality predicted reported adherence to airway clearance and use of aerosolized medications among child and adolescent patients (DeLambo et al., 2008).

Family and Adolescent Control: Responsibility for Illness Management

Adherence to medication and other treatment regimens for children and adolescents depends, to a great extent, on the help of parents/guardians and other family members (DeLambo et al., 2008). With the onset of adolescence, there are often changes in the allocation of treatment-related responsibilities among adolescent patients and their caregivers. Yet, although adolescents can be given increased responsibility for their care compared to what they had as children, research shows that adolescents need help from their parents as well as scheduled support and help from their health professionals. Data suggest that there are predictable differences in treatment-related expectations for adherence behaviors among children versus adolescent. For example, children age 7–10 will likely have different and fewer responsibilities compared to those 11–15 years of age (Modi, Marciel, Slater, Drotar, & Quittner, 2008; Walders, Drotar, & Kercsmar, 2000). Yet, the division of illness-related responsibilities between an adolescent and his or her parents/caregivers needs to be optimal and reflect the adolescent's unique abilities (Lewandowski & Drotar, 2007; Miller & Drotar, 2003). There is no significant relationship between adolescent chronological age and the ability to take responsibility for asthma management (Walders et al., 2000). This study shows that when caretakers reduce their involvement in asthma management based on their child's chronological age, they might operate under the false premise that adolescents are consistently able and/or willing to take on increasing accountability for asthma management (Walders et al., 2000).

It is, therefore, necessary for families to help, and for parents to supervise. Yet, one study of cystic fibrosis patients found that by age 15, adolescents were completing nearly 90 % of their daily treatments on their own—although this was often done at the cost of poor adherence (Modi et al., 2008). In addition, adolescents who spent more of their treatment time supervised by their parents had better adherence (Modi et al., 2008). Walders et al. (2000) examined family management patterns among African-American adolescents with asthma. They found a relationship between caretakers' overestimation of adolescent responsibility for important self-care tasks and increased nonadherence and functional morbidity (Walders et al., 2000). These studies demonstrated that parents and adolescents need anticipatory guidance on how and when to transition responsibility for daily treatment regimens and that family interventions are essential for improving adherence among adolescents with chronic illness (Modi et al., 2008).

Should adolescents make their own decisions about their treatments, and take complete responsibility for them? Probably not. Lewandowski and Drotar (2007) found that adolescent decision-making autonomy did not help adherence; it was not necessarily a good thing to have adolescents making their own decisions about care. Instead, decision-making responsibility and disease management were better negotiated and agreed upon by parents and their adolescents. A discrepancy in expectations about who will make decisions is a problem; parent/adolescent conflict can lead to resistance to adherence. In diabetes treatment, increased levels of mother–adolescent conflict have been found to be associated with poorer treatment adherence and mother-reported diabetes-related conflict and disagreements about decision-making autonomy predicted poor glycemic control (Lewandowski & Drotar, 2007).

One study examined decision-making competence in a sample of parents and their adolescents with type 1 diabetes (Miller & Drotar, 2007). Parent–adolescent communication during a problem-solving task was assessed, along with the adaptiveness of adolescent decision-making, adherence to treatment, and metabolic control (Miller & Drotar, 2007). Parent–adolescent communication was associated with adherence to treatment, but not with the quality of adolescent decision-making (Miller & Drotar, 2007). Poorer decision-making was associated with lower adherence (measured by parent report), and decision-making competence did not mediate the relationships between parent–adolescent communication and adherence (Miller & Drotar, 2007).

Parent–Adolescent Collaboration

Data suggest that full responsibility by parents may not be the best course of action for adolescent care, for several reasons. In some research, parents made significant errors in the timing of medication and some even encouraged premature discontinuation of medication because symptoms "seemed" to improve (Dawson & Newell, 1994). Parents with low health literacy have been found to struggle to help their children adhere to complex treatment regimens (Janisse et al., 2010). Family habits have sometimes been found to jeopardize adherence to the treatment regimen (Nock & Kazdin, 2005). In order to optimize the efficacy of asthma management, for example, researchers suggest that family-based treatment plans should be collaboratively developed between physicians and family members (Walders et al., 2000). Effective illness management requires good communication between adolescent, parents, and health professionals in order to have an appropriate and effective division of illness-related responsibilities.

Validated Interventions to Improve Adolescent Adherence

Several interventions to improve adolescent adherence have been shown to be effective; each emphasizes at least one component of the IMS model, and most are multifactorial—incorporating some combination of all of the factors. Interventions that target, in an integrated way, the many elements that affect patient adherence are most likely to be successful (DiMatteo et al., 2012).

In a pilot study with ten adolescents with type 1 diabetes and HbA1c levels greater than 7 %, Salamon et al. (2010) assessed a cognitive–behavioral intervention geared toward challenging and restructuring negative social attributions that can contribute to nonadherence. One hour intervention sessions to boost understanding and motivation were combined with three weekly phone calls that focused on cognitive restructuring and on problem-solving training to improve strategizing (Salamon et al., 2010). Problem-solving that was geared toward dealing with social situations (in which adolescents likely experience the greatest pressure to be nonadherent) was the most helpful.

Nock and Kazdin (2005) used a brief adjunctive intervention (called PEI training) which provided parents of adolescents with knowledge, motivation, and tools toward the goal of overcoming conduct problems and barriers to treatment participation. PEI therapists helped parents develop specific plans to overcome each barrier through the use of a change plan worksheet (Nock & Kazdin, 2005). When parents received the training, their adolescents had better attendance at treatment sessions and showed greater adherence to treatment recommendations.

Dean, Walters, and Hall (2010) conducted a comprehensive search of the literature and reviewed 17 studies that offered empirical data on interventions to improve long-term medication adherence in children and adolescents with chronic disease. They examined educational interventions, behavior interventions (that may have also included education), and educational approaches combined with another intervention. Of seven (primarily) educational interventions, only one (Jay, DuRant, Shoffitt, Linder, & Litt, 1984) targeted adolescents only, and found that an educational intervention with peer counselors significantly increased adolescent girls' adherence to their oral contraceptives for 1–2 months, although the significant effect did not last over the 4 months of the study. Four studies involved both children and adolescents, but did not allow separate analyses. Three of these four were with asthma. One study (Hughes, McLeod, Garner, & Goldbloom, 1991) found that home visits and education about asthma management did not affect adherence as measured by medication diary, but did lead to significantly better asthma control. Another (Farber & Oliveria, 2004) provided single-session education with video and discussion, and found adherence significantly higher in the intervention group, but only for preventer mediation (not the rescue bronchodilator). The intervention group had lower rates of corticosteroid undertreatment. In the treatment of HIV in children and adolescents, home visits involving education and strategies to resolve adherence barriers resulted in significantly greater self-reported adherence as well as increased dose frequency (Berrien, Salazar, Reynolds, & Mckay, 2004). In this review, there were seven studies using behavioral interventions, five of which were with both adolescents and children (not separated) and one studying only adolescents. In the latter, behavioral management (including advice with contingency contracting, advising about problems, goal setting, development of habits and routines, and family involvement) prevented missed doses of tuberculosis medication (as self-reported in face-to-face interviews) significantly more often than both control treatment and an intervention to improve self-esteem (Hovell et al., 2003). Of the five studies of children and adolescents, all showed significant improvements in adherence to some or all medications when the intervention involved behavioral management. These behavioral interventions included monitoring and goal setting, reinforcing medication-taking with rewards, contingency contracting, problem-solving, and linking medication taking with established routines to establish habits. Van Es, Nagelkerke, Colland, Scholten, and Bouter (2001) found that adolescents with asthma demonstrated better treatment adherence if they received both education and group therapy exploring treatment and disease-focused issues including their attitudes, coping skills, and management of peers. (Two other interventions cited by Dean et al. (2010) showed no benefit of education combined with cognitive behavioral therapy or stress management.) No studies were found to demonstrate the effectiveness of intervention to reverse nonadherence among young people once nonadherence has been established.

Future Research on Interventions

Currently validated interventions exist to promote adherence among adolescents with chronic disease. The empirical data available so far is limited but does suggest that multifaceted interventions work better than do single-issue interventions. The best combination of elements to produce the greatest improvements in adherence with the greatest efficiency is not yet evident, but it does appear that a combination of education, information, methods for increasing motivation, and problem-solving strategies and supports may offer the greatest opportunities for success (Dean et al., 2010). While there is no clear message from the literature about why various factors may be effective, some of the more theoretical and empirical work in adult adherence notes that multifaceted solutions, targeting many factors that affect adherence, may be essential. Future research attention to intervention studies should seek to determine the mediating and moderating factors of successful interventions, so that effective elements can be preserved in exportable interventions that can be used on a wide scale. Further, as Dean et al. (2010) conclude, some studies do not provide data for calculation of effect sizes that are necessary for meta-analyses; meta-analytic work is essential to moving this field forward. Also, many studies combine data from children and adolescents, making it difficult to determine the unique effectiveness of interventions for adolescent populations. Thus, future research should focus on adolescents, and in publication should offer as much data as possible for extracting or calculating effect sizes, in order to allow meta-analyses of the growing literature on adolescent adherence to treatment.

Clinical Implications

Research on the challenges of adolescent treatment adherence suggests some important clinical recommendations. First, it is essential for medical teams (consisting of physicians, nurses, nurse practitioners, physician-assistants, pharmacists, case managers, etc.) to coordinate their efforts and share information toward the goal of helping patients achieve adherence. Second, clinicians on the medical team should regularly ask patients and their families about adherence. Assessing adherence accurately is central to the enhancement of treatment choices and to the prediction and optimization of health outcomes (Sherbourne et al., 1992). Assessing adherence accurately is not easy, of course (Hays & DiMatteo, 1987), but there exist many methods to collect accurate self-reports from patients in ways that encourage truthfulness (see measures in DiMatteo, Hays, & Sherbourne, 1992). Third, clinicians on the medical team should help family members work together in treatment management, helping each member of the family to be clear about their responsibilities in the treatment regimen. Discrepancies between parents' and adolescents' perceptions of disease-related decision-making autonomy can contribute to nonadherence; identifying and solving these discrepancies can be a potentially important area for clinical intervention (Miller & Drotar, 2003). Fourth, as Dean et al. (2010) note, there is no research to date offering effective interventions to reverse adolescent nonadherence once it becomes habitual; until evidence-based offerings are available, preventing nonadherence should be a clinical priority. Finally, the medical team should approach adherence in an organized fashion, with a focus on three broad elements of care: providing *information*, building *motivation*, and assisting with *strategy*. Working on these goals in the context of effective communication can result in substantial and significant improvements in adherence and, ultimately, in better adolescent health care outcomes.

References

Bearman, K. J., & La Greca, A. M. (2002). Assessing friend support of adolescents' diabetes care: The diabetes social questionnaire—Friends version. *Journal of Pediatric Psychology, 27*(5), 417–428.

Berrien, V. M., Salazar, J. C., Reynolds, E., & Mckay, K. (2004). Adherence to antiretroviral therapy in HIV-infected pediatric patients improves with home-based intensive nursing intervention. *AIDS Patient Care and STDs, 18*(6), 355–363.

Blotcky, A. D., Cohen, D. G., Conaster, C., & Klopovich, P. (1985). Psychosocial characteristics of adolescents who refuse cancer treatment. *Journal of Consulting and Clinical Psychology, 53*, 729–731.

Brownbridge, B., & Fielding, D. (1989). An investigation of psychological factors influencing adherence to medial regime in children and adolescents undergoing haemodialysis and CAPD. *International Journal of Adolescent Medicine and Health, 4*, 7–18.

Chappuy, H., Treluyer, J. M., Faesch, S., Giraud, C., & Cheron, G. (2009). Length of the treatment and number of doses per day as major determinants of child adherence to acute treatment. *Acta Paediatrica, 99*(3), 433–437.

Chmelik, F., & Doughty, A. (1994). Objective measurements of compliance in asthma treatment. *Annals of Allergy, 73*, 527–532.

Christian, B. J., & D'Auria, J. P. (1997). The child's eye: Memories of growing up with cystic fibrosis. *Journal of Pediatric Nursing, 12*(1), 3–12.

Coutts, J. A., Gibson, N. A., & Paton, J. Y. (1992). Measuring compliance with inhaled medication in asthma. *Archives of Disease in Childhood, 67*(3), 332–333.

Cox, D. J., & Gonder-Frederick, L. (1992). Major developments in behavioral diabetes research. *Journal of Consulting and Clinical Psychology, 60*, 628–638.

Dawson, A., & Newell, R. (1994). The extent of parental compliance with timing of administration of their children's antibiotics. *Journal of Advanced Nursing, 20*, 483–490.

Dean, A. J., Walters, J., & Hall, A. (2010). A systematic review of interventions to enhance medication adherence in children and adolescents with chronic illness. *Archives of Disease in Childhood, 95*, 717–723.

DeLambo, K. E., Ievers-Landis, C. E., Drotar, D., & Quittner, A. L. (2008). Evidence-based assessment of Adherence to Medical Treatments in Pediatric Psychology. *Journal of Pediatric Psychology, 33*(9), 916–936.

DiGirolmo, A. M., Quittner, A. L., Ackerman, V., & Stevens, J. (1997). Identification and assessment of ongoing stressors in adolescents with a chronic illness: An application of the behavior analytic model. *Journal of Clinical Child Psychology, 26*, 53–66.

DiMatteo, M. R. (2004a). Variations in patients' adherence to medical recommendations: A quantitative review of 50 years of research. *Medical Care, 42*(3), 200–209.

DiMatteo, M. R. (2004b). Social support and patient adherence to medical treatment: a meta-analysis. *Health Psychology, 23*(2), 207–218.

DiMatteo, M. R., Giordani, P. J., Lepper, H. S., & Croghan, T. W. (2002). Patient adherence and medical treatment outcomes: A meta-analysis. *Medical Care, 40*(9), 794–811.

DiMatteo, M. R., Haskard-Zolnierek, K. B., & Martin, L. R. (2012). Improving patient adherence: A three-factor model to guide practice. *Health Psychology Review, 6*(1), 74–91.

DiMatteo, M. R., Hays, R. D., & Sherbourne, C. D. (1992). Adherence to cancer regimens: Implications for treating the older patient. *Oncology, 6*, 50–57.

DiMatteo, M. R., Lepper, H. S., & Croghan, T. W. (2000). Depression is a risk factor for noncompliance with medical treatment: Meta-analysis of the effects of anxiety and depression on patient adherence. *Archives of Internal Medicine, 160*(14), 2101–2107.

DiMatteo, M. R., Sherbourne, C. D., Hays, R. D., Ordway, L., Kravitz, R. L., McGlynn, E. S., et al. (1993). Physicians' characteristics influence patients' adherence to medical treatment: Results from the Medical Outcomes Study. *Health Psychology, 12*(2), 93–102.

Drotar, D. (2009). Physician behavior in the care of pediatric chronic illness: Association with health outcomes and treatment adherence. *Journal of Developmental and Behavioral Pediatrics, 30*(3), 254.

Farber, H. J., & Oliveria, L. (2004). Trial of an asthma education program in an inner-city pediatric emergency department. *Pediatric Asthma, Allergy & Immunology, 17*(2), 107–115.

Friedman, I. M., Litt, I. F., King, D. R., Henson, R., Holtzman, D., Halverson, D., et al. (1986). Compliance with anticonvulsant therapy by epileptic youth. *Journal of Adolescent Health Care, 7*, 12–17.

Golin, C. E., DiMatteo, M. R., & Gelberg, L. (1996). The role of patient participation in the doctor visit. Implications for adherence to diabetes care. *Diabetes Care, 19*(10), 1153–1164.

Hampson, S. E., Glasgow, R. E., & Toobert, D. J. (1990). Personal models of diabetes and their relations to self-care activities. *Health Psychology, 9*, 516–528.

Haskard-Zolnierek, K. B., & DiMatteo, M. R. (2009). Physician communication and patient adherence to treatment: A meta-analysis. *Medical Care, 47*(8), 826–834.

Hays, R. D., & DiMatteo, M. R. (1987). Key issues and suggestions for patient compliance assessment: Sources of information focus of measures, and nature of response options. *The Journal of Compliance in Health Care, 2*, 37–53.

Hovell, M. F., Sipan, C. L., Blumberg, E. J., Hofstetter, C. R., Slymen, D., Friedman, L., et al. (2003). Increasing Latino adolescents' adherence to treatment for latent tuberculosis infection: A controlled trial. *American Journal of Public Health, 93*(11), 1871–1877.

Hughes, D. M., McLeod, M., Garner, B., & Goldbloom, R. B. (1991). Controlled trial of a home and ambulatory program for asthmatic children. *Pediatrics, 87*(1), 54–61.

Ievers, C. E., Brown, R. T., Drotar, D., Caplan, D., Pishevar, B. S., & Lambert, R. G. (1999). Knowledge of physician prescriptions and adherence to treatment among children with cystic fibrosis and their mothers. *Journal of Developmental and Behavioral Pediatrics, 20*(5), 335–343.

Ingerski, L. M., Baldassano, R. N., Denson, L. A., & Hommel, K. A. (2010). Barriers to oral medication adherence for adolescents with inflammatory bowel disease. *Journal of Pediatric Psychology, 35*(6), 683–691.

Jahng, K. H., Martin, L. R., Golin, C. E., & DiMatteo, M. R. (2005). Preferences for medical collaboration: Patient-physician congruence and patient outcomes. *Patient Education and Counseling, 57*, 308–314.

Janisse, H. C., Naar-King, S., & Ellis, D. (2010). Brief report: Parent's health literacy among high-risk adolescents with insulin dependent diabetes. *Journal of Pediatric Psychology, 35*(4), 436–440.

Jay, M. S., DuRant, R. H., Shoffitt, T., Linder, C. W., & Litt, I. F. (1984). Effect of peer counselors in adolescent compliance in use of oral contraceptives. *Pediatrics, 73*(2), 126–131.

Kovacs, M., Goldston, D., Obrosky, D. S., & Iyengar, S. (1992). Prevalence and predictors of pervasive noncompliance with medical treatment among youths with insulin-dependent diabetes mellitus. *Journal of the American Academy of Child and Adolescent Psychiatry, 31*, 1112–1119.

Kravitz, R. L., Hays, R. D., Sherbourne, C. D., DiMatteo, M. R., Rogers, W. H., Ordway, L., et al. (1993). Recall of recommendations and adherence to advice among patients with chronic medical conditions. *Archives of Internal Medicine, 153*(16), 1869–1878.

La Greca, A. M., Bearman, K. J., & Moore, H. (2002). Peer relations of youth with pediatric conditions and health risks: Promoting social support and healthy lifestyles. *Journal of Developmental and Behavioral Pediatrics, 23*(4), 271–280.

La Greca, A. M., & Hanna, N. (1983). Diabetes-related health beliefs in children and their mothers: Implications for treatment. *Diabetes, 32*(Suppl. 1), 66.

Lewandowski, A., & Drotar, D. (2007). The relationship between parent-reported social support and adherence to medical treatment in families of adolescents with type 1 diabetes. *Journal of Pediatric Psychology, 32*, 427–436.

Lewis, C. C., Pantell, R. H., & Sharp, L. (1991). Increasing patient knowledge, satisfaction, and involvement: Randomized trial of communication intervention. *Pediatrics, 88*(2), 351–358.

Manning, W., & Wells, K. B. (1992). The effect of psychological distress and psychological well-being on use of medical services. *Medical Care, 30*, 541–553.

Martin, L. R., Haskard-Zolnierek, K. B., & DiMatteo, M. R. (2010). *Health behavior change and treatment adherence: Evidence-based guidelines for improving healthcare*. New York: Oxford University Press.

Miller, V. A., & Drotar, D. (2003). Discrepancies between mother and adolescent perceptions of diabetes-related decision-making autonomy and their relationship to diabetes-related conflict and adherence to treatment. *Journal of Pediatric Psychology, 28*(4), 265–274.

Miller, V. A., & Drotar, D. (2007). Decision-making competence and adherence to treatment in adolescents with diabetes. *Journal of Pediatric Psychology, 32*(2), 178–188.

Modi, A. C., Marciel, K. K., Slater, S. K., Drotar, D., & Quittner, A. L. (2008). The influence of parental supervision on medical adherence in adolescents with cystic fibrosis: Developmental shifts from early to late adolescence. *Children's Health Care, 37*, 78–92.

Murphy, D. A., Lam, P., Naar-King, S., Harris, D. R., Parsons, J. T., & Muenz, L. R. (2010). Health literacy and antiretroviral adherence among HIV-infected adolescents. *Patient Education and Counseling, 79*, 25–29.

New England Healthcare Institute. (2010, December 22). *Thinking outside the pillbox: A system wide approach to improving patient medication adherence for chronic disease*. Retrieved from http://www.nehi.net/publications/44/thinking_outside_the_pillbox_a_systemwide_approach_to_improving_patient_medication_adherence_for_chronic_disease.

Nock, M. K., & Kazdin, A. E. (2005). Randomized controlled trial of a brief intervention for increasing participation in parent management training. *Journal of Consulting and Clinical Psychology, 73*(5), 872–879.

Orban, L. A., Stein, R., Koenig, L. J., Conner, L. C., Rexhouse, E. L., Lewis, J. V., et al. (2010). Coping strategies of adolescents living with HIV: Disease-specific stressors and responses. *AIDS Care, 22*(4), 420–430.

Phelan, P. D. (1984). Compliance with medication in children. *Journal of Paediatrics and Child Health, 20*(5), 1440–1754.

Prochaska, J. O., DiClemente, C. C., & Norcross, J. C. (1992). In search of how people change. Applications to addictive behaviors. *American Psychologist, 47*, 1102–1114.

Rapoff, M. A. (1999). *Adherence to pediatric medical regimens*. Dordrecht, Netherlands: Kluwer Academic Publishers.

Riekert, K. A., & Drotar, D. (1999). Who participates in research on adherence to treatment in insulin-dependent diabetes mellitus? Implications and recommendations for research. *Journal of Pediatric Psychology, 24*(3), 253–258.

Rohan, J., Drotar, D., McNally, K., Schluchter, M., Riekert, K., Vavrek, P., et al. (2010). Adherence to pediatric asthma treatment in economically disadvantaged African-American children and adolescents: An application of growth curve analysis. *Journal of Pediatric Psychology, 35*(4), 394–404.

Rudy, B. J., Murphy, D. A., Harris, D. R., Muenz, L., & Ellen, J. (2009). Patient-related risks for nonadherence to antiretroviral therapy among HIV infected youth in the United States: A study of prevalence and interactions. *AIDS Patient Care and STDs, 23*(3), 185–194.

Salamon, K. S., Hains, A. A., Fleischman, K. M., Davies, W. H., & Kichler, J. (2010). Improving adherence in social situations for adolescents with type 1 diabetes mellitus (T1DM): A pilot study. *Primary Care Diabetes, 4*(1), 47–55.

Schrag, S. J., Peña, C., Fernández, J., Sánchez, J., Gómez, V., Pérez, E., et al. (2001). Effect of short-course, high-dose amoxicillin therapy on resistant pneumococcal carriage: a randomized trial. *JAMA: The Journal of the American Medical Association, 286*(1), 49–56.

Sherbourne, C. D., Hays, R. D., Ordway, L., DiMatteo, M. R., & Kravitz, R. L. (1992). Antecedents of adherence to medical recommendations: Results from the medical outcomes study. *Journal of Behavioral Medicine, 15*(5), 447–468.

Sherbourne, C. D., Wells, K. B., Meredith, L. S., Jackson, C. A., & Camp, P. (1996). Comorbid anxiety disorder and the functioning and well-being of chronically ill patients of general medical providers. *Archives of General Psychiatry, 53*, 889–895.

Simmons, L. E., Logan, D. E., Chastain, L., & Cerullo, M. (2010). Engagement in multidisciplinary interventions for pediatric chronic pain: Parental expectations, barriers, and child outcomes. *The Clinical Journal of Pain, 26*(4), 291–299.

Simon, G., Ormel, J., VonKorff, M., & Barlow, W. (1995). Health care costs associated with depressive and anxiety disorders in primary care. *The American Journal of Psychiatry, 152*, 352–357.

Thomas, A. M., Peterson, L., & Goldstein, D. (1997). Problem solving and diabetes regimen adherence by children and adolescents with IDDM in social pressure situations: A reflection of normal development. *Journal of Pediatric Psychology, 22*(4), 541–561.

Van Es, S. M., Nagelkerke, A. F., Colland, V. T., Scholten, R. J. P. M., & Bouter, L. M. (2001). An intervention programme using the ASE-model aimed at enhancing adherence in adolescents with asthma. *Patient Education and Counseling, 44*(3), 193–203.

Walders, N. W., Drotar, D., & Kercsmar, C. (2000). An interdisciplinary intervention for undertreated pediatric asthma. *Chest, 129*, 292–299.

Weissberg-Benchell, J., Glasgow, A. M., Tynan, W. D., Wirtz, P., Turek, J., & Ward, J. (1995). Adolescent diabetes management and mismanagement. *Diabetes Care, 18*, 77–82.

World Health Organization. (2003). *Adherence to long-term therapies evidence for action.* Geneva, Switzerland: Eduardo Sabaté.

Wysocki, T., Greco, P., & Buckloh, L. M. (2003). Childhood diabetes in psychological context. In M. C. Roberts (Ed.), *Handbook of pediatric psychology* (3rd ed.). New York: Guilford Publications, Inc.

Part IV

Mental Health in Adolescent Health Psychology

Smoking in Adolescence

Judith S. Brook, Kerstin Pahl, David W. Brook, and Elaine N. Brown

Rates of adult smoking in the United States have declined in recent years (Centers for Disease Control and Prevention [CDC], 2009; Lee et al., 2007). National antismoking efforts are credited with similar "substantial reductions" in cigarette smoking by adolescents in the last decade (Lopez, Compton, & Volkow, 2009). Unfortunately, according to a national report, this decline in adolescent smoking has diminished in the last few years (CDC, 2010a), and it only continues among specific populations (CDC, 2010b).

Recent estimates indicate that large numbers of adolescents continue to initiate smoking and become regular cigarette smokers. Approximately 1.5 million adolescents smoked cigarettes for the first time in 2009 (Substance Abuse and Mental Health Services Administration [SAMHSA], 2010). Additionally, 403,000 adolescents are estimated to have initiated daily smoking in the past year, or an average of 1,100 per day (SAMHSA, 2010). The prevalence of current smoking among adolescents is approximately 9 % according to one national study (SAMHSA, 2010). Another estimates that 5 % of middle school students and 17 % of high school students were current cigarette smokers in 2009 (CDC, 2010b). These numbers do not account for the use of additional tobacco products such as cigars and smokeless tobacco; 14 % and 9 % of high school students, respectively, reported current use of these products in 2009 (CDC, 2010c).

The initiation of smoking in adolescence is associated with an increased likelihood of smoking in adulthood (Hu, Davies, & Kandel, 2006). This puts adolescent smokers at greater risk of experiencing the health consequences of smoking in adulthood, including heart disease, stroke, respiratory disease (Fagerström, 2002), and at least 15 types of cancer (American Cancer Society, 2010). Nationally, an estimated 443,000 deaths are attributable to tobacco use each year (CDC, 2008). In fact, tobacco use is the leading *preventable* cause of death in the United States (CDC, 2010d). As a result, the persistence of tobacco use among adolescents remains one of the most important public health challenges of our time.

For adolescents, motivations for taking a first cigarette, cigar, or other form of tobacco are manifold. Tobacco use can be an act of rebellion, a way of mimicking adult behaviors, a means for managing one's weight, or an attempt to "fit in" with one's peers. Regardless of these motivational factors, smoking in adolescents is a troubling public health problem because of its adverse effects on the developing adolescent brain and body, which may increase the chance of long-term smoking addiction. Clearly, effective programs are needed to prevent more young people from trying tobacco and to help those who are currently smoking to quit.

J.S. Brook, Ed.D. (✉) • K. Pahl, Ph.D.
D.W. Brook, M.D. • E.N. Brown, B.A.
Department of Psychiatry, New York University
School of Medicine, 215 Lexington Avenue, 15th Floor, New York, NY 10016, USA
e-mail: judith.brook@med.nyu.edu

W.T. O'Donohue et al. (eds.), *Handbook of Adolescent Health Psychology*,
DOI 10.1007/978-1-4614-6633-8_25, © Springer Science+Business Media New York 2013

Developmental Course of Smoking

Recent research has identified prototypical patterns of cigarette use in the form of differential longitudinal trajectories of smoking from adolescence into adulthood (e.g., Brook, Pahl, & Ning, 2006; Brook, Zhang, Brook, & Finch, 2010; Chassin et al., 2008; Costello, Dierker, Jones, & Rose, 2008; Orlando, Tucker, Ellickson, & Klein, 2004). This research suggests that there are different classes of smokers which are characterized by differential developmental patterns of tobacco use over time. Researchers have found between three and six different trajectories, typically including a continuous nonsmoking group, an early-starting group of continuous heavy smokers, and a group of quitters (Chassin et al., 2008; Orlando et al., 2004). It is likely that adolescents in classes of smoking characterized by early initiation and high frequency of use will become dependent on nicotine.

Adolescent Nicotine Dependence

Epidemiology

Nicotine dependence is one of the major risks of tobacco use. Many people continue to smoke, despite concomitant health and social problems, because of their dependence on nicotine. Among adolescents, a recent large-scale community study found that 3.5 % of the sample met CIDI criteria for nicotine dependence (Palmer et al., 2009). When estimates of nicotine dependence are restricted to the smoking population, 36 % of adolescents who smoked in the past month were estimated to be nicotine dependent (SAMHSA, 2008).

Comparisons of rates of nicotine dependence indicate that far fewer adolescent smokers than adult smokers are nicotine dependent (Colby, Tiffany, Shiffman, & Niaura, 2000; SAMHSA, 2008). However, it is important to note that some researchers have argued for the use of a more liberal measure of addiction among adolescent smokers than meeting DSM-IV criteria for dependence. Loss of autonomy over cigarette use, a defining symptom of nicotine addiction, has been reported by adolescent smokers who have not progressed beyond an average rate of consumption of two cigarettes per week (DiFranza, Riggs, & Pentz, 2008).

Transition from Smoking to Nicotine Dependence

It has been suggested that adolescents are more vulnerable to the addictive properties of nicotine than adults (Caraballo, Novak, & Asman, 2009; DiFranza, Savageau, Fletcher, et al., 2002). This may be due to the neurodevelopmental changes that occur during adolescence (Barron et al., 2005; Chambers, Taylor, & Potenza, 2003). According to Gervais and colleagues (2006), adolescents develop symptoms of nicotine dependence soon after they initiate smoking. They can develop nicotine dependence at what are commonly considered infrequent or experimental levels of use (Rose, Dierker, & Donny, 2010). This finding supports the recent call by Fagan and Rigotti (2009) for increased research and policy implementations with regard to light and intermittent smoking worldwide.

Research suggests that genetic factors may also play a role in the transition to dependence. Volkow (April, 2007a) reported on the recent identification of as many as 80 single nucleotide polymorphisms (SNPs), or locations on the human genome, where variations in DNA are highly correlated with nicotine dependence.

Assessment of Nicotine Dependence

Given the recent attention to the criteria used to determine addiction to nicotine among adolescents, it is important to take into consideration a range of diagnostic instruments and their applicability to an adolescent population. According to the Diagnostic and Statistical Manual of Mental Disorders (DSM-IV-TR), published by the American Psychiatric

Association (2000), in order to receive a diagnosis of nicotine dependence, a person must meet a minimum of three out of the following seven criteria: (1) tolerance; (2) withdrawal; (3) greater intake of nicotine or use over a longer period of time than intended; (4) persistent desire or unsuccessful attempts to cut down; (5) spending a great deal of time in activities related to obtaining or using nicotine (e.g., chain-smoking); (6) giving up or reducing important social, occupational, or recreational activities because of nicotine use (e.g., avoiding places where smoking is prohibited); and (7) continued use of nicotine despite knowledge of its having persistent negative physiological or psychological effects.

DiFranza and colleagues (DiFranza et al., 2002) have developed a measure, the ten-item "Hooked on Nicotine Checklist" (HONC), for use with adolescents, which reflects the idea that the single most important feature of dependence is impaired control or the loss of autonomy over the use of the substance. Following are some sample items from the HONC: (1) Have you ever tried to quit, but couldn't? (2) Is it hard to keep from smoking in places where you are not supposed to, like school? (3) Did you feel nervous, restless, or anxious because you couldn't smoke? (DiFranza et al., 2002). According to DiFranza et al. (2002) the onset of dependence can be defined as the moment when an individual loses full exercise of choice over the use of tobacco. Researchers who wish to assess nicotine dependence in adolescents may consider employing the HONC, or the Fagerström Test of Nicotine Dependence (Fagerström, 1978), in addition to the more commonly used DSM-based measures.

Demographic Correlates of Adolescent Smoking

Research in industrialized countries has demonstrated an inverse association between SES and nicotine dependence (Siahpush, McNeill, Borland, & Fong, 2006), and recent studies suggest that this effect extends to the offspring. That is, lower parental SES is linked with greater offspring smoking from adolescence through adulthood (e.g., Fagan, Brook, Rubenstone, & Zhang, 2005; Najman et al., 2004). Low SES may be linked, in part, to adolescents' tobacco use by exposing adolescents to contexts (e.g., neighborhoods) where more people smoke (Fite, Wynn, Lochman, & Wells, 2009).

According to the most recent findings obtained by the Monitoring the Future study (Johnston, O'Malley, Bachman, & Schulenberg, 2010), slightly fewer girls than boys in 8th, 10th, and 12th grades reported smoking in the past 30 days (6.0 % vs. 6.7 %, 12.5 % vs. 13.7 %, and 17.6 % vs. 22.1 %, respectively). There seems to have been a small decrease in smoking among adolescent girls between 2008 and 2009, while the percentage of boys who reported smoking in 10th and 12th grades increased somewhat (there was no change among 8th-grade boys).

The Youth Risk Behavior Surveillance 2009 (CDC, 2010c) found that the prevalence of current smoking among males and females age 12–18 years differed by ethnicity: among Latino and Black adolescents, slightly more males than females reported currently using tobacco (19.4 % vs. 16.7 % and 10.7 % vs. 8.4 %, respectively), while there were virtually no gender differences among White adolescents (22.3 % of boys vs. 22.8 % of girls). With regard to heavy smoking (10+ cigarettes a day), among those who smoked, a greater percentage of males than females reported heavy use across all three ethnic/racial groups (11.0 % of White boys vs. 4.3 % of White girls, 9.3 % of Black boys vs. 1.3 % of Black girls, and 7.9 % of Latino boys vs. 4.4 % of Latina girls).

Risk Factors for Adolescent Smoking

Individual-Level Factors

Personal Attributes

There has been a considerable amount of research examining the types of personal attributes related to adolescent smoking. Personal attributes reflecting unconventionality (e.g., rebelliousness, tolerance of deviance, delinquency) are associated with adolescent smoking initiation, maintenance, and nicotine dependence (Brook, Pahl, Balka, & Fei, 2004; Pahl, Brook, Morojele, & Brook, 2010; Turbin, Jessor, & Costa, 2000). Adolescents who are unconventional are also more likely to associate with friends who smoke cigarettes (Brook, Brook, Gordon, Whiteman, & Cohen, 1990; Brook, Pahl, et al., 2006; Oetting & Donnermeyer, 1998).

Personal attributes reflecting low levels of emotional and behavioral control (e.g., impulsivity) have repeatedly been found related to adolescent smoking (Brook et al., 2004; Mâsse & Tremblay, 1997). For example, a study by Mâsse and Tremblay (1997) found that novelty-seeking occurred more frequently in adolescent smokers than nonsmokers.

Since nicotine is a central nervous system (CNS) stimulant, smokers may use cigarettes in order to control their negative mood states (Shiffman, 1989). Indeed, Orlando et al. (2001) postulate that smoking may be used to ameliorate negative affect such as depression.

Individuals who smoke are also less likely to engage in responsible behavior, are less confident and resourceful, and report lower levels of self-esteem (Etter, 2010).

Weight Concerns

Smoking is often used as a weight reduction and management strategy, especially among adolescent girls and women (Jasuja, Chou, Riggs, & Pentz, 2008; Strauss & Mir, 2001). Although the association of smoking cessation with weight gain has been well documented (Eisenberg & Quinn, 2006; Janzon, Hedblad, Berglund, & Engstrom, 2004), the relationship of current smoking to body weight or body mass index (BMI) is less clear. Some investigations have found that smokers weigh less than nonsmokers (Brook et al., 2010; Jasuja, Chou, Riggs, & Pentz, 2008). In general, adolescents who are overweight may turn to smoking as a method of weight reduction. However, as noted by Jasuja et al. (2008), smoking prevention programs should de-emphasize the benefits of smoking as a means of weight control and emphasize the benefits of healthy eating and exercise instead.

Contextual-Level Factors

Familial Smoking

Family smoking, and especially parental smoking, has been implicated in the development of adolescent smoking (Gilman et al., 2009). Several mechanisms underlying the association between family smoking and tobacco use have been postulated. Behavioral genetic studies suggest that this association may be attributed to genetic influences (Sullivan & Kendler, 1999). There is also the possibility that adolescents model their parents' behavior (Bandura, 1986), although this mechanism is thought to have a greater effect on smoking initiation than smoking persistence (Griesler, Kandel, & Davies, 2002). Several investigators who have examined smoking trajectories over time note that parental smoking is associated with smoking trajectories characterized by early onset and a progression to high levels of smoking over time (Brook, Pahl, et al., 2006; Chassin, Presson, Pitts, & Sherman, 2000).

Maternal smoking during pregnancy has been found to be related to offspring smoking during adolescence (Agrawal et al., 2010). At present, the mechanisms that underlie this association require further study. Nicotine exposure in utero may affect the nicotine receptors of the fetal brain (Ernst, Moolchan, & Robinson, 2001), or it may increase the probability of behavioral dysregulation (e.g., ADHD: Braun, Kahn, Froelich, Auinger, & Lanphear, 2006) and ultimately offspring smoking (Shenassa et al., 2003). Another possibility is that mothers who smoke may have high rates of psychopathology as a result of smoking (e.g., depression), which is transmitted to the child and makes him/her more likely to smoke during adolescence (Shenassa et al., 2003).

Peer Smoking

Brook, Saar, Zhang, and Brook (2009) recently reported that peer smoking was an important factor which mediated the path from parental smoking to the individual's smoking behavior. Indeed, social networks, including friends as well as classmates, have been linked to adolescent smoking behavior. One recent study noted that a 10 % increase in the proportion of classmates who smoke increased the likelihood of smoking by more than 3 %; similarly, an increase of 10 % in the proportion of close friends who smoke resulted in a 5 % increase in an adolescent smoking (Ali & Dwyer, 2009). It is not entirely clear whether the high correlations found between reports of self and peer smoking are due to social influences or to assortative peer selection (i.e., the tendency to select social groups that are similar to oneself; Hoffman, Monge, Chou, & Valente, 2007).

Neighborhood and School Contexts

Characteristics of schools and neighborhoods may also influence adolescent smoking (Ennett et al., 2010; Wen, Van Duker, & Olson, 2009). For example, exposure to models of smoking in the school context is related to adolescent smoking (Ennett et al., 2010). Similarly, Henriksen et al. (2008) found that social norms and the availability of tobacco products in the neighborhood context influence adolescent tobacco use. On the other hand, neighborhoods which are characterized by closeness and which provide social regulation can be deterrents to youth deviance, including tobacco use (Ennett et al., 2010; Sampson, 2006).

Many adolescents of color are subject to high levels of ethnicity-based/racial discrimination, particularly within school settings (e.g., Fisher, Wallace, & Fenton, 2000; Greene, Way, & Pahl, 2006). A growing body of research has linked the experience of ethnicity-based/racial discrimination with tobacco use among adolescents (e.g., Brook, Morojele, Brook, Zhang, & Whiteman, 2006; Gibbons, Gerrard, Cleveland, Wills, & Brody, 2004; Landrine, Klonoff, Corral, Fernandez, & Roesch, 2006). It is likely that stress, caused by racial discrimination, is a main factor leading to higher levels of tobacco use (Williams, Neighbors, & Jackson, 2003).

Media Influences

The media is a significant macro-contextual influence on adolescent smoking (Colby et al., 2000). Individuals in the developmental periods of early and mid-adolescence are particularly vulnerable to tobacco product placement as their recall of tobacco products, including specific cigarette brands, is superior to that of older age groups (Mekemson & Glantz, 2002). It is possible that adolescents' exposure to positive images of smoking is especially powerful in its effect on smoking behavior because adolescents are in the process of developing personal identities and are seeking behavioral role models (Chen, Cruz, Schuster, Unger, & Johnson, 2002).

Exposure to media models of smoking is linked with smoking initiation (Dalton et al., 2003; Sargent et al., 2001), and greater frequency of smoking (Tickle, Sargent, Dalton, Beach, & Heatherton, 2001). Distefan and colleagues (2004) reported that having a favorite movie star who had appeared smoking on-screen in the previous 2 years was independently related to higher odds of smoking initiation. Brook, Pahl, and Morojele (2009) found that adolescents' receptivity to media models of smoking was also related to higher levels of nicotine dependence.

A growing body of research has also linked the use of electronic media, including the Internet and cell phones, to adolescent tobacco use (e.g., Iannotti, Kogan, Janssen, & Boyce, 2009; Ko et al., 2006; Koivusilta, Lintonen, & Rimpelä, 2003; Sánchez-Martínez & Otero, 2009; Steggles & Jarvis, 2003; Sun et al., 2005). The nature of this relationship deserves to be investigated more closely in future research.

Comorbidity of Tobacco Use and Psychopathology

Several investigators have reported high rates of smoking among psychiatric outpatients and inpatients (Brook, Richter, & Rubenstone, 2000; Volkow, Feb., 2007b). Furthermore, research has shown that, among adults, nicotine dependence frequently co-occurs with several psychiatric disorders such as drug and alcohol abuse and dependence (Hasin, Stinson, Ogburn, & Grant, 2007), anxiety (Stinson et al., 2007), and personality disorders (Pulay et al., 2010). The relationship between nicotine dependence and psychiatric disorders may work in two directions: Those with preexisting psychiatric disorders may smoke to decrease some of the negative affect associated with the disorder, and the use of nicotine may serve as a cue for the use of other substances or may induce non-substance-related psychiatric disorders.

Griesler and colleagues (2008), reporting on the co-occurrence of psychiatric disorders with nicotine dependence within an adolescent sample, found support for the role of psychiatric disorders as a risk factor for nicotine dependence. The authors found that, while lifetime psychiatric disorders predicted nicotine dependence in mid-adolescence, nicotine dependence did not predict the onset of psychiatric disorder within adolescence. These results suggest that, in adolescence, nicotine dependence may be operating as a means of self-medication (Khantzian & Albanese, 2008; Upadhyaya, Deas, Brady, & Kruesi, 2002). Indeed, Bizzarri et al. (2007) reported that those with comorbid substance use and mood or anxiety disorders reported higher scores for purposeful "self-medication" compared to those with only substance use disorders. The use of smoking for self-medication can relieve some symptoms temporarily. In the case of individuals with depressive disorders, smoking serves a function similar to that of antidepressants by inhibiting MAO activity (Herraiz & Chaparro, 2005).

Tobacco Use and Health Problems

Bloch, Haverkos, and Jobe (2008) recently called attention to the comorbidity of smoking with serious chronic illnesses among adolescents. Rates of smoking among adolescents with asthma, for example, are equal to or greater than rates of smoking among those without asthma (Tyc & Throckmorton-Belzer, 2006). Even when rates of smoking among adolescents with chronic illnesses such as cancer are less than the rates of the general population, the health complications from smoking while undergoing treatments which already compromise the cardiopulmonary system can be acute (Tyc & Throckmorton-Belzer, 2006). Smoking is likely used as a coping mechanism for stress associated with chronic illness; adolescents with asthma are more likely to initiate smoking if they report using maladaptive coping strategies and a poorer quality of life (Van De Ven, Engels, & Sawyer, 2009).

Prevention and Treatment

Smoking is associated with a host of adverse effects and high morbidity and mortality (e.g., Ezzati, Henley, Thun, & Lopez, 2005; Teo et al., 2006). Because nicotine is a highly addictive substance, it is more promising and more cost-effective to prevent the onset of smoking than to provide smoking cessation treatment.

Smoking Prevention Programs

Strategies for the prevention of adolescent smoking are similar to those used to prevent other adolescent substance use. Preventive interventions at the individual level may target the enhancement of general problem-solving and coping skills, social competence, behavioral self-management, life skills, and specific cigarette refusal skills (Dierker, Merikangas, & Essau, 1997). At the contextual level, giving youth the opportunity for involvement in alternative activities, effecting organizational changes in schools, and training community leaders to organize smoking and drug use prevention task forces can be effective means for smoking prevention (Dierker et al., 1997). A comprehensive approach focusing on different sources of social influence, as well as individual-level factors, seems the most promising.

Macro-Level Prevention Strategies

In addition to antismoking strategies in the home, the school, and the community, public health policies are useful tools in preventing adolescents from smoking. These include educating adolescents about the adverse health effects of smoking and the addictive properties of nicotine, antismoking advertising (Biener et al., 2006; Pechmann & Reibling, 2006), legal and other regulatory efforts (Jason, Berk, Schnopp-Wyatt, & Talbot, 1999; Levy & Friend, 2003), and economic approaches (Frieden et al., 2005; Ross & Chaloupka, 2003). The institutionalization of rules against smoking may motivate people to refrain from smoking initiation or to stop smoking.

The general downward trend in smoking prevalence observed among youth since the late 1990s mirrors the United States' increasing adoption of antismoking legislation, including policies restricting youth access to tobacco products, introducing clean indoor air laws, and imposing additional excise taxes (Nelson et al., 2008).

For example, a study of smoking in 39 states with smoking control policies revealed that, while a relatively small number of high school students purchased cigarettes at stores, stringent restrictions prohibiting sales of cigarettes to minors reduce the likelihood that adolescents will transition from experimental smoking to established smoking (Botello-Harbaum et al., 2009). Retailer compliance with laws limiting sales to minors has been demonstrated to be an important factor in reducing access to cigarettes among youth (Cummings, Hyland, Perla, & Giovino, 2003).

In addition, indirect policies like clean indoor air laws that designate smoke-free stores, recreational facilities, schools, and worksites have proven another effective tool to prevent adolescent smoking. An increase in clean indoor air laws in several states has been shown to be inversely related to the number of youth who smoke in these states (McMullen, Brownson, Luke, & Chriqui, 2005).

As part of an economic approach to smoking prevention, additional excise taxes on cigarettes, resulting in higher retail prices, have been shown to deter initiation of smoking and to lower levels of consumption. In fact, increasing the price of cigarettes may be even more effective in preventing tobacco use among youth than among adults. Increased prices not only decrease cigarette purchases directly but also indirectly by restricting the possibility of "bumming" cigarettes from friends, who are less likely to share when prices run high (Chaloupka, 2003; Liang, Chalpoupka, Nichter, & Clayton, 2003).

Smoking Cessation Treatment

This section will discuss briefly a number of approaches used in the treatment of tobacco dependence. The term tobacco dependence is commonly used, but tobacco is addicting because of its nicotine content, although the psychosocial concomitants of smoking also contribute to dependence. Nicotine, a CNS stimulant, is among the most addictive substances (U.S. Department of Health and Human Services, 2010). Nicotine stimulates dopamine release in the nucleus accumbens, a component of the brain reward system, thus reinforcing smoking behavior (Fu, Matta, Gao, Brower, & Sharp, 2000). As a result, it is difficult to achieve lasting smoking cessation for most people. Repeated quit attempts are commonly needed, and an interim goal of decreasing the number of cigarettes smoked (a harm reduction approach) may be helpful. Methods of treating tobacco dependence which combine psychosocial treatment techniques and psychopharmacological treatments are most effective (Ingersoll & Cohen, 2005).

Psychosocial Treatments

Many methods to achieve cessation involve the use of educational materials and advice given by physicians and other healthcare professionals. These types of interventions can be helpful in smoking cessation (Pbert et al., 2008). In addition, therapeutic approaches, both for individuals and groups, have been developed to motivate smokers to quit. Treatment may include individual or group sessions, which often employ a cognitive-behavioral approach. Smoking cessation groups for adolescents can provide mutual support, education about smoking and cessation, and behavioral skills training to quit smoking and maintain abstinence (Carmody, 2002). Several public and private agencies such as the American Cancer Society and the American Lung Association offer smoking cessation programs for adolescents. Unfortunately, many smokers who want to quit do not join smoking cessation treatment programs.

In both individual and group therapy, smoking cessation involves three phases: (1) evaluating the adolescent's desire to stop smoking, (2) providing the adolescent with practical assistance to quit, and (3) monitoring the adolescent's success in quitting. For those adolescents who do not want to stop smoking in phase 1, a motivational intervention may be implemented in which the adolescent is encouraged to consider the adverse health and social consequences of smoking, as well as the positive effects of stopping smoking. The difficulties the adolescent will confront in the process of quitting are discussed and techniques that can be used to deal with these barriers are presented. In phase 2, therapists and group members talk about methods of stopping and determine "quit dates." On the quit date, the group offers support and methods for coping without cigarettes.

In phase 3, relapse prevention sessions help adolescent group members maintain abstinence. Cognitive-behavioral techniques and coping skills training are helpful not only in prevention and treatment but also in relapse prevention. Relapse prevention methods identify risky "people, places, and things," and help adolescent members cope with these risks. Examples of risky situations include the presence of other people smoking, or being in a store where cigarettes are offered for sale. The concurrent treatment of depression is essential in smoking cessation. Group support and antidepressant medication (e.g., bupropion) have been shown to contribute to success in smoking cessation.

Psychopharmacological Treatments

There are a number of medications now available for the treatment of tobacco dependence. We summarize these in the table below.

Tobacco dependence medications

Classification	Examples
Nicotinic receptor agonists	Nicotine oral inhaler
	Nicotine nasal spray
	Nicotine polacrilex (gum or lozenge)
	Nicotine transdermal patch
Dopaminergic–noradrenergic reuptake inhibitor (DNRI)	Bupropion
Nicotinic receptor partial agonist	Varenicline

Concluding Remarks

Adolescent smoking is a considerable public health problem in the USA today, as a substantial number of teenagers continue to engage in tobacco use (SAMHSA, 2010). Despite a downward trend in adolescent smoking since the 1990s, 20% of 12th graders reported daily tobacco use in 2009. Thus, existing prevention initiatives do not seem to reach a fifth of all US adolescents. Identifying and targeting the most important risk factors for adolescent tobacco use is therefore a crucial concern for public health.

Most smokers initiate tobacco use in adolescence (Johnston, O'Malley, Bachman, & Schulenberg, 2009), and research shows that early initiation is linked with lifelong patterns of heavy smoking and dependence on nicotine (Hu et al., 2006). The percentage of adolescents who smoke on a regular basis increases throughout the high school years (Johnston et al., 2010). Thus, a substantial number of adolescents are dependent on nicotine by late adolescence. Over time, smoking initiated in adolescence will result in a staggering health cost and economic burden.

Research has shown that a broad constellation of developmental domains influence adolescent tobacco use. These domains include the school and neighborhood contexts, family SES, parental tobacco use, peer factors, media use, and macrocontextual factors such as tobacco policies (e.g., Ennett et al., 2010; Fagan et al., 2005; Hoffman et al., 2007; Nelson et al., 2008; Peretti-Watel, Legleye, & Beck, 2002; Sánchez-Martínez & Otero, 2009; Steggles & Jarvis, 2003; Sun et al., 2005).

It would be of great value to gain a better understanding of how these factors interact with one another to influence adolescent tobacco use. Research which examines the contributions of multiple individual-level and contextual-level factors to adolescent smoking simultaneously is needed. Such research can inform policy makers and intervention specialists about the most proximal and powerful determinants of adolescent smoking, and thus guide resource allocation.

In addition, large controlled clinical trials are needed to assess underlying genetic predispositions for tobacco use and nicotine dependence, and to examine gene–environment interactions. A greater understanding of the complex interactions of the biopsychosocial factors implicated in the etiology of adolescent tobacco use and dependence is essential for the development of more effective treatments.

In sum, future research into the biological and psychosocial etiology of adolescent tobacco use and nicotine dependence is needed using a comprehensive biobehavioral approach. Both pharmacological and psychosocial approaches to prevention and treatment focused on smoking cessation deserve research and clinical attention.

References

Agrawal, A., Scherrer, J. F., Grant, J. D., Sartor, C. E., Pergadia, M. L., Duncan, A. E., et al. (2010). The effects of maternal smoking during pregnancy on offspring outcomes. *Preventive Medicine, 50*, 13–18.

Ali, M. M., & Dwyer, D. S. (2009). Estimating peer effects in adolescent smoking behavior: A longitudinal analysis. *Journal of Adolescent Health, 45*, 402–408.

American Cancer Society. (2010). *Cancer facts & figures 2010*. Atlanta, GA: American Cancer Society.

American Psychiatric Association. (2000). *Diagnostic and statistical manual of mental disorders: Revised* (4th ed.). Washington, DC: American Psychiatric Association.

Bandura, A. (1986). *Social foundations of thought and action: A social cognitive theory*. Englewood Cliffs, NJ: Prentice Hall.

Barron, S., White, A., Swartzwelder, H. S., Bell, R. L., Rodd, Z. A., Slawecki, C. J., et al. (2005). Adolescent vulnerabilities to chronic alcohol or nicotine exposure: Findings from rodent models. *Alcoholism, Clinical and Experimental Research, 29*, 1720–1725.

Biener, L., Reimer, R. L., Wakefield, M., Szczypka, G., Rigotti, N. A., & Connolly, G. (2006). Impact of smoking cessation aids and mass media among recent quitters. *American Journal of Preventive Medicine, 30*, 217–224.

Bizzarri, J. V., Rucci, P., Sbrana, A., Gonnelli, C., Massei, G. J., Ravani, L., et al. (2007). Reasons for substance use and vulnerability factors in patients with substance use disorder and anxiety or mood disorders. *Addictive Behaviors, 32*, 384–391.

Bloch, M., Haverkos, L., & Jobe, J. B. (2008). Tobacco use and secondhand smoke exposure of children and youth with serious chronic illness: Establishing an agenda for research and action. *Journal of Pediatric Psychology, 33*, 111–112.

Botello-Harbaum, M., Haynie, D., Iannotti, R., Wang, J., Gase, L., & Simons-Morton, B. (2009). Tobacco control policy and adolescent smoking status in the United States. *Nicotine & Tobacco Research, 11*, 875–885.

Braun, J., Kahn, R. S., Froelich, T., Auinger, P., & Lanphear, B. P. (2006). Exposure to environmental toxicants and Attention Deficit Hyperactivity Disorder in US children. *Environmental Health Perspectives, 114*, 1904–1909.

Brook, D. W., Zhang, C., Brook, J. S., & Finch, S. J. (2010). Trajectories of cigarette smoking from adolescence to young adulthood as predictors of obesity in the mid-30s. *Nicotine & Tobacco Research, 12*, 263–270.

Brook, J. S., Brook, D. W., Gordon, A., Whiteman, M., & Cohen, P. (1990). The psychosocial etiology of adolescent drug use: A family interactional approach. *Genetic, Social, and General Psychology Monographs, 116*, 111–267.

Brook, J. S., Morojele, N. K., Brook, D. W., Zhang, C., & Whiteman, M. (2006). Personal, interpersonal, and cultural predictors of stages of cigarette smoking among adolescents in Johannesburg, South Africa. *Tobacco Control, 15*, i48–i53.

Brook, J. S., Pahl, K., Balka, E. B., & Fei, K. (2004). Smoking among New Yorican adolescents: Time 1 predictors of time 2 tobacco use. *Journal of Genetic Psychology, 165*, 310–323.

Brook, J. S., Pahl, K., & Morojele, N. K. (2009). The relationship between receptivity to media models of smoking and nicotine dependence among South African adolescents. *Addiction Research and Theory, 17*, 493–503.

Brook, J. S., Pahl, K., & Ning, Y. (2006). Peer and parent influences on longitudinal trajectories of smoking among African Americans and Puerto Ricans. *Nicotine & Tobacco Research, 8*, 639–651.

Brook, J. S., Richter, L., & Rubenstone, E. (2000). Consequences of adolescent drug use on psychiatric disorders in early adulthood. *Annals of Medicine, 32*, 401–407.

Brook, J. S., Saar, N. S., Zhang, C., & Brook, D. W. (2009). Familial and non-familial smoking: Effects on smoking and nicotine dependence. *Drug and Alcohol Dependence, 101*, 62–68.

Caraballo, R. S., Novak, S. P., & Asman, K. (2009). Linking quantity and frequency profiles of cigarette smoking to the presence of nicotine dependence symptoms among adolescent smokers: Findings from the 2004 National Youth Tobacco Survey. *Nicotine & Tobacco Research, 11*, 49–57.

Carmody, T. P. (2002). Smoking cessation treatment groups. In D. W. Brook & H. I. Spitz (Eds.), *The group therapy of substance abuse* (pp. 351–368). New York: Haworth Press.

Centers for Disease Control and Prevention. (2008, November). Smoking-attributable mortality, years of potential life lost, and productivity losses—United States, 2000–2004. *Morbidity and Mortality Weekly Report, 57*(45), 1226–1228.

Centers for Disease Control and Prevention. (2009, November). Cigarette smoking among adults and

trends in smoking cessation—United States, 2008. *Morbidity and Mortality Weekly Report, 58*(44), 1227–1232.
Centers for Disease Control and Prevention. (2010a). Cigarette use among high school students—United States, 1991–2009. *Morbidity and Mortality Weekly Report, 59*(26), 797–801.
Centers for Disease Control and Prevention. (2010b). Tobacco use among middle and high school students—United States, 2000–2009. *Morbidity and Mortality Weekly Report, 59*(33), 1063–1068.
Centers for Disease Control and Prevention. (2010c). Youth risk behavior surveillance—United States, 2009. *Morbidity and Mortality Weekly Report, 59*(SS-5), 1–13.
Centers for Disease Control and Prevention. (2010d). Vital signs: Current cigarette smoking among adults aged ≥18 years—United States, 2009. *Morbidity and Mortality Weekly Report, 59*(35), 1135–1140.
Chaloupka, F. J. (2003). Contextual factors and youth tobacco use: Policy linkages. *Addiction, 98*(Suppl. 1), 147–149.
Chambers, R. A., Taylor, J. R., & Potenza, M. N. (2003). Developmental neurocircuitry of motivation in adolescence: A critical period of addiction vulnerability. *The American Journal of Psychiatry, 160*, 1041–1052.
Chassin, L., Presson, C. C., Pitts, S. C., & Sherman, S. J. (2000). The natural history of cigarette smoking from adolescence to adulthood in a Midwestern community sample: Multiple trajectories and their psychosocial correlates. *Health Psychology, 19*, 223–231.
Chassin, L., Presson, C., Seo, D.-C., Sherman, S. J., Macy, J., Wirth, R. J., et al. (2008). Multiple trajectories of cigarette smoking and the intergenerational transmission of smoking: A multigenerational, longitudinal study of a Midwestern community sample. *Health Psychology, 27*, 819–828.
Chen, X., Cruz, T. S., Schuster, D. V., Unger, J. B., & Johnson, C. A. (2002). Receptivity to pro-tobacco media and its impact on cigarette smoking among ethnic minority youth in California. *Journal of Health Communication, 7*, 95–111.
Colby, S. M., Tiffany, S. T., Shiffman, S., & Niaura, R. S. (2000). Are adolescent smokers dependent on nicotine? A review of the evidence. *Drug and Alcohol Dependence, 59*(Suppl. 1), S83–S95.
Costello, D. M., Dierker, L. C., Jones, B. L., & Rose, J. S. (2008). Trajectories of smoking from adolescence to early adulthood and their psychosocial risk factors. *Health Psychology, 27*, 811–818.
Cummings, K. M., Hyland, A., Perla, J., & Giovino, G. A. (2003). Is the prevalence of youth smoking affected by efforts to increase retailer compliance with minors' access law? *Nicotine & Tobacco Research, 5*, 465–471.
Dalton, M. A., Sargent, J. D., Beach, M. L., Titus-Ernstoff, L., Gibson, J. J., Ahrens, M. B., et al. (2003). Effect of viewing smoking in movies on adolescent smoking initiation: A cohort study. *Lancet, 362*, 281–285.
Dierker, L., Merikangas, K. R., & Essau, C. A. (1997). Substance use disorders. In C. A. Essau & F. Petermann (Eds.), *Developmental psychopathology: Epidemiology, diagnostics and treatment* (pp. 311–344). Australia: Harwood Academic Publishers.
DiFranza, J. R., Riggs, N., & Pentz, M. A. (2008). Time to re-examine old definitions of nicotine dependence. *Nicotine & Tobacco Research, 10*, 1109–1111.
DiFranza, J. R., Savageau, J. A., Fletcher, K., Ockene, J. K., Rigotti, N. A., McNeill, A., et al. (2002). Measuring the loss of autonomy over nicotine use in adolescents: The DANDY (Development and Assessment of Nicotine Dependence in Youths) study. *Archives of Pediatrics & Adolescent Medicine, 156*, 397–403.
Distefan, J. M., Pierce, J. P., & Gilpin, E. A. (2004). Do favorite movie stars influence adolescent smoking initiation? *American Journal of Public Health, 94*, 1239–1244.
Eisenberg, D., & Quinn, B. C. (2006). Estimating the effect of smoking cessation on weight gain: An instrumental variable approach. *Health Services Research, 41*, 2255–2266.
Ennett, S. T., Foshee, V. A., Bauman, K. E., Hussong, A., Faris, R., Hipp, J. R., et al. (2010). A social contextual analysis of youth cigarette smoking development. *Nicotine & Tobacco Research, 12*, 950–962.
Ernst, M., Moolchan, E., & Robinson, M. (2001). Behavioral and neural consequences of prenatal exposure to nicotine. *Journal of the American Academy of Child and Adolescent Psychiatry, 40*, 630–641.
Etter, J.-F. (2010). Smoking and Cloninger's temperament and character inventory. *Nicotine & Tobacco Research Advance Access, 12*, e1–e8.
Ezzati, M., Henley, S. J., Thun, M. J., & Lopez, A. D. (2005). Role of smoking in global and regional cardiovascular mortality. *Circulation, 112*(4), 489–497.
Fagan, P., Brook, J. S., Rubenstone, E., & Zhang, C. (2005). Parental occupation, education, and smoking as predictors of offspring tobacco use in adulthood: A longitudinal study. *Addictive Behaviors, 30*, 514–529.
Fagan, P., & Rigotti, N. A. (2009). Light and intermittent smoking: The road less traveled. *Nicotine & Tobacco Research, 11*, 107–110.
Fagerström, K. O. (1978). Measuring degree of physical dependence to tobacco smoking with reference to individualization of treatment. *Addictive Behaviors, 3*, 235–241.
Fagerström, K. (2002). The epidemiology of smoking: Health consequences and benefits of cessation. *Drugs, 62*, 1–9.
Fisher, C. B., Wallace, S. A., & Fenton, R. E. (2000). Discrimination distress during adolescence. *Journal of Youth and Adolescence, 29*, 679–695.
Fite, P. J., Wynn, P., Lochman, J. E., & Wells, K. C. (2009). The influence of neighborhood disadvantage and perceived disapproval on early substance use initiation. *Addictive Behaviors, 34*, 769–771.
Frieden, T. R., Mostashari, F., Kerker, B. D., Miller, N., Hajat, A., & Frankel, M. (2005). Adult tobacco use levels after intensive tobacco control measures: New York City, 2002–2003. *American Journal of Public Health, 95*, 1016–1023.

Fu, Y., Matta, S. G., Gao, W., Brower, V. G., & Sharp, B. M. (2000). Systemic nicotine stimulates dopamine release in nucleus accumbens: Re-evaluation of the role of *N*-methyl-D-aspartate receptors in the ventral tegmental area. *Journal of Pharmacology and Experimental Therapeutics, 294*, 458–465.

Gervais, A., O'Loughlin, J., Meshefedjian, G., Bancej, C., & Tremblay, M. (2006). Milestones in the natural course of onset of cigarette use among adolescents. *Canadian Medical Association Journal, 175*, 255–263.

Gibbons, F. X., Gerrard, M., Cleveland, M. J., Wills, T. A., & Brody, G. (2004). Perceived discrimination and substance use in African American parents and their children: A panel study. *Journal of Personality and Social Psychology, 86*, 517–529.

Gilman, S. E., Rende, R., Boergers, J., Abrams, D. B., Buka, S. L., Clark, M. A., et al. (2009). Parental smoking and adolescent smoking initiation: An intergenerational perspective on tobacco control. *Pediatrics, 123*, e274–e281.

Greene, M. L., Way, N., & Pahl, K. (2006). Trajectories of perceived adult and peer discrimination among Black, Latino, and Asian American adolescents: Patterns and psychological correlates. *Developmental Psychology, 42*, 218–238.

Griesler, P. C., Hu, M.-C., Schaffran, C., & Kandel, D. B. (2008). Comorbidity of psychiatric disorders and nicotine dependence among adolescents: Findings from a prospective, longitudinal study. *Journal of the American Academy of Child and Adolescent Psychiatry, 47*, 1340–1350.

Griesler, P. C., Kandel, D. B., & Davies, M. (2002). Ethnic differences in predictors of initiation and persistence of adolescent cigarette smoking in the National Longitudinal Survey of Youth. *Nicotine & Tobacco Research, 4*, 79–93.

Hasin, D. S., Stinson, F. S., Ogburn, E., & Grant, B. F. (2007). Prevalence, correlates, disability, and comorbidity of DSM-IV alcohol abuse and dependence in the United States: Results from the National Epidemiologic Survey on Alcohol and Related Conditions. *Archives of General Psychiatry, 64*, 830–842.

Henriksen, L., Feighery, E. C., Schleicher, N. C., Cowling, D. W., Kline, R. S., & Fortmann, S. P. (2008). Is adolescent cigarette smoking related to the density and proximity of tobacco outlets and retail cigarette advertising near schools? *Preventive Medicine, 47*, 210–214.

Herraiz, T., & Chaparro, C. (2005). Human monoamine oxidase is inhibited by tobacco smoke: β-Carboline alkaloids act as potent and reversible inhibitors. *Biochemical and Biophysical Research Communications, 326*, 378–386.

Hoffman, B. R., Monge, P. R., Chou, C.-P., & Valente, T. W. (2007). Perceived peer influence and peer selection on adolescent smoking. *Addictive Behaviors, 32*, 1546–1554.

Hu, M.-C., Davies, M., & Kandel, D. B. (2006). Epidemiology and correlates of daily smoking and nicotine dependence among young adults in the United States. *American Journal of Public Health, 96*, 299–308.

Iannotti, R. J., Kogan, M. D., Janssen, I., & Boyce, W. F. (2009). Patterns of adolescent physical activity, screen-based media use, and positive and negative health indicators in the U.S. and Canada. *Journal of Adolescent Health, 44*, 493–499.

Ingersoll, K. S., & Cohen, J. (2005). Combination treatment for nicotine dependence: State of the science. *Substance Use & Misuse, 40*, 1923–1943.

Janzon, E., Hedblad, B., Berglund, G., & Engstrom, G. (2004). Changes in blood pressure and body weight following smoking cessation in women. *Journal of Internal Medicine, 255*, 266–272.

Jason, L. A., Berk, M., Schnopp-Wyatt, D. L., & Talbot, B. (1999). Effects of enforcement of youth access laws on smoking prevalence. *American Journal of Community Psychology, 27*, 143–160.

Jasuja, G. K., Chou, C.-P., Riggs, N. R., & Pentz, M. A. (2008). Early cigarette use and psychological distress as predictors of obesity risk in adulthood. *Nicotine & Tobacco Research, 10*, 325–355.

Johnston, L. D., O'Malley, P. M., Bachman, J. G., & Schulenberg, J. E. (2009). *Monitoring the future national survey results on drug use, 1975–2008* (College students and adults ages 19–50, Vol. 2). Bethesda, MD: National Institute on Drug Abuse (NIH Publication No. 09-7403).

Johnston, L. D., O'Malley, P. M., Bachman, J. G., & Schulenberg, J. E. (2010). *Monitoring the future national survey results on drug use, 1975–2009* (Secondary school students, Vol. 1). Bethesda, MD: National Institute on Drug Abuse (NIH Publication No.10-7584).

Khantzian, E. J., & Albanese, M. J. (2008). *Understanding addiction as self medication: Finding hope behind the pain*. Plymouth, UK: Rowman & Littlefield.

Ko, C.-H., Yen, J.-Y., Chen, C.-C., Chen, S.-H., Wu, K., & Yen, C.-F. (2006). Tridimensional personality of adolescents with internet addiction and substance use experience. *Canadian Journal of Psychiatry, 51*, 887–894.

Koivusilta, L., Lintonen, T., & Rimpelä, A. (2003). Mobile cell phone use has not replaced smoking in adolescence. *British Medical Journal, 326*, 161.

Landrine, H., Klonoff, E. A., Corral, I., Fernandez, S., & Roesch, S. (2006). Conceptualizing and measuring ethnic discrimination in health research. *Journal of Behavioral Medicine, 29*, 79–94.

Lee, D. J., Fleming, L. E., Arheart, K. L., LeBlanc, W. G., Caban, A. J., Chung-Bridges, K., et al. (2007). Smoking rate trends in U.S. occupational groups: The 1987 to 2004 National Health Interview Survey. *Journal of Occupational and Environmental Medicine, 49*, 75–81.

Levy, D. T., & Friend, K. B. (2003). The effects of clean indoor air laws: What do we know and what do we need to know? *Health Education Research, 18*, 592–609.

Liang, L., Chalpoupka, F., Nichter, M., & Clayton, R. (2003). Prices, policies and youth smoking. *Addiction, 98*(Suppl. 1), 105–122.

Lopez, M. F., Compton, W. M., & Volkow, N. D. (2009). Changes in cigarette and illicit drug use among US teenagers. *Archives of Pediatric and Adolescent Medicine, 163*, 869.

Mâsse, L., & Tremblay, R. (1997). Behavior of boys in kindergarten and onset of substance use during adolescence. *Archives of General Psychiatry, 54*, 62–68.

McMullen, K. M., Brownson, R. C., Luke, D., & Chriqui, J. (2005). Strength of clean indoor air laws and smoking related outcomes in the USA. *Tobacco Control, 14*, 43–48.

Mekemson, C., & Glantz, S. A. (2002). How the tobacco industry built its relationship with Hollywood. *Tobacco Control, 11*(Suppl. 1), I81–I191.

Najman, J. M., Aird, R., Bor, W., O'Callaghan, M., Williams, G. M., & Shuttlewood, G. J. (2004). The intergenerational transmission of socioeconomic inequalities in child cognitive development and emotional health. *Social Science & Medicine, 58*, 1147–1158.

Nelson, D. E., Mowery, P., Asman, K., Pederson, L. L., O'Malley, P. M., Malarcher, A., et al. (2008). Long-term trends in adolescent and young adult smoking in the United States: Metapatterns and implications. *American Journal of Public Health, 98*, 905–915.

Oetting, E. R., & Donnermeyer, J. F. (1998). Primary socialization theory: The etiology of drug use and deviance. I. *Substance Use & Misuse, 33*, 995–1026.

Orlando, M., Ellickson, P. L., & Jinnett, K. (2001). The temporal relationship between emotional distress and cigarette smoking during adolescence and young adulthood. *Journal of Consulting and Clinical Psychology, 69*, 959–970.

Orlando, M., Tucker, J. S., Ellickson, P. L., & Klein, D. J. (2004). Developmental trajectories of cigarette smoking and their correlates from early adolescence to young adulthood. *Journal of Consulting and Clinical Psychology, 72*, 400–410.

Pahl, K., Brook, D. W., Morojele, N. K., & Brook, J. S. (2010). Nicotine dependence and problem behaviors among urban South African adolescents. *Journal of Behavioral Medicine, 33*, 101–109.

Palmer, R. H. C., Young, S. E., Hopfer, C. J., Corley, R. P., Stallings, M. C., Crowley, T. J., et al. (2009). Developmental epidemiology of drug use and abuse in adolescence and young adulthood: Evidence of generalized risk. *Drug and Alcohol Dependence, 102*, 78–87.

Pbert, L., Flint, A. J., Fletcher, K. E., Young, M. H., Druker, S., & DiFranza, J. R. (2008). Effect of a pediatric practice-based smoking prevention and cessation intervention for adolescents: A randomized, controlled trial. *Pediatrics, 121*, e738–e747.

Pechmann, C., & Reibling, E. T. (2006). Antismoking advertisements for youths: An independent evaluation of health, counter-industry, and industry approaches. *American Journal of Public Health, 96*, 906–913.

Peretti-Watel, P., Legleye, S., & Beck, F. (2002). Cigarettes and mobile phones: Are they complementary or substitutable products? *Drugs: Education, Prevention, and Policy, 9*, 339–343.

Pulay, A. J., Stinson, F. S., Ruan, W. J., Smith, S. M., Pickering, R. P., Dawson, D. A., et al. (2010). The relationship of DSM-IV personality disorders to nicotine dependence—Results from a national survey. *Drug and Alcohol Dependence, 108*, 141–145.

Rose, J. S., Dierker, L. C., & Donny, E. (2010). Nicotine dependence symptoms among recent onset adolescent smokers. *Drug and Alcohol Dependence, 106*, 126–132.

Ross, H., & Chaloupka, F. J. (2003). The effect of cigarette prices on youth smoking. *Health Economics, 12*, 217–230.

Sampson, R. J. (2006). Collective efficacy theory: Lessons learned and directions for future inquiry. In F. T. Cullen, J. P. Wright, & K. R. Blevins (Eds.), *Taking stock: The status of criminological theory* (pp. 149–167). New Brunswick, NJ: Transaction Publishers.

Sánchez-Martínez, M., & Otero, A. (2009). Factors associated with cell phone use in adolescents in the community of Madrid (Spain). *Cyberpsychology & Behavior, 12*, 131–137.

Sargent, J. D., Tickle, J. J., Beach, M. L., Dalton, M. A., Ahrens, M. B., & Heatherton, T. F. (2001). Brand appearance in contemporary cinema films and contribution to global marketing of cigarettes. *Lancet, 357*, 29–32.

Shenassa, E. D., McCaffery, J. M., Swan, G. E., Khroyan, T. V., Shakib, S., Lerman, C., et al. (2003). Intergenerational transmission of tobacco use and dependence: A transdisciplinary approach. *Nicotine & Tobacco Research, 5*(Suppl. 1), S55–S69.

Shiffman, S. (1989). Tobacco "chippers"—Individual differences in tobacco dependence. *Psychopharmacology, 97*, 539–547.

Siahpush, M., McNeill, A., Borland, R., & Fong, G. T. (2006). Socioeconomic variations in nicotine dependence, self-efficacy, and intention to quit across four countries: Findings from the International Tobacco Control (ITC) Four Country Survey. *Tobacco Control, 15*(Suppl 3), iii71–iii75.

Steggles, N., & Jarvis, M. J. (2003). Do mobile phones replace cigarette smoking among teenagers? *Tobacco Control, 12*, 339–340.

Stinson, F. S., Dawson, D. A., Chou, S. P., Smith, S., Goldstein, R. B., Ruan, W. J., et al. (2007). The epidemiology of DSM-IV specific phobia in the USA: Results from the National Epidemiologic Survey on Alcohol and Related Conditions. *Psychological Medicine, 37*, 1047–1059.

Strauss, R. S., & Mir, H. M. (2001). Smoking and weight loss attempts in overweight and normal-weight adolescents. *International Journal of Obesity and Related Metabolic Disorders, 25*, 1381–1385.

Substance Abuse and Mental Health Services Administration. (2008). *NSDUH Report, Nicotine dependence: 2006*. Rockville, MD: Office of Applied Studies.

Substance Abuse and Mental Health Services Administration. (2010). *Results from the 2009 national survey on drug use and health* (Summary of national findings, Vol. 1). Rockville, MD: Office of Applied

Studies. NSDUH Series H-38A, HHS Publication No. SMA 10-4586Findings.

Sullivan, P. F., & Kendler, K. S. (1999). The genetic epidemiology of smoking. *Nicotine & Tobacco Research, 1*, S51–S57.

Sun, P., Unger, J. B., Palmer, P. H., Gallaher, P., Chou, C.-P., Baezconde-Garbanati, L., et al. (2005). Internet accessibility and usage among urban adolescents in Southern California: Implications for web-based health research. *Cyberpsychology & Behavior, 8*, 441–453.

Teo, K. K., Ounpuu, S., Hawken, S., Pandey, M. R., Valentin, V., Hunt, D., et al. (2006). Tobacco use and risk of myocardial infarction in 52 countries in the INTERHEART study: A case-control study. *Lancet, 368*, 647–658.

Tickle, J. J., Sargent, J. D., Dalton, M. A., Beach, M. L., & Heatherton, T. F. (2001). Favourite movie stars, their tobacco use in contemporary movies, and its association with adolescent smoking. *Tobacco Control, 10*, 16–22.

Turbin, M., Jessor, R., & Costa, F. (2000). Adolescent cigarette smoking: Health-related behavior or normative transgression? *Prevention Science, 1*, 115–124.

Tyc, V. L., & Throckmorton-Belzer, L. (2006). Smoking rates and the state of smoking interventions for children and adolescents with chronic illness. *Pediatrics, 118*, e471–e487.

U.S. Department of Health and Human Services. (2010). *How tobacco smoke causes disease: The biology and behavioral basis for smoking-attributable disease: A report of the surgeon general*. Atlanta, GA: U.S. Department of Health and Human Services, Centers for Disease Control and Prevention, National Center for Chronic Disease Prevention and Health Promotion, Office on Smoking and Health.

Upadhyaya, H. P., Deas, D., Brady, K. T., & Kruesi, M. (2002). Cigarette smoking and psychiatric comorbidity in children and adolescents. *Journal of the American Academy of Child and Adolescent Psychiatry, 41*, 1294–1305.

Van De Ven, M. O. M., Engels, R. C. M. E., & Sawyer, S. M. (2009). Asthma-specific predictors of smoking onset in adolescents with asthma: A longitudinal study. *Journal of Pediatric Psychology, 34*, 118–128.

Volkow, N. D. (April 2007). Director's perspective: Genes and smoking. *NIDA Notes, 21*(3).

Volkow, N. D. (Feb. 2007). Director's perspective: Addiction and co-occurring mental disorders. *NIDA Notes, 21*(2).

Wen, M., Van Duker, H., & Olson, L. M. (2009). Social contexts of regular smoking in adolescence: Towards a multidimensional ecological model. *Journal of Adolescence, 32*, 671–692.

Williams, D. R., Neighbors, H. W., & Jackson, J. S. (2003). Racial/ethnic discrimination and health: Findings from community studies. *American Journal of Public Health, 93*, 200–208.

Adolescent Substance Abuse

Brad Donohue, Jessica Urgelles, and Jasmine Fayeghi

Adolescent Substance Abuse

Adolescent substance use disorders (SUDs) have great implications in public health. Indeed, very few disorders have been associated with greater physical, mental, and emotional consequences. In this chapter we will review (1) the diagnostic symptoms of substance abuse and dependence, (2) the prevalence of illicit substances that are commonly abused by adolescents, (3) common coexisting problem disorders, (4) etiological theories that assist in explaining how SUDs develop, and (5) evidence-based methods of assessing and treating this pandemic problem. Throughout this chapter, we highlight contextual factors that act to influence SUDs in adolescents, including "real-life" examples, cultural and developmental considerations, and future directions.

Description of Substance Abuse and Dependence

In the fourth edition of the Diagnostic and Statistical Manual (DSM-IV-TR; American Psychiatric Association, 2000), substance abuse is reported to be a maladaptive pattern of substance use that leads to clinically significant impairment or distress. The condition is marked by one of four problematic patterns of use within a 12-month period. These patterns include failure to fulfill major role obligations, use in physically hazardous situations, use resulting in legal problems, and use despite continued interpersonal problems. Relative to adults, adolescents may be particularly vulnerable to substance abuse because, as will be underscored later, they are more prone to act without consideration of consequences, evidence decreased tolerance, and generally lack insight and problem-solving abilities. Examples of how common role obligations may go unfulfilled include, poor academic performance, poor work performance, or quitting established activities, such as sport leagues, choir, or clubs. There are numerous scenarios in which youths may use substances in physically hazardous situations. However, a few examples include cutting wood with a gas saw when intoxicated, driving a motorcycle while intoxicated, or ingesting Freon from an air conditioner located on the roof of a house. Adolescents are especially vulnerable to experiencing legal problems due to their use because all illicit drugs and alcohol are illegal for them to consume. However, substance use may compound their chances of engaging in criminal activity (e.g., rape, stealing) because the intoxicating effects of substances decrease impulse control and rational thinking.

Substance dependence is a more severe disorder that, while also associated with general

B. Donohue, Ph.D. (✉) • J. Urgelles, M.A.
J. Fayeghi, B.A.
Psychology Department, University of Nevada, Las Vegas, 4505 S. Maryland Parkway, Box 455030, Las Vegas, NV 89154, USA
e-mail: bradley.donohue@unlv.edu; urgelles@unlv.nevada.edu; jasminefayeghi@gmail.com

W.T. O'Donohue et al. (eds.), *Handbook of Adolescent Health Psychology*,
DOI 10.1007/978-1-4614-6633-8_26, © Springer Science+Business Media New York 2013

impairments, is indicated when three or more of the following behavioral patterns occur: (1) tolerance (need for increased amounts of the substance to achieve intoxication or the desired effect, or diminished effect with continued use of the same amount); (2) withdrawal (physiological reactions that are usually perceived to be negative upon rapid cessation of the substance or use to minimize withdrawal symptoms); (3) used in relatively greater amounts or for a longer period of time than was originally intended; (4) persistent desire or unsuccessful efforts to cut down or control substance use; (5) excessive activities necessary to obtain, use, or recover, from the respective substance; (6) giving up important activities due to substance use; and (7) continued use despite ongoing problems that are likely to have been influenced by substance use. Adolescents often demonstrate less physiological dependence, as compared with their adult counterparts (Sussman, Skara, & Ames, 2008). However, the frequency and severity of use is usually more erratic and experimental than adults, resulting in more fatalities due to substance abuse overdose (Schramm-Sapyta, Walker, Caster, Levin, & Kuhn, 2009). When substance dependence is found to occur in adolescents, it is often predicted by early onset of use (Dennis, Babor, Roebuck, & Donaldson, 2002; Odgers et al., 2008).

Consequences of Substance Abuse and Dependence

Although symptoms of substance abuse and dependence are reported to be diagnostically the same between adults and children, as this chapter will clearly reveal, the contributing factors and overall context in which substances are abused changes with age. Indeed, adolescent substance abusers are three times more likely to experience adverse psychological or health problems than adults (Dennis et al., 2002). The negative consequences of SUDs are especially damaging to the emotional, physical, and mental health development of youth. For example, youths with SUDs evidence relatively high rates of psychiatric symptoms, distress, problems relating with others, job instability, and deficits in cognitive, emotional, and social development (e.g., Newcomb & Bentler, 1988). Youths with SUDs are also prone to physical health problems, such as serious cardiac, neural, and renal disorders (Baigent, 2003); teen pregnancy; poor academic performance; and illicit conduct and violence (Sussman et al., 2008). Substance intoxication has also been shown to influence decreased condom use and increased sexual promiscuity, resulting in an elevated risk of contracting sexually transmitted diseases (e.g., Kingree, Braithwaite, & Woodring, 2000; Tubman, Wagner, & Langer, 2003). Substance intoxication also contributes to serious injuries and fatalities through inappropriate risk-taking behavior (Usher, Jackson, & O'Brien, 2007). As indicated by Usher et al. (2007), the effects of adolescent substance abuse affect the entire family through arguments, noncompliance, general tone in the relationship development, and so on. Without intervention these problem behaviors are likely to continue into adulthood (see Odgers et al., 2008).

Extent of the Problem

Recent polls indicate that nearly half of the teenagers in America have used an illicit drug, with more than 20 % of these youths having used by the 8th grade (Johnston, O'Malley, Bachman, & Schulenberg, 2010). The age of onset has been decreasing since the 1970s (Dennis et al., 2002), which is particularly problematic because earlier onset is associated with family dysfunction, poor academic functioning, criminal activity, antisocial behavior (e.g., bullying, cruelty), and high-risk sexual behaviors (Gordon, Kinlock, & Battjes, 2004). Most adolescents presenting to outpatient treatment centers for substance abuse are male (73 %), between the ages 15 and 17 (82 %), Caucasian (64 %), referred by the criminal justice system (51 %), and started using illicit drugs before their 15th birthday (86 %) (Dennis et al., 2002). Tarter (2002) reported that substance use disorders negatively affect approximately 5 % of adolescents, and information gained from the *Monitoring the Future Survey* as summarized by Johnston et al. (2010) indicates illicit drug use among American teens has been rising during the very recent past after an extended period of decreased frequency of use. As summarized from Johnston et al. (2010), increases in drug use are slightly pronounced in younger age groups, as compared with older groups. For instance, in 2007 the percentage of 8th graders reporting use of any illicit drug was 13 %. This increased to 16 % in 2010, whereas older age groups increased their drug use by 2 % during this same time period. Drug use generally increases with age. For instance, the percentage of youths who used illicit drugs in 2010 is 16 % and 38 % for 8th and 12th graders, respectively. As the most frequently used substance other than alcohol (which is used by almost a third of teenagers during the past month), marijuana use was found to increase in 2010, with 6 % of 12th graders reporting almost daily use. Specific to illicit drugs other than marijuana, there has been a general decline in use with the exception of a spike in the use of these substances during 2010. The current rate of illicit drug use other than marijuana during the past year is 7 % and 17 % in grades 8 and 12, respectively. However, there is great variability in rates of use across the substance classes. For instance, the use of prescription drugs had been rising steadily since the mid-1990s, leveling off in the late 2000s. In 12th graders, the current use of prescription amphetamines, such as Ritalin and Adderall, is 6.6 % and 4.8 %. The use of narcotics other than heroine, such as analgesics (pain killers), has been increasing since the early 1990s, with current use among 12th graders at about 9 %. The mostly widely used analgesics among adolescents are Vicodin and OxyContin. Annual prevalence rates for Vicodin in 2010 were 2.7 % and 8.0 % in 8th and 12th grade, respectively. The current annual rates for OxyContin were found to be a little lower than Vicodin. Frequently abused "over-the-counter" medications include cough and cold medicines containing dextromethorphan. Annual prevalence rates in 2010 were 3.2 % and 6.6 % in grades 8 and 12, respectively. The use of prescription drugs is extremely dangerous for young adolescents, relative to older adolescents and adults, because they are often unaware of their negative effects, and these youths have a tendency to underestimate the potentially lethal effects of use when concurrently used with alcohol. Other notoriously dangerous illicit drugs that are used by teenagers include anabolic steroids. Although these drugs appear to have declined since the early 2000s, they are still problematic, particularly in 12th grade boys (i.e., 2.5 % in 2010) and relevant subgroups (e.g., athletes, body builders).

Mental Health Disorders That Often Coexist with Substance Abuse and Dependence

As emphasized by Roberts and Corcoran (2005), adolescents with a dual diagnosis (i.e., evidencing at least one mental health disorder in addition to substance abuse or dependence) are actually the norm and not a special subpopulation among adolescents seeking services. For instance, approximately 60 % of adolescents with substance use, abuse, or dependence have a comorbid diagnosis (Armstrong & Costello, 2002). Therefore, mental health practitioners (MHPs) should be prepared to assess and subsequently address commonly evidenced comorbid problems that typically exacerbate treatment outcomes. Indeed, adolescent substance abusers who evidence coexisting mental health problems, as compared with youth SUDs without coexisting mental health disorders, are more likely to experience problems in family relationships and school functioning, and engage in criminal activity (Grella, Hser, Joshi, & Rounds-Bryant, 2001). They are also more likely to relapse after treatment (McCarthy, Tomlinson, Anderson, Marlatt, & Brown, 2005; Tomlinson, Brown, & Abrantes, 2004).

The most common comorbid diagnoses with SUDs are disruptive behavior disorders (i.e., conduct disorders). Median prevalence for disruptive behavior disorders in SUDs is 46 %, in comparison to 12 % in youth samples without SUDs (Armstrong & Costello, 2002). When behaviors related to substance use are included in the diagnosis of conduct disorder (CD), the incidence of comorbid CD jumps to 95 % (Brown, Gleghorn, Schuckit, Myers, & Mott, 1996).

A dual diagnosis of CD and substance abuse is more often seen in adolescent males (72 %) than females (47 %) (Latimer, Stone, Voight, Winters, & August, 2002). Finally, CD may complicate adolescent substance abuse treatment more than any other coexisting mental health condition (Weinberg, Rahdert, Colliver, & Glantz, 1998).

The second most common comorbid mental health condition in adolescents who evidence substance abuse is depression. Depressive disorders are seen in about 5 % of non-substance-using adolescents, and about 24 % in adolescents who use alcohol at least once a week, or an illicit drug at least once a year (Kandel et al., 1997). Adolescent females evidence comorbid depressive and substance use disorders (44.1 %) more than males (16.8 %) (Latimer et al., 2002). Substance abuse may develop in adolescents who evidence depression as a means of self-medication (Deykin, Levy, & Wells, 1987) or due to commonly shared risk factors (Clark & Bukstein, 1998). A history of childhood maltreatment, including sexual abuse, is often seen in adolescents with comorbid depression and substance use (see Tubman et al., 2003), and individuals with this clinical presentation are particularly at risk to develop anxiety disorders.

Attention deficit hyperactivity disorder (ADHD) is often seen in adolescents with SUDs, with up to 50 % of adolescents in addiction treatment settings meeting criteria for both diagnoses (Gordon, Tulak, & Troncale, 2004; Horner & Scheibe, 1997). This is striking when considering that ADHD only occurs in 5 % of youths in the general population (Cantwell, 1996). The rate of ADHD and substance abuse or dependence in males (46 %) is nearly twice that in females (24 %) (Latimer et al., 2002). The presence of ADHD may increase vulnerability to drug use in children who evidence other risk factors. For instance, Molina, Smith, and Pelham (1999) found that only 36 % of conduct-disordered adolescents who did not evidence ADHD reported alcohol or drug use during the past 3 months, compared with 73 % of conduct-disordered adolescents who were diagnosed with ADHD. Interestingly, children with ADHD are also more likely to associate with deviant peers, making them more vulnerable to substance use disorders (Marshal, Molina, & Pelham, 2003). Youths who are diagnosed with SUDS also appear to evidence higher rates of some anxiety disorders than normative populations when entering treatment (Azrin et al., 2001).

Etiological Considerations

From a behavioral perspective, adolescents use illicit substances due to numerous and often complicated interactions that occur between antecedent stimuli that act to predispose, permit, or facilitate substance use to occur, and positive and negative reinforcement. Antecedent stimuli may occur prior to birth (e.g., inheritance of genes, in utero exposure to substances), or include emotions (e.g., anger/upset, depression, excitement), environmental situations and events (e.g., boredom, celebrations, parties, anniversaries), social scenarios (e.g., encouragement from friends to use drugs, poor drug refusal and conflict resolution skills, arguments with parents), aversive environments (e.g., child maltreatment, being excessively teased at school), neurological impairments (e.g., poor impulse control due to dysfunction in the frontal lobe), physical pain, irritability, easy access to substances, and locations and people associated with substance use. Many of these stimuli may elicit strong physiological cravings or desires for substance use. For instance, when adolescents perceive their environment as aversive, they may seek substance use to "numb" or distort undesired feeling states through substance intoxication. Of course, the immediate removal of aversive stimuli (e.g., depressive and worrisome thoughts, physical pain) consequent to substance use may increase future use through the process of negative reinforcement. Common positive reinforcers for substance use include social acknowledgment, positive attention, social approval, perceived insight, and pleasurable physical feelings.

The relative influence of environmental stimuli is impossible to determine because the environment is dynamic, multiply interactive, and thus unpredictable. For instance, Tarter (2002) outlines a developmental perspective in which the degree of risk for SUDs is determined by a unique set of behavioral, biological, and environmental factors. According to his perspective, risk for SUDs changes over time in relation to the environment and quality of interpersonal relationships. Because maturation and socialization factors interact with these variables, the number of variables that interact in a given situation is nearly infinite, making the prediction of outcome difficult. Developmental factors include tolerance. For instance, the consumption of larger amounts of drug to receive desired effects may result in brain injury to a young, still-maturing brain. In turn, these brain injuries may go on to disrupt psychosocial adjustment and psychological development, especially if they are initially unrecognized. Additionally, hormonal changes during puberty may result in difficulties with emotional self-regulation and social adjustment. During this time of intense emotion, there may be signs of negative affect, irritability, and moodiness, all of which are associated with increased risk for SUDs. Also as reviewed by Tarter (2002), differences in the sleep-wake cycle between adolescents and adults may put adolescents at increased risk for SUDs. That is, adolescents go to sleep later and wake up later than children and adults. They also require more sleep than adults. However, school schedules require adolescents to wake up early, possibly resulting in sleep deprivation. Chronic sleep deprivation is associated with psychopathology, low academic performance, disciplinary problems, and impaired concentration in the classroom, all of which have been associated with substance abuse problems.

Adolescents often engage in risk-taking behavior, which puts them at risk for substance abuse problems. According to Spear (2000), this behavior may be due to changes in the brain that occur during adolescence. These changes include decreased GABA and glutamate concentrations in the prefrontal cortex and increased concentrations of dopamine. Therefore, adolescents have difficulty with behavioral and affective self-regulation due to underdeveloped executive cognitive functioning capacity, which can lead to poor decision-making. Deficits in executive cognitive functioning are also seen in those with ADHD and CD. Adolescents low in self-regulation are more likely to spend time with peers who are also low in self-regulation, creating a social environment with increased opportunities to engage in substance abuse.

Tarter (2002) discusses etiology within an ontogenetic framework considering SUD liability across different developmental stages, such as gestation, neonatal and infancy period, preschool period, primary school period, and high school period. During the gestation period, exposure to nicotine can increase tolerance. Intrauterine exposure to nicotine during fetal development can also lead to cross-tolerance to other substances, leading to drug tolerance and predisposing the individual to drug dependence. During the neonatal/infancy period, biobehavioral characteristics, such as a child's temperament, may predispose the child to substance use. Internalizing (e.g., depression, anxiety) and externalizing (e.g., conduct disorders, ADHD) behaviors apparent in the preschool period may be precursors to problems with substance abuse. Experimentation with substance use can start in the later primary school period. This is more likely to happen in a family environment in which parent-child attachment is weak, supervision is low, and rules are few or not enforced. During the high school period opportunities for substance use increase dramatically and adolescents in this stage place great importance in adopting behaviors, attitudes, and values that are consistent with those of their peers.

Based on animal studies, there is evidence that suggests adolescents may experience the rewarding and aversive effects of drugs differently than adults, potentially putting them at risk for increased experimentation (Schramm-Sapyta et al., 2009). The imbalance is such that adolescents tend to experience the rewarding effects more than the aversive. They are less sensitive to withdrawal symptoms, which may lead to increased use in the early stages.

There are also differences in the relapse patterns of adolescents and adults. Adolescent relapses are more often associated with social pressure as compared to adults (Brown, Vik, & Creamer, 1989). Ramo and Brown (2008) found that 67 % of adults relapsed in social situations in which they felt urges and temptations and 33% relapsed when trying to cope with negative emotion while also experiencing urges and temptations. On the other hand, adolescents primarily relapsed in social situations while trying to enhance a positive emotional state (69 %) or when trying to manage interpersonal conflicts while also being in a negative emotional state and attempting to cope with urges and social pressures to use (31 %). Similarly, adolescents are five times more likely to relapse while in a positive emotional state than adults (Ramo & Brown, 2008). These findings have direct implications for assessment and treatment.

Assessment of Substance Abuse and Dependence

The need for evidence-based treatments in community settings has resulted in the development and implementation of psychometrically valid measures to assist in the assessment of adolescent SUDs (Allen, Donohue, Sutton, Haderlie, & Lapota, 2009). Along these lines, exclusive use of straightforward self-report measures with face validity is often insufficient to bring about accurate diagnostic information because adolescents are often guarded to deny substance use due to perceived, or actual, consequences for doing so, and because their memory may be distorted due to excessive substance use. Therefore, particularly when there is concern about the honesty and accuracy of the informant's responses, self-report measures should include "lie scales." Lie scales include queries about undesired behaviors that most people would endorse (e.g., "Have you lied more than once"). Denial of a significant number of such items could indicate an attempt to present oneself favorably (i.e., denial of pathology). Because SUDs are often associated with other pathologies, mental health practitioners should administer comprehensive batteries capable of assessing coexisting conditions that are common in SUDs. For instance, it is important to assess medical status and psychosocial functioning (Sussman et al., 2008), as medical conditions may mask, exacerbate, or mimic the symptoms of alcohol or drug abuse (Donohue, Karmely, & Strada, 2006). Of course, gathering an appreciation of social support systems, attitudes towards substance use, and motivation towards abstinence all assist in determining prognosis and readiness for treatment planning (Gans, Falco, Schackman, & Winters, 2010). Inclusion of standardized, evidence-supported assessment measures better enable mental health practitioners to identify clinical problems, structure appropriate treatment, and evaluate treatment outcomes (Barlow, 2005). Along these lines, the multi-informant (e.g., parents, teachers, probation officers, ministers, siblings, coaches, friends, physicians) and multi-assessment method is becoming increasingly utilized in community settings (Winters & Kaminer, 2008). Assessment methods most often include behavioral interviews, functional analysis, standardized questionnaires, behavioral observation, behavioral role-playing, self-monitoring, and biological testing (e.g., urinalysis testing, hair follicle).

Behavioral Interviews

Unstructured Interviews

Most mental health practitioners initiate assessment with a behavioral interview. There are three major interview formats: (1) unstructured, (2) structured, and (3) semi-structured. In unstructured interviews, the method of assessing content is determined solely by the interviewer. Unstructured interviews for adolescent SUDs emphasize queries that are relevant to understanding the function of substance use behaviors and its associated behaviors. Commonly assessed areas include the onset, severity, frequency, precursors, and consequences of both substance use and nonuse; medical, psychiatric, mental health, and psychosocial history; mental status; suicidal and homicidal ideation and intent; level of development (i.e., social, emotional, cognitive); intellectual and academic functioning; and motivation for treatment. Interviewers are free to determine the extent to which particular domains are emphasized. Thus, unstructured interviewers offer flexibility in the method and extent of questioning, but lack reliability since this format cannot be replicated with precision by others. Indeed, some domains may be overlooked or overemphasized based on interviewer biases.

Structured Interviews

The method of assessing content in structured interviews is predetermined. Structured interviews assure that each respondent is asked exactly the same set of questions, and in the same order. Questions are usually read verbatim from interview forms, and youth responses are recorded according to standard response formats, such as Likert scales (e.g., 1 = does not meet the diagnostic criterion, 2 = meets diagnostic criterion) or dichotomous scales (e.g., yes, no). Thus, structured interviews are almost exclusively utilized to assist in standardizing assessment protocols when conducting research (e.g., assuring an accurate SUDs diagnosis in a treatment outcome study).

The Structured Clinical Interview for DSM-IV-TR (SCID-IV; First, Spitzer, Gibbon, & Williams, 1996) is widely used in research settings. It requires up to 2 h to complete, and assesses Axis I disorders, such as SUDs. Use of the SCID-IV requires extensive training, but has very good reliability and validity (Kranzler, Kadden, Babor, & Tennen, 1996; Lobbestael, Leurgans, & Arntz, 2012). Utilization of the SCID-IV may be particularly useful when it is necessary to determine DSM disorders that coexist in SUDs. Although the SCID-IV has been utilized successfully in samples involving adolescents with SUDs (e.g., Azrin et al., 2001), the adolescent version is recommended (Martin & Kaczynski, 1995).

The Teen-Addiction Severity Index (T-ASI; Kaminer, Bukstein, & Tarter, 1991) is a structured interview that may be utilized to assess seven domains (i.e., chemical use, school status, employment-support status, family relationships, peer-social relationships, legal status, psychiatric status). However, the T-ASI permits additional probing, whenever indicated. There is a computerized version, and a revised format is currently under investigation (Brodey et al., 2008).

Semi-structured Interviews

Balancing the extent of structure between unstructured and structured interviews, semi-structured interviews permit interviewers to choose from a set of predetermined questions. It is also within the interviewer's discretion to ask questions that may not be included in the standard format. Similarly, response sets in semi-structured interviews are flexible to permit interviewees to record verbatim responses or utilize standardized response sets. The Global Appraisal of Individual Needs (GAIN; Dennis, Funk, Godley, Godley, & Waldron, 2004) is a semi-structured interview that is specific for adolescent SUDs, and this tool may be utilized to assess background, substance use, physical health, risk behaviors, mental health, environment, and legal and vocational domains. The GAIN is comprehensive; thus it requires training (Winters & Kaminer, 2008).

A reliable semi-structured interview for assessing illicit drug and alcohol use frequency is the Timeline Follow-back interview (TLFB; Sobell, Sobell, Klajner, Pavan, & Basian, 1986). It has a structured format, but allows for some flexibility in the determination of factors that are assessed. Substance use frequency and other variables of interest (e.g., HIV risk behaviors, police contacts) are retrospectively assessed month by month for a specified period of time (i.e., 4 months) using a calendar. There are techniques for aiding memory recall when administering the TLFB, such as marking significant memory anchor points (e.g., birthdays, holidays) on the calendar. The respondent is asked to specify on the calendar which days drug and alcohol use occurred. Information may be reliably and independently obtained from an additional informant (e.g., parent) utilizing separate calendars.

The Semi-Structured Interview for Consideration of Ethnic Culture in Therapy (SSICECTS; Donohue, Strada, et al., 2006) was empirically developed to enhance the cultural competence of interviewers. It is a 6-item scale that was psychometrically validated in a sample of 279 individuals of various ethnicities. Ethnic minority participants have demonstrated significantly higher scores than Caucasians, suggesting this scale may be particularly applicable in ethnic minority populations. In a controlled trial (Donohue, Strada, et al., 2006), implementation of this interview was found to improve participant ratings of perceived clinical skills, and relative to a control group, interviewers who administered the SSICECTS were perceived by the participants as having greater knowledge and respect for the participants' ethnic culture.

Other interviews useful for diagnosing adolescents with substance abuse problems include the Customary Drinking and Drug Use Record (CDDR; Brown, Creamer, & Stetson, 1987), the Structured Clinical Interview for Adolescents (SCI; Brown, Vik, & Creamer, 1989), the Adolescent Diagnostic Interview (ADI; Winters & Henly, 1993), the National Institute of Mental Health Diagnostic Interview Schedule for Children (NIMH DISC-IV; Shaffer, Fisher, Lucas, Dulcan, & Schwab-Stone, 2000), and the Adolescent Drug Abuse Diagnosis (ADAD; Friedman & Utada, 1989).

Functional Analysis

In determining behaviors and thoughts that act to maintain substance use, the functional analysis, or ABC model, is an invaluable tool. As the name of this method implies, its purpose is to assist in understanding the *function* of substance use. The "A" represents antecedent stimuli that precede substance use. Most behavioral practitioners limit these stimuli to specific actions, places, objects, and situations or circumstances, such as getting into a fight with a parent or celebrations. In this model, thoughts and feeling states (e.g., boredom) can usually be reduced to behavioral precursors (e.g., at home watching television). Other antecedent stimuli include community factors, such as cultural influences, neighborhood characteristics, and availability of drugs in the community. The "B" represents the target behavior (i.e., substance use), and the "C" represents the behavioral consequences that occur after substance use. Consequences may be positive reinforcers (e.g., praise) or negative reinforcers (e.g., reduction of anxiety). If the informant is insightful and honest, and the MHP does a good job comprehensively assessing antecedents and consequences, important treatment targets will be identified. Adolescents with SUDs may be taught to avoid antecedent stimuli that have been identified to lead to substance use, and consequences may be altered to reward behaviors that are incompatible with drug use behavior. For instance, if boredom is found to precede substance use, youths may be taught to engage in pleasant, non-substance-associated activities when boredom is initially perceived. If substance use results in relaxation, youths can be taught alternative relaxation exercises. Toneatto (2008) developed a functional analysis model to assist MHPs in determining how the symptoms of substance use reduce negative symptoms that are caused by comorbid disorders. For instance, a stimulant drug (e.g., cocaine) may have energizing effects on depression-induced fatigue, and a depressive drug (benzodiazepine) may have calming effects when depression-induced agitation occurs. Knowing this information, the MHP and youth may work together to define the relationship between symptoms and substances so that better coping strategies for comorbid mental health symptoms can be developed.

Self-Report Questionnaires

Self-report questionnaires are cost- and time-effective, and easy to administer. Thus, they do not require much training. These measures are usually in a "paper-and-pencil" format, though some computerized versions are available. The person conducting the assessment usually reads questions (e.g., "Have you used alcohol at parties in the past?") or comments (e.g., "I enjoy using at parties."), and the interviewee provides the most accurate response from a forced-choice dichotomous scale (e.g., yes, no) or Likert-type scale (e.g., 1 = strongly disagree, 7 = strongly agree). Forced-choice responses to self-report questionnaires may be scored according to standardized procedures, and the resulting scores may be compared with the responses of normative groups, permitting percentile ranks and clinical cutoff scores to be derived. Interviewees may also respond in an open-ended format (e.g., free to respond however they feel). Open-ended responses provide valuable information that is not possible in forced-choice formats. However, interpretation is usually more difficult, as responses may vary between interviewees.

The Achenbach System of Empirically Based Assessment (ASEBA; Achenbach, 1991) provides a comprehensive assessment of problem behaviors and competence. Problems are classified into internalizing, externalizing, social, thought, and attention. The Youth Self Report (YSR) is administered to adolescents, the Child Behavior Checklist (CBCL) is administered to the youth's parents, and the Teacher's Report Form (TRF) is administered to the youth's teachers. These questionnaires assist in DSM diagnosis, and normative data is available in which to compare youth responses. The ASEBA does not assess SUD symptoms, but is a good choice for understanding disorders that coexist with SUDs.

The Personal Experience Screening Questionnaire (PESQ; Winters, 1992) is a self-report screening instrument for adolescent substance abuse problems. It includes norms for nonclinical, juvenile offender, and drug-abusing populations. The PESQ includes a problem severity scale, and items measuring drug use history, psychosocial problems, defensiveness (faking good), and infrequency (faking bad). An interesting innovation is the construction of items that measure distortion tendencies to assist in determining if a respondent is experiencing difficulty reading questions or responding to questions at random.

Examples of other self-report questionnaires that are useful in assessing adolescent SUDs include the Adolescent Alcohol Involvement Scale (AAIS; Mayer & Filstead, 1979), Adolescent Drinking Index (ADI; Harrell & Wirtz, 1989), Adolescent Obsessive-Compulsive Drinking Scale (A-OCDS; Deas, Roberts, Randall, & Anton, 2001), Rutgers Alcohol Problem Index (RAPI; White & Labouvie, 1989), Adolescent Drug Involvement Scale (ADIS; Moberg & Hahn, 1991), Drug Use Screening Inventory-Revised (DUSI-R; Tarter, 1990), Client Substance Index (CSI; Moore, 1983), Personal Experience Inventory (PEI; Winters & Henly, 1989), Problem Oriented Screening Instrument for Teenagers (POSIT; Rahdert, 1991), and the Substance Abuse Subtle Screening Inventory, adolescent form (SASSI-A; Miller, 1985, 1999).

Self-Monitoring

This assessment method involves the explicit tracking of target behaviors and thoughts in relation to specified times and events. This assessment strategy is primarily utilized during treatment. Monitored behaviors need to be observable and objective, such as the frequency of interactions with non-drug-using friends, number of days attending school, frequency of drinks, or days using drugs. Thoughts need to be recorded verbatim to help provide insight into the maintenance of the adolescent's substance use problem (e.g., "I need to go to the party"). Contextual factors include associated times, locations, feelings, and associated events in which target responses occur. The chief advantage of this assessment tool is its direct applicability to treatment (e.g., relapse prevention; McGovern, Wrisley, & Drake, 2005) and potential accuracy if completed in a timely manner.

Behavioral Observation

This assessment strategy may occur spontaneously and informally, such as witnessing youth interactions with family members in the waiting room prior to a therapy session, or observation may be highly structured and guided by checklists and specified criteria, such as recording the number of critical comments made by a parent during a 20-min sampling of the family at dinner. Such observation assists in decreasing self-report biases that often occur in SUDs (i.e., social desirability). During treatment sessions behavioral observations may provide insights regarding maladaptive parent-child interactions and parenting skills that should be targeted in treatment. Behavioral observation is also a good way to gather information regarding interpersonal skills, such as how the adolescent interacts with peers during group therapy. The presence of behavioral markers of substance abuse or dependence can help to corroborate results from an interview or questionnaire (Fisher & Harrison, 1992). Some of these markers may include excessive restlessness, poor short-tem memory, mood swings, or anorexic appearance. Informal behavioral data can be collected from various sources, such as parents and teachers. Of course, individuals may respond unnaturally when they know they are being observed by others, particularly when first observed. With continued observation, however, this type of response reactivity typically goes away.

Behavioral Role-Playing

As summarized by Donohue, Van Hasselt, Hersen, and Perrin (1998), behavioral role-playing is an inexpensive and easy-to-employ assessment method that may be utilized to evaluate social skill functioning in simulated scenarios that represent "real-life" social interactions. In brief, the individual targeted for assessment is read a social scenario that is relevant to the presenting problem, and subsequently prompted by the assessor to demonstrate the targeted skill. The number and content of prompts may be determined prior to the role-play, or may fluctuate during the role-play. The following dialogue depicts a role-play assessment designed to assess drug refusal skills utilizing two prompts that were determined a priori.

> Assessor: "I'm going to read you a situation in which your friend wants to go to a party where marijuana will be present. You don't want to go. Show me how you will avoid going to the party with your friend. I'm going to pretend like I'm your friend. Let's get started. So, let's go to the party."
> Client: "No, I'm not in the mood."
> Assessor: "Come on it will be fun."
> Client: "No, I have to go home."

After role-plays the assessor can query additional questions, such as thoughts that may have occurred during the role-play performance, and alternative options that may have been considered, or the assessor can provide feedback to the youth to enhance future performance. During treatment, target skills can be practiced in role-play scenarios until performance is perfected. Role-play assessment provides opportunities to observe behaviors, mannerisms, and statements from the adolescent that can be targeted in treatment. Role-playing of substance abuse-related behaviors typically involves (a) querying situations related to recent use of substances, (b) identifying a key person who influenced the drug-associated behavior, (c) simulating the scenario while playing the role of the key person involved in the role-play scenario (while the client attempts the target skill), and (d) querying thoughts and feelings that may have occurred during the role-play (Donohue et al., 2006). The predominant disadvantage of role-play assessment is that it is not possible to determine if target behaviors are representative of in vivo environments, or if the individual will be able to subsequently demonstrate learned skills at home. To increase generalizability, it is important to practice skills in various problem scenarios. Such practice assists in reducing anxiety associated with the demonstration of skill sets at home.

The Parent Situation Inventory (PSI; McGillicuddy, Rychtarik, & Morsheimer, 2004) requires parents to respond to problem situation vignettes as they normally would, while the assessor portrays the youth client. The parent's performance is subsequently rated on a 6-point effectiveness scale. Parents also rate how similar the event was to a real-life situation that occurred during the past year utilizing a 5-point scale. Relevant skills that are poorly rated in their effectiveness and rated high in their occurrence are targeted in treatment.

Biological Testing

The presence of illicit drugs and alcohol may be tested through urine, saliva, blood, and hair follicles. The primary advantage of biological testing is, of course, objectivity, which is particularly valuable when results of self-reported information are questionable. Indeed, as mentioned earlier, there are potentially severe consequences for admitting substance use. However, there are also problems with biological testing. First, it is relatively intrusive and requires careful monitoring. For instance, the youth may insert containers of "clean" urine in their pants or skirts and attempt to provide these samples to the trained monitor, dip the sample container in the toilet and attempt to pass on the toilet water as their urine, or drink excessive amounts of water. These problems may be managed by observing temperature strips on the urine sample to assure that the urine is at body temperature, and testing creatinine levels to assure the urine sample is not diluted. Other problems include the youth touching the urine sample with a finger that has been soaked in bleach (although this is detectable, the test results will be invalidated), and using adulterants that may lead positive results to appear negative. It is also difficult to identify the use of many illicit drugs and alcohol from urinalysis testing if (1) these substances were used outside the possibility of substance-specific detection (e.g., alcohol will be out of the system within 24 h, whereas marijuana may be detected for up to a month), (2) if the adolescent has a fast metabolism, and (3) if the adolescent exercises regularly. Hair follicle tests may assess substance use a few months from the time of testing. However, these tests are expensive, and it is difficult to determine when, specifically, the use occurred. The ability to detect substances will vary according to the metabolic rate of the specific substances.

Enlistment and Engagement

Most adolescents with SUDs attend therapy at the urging or mandate of others (e.g., court, school, parent). Although nonattendance to therapeutic sessions is usually most problematic during the initial sessions, a very high percentage of youth who enroll in therapy will terminate treatment prematurely (see Lefforge, Donohue, & Strada, 2007). Assuming therapy is evidence-based, the implementation of intervention programs designed to improve therapy session attendance is imperative in the recovery of adolescent SUDs, and parental support appears to be important in this process (Austin, Hospital, Wagner, & Morris, 2010). Moreover, motivation for substance use change has been linked to the implementation of engagement strategies (Broome, Joe, & Simpson, 2001), and attendance improvement interventions result in better treatment outcomes (Breda & Heflinger, 2007). At an administrative level, engagement can occur through greater accessibility to services, assuring staff members maintain a positive perspective when service utilization is attempted, and adopting culturally sensitive, flexible services for adolescents and their families (Henggeler, Pickrel, Brondino, & Crouch, 1996). Many of the strategies and procedures involved in attendance improvement interventions have been pioneered by Jose Szapocznik and his colleagues during the past two decades (e.g., Briones, Robbins, & Szapocznik, 2008; Szapocznik et al., 1988). When they initiated their work it was uncommon for counselors to visit homes of adolescent with SUDs or actively attempt to motivate youth and their families to attend sessions. These investigators assisted in changing these norms. For instance, counselors were taught to visit families outside the office (e.g., home, restaurants) to help family members feel more comfortable, actively listen to the concerns of family, call family members several times between treatment sessions, and so on. Other strategies to improve session attendance in adolescents include orienting both parents and youth about treatment, reviewing directions to the clinic if outpatient therapy is initiated, offering token gifts and refreshments, facilitating written commitments, and appointment reminder calls to both the youth and the parent (see Lefforge et al., 2007 for a comprehensive review of attendance interventions).

Treatment

Whereas two decades ago it was difficult for community practitioners to identify adolescent substance abuse treatments with established effectiveness, the descriptions and research-base for these programs are now widely accessible and easily interpreted in national registries, such as the Substance Abuse and Mental Health

Administration's National Registry of Evidence-Based Practices and Programs (SAMHSA's NREPP; www.nrepp.samhsa.gov). Some of these interventions have been extensively evaluated both in controlled efficacy and effectiveness trials, and have extensively developed dissemination tools, including interactive computer-based training guides, access to videos depicting exemplary implementation of treatments, and dedicated websites in which to electronically gather updated treatment forms. Most of the evidence-based treatment programs include parsimonious methods of assessing treatment integrity; treatment manuals that depict how, specifically, to implement the interventions; and standardized interviews and formats to assess agency needs relevant to adoption of evidence-based treatment. The interventions are also now more sophisticated than in past years. Indeed, many of the evidence-based treatments are capable of simultaneously addressing various behavior problems and conditions that coexist in SUDs, and some clinical trials are showing enhanced effectiveness when evidence-based treatments are combined (see Stanger, Budney, Kamon, & Thostensen, 2009 as an exemplary). Most of the programs owe their theoretical underpinnings to behavioral therapy and family systems. However, methods of application vary considerably.

Behavioral and Cognitive-Behavioral Therapies (BT, CBT) for substance abuse involve multiple interventions that are designed to eliminate substance use and its associated problem behaviors through self-monitoring desired behaviors; increasing the quality and frequency of praise and rewards for desired behaviors through the development of contingency systems involving parents and youth; teaching youth to recognize, manage, and avoid cues that often lead to undesired behaviors; and skills training. In treating substance use, most BT and CBT MHPs attempt to determine behavioral and cognitive cues in the environment that influence or permit substance use to occur. BT and CBT approaches are employed to replace these antecedent stimuli to drug use with non-drug associated actions. For instance, if tension is found to influence substance use, behavioral relaxation exercises with abstinent friends might be encouraged. If worrisome depressive thoughts are found to influence substance use, cognitive restructuring exercises might target the acquisition of objective thinking patterns, problem-solving skill training might be utilized to generate potential solutions to achieving greater satisfaction in life, and behavioral coping strategies could be utilized to manage stressful situations that bring about anxiety. BT and CBT MHPs also attempt to modify the environment to disallow or interfere with positive and negative stimuli that influence or permit substance use. However, they are also focused on restructuring the environment to eliminate stimuli that positively and negatively reinforce substance use, and increase non-drug-associated behaviors and thoughts that are likely to bring about reinforcement. Positive reinforcers for drug use often include social approval, recognition, and pleasant physiological sensations, whereas negative reinforcers include tension in muscles, stress, upset, and anxious thoughts (i.e., substance use results in their withdrawal). The specific methods of accomplishing the aforementioned strategies differ between the various BT and CBT programs. However, modeling, behavior rehearsal, feedback, and homework assignments are hallmark characteristics of BT and CBT for adolescent SUDs. Most treatment programs are scheduled to include 12–16 h of therapy, with treatment being implemented in individual, group, and family formats. What follows is a brief summary of several BT and CBT programs that are specific to adolescent SUDs to assist in understanding how these interventions are applied. Readers are referred elsewhere for comprehensive and critical reviews of BT and CBT approaches (e.g., Bukstein & Horner, 2010; Deas & Clark, 2009; MacGowan & Engle, 2010; Strada, Donohue, & Lefforge, 2006; Waldron & Turner, 2008).

In very well-controlled trials with relatively high participant numbers, investigators have found cost-effective group Cognitive Behavior Therapies (CBT) to demonstrate significant improvements in substance use and comorbid problems, although the group CBT effects are relatively less impressive when compared with active evidence-supported treatment conditions (e.g., Kaminer, Burleson, Blitz, Sussman, & Rounsaville, 1998; Kaminer, Burleson, & Goldberger, 2002; Liddle et al., 2001). These group-based treatments generally include skill-based training (e.g., communication, self-control, problem-solving). Interestingly, when group CBT is combined with family-based treatment, motivational interviewing, an extended number of treatment sessions (24), and target relatively more skill sets (e.g., school-related skills, negative mood management, social support, relapse prevention) efficacy appears to be substantially improved (Waldron, Slesnick, Brody, Turner, & Peterson, 2001). Latimer, Winters, D'Zurilla, and Nichols (2003) formally demonstrated positive effects in a specified group CBT they coined Integrated Family and Cognitive Behavioral Therapy (IFCBT). This treatment combines CBT with Rational Emotive Therapy (RET), Problem Solving Therapy (PST), Learning Strategy Training (LST), and Problem-Focused Family Therapy (PFFT). RET sessions focus on discovering and combating irrational thoughts associated with drug use and other psychopathology. PST is used to develop skills to better handle situations that put the adolescent at risk for drug use, whereas LST takes the adolescent's cognitive strengths and limitations in consideration to develop learning strategy systems for school learning. There is evidence that treatment with IFCBT leads to decreased alcohol and drug use, improved problem-solving skills, and better parenting practices (Latimer et al., 2003).

The Adolescent Community Reinforcement Approach (ACRA) is a comprehensive outpatient, family-assisted behavioral intervention that aims to eliminate marijuana and alcohol use by teaching adolescents to restructure their environment to include activities with abstinent peers and family, and eliminating stressors that act to facilitate substance use. A functional analysis is utilized to assist in identifying behaviors that lead to substance use, as well as consequences that act to reinforce substance use. Problems within the family are conceptualized to be reciprocally determined and based on skill deficits specific to conflict resolution and inequity in the exchange of reinforcement. There are more than a dozen interventions for therapists to choose from, including youth, parent, and parent and youth treatment protocols. Thus, relationships with family and friends are repaired through communication skills training. Other youth-based treatments are focused on learning to solicit and do well in job interviews and substance refusal skills training. Parents are assisted in learning parenting and problem-solving skills. Treatment sessions are usually with the adolescent, parents, and with the adolescent and parents together. Thus, ACRA includes multiple goal-oriented components that are flexible, and straightforward. This intervention is also cost-effective and has demonstrated improved outcomes in substance use, social stability, symptoms of depression, and other internalizing problems (see Dennis et al., 2004; Godley, Godley, Dennis, Funk, & Passetti, 2007). ACRA is one of the very few programs that has demonstrated positive results in severely troubled samples, such as the homeless (Slesnick, Prestopnik, Meyers, & Glassman, 2007). A contingency management intervention may be incorporated to enhance session attendance (Ledgerwood, Alessi, Hanson, Godley, & Petry, 2008).

Family Behavior Therapy (FBT) is an outpatient behavioral treatment that resembles ACRA. FBT sessions for adolescents and their families are focused on a program orientation, establishing contingent rewards for youth from family members when behavioral goals are accomplished, self-control skills training to reduce the intensity of problematic impulsive behaviors, problem-solving exercises and imagery trials focused on receiving rewards for drug-incompatible prosocial behaviors, adjusting the environment to facilitate drug-free behavior (stimulus control), communication skills training, and vocational assistance. In a meta-analysis conducted by Bender, Springer, and Kim (2006), FBT was found to be one of only two treatments reviewed to produce large effect sizes in dually diagnosed adolescents across externalizing, internalizing, and substance abuse domains. In controlled trials, FBT has demonstrated improved outcomes in drug and alcohol use, family relationships, depression, school/work attendance, problem-solving skills, parental satisfaction, and CD symptoms (Azrin et al., 1996, 2001; Azrin, Donohue, Besalel, Kogan, & Acierno, 1994; Azrin, McMahon, et al., 1994). FBT also includes a telephone intervention that has demonstrated a 30 % improvement in session attendance relevant to a control condition in conduct-disordered and drug-abusing youth (Donohue, Azrin, et al., 1998).

Other emerging adolescent substance abuse treatments with BT and CBT underpinnings include Multidimensional Treatment Foster Care (MTFC; Smith, Chamberlain, & Eddy, 2010), Seeking Safety (SS; Najavits, Gallop, & Weiss, 2006), and Teen Intervene (TI; Winters & Leitten, 2007). These interventions are welcome additions to adolescent substance abuse treatment, as each of these interventions is focused on particular subpopulations that are often neglected in this field. For instance, MTFC has an established track record in treating severe problems that frequently coexist with adolescent substance abuse (e.g., violence, delinquency), and provides practitioners an opportunity to implement evidence-based treatment in youths who are mandated to out-of-home placements. In addition to reductions in substance use, the SS program emphasizes treatment of traumatic experiences that often exacerbate treatment outcomes, and TI may be implemented in the school system, which has been relatively neglected in treatment development.

Family Systems-Based Therapies

Brief Strategic Family Therapy (BSFT) is a family-based treatment in which maladaptive patterns of interaction within the family are conceptualized to influence adolescent SUDs. Therefore, MHPs build a therapeutic alliance with the family, and carefully observe family member interactions during treatment sessions (about 24) to assist in understanding how maladaptive interactions are related to substance use behaviors. The MHP then attempts to restructure these interactions to encourage abstinence from drugs, alcohol, and problem behaviors. Restructuring techniques include staying focused in the present, reframing perspectives to be less negative, encouraging family members to attempt new patterns of behavior, realigning maladaptive alliances, encouraging family members to resolve conflicts as dyads, opening up closed systems and covert emotional issues to address conflicts, and family-focused homework assignments. BSFT MHPs meet family members in nontraditional settings (e.g., home) and utilize evidence-supported engagement strategies to recruit important family members in therapy. BSFT is well-adapted to treat Hispanic families, and has demonstrated improved outcomes in conduct problems, socialized aggression, substance use, and family functioning across many controlled clinical trials (Coatsworth, Santisteban, McBride, & Szapocznik, 2001; Nickel et al., 2006; Santisteban et al., 1996, 1997, 2003; Szapocznik et al., 1988, 1989).

Functional Family Therapy (FFT) may be implemented in 12 sessions over a 3–4-month period, and sessions can be held where needed. The engagement phase consists of several activities that the MHP can use to increase family willingness to attend and develop a positive reaction to the MHP. During the motivation to change phase family members are taught to reduce behaviors that act to increase negativity and restrict opportunities to change and instead increase change-enhancing hopefulness. The relational/interpersonal assessment phase involves assessing interpersonal processes in intrafamilial and extrafamilial contexts. In the behavior change phase, family members are taught to change habitual problematic interactions and other coping patterns utilizing functional behaviors and communication patterns. Lastly, the generalization phase consists of supporting continued positive family interactions, relapse prevention, and provision of community resources. When Alexander and Parsons (1973) pioneered FFT, there were essentially no other structured interventions for adolescent SUDs. Thus, this treatment acted as an exemplary model in which to develop other treatments. FFT has shown to significantly improve outcomes in drug and alcohol use, criminal behavior, and family communication and interaction (e.g., Gordon, Graves, & Arbuthnot, 1995; Sexton & Turner, 2010; Waldron et al., 2001).

Multidimensional Family Therapy (MDFT) is a well-studied adolescent substance abuse treatment that acts to influence various systems, such as individual, family, peer, and community factors. It is typically completed in 12–16 sessions, which can be held in a clinic, or any other convenient location. MDFT includes interventions for the identified youth, parents, parent-child interaction, other family members, and extra-familial systems. Youths learn skills that are relevant to communicating their feelings and thoughts in a nonconfrontational and effective manner. Consistent with other treatments for adolescent SUDs, youths are taught problem-solving and job skills, and parents are taught parenting skills with an emphasis on self-evaluation and making adjustments on their child management style. Additionally, parents are taught to accept that they do not have to be "perfect" while attempting to "influence" their children, rather than controlling them. The research has shown that MDFT consistently results in decreased substance use and associated behavior problems, and improved family functioning (e.g., Liddle et al., 2001; Liddle, Dakof, Turner, Henderson, & Greenbaum, 2008; Liddle, Rowe, Dakof, Henderson, & Greenbaum, 2009). Importantly, this intervention has developed strategies that have been shown to improve treatment retention, school performance, and better cost-effectiveness (Liddle et al., 2001, 2008, 2009; Liddle, Rowe, Dakof, Ungaro, & Henderson, 2004).

Multisystemic Therapy (MST) is used to comprehensively address youth problem behaviors within the context of various systems (i.e., family, peer, school, neighborhoods). MST sessions are typically held in the home, or wherever convenient. Treatment usually lasts 4 months, with contacts between the family and the MST therapist occurring multiple times a week. Therapists are guided by nine therapeutic principles, including (1) understanding how youth problems "fit" into the environment; (2) focusing on positives and strengths; (3) promoting responsible behavior in family members; (4) being present focused, action oriented, and well defined; (5) targeting sequences of behavior within and between the various interacting elements of the adolescent's life; (6) being developmentally appropriate; (7) insisting on continuous effort in family members; (8) continuously evaluating treatment effectiveness; and (9) designing interventions that will be sustainable after the therapist leaves. MST therapists are available to their clients 24 h a day, 7 days a week, if the family is in need of assistance. MST therapists emphasize harm-reduction methods (i.e., attempting to keep youth out of stressful situations, such as jail) at all times. Parents are taught to improve their parenting skills, dissociate their child from antisocial peers, and alternatively initiate relationships with pro-social peers. Parents are also encouraged to become more involved with teachers and community professionals. Cognitive behavioral techniques, such as contingency management, are well-integrated into MST. MST has been shown to produce significantly improved outcomes in criminal activity, alcohol and drug use, family functioning, peer aggression, and other problem behaviors (e.g., Henggeler, Clingempeel, Brondino, & Pickrel, 2002; Henggeler et al., 2006; Henggeler, Melton, Brondino, Scherer, & Hanley, 1997; Henggeler, Melton, Smith, Schoenwald, & Hanley, 1993; Schaeffer & Borduin, 2005).

Concluding Remarks

After approximately three decades, the scientific base for adolescent substance abuse is now relatively strong. Indeed, as underscored in this chapter, the symptoms of substance abuse and dependence are now somewhat uniform, and we have a better understanding of the factors that influence these symptoms to occur. There is also a greater understanding of the relationship between symptoms of adolescent SUDs and coexisting conditions. Dozens of validated methods of assessment and treatment for adolescent SUDs are now available, and controlled clinical trials have assisted in determining optimal training methods involved in the dissemination of these methods for use by community practitioners to some small extent. The integration of evidence-based treatments will continue to occur, and clinical trials will assist in parsimoniously eliminating unnecessary intervention components and adopting effective ones. Of course, dissemination-oriented studies (or effectiveness trials) that emphasize development and evaluation of training programs for community practitioners will occur more frequently in the upcoming years. However, one of the relatively unexplored areas of study that will need to be addressed concerns the training of students at the graduate school level, that is, prior to them becoming "community practitioners." Indeed, most MHPs who are qualified to conduct treatment with adolescents who evidence SUDs have a master's or doctorate degree. However, most graduate training programs in the United States fail to incorporate evidence-based treatment protocols into student clinical practicum, and their coursework is broad based and usually non-applied. In this traditional format, students learn a lot of information about many theories and approaches, but are not provided opportunities to intensively learn one or two comprehensive evidence-based treatments. In many cases, students are exposed to treatments that are not empirically validated. This approach results in students learning most of their hands-on work in their internships or community vocations where they are likely to be unprepared to *hit the ground running* or not offered training in evidence-based treatment. Indeed, many internships include rotations with different supervisors, thus limiting their opportunities to gain extensive knowledge in a particular evidence-based treatment. It would seem to make more sense to target intensive dissemination of evidence-based treatments for adolescent substance abuse during graduate training through coursework that is interconnected directly with opportunities to practice the evidence-based therapies in concurrently attended practicum sites. Although this paradigm shift away from traditional graduate school training models may appear to be a daunting task, this approach is already being implemented in several schools that actively profess evidence-based treatment, such as the Psychology Department at the University of Wisconsin, Milwaukee.

References

Achenbach, T. M. (1991). *Integrative guide for the 1991 CBCL/4-18, YSR, and TRF profiles*. Burlington, VT: Department of Psychiatry, University of Vermont.

Alexander, J. F., & Parsons, B. V. (1973). Short term behavioral intervention with delinquent families: Impact on family process and recidivism. *Journal of Abnormal Psychology, 81*(3), 219–225.

Allen, D., Donohue, B., Sutton, G., Haderlie, M., & Lapota, H. (2009). Application of a standardized assessment methodology within the context of an evidence-based treatment for substance abuse and its associated problems. *Behavior Modification, 33*, 618–654.

American Psychiatric Association. (2000). *Diagnostic and statistical manual of mental disorders* (4th ed., text rev.). Washington, DC: Author.

Armstrong, T. D., & Costello, E. (2002). Community studies on adolescent substance use, abuse, or dependence and psychiatric co morbidity. *Journal of Consulting and Clinical Psychology, 70*, 1224–1239.

Austin, A., Hospital, M., Wagner, E. F., & Morris, S. (2010). Motivation for reducing substance use among minority adolescents: Targets for intervention. *Journal of Substance Abuse Treatment, 39*, 399–407.

Azrin, N. H., Acierno, R., Kogan, E. S., Donohue, B., Besalel, V. A., & McMahon, P. T. (1996). Follow-up results of supportive versus behavioral therapy for illicit drug use. *Behavior Research and Therapy, 34*, 41–46.

Azrin, N. H., Donohue, B., Besalel, V. A., Kogan, E., & Acierno, R. (1994). Youth drug abuse treatment: A controlled outcome study. *Journal of Child & Adolescent Substance Abuse, 3*, 1–16.

Azrin, N. H., Donohue, B., Teichner, G. A., Crum, T., Howell, J., & DeCato, L. A. (2001). A controlled evaluation and description of individual-cognitive problem solving and family-behavior therapies in dually-diagnosed conduct-disordered and substance-dependent youth. *Journal of Child & Adolescent Substance Abuse, 11*, 1–43.

Azrin, N. H., McMahon, P. T., Donohue, B., Besalel, V. A., Lapinski, K. J., Kogan, E. S., et al. (1994). Behavior therapy for drug abuse: A controlled treatment outcome study. *Behavior Research and Therapy, 33*, 857–866.

Baigent, M. F. (2003). Physical complications of substance abuse: What the psychiatrist needs to know. *Current Opinion in Psychiatry, 16*, 291–295.

Barlow, D. H. (2005). What's new about evidence-based assessment? *Psychological Assessment, 17*, 308–311.

Bender, K., Springer, D. W., & Kim, J. S. (2006). Treatment effectiveness with dually diagnosed adolescents: A systematic review. *Brief Treatment and Crisis Intervention, 6*, 177–205.

Breda, C., & Heflinger, C. (2007). The impact of motivation to change on substance use among adolescents in treatment. *Journal of Child & Adolescent Substance Abuse, 16*, 109–124.

Briones, E., Robbins, M. S., & Szapocznik, J. (2008). Brief strategic family therapy: Engagement and treatment. *Alcoholism Treatment Quarterly, 26*, 81–103.

Brodey, B., McMullin, D., Kaminer, Y., Winters, K., Mosshart, E., Rosen, C., et al. (2008). Psychometric characteristics of the Teen Addiction Severity Index-Two (T-ASI-2). *Substance Abuse, 29*, 19–32.

Broome, K. M., Joe, G. W., & Simpson, D. (2001). Engagement models for adolescents in DATOS-A. *Journal of Adolescent Research, 16*, 608–624.

Brown, S. A., Vik, P. W., & Creamer, V. A. (1989). Characteristics of relapse following adolescent substance abuse treatment. *Addictive Behavior, 14*, 291–300.

Brown, S. A., Creamer, V. A., & Stetson, B. A. (1987). Adolescent alcohol expectancies in relation to personal and parental drinking patterns. *Journal of Abnormal Psychology, 96*, 117–121.

Brown, S. A., Gleghorn, A. A., Schuckit, M. A., Myers, M. G., & Mott, M. A. (1996). Conduct disorder among adolescent alcohol and drug abusers. *Journal of Studies on Alcohol, 57*, 314–324.

Bukstein, O. G., & Horner, M. S. (2010). Management of the adolescent with substance use disorders and co morbid psychopathology. *Child and Adolescent Psychiatric Clinics of North America, 19*, 609–623.

Cantwell, D. P. (1996). Attention deficit disorder: A review of the past 10 years. *Journal of the American Academy of Child and Adolescent Psychiatry, 35*, 978–987.

Clark, D. B., & Bukstein, O. G. (1998). Psychopathology in adolescent alcohol abuse and dependence. *Alcohol Health and Research World, 22*, 117–121.

Coatsworth, J., Santisteban, D. A., McBride, C. K., & Szapocznik, J. (2001). Brief strategic family therapy versus community control: Engagement, retention, and an exploration of the moderating role of adolescent symptom severity. *Family Process, 40*, 313–332.

Deas, D., & Clark, A. (2009). Current state of treatment for alcohol and other drug use disorders in adolescents. *Alcohol Research & Health, 32*, 76–82.

Deas, D., Roberts, J., Randall, C., & Anton, R. (2001). Adolescent obsessive-compulsive drinking scale: An assessment tool for problem drinking. *Journal of the National Medical Association, 93*, 92–103.

Dennis, M., Babor, T., Roebuck, M., & Donaldson, J. (2002). Changing the focus: The case for recognizing and treating cannabis use disorders. *Addiction, 97*, 4–15.

Dennis, M. L., Funk, R., Godley, S., Godley, M. D., & Waldron, H. (2004). Cross-validation of the alcohol and cannabis use measures in the Global Appraisal of Individual Needs (GAIN) and Timeline Follow Back (TLFB; Form 90) among adolescents in substance abuse treatment. *Addiction, 99*, 120–128.

Deykin, E. Y., Levy, J. C., & Wells, V. (1987). Adolescent depression, alcohol and drug abuse. *American Journal of Public Health, 77*, 178–182.

Donohue, B., Azrin, N. H., Lawson, H., Friedlander, J., Teichner, G., & Rindsberg, J. (1998). Improving initial session attendance of substance abusing and conduct disordered adolescents: A controlled study. *Journal of Child & Adolescent Substance Abuse, 8*, 1–13.

Donohue, B. C., Karmely, J., & Strada, M. J. (2006). Alcohol and drug abuse. In M. Hersen & M. Hersen (Eds.), *Clinician's handbook of child behavioral assessment* (pp. 337–375). San Diego, CA: Elsevier Academic.

Donohue, B., Strada, M., Rosales, R., Taylor-Caldwell, A., Hise, D., Ahman, S., et al. (2006). The semistructured interview for consideration of ethnic culture in therapy scale: Initial psychometric and outcome support. *Behavior Modification, 30*, 867–891.

Donohue, B., Van Hasselt, V., Hersen, M., & Perrin, S. (1998). Role-play assessment of social skills in conduct disordered and substance abusing adolescents: An empirical review. *Journal of Child & Adolescent Substance Abuse, 8*, 1–28.

First, M. B., Spitzer, R. L, Gibbon, M, & Williams, J. B. W. (1996). *Structured Clinical Interview for DSM-IV-TR Axis I Disorders, Research Version (SCID-I)*. New York, NY: Biometrics Research, New York State Psychiatric Institute.

Fisher, G. L., & Harrison, T. C. (1992). Assessment of alcohol and other drug abuse with referred adolescents. *Psychology in the Schools, 29*, 172–178.

Friedman, A. S., & Utada, A. A. (1989). A method for diagnosing and planning the treatment of adolescent drug abusers. *Journal of Drug Education, 19*, 285–312.

Gans, J., Falco, M., Schackman, B. R., & Winters, K. C. (2010). An in-depth survey of the screening and assessment practices of highly regarded adolescent substance abuse treatment programs. *Journal of Child & Adolescent Substance Abuse, 19*, 33–47.

Godley, M. D., Godley, S. H., Dennis, M. L., Funk, R. R., & Passetti, L. L. (2007). The effect of assertive continuing care on continuing care linkage, adherence and abstinence following residential treatment for adolescents with substance use disorders. *Addiction, 102*, 81–93.

Gordon, D. A., Graves, K., & Arbuthnot, J. (1995). The effect of functional family therapy for delinquents on adult criminal behavior. *Criminal Justice and Behavior, 22*, 60–73.

Gordon, M. S., Kinlock, T. W., & Battjes, R. J. (2004). Correlates of early substance use and crime among adolescents entering outpatient substance abuse treatment. *The American Journal of Drug and Alcohol Abuse, 30*, 39–59.

Gordon, S., Tulak, F., & Troncale, J. (2004). Prevalence and characteristics of adolescent patients with co-occurring ADHD and substance dependence. *Journal of Addictive Diseases, 23*, 31–40.

Grella, C., Hser, Y., Joshi, V., & Rounds-Bryant, J. (2001). Drug treatment outcomes for adolescents with co morbid mental and substance use disorders. *The Journal of Nervous and Mental Disease, 189*, 384–392.

Harrell, A. V., & Wirtz, P. W. (1989). Screening for adolescent problem drinking: Validation of a multidimensional instrument for case identification. *Psychological Assessment, 1*, 61–63.

Henggeler, S. W., Clingempeel, W., Brondino, M. J., & Pickrel, S. G. (2002). Four-year follow-up of multisystemic therapy with substance-abusing and substance-dependent juvenile offenders. *Journal of the American Academy of Child and Adolescent Psychiatry, 41*, 868–874.

Henggeler, S. W., Halliday-Boykins, C. A., Cunningham, P. B., Randall, J., Shapiro, S. B., & Chapman, J. E. (2006). Juvenile drug court: Enhancing outcomes by integrating evidence-based treatments. *Journal of Consulting and Clinical Psychology, 74*, 42–54.

Henggeler, S. W., Melton, G. B., Brondino, M. J., Scherer, D. G., & Hanley, J. H. (1997). Multisystemic therapy with violent and chronic juvenile offenders and their families: The role of treatment fidelity in successful dissemination. *Journal of Consulting and Clinical Psychology, 65*, 821–833.

Henggeler, S. W., Melton, G. B., Smith, L. A., Schoenwald, S. K., & Hanley, J. H. (1993). Family preservation using multisystemic treatment: Long-term follow-up to a clinical trial with serious juvenile offenders. *Journal of Child and Family Studies, 3*, 283–293.

Henggeler, S., Pickrel, S., Brondino, M., & Crouch, J. (1996). Eliminating (almost) treatment dropout of substance abusing or dependent delinquents through home-based multisystemic therapy. *The American Journal of Psychiatry, 153*, 427–428.

Horner, B. R., & Scheibe, K. E. (1997). Prevalence and implications of attention-deficit hyperactivity disorder among adolescents in treatment for substance abuse. *Journal of the American Academy of Child and Adolescent Psychiatry, 36*, 30–36.

Johnston, L. D., O'Malley, P. M., Bachman, J. G., & Schulenberg, J. E. (2010, December 14). *National press release, Marijuana use is rising; ecstasy use is beginning to rise; and alcohol use is declining among U.S. teens* (p. 65). Ann Arbor, MI: University of Michigan News Service.

Kaminer, Y., Bukstein, O., & Tarter, R. (1991). The teen-addiction severity index: Rationale and reliability. *International Journal of the Addictions, 26*, 219–226.

Kaminer, Y., Burleson, J. A., Blitz, C., Sussman, J., & Rounsaville, B. J. (1998). Psychotherapies for adolescent substance abusers: A pilot study. *The Journal of Nervous and Mental Disease, 186*, 684–690.

Kaminer, Y., Burleson, J. A., & Goldberger, R. (2002). Cognitive-behavioral coping skills and psycho education therapies for adolescent substance abuse. *The Journal of Nervous and Mental Disease, 190*, 737–745.

Kandel, D., Johnson, J., Bird, H., Canino, G., Goodman, S., Lahey, B., et al. (1997). Psychiatric disorders associated with substance use among children and adolescents: Findings from the methods for the epidemiology of child and adolescent mental disorders (MECA) study. *Journal of Abnormal Child Psychology, 25*, 121–132.

Kingree, J., Braithwaite, R., & Woodring, T. (2000). Unprotected sex as a function of alcohol and marijuana use among adolescent detainees. *Journal of Adolescent Health, 27*, 179–185.

Kranzler, H. R., Kadden, R. M., Babor, T. F., & Tennen, H. (1996). Validity of the SCID in substance abuse patients. *Addiction, 91*, 859–868. doi:10.1111/j.1360-0443.1996.tb03580.x.

Latimer, W. W., Stone, A. L., Voight, A., Winters, K. C., & August, G. J. (2002). Gender differences in psychiatric co morbidity among adolescents with substance use disorders. *Experimental and Clinical Psychopharmacology, 10*, 310–315.

Latimer, W., Winters, K., D'Zurilla, T., & Nichols, M. (2003). Integrated family and cognitive-behavioral therapy for adolescent substance abusers: A stage I efficacy study. *Drug and Alcohol Dependence, 71*, 303–317.

Ledgerwood, D. M., Alessi, S. M., Hanson, T., Godley, M. D., & Petry, N. M. (2008). Contingency management for attendance to group substance abuse treatment administered by clinicians in community clinics. *Journal of Applied Behavior Analysis, 41*, 517–526.

Lefforge, N. L., Donohue, B., & Strada, M. J. (2007). Improving session attendance in mental health and substance abuse settings: A review of controlled studies. *Behavior Therapy, 38*, 1–22.

Liddle, H. A., Dakof, G. A., Parker, K., Diamond, G. S., Barrett, K., & Tejeda, M. (2001). Multidimensional family therapy for adolescent drug abuse: Results of a randomized clinical trial. *The American Journal of Drug and Alcohol Abuse, 27*, 651–688.

Liddle, H. A., Dakof, G. A., Turner, R. M., Henderson, C. E., & Greenbaum, P. E. (2008). Treating adolescent drug abuse: A randomized trial comparing multidimensional family therapy and cognitive behavior therapy. *Addiction, 103*, 1660–1670.

Liddle, H. A., Rowe, C. L., Dakof, G. A., Henderson, C. E., & Greenbaum, P. E. (2009). Multidimensional family therapy for young adolescent substance abuse: Twelve-month outcomes of a randomized controlled trial. *Journal of Consulting and Clinical Psychology, 77*, 12–25.

Liddle, H. A., Rowe, C. L., Dakof, G. A., Ungaro, R. A., & Henderson, C. (2004). Early intervention for adolescent substance abuse: Pretreatment to post treatment outcomes of a randomized controlled trial comparing multidimensional family therapy and peer group treatment. *Journal of Psychoactive Drugs, 36*, 49–63.

Lobbestael, J., Leurgans, M., & Arntz, A. (2011). Interrater reliability of the structured clinical interview for DSM-IV Axis I disorders (SCID I) and Axis II disorders (SCID II). *Clinical Psychology & Psychotherapy, 18*, 75–79. doi:10.1002/cpp.693.

Macgowan, M. J., & Engle, B. (2010). Evidence for optimism: Behavior therapies and motivational interviewing in adolescent substance abuse treatment. *Child and Adolescent Psychiatric Clinics of North America, 19*, 527–545.

Marshal, M. P., Molina, B. G., & Pelham, W. R. (2003). Childhood ADHD and adolescent substance use: An examination of deviant peer group affiliation as a risk factor. *Psychology of Addictive Behaviors, 17*, 293–302.

Martin, C. S., & Kaczynski, N. A. (1995). Patterns of DSM-IV alcohol abuse and dependence symptoms in adolescent drinkers. *Journal of Studies on Alcohol, 56*, 672–680.

Mayer, J. E., & Filstead, W. J. (1979). The adolescent alcohol involvement scale: An instrument for measuring adolescent's use and misuse of alcohol. *Journal of Studies on Alcohol, 40*, 291–300.

McCarthy, D. M., Tomlinson, K. L., Anderson, K. G., Marlatt, G., & Brown, S. A. (2005). Relapse in alcohol- and drug-disordered adolescents with co morbid psychopathology: Changes in psychiatric symptoms. *Psychology of Addictive Behaviors, 19*, 28–34.

McGillicuddy, N. B., Rychtarik, R. G., & Morsheimer, E. T. (2004). Psychometric evaluation of the parent situation inventory: A role-play measure of coping in parents of substance-using adolescents. *Psychological Assessment, 16*, 386–390.

McGovern, M., Wrisley, B., & Drake, R. (2005). Relapse of substance use disorder and its prevention among persons with co-occurring disorders. *Psychiatric Services, 56*, 1270–1273.

Miller, G. A. (1985, 1999). *The substance abuse subtle screening inventory (SASSI): manual* (2nd ed.). Springfield, IN: SASSI Institute.

Moberg, D., & Hahn, L. (1991). The adolescent drug involvement scale. *Journal of Adolescent Chemical Dependency, 2*, 75–88.

Molina, B. G., Smith, B. H., & Pelham, W. E. (1999). Interactive effects of attention deficit hyperactivity disorder and conduct disorder on early adolescent substance use. *Psychology of Addictive Behaviors, 13*, 348–358.

Moore, D. D. (1983). *Client substance index*. Olympia, WA: Olympic Counseling Services.

Najavits, L. M., Gallop, R. J., & Weiss, R. D. (2006). Seeking safety therapy for adolescent girls with PTSD and substance use disorder: A randomized controlled trial. *The Journal of Behavioral Health Services & Research, 33*, 453–463.

Newcomb, M. D., & Bentler, P. M. (1988). Impact of adolescent drug use and social support on problems of young adults: A longitudinal study. *Journal of Abnormal Psychology, 97*, 64–75.

Nickel, M., Luley, J., Krawczyk, J., Nickel, C., Widermann, C., Lahmann, C., et al. (2006). Bullying girls—changes after brief strategic family therapy: A randomized, prospective, controlled trial with one-year follow-up. *Psychotherapy and Psychosomatics, 75*, 47–55.

Odgers, C. L., Caspi, A., Nagin, D. S., Piquero, A. R., Slutske, W. S., Milne, B. J., et al. (2008). Is it important to prevent early exposure to drugs and alcohol among adolescents? *Psychological Science (Wiley-Blackwell), 19*, 1037–1044.

Rahdert, E. (Ed.). (1991). *The adolescent assessment/referral system manual*. Rockville, MD: U.S. Department of Health and Human Services, ADAMHA, National Institute on Drug Abuse. DHHS Pub. No. (ADM) 91-1735.

Ramo, D. E., & Brown, S. A. (2008). Classes of substance abuse relapse situations: A comparison of adolescents and adults. *Psychology of Addictive Behaviors, 22*, 372–379.

Roberts, A. R., & Corcoran, K. (2005). Adolescents growing up in stressful environments, dual diagnosis, and sources of success. *Brief Treatment and Crisis Intervention, 5*, 1–8.

Santisteban, D. A., Coatsworth, J. D., Perez-Vidal, A., Kurtines, W. M., Schwartz, S., LaPerriere, A., et al. (2003). The efficacy of brief strategic family therapy in modifying Hispanic adolescent behavior problems and substance use. *Journal of Family Psychology, 17*, 121–133.

Santisteban, D. A., Coatsworth, J., Perez-Vidal, A., Mitrani, V., Jean-Gilles, M., & Szapocznik, J. (1997). Brief structural/strategic family therapy with African American and Hispanic high-risk youth. *Journal of Community Psychology, 25*, 453–471.

Santisteban, D. A., Szapocznik, J., Perez-Vidal, A., Kurtines, W. M., Murray, E. J., & LaPerriere, A. (1996). Efficacy of intervention for engaging youth and families into treatment and some variables that may contribute to differential effectiveness. *Journal of Family Psychology, 10*, 35–44.

Schaeffer, C. M., & Borduin, C. M. (2005). Long-term follow-up to a randomized clinical trial of multisystemic therapy with serious and violent juvenile offenders. *Journal of Consulting and Clinical Psychology, 73*, 445–453.

Schramm-Sapyta, N. L., Walker, Q., Caster, J. M., Levin, E. D., & Kuhn, C. M. (2009). Are adolescents more vulnerable to drug addiction than adults? Evidence from animal models. *Psychopharmacology, 206*, 1–21.

Sexton, T., & Turner, C. W. (2010). The effectiveness of functional family therapy for youth with behavioral problems in a community practice setting. *Journal of Family Psychology, 24*, 339–348.

Shaffer, D., Fisher, P., Lucas, C. P., Dulcan, M. K., & Schwab-Stone, M. E. (2000). NIMH diagnostic interview schedule for children version IV (NIMH DISC-IV): Description, differences from previous versions, and reliability of some common diagnoses. *Journal of the American Academy of Child and Adolescent Psychiatry, 39*, 28–38.

Slesnick, N. N., Prestopnik, J. L., Meyers, R. J., & Glassman, M. (2007). Treatment outcome for street-living, homeless youth. *Addictive Behavior, 32*, 1237–1251.

Smith, D., Chamberlain, P., & Eddy, J. (2010). Preliminary support for multidimensional treatment foster care in reducing substance use in delinquent boys. *Journal of Child & Adolescent Substance Abuse, 19*, 343–358.

Sobell, M. B., Sobell, L. C., Klajner, F. F., Pavan, D. D., & Basian, E. E. (1986). The reliability of a timeline method for assessing normal drinker college students' recent drinking history: Utility for alcohol research. *Addictive Behaviors, 11*, 149–161.

Spear, L. P. (2000). The adolescent brain and age-related behavioral manifestations. *Neuroscience and Biobehavioral Review, 24*, 417–463.

Stanger, C., Budney, A., Kamon, J., & Thostensen, J. (2009). A randomized trial of contingency management for adolescent marijuana abuse and dependence. *Drug and Alcohol Dependence, 105*, 240–247.

Strada, M. J., Donohue, B., & Lefforge, N. L. (2006). Examination of ethnicity in controlled treatment outcome studies involving adolescent substance abusers: A comprehensive literature review. *Psychology of Addictive Behaviors, 20*, 11–27.

Sussman, S., Skara, S., & Ames, S. L. (2008). Substance abuse among adolescents. *Substance Use & Misuse, 43*, 1802–1828.

Szapocznik, J., Perez-Vidal, A., Brickman, A. L., Foote, F. H., Santisteban, D., Hervis, O., et al. (1988). Engaging adolescent drug abusers and their families in treatment: A strategic structural systems approach. *Journal of Consulting and Clinical Psychology, 56*, 552–557.

Szapocznik, J., Rio, A., Murray, E., Cohen, R., Scopetta, M., Rivas-Vazquez, A., et al. (1989). Structural family versus psychodynamic child therapy for problematic Hispanic boys. *Journal of Consulting and Clinical Psychology, 57*, 571–578.

Tarter, R. E. (1990). Evaluation and treatment of adolescent substance abuse: A decision tree method. *American Journal of Drugs and Alcohol Abuse, 16*, 1–46.

Tarter, R. E. (2002). Etiology of adolescent substance abuse: A developmental perspective. *The American Journal on Addictions, 11*, 171–191.

Tomlinson, K. L., Brown, S. A., & Abrantes, A. (2004). Psychiatric co morbidity and substance use treatment outcomes of adolescents. *Psychology of Addictive Behaviors, 18*, 160–169.

Toneatto, T. (2008). Screening and assessment of co-occurring disorders: Towards a phenomenological approach. *International Journal of Mental Health and Addiction, 6*, 37–44.

Tubman, J., Wagner, E., & Langer, L. (2003). Patterns of depressive symptoms, drinking motives, and sexual behavior among substance abusing adolescents: Implications for health risk. *Journal of Child & Adolescent Substance Abuse, 13*, 37–57.

Usher, K., Jackson, D., & O'Brien, L. (2007). Shattered dreams: Parental experiences of adolescent substance abuse. *International Journal of Mental Health Nursing, 16*, 422–430.

Waldron, H., Slesnick, N., Brody, J. L., Turner, C. W., & Peterson, T. R. (2001). Treatment outcomes for adolescent substance abuse at 4- and 7-month assessments. *Journal of Consulting and Clinical Psychology, 69*, 802–813.

Waldron, H., & Turner, C. W. (2008). Evidence-based psychosocial treatments for adolescent substance abuse. *Journal of Clinical Child and Adolescent Psychology, 37*, 238–261.

Weinberg, N. Z., Rahdert, E., Colliver, J. D., & Glantz, M. D. (1998). Adolescent substance abuse: A review of the past 10 years. *Journal of the American Academy of Child and Adolescent Psychiatry, 37*, 252–261.

White, H., & Labouvie, E. (1989). Towards the assessment of adolescent problem drinking. *Journal of Studies on Alcohol, 50*, 30–37.

Winters, K. C. (1992). Development of an adolescent alcohol and other drug abuse screening scale: Personal Experience Screening Questionnaire. *Addictive Behaviors, 17*, 479–490.

Winters, K. C., & Henly, G. (1989). *The personal experience inventory*. Los Angeles, CA: Western Psychological Services.

Winters, K. C., & Henly, G. (1993). *Adolescent diagnostic interview schedule and manual*. Los Angeles, CA: Western Psychological Services.

Winters, K. C., & Kaminer, Y. (2008). Screening and assessing adolescent substance use disorders in clinical populations. *Journal of the American Academy of Child and Adolescent Psychiatry, 47*, 740–744.

Winters, K. C., & Leitten, W. (2007). Brief intervention for drug-abusing adolescents in a school setting. *Psychology of Addictive Behaviors, 21*, 249–254.

Attention-Deficit/Hyperactivity Disorder in Adolescence

John T. Mitchell and Scott H. Kollins

Attention-deficit/hyperactivity disorder (ADHD) is a developmental disorder characterized by symptoms of inattention, hyperactivity, and impulsivity (American Psychiatric Association, 2000). ADHD affects approximately 3–7 % of school-aged children (Faraone, Sergeant, Gillberg, & Biederman, 2003; Polanczyk, de Lima, Horta, Biederman, & Rohde, 2007) and is one of the most common mental disorders in childhood (Olfson, 1992). Though traditionally children with ADHD were believed to outgrow the diagnosis (Bawkin & Bawkin, 1966), longitudinal studies demonstrate that the disorder persists for the majority of cases into adulthood (Barkley, Murphy, & Fischer, 2008; Mannuzza, Klein, Bessler, Malloy, & LaPadula, 1993; Weiss & Hechtman, 1993). How ADHD is manifested at different developmental points varies, particularly in adolescence (Barkley, 2006). As noted within this handbook, various physical, psychological, and social changes occur during this developmental period that makes adolescence quite a challenging point in life. For adolescents with ADHD, navigating through this developmental period is particularly challenging. The purpose of this chapter is to address the phenomenology of this disorder among adolescents, including diagnostic and treatment issues.

ADHD is typically diagnosed in accordance with the *Diagnostic and Statistical Manual, Fourth Edition, Text Revision* (*DSM-IV TR*) criteria (American Psychiatric Association, 2000). These criteria include (a) six or more of inattention or hyperactive–impulsive symptoms (see Table 1); (b) symptom onset prior to age seven; (c) some impairment from current symptoms in two or more settings; (d) clinically significant functional impairment in social, academic, or occupational domains; and (e) evidence that symptoms are not better accounted for by another psychiatric disorder. The *DSM-IV TR* classifies those that meet criteria for the disorder based on symptom presentation into different subtypes: ADHD predominantly inattentive type for those with greater than six inattentive symptoms and fewer than six hyperactive–impulsive symptoms, ADHD predominantly hyperactive–impulsive type for those with fewer than six inattentive symptoms and greater than six hyperactive–impulsive symptoms, and ADHD combined type for those with six or more of both inattentive and hyperactive–impulsive symptoms. The *International Classification of Diseases-10* criteria (World Health Organization, 1992) are more commonly used to diagnose ADHD outside of the United States and differ to some

J.T. Mitchell, Ph.D. (✉) • S.H. Kollins, Ph.D.
Duke ADHD Program, Department of Psychiatry and Behavioral Sciences, Duke University Medical Center, 2608 Erwin Road, Pavilion East, Suite 300, Durham, NC 27705, USA
e-mail: john.mitchell@duke.edu; scott.kollins@duke.edu

W.T. O'Donohue et al. (eds.), *Handbook of Adolescent Health Psychology*,
DOI 10.1007/978-1-4614-6633-8_27, © Springer Science+Business Media New York 2013

Table 1 ADHD symptoms

Inattention
(a) Often fails to give close attention to details or makes careless mistakes in schoolwork, work, or other activities
(b) Often has difficulty sustaining attention in tasks or play activities
(c) Often does not seem to listen when spoken to directly
(d) Often does not follow through on instructions and fails to finish schoolwork, chores, or duties in the workplace (not due to oppositional behavior or failure to understand instructions)
(e) Often has difficulty organizing tasks and activities
(f) Often avoids, dislikes, or is reluctant to engage in tasks that require sustained mental effort (such as school work or homework)
(g) Often loses things necessary for tasks or activities (e.g., toys, school assignments, pencils, books, or tools)
(h) Is often easily distracted by extraneous stimuli
(i) Is often forgetful in daily activities
Hyperactivity–impulsivity
(a) Often fidgets with hands or feet or squirms in seat
(b) Often leaves seat in classroom or in other situations in which remaining seated is expected
(c) Often runs about or climbs excessively in situations in which it is inappropriate (in adolescents or adults, may be limited to subjective feelings of restlessness)
(d) Often has difficulty playing or engaging in leisure activities quietly
(e) Is often "on the go" or often acts as if "driven by a motor"
(f) Often talks excessively
Impulsivity
(g) Often blurts out answers before the questions have been completed
(h) Often has difficulty awaiting turn
(i) Often interrupts or intrudes on others (e.g., butts into conversations or games)

degree (e.g., several symptoms of inattention, hyperactivity, *and* impulsivity are required for an ADHD diagnosis). The majority of studies in this chapter involve samples classified using versions of the *DSM* criteria.

ADHD into Adolescence

Longitudinal studies demonstrate that ADHD is a disorder that children do not simply outgrow as they reach adolescence (Biederman et al., 1996; Fischer, Barkley, Edelbrock, & Smallish, 1990; Mannuzza, Klein, Bessler, Malloy, & LaPadula, 1998; Rasmussen & Gillberg, 2000; Weiss & Hechtman, 1993). It is estimated that the diagnosis persists in 50–80 % of cases (August, Stewart, & Holmes, 1983; Barkley, Fischer, Smallish, & Fletcher, 2002; Biederman et al., 1996; Gittelman, Mannuzza, Shenker, & Bonagura, 1985; Ingram, Hechtman, & Morgenstern, 1999; Mannuzza et al., 1993).[1] Studies of clinically referred adolescents with ADHD also indicate that the disorder continues into adolescence and is associated with various functional impairments in comparison to non-diagnosed peers, including social competence, behavioral and emotional adjustment, school performance, and general quality of life (Barkley, Anastopoulos, Guevremont, & Fletcher, 1991; Topolski et al., 2004).

Although ADHD as a disorder is continuous from childhood into adolescence (Faraone, Biederman, & Monuteaux, 2002), the development of ADHD into adolescence needs to be considered in the context of adolescence as a period of devel-

[1] One caveat to these findings involves ADHD subtypes. To date, no longitudinal studies have assessed rates of persistence for those meeting criteria for ADHD predominantly inattentive type. See the special issue of *Clinical Psychology: Science and Practice* (2001); 8(4) for classification issues involving the inattentive subtype.

opment in which there are many changes at multiple levels, including physical, psychological, and social changes. During this developmental period, adolescents typically experience an increased influence of peers and independence from family members (Barkley, 2006). For adolescents with a disorder like ADHD in which social and emotional impairment is common (Wehmeier, Schacht, & Barkley, 2010), this transitional period may be particularly difficult. Cognitive demands increase along with greater independence from adult supervision (e.g., multiple teachers, amount of homework) as children enter into middle and high school (Barkley et al., 1991), which requires greater self-regulation that is often impaired in ADHD.

Neuronal and hormonal developmental changes occur for adolescents as well which can further impact how symptoms are expressed (Barkley, 2006). Related to such biologically based changes, adolescence is a critical period neurobiologically in which adolescents are at risk for elevations in risk-taking behavior and drug and alcohol use which correspond with notable changes in motivational and reward-related brain regions. Such elevations can be problematic as adolescents are naturally more sensitive to positive rewarding properties of various drugs and natural stimuli, and less sensitive to the aversive properties of these stimuli (Doremus-Fitzwater, Varlinskaya, & Spear, 2010). These behavioral and neurobiological developmental changes in concert with social, hormonal, and physiological changes place adolescents at high risk for substance use (Masten, Faden, Zucker, & Spear, 2008; Windle et al., 2008). ADHD is a risk factor for such substance use behavior (reviewed in greater detail below) and thus places adolescents with ADHD at a heightened risk during this critical developmental period.

Given such developmental changes, the presentation of ADHD changes into adolescence as well, including symptom presentation. That is, although inattentive symptoms continue to be involved in the clinical presentation of the majority of presenting cases, hyperactive symptoms decline in severity for many (Barkley et al., 2002; Barkley, Fischer, Edelbrock, & Smallish, 1990; Hart, Lahey, Loeber, Applegate, & Frick, 1995; Milich & Loney, 1979). Such symptom presentation continues to be functionally impairing in domains typically impaired in childhood, including academics (Mannuzza, Klein, Bessler, Malloy, & Hynes, 1997). However, different areas of functional impairment emerge during adolescence as well in which those with ADHD are at heightened risk. Driving is one example. In North America, motor vehicle accidents are the leading cause of death among adolescents (World Health Organization, 2002). ADHD drivers are at significantly higher risk for poor driving outcome, including increased traffic citations (particularly speeding), accidents which are their fault, repeated and more severe accidents, driving-related morbidity, and license suspensions and revocations (Barkley, 2004b). Such findings were not better accounted for by comorbidity or intelligence. Given that substance use is not uncommon in ADHD, the risks associated with drug and alcohol use should also be considered (Cox, Merkel, Penberthy, Kovatchev, & Hankin, 2004). In terms of clinical implications of such findings, stimulant medications have demonstrated to improve driving performance in ADHD drivers (Barkley & Cox, 2007; Barkley, Murphy, & Kwasnik, 1996; Jerome, Habinski, & Segal, 2006). The method of stimulant delivery is also an important factor. In one study, adolescent ADHD drivers drove better throughout the day on a driving simulator after taking an extended, controlled release stimulant in comparison to immediate release (Cox et al., 2004).

Issues related to sexual behavior begin to emerge in adolescence as well and risky sexual behavior appears to be associated with ADHD. In one longitudinal study of males diagnosed with ADHD in childhood, childhood ADHD predicted earlier initiation of sexual activity and intercourse, more sexual partners, more casual sex, and more partner pregnancies (Flory, Molina, Pelham, Gnagy, & Smith, 2006). These findings were not better accounted for by comorbid childhood conduct problems and suggest that childhood ADHD may be a valuable predictor of vulnerability to risky sexual behavior. Although this study involved only males, the association between ADHD and risky sexual behavior does not appear to be restricted to males only. In one study of adolescents followed from age 13 to 15, higher levels of ADHD symptoms were a significant predictor of earlier initial sexual activity in both males and females (Price & Hyde, 2009).

Comorbidity

Comorbidity within ADHD adolescent samples is typically the norm rather than the exception. For example, in one clinical sample of 6–18-year-olds, over half met criteria for at least one comorbid disorder (Elia, Ambrosini, & Berrettini, 2008). Disruptive behavior disorders, including oppositional defiant disorder (ODD) and conduct disorder (CD), are particularly common (Loeber, Burke, Lahey, Winters, & Zera, 2000). In general population studies, ADHD increases the odds of ODD or CD by 10.7-fold (Angold, Costello, & Erkanli, 1999). Some studies have estimated that between 25 and 75 % of adolescents with ADHD meet diagnostic criteria for ODD or CD [reviewed in (Barkley, 2006)]. In another study of clinically referred 7–15-year-olds, ODD was comorbid among 54–67 % (Elia et al., 2008). In this study, differences in subtypes also emerged. ODD was significantly more common among combined and hyperactive–impulsive ADHD subtypes (50.7 % and 41.9 %, respectively) than the inattentive subtype (20.8 %). Such rates are not only concerning because of characteristics of these comorbid disruptive behavior disorders (e.g., delinquency) that are dealt with in adolescence but also that CD is a precursor to antisocial personality disorder into adulthood. Given that CD (a) is commonly comorbid with ADHD and (b) is a precursor to antisocial personality disorder, it is not surprising that rates of antisocial personality disorder (among additional forms of Axis II psychopathology) are elevated in adult ADHD samples (Fischer, Barkley, Smallish, & Fletcher, 2002; Mannuzza et al., 1993; Miller, Nigg, & Faraone, 2007; Rasmussen & Gillberg, 2000; Weiss & Hechtman, 1993).

Substance use disorders (SUDs) are common in ADHD adolescents as well. In longitudinal studies of hyperactive children, the risk for SUDs ranges from 12 to 24 % into adulthood (Fischer et al., 2002; Gittelman et al., 1985; Mannuzza et al., 1993). Given that adolescence is when initial exposure to substances emerges and is a developmental period in which susceptibility to the reinforcing effects of substances is heightened (Doremus-Fitzwater et al., 2010; Masten et al., 2008; Windle et al., 2008), substance use in adolescence is both a concern as an outcome of current use and continued risk for future use. This risk is further elevated among adolescents with ADHD. Individuals with ADHD engage in experimentation earlier than children without ADHD (Carroll & Rounsaville, 1993; Wilens, Biederman, Mick, Faraone, & Spencer, 1997). Although such findings indicate that the relationship between ADHD and SUDs is independent of comorbidity, CD comorbidity is a strong predictor of risk for substance use disorders among ADHD children when they reach adolescence and adulthood (Burke, Loeber, & Lahey, 2001; Molina, Smith, & Pelham, 1999; White, Xie, Thompson, Loeber, & Stouthamer-Loeber, 2001). In addition, prospective studies indicate that childhood ADHD with co-occurring CD or bipolar disorder is at a higher risk for SUDs during adolescence (Biederman et al., 1997; Molina & Pelham, 2003; Satterfield, Hoppe, & Schell, 1982).

In terms of cigarette smoking, adolescents with ADHD smoke at significantly higher rates than non-diagnosed peers. Prevalence rates range from 10 to 46 % for ADHD adolescents versus 10 to 24 % for non-ADHD peers (Lambert & Hartsough, 1998; Milberger, Biederman, Faraone, Chen, & Jones, 1997; Molina & Pelham, 2003; Pomerleau, Downey, Stelson, & Pomerleau, 1995). Even among nonclinical samples there is a linear relationship between number of ADHD symptoms, lifetime risk of smoking, and age of onset of regular smoking (Kollins, McClernon, & Fuemmeler, 2005; Tercyak, Lerman, & Audrain, 2002). Additional studies have demonstrated that ADHD samples initiate smoking earlier, exhibit a higher level of nicotine dependence, have greater difficulty quitting in comparison to non-ADHD smoking samples, and are at an increased risk for becoming a regular cigarette smoker (Covey, Manubay, Jiang, Nortick, & Palumbo, 2008; Fuemmeler, Kollins, & McClernon, 2007; Hartsough & Lambert, 1987; Humfleet et al., 2005; Milberger et al., 1997; Pomerleau et al., 1995; Rohde, Kahler, Lewinsohn, & Brown, 2004). In addition, the relationship between ADHD and tobacco use has remained significant as an independent risk factor after accounting for comorbidity, including CD (Milberger et al., 1997; Molina & Pelham, 2003) [see (Glass & Flory, 2010; McClernon & Kollins, 2008) for reviews].

Mood disorders are also common among adolescents with ADHD (Cuffe et al., 2001). For example, in one study, a depressive disorder was comorbid in 21.6 % of an ADHD sample of 6–18-year-olds (Elia et al., 2008). Given that the combination of a major depressive disorder and a comorbid disruptive behavior disorder is a risk factor for suicidal behavior (Lewinsohn, Rohde, & Seeley, 1995), both common comorbidities in ADHD, considering comorbidity in adolescent ADHD samples has clear implications. Indeed, one longitudinal study assessing childhood ADHD reported the diagnosis in children predicted adolescent depression and/or suicide attempts. In addition, female sex, maternal depression, and concurrent ADHD symptoms in childhood predicted which children with ADHD were at greatest risk for these outcomes (Chronis-Tuscano et al., 2010).

Bipolar disorder is another commonly comorbid disorder with ADHD. Studies have estimated that it co-occurs among 10–20 % of children and adolescents with ADHD (Carlson, 1990; Wozniak et al., 1995; Wozniak & Biederman, 1995). Longitudinal studies of hyperactive children indicate no significant differences by adulthood (Fischer et al., 2002; Mannuzza et al., 1993; Weiss & Hechtman, 1993), although another longitudinal study of ADHD children reported higher rates into adolescence (12 %) (Biederman, Faraone, et al., 1999). In some cases, ADHD may be indicative of more severe bipolar. For instance, ADHD is more common in childhood-onset cases of bipolar disorder, which suggested that in some cases ADHD may signal an earlier onset, more chronic bipolar disorder (Faraone et al., 1997; Masi et al., 2006). Regarding anxiety disorders, longitudinal studies of hyperactive children do not report significant elevations in comorbid anxiety disorders (Fischer et al., 2002; Mannuzza et al., 1993; Weiss & Hechtman, 1993). However, anxiety disorders have been reported to be comorbid in 10–40 % of clinic-referred children and adolescents with ADHD (Biederman, Newcorn, & Sprich, 1991; Elia et al., 2008; Pliszka, 1992; Tannock, 2000). These studies in general demonstrate that comorbidity is typical among adolescents with ADHD and further complicates its clinical presentation in adolescence. In addition to concerns about prognosis, such comorbidities can easily complicate issues related to assessment, which we review below (Table 2).

Assessment

Empirically based assessments of ADHD typically involve structured clinical interviews, standardized questionnaires, and record review following diagnostic criteria (Anastopoulos & Shelton, 2001; Barkley, 2006). Cognitive test performance may also provide additive value in some cases to assess different ADHD subtypes (Clarke et al., 2007). Although there is diagnostic continuity of ADHD from childhood to adolescence (Faraone, Biederman, & Monuteaux, 2002), assessing ADHD into adolescence needs to be considered in the context of complicating factors. One such factor involves comorbidity. As reviewed above, comorbidity is common in adolescents with ADHD. Such conditions can co-occur with ADHD or mimic ADHD symptoms. Regarding the latter, diminished ability to concentrate can also be a symptom of a major depressive episode, distractibility and being overly talkative can also be symptoms of a manic or hypomanic episode, and restlessness and difficulty in concentrating can be symptoms of generalized anxiety disorder or post-traumatic stress disorder (American Psychiatric Association,

Table 2 Summary of adolescent developmental factors, emergent domains of impairment, and comorbid disorders among adolescents with ADHD

Adolescent developmental factors and new domains of impairment	
Cognitive demands increase along with greater independence from adult supervision (e.g., multiple teachers, amount of homework) as children enter into middle and high school	Barkley et al. (1991)
Inattentive symptoms continue, although overt hyperactive symptoms from childhood decline in severity	Barkley et al. (1990, 2002), Hart et al. (1995), Milich and Loney (1979)
Driving difficulties emerge (e.g., traffic citations, motor vehicle accidents)	Barkley (2004b), Barkley et al. (1996), Cox et al. (2004)
Increase in risky sexual behavior	Flory et al. (2006), Price and Hyde (2009)
Comorbid disorders	
Disruptive behavior disorders (ODD/CD)	Angold et al. (1999), Elia et al. (2008), Loeber et al. (2000)
Substance use disorders	Carroll and Rounsaville (1993), Covey et al. (2008), Fischer et al. (2002), Fuemmeler et al. (2007), Gittelman et al. (1985), Hartsough and Lambert (1987), Humfleet et al. (2005), Lambert and Hartsough (1998), Mannuzza et al. (1993), Milberger et al. (1997), Molina and Pelham (2003), Pomerleau et al. (1995), Rohde et al. (2004), Wilens et al. (1997)
Depressive disorders	Cuffe et al. (2001), Elia et al. (2008), Lewinsohn et al. (1995), Chronis-Tuscano et al. (2010)
Bipolar disorder	Carlson (1990), Wozniak and Biederman (1995), Wozniak et al. (1995), Biederman, Faraone, et al. (1999)
Anxiety disorders	Biederman et al. (1991), Elia et al. (2008), Pliszka (1992), Tannock (2000)

2000). Further, substance use can confound assessment for ADHD as alcohol and illicit drug use can create cognitive impairments common in ADHD (Ehrenreich et al., 1999; Fried, Watkinson, James, & Gray, 2002; Kempel, Lampe, Parnefjord, Hennig, & Kunert, 2003; Parrott, 2003).

An additional factor that emerges in adolescent ADHD assessments involves reporting source. In childhood ADHD assessments, parents and teachers are typical reporters (Barkley, 2006). However, into adolescence, adolescents spend more time with peers and less with parents. Further, as opposed to elementary school, adolescents have multiple teachers who spend less time with them during the school day and thus have fewer opportunities to observe their student's behavior. Self-report methods can be incorporated into adolescent ADHD assessments as well. However, adolescents with ADHD have a tendency to underreport the severity of their symptoms [(Barkley et al., 2002), see (Willoughby, 2003) for a review], which should be considered in any assessment. In ADHD, self-report concerns involve not just report of ADHD symptoms but past delinquent behaviors as well. In one study, adolescents and young adults with ADHD were less likely than non-ADHD peers to report accurately on delinquent behaviors they engaged in 1 year earlier (Sibley et al., 2010). Such inaccurate reporting of behavior in ADHD is consistent with findings that those with ADHD have a tendency towards a positive illusory bias view of their behavior (Hoza, Pelham, Dobbs, Owens, & Pillow, 2002; Owens, Goldfine, Evangelista, Hoza, & Kaiser, 2007; Owens & Hoza, 2003) and theories of ADHD that argue that problems with self-awareness emerge from working memory impairments [e.g., (Barkley, 1997)]. Another factor in adolescent ADHD assessments that has implications for self-report involves developmental changes in ADHD symptom presentation. In particular, we are referring to the decline in overt hyperactive symptoms into adolescence (Barkley et al., 1990, 2002; Hart et al., 1995; Milich & Loney, 1979), which makes inattentive symptoms become more prominent. As a clinical observation, inattentive features common in ADHD can be experienced more subjectively (e.g., daydreaming) than more overt hyperactive behaviors (e.g., getting out of one's seat at inappropriate times), thus making self-report more relevant in this age group.

Finally, the appropriateness of diagnostic criteria for ADHD is a complicating issue involved in adolescent assessment as well. Specially, the *DSM-IV TR* lists that an age of symptom onset must have occurred by age seven in order to qualify for an ADHD diagnosis (American Psychiatric Association, 2000). However, studies addressing the empirical basis for this criterion have called it into question and recommend a revision to include childhood onset at or prior to age 12 (Applegate et al., 1997; Barkley & Biederman, 1997; Faraone, Kunwar, Adamson, & Biederman, 2009; Rohde, 2008; Todd, Huang, & Henderson, 2008). One study assessing the implications of this diagnostic revision in a large longitudinal sample found that the prevalence estimate, correlates, and risk factors of ADHD would not be affected if the new diagnostic criterion was adopted (Polanczyk et al., 2010). Thus, although it is recommended to follow diagnostic criteria in adolescent ADHD assessments, incorporating such findings may be crucial in making a diagnosis (Table 3).

Table 3 Summary of factors to consider in adolescent ADHD assessments

Comorbid disorders can mimic or co-occur with ADHD symptoms
Reporting sources may change, including (a) an increase in self-report and peer perspectives and (b) a decrease in parent and teacher report perspectives
Change in symptom presentation (i.e., decrease in overt hyperactive symptoms)
Appropriateness of the age of onset criterion

Treatment

Relatively less research is devoted to efficacious treatments for adolescents with ADHD in comparison to children with ADHD (Smith, Waschbusch, Willoughby, & Evans, 2000). Despite diagnostic continuity (Faraone, Biederman & Monuteaux, 2002), given the physical, social, and psychological changes that occur in adolescents with ADHD, it is somewhat difficult to simply extend childhood treatments to this group. Adolescents ADHD treatments are more likely to require more extensive and costly intervention (Smith et al., 2000). Further, treating adolescents is particularly challenging as they are less likely than children to receive mental health services in the first place (Jensen, Martin, & Cantwell, 1997).

ADHD treatment is focused on symptom management and the reduction of downstream effects of unmanaged ADHD, such as school failure, automobile accidents, and peer rejection (Barkley, 2004a). Symptom management is analogous to symptom management for any lifelong condition, such as poor eyesight, diabetes, or asthma. Such comparisons that emphasize that ADHD is not the fault of the person with the disorder, but rather a neurobiological condition, are also helpful to deal with any stigmatization associated with a psychiatric disorder (Wolraich et al., 2005).

Among children with ADHD, psychoeducation about ADHD, psychopharmacology (primarily stimulants), parent training in behavior management methods, classroom behavioral modification and academic interventions, and special educational placement are most efficacious or promising (Barkley, 2004a). However, the empirical literature extending these treatments into adolescence is much more sparse. That is, adolescent ADHD treatment options may be available, although not all are equally efficacious and in many cases well-controlled studies are often lacking (Barkley, 2004a; Ingersoll & Goldstein, 1993). However, there are some empirically supported treatments for adolescents with ADHD and their families, particularly pharmacotherapy and specific psychosocial treatment approaches (Barkley, 2004a).

Pharmacotherapy

Stimulants and noradrenergic agonists are ADHD psychotropic treatments approved by the US Food and Drug Administration for use in adolescents [also see (Barkley, 2004a) for a general review]. Stimulants include methylphenidate (e.g., Ritalin,

Concerta, Metadate ER) and amphetamine compounds (e.g., Adderall, Dexedrine, and DextroStat), and have a long-standing history in the treatment of ADHD (Conners, 2002). Both classes of stimulants have slightly differing mechanisms of action. Whereas both block the reuptake of dopamine and norepinephrine into the presynaptic neuron and thereby increase neurotransmitter concentrations, amphetamine compounds also increase the release of dopamine from presynaptic cytoplasmic storage vesicles (Connor, 2006). Stimulants are effective in approximately 70 % of adolescents with ADHD (Biederman, Spencer, & Wilens, 2004; Evans et al., 2001; Wilens & Spencer, 2000). At least seven randomized controlled trials have been conducted among adolescents with ADHD—all but one support the efficacy of stimulants [reviewed in (Connor, 2006)]. Consistent with findings that there is diagnostic continuity of ADHD from childhood to adolescence (Faraone, Biederman, & Monuteaux, 2002), the efficacy of stimulants (specifically, methylphenidate) is largely equal from childhood to adolescence (Smith, Pelham, Gnagy, & Yudell, 1998). In a meta-analysis of children and adolescents comparing the comparative efficacy of the two broad class of stimulants (i.e., methylphenidate and amphetamine compounds), amphetamine compounds had a small yet statistically significant advantage over a standard-release form of methylphenidate for parent and clinician ratings of ADHD symptoms and global ratings (but not for teacher ratings) (Faraone, Biederman, & Roe, 2002). Although stimulants such as methylphenidate are efficacious in acutely reducing ADHD symptoms, medication side effects (e.g., decreased appetite) are common and have prompted consideration of other pharmacological interventions (Schachter, Pham, King, Langford, & Moher, 2001).

Noradrenergic agonists approved for use in ADHD children and adolescents by the US Food and Drug Administration include guanfacine extended release (Intuniv) and clonidine modified release [see (Bidwell, Dew, & Kollins, 2010) for a review]. Though the precise mechanism of action for treating ADHD is unclear, these medications likely facilitate dopamine and noradrenaline neurotransmission thought to play a role in the pathophysiology of ADHD (Arnsten, 2009; Bidwell et al., 2010). In 2009, guanfacine extended release was the first α-2 agent to be approved by the US Food and Drug Administration for use in treatment of ADHD in children and adolescents. According to one randomized controlled trial in children and adolescents with ADHD, guanfacine performed better than a placebo in reducing teacher-rated ADHD symptoms, but not parent-rated ADHD symptoms (Scahill et al., 2001). In three double-blind, placebo-controlled trials involving child and adolescent participants, guanfacine extended release performed significantly better than placebo in reducing symptoms (Biederman, Melmed, Patel, McBurnett, Konow, et al., 2008; Kollins, Spencer, Findling, et al., 2009; Sallee et al., 2009). A 2-year, open-label, follow-up study of guanfacine extended release in children and adolescents, with or without coadministration of stimulants, demonstrated continued efficacy as that seen in short-term randomized controlled trials (Sallee, Lyne, Wigal, & McGough, 2009). Such findings emerged in a similar study (Biederman, Melmed, Patel, McBurnett, Donahue, et al., 2008), although the attrition rate in both studies was greater than 75 % and therefore limits generalizability. Two randomized, double-blind, placebo-controlled studies evaluating the efficacy of clonidine modified release in children and adolescents with ADHD have been conducted. One assessed clonidine modified release as a monotherapy, while another studied it as an add-on agent in patients on a nonoptimal stimulant drug regimen. In both trials, clonidine modified release significantly reduced ADHD symptoms from baseline and was well tolerated (Jain, Kollins, Baily, et al., 2008; Kollins, Findling, Wigal, et al., 2009).

Atomoxetine (Strattera) is another noradrenergic agonist approved for use in adolescents with ADHD [see (Cheng, Chen, Ko, & Ng, 2007; Thomason & Michelson, 2004; Wilens, Newcorn, et al., 2006) for reviews and meta-analyses] and has comparable efficacy with methylphenidate in reducing core ADHD symptoms in children and adolescents (Hazell et al., 2011). In one randomized, placebo-controlled, dose–response study of atomoxetine in children and adolescents with ADHD, atomoxetine was consistently associated with a significant reduction of ADHD symptoms (Michelson et al., 2001). Social and family functioning also improved among those taking atomoxetine with statistically significant improvements in measures of ability to meet psychosocial role expectations and parental impact. In a randomized, placebo-controlled study of atomoxetine among children and adolescents with ADHD, atomoxetine-treated participant reductions in ADHD symptoms were superior to those of the placebo treatment group as assessed by investigator, parent, and teacher ratings (Michelson et al., 2002). Additional trials have demonstrated the efficacy and tolerability of this medication in children and adolescents with ADHD (Buitelaar et al., 2004; Kratochvil et al., 2007; Michelson et al., 2007; Newcorn, Spencer, Biederman, Milton, & Michelson, 2005; Prasad et al., 2007; Wehmeier et al., 2008). Although these studies included children and adolescents, acute atomoxetine treatment appears to be equally effective and tolerated in children and adolescents (Wilens, Kratochvil, Newcorn, & Gao, 2006). Such findings suggest that pharmacological differences in tolerability or ADHD symptom response are negligible between children and adolescents.

When considering pharmacotherapy, one issue relevant to adolescents with ADHD involves treatment discontinuation. The prevalence of prescribing by general practitioners to patients with ADHD drops significantly in adolescence (Charach, Ickowicz, & Schachar, 2004). Further, this decrease is greater than the reported age-related decrease in symptoms, indicating that treatment is prematurely discontinued in many cases where symptoms persist (McCarthy et al., 2009). In one longitudinal study, 48 % of children between the ages of 9 and 15 had discontinued ADHD medication. Age was a significant moderator of medication adherence such that adolescents were less likely to continue their medication (Thiruchelvam, Charach, & Schachar, 2001). Thus, in addition to a need for continued research devoted to efficacious treatments for adolescents with ADHD (Smith et al., 2000), unique barriers to treatment such as premature discontinuation needs to be addressed.

Psychosocial Treatments

In terms of psychosocial treatments for adolescents with ADHD, the empirical literature is sparse in comparison to pharmacotherapy options. In addition, due to the many developmental and environmental changes that occur during transition into adolescence, childhood treatments are not easily translated for this age group (Chronis, Jones, & Raggi, 2006). Among the developmental changes that have implications for treatment, adolescents have a greater cognitive capacity for abstraction, behavioral self-awareness, identity formation and need for independence, peer influence, variability in daily school routines, and physiological changes (e.g., development of secondary sex characteristics) (Smith et al., 2000). Thus, treatments are recommended to include increased involvement of the teenager, behavioral contingencies that involve more opportunities to socialize with peers and exert independence, collaboration with multiple teachers, homework issues (particularly time management and organizational skills), and self-monitoring strategies (Chronis et al., 2006). Among studies that have considered psychosocial treatments for adolescents with ADHD, family-based and school-based approaches are the most promising (Chronis et al., 2006; Pelham & Fabiano, 2008).

Three studies have involved family-based interventions. One study randomized 12–18-year-olds to 8–10 sessions of behavior management training, problem-solving and communication training, or structural family therapy (Barkley, Guevremont, Anastopoulos, & Fletcher, 1992). All conditions resulted in significant improvement in negative communication, conflict, anger during conflicts, school adjustment, internalizing and externalizing symptoms, and maternal depressive symptoms at posttreatment and were largely maintained for a 3-month follow-up. However, only 5–20 % in each condition demonstrated clinically significant reliable change following treatment. Another study compared parent behavior management training to parent behavior management training/

problem-solving and communication therapy (Barkley, Edwards, Laneri, Fletcher, & Metevia, 2001). Both treatments demonstrated significant improvement in parent–teen conflicts, but were not statistically different from one another. Although such group-level analysis and normalization rates supported the efficacy of these treatments, reliable change indices were similar to Barkley et al. (1992). Another study evaluated a behavior management, problem-solving, and education group for parents of adolescents with ADHD (McCleary & Ridley, 1999). Pre- and post-treatment comparisons indicated statistically significant decreases in the frequency and intensity of self-reported parent–adolescent conflict and in parent-reported problem behavior, and positive effects on parent skills and confidence. Although these studies are promising, they did not produce much clinically significant reliable change or are limited by methodological design (i.e., lack of a control or alternative treatment group). In terms of clinical implications, multimodal, long-term treatment may be useful to assist parents in their interactions with their teens to manage parental and family distress (Robin, 2006), as opposed to simply reducing ADHD symptom severity.

Academic functioning is one of the most common concerns of parents of adolescents with ADHD (Robin, 2006). Interventions targeting academic impairment in adolescents with ADHD are promising (Raggi & Chronis, 2006). One school-based intervention involving directed note taking through group-based didactic and modeling yielded statistically significant improvement in on-task behavior, material comprehension, and daily assignment scores in an adolescent ADHD sample (Evans, Pelham, & Grudberg, 1995). A more comprehensive treatment, called the Challenging Horizons Program (Evans, Axelrod, & Langberg, 2004), involving (a) after-school academic training incorporating behavioral strategies in a group and individual setting and (b) monthly group parent training has yielded moderate to large effect sizes on parent and teacher-rated academic functioning and classroom disturbance in comparison to a community care group among middle school students with ADHD (Evans, Langberg, Raggi, Allen, & Buvinger, 2005). Although effect sizes were less promising for social functioning and methodological designs limited the generalizability of these findings (e.g., quasi-experimental design, small sample size), a 3-year treatment outcome study of this program indicated cumulative long-term benefits for the treatment group in comparison to a community care control group for parent ratings of ADHD symptoms and social functioning (Evans, Serpell, Schultz, & Pastor, 2007). However, this latter study did not indicate any academic benefits of the treatment. Single-subject design studies also indicate the beneficial impact of behavioral techniques (e.g., self-monitoring and functional analysis) in improving goal-oriented behavior in the classroom while decreasing disruptive behavior among adolescents with ADHD (Ervin, DuPaul, Kern, & Friman, 1998; Stewart & McLaughlin, 1992), which deserves additional consideration in future research.

A variant of the interventions discussed above targeting academic behavior in adolescents with ADHD is also emerging. That is, the Homework Intervention Program is a behaviorally based parent training program targeting homework in middle school students. In a pilot study of a small sample of middle school students diagnosed with ADHD ($n = 11$), multiple-baseline design analyses indicated an improvement in parent-reported homework problems and ADHD symptoms, overall grade point average, and teacher-reported productivity (Raggi, Chronis-Tuscano, Fishbein, & Groomes, 2009).

Overall, comprehensive school-based interventions are promising and, similar to family-based interventions, warrant future research. Psychosocial treatment development for adolescents with ADHD is a small, yet developing field of research. Current treatments need to be more thoroughly assessed. For example, social impairment continues into adolescence (Bagwell, Molina, Pelham, & Hoza, 2001) and needs to be assessed more thoroughly. Further, social impairment with ADHD increases the risk for substance use and related problems (Greene et al., 1999), which demonstrates the need to also target social functioning in adolescent ADHD interventions. Treatments need to also consider ADHD adolescents and how to individualize treatment for the various comorbidities that can be presented. In addition, treatments that complement existing psychosocial treatment approaches should also be considered to target the multidimensional challenges that adolescents with ADHD face (Smith et al., 2000). Some potentially complimentary treatments have yielded promising results. For example, attention training in cognitive training programs (Epstein & Tsal, 2010), mindfulness meditation (Zylowska et al., 2008), and physical exercise to reduce disruptive behaviors (Allison, Faith, & Franklin, 1995) have potential, although more methodologically rigorous trials are required.

Special Considerations

Stimulant Use and Long-Term Consequences

Although stimulant medications are efficacious in targeting ADHD symptoms, there are several controversial topics that are common about this particular type of pharmacotherapy. One concern involves the non-prescribed use of stimulants. One study assessing poison control center calls among 13–19-year-olds indicates that the rates of stimulant medication abuse in adolescents are rising (Setlik, Bond, & Ho, 2009). In one longitudinal sample, 11 % of an ADHD group reported selling their medications in comparison to no subjects in a control group taking other medications (Wilens, Gignac, Swezey, Monuteaux, & Biederman, 2006). Also, significantly more participants with ADHD reported misusing their stimulant medications (22 %). Those with comorbid CD or a substance use disorder accounted for this trend, which further demonstrates the necessity to understand and consider the role of comorbidity in clinical settings. In another study among junior and senior high school students who were prescribed stimulants, 7 % had sold their medications (Michelson et al., 2001). In a sample of college students taking ADHD medications, 31 % had misused their medication by taking larger or more frequent doses than prescribed or by using someone else's medication (Rabiner et al., 2009). In addition, 8 % engaged in intranasal use and 26 % had diverted their medications to peers. Although nonacademic reasons for misuse were reported, enhancing ability to study outside of class was the primary motive for misuse. These findings indicate the need to monitor medication use in adolescents with ADHD, particularly those with comorbid CD or substance use disorders, and to consider treatments that have a lower likelihood of misuse or diversion (Wilens, Gignac, et al., 2006). In cases in which the primary motive of misuse is to assist in studying and other academic behavior, concerns about inadequate dosing and the need to improve communication between adolescents and their prescribing physicians need to be addressed.

Another issue regarding stimulant medication use involves its suppressive impact on physical growth. Reviews indicate that treatment with stimulant medication does lead to subsequent delays in height (approximately amounted to 1 cm/year during the first 3 years) and weight (Faraone, Biederman, Morley, & Spencer, 2008; Ptacek, Kuzelova, & Paclt, 2009). These reviews also indicate that the effect of stimulants on growth suppression reduces over time, growth deficits may be dose dependent, growth suppression effects may not differ between methylphenidate and amphetamine, stimulant discontinuation may lead to growth normalization, and ADHD may itself be associated with dysregulated growth. In one longitudinal study, methylphenidate treatment was associated with small yet significant delays in height, weight, and body mass index (Faraone & Giefer, 2007). Within the ADHD sample, those who had not received prior stimulant therapy and those who entered the study with an above average height, weight, and body mass index were most likely to experience growth deficits while taking stimulants. Further, the impact on all growth indices was most apparent during the first year of treatment and attenuated over time. In another longitudinal study evaluating the effect of stimulant medication on physical growth, a newly medicated group exhibited decreases in size after 3 years of treatment relative to a non-medicated group—the newly medicated group was 2.0 cm shorter and weighed 2.7 kg less (Swanson et al., 2007).

Other studies have considered non-stimulant ADHD medications as well and have reported a relationship with growth suppression. In one study, for example, lisdexamfetamine dimesylate treatment lead to statistically significant reductions in expected height, weight, and body mass index (Faraone, Spencer, Kollins, & Glatt, 2010). These findings indicate that in clinical settings, the potential benefits in symptom reduction and daily functioning need to be contrasted with the small but significant effects of pharmacotherapy (particularly stimulants) on growth. In most cases, growth suppression effects do not appear to be a clinical concern for most children treated with stimulants (Faraone et al., 2008). Although future studies are required to clarify the effects of continuous pharmacotherapy into adulthood to attain a better perspective of the long-term impact on growth, these findings suggest that growth rate should be monitored during treatment for ADHD.

Another controversial issue regarding the use of stimulants is whether they increase risk for substance use later in life. While some studies have reported that nicotine and cocaine abuse were associated with previous stimulant treatment in children with ADHD (Lambert, 1998, 2002; Lambert & Hartsough, 1998; Lambert, McLeod, & Schenk, 2006), others have found that stimulant treatment does not increase risk for substance use disorders (Barkley, Fischer, Smallish, & Fletcher, 2003; Biederman, Monuteaux, et al., 2008; Faraone, Biederman, Wilens, & Adamson, 2007; Katusic et al., 2005; Mannuzza, Klein, & Moulton, 2003; Paternite, Loney, Salisbury, & Whaley, 1999). Further, some studies have reported that stimulant pharmacotherapy may have a protective effect against later substance use disorders (Biederman, Wilens, Mick, Spencer, & Faraone, 1999; Whalen, Jamner, Henker, Gehricke, & King, 2003).

In a meta-analysis of six studies assessing the relationship between stimulant pharmacotherapy and later substance use disorder, a 1.9-fold reduction in risk for a substance use disorder was reported for youths treated with stimulants (Wilens, Faraone, Biederman, & Gunawardene, 2003). This protective effect was particularly strong in adolescence. Stimulant therapy was also reported to reduce risk for substance use disorders by 50 %, which reduced risk for this comorbidity in ADHD individuals to normal population risk levels (Faraone & Wilens, 2003). Given the contradictory findings assessing the relationship between stimulant and subsequent substance use, future studies need to assess methodological issues that limit these findings. In particular, future studies should further consider the developmental period assessed that confers differing risk for substance use (e.g., adolescence, young adulthood), comorbidity that also predicts substance use (particularly CD), sample composition that limits generalizability (e.g., gender, race, ADHD diagnostic criteria), different substances of abuse and substance use outcomes (e.g., substance use vs. substance use disorder), and naturalistic designs using retrospective reporting of stimulant treatment (including dose and medication adherence) and substance use.

Emotion Dysregulation

Consistent with findings that adolescents with ADHD appear more emotionally immature relative to non-diagnosed peers (Hoy, Weiss, Minde, & Cohen, 1978), recent reviews argue that emotion dysregulation is an additional feature of ADHD (in addition to the core symptoms of inattention and hyperactivity–impulsivity) that should be incorporated into theoretical conceptualizations and *DSM-V* diagnostic criteria (Barkley, 2010; Martel, 2009; Skirrow, McLoughlin, Kuntsi, & Asherson, 2009).

Despite that there is no consistently agreed upon definition of emotion dysregulation (Putnam & Silk, 2005), most accounts describe it as a multidimensional construct (Gratz & Roemer, 2004) that includes (a) the inhibition of behavior associated with strong negative or positive emotion and (b) subsequent engagement in self-regulatory actions, including self-soothing, refocusing attention, moderating the initial emotion, and organizing for coordinated action in the service of goal-directed behavior (Barkley, 2010; Gottman & Katz, 1989; Hinshaw, 2003; Martel, 2009; Melnick & Hinshaw, 2000). According to one account of emotion dysregulation in ADHD (Barkley, 2010), those with the disorder are less likely to inhibit their emotions, particularly those pertaining to frustration, impatience, and anger, as a result of deficient cognitive control. The outcome of this poor inhibitory process is emotional impulsivity, which "refers to the quickness or speed with which and the greater likelihood that an individual with ADHD will react with negative emotions in response to events relative to others of the same developmental level or age without ADHD" [p. 5, (Barkley, 2010)]. In other words, deficient emotion regulation involves a failure to inhibit negative emotions that leads to negative affectively driven impulsive behavior in ADHD. Much like other emotion dysregulation definitions, this is not the same as emotional intensity or reactivity (Gratz & Roemer, 2004); rather emotions are less moderated by top-down, effortful executive control (Barkley, 2010).

Empirical support for the inclusion of emotion dysregulation as a feature of the disorder comes from several sources. First, neuroanatomical networks associated with ADHD also underlie emotional functioning [see (Barkley, 2010) for a review]. For example, the anterior cingulated cortex and the lateral prefrontal cortex are identified in studies of ADHD (Bush, Valera, & Seidman, 2005; Paloyelis, Mehta, Kuntsi, & Asherson, 2007; Valera, Faraone, Murray, & Seidman, 2007) and emotion regulation (Ochsner & Gross, 2005). Emotion dysregulation may emerge in ADHD because of structural and functional deficits in top-down emotion regulation in these regions that support goal-directed (Bush, Luu, & Posner, 2000).

Second, several studies involving behavioral observations, rating scales, and clinician ratings have supported overlap between the construct of emotion dysregulation and ADHD among children and adults (Anastopoulos et al., 2011; Barkley & Fischer, 2010; Barkley & Murphy, 2010; Maedgen & Carlson, 2000; Melnick & Hinshaw, 2000; Mitchell, Robertson, Anastopolous, Nelson-Gray, & Kollins, 2012; Reimherr et al., 2005, 2010; Walcott & Landau, 2004). For instance, a recent study reported that emotion dysregulation is higher in children with ADHD and that it plays an important role in determining functional impairment and comorbidity outcomes (Anastopoulos et al., 2011). Another study in adults with ADHD found that symptoms of emotional impulsivity thought to be involved in ADHD (a) were higher in a group of adults with ADHD than in clinical and community control groups and (b) added explanatory and predictive power to various forms of impairment (e.g., occupational, educational, criminal history, driving outcomes, marital satisfaction) above and beyond core inattentive and hyperactive–impulsive symptoms (Barkley & Murphy, 2010). In a longitudinal sample of hyperactive children followed into adulthood, these findings were replicated in similar domains of impairment among those meeting ADHD criteria into adulthood (Barkley & Fischer, 2010). In addition, clinician-rated emotion dysregulation symptoms of ADHD (i.e., items assessing emotional overreactivity, temper, and affective lability) were higher among adults with ADHD than non-diagnosed individuals (Reimherr et al., 2005, 2010). These emotion dysregulation symptoms were responsive to both stimulant and non-stimulant ADHD pharmacological treatments. Finally, evidence from studies indicating that ADHD is associated with other emotion-related abilities (Miller, Hanford, Fassbender, Duke, & Schweitzer, 2011) and emotion-related constructs (Martel, Nigg, & von Eye, 2009; Mitchell & Nelson-Gray, 2006; Nigg et al., 2002) indirectly suggest a relationship between ADHD and emotion dysregulation.

It is noteworthy that emotion dysregulation is functionally impairing above and beyond the hallmark symptoms of ADHD (Barkley & Fischer, 2010; Barkley & Murphy, 2010). Similar findings may emerge among adolescent samples, although such studies have yet to be conducted. Delineating the role of emotion dysregulation may be crucial as it has also been linked to various forms of substance use (Bonn-Miller, Vujanovic, & Zvolensky, 2008; Weinstein, Mermelstein, Shiffman, & Flay, 2008) and may be a contributory factor in the highly comorbid relationship between ADHD and substance use. Further, emotion dysregulation in adolescents with ADHD may be an additional symptom set that should be targeted in treatment.

Persistence into Adulthood

Although this chapter has focused on ADHD during adolescence, which is an important period of development in which many unique challenges emerge, it is important to consider adolescence as both an outcome (as we have in this chapter) and an antecedent to another relevant developmental period: young adulthood. Continuation of ADHD into adulthood is a highly relevant issue for anyone studying adolescent ADHD as most who carry the diagnosis into adolescence will meet criteria for ADHD in adulthood (Barkley et al., 2008). Various domains are negatively impacted among those who continue to meet diagnostic criteria into adulthood, including driving, financial, occupational, educational, criminal, and relational (Barkley et al., 2008; Biederman et al., 2006; Mannuzza et al., 1993, 1998; Weiss & Hechtman, 1993). Similar to adolescence, comorbidity in adults with ADHD is common (Miller et al., 2007). Continued empirically guided treatment to target such domains is crucial for adaptive developmental outcome. Although empirically supported treatments including pharmacotherapy and cognitive-behavioral therapy are available (Price, Wilens, Spencer, & Biederman, 2006; Safren et al., 2010; Solanto et al., 2010), they may not necessarily be disseminated or utilized. In particular, health care coverage may pose a barrier to young adults with ADHD seeking treatment. The percentage of those without health insurance coverage increases from 12 % among those under age 18 to approximately 32 % among those 18–24 years of age (White, 2002). Consistent with this trend, young adults aged 18–24 years are more likely than any other age group to be uninsured (Newacheck, Park, Brindis, Biehl, & Irwin, 2004). For someone with ADHD, health care coverage is important as the median costs of health care for those with ADHD are twice that of non-ADHD peers (Leibson, Katusic, Barbaresi, Ransom, & O'Brien, 2001). Given the importance of continued treatment to manage ADHD symptoms, health coverage is a particularly relevant topic for adolescents as they enter into adulthood. This area deserves attention in future research.

Conclusion

Adolescence is a unique period of development in one's life that is occasioned by many unique changes at various levels (e.g., physical, psychological, and social). Those who enter into this developmental period with ADHD face a number of additional unique challenges. Among children who meet diagnostic criteria for ADHD, many will carry the diagnosis into adolescence. Also, ADHD in adolescence confers a risk factor for various negative outcomes in domains that become more relevant into adolescence, including driving and risky sexual behavior. In addition, comorbid psychiatric disorders are quite common for this group, which themselves confer additional developmental concerns.

Assessing ADHD is also somewhat different in adolescence in comparison to assessment procedures among children. Such differences are attributable to normative developmental changes that occur in adolescence which add complex layers to empirically guided assessments. The treatment literature for ADHD in adolescence is small in comparison to treatment studies for children with ADHD. However, this literature does demonstrate that stimulant and noradrenergic agonists are efficacious. The psychosocial treatment literature is a comparatively smaller literature than studies assessing pharmacotherapy options, but certain family- and school-based interventions are promising and deserve further empirical attention. In most cases, due to the complex presentation in most adolescents with ADHD (partly as a function of normative developmental changes that occur into adolescence), multimodal treatment options will likely be preferable. Finally, particular areas that have important clinical implications among adolescents with ADHD were reviewed. Though there is a growing research literature addressing issues relevant to adolescents with ADHD, there are many avenues for future research to assist this population during a particularly important developmental period in life.

References

Allison, D. B., Faith, M. S., & Franklin, R. D. (1995). Antecedent exercise in the treatment of disruptive behavior: A meta-analytic review. *Clinical Psychology: Science and Practice, 2*, 279–304.

American Psychiatric Association. (2000). *Diagnostic and statistical manual of mental disorders* (4th ed.). Washington, DC: American Psychiatric Association. Text revision (DSM-IV-TR).

Anastopoulos, A. D., & Shelton, T. L. (2001). *Assessing attention-deficit/hyperactivity disorder*. New York: Kluwer Academic/Plenum Publishers.

Anastopoulos, A. D., Smith, T. F., Garrett, M. E., Morrissey-Kane, E., Schatz, N. K., Sommer, J. L., et al. (2011). Self-regulation of emotion, functional impairment, and comorbidity among children with AD/HD. *Journal of Attention Disorders, 15*(7), 583–592. doi:10.1177/1087054710370567.

Angold, A., Costello, E. J., & Erkanli, A. (1999). Comorbidity. *Journal of Child Psychology and Psychiatry, 40*(1), 57–87.

Applegate, B., Lahey, B. B., Hart, E. L., Biederman, J., Hynd, G. W., Barkley, R. A., et al. (1997). Validity of the age-of-onset criterion for ADHD: A report from the DSM-IV field trials. *Journal of the American Academy of Child and Adolescent Psychiatry, 36*(9), 1211–1221.

Arnsten, A. F. (2009). Toward a new understanding of attention-deficit hyperactivity disorder pathophysiology: An important role for prefrontal cortex dysfunction. *CNS Drugs, 23*(Suppl 1), 33–41. doi:10.2165/00023210-200923000-00005.

August, G. J., Stewart, M. A., & Holmes, C. S. (1983). A four-year follow-up of hyperactive boys with and without conduct disorder. *The British Journal of Psychiatry, 143*, 192–198.

Bagwell, C. L., Molina, B. S., Pelham, W. E., Jr., & Hoza, B. (2001). Attention-deficit hyperactivity disorder and problems in peer relations: Predictions from childhood to adolescence. *Journal of the American Academy of Child and Adolescent Psychiatry, 40*(11), 1285–1292. doi:10.1097/00004583-200111000-00008.

Barkley, R. A. (1997). Behavioral inhibition, sustained attention, and executive functions: Constructing a unifying theory of ADHD. *Psychological Bulletin, 121*(1), 65–94. doi:10.1037/0033-2909.121.1.65.

Barkley, R. A. (2004a). Adolescents with attention-deficit/hyperactivity disorder: An overview of empirically based treatments. *Journal of Psychiatric Practice, 10*(1), 39–56. doi:00131746-200401000-00005.

Barkley, R. A. (2004b). Driving impairments in teens and adults with attention-deficit/hyperactivity disorder. *Psychiatric Clinics of North America, 27*(2), 233–260. doi:10.1016/S0193-953X(03)00091-1.

Barkley, R. A. (2006). *Attention deficit hyperactivity disorder: A handbook for diagnosis and treatment*. New York: Guilford Press.

Barkley, R. A. (2010). Deficient emotional self-regulation is a core component of attention-deficit/hyperactivity disorder. *Journal of ADHD & Related Disorders, 1*(2), 5–37.

Barkley, R. A., Anastopoulos, A. D., Guevremont, D. C., & Fletcher, K. E. (1991). Adolescents with ADHD: Patterns of behavioral adjustment, academic functioning, and treatment utilization. *Journal of the American Academy of Child and Adolescent Psychiatry, 30*(5), 752–761.

Barkley, R. A., & Biederman, J. (1997). Toward a broader definition of the age-of-onset criterion for attention-deficit hyperactivity disorder. *Journal of the American Academy of Child and Adolescent Psychiatry, 36*(9), 1204–1210. doi:10.1097/00004583-199709000-00012.

Barkley, R. A., & Cox, D. (2007). A review of driving risks and impairments associated with attention-deficit/hyperactivity disorder and the effects of stimulant medication on driving performance. *Journal of Safety Research, 38*(1), 113–128. doi:10.1016/j.jsr.2006.09.004.

Barkley, R. A., Edwards, G., Laneri, M., Fletcher, K., & Metevia, L. (2001). The efficacy of problem-solving communication training alone, behavior management training alone, and their combination for parent-adolescent conflict in teenagers with ADHD and ODD. *Journal of Consulting and Clinical Psychology, 69*(6), 926–941. doi:10.1037/0022-006X.69.6.926.

Barkley, R. A., & Fischer, M. (2010). The unique contribution of emotional impulsiveness to impairment in major life activities in hyperactive children as adults. *Journal of the American Academy of Child and Adolescent Psychiatry, 49*(5), 503–513. doi:00004583-201005000-00011.

Barkley, R. A., Fischer, M., Edelbrock, C. S., & Smallish, L. (1990). The adolescent outcome of hyperactive children diagnosed by research criteria: I. An 8-year prospective follow-up study. *Journal of the American Academy of Child and Adolescent Psychiatry, 29*(4), 546–557. doi:10.1097/00004583-199007000-00007.

Barkley, R. A., Fischer, M., Smallish, L., & Fletcher, K. (2002). The persistence of attention-deficit/hyperactivity disorder into young adulthood as a function of reporting source and definition of disorder. *Journal of Abnormal Psychology, 111*(2), 279–289. doi:10.1037/0021-843X.111.2.279.

Barkley, R. A., Fischer, M., Smallish, L., & Fletcher, K. (2003). Does the treatment of attention-deficit/hyperactivity disorder with stimulants contribute to drug use/abuse? A 13-year prospective study. *Pediatrics, 111*(1), 97–109.

Barkley, R. A., Guevremont, D. C., Anastopoulos, A. D., & Fletcher, K. E. (1992). A comparison of three family therapy programs for treating family conflicts in adolescents with attention-deficit hyperactivity disorder. *Journal of Consulting and Clinical Psychology, 60*(3), 450–462.

Barkley, R. A., & Murphy, K. R. (2010). Deficient emotional self-regulation in adults with attention-deficit/hyperactivity disorder (ADHD): The relative contributions of emotional impulsiveness and ADHD symptoms to adaptive impairments in major life activities. *Journal of ADHD & Related Disorders, 1*(4), 5–28.

Barkley, R. A., Murphy, K. R., & Fischer, M. (2008). *ADHD in adults: What the science says*. New York: Guilford Press.

Barkley, R. A., Murphy, K. R., & Kwasnik, D. (1996). Motor vehicle driving competencies and risks in teens and young adults with attention deficit hyperactivity disorder. *Pediatrics, 98*(6 Pt 1), 1089–1095.

Bawkin, H., & Bawkin, R. (1966). *Clinical management of behavior disorders in children*. Philadelphia, PA: WB Saunders.

Bidwell, C. L., Dew, R. E., & Kollins, S. H. (2010). Alpha-2 adrenergic receptors and attention-deficit/hyperactivity disorder. *Current Psychiatry Reports, 12*(5), 366–373. doi:10.1007/s11920-010-0136-4.

Biederman, J., Faraone, S. V., Mick, E., Williamson, S., Wilens, T. E., Spencer, T. J., et al. (1999). Clinical correlates of ADHD in females: Findings from a large group of girls ascertained from pediatric and psychiatric referral sources. *Journal of the American Academy of Child and Adolescent Psychiatry, 38*(8), 966–975. doi:10.1097/00004583-199908000-00012.

Biederman, J., Faraone, S., Milberger, S., Guite, J., Mick, E., Chen, L., et al. (1996). A prospective 4-year follow-up study of attention-deficit hyperactivity and related disorders. *Archives of General Psychiatry, 53*(5), 437–446.

Biederman, J., Faraone, S. V., Spencer, T. J., Mick, E., Monuteaux, M. C., & Aleardi, M. (2006). Functional impairments in adults with self-reports of diagnosed ADHD: A controlled study of 1001 adults in the community. *The Journal of Clinical Psychiatry, 67*(4), 524–540.

Biederman, J., Melmed, R. D., Patel, A., McBurnett, K., Donahue, J., & Lyne, A. (2008). Long-term, open-label extension study of guanfacine extended release in children and adolescents with ADHD. *CNS Spectrums, 13*(12), 1047–1055.

Biederman, J., Melmed, R. D., Patel, A., McBurnett, K., Konow, J., Lyne, A., et al. (2008). A randomized, double-blind, placebo-controlled study of guanfacine extended release in children and adolescents with attention-deficit/hyperactivity disorder. *Pediatrics, 121*(1), e73–e84. doi:10.1542/peds.2006-3695.

Biederman, J., Monuteaux, M. C., Spencer, T., Wilens, T. E., Macpherson, H. A., & Faraone, S. V. (2008). Stimulant therapy and risk for subsequent substance use disorders in male adults with ADHD: A naturalistic controlled 10-year follow-up study. *The American Journal of Psychiatry, 165*(5), 597–603. doi:10.1176/appi.ajp. 2007.07091486.

Biederman, J., Newcorn, J., & Sprich, S. (1991). Comorbidity of attention deficit hyperactivity disorder with conduct, depressive, anxiety, and other disorders. *The American Journal of Psychiatry, 148*(5), 564–577.

Biederman, J., Spencer, T., & Wilens, T. (2004). Evidence-based pharmacotherapy for attention-deficit hyperactivity disorder. *The International Journal of Neuropsychopharmacology, 7*(1), 77–97. doi:10.1017/S1461145703003973.

Biederman, J., Wilens, T., Mick, E., Faraone, S. V., Weber, W., Curtis, S., et al. (1997). Is ADHD a risk factor for psychoactive substance use disorders? Findings from a four-year prospective follow-up study. *Journal of the American Academy of Child and Adolescent Psychiatry, 36*(1), 21–29. doi:10.1097/00004583-199701000-00013.

Biederman, J., Wilens, T., Mick, E., Spencer, T., & Faraone, S. V. (1999). Pharmacotherapy of attention-deficit/hyperactivity disorder reduces risk for substance use disorder. *Pediatrics, 104*(2), e20.

Bonn-Miller, M. O., Vujanovic, A. A., & Zvolensky, M. J. (2008). Emotional dysregulation: Association with coping-oriented marijuana use motives among current marijuana users. *Substance Use & Misuse, 43*(11), 1653–1665. doi:10.1080/10826080802241292.

Buitelaar, J. K., Danckaerts, M., Gillberg, C., Zuddas, A., Becker, K., Bouvard, M., et al. (2004). A prospective, multicenter, open-label assessment of atomoxetine in non-North American children and adolescents with ADHD. *European Child & Adolescent Psychiatry, 13*(4), 249–257. doi:10.1007/s00787-004-0401-3.

Burke, J. D., Loeber, R., & Lahey, B. B. (2001). Which aspects of ADHD are associated with tobacco use in early adolescence? *Journal of Child Psychology and Psychiatry, 42*(4), 493–502.

Bush, G., Luu, P., & Posner, M. I. (2000). Cognitive and emotional influences in anterior cingulate cortex. *Trends in Cognitive Sciences, 4*(6), 215–222. doi:10.1016/S1364-6613(00)01483-2.

Bush, G., Valera, E. M., & Seidman, L. J. (2005). Functional neuroimaging of attention-deficit/hyperactivity disorder: A review and suggested future directions. *Biological Psychiatry, 57*(11), 1273–1284. doi:10.1016/j.biopsych.2005.01.034.

Carlson, G. A. (1990). Child and adolescent mania—Diagnostic considerations. *Journal of Child Psychology and Psychiatry, 31*(3), 331–341.

Carroll, K. M., & Rounsaville, B. J. (1993). History and significance of childhood attention deficit disorder in treatment-seeking cocaine abusers. *Comprehensive Psychiatry, 34*(2), 75–82. doi:10.1016/0010-440X(93)90050-E.

Charach, A., Ickowicz, A., & Schachar, R. (2004). Stimulant treatment over five years: Adherence, effectiveness, and adverse effects. *Journal of the American Academy of Child and Adolescent Psychiatry, 43*(5), 559–567. doi:10.1097/00004583-200405000-00009.

Cheng, J. Y., Chen, R. Y., Ko, J. S., & Ng, E. M. (2007). Efficacy and safety of atomoxetine for attention-deficit/hyperactivity disorder in children and adolescents-meta-analysis and meta-regression analysis. *Psychopharmacology, 194*(2), 197–209. doi:10.1007/s00213-007-0840-x.

Chronis, A. M., Jones, H. A., & Raggi, V. L. (2006). Evidence-based psychosocial treatments for children and adolescents with attention-deficit/hyperactivity disorder. *Clinical Psychology Review, 26*(4), 486–502. doi:10.1016/j.cpr.2006.01.002.

Chronis-Tuscano, A., Molina, B. S., Pelham, W. E., Applegate, B., Dahlke, A., Overmyer, M., et al. (2010). Very early predictors of adolescent depression and suicide attempts in children with attention-deficit/hyperactivity disorder. *Archives of General Psychiatry, 67*(10), 1044–1051. doi:10.1001/archgenpsychiatry.2010.127.

Clarke, S. D., Kohn, M. R., Hermens, D. F., Rabbinge, M., Clark, C. R., Gordon, E., et al. (2007). Distinguishing symptom profiles in adolescent ADHD using an objective cognitive test battery. *International Journal of Adolescent Medicine and Health, 19*(3), 355–367.

Conners, C. K. (2002). Forty years of methylphenidate treatment in attention-deficit/hyperactivity disorder. *Journal of Attention Disorders, 6*(Suppl 1), S17–S30.

Connor, D. F. (2006). Stimulants. In R. A. Barkley (Ed.), *Attention-deficit hyperactivity disorder: A handbook for diagnosis and treatment* (3rd ed., pp. 608–647). New York: Guilford Press.

Covey, L. S., Manubay, J., Jiang, H., Nortick, M., & Palumbo, D. (2008). Smoking cessation and inattention or hyperactivity/impulsivity: A post hoc analysis. *Nicotine & Tobacco Research, 10*(12), 1717–1725. doi:10.1080/14622200802443536.

Cox, D. J., Merkel, R. L., Penberthy, J. K., Kovatchev, B., & Hankin, C. S. (2004). Impact of methylphenidate delivery profiles on driving performance of adolescents with attention-deficit/hyperactivity disorder: A pilot study. *Journal of the American Academy of Child and Adolescent Psychiatry, 43*(3), 269–275. doi:10.1097/00004583-200403000-00007.

Cuffe, S. P., McKeown, R. E., Jackson, K. L., Addy, C. L., Abramson, R., & Garrison, C. Z. (2001). Prevalence of attention-deficit/hyperactivity disorder in a community sample of older adolescents. *Journal of the American Academy of Child and Adolescent Psychiatry, 40*(9), 1037–1044. doi:10.1097/00004583-200109000-00012.

Doremus-Fitzwater, T. L., Varlinskaya, E. I., & Spear, L. P. (2010). Motivational systems in adolescence: Possible implications for age differences in substance abuse and other risk-taking behaviors. *Brain and Cognition, 72*(1), 114–123. doi:10.1016/j.bandc.2009.08.008.

Ehrenreich, H., Rinn, T., Kunert, H. J., Moeller, M. R., Poser, W., Schilling, L., et al. (1999). Specific attentional dysfunction in adults following early start of cannabis use. *Psychopharmacology, 142*(3), 295–301. doi:10.1007/s002130050892.

Elia, J., Ambrosini, P., & Berrettini, W. (2008). ADHD characteristics: I. Concurrent co-morbidity patterns in children & adolescents. *Child and Adolescent Psychiatry and Mental Health, 2*(1), 15. doi:10.1186/1753-2000-2-15.

Epstein, J. N., & Tsal, Y. (2010). Evidence for cognitive training as a treatment strategy for children with attention-deficit/hyperactivity disorder. *Journal of ADHD & Related Disorders, 1*(2), 49–64.

Ervin, R. A., DuPaul, G. J., Kern, L., & Friman, P. C. (1998). Classroom-based functional and adjunctive assessments: Proactive approaches to intervention selection for adolescents with attention deficit hyperactivity disorder. *Journal of Applied Behavior Analysis, 31*(1), 65–78. doi:10.1901/jaba.1998.31-65.

Evans, S. W., Axelrod, J., & Langberg, J. M. (2004). Efficacy of a school-based treatment program for middle school youth with ADHD: Pilot data. *Behavior Modification, 28*(4), 528–547. doi:10.1177/0145445503259504.

Evans, S. W., Langberg, J., Raggi, V., Allen, J., & Buvinger, E. C. (2005). Development of a school-based treatment program for middle school youth with ADHD. *Journal of Attention Disorders, 9*(1), 343–353. doi:10.1177/1087054705279305.

Evans, S. W., Pelham, W. E., & Grudberg, M. V. (1995). The efficacy of notetaking to improve behavior and comprehension of adolescents with attention-deficit hyperactivity disorder. *Exceptionality, 5*(1), 1–17.

Evans, S. W., Pelham, W. E., Smith, B. H., Bukstein, O., Gnagy, E. M., Greiner, A. R., et al. (2001). Dose-response effects of methylphenidate on ecologically valid measures of academic performance and classroom behavior in adolescents with ADHD. *Experimental and Clinical Psychopharmacology, 9*(2), 163–175. doi:10.1037/1064-1297.9.2.163.

Evans, S. W., Serpell, Z. N., Schultz, B. K., & Pastor, D. A. (2007). Cumulative benefits of secondary school-based treatment of students with attention deficit hyperactivity disorder. *School Psychology Review, 36*(2), 256–273.

Faraone, S., Biederman, J., & Monuteaux, M. C. (2002). Further evidence for the diagnostic continuity between child and adolescent ADHD. *Journal of Attention Disorders, 6*(1), 5–13. doi:10.1177/108705470200600102.

Faraone, S. V., Biederman, J., Morley, C. P., & Spencer, T. J. (2008). Effect of stimulants on height and weight: A review of the literature. *Journal of the American Academy of Child and Adolescent Psychiatry, 47*(9), 994–1009. doi:10.1097/CHI.ObO13e31817eOea7.

Faraone, S. V., Biederman, J., & Roe, C. (2002). Comparative efficacy of adderall and methylphenidate in attention-deficit/hyperactivity disorder: A meta-analysis. *Journal of Clinical Psychopharmacology, 22*(5), 468–473.

Faraone, S. V., Biederman, J., Wilens, T. E., & Adamson, J. (2007). A naturalistic study of the effects of pharmacotherapy on substance use disorders among ADHD adults. *Psychological Medicine, 37*(12), 1743–1752. doi:10.1017/S0033291707000335.

Faraone, S. V., Biederman, J., Wozniak, J., Mundy, E., Mennin, D., & O'Donnell, D. (1997). Is comorbidity with ADHD a marker for juvenile-onset mania? *Journal of the American Academy of Child and Adolescent Psychiatry, 36*(8), 1046–1055. doi:10.1097/00004583-199708000-00012.

Faraone, S. V., & Giefer, E. E. (2007). Long-term effects of methylphenidate transdermal delivery system treatment of ADHD on growth. *Journal of the American Academy of Child and Adolescent Psychiatry, 46*(9), 1138–1147. doi:10.1097/chi.0b013e31806ad1d7.

Faraone, S. V., Kunwar, A., Adamson, J., & Biederman, J. (2009). Personality traits among ADHD adults: Implications of late-onset and subthreshold diagnoses. *Psychological Medicine, 39*(4), 685–693. doi:10.1017/S0033291708003917.

Faraone, S. V., Sergeant, J., Gillberg, C., & Biederman, J. (2003). The worldwide prevalence of ADHD: Is it an American condition? *World Psychiatry, 2*(2), 104–113.

Faraone, S. V., Spencer, T. J., Kollins, S. H., & Glatt, S. J. (2010). Effects of lisdexamfetamine dimesylate treatment for ADHD on growth. *Journal of the American Academy of Child and Adolescent Psychiatry, 49*(1), 24–32. doi:10.1016/j.jaac.2009.10.003.

Faraone, S. V., & Wilens, T. (2003). Does stimulant treatment lead to substance use disorders? *The Journal of Clinical Psychiatry, 64*(Suppl 11), 9–13.

Fischer, M., Barkley, R. A., Edelbrock, C. S., & Smallish, L. (1990). The adolescent outcome of hyperactive children diagnosed by research criteria: II. Academic, attentional, and neuropsychological status. *Journal of Consulting and Clinical Psychology, 58*(5), 580–588. doi:10.1037/0022-006X.58.5.580.

Fischer, M., Barkley, R. A., Smallish, L., & Fletcher, K. (2002). Young adult follow-up of hyperactive children: Self-reported psychiatric disorders, comorbidity, and the role of childhood conduct problems and teen CD. *Journal of Abnormal Child Psychology, 30*(5), 463–475. doi:10.1023/A:1019864813776.

Flory, K., Molina, B. S., Pelham, W. E., Jr., Gnagy, E., & Smith, B. (2006). Childhood ADHD predicts risky sexual behavior in young adulthood. *Journal of Clinical Child and Adolescent Psychology, 35*(4), 571–577. doi:10.1207/s15374424jccp3504_8.

Fried, P., Watkinson, B., James, D., & Gray, R. (2002). Current and former marijuana use: Preliminary findings of a longitudinal study of effects on IQ in young adults. *Canadian Medical Association Journal, 166*(7), 887–891.

Fuemmeler, B. F., Kollins, S. H., & McClernon, F. J. (2007). Attention deficit hyperactivity disorder symptoms predict nicotine dependence and progression to regular smoking from adolescence to young adulthood. *Journal of Pediatric Psychology, 32*(10), 1203–1213. doi:10.1093/jpepsy/jsm051.

Gittelman, R., Mannuzza, S., Shenker, R., & Bonagura, N. (1985). Hyperactive boys almost grown up. I. Psychiatric status. *Archives of General Psychiatry, 42*(10), 937–947.

Glass, K., & Flory, K. (2010). Why does ADHD confer risk for cigarette smoking? A review of psychosocial mechanisms. *Clinical Child and Family Psychology Review, 13*(3), 291–313. doi:10.1007/s10567-010-0070-3.

Gottman, J. M., & Katz, L. F. (1989). Effects of marital discord on young children's peer interaction and health. *Developmental Psychology, 25*, 373–381.

Gratz, K. L., & Roemer, L. (2004). Multidimensional assessment of emotion regulation and dysregulation: Development, factor structure, and initial validation of the difficulties in emotion regulation scale. *Journal of Psychopathology and Behavioral Assessment, 26*, 41–54.

Greene, R. W., Biederman, J., Faraone, S. V., Wilens, T. E., Mick, E., & Blier, H. K. (1999). Further validation of social impairment as a predictor of substance use disorders: Findings from a sample of siblings of boys with and without ADHD. *Journal of Clinical Child Psychology, 28*(3), 349–354.

Hart, E. L., Lahey, B. B., Loeber, R., Applegate, B., & Frick, P. J. (1995). Developmental change in attention-deficit hyperactivity disorder in boys: A four-year longitudinal study. *Journal of Abnormal Child Psychology, 23*(6), 729–749. doi:DOI: 10.1007/BF01447474.

Hartsough, C. S., & Lambert, N. M. (1987). Pattern and progression of drug use among hyperactives and controls: A prospective short-term longitudinal study. *Journal of Child Psychology and Psychiatry, 28*(4), 543–553. doi:10.1111/j.1469-7610.1987.tb00222.x.

Hazell, P. L., Kohn, M. R., Dickson, R., Walton, R. J., Granger, R. E., & van Wyk, G. W. (2011). Core ADHD symptom improvement with atomoxetine versus methylphenidate: A direct comparison meta-analysis. *Journal of Attention Disorders, 15*, 674–683. doi:10.1177/1087054710379737.

Hinshaw, S. P. (2003). Impulsivity, emotion regulation, and developmental psychopathology: Specificity versus generality of linkages. *Annals of the New York Academy of Sciences, 1008*, 149–159. doi:10.1196/annals.1301.016.

Hoy, E., Weiss, G., Minde, K., & Cohen, N. (1978). The hyperactive child at adolescence: Cognitive, emotional, and social functioning. *Journal of Abnormal Child Psychology, 6*(3), 311–324.

Hoza, B., Pelham, W. E., Jr., Dobbs, J., Owens, J. S., & Pillow, D. R. (2002). Do boys with attention-deficit/hyperactivity disorder have positive illusory self-concepts? *Journal of Abnormal Psychology, 111*(2), 268–278. doi:10.1037//0021-843X.111.2.268.

Humfleet, G. L., Prochaska, J. J., Mengis, M., Cullen, J., Munoz, R., Reus, V., et al. (2005). Preliminary evidence of the association between the history of childhood attention-deficit/hyperactivity disorder and smoking treatment failure. *Nicotine & Tobacco Research, 7*(3), 453–460. doi:10.1080/14622200500125310.

Ingersoll, B. D., & Goldstein, S. (1993). *Attention deficit disorder and learning disabilities: Realities, myths, and controversial treatments*. New York: Doubleday.

Ingram, S., Hechtman, L., & Morgenstern, G. (1999). Outcome issues in ADHD: Adolescent and adult long-term outcome. *Mental Retardation and Developmental Disabilities Research Review, 5*, 243–250. doi:10.1002/(SICI)1098-2779.

Jain, R., Kollins, S. H., Baily, C., et al. (2008). *Developing a sustained release formulation of clonidine for the treatment of children and adolescents with attention-deficit hyperactivity disorder (ADHD)*. Paper presented at the 47th Annual Meeting of the American College of Neuropsychopharmacology, Scottsdale, AZ.

Jensen, P. S., Martin, D., & Cantwell, D. P. (1997). Comorbidity in ADHD: Implications for research, practice, and DSM-V. *Journal of the American Academy of Child and Adolescent Psychiatry, 36*(8), 1065–1079. doi:10.1097/00004583-199708000-00014.

Jerome, L., Habinski, L., & Segal, A. (2006). Attention-deficit/hyperactivity disorder (ADHD) and driving risk: A review of the literature and a methodological critique. *Current Psychiatry Reports, 8*(5), 416–426.

Katusic, S. K., Barbaresi, W. J., Colligan, R. C., Weaver, A. L., Leibson, C. L., & Jacobsen, S. J. (2005). Psychostimulant treatment and risk for substance abuse among young adults with a history of attention-deficit/hyperactivity disorder: A population-based, birth cohort study. *Journal of Child and Adolescent Psychopharmacology, 15*(5), 764–776. doi:10.1089/cap.2005.15.764.

Kempel, P., Lampe, K., Parnefjord, R., Hennig, J., & Kunert, H. J. (2003). Auditory-evoked potentials and selective attention: Different ways of information processing in cannabis users and controls. *Neuropsychobiology, 48*(2), 95–101. doi:10.1159/000072884.

Kollins, S. H., Findling, R. L., Wigal, S. B., et al. (2009). *Modified-release clonidine for the treatment of children/adolescents with ADHD*. Paper presented at the 56th Annual Meeting of the American Academy of Child and Adolescent Psychiatry, Honolulu, HI.

Kollins, S. H., McClernon, F. J., & Fuemmeler, B. F. (2005). Association between smoking and attention-deficit/hyperactivity disorder symptoms in a population-based sample of young adults. *Archives of General Psychiatry, 62*(10), 1142–1147. doi:62/10/1142.10.1001/archpsyc.62.10.1142.

Kollins, S. H., Spencer, T. J., Findling, R. L., et al. (2009). *Effects of guanfacine extended release in children aged 6 to 12 with oppositional symptoms and a diagnosis of ADHD*. Paper presented at the 56th Annual Meeting of the American Academy of Child and Adolescent Psychiatry, Honolulu, HI.

Kratochvil, C. J., Michelson, D., Newcorn, J. H., Weiss, M. D., Busner, J., Moore, R. J., et al. (2007). High-dose atomoxetine treatment of ADHD in youths with limited response to standard doses. *Journal of the American Academy of Child and Adolescent Psychiatry, 46*(9), 1128–1137. doi:10.1097/chi.0b013e318074eeb3.

Lambert, N. M. (1998). *Stimulant treatment as a risk factor for nicotine use and substance abuse. NIH Consensus Development Conference Diagnosis and Treatment of Attention Deficit Hyperactivity Disorder* (pp. 191–198). Bethesda, MD: NIH.

Lambert, N. M. (2002). Stimulant treatment as a risk factor for nicotine and substance abuse. In P. S. Jensen & J. Cooper (Eds.), *Attention deficit hyperactivity disorder: State of the science, best practices* (pp. 1–24). Kingston, NJ: Civic Research Institute.

Lambert, N. M., & Hartsough, C. S. (1998). Prospective study of tobacco smoking and substance dependencies among samples of ADHD and non-ADHD participants. *Journal of Learning Disabilities, 31*(6), 533–544.

Lambert, N. M., McLeod, M., & Schenk, S. (2006). Subjective responses to initial experience with cocaine: An exploration of the incentive-sensitization theory of drug abuse. *Addiction, 101*(5), 713–725. doi:10.1111/j.1360-0443.2006.01408.x.

Leibson, C. L., Katusic, S. K., Barbaresi, W. J., Ransom, J., & O'Brien, P. C. (2001). Use and costs of medical care for children and adolescents with and without attention-deficit/hyperactivity disorder. *Journal of the American Medical Association, 285*(1), 60–66. doi:10.1001/jama.285.1.60.

Lewinsohn, P. M., Rohde, P., & Seeley, J. R. (1995). Adolescent psychopathology: III. The clinical consequences of comorbidity. *Journal of the American Academy of Child and Adolescent Psychiatry, 34*(4), 510–519.

Loeber, R., Burke, J. D., Lahey, B. B., Winters, A., & Zera, M. (2000). Oppositional defiant and conduct disorder: A review of the past 10 years, part I. *Journal of the American Academy of Child and Adolescent Psychiatry, 39*(12), 1468–1484. doi:10.1097/00004583-200012000-00007.

Maedgen, J. W., & Carlson, C. L. (2000). Social functioning and emotional regulation in the attention deficit hyperactivity disorder subtypes. *Journal of Clinical Child Psychology, 29*(1), 30–42.

Mannuzza, S., Klein, R. G., Bessler, A., Malloy, P., & Hynes, M. E. (1997). Educational and occupational outcome of hyperactive boys grown up. *Journal of the American Academy of Child and Adolescent Psychiatry, 36*(9), 1222–1227. doi:10.1097/00004583-199709000-00014.

Mannuzza, S., Klein, R. G., Bessler, A., Malloy, P., & LaPadula, M. (1993). Adult outcome of hyperactive boys. Educational achievement, occupational rank, and psychiatric status. *Archives of General Psychiatry, 50*(7), 565–576.

Mannuzza, S., Klein, R. G., Bessler, A., Malloy, P., & LaPadula, M. (1998). Adult psychiatric status of hyperactive boys grown up. *The American Journal of Psychiatry, 155*(4), 493–498.

Mannuzza, S., Klein, R. G., & Moulton, J. L., III. (2003). Does stimulant treatment place children at risk for adult substance abuse? A controlled, prospective follow-up study. *Journal of Child and Adolescent Psychopharmacology, 13*(3), 273–282. doi:10.1089/104454603322572606.

Martel, M. M. (2009). Research review: A new perspective on attention-deficit/hyperactivity disorder: Emotion dysregulation and trait models. *Journal of*

Child Psychology and Psychiatry, 50(9), 1042–1051. doi:10.1111/j.1469-7610.2009.02105.x.

Martel, M. M., Nigg, J. T., & von Eye, A. (2009). How do trait dimensions map onto ADHD symptom domains? *Journal of Abnormal Child Psychology, 37*(3), 337–348. doi:10.1007/s10802-008-9255-3.

Masi, G., Perugi, G., Toni, C., Millepiedi, S., Mucci, M., Bertini, N., et al. (2006). Attention-deficit hyperactivity disorder—Bipolar comorbidity in children and adolescents. *Bipolar Disorders, 8*(4), 373–381. doi:10.1111/j.1399-5618.2006.00342.x.

Masten, A. S., Faden, V. B., Zucker, R. A., & Spear, L. P. (2008). Underage drinking: A developmental framework. *Pediatrics, 121*(Suppl 4), S235–S251. doi:10.1542/peds.2007-2243A.

McCarthy, S., Asherson, P., Coghill, D., Hollis, C., Murray, M., Potts, L., et al. (2009). Attention-deficit hyperactivity disorder: Treatment discontinuation in adolescents and young adults. *The British Journal of Psychiatry, 194*(3), 273–277. doi:10.1192/bjp.bp. 107.045245.

McCleary, L., & Ridley, T. (1999). Parenting adolescents with ADHD: Evaluation of a psychoeducation group. *Patient Education and Counseling, 38*(1), 3–10. doi:10.1016/S0738-3991(98)00110-4.

McClernon, F. J., & Kollins, S. H. (2008). ADHD and smoking: From genes to brain to behavior. *Annals of the New York Academy of Sciences, 1141*, 131–147. doi:NYAS1141016.10.1196/annals.1441.016.

Melnick, S. M., & Hinshaw, S. P. (2000). Emotion regulation and parenting in AD/HD and comparison boys: Linkages with social behaviors and peer preference. *Journal of Abnormal Child Psychology, 28*(1), 73–86. doi:10.1023/A:1005174102794.

Michelson, D., Allen, A. J., Busner, J., Casat, C., Dunn, D., Kratochvil, C., et al. (2002). Once-daily atomoxetine treatment for children and adolescents with attention deficit hyperactivity disorder: A randomized, placebo-controlled study. *The American Journal of Psychiatry, 159*(11), 1896–1901.

Michelson, D., Faries, D., Wernicke, J., Kelsey, D., Kendrick, K., Sallee, F. R., et al. (2001). Atomoxetine in the treatment of children and adolescents with attention-deficit/hyperactivity disorder: A randomized, placebo-controlled, dose-response study. *Pediatrics, 108*(5), E83. doi:10.1542/peds.108.5.e83.

Michelson, D., Read, H. A., Ruff, D. D., Witcher, J., Zhang, S., & McCracken, J. (2007). CYP2D6 and clinical response to atomoxetine in children and adolescents with ADHD. *Journal of the American Academy of Child and Adolescent Psychiatry, 46*(2), 242–251. doi:10.1097/01.chi.0000246056.83791.b6.

Milberger, S., Biederman, J., Faraone, S. V., Chen, L., & Jones, J. (1997). ADHD is associated with early initiation of cigarette smoking in children and adolescents. *Journal of the American Academy of Child and Adolescent Psychiatry, 36*(1), 37–44. doi:10.1097/00004583-199701000-00015.

Milich, R., & Loney, J. (1979). The role of hyperactivity and aggressive symptomatology in predicting adolescent outcome among hyperactive children. *Journal of Pediatric Psychology, 4*, 93–112.

Miller, M., Hanford, R. B., Fassbender, C., Duke, M., & Schweitzer, J. B. (2011). Affect recognition in adults with ADHD. *Journal of Attention Disorders, 15*(6), 452–460.

Miller, T. W., Nigg, J. T., & Faraone, S. V. (2007). Axis I and II comorbidity in adults with ADHD. *Journal of Abnormal Psychology, 116*(3), 519–528. doi:10.1037/0021-843X.116.3.519.

Mitchell, J. T., & Nelson-Gray, R. O. (2006). Attention-deficit/hyperactivity disorder symptoms in adults: Relationship to Gray's behavioral approach system. *Personality and Individual Differences, 40*, 749–760. doi:10.1016/j.paid.2005.08.011.

Mitchell, J. T., Robertson, C. D., Anastopolous, A. D., Nelson-Gray, R. O., & Kollins, S. H. (2012). Emotion dysregulation and emotional impulsivity among adults with attention-deficit/hyperactivity disorder: Results of a preliminary study. *Journal of Psychopathology and Behavioral Assessment, 34*, 510–519.

Molina, B. S., & Pelham, W. E., Jr. (2003). Childhood predictors of adolescent substance use in a longitudinal study of children with ADHD. *Journal of Abnormal Psychology, 112*(3), 497–507. doi:10.1037/0021-843X.112.3.497.

Molina, B. S. G., Smith, B. H., & Pelham, W. E. (1999). Interactive effects of attention deficit hyperactivity disorder and conduct disorder on early adolescent substance use. *Psychology of Addictive Behaviors, 13*, 348–358. doi:10.1037/0893-164X.13.4.348.

Newacheck, P. W., Park, M. J., Brindis, C. D., Biehl, M., & Irwin, C. E., Jr. (2004). Trends in private and public health insurance for adolescents. *Journal of the American Medical Association, 291*(10), 1231–1237. doi:10.1001/jama.291.10.1231.

Newcorn, J. H., Spencer, T. J., Biederman, J., Milton, D. R., & Michelson, D. (2005). Atomoxetine treatment in children and adolescents with attention-deficit/hyperactivity disorder and comorbid oppositional defiant disorder. *Journal of the American Academy of Child and Adolescent Psychiatry, 44*(3), 240–248. doi:10.1097/00004583-200503000-00008.

Nigg, J. T., John, O. P., Blaskey, L. G., Huang-Pollock, C. L., Willcutt, E. G., Hinshaw, S. P., et al. (2002). Big five dimensions and ADHD symptoms: Links between personality traits and clinical symptoms. *Journal of Personality and Social Psychology, 83*(2), 451–469. doi:10.1037//0022-3514.83.2.451.

Ochsner, K. N., & Gross, J. J. (2005). The cognitive control of emotion. *Trends in Cognitive Sciences, 9*(5), 242–249. doi:10.1016/j.tics.2005.03.010.

Olfson, M. (1992). Diagnosing mental disorders in office-based pediatric practice. *Journal of Developmental and Behavioral Pediatrics, 13*(5), 363–365.

Owens, J. S., Goldfine, M. E., Evangelista, N. M., Hoza, B., & Kaiser, N. M. (2007). A critical review of self-perceptions and the positive illusory bias in children with ADHD. *Clinical Child and Family Psychology Review, 10*(4), 335–351. doi:10.1007/s10567-007-0027-3.

Owens, J. S., & Hoza, B. (2003). The role of inattention and hyperactivity/impulsivity in the positive illusory bias. *Journal of Consulting and Clinical Psychology, 71*(4), 680–691. doi:10.1037/0022-006X.71.4.680.

Paloyelis, Y., Mehta, M. A., Kuntsi, J., & Asherson, P. (2007). Functional MRI in ADHD: A systematic literature review. *Expert Review of Neurotherapeutics, 7*(10), 1337–1356. doi:10.1586/14737175.7.10.1337.

Parrott, A. (2003). Cognitive deficits and cognitive normality in recreational cannabis and Ecstasy/MDMA users. *Human Psychopharmacology, 18*(2), 89–90. doi:10.1002/hup. 449.

Paternite, C. E., Loney, J., Salisbury, H., & Whaley, M. A. (1999). Childhood inattention-overactivity, aggression, and stimulant medication history as predictors of young adult outcomes. *Journal of Child and Adolescent Psychopharmacology, 9*(3), 169–184.

Pelham, W. E., Jr., & Fabiano, G. A. (2008). Evidence-based psychosocial treatments for attention-deficit/hyperactivity disorder. *Journal of Clinical Child and Adolescent Psychology, 37*(1), 184–214. doi:10.1080/15374410701818681.

Pliszka, S. R. (1992). Comorbidity of attention-deficit hyperactivity disorder and overanxious disorder. *Journal of the American Academy of Child and Adolescent Psychiatry, 31*(2), 197–203. doi:10.1097/00004583-199203000-00003.

Polanczyk, G., Caspi, A., Houts, R., Kollins, S. H., Rohde, L. A., & Moffitt, T. E. (2010). Implications of extending the ADHD age-of-onset criterion to age 12: Results from a prospectively studied birth cohort. *Journal of the American Academy of Child and Adolescent Psychiatry, 49*(3), 210–216. doi:10.1016/j.jaac.2009.12.014.

Polanczyk, G., de Lima, M. S., Horta, B. L., Biederman, J., & Rohde, L. A. (2007). The worldwide prevalence of ADHD: A systematic review and metaregression analysis. *The American Journal of Psychiatry, 164*(6), 942–948. doi:10.1176/appi.ajp. 164.6.942.

Pomerleau, O. F., Downey, K. K., Stelson, F. W., & Pomerleau, C. S. (1995). Cigarette smoking in adult patients diagnosed with attention deficit hyperactivity disorder. *Journal of Substance Abuse, 7*(3), 373–378. doi:10.1016/0899-3289(95)90030-6.

Prasad, S., Harpin, V., Poole, L., Zeitlin, H., Jamdar, S., & Puvanendran, K. (2007). A multi-centre, randomised, open-label study of atomoxetine compared with standard current therapy in UK children and adolescents with attention-deficit/hyperactivity disorder (ADHD). *Current Medical Research and Opinion, 23*(2), 379–394. doi:10.1185/030079906X167309.

Price, M. N., & Hyde, J. S. (2009). When two isn't better than one: Predictors of early sexual activity in adolescence using a cumulative risk model. *Journal of Youth and Adolescence, 38*(8), 1059–1071. doi:10.1007/s10964-008-9351-2.

Price, J. B., Wilens, T. E., Spencer, T. J., & Biederman, J. (2006). Pharmacotherapy of ADHD in adults. In R. A. Barkley (Ed.), *Attention-deficit hyperactivity disorder: A handbook for diagnosis and treatment* (Vol. 3, pp. 704–736). New York: Guilford Press.

Ptacek, R., Kuzelova, H., & Paclt, I. (2009). Effect of stimulants on growth of ADHD children: A critical review. *Activitas Nervosa Superior, 51*(4), 140–146.

Putnam, K. M., & Silk, K. R. (2005). Emotion dysregulation and the development of borderline personality disorder. *Development and Psychopathology, 17*(4), 899–925.

Rabiner, D. L., Anastopoulos, A. D., Costello, E. J., Hoyle, R. H., McCabe, S. E., & Swartzwelder, H. S. (2009). The misuse and diversion of prescribed ADHD medications by college students. *Journal of Attention Disorders, 13*(2), 144–153. doi:10.1177/1087054708320414.

Raggi, V. L., & Chronis, A. M. (2006). Interventions to address the academic impairment of children and adolescents with ADHD. *Clinical Child and Family Psychology Review, 9*(2), 85–111. doi:10.1007/s10567-006-0006-0.

Raggi, V. L., Chronis-Tuscano, A., Fishbein, H., & Groomes, A. (2009). Development of a brief, behavioral homework intervention for middle school students with attention-deficit/hyperactivity disorder. *School Mental Health, 1*(2), 61–77. doi:10.1007/s12310-009-9008-7.

Rasmussen, P., & Gillberg, C. (2000). Natural outcome of ADHD with developmental coordination disorder at age 22 years: A controlled, longitudinal, community-based study. *Journal of the American Academy of Child and Adolescent Psychiatry, 39*(11), 1424–1431. doi:10.1097/00004583-200011000-00017.

Reimherr, F. W., Marchant, B. K., Olsen, J. L., Halls, C., Kondo, D. G., Williams, E. D., et al. (2010). Emotional dysregulation as a core feature of adult ADHD: Its relationship with clinical variables and treatment response in two methylphenidate trials. *Journal of ADHD & Related Disorders, 1*(4), 53–64.

Reimherr, F. W., Marchant, B. K., Strong, R. E., Hedges, D. W., Adler, L., Spencer, T. J., et al. (2005). Emotional dysregulation in adult ADHD and response to atomoxetine. *Biological Psychiatry, 58*, 125–131. doi:10.1016/j.biopsych.2005.04.040.

Robin, A. L. (2006). Treating families with adolescents with ADHD. In R. A. Barkley (Ed.), *Attention deficity hyperactivity disorder: A handbook for diagnosis and treatment* (Vol. 3, pp. 499–546). New York: Guilford Press.

Rohde, L. A. (2008). Is there a need to reformulate attention deficit hyperactivity disorder criteria in future nosologic classifications? *Child and Adolescent Psychiatric Clinics of North America, 17*(2), 405–420. doi:10.1016/j.chc.2007.11.007.

Rohde, P., Kahler, C. W., Lewinsohn, P. M., & Brown, R. A. (2004). Psychiatric disorders, familial factors, and cigarette smoking: II. Associations with progression to daily smoking. *Nicotine & Tobacco Research, 6*(1), 119–132. doi:10.1080/14622200310001656948.

Safren, S. A., Sprich, S., Mimiaga, M. J., Surman, C., Knouse, L., Groves, M., et al. (2010). Cognitive behavioral therapy vs. relaxation with educational support for medication-treated adults with ADHD and persistent symptoms: A randomized controlled trial. *Journal of the American Medical Association, 304*(8), 875–880. doi:10.1001/jama.2010.1192.

Sallee, F. R., Lyne, A., Wigal, T., & McGough, J. J. (2009). Long-term safety and efficacy of guanfacine extended release in children and adolescents with attention-deficit/hyperactivity disorder. *Journal of Child and Adolescent Psychopharmacology, 19*(3), 215–226. doi:10.1089/cap. 2008.0080.

Sallee, F. R., McGough, J., Wigal, T., Donahue, J., Lyne, A., & Biederman, J. (2009). Guanfacine extended release in children and adolescents with attention-deficit/hyperactivity disorder: A placebo-controlled trial. *Journal of the American Academy of Child and Adolescent Psychiatry, 48*(2), 155–165. doi:10.1097/CHI.0b013e318191769e.

Satterfield, J. H., Hoppe, C. M., & Schell, A. M. (1982). A prospective study of delinquency in 110 adolescent boys with attention deficit disorder and 88 normal adolescent boys. *The American Journal of Psychiatry, 139*(6), 795–798.

Scahill, L., Chappell, P. B., Kim, Y. S., Schultz, R. T., Katsovich, L., Shepherd, E., et al. (2001). A placebo-controlled study of guanfacine in the treatment of children with tic disorders and attention deficit hyperactivity disorder. *The American Journal of Psychiatry, 158*(7), 1067–1074.

Schachter, H. M., Pham, B., King, J., Langford, S., & Moher, D. (2001). How efficacious and safe is short-acting methylphenidate for the treatment of attention-deficit disorder in children and adolescents? A meta-analysis. *Canadian Medical Association Journal, 165*(11), 1475–1488.

Setlik, J., Bond, G. R., & Ho, M. (2009). Adolescent prescription ADHD medication abuse is rising along with prescriptions for these medications. *Pediatrics, 124*(3), 875–880. doi:10.1542/peds.2008-0931.

Sibley, M. H., Pelham, W. E., Molina, B. S., Waschbusch, D. A., Gnagy, E. M., Babinski, D. E., et al. (2010). Inconsistent self-report of delinquency by adolescents and young adults with ADHD. *Journal of Abnormal Child Psychology, 38*(5), 645–656. doi:10.1007/s10802-010-9404-3.

Skirrow, C., McLoughlin, G., Kuntsi, J., & Asherson, P. (2009). Behavioral, neurocognitive and treatment overlap between attention-deficit/hyperactivity disorder and mood instability. *Expert Review of Neurotherapeutics, 9*(4), 489–503. doi:10.1586/ern.09.2.

Smith, B. H., Pelham, W. E., Gnagy, E., & Yudell, R. S. (1998). Equivalent effects of stimulant treatment for attention-deficit hyperactivity disorder during childhood and adolescence. *Journal of the American Academy of Child and Adolescent Psychiatry, 37*(3), 314–321. doi:10.1097/00004583-199803000-00017.

Smith, B. H., Waschbusch, D. A., Willoughby, M. T., & Evans, S. (2000). The efficacy, safety, and practicality of treatments for adolescents with attention-deficit/hyperactivity disorder (ADHD). *Clinical Child and Family Psychology Review, 3*(4), 243–267. doi:10.1023/A:1026477121224.

Solanto, M. V., Marks, D. J., Wasserstein, J., Mitchell, K., Abikoff, H., Alvir, J. M., et al. (2010). Efficacy of meta-cognitive therapy for adult ADHD. *The American Journal of Psychiatry, 167*, 958–968. doi:10.1176/appi.ajp. 2009.09081123.

Stewart, K. G., & McLaughlin, T. F. (1992). Self-recording: Effects of reducing off-task behavior with a high school student with an attention deficit hyperactivity disorder. *Child & Family Behavior Therapy, 14*(3), 53–59.

Swanson, J. M., Elliott, G. R., Greenhill, L. L., Wigal, T., Arnold, L. E., Vitiello, B., et al. (2007). Effects of stimulant medication on growth rates across 3 years in the MTA follow-up. *Journal of the American Academy of Child and Adolescent Psychiatry, 46*(8), 1015–1027. doi:10.1097/chi.0b013e3180686d7e.

Tannock, R. (2000). Attention-deficit/hyperactivity disorder with anxious disorders. In T. E. Brown (Ed.), *Attention deficit disorders and comorbidities in children, adolescents, and adults* (Vol. 125–170). Washington, DC: American Psychiatric Association.

Tercyak, K. P., Lerman, C., & Audrain, J. (2002). Association of attention-deficit/hyperactivity disorder symptoms with levels of cigarette smoking in a community sample of adolescents. *Journal of the American Academy of Child and Adolescent Psychiatry, 41*(7), 799–805. doi:10.1097/00004583-200207000-00011.

Thiruchelvam, D., Charach, A., & Schachar, R. J. (2001). Moderators and mediators of long-term adherence to stimulant treatment in children with ADHD. *Journal of the American Academy of Child and Adolescent Psychiatry, 40*(8), 922–928. doi:10.1097/00004583-200108000-00014.

Thomason, C., & Michelson, D. (2004). Atomoxetine—Treatment of attention deficit hyperactivity disorder: Beyond stimulants. *Drugs of Today (Barcelona, Spain), 40*(5), 465–473. doi:10.1358/dot.2004.40.5.850493.

Todd, R. D., Huang, H., & Henderson, C. A. (2008). Poor utility of the age of onset criterion for DSM-IV attention deficit/hyperactivity disorder: Recommendations for DSM-V and ICD-11. *Journal of Child Psychology and Psychiatry, 49*(9), 942–949. doi:10.1111/j.1469-7610.2008.01892.x.

Topolski, T. D., Edwards, T. C., Patrick, D. L., Varley, P., Way, M. E., & Buesching, D. P. (2004). Quality of life of adolescent males with attention-deficit hyperactivity disorder. *Journal of Attention Disorders, 7*(3), 163–173. doi:10.1177/108705470400700304.

Valera, E. M., Faraone, S. V., Murray, K. E., & Seidman, L. J. (2007). Meta-analysis of structural imaging findings in attention-deficit/hyperactivity disorder. *Biological Psychiatry, 61*(12), 1361–1369. doi:10.1016/j.biopsych.2006.06.011.

Walcott, C. M., & Landau, S. (2004). The relation between disinhibition and emotion regulation in boys with attention deficit hyperactivity disorder. *Journal of Clinical Child and Adolescent Psychology, 33*(4), 772–782. doi:10.1207/s15374424jccp3304_12.

Wehmeier, P. M., Schacht, A., & Barkley, R. A. (2010). Social and emotional impairment in children and adolescents with ADHD and the impact on quality of life. *Journal of Adolescent Health, 46*(3), 209–217. doi:10.1016/j.jadohealth.2009.09.009.

Wehmeier, P. M., Schacht, A., Lehmann, M., Dittmann, R. W., Silva, S. G., & March, J. S. (2008). Emotional well-being in children and adolescents treated with atomoxetine for attention-deficit/hyperactivity disorder: Findings from a patient, parent and physician perspective using items from the pediatric adverse event rating scale (PAERS). *Child and Adolescent Psychiatry and Mental Health, 2*(1), 11. doi:10.1186/1753-2000-2-11.

Weinstein, S. M., Mermelstein, R., Shiffman, S., & Flay, B. (2008). Mood variability and cigarette smoking escalation among adolescents. *Psychology of Addictive Behaviors, 22*(4), 504–513. doi:10.1037/0893-164X.22.4.504.

Weiss, G., & Hechtman, L. T. (1993). *Hyperactive children grown up* (2nd ed.). New York: Guilford Press.

Whalen, C. K., Jamner, L. D., Henker, B., Gehricke, J. G., & King, P. S. (2003). Is there a link between adolescent cigarette smoking and pharmacotherapy for ADHD? *Psychology of Addictive Behaviors, 17*(4), 332–335. doi:10.1037/0893-164X.17.4.332.

White, P. H. (2002). Access to health care: Health insurance considerations for young adults with special health care needs/disabilities. *Pediatrics, 110*(6 Pt 2), 1328–1335.

White, H. R., Xie, M., Thompson, W., Loeber, R., & Stouthamer-Loeber, M. (2001). Psychopathology as a predictor of adolescent drug use trajectories. *Psychology of Addictive Behaviors, 15*(3), 210–218. doi:10.1037/0893-164X.15.3.210.

Wilens, T. E., Biederman, J., Mick, E., Faraone, S. V., & Spencer, T. (1997). Attention deficit hyperactivity disorder (ADHD) is associated with early onset substance use disorders. *The Journal of Nervous and Mental Disease, 185*(8), 475–482.

Wilens, T. E., Faraone, S. V., Biederman, J., & Gunawardene, S. (2003). Does stimulant therapy of attention-deficit/hyperactivity disorder beget later substance abuse? A meta-analytic review of the literature. *Pediatrics, 111*(1), 179–185. doi:10.1542/peds.111.1.179.

Wilens, T. E., Gignac, M., Swezey, A., Monuteaux, M. C., & Biederman, J. (2006). Characteristics of adolescents and young adults with ADHD who divert or misuse their prescribed medications. *Journal of the American Academy of Child and Adolescent Psychiatry, 45*(4), 408–414. doi:10.1097/01.chi.0000199027.68828.b3.

Wilens, T. E., Kratochvil, C., Newcorn, J. H., & Gao, H. (2006). Do children and adolescents with ADHD respond differently to atomoxetine? *Journal of the American Academy of Child and Adolescent Psychiatry, 45*(2), 149–157. doi:10.1097/01.chi.0000190352.90946.0b.

Wilens, T. E., Newcorn, J. H., Kratochvil, C. J., Gao, H., Thomason, C. K., Rogers, A. K., et al. (2006). Long-term atomoxetine treatment in adolescents with attention-deficit/hyperactivity disorder. *Journal of Pediatrics, 149*(1), 112–119. doi:10.1016/j.jpeds.2006.01.052.

Wilens, T. E., & Spencer, T. J. (2000). The stimulants revisited. *Child and Adolescent Psychiatric Clinics of North America, 9*(3), 573–603. viii.

Willoughby, M. T. (2003). Developmental course of ADHD symptomatology during the transition from childhood to adolescence: A review with recommendations. *Journal of Child Psychology and Psychiatry, 44*(1), 88–106. doi:10.1111/1469-7610.t01-1-00104.

Windle, M., Spear, L. P., Fuligni, A. J., Angold, A., Brown, J. D., Pine, D., et al. (2008). Transitions into underage and problem drinking: Developmental processes and mechanisms between 10 and 15 years of age. *Pediatrics, 121*(Suppl 4), S273–S289. doi:10.1542/peds.2007-2243C.

Wolraich, M. L., Wibbelsman, C. J., Brown, T. E., Evans, S. W., Gotlieb, E. M., Knight, J. R., et al. (2005). Attention-deficit/hyperactivity disorder among adolescents: A review of the diagnosis, treatment, and clinical implications. *Pediatrics, 115*(6), 1734–1746. doi:10.1542/peds.2004-1959.

World Health Organization. (1992). *The ICD-10 classification of mental and behavioural disorders. Clinical descriptions and diagnostic guidelines*. Geneva: World Health Organization.

World Health Organization. (2002). *Injury: A leading cause of the global burden of disease*. Geneva: World Health & Organization.

Wozniak, J., & Biederman, J. (1995). Prepubertal mania exists (and co-exists with ADHD). *The ADHD Report, 2*, 5–6.

Wozniak, J., Biederman, J., Kiely, K., Ablon, J. S., Faraone, S. V., Mundy, E., et al. (1995). Mania-like symptoms suggestive of childhood-onset bipolar disorder in clinically referred children. *Journal of the American Academy of Child and Adolescent Psychiatry, 34*(7), 867–876. doi:10.1097/00004583-199507000-00010.

Zylowska, L., Ackerman, D. L., Yang, M. H., Futrell, J. L., Horton, N. L., Hale, T. S., et al. (2008). Mindfulness meditation training in adults and adolescents with ADHD: A feasibility study. *Journal of Attention Disorders, 11*(6), 737–746. doi:10.1177/1087054707308502.

Social and Biological Changes During Adolescence That Precipitate the Onset of Antisocial Behavior

Lisa M. Gatzke-Kopp, David DuPuis, and Robert L. Nix

Adolescence is a period of development anecdotally synonymous with rebellion, defiance, and a vpropensity to engage in behaviors that call into question the existence of a human instinct to survive. Although these behaviors evolve from a normative motivation to establish independence and develop a personal and sexual identity, adolescence is a vulnerable time period for the development of pathological behavior. Criminological data indicate a nearly tenfold increase in crime during the adolescent period, a rate that substantially declines over the course of adulthood.

The observed rise in antisocial behavior during adolescence led to the proposal of classes of antisocial individuals that were considered to be taxonomically distinct (Moffitt, 1993). It was originally proposed that the behaviors associated with delinquency were relatively normative in adolescence, and thus carried less risk when onset occurred in adolescence versus in childhood. Onset of antisocial behavior during early childhood was significantly more predictive of chronicity of symptoms, whereas onset in adolescence appeared to be a more transient form of antisocial behavior, often remitting in adulthood in conjunction with the increase in responsibility associated with independence (Moffitt, 1993). Reflecting the differential prognostic value between the two categories, the terms "life course persistent" and "adolescent limited" were coined as labels for the two subgroups.

In the past two decades, however, evidence has amassed that these labels oversimplify the categorization of antisocial individuals. Specifically, onset in adolescence does not appear to be entirely normative, nor is it a relatively innocuous or necessarily temporary condition (Moffitt & Caspi, 2005; Roisman, Aguilar, & Egeland, 2004). Regardless of age of onset, individuals with elevated levels of antisocial behavior in adolescence are distinguishable from non-antisocial peers both in terms of their early risk factors (Roisman et al., 2010) and their adult outcomes (Woodward, Fergusson, & Horwood, 2002). Furthermore, antisocial individuals evidence common individual risk factors, such as poor fear conditioning, regardless of age of onset (Fairchild, Van Goozen, Stollery, & Goodyer, 2008). Therefore onset of antisocial behavior in adolescence appears to be along the continuum of risk associated with onset in childhood, and

L.M. Gatzke-Kopp, Ph.D. (✉)
Department of Human Development and Family Studies and Neuroscience, The Pennsylvania State University, 315 HHD East, University Park, PA 16802, USA
e-mail: lisakopp@psu.edu

D. DuPuis
Department of Human Development and Family Studies, The Pennsylvania State University, 315 HHD East, University Park, PA 16802, USA
e-mail: dud164@psu.edu; lisakopp@psu.edu

R.L. Nix, Ph.D.
The Prevention Research Center, The Pennsylvania State University, 316A Biobehavioral Health Building, University Park, PA 16802, USA
e-mail: rnix@psu.edu

W.T. O'Donohue et al. (eds.), *Handbook of Adolescent Health Psychology*,
DOI 10.1007/978-1-4614-6633-8_28,

the risky behaviors associated with this disorder can result in lifelong consequences to the individual, diverting them into an adverse developmental trajectory (Molero, Hodgins, Larsson, Larm, & Tengstrom, 2010; Odgers et al., 2008; Roisman et al., 2010).

This chapter will focus on the social and biological changes associated with adolescence that heighten the risk for the onset of antisocial behaviors during this period. Consistent with the notion of a continuum, increases in the severity, chronicity, or accumulation of contextual and individual risk factors decrease the latency to symptom onset. For individuals in the moderate range of risk exposure, symptom onset may not be evident until later in development, when the underlying vulnerability is amplified by developmentally normative changes in neural structure and function that occur across the adolescent period. Metaphorically, for some individuals, the flux of social and biological changes during this period represent the gasoline on a previously contained campfire.

Definitions

It is important to first address the different permutations and definitions of the broad category of antisocial behavior. Following from the American Psychiatric Association's diagnostic manual (American Psychiatric Association, 2000), the two most pertinent disorders to this discussion are oppositional defiant disorder (ODD) and conduct disorder (CD). ODD consists of a pattern of easy loss of temper, arguing (particularly with adults or authority figures), failing to abide by rules, deliberate attempts to annoy others, being angry or spiteful, and displacing blame for one's actions onto others. In an effort to avoid over-pathologizing developmentally normative behavior associated with toddlerhood and adolescence, diagnosis is reserved for individuals with four or more symptoms causing significant interpersonal impairment for a period of 6 months or longer (DSM-IV-TR, 2000). Symptoms classified in conjunction with CD tend to represent more severe behaviors along this continuum, including destruction of property, such as fire-setting; physically violent or cruel actions; theft or fraud; and statutory crimes, like regularly skipping school. Again, to avoid diagnosing sporadic or situation-specific behaviors, symptoms must be present over the preceding 12-month period in order to meet diagnostic threshold.

Comorbidity between ODD and CD exceeds the predicted rates that would occur if each diagnosis were truly independent of the other. This has led some researchers to argue that the distinction between the two is artificial, and that the criteria simply represent antisocial behavior at different developmental stages (see Biederman, Newcorn, & Sprich, 1991). For instance, young children can easily engage in deliberately annoying behavior and defying adult instruction; however, a certain degree of physical maturity is required before they can successfully engage in crimes like armed robbery or sexual assault. Thus ODD is often considered a developmental precursor for CD. However, the majority of individuals who obtain an ODD diagnosis in childhood will not go on to meet the criteria for CD, suggesting value in retaining the two diagnoses as separate entities. The interrelated nature of ODD and CD has led the American Psychiatric Association to establish a hierarchical structure between these disorders. Because ODD is frequently considered to be a developmental antecedent of CD or a less severe manifestation of the same underlying pathology, ODD is not diagnosed in the presence of CD (DSM-IV-TR, 2000).

In addition to these formal diagnoses, many other terms are used to characterize pathological behavior of this nature. Developmentally, problem behaviors defined by their outward manifestation and impact on others are often referred to as "externalizing" behaviors. Researchers often examine correlates of symptoms in this domain without requiring that full diagnostic criteria be met. Additionally, some researchers focus more specifically on sociological—rather than psychological—constructs, such as the development of delinquent and/or criminal behavior as defined legally. Other researchers focus on the personality constructs that underlie complex psychiatric syndromes, such as impulsivity. Generally speaking, researchers across different disciplines acknowledge the conceptual overlap between these various approaches, often reviewing literature in one domain to inform another. To this end, the term "antisocial behavior" is often used to subsume the various instantiations of pathological behavior.

Common Vulnerability

An inclusive approach to studying these related behavioral profiles is supported by behavioral genetics research, which indicates that demarcation between disorders such CD, ODD, and even attention deficit hyperactivity disorder (ADHD) may be artificial. These disorders appear to be influenced by similar physiological and environmental risk factors, leading to their frequently comorbid presentation (Burt, Krueger, McGue, & Iacono, 2001; Hofvander, Ossowski, Lundstrom, & Anckarsater, 2009). In a study of twins followed longitudinally, externalizing disorders measured across childhood (CD), adolescence (delinquency), and adulthood (antisocial behavior and substance dependence), as well as non-pathological constructs such as disinhibited personality, could be explained primarily by a common latent vulnerability that is highly heritable (Krueger et al., 2002). This kind of common vulnerability has important implications for research and treatment of antisocial behavior over time. Rather than consider these diagnoses as independent contributions to adverse outcomes that may or may not be present in any given individual, this model proposes that any individual with one externalizing disorder is inherently at risk for the others.

The realization of this risk appears to be predicated on environmental exposures. For instance, although an individual displaying age-inappropriate oppositionality and a willingness to violate rules and social norms is at high risk for developing substance dependence, doing so requires exposure to substances of abuse, a phenomenon correlated with environmental factors such as neighborhood, peer, and family factors that make substances of abuse accessible. Thus, an individual's propensity to develop a psychological disorder may not manifest until, or unless, the right environmental circumstances interact with individual risk. It follows logically then, that the increase in manifestation of antisocial behavior in adolescence reflects the expansion of environments that the individual is exposed to. The identification of the environmental processes that contribute to the progression from disinhibited personality to a specific form of psychopathology is invaluable in identifying appropriate targets for intervention.

Epidemiologically, boys are more likely to garner a CD diagnosis than girls (DSM-IV-TR, 2000). This has led to some controversy regarding approaches to research and diagnosis of these disorders with respect to sex differences. This is consistent with males' tendency to be more aggressive in most mammalian species (Archer, 2009). However, some researchers have argued that the diagnostic discrepancy is an artifact of the gender-stereotyped behaviors listed as symptoms for CD, which favor behavior more typical of boys. In response, researchers have argued that females engage in aggressive behavior toward peers, but are less likely to do so in a physical domain, instead focusing on the use of gossip and slander to manipulate social status as a mechanism of harming peers (Crick, Bigbee, & Howes, 1996). Although this profile of behavior, termed "relational aggression," is more prototypical of females, it is likely a construct unrelated to CD. Furthermore, although the criteria for CD may contain legitimately sexually dimorphic symptoms, such as aggression (see Archer, 2009), females are quite capable of meeting the existing criteria for CD. However, they tend to do so by exhibiting different profiles of behavior than males. Females with CD are less likely to engage in physical fighting, but rather to express their impulsivity and proclivity for law breaking through behaviors such as truancy, lying, stealing (without confronting the victim), using drugs, and engaging in promiscuous sex, possibly for money (Vera, Ezpeleta, Granero, & de la Osa, 2010). Indeed, much of the research regarding risk factors for antisocial behavior does not support a sexually divergent model (Fontaine, Carbonneau, Vitaro, Barker, & Tremblay, 2009).

Family Processes

Parents represent the first socializing influence on children and, as such, play a fundamental role in the development of behavioral and emotional regulation. However, as children grow into adolescence, both parents and children struggle with the changing need for autonomy. Although parents might welcome adolescents' increased self-sufficiency, they often worry about what they do not know of their adolescents' independent lives. Parents continue to play an important role during this transitional period, even if an unwelcome one on the part of the child.

Research on general parenting styles reveals an association between an authoritative approach to child-rearing and adolescent adjustment (Steinberg, 2001; Steinberg, Mounts, Lamborn, & Dornbusch, 1991). Parents who are authoritative display high levels of sensitivity and responsiveness to their adolescents' needs but also expectations for respectful and responsible behavior. These parents tend to rely on more democratic means of control and encourage their adolescents to express themselves. In contrast, factors consistently associated with antisocial outcomes and early substance experimentation in youths include a lack of parental supervision, harsh punishment practices, and lack of emotional support (Murray & Farrington, 2010).

In addition to broad parenting domains, research has also revealed specific coercive cycles of exchanges that can take place between parents and young children or adolescents that contribute to the escalation of antisocial behavior (Granic & Patterson, 2006; Patterson, 1982). For instance, a single cycle might begin with a mother asking her son to clean his room. The child might resist by passively ignoring the instruction, actively defying it, or engaging in aversive behaviors such as whining. If the parent is feeling tired or stressed, she might decide not to follow through on the request. Because the child's behavior was aversive, the parent's decision to escape the argument is negatively reinforced and thus more likely to occur again. Likewise, the parent's withdrawal of her request negatively reinforces the child's aversive response. Thus both parent and child have reinforced each other in the exchange, which has failed to result in a satisfying and appropriate resolution. In future episodes, the parent is more likely to be exacerbated by the child's defiance and escalate her demand with yelling and threats of punishment. Over time, the child learns that anger, threats, and dominance are an effective means to accomplish goals.

This kind of coercive cycle of exchanges may be especially likely to occur in adolescence, when the newly developed need for autonomy leads most youths to experiment with more defiant responses to parental control. Parents may be inclined to avoid unpleasant arguments with irritable adolescents and retreat from a more active role in their adolescents' daily lives. Coercive exchanges that have undermined positive relationships and induced parents to withdraw and adolescents to withhold information may be particularly detrimental for high-risk adolescents, who often use unsupervised time to engage with deviant peer groups (Dishion, Nelson, & Bullock, 2004). As such, parenting practices and family interactions likely contribute to the confluence of risk factors that promote a rise in antisocial behavior during adolescence.

Peer Processes and the Moderating Influences of Parents

Friendship is a normative and fundamental aspect of adolescent development that exposes the individual to a world of social behaviors and expectations beyond that of the family context. However, the increasing influence of peers during adolescent development can introduce new contexts for psychopathological risk.

Association with deviant peers has been shown to have a facilitatory effect on individual delinquency (Brendgen, Vitaro, & Bukowski, 2000; Lacourse, Nagin, Tremblay, Vitaro, & Claes, 2003). This is likely a product of the tendency for antisocial individuals to associate with other deviant peers (Cairns, Leung, Buchanan, & Cairns, 1996), forming relationships in which peers mutually exacerbate each other's antisocial behavior (Dishion, Bullock, & Granic, 2002). This phenomenon has been observed across developmental time and irrespective of age of onset of delinquency (Lacourse et al., 2003). Process-oriented research has determined that friendship interactions can increase antisocial behavior through mutually reinforcing responses to deviant talk (Dishion, Nelson, Winter, & Bullock, 2004). In fact, evidence from clinical interventions conducted in a group format has identified adverse outcomes of increased delinquency due to the introduction of deviant peers to each other (Dishion, Bullock, et al., 2002; Dishion, McCord, & Poulin, 1999; Poulin, Dishion, & Burraston, 2001). These findings support the notion of a causal role for peer influence in the development and exacerbation of delinquency, and indicate the powerful effect of social influences on deviance, even in a seemingly therapeutic context.

Despite the significant effect peers have on exacerbating antisocial tendencies, exertion of parental influence over adolescent friendships appears to have protective effects. There is some evidence that parenting practices, such as encouragement of achievement, influence adolescent adjustment, such as school grade point average, which in turn affects the peers adolescents tend to spend time with (Brown, Mounts, Lamborn, & Steinberg, 1993). Intervention research in which participants were randomly assigned to therapeutic resources during the middle school period indicates that strengthening parenting skills and parental monitoring of friendships resulted in a significant decline in deviant peer associations and delinquent behavior (Dishion, Bullock, et al., 2002).

However, as noted above, parent-child relationships are likely to become strained through the transition to adolescence as parental authority is met with adolescent autonomy needs. Research highlights the importance of warm, supportive family interactions that make adolescents comfortable disclosing what is happening in their lives (Kerr & Stattin, 2000; Stattin & Kerr, 2000) and allow parents to provide guidance regarding peer relationships (Mounts, 2000). Although supervision of adolescent's peer group is important, parents' approach to this responsibility cannot be overlooked (Steinberg, 2001). Authoritarian prohibition of a deviant friend can have the effect of increasing adolescent defiance of the parent, eroding the parent-child relationship, and strengthening the deviant peer friendship. Alternatively, parental prohibition of a specific friend that is delivered in an autonomy granting way, supporting the adolescent's perspective and providing a clear rationale, promoted acceptance of the parent's prohibition, and reduced the association with that deviant friend (Soenens, Vansteenkiste, & Niemiec, 2009).

Neural Correlates of Pathological Antisocial Behavior

Most research on antisocial behavior has focused on family and peer influences because of the desire to understand better those processes that might be amenable to intervention. However, in recent decades, more research has focused on individual variability in vulnerability to those influences. Although no specific brain region can be implicated in a complex behavioral syndrome, individual differences in neural function underlie traits such as emotional arousal, fear conditioning, and the ability to regulate behavior in the service of long-term goals. These systems are implicated in symptoms of conduct disorder, such as extreme anger and arousal that lead to fighting and aggressive behavior. Deficits in fear conditioning have also been implicated in covert delinquent behaviors, such as lying and cheating, and overt cruel behaviors, such as bullying. Variation in these systems interacts with environmental factors to establish patterns of behavior that become self-sustaining over time. Understanding the source of individual vulnerability may help refine intervention programs to more directly address the needs of individual adolescents.

Perhaps the most consistent findings associated with antisocial behavior are deficits in the structure and/or function of the prefrontal cortex (Raine, 2008; Yang & Raine, 2009). The prefrontal cortex in humans represents a large and functionally diverse region which is attributed the higher order cognitive functions that make humans unique.

Among these functions are the abilities to resolve competition between goals with conflicting timescales, to retain appropriate information in active memory while executing a behavior, and to update behavioral goals based on feedback from the environment. These actions often require the suppression of lower order brain regions that subserve emotions and otherwise would result in impulsive and reactive behavior. The evolutionarily older limbic system, including the nucleus accumbens, amygdala, and anterior cingulate cortex, is responsible for generating basic emotional drives such as fear, anger, and reward seeking, and has also been implicated in pathological behavior.

Several researchers have proposed a dynamic model of neural processing in which the prefrontal cortex and limbic nuclei each contribute to the execution of behavior, but do so adaptively under different circumstances (Lewis & Todd, 2007; Metcalfe & Mischel, 1999; Seeley et al., 2007). Under normal conditions, the prefrontal cortex is an invaluable resource in processing the complexities of judgment in social situations. To do this, the brain must integrate information from past experiences to generate a range of possible actions or responses and make predictions about their probable consequences; it then must select the action that has the highest likelihood of being effective. Although these computations take place quickly, they are far slower and more metabolically costly than the impulsive decisions executed by the limbic system. Under conditions of perceived threat, it is more advantageous to react immediately without concern for consequences. For instance, if one were to come across something that looks like a snake during a hike, it would be more reasonable to jump back immediately than to pause and notice upon closer inspection that the stimulus is in fact a twisted branch. Thus, under conditions of threat, emotional impulse overrides deliberate and possibly rational behavior. Metcalfe and Mischel (1999) coined the terms "cold" and "hot" cognitive processing to distinguish between the slow and methodical responses generated in the prefrontal cortex and the rapid and potentially irrational responses of the limbic nuclei. The balance between these systems is thus dynamic and contextually determined.

Neuroimaging research indicates reduced connectivity between the prefrontal and limbic regions in adolescent boys with CD (Shannon, Sauder, Beauchaine, & Gatzke-Kopp, 2009). This suggests that antisocial individuals may have difficulty modulating the relative balance between these two systems. This is consistent with findings revealing pathological disruptions in neurotransmitter systems that facilitate inhibitory control of limbic regions (Siever, 2008). Developmental research indicates that disruptions in neurotransmission in these regions is not sufficient to predispose an individual to aggressive behavior; however, such disruptions render an individual especially sensitive to environmental adversity that more readily programs hostility and aggression in response to provocation (see Buckholtz & Meyer-Lindenberg, 2008).

The confluence of these structural and functional deficiencies results in the individual's experiencing social-emotional cues differently than developmentally typical adolescents. It has long been observed that highly aggressive individuals show an increased tendency to infer hostile intent in others, especially when social situations are ambiguous (Dodge, 1986). By adolescence, most students who are bumped in a crowded hallway would dismiss the incident without much regard, presuming the contact to have been accidental, and noting only a minor physical annoyance. However, individuals characterized by psychopathology are more likely to suppose a purposeful and aggressive intention on the part of the bumping student. This attribution of hostility essentially engages the limbic system in the brain, eliciting a rapid, emotional, and defensive act of self-protection. This overidentification of threat results in a defensive override of appropriate judgment in the heat of the moment. This phenomenon explains why children and adolescents can often identify appropriate social responses to minor social threat in a hypothetical context, but frequently have difficulty enacting them in the real world, when the youths are more likely to be emotionally aroused.

Individuals with antisocial behavior may be more likely to attribute hostile intent in ambiguous or benign situations due to abnormalities in processing emotional cues from facial expression. Adolescents with a history of CD show greater limbic activation in response to pictures with negative emotional content than age-matched controls, suggesting an over-reactive emotion response (Herpertz et al., 2008). However, eye tracking technology reveals that aggressive early adolescents do not focus on hostile social cues preferentially, but rather appear to be regulated by a preexisting social schema that construes social cues so they are consistent with expectations (Horsley, de Castro, & Van der Schoot, 2010). Thus, over-activation of emotion-processing regions of the brain appears to represent a functionally appropriate response to distorted cognitive interpretations, suggesting the importance of targeting these interpretive processes in intervention (Dodge, 2011).

Antisocial adolescents also appear to have deficits in processing reward-related information, even outside of the social context. This has important implications for understanding antisocial behavior, as reward and punishment contingencies are the driving forces behind behavior modification. Similar to individuals with acquired brain damage, adolescents and adults with antisocial behavior or substance abuse disorders have been documented to engage in poor decision-making in monetary tasks (Ernst et al., 2003; Stadler et al., 2007). Recently, researchers have examined the neural correlates of risky decision making in antisocial adolescents and found a consistent pattern of under-activation in the prefrontal and limbic regions during the decision-making process, suggesting a deficient recognition of the relative risk between decisions (Crowley et al., 2010). Furthermore, antisocial adolescents showed less activation during monetary wins than normally developing controls, and more activation during monetary loss (Crowley et al., 2010). These findings suggest that antisocial adolescents respond atypically to cues of reward and punishment; this difference likely contributes to the challenges of appropriately shaping these adolescents' prosocial behavior. Some researchers have suggested that externalizing disorders are characterized by deficient processing of reward cues, requiring larger, and more immediate, reinforcement to effectively shape behavior (Beauchaine, Gatzke-Kopp, & Mead, 2007; Sagvolden, Johansen, Aase, & Russell, 2005).

Additional research indicates that adolescents with CD have deficits in processing changes in reward contingencies. During a monetary incentive task, adolescents with CD and ADHD were compared to developmentally normative peers (Gatzke-Kopp et al., 2009). In this task, participants were asked to complete a simple game while undergoing a functional imaging scan. During some blocks of this game, correct answers resulted in the administration of a monetary reward, which accumulated across trials in the center of the screen for the participant to watch. During other blocks, the monetary reward was reset to zero, with no reward for correct responses although the participant was instructed to continue responding. The simplicity of the task ensured equivalent performance across groups, allowing for the examination of how adolescents with and without externalizing disorders reacted to the same levels of reward incentives. Individuals in both the CD and developmentally normative groups showed a robust activation in the caudate nucleus during blocks in which correct answers were rewarded, consistent with the neural networks associated with behavioral responding for reward. However, when participants engaged in blocks in which the same performance was no longer accompanied by reward, the two groups differed significantly in the regional brain activation they demonstrated. Developmentally normative adolescents evidenced a shift of activation from the caudate to the anterior cingulate cortex. However, adolescents with a diagnosis of CD and/or ADHD did not show this typical shift in processing the contingency change. In fact, these adolescents continued to activate the caudate nucleus, with no significant difference between the reward and non-reward conditions (Gatzke-Kopp et al., 2009).

The failure of adolescents with CD to recognize the experimentally induced change in feedback suggests that they may be especially insensitive to cues of behavioral ineffectiveness. In normally developing adolescents, behavior that may have been successful in the past but now consistently fails to yield desired results will extinguish naturally. It has been proposed that failure in this process to use feedback to make adjustments to behavior is due to deficits in dopamine (Sagvolden et al., 2005). Support for this hypothesis has also been reported with electroencephalographic techniques, which measure brain response to error feedback in real time. Individuals with externalizing symptoms showed reduced brain activation in response to error commission, indicating a reduction in monitoring behavioral success (Hall, Bernat, & Patrick, 2007). Thus individuals with antisocial behavior disorders may appear to perseverate in behaviors despite their obvious lack of success in achieving goals.

In addition to deficits in reinforcement and extinction that mediate behavioral change in normally developing individuals, antisocial individuals have also been shown to have deficient response to punishment. Antisocial behavior has frequently been associated with deficits in fear conditioning, which is thought to contribute to the relative ineffectiveness of punishment threat in deterring antisocial behavior. Research has consistently demonstrated low levels of physiological arousal in antisocial individuals (Gatzke-Kopp, Raine, Loeber, Stouthamer-Loeber, & Steinhauer, 2002). Physiological arousal has been proposed to play a fundamental role in the development of conscience and internalization of rule structures that guide behavior. Researchers propose that the experience of punishment or negative performance feedback elicits a physiological response (typically measured through skin conductance) that provides an internal marker or cue of the negative experience. Over time this results in a conditioned response whereby the individual is able to use situational cues to avoid punishing consequence (Bechara, Damasio, & Damasio, 2000). For normally developing children, a simple scolding of an unwanted behavior, such as touching an electrical outlet, establishes a physiological code—coupled with the emotional experience of the mildly punishing parental admonishment—that the behavior is inappropriate. In time the child learns to avoid the cueing stimulus (e.g., the electrical outlet), thus internalizing the situational rule and regulating his or her own behavior outside of parent supervision. Children with antisocial behavior regularly fail to internalize cues of punishment and continually engage in behaviors that result in negative consequences. Adolescents with CD, regardless of the age of onset, show deficits in fear conditioning, indicating an inability to pair negative experience in a manner contingent with environmental cues (Fairchild et al., 2008).

No research has yet identified a single necessary or sufficient neuropathology that underlies antisocial behavior. It seems most likely that individuals meeting criteria for CD represent a heterogeneous class (Jones & Westen, 2010). However, evidence has amassed to implicate profiles of psychological dysfunction that likely contribute to some individuals developing antisocial symptoms. Specifically, heightened sensitivity to emotional cues in social contexts appears to lead some children to experience emotional arousal disproportionate to the situation, which may be difficult for them to regulate appropriately and which may result in inappropriate and unnecessary behavioral retaliation. In addition, some antisocial individuals appear to be characterized by an increased drive to seek reward and excitement, accompanied by a tendency not to respond to punishment. Because punishment is not as effective in preemptively deterring behavior and because extinction learning is not as effective in eliminating unsuccessful behavior, it can be especially challenging to successfully change the behavior of adolescents with CD.

Normative Brain Changes in Adolescence

Although a significant amount of research indicates pathological neural processing in adolescents with antisocial behavior, normative developmental changes in adolescence may also serve as a catalyst for vulnerable individuals who experience onset of antisocial behavior during this time. Just as adolescence is defined by the robust physical changes in body shape, size, and reproductive function, dramatic changes occur in neural development during this time as well. Increasing research on adolescent brain development indicates that, in some domains, adolescents exist midway along a continuum from childhood to adulthood, with a steady linear increase in function and ability. In other domains, however, adolescence represents a unique stage of development, deviating both from the previous state of childhood as well as the future state of adulthood. This likely contributes to the dramatic rise in antisocial behavior during adolescence, when moderate levels of environmental risk are met with developmental changes in impulsivity, culminating in antisocial behaviors not previously seen.

Poor judgment in adolescence has often been attributed to the prolonged maturation of the prefrontal cortex. This region, responsible for higher order processing of information, decision-making, and regulatory control over other brain regions, is among the last region of the brain to reach full maturity (Colby, Van Horn, & Sowell, 2011; Sowell et al., 2003). This is reflected in the linear increase from childhood to adulthood observed for performance on a number of cognitive tasks (Levin et al., 1991; Swanson, 1999; Williams, Ponesse, Schachar, Logan, & Tannock, 1999). However, risky decision making does not demonstrate a parallel linear decrease across this developmental span, suggesting that the increase of these types of behaviors in adolescence is not solely attributable to delayed prefrontal maturation. Recently, researchers have focused on the relative balance between the prefrontal and limbic regions to understand the nonlinear development in reward processing and decision-making. Unlike the prefrontal cortex, limbic regions show adultlike activation patterns by adolescence (Galvan et al., 2006). This has led to the proposal that during childhood, both the prefrontal and limbic systems are relatively immature, and during adulthood, both have reached appropriate maturation. It is during adolescence, when the maturity of these two systems is out of balance, that there is a spike in impulsive, emotionally charged, reward-focused behaviors that originate in the relatively more developed limbic system and that are not mollified by the relatively less mature prefrontal cortex (Ernst & Fudge, 2009; Somerville & Casey, 2010).

In addition, hormonal changes that accompany the onset of puberty have been implicated in exacerbating vulnerability in some individuals, leading to an increase in antisocial behavior (Susman et al., 2010). In particular, the timing of pubertal onset relative to peers appears to play a role in increasing antisocial behaviors. Girls with early-onset menarche are at a higher risk for CD than their peers. Early-onset menarche has been shown to be more common in girls with high levels of familial stress and, in particular, the experience of sexual abuse (Zabin, Emerson, & Rowland, 2005). Although the presence of these risk factors likely contributes independently to the risk for antisocial behaviors, research suggests that early menarche also may increase risk for girls by altering aspects of their social development. Girls with visible bodily changes associated with puberty well in advance of their peers often feel isolated from age-comparable peers and are more likely to receive the attention of older boys. Furthermore, those boys who are less successful in cultivating romantic relationships with girls their own age may be more likely to seek out younger girls. Thus, early-onset puberty appears to become a mechanism by which young girls begin an association with deviant peer groups, thus exacerbating their own risk (Burt, McGue, DeMarte, Krueger, & Iacono, 2006). In homes with low parental supervision, these emerging social relationships are likely to significantly contribute to female delinquency and other risk behaviors, illustrating the synergistic effects of parental, peer, and biological mechanisms in precipitating risk.

Interestingly, similar phenomena have been observed for boys. Pubertal development significantly out of sync with age-matched peers appears to exacerbate risk in vulnerable boys. However, pubertal onset was not a sufficient predictor of risk; rather it interacted with biological measures of trait stress reactivity to predict risk. Only boys with late-onset pubertal development who were characterized by low levels of salivary alpha amylase (thought to reflect low levels of reactive arousal) demonstrated an increased propensity toward antisocial behavior (Susman et al., 2010). Alternatively, boys with early-onset pubertal development were at risk only if additionally characterized by high levels of cortisol reactivity (thought to reflect stress; Susman et al., 2010). Each of these biological predispositions may reflect vulnerability for antisocial behavior through mechanisms such as poor fear conditioning or hypersensitivity to threat. It may be that the resultant social stresses involved in being physically different from peers during this sensitive period of development interact with these predisposing traits to increase risk for antisocial behavior.

Prevention and Intervention

Regardless of the etiology or age of onset of antisocial behavior, engaging in illegal and dangerous acts carries substantial risk for consequences that may permanently alter an adolescent's developmental trajectory. For instance, experimentation with drugs of abuse is common in this time period, with 46 % of high school seniors reporting having used an illicit drug at least once and 56 % reporting having been drunk at some point (Johnston, O'Malley, Bachman, & Schulenberg, 2009). Although research in substance dependence suggests that not all individuals are equally vulnerable to the transition between initiation of use and development of addiction, even nonaddictive substance experimentation can carry substantial risks. Overdose of a single drug, lethal combinations of multiple drugs, accidental death, and victimization are among the life-altering consequences of even experimental use. Relatively minor illegal acts committed for the first time can go awry and result in incarceration, and risky decisions related to sexual behavior can have life-altering consequences. The severity of these potential consequences suggests that prevention and intervention efforts are important, regardless of the severity of the symptoms expressed.

Prevention programs may alleviate some of the social risk factors that contribute to antisocial behavior, and successfully redirect development along a more positive trajectory. Several of the most effective antisocial behavior prevention programs deliver services to adolescents and their families. The Strengthening Families Program is a universal prevention program designed to address issues parents and children face in the transition to adolescence (Spoth, Redmond, & Shin, 2001). The program is administered in seven weekly sessions with concurrent parent and child components, followed by a structured family interaction time. The program focuses on providing parents with strategies to improve monitoring of child behavior, support open communication and bonding, and implement effective discipline strategies. Children are also guided in communicating with parents and managing challenges in peer relationships.

Randomized clinical trials demonstrated that the Strengthening Families Program significantly reduced the onset of adolescent substance use through high school, suggesting that effects are maintained over the course of several years (Spoth, Guyll, & Shin, 2009; Spoth et al., 2001). Moreover, it appears that this reduction in use is due to limited exposure. Thus, parental supervision, communication, and support appear to guide adolescents into friendships with peers who are less likely to seek out drugs and alcohol (Spoth et al., 2001, 2009). This is an excellent example of how preventing exposure to substances during this sensitive period of brain development may divert otherwise at-risk youth from potential addiction and the adverse consequences of experimental use.

Often antisocial behavior involves criminal activity that requires legal intervention. Although it is usually adolescents with life-course-persistent antisocial behavior who engage in more serious criminal activity, this is not always the case. Behavior of this sort is often met with punitive rather than therapeutic responses. However, as described above, punitive responses, whether in school or through the justice system, have little impact in deterring or redirecting antisocial behavior. Equally important, punitive responses may further alienate individuals from prosocial influences, increase their exposure to antisocial peers, and reduce the academic and skill development that would support a positive outcome.

One program that appears effective in reducing the recidivism of adolescents engaged in criminal activity is Functional Family Therapy (Sexton &

Alexander, 1999). Initially developed for first-time status offenders from mostly middle-income families, Functional Family Therapy is a short-term intervention that integrates social-learning and systems theories to motivate family members to change by identifying and building upon unique strengths and offering families specific ways to improve. Like many family interventions, Functional Family Therapy helps enhance parenting skills, promote supportive communication, and reduce negative exchanges, including blaming.

Functional Family Therapy has been replicated independently in several clinical trials with diverse samples, including adolescents who have committed multiple serious offenses. These trials indicate that Functional Family Therapy reduces dramatically the likelihood of being convicted of another crime compared to normal practices in the criminal justice system, such as probation or placement in residential treatment, or other forms of therapy. In one follow-up study, Functional Family Therapy, compared to probation, accounted for an 83 % reduction in recidivism during the remainder of adolescence (11.1 % versus 66.7 % across 2.5 years) and a 79 % reduction during early adulthood (8.7 % versus 40.9 % across 3 years; Gordon, Graves, & Arbuthnot, 1995). There is even some intriguing evidence that Functional Family Therapy can reduce the likelihood that younger siblings in the family will become involved in criminal activity in the first place (Klein, Alexander, & Parsons, 1977).

Adolescents who are involved in the criminal justice system are often mired in an array of risk-exacerbating factors, including low academic achievement (possibly due to low IQ or unaddressed learning disabilities); an antisocial peer network; potential use or dependence on illicit substances; a harsh, hostile, or abusive home environment; and parental antisocial behavior or substance dependence. Multisystemic Therapy (MST) was designed to address the compounding effect of multiple risk factors by focusing on adolescents and the family, peer, school, and community systems within which they are embedded (Henggeler, Cunningham, Schoenwald, Borduin, & Rowland, 2009). MST provides short-term, but intensive, in-home treatment that is problem-focused and highly individualized, based on the resources individual adolescents have access to and the particular challenges they face.

Despite the fact that MST tends to serve adolescents exhibiting serious antisocial behavior, one randomized study showed that—compared to treatment as usual in the Department of Youth Services—it reduced subsequent arrests by 43 % (0.87 versus 1.52), reduced incarceration by 10.4 weeks on average, and improved family cohesion (Henggeler, Melton, & Smith, 1992). In an independent replication, MST, compared to individual therapy, reduced the likelihood of recidivism across 4 years by 63 % (26.1 % versus 71.4 %).

With any intervention program, participation is a critical factor in success. Unfortunately, the investment in terms of both time and mental commitment are high, often serving as a barrier to success for many families. Even when available at no cost, attendance in weekly sessions can be a low priority for busy families. This might be especially true for programs that provide preventive services before serious problems have developed. In the Strengthening Families Program, as many as one-half of the participants assigned to the intervention did not participate in the weekly sessions, indicating that intensive therapeutic programs do not serve the needs of a large number of families (Spoth et al., 2001). Not surprisingly, those families who fail to participate or who drop out of therapeutic programs are often the families with the most risk factors and the greatest need for intervention (Kazdin, Mazurick, & Bass, 1993).

Addressing the diversity of parental needs and motivating drives requires a flexible approach to delivering intervention. In order to accommodate individual and cultural variation in acceptance of mental health intervention, an adaptive program called the Family Check-Up (FCU) was developed (Dishion & Kavanagh, 2003). The FCU model addresses the intervention process in stages, working with each family to deliver the intervention service that best matches expectations and best meets individual needs. After a comprehensive assessment, feedback is delivered to the family and potential goals for treatment are identified and discussed. The clinician then describes a range of empirically supported treatment options that target the family's most salient concerns, and the family selects to participate in specific services from available resources. Not all families select the same level of intervention, and some families forego the intervention most likely to succeed. However, by involving families in the decision-making process, participation is enhanced and some level of intervention is delivered for families who may have otherwise refused treatment. In this way, the dynamic and client-oriented approach to therapy maximizes client buy-in and appears to result in treatment effects on the reduction of substance use that are as large or larger than other prevention programs (Dishion, Kavanagh, Schneiger, Nelson, & Kaufman, 2002).

Despite the effectiveness in increasing intervention participation that the FCU approach has had, biases against seeking mental health support as well as cost, time, and the availability of appropriately trained clinicians still represent significant barriers to access for many families. To address this, researchers have begun to explore alternative dissemination strategies for reaching parents on a global scale. By documenting families engaged in a therapeutic program in a six-part reality TV series, researchers were able to effectively disseminate information related to normative and nonnormative child development, destigmatize and model the value of seeking mental health assistance to deal with problem behaviors, and provide information about where to locate those additional targeted services. Findings suggest that such an approach can result in significant improvements in child behavior and parental reports of their own anger and depression (Calam, Sanders, Miler, Sadhnani, & Carmont, 2008). Web-based programming to supplement the television program was assigned to half of the intervention group, although treatment effects were evident even at the viewing-only level (Sanders, Calam, Durand, Liversidge, & Carmont, 2008; Sanders & Prinz, 2008). Capitalizing on technological advances and integrating educational missions within entertainment media may prove to diversify access to therapeutic strategies and educational information about parenting.

Summary and Conclusions

Although adolescence is a time of significant experimentation and risky decision making, it is not a pathological condition. However, individuals with certain patterns of emotional reactivity and/or deficits in social reinforcement learning may be especially vulnerable during this period. If family relationships are characterized by ongoing and escalating coercive exchanges, adolescents might not have the close relationships necessary for parents to positively influence behavior and provide appropriate guidance. Moreover, this breakdown in family relationships occurs as adolescents spend more unsupervised time, often with similar adolescents who share a propensity for antisocial behavior. Although the limbic system appears to be more advanced than the prefrontal cortex in all adolescents, these more vulnerable adolescents may be especially predisposed to exhibit impulsive, sensation-seeking, reward-focused actions that are less modulated by deliberative consideration of long-term consequences.

There are clear differences between individuals who first display serious antisocial behavior during early childhood and those who first display antisocial behavior during adolescence. However, those differences appear to be ones of degree, not kind. Individuals who first display serious antisocial behavior during early childhood experience a well-documented array of risk factors. Individuals who display antisocial behavior during adolescence may not experience as many of these risk factors at such intense levels. For these vulnerable individuals, however, the changes in family and peer relationships and cognitive and physical maturation that are defining features of normal adolescence might also change dynamics just enough to precipitate the onset of antisocial behavior.

References

American Psychiatric Association. (2000). *Diagnostic and statistical manual of mental disorders* (Revised 4th ed.). Washington, DC: American Psychiatric Association.

Archer, J. (2009). Does sexual selection explain human sex differences in aggression? *The Behavioral and Brain Sciences, 32*, 249–311.

Beauchaine, T. P., Gatzke-Kopp, L., & Mead, H. (2007). Polyvagal theory and developmental psychopathology. Emotion dysregulation and conduct problems from preschool to adolescence. *Biological Psychology, 74*, 174–184.

Bechara, A., Damasio, H., & Damasio, A. R. (2000). Emotion, decision making and the orbitofrontal cortex. *Cerebral Cortex, 10*, 295–307.

Biederman, J., Newcorn, J., & Sprich, S. (1991). Comorbidity of attention deficit hyperactivity disorder with conduct, depressive, anxiety, and other disorders. *The American Journal of Psychiatry, 148*, 564–577.

Brendgen, M., Vitaro, F., & Bukowski, W. M. (2000). Stability and variability of adolescents' affiliation with delinquent friends: Predictors and consequences. *Social Development, 9*, 205–225.

Brown, B. B., Mounts, N., Lamborn, S. D., & Steinberg, L. (1993). Parenting practices and peer group affiliation in adolescence. *Child Development, 64*, 467–482.

Buckholtz, J. W., & Meyer-Lindenberg, A. (2008). MAOA and the neurogenetic architecture of human aggression. *Trends in Neuroscience, 31*, 120–129.

Burt, S. A., Krueger, R. F., McGue, M., & Iacono, W. G. (2001). Sources of covariation among attention-deficit/hyperactivity disorder, oppositional defiant disorder, and conduct disorder: The importance of shared environment. *Journal of Abnormal Psychology, 110*, 516–525.

Burt, S. A., McGue, M., DeMarte, J. A., Krueger, R. F., & Iacono, W. G. (2006). Timing of menarche and the origins of conduct disorder. *Archives of General Psychiatry, 63*, 890–896.

Cairns, R. B., Leung, M., Buchanan, L., & Cairns, B. (1996). Friendships and social networks in childhood and adolescence: Fluidity, reliability, and interrelations. *Social Development, 66*, 1330–1345.

Calam, R., Sanders, M. R., Miler, C., Sadhnani, V., & Carmont, S.-A. (2008). Can technology and the media help reduce dysfunctional parenting and increase engagement with preventative parenting interventions? *Child Maltreatment, 13*, 347–361.

Colby, J. B., Van Horn, J. D., & Sowell, E. R. (2011). Quantitative in vivo evidence for broad regional gradients in the timing of white matter maturation during adolescence. *NeuroImage, 54*, 25–31.

Crick, N. R., Bigbee, M. A., & Howes, C. (1996). Gender differences in children's normative beliefs about aggression: How do I hurt thee? Let me count the ways. *Child Development, 67*, 1003–1014.

Crowley, T. J., Dalwani, M. S., Mikulich-Gilbertson, S. K., Du, Y. P., Lejuez, C. W., Raymond, K. M., et al. (2010). Risky decision and their consequences: Neural processing by boys with antisocial substance disorder. *PLoS One, 5*, e12835.

Dishion, T. J., Bullock, B. M., & Granic, I. (2002). Pragmatism in modeling peer influence: Dynamics, outcomes, and change processes. *Development and Psychopathology, 14*, 969–981.

Dishion, T. J., & Kavanagh, K. (2003). *Intervening in adolescent problem behavior: A family-centered approach*. New York: Guilford Press.

Dishion, T. J., Kavanagh, K., Schneiger, A., Nelson, S., & Kaufman, N. K. (2002). Preventing early adolescent substance use: A family-centered strategy for the public middle school. *Prevention Science, 3*, 191–201.

Dishion, T. J., McCord, J., & Poulin, F. (1999). When interventions harm: Peer groups and problem behavior. *American Psychologist, 54*, 755–764.

Dishion, T. J., Nelson, S. E., & Bullock, B. M. (2004). Premature adolescent autonomy: Parent disengagement and deviant peer process in the amplification of problem behavior. *Journal of Adolescence, 27*, 515–530.

Dishion, T. J., Nelson, S. E., Winter, C. E., & Bullock, B. M. (2004). Adolescent friendship as a dynamic system: Entropy and deviance in the etiology and course of male antisocial behavior. *Journal of Abnormal Child Psychology, 32*, 651–663.

Dodge, K. A. (1986). A social information processing model of social competence in children. In M. Perlmutter (Ed.), *Minnesota symposium in child psychology* (pp. 77–125). Hillsdale, NJ: Lawrence Erlbaum.

Dodge, K. A. (2011). Social information processing as mediators of the interaction between genetic factors and life experiences in the development of aggressive behavior. In P. R. Shaver & M. Mikulincer (Eds.), *Human aggression and violence: Causes, manifestations, and consequences* (pp. 165–185). Washington, DC: American Psychological Association.

Ernst, M., & Fudge, J. L. (2009). A developmental neurobiological model of motivated behavior: Anatomy, connectivity and ontogeny of the triadic nodes. *Neuroscience and Biobehavioral Reviews, 33*, 367–382.

Ernst, M., Grant, S. J., London, E. D., Contoreggi, C. S., Kimes, A. S., & Spurgeon, L. (2003). Decision making in adolescents with behavior disorders and adults with substance abuse. *The American Journal of Psychiatry, 160*, 33–40.

Fairchild, G., Van Goozen, S. H., Stollery, S. J., & Goodyer, I. M. (2008). Fear conditioning and affective modulation of the startle reflex in male adolescents with early-onset or adolescence-onset conduct disorder and healthy control subjects. *Biological Psychiatry, 63*, 279–285.

Fontaine, N., Carbonneau, R., Vitaro, F., Barker, E. D., & Tremblay, R. E. (2009). Research review: A critical review of studies on the developmental trajectories of antisocial behavior in females. *Journal of Child Psychology and Psychiatry, 50*, 363–385.

Galvan, A., Hare, T. A., Parra, C. E., Penn, J., Voss, H., Glover, G., et al. (2006). Earlier development of the accumbens relative to orbitofrontal cortex might underlie risk-taking behavior in adolescents. *Journal of Neuroscience, 26*, 6885–6892.

Gatzke-Kopp, L. M., Beauchaine, T. P., Shannon, K. E., Chipman, J., Fleming, A. P., Crowell, S. E., et al. (2009). Neurological correlates of reward responding in adolescents with conduct disorder and/or attention-deficit/hyperactivity disorder. *Journal of Abnormal Psychology, 118*, 203–213.

Gatzke-Kopp, L. M., Raine, A., Loeber, S., Stouthamer-Loeber, M., & Steinhauer, S. R. (2002). Serious delinquent behavior, sensation-seeking and electrodermal arousal. *Journal of Abnormal Child Psychology, 30*(5), 477–486.

Gordon, D. A., Graves, K., & Arbuthnot, J. (1995). The effect of functional family therapy for delinquents on adult criminal behavior. *Criminal Justice and Behavior, 22*, 60–73.

Granic, I., & Patterson, G. R. (2006). Toward a comprehensive model of antisocial development: A dynamic systems approach. *Psychological Review, 113*, 101–131.

Hall, H. R., Bernat, E. M., & Patrick, C. J. (2007). Externalizing psychopathology and the error-related negativity. *Psychological Science, 18*, 326–333.

Henggeler, S. W., Cunningham, P. B., Schoenwald, S. K., Borduin, C. M., & Rowland, M. D. (2009). *Multisystemic therapy for antisocial behavior in children and adolescents* (2nd ed.). New York: Guilford Press.

Henggeler, S. W., Melton, G. B., & Smith, L. A. (1992). Family preservation using multisystemic therapy: An effective alternative to incarcerating serious juvenile offenders. *Journal of Consulting and Clinical Psychology, 60*, 953–961.

Herpertz, S. C., Huebner, T., Marx, I., Vloet, T. D., Fink, G. R., Stoecker, T., et al. (2008). Emotional processing in male adolescents with childhood-onset conduct disorder. *Journal of Child Psychology and Psychiatry, 49*, 781–791.

Hofvander, B., Ossowski, D., Lundstrom, S., & Anckarsater, H. (2009). Continuity of aggressive antisocial behavior from childhood to adulthood: The question of phenotype definition. *International Journal of Law and Psychiatry, 32*, 224–234.

Horsley, T. A., de Castro, B. O., & Van der Schoot, M. (2010). In the eye of the beholder: Eye-tracking assessment of social information processing in aggressive behavior. *Journal of Abnormal Child Psychology, 38*, 587–599.

Johnston, L. D., O'Malley, P. M., Bachman, J. G., & Schulenberg, J. E. (2009). *Monitoring the future: National results on adolescent drug use*. Bethesda, MD: National Institute on Drug Abuse.

Jones, M., & Westen, D. (2010). Diagnosis and subtypes of adolescent antisocial personality disorder. *Journal of Personality Disorders, 24*, 217–243.

Kazdin, A. E., Mazurick, J. L., & Bass, D. (1993). Risk for attrition in treatment of antisocial children and families. *Journal of Clinical Child Psychology, 22*, 1–16.

Kerr, M., & Stattin, H. (2000). What parents know, how they know it, and several forms of adolescent adjustment: Further support for a reinterpretation of monitoring. *Developmental Psychology, 36*, 366–380.

Klein, N. C., Alexander, J. F., & Parsons, B. V. (1977). Impact of family systems intervention on recidivism and sibling delinquency: A model of primary prevention and program evaluation. *Journal of Consulting and Clinical Psychology, 45*, 469–474.

Krueger, R. F., Hicks, B. M., Patrick, C. J., Carlson, S. R., Iacono, W. G., & McGue, M. (2002). Etiologic connections among substance dependence, antisocial behavior, and personality: Modeling the externalizing spectrum. *Journal of Abnormal Psychology, 111*, 411–424.

Lacourse, E., Nagin, D., Tremblay, R. E., Vitaro, F., & Claes, M. (2003). Developmental trajectories of boys' delinquent group membership and facilitation of violent behaviors during adolescence. *Development and Psychopathology, 15*, 183–197.

Levin, H. S., Culhaneb, K. A., Hartmannb, J., Evankovichb, K., Mattsonb, A. J., Harward, H., et al. (1991). Developmental changes in performance on tests of purported frontal lobe functioning. *Developmental Neuropsychology, 7*, 377–395.

Lewis, M. D., & Todd, R. M. (2007). The self-regulating brain: Cortical-subcortical feedback and the development of intelligent action. *Cognitive Development, 22*, 406–430.

Metcalfe, J., & Mischel, W. (1999). A hot/cool systems analysis of delay of gratification: Dynamics of willpower. *Psychological Review, 106*, 3–19.

Moffitt, T. E. (1993). Adolescence-limited and life-course-persistent antisocial behavior: A developmental taxonomy. *Psychological Review, 100*, 674–701.

Moffitt, T. E., & Caspi, A. (2005). Life-course persistent and adolescence-limited antisocial males: Longitudinal follow up to adulthood. In D. M. Stoff & E. J. Susman (Eds.), *Developmental psychobiology of aggression* (pp. 161–186). New York: Cambridge University Press.

Molero, S. Y., Hodgins, S., Larsson, A., Larm, P., & Tengstrom, A. (2010). Adolescent antisocial behavior as predictor of adverse outcomes to age 50: A follow up study of 1,974 individuals. *Criminal Justice and Behavior, 37*, 158–174.

Mounts, N. S. (2000). Parental management of adolescent peer relationships: What are its effects on friend selection. In K. A. Kerns, J. M. Contreras, & A. M. Neal-Barnett (Eds.), *Family and peers: Linking two social worlds* (pp. 169–193). Westport, CT: Praeger.

Murray, J., & Farrington, D. P. (2010). Risk factors for conduct disorder and delinquency: Key findings from longitudinal studies. *Canadian Journal of Psychiatry, 55*, 633–642.

Odgers, C. L., Moffitt, T. E., Broadbent, J. M., Dickson, N., Hancox, R. J., Harrington, H., et al. (2008). Female and male antisocial trajectories: From childhood origins to adult outcomes. *Development and Psychopathology, 20*, 673–716.

Patterson, G. R. (1982). *Coercive family process*. Eugene, OR: Castalia.

Poulin, F., Dishion, T. J., & Burraston, B. (2001). 3-year iatrogenic effects associated with aggregating high-risk adolescents in cognitive-behavioral preventive interventions. *Applied Developmental Science, 5*, 214–224.

Raine, A. (2008). From genes to brain to antisocial behavior. *Current Directions in Psychological Science, 17*, 323–328.

Roisman, G. I., Aguilar, B., & Egeland, B. (2004). Antisocial behavior in the transition to adulthood: The independent and interactive roles of developmental history and emerging developmental tasks. *Development and Psychopathology, 21*, 417–439.

Roisman, G. I., Monahan, K. C., Campbell, S. B., Steinberg, L., Cauffman, E., & The National Institute of Child Health and Human Development Early Child Care Research Network. (2010). Is adolescence-onset antisocial behavior developmentally normative? *Development and Psychopathology, 22*, 295–311.

Sagvolden, T. A., Johansen, E. B., Aase, H., & Russell, V. A. (2005). A dynamic developmental theory of attention-deficit/hyperactivity disorder (ADHD) predominantly hyperactive/impulsive and combined subtypes. *The Behavioral and Brain Sciences, 28*, 397–419.

Sanders, M. R., Calam, R., Durand, M., Liversidge, T., & Carmont, S. A. (2008). Does self-directed and web-based support for parents enhance the effects of viewing a reality television series based on the Tripe P-Positive Parenting Programme? *Journal of Child Psychology and Psychiatry, 49*, 924–932.

Sanders, M. R., & Prinz, R. J. (2008). Using the mass media as a population level strategy to strengthen parenting skills. *Journal of Clinical Child and Adolescent Psychology, 37*, 609–621.

Seeley, W. W., Menon, V., Schatzberg, A. F., Keller, J., Glover, G. H., Kenna, H., et al. (2007). Dissociable intrinsic connectivity networks for salience processing and executive control. *Journal of Neuroscience, 27*, 2349–2356.

Sexton, T. L., & Alexander, J. F. (1999). *Functional family therapy: Principles of clinical intervention, assessment, and implementation*. Henderson, NV: RCH Enterprises.

Shannon, K. E., Sauder, C., Beauchaine, T. P., & Gatzke-Kopp, L. M. (2009). Disrupted effective connectivity between the medial frontal cortex and the caudate in adolescent boys with externalizing behavior disorders. *Criminal Justice and Behavior, 36*, 1141–1157.

Siever, L. J. (2008). Neurobiology of aggression and violence. *The American Journal of Psychiatry, 165*, 429–442.

Soenens, B., Vansteenkiste, M., & Niemiec, C. P. (2009). Should parental prohibition of adolescents' peer relationships be prohibited? *Personal Relationships, 16*, 507–530.

Somerville, J. H., & Casey, B. J. (2010). Development neurobiology of cognitive control and motivational systems. *Current Opinion in Neurobiology, 20*, 236–241.

Sowell, E. R., Peterson, B. S., Thompson, P. M., Welcome, S. E., Henkenius, A. L., & Toga, A. W. (2003). Mapping cortical change across the human life span. *Nature Neuroscience, 6*, 309–315.

Spoth, R., Guyll, M., & Shin, C. (2009). Universal intervention as a protective shield against exposure to substance use: Long-term outcomes and public health significance. *American Journal of Public Health, 99*, 2026–2033.

Spoth, R. L., Redmond, C., & Shin, C. (2001). Randomized trial of brief family interventions for general populations: Adolescent substance use outcomes 4 years following baseline. *Journal of Consulting and Clinical Psychology, 69*, 627–642.

Stadler, C., Sterzer, P., Schmeck, K., Krebs, A., Kleinschmidt, A., & Poustka, F. (2007). Reduced anterior cingulate activation in aggressive children and adolescents during affective stimulation: Association with temperament traits. *Journal of Psychiatric Research, 41*, 410–417.

Stattin, H., & Kerr, M. (2000). Parental monitoring: A reinterpretation. *Child Development, 71*, 1072–1085.

Steinberg, L. (2001). We know some things: Parent-adolescent relationships in retrospect and prospect. *Journal of Research on Adolescence, 11*, 1–19.

Steinberg, L., Mounts, N. S., Lamborn, S. D., & Dornbusch, S. M. (1991). Authoritative parenting and adolescent adjustment across varied ecological niches. *Journal of Research on Adolescence, 1*, 19–36.

Susman, E. J., Dockray, S., Granger, D. A., Blades, K. T., Randazzo, W., Heaton, J. A., et al. (2010). Cortisol and alpha amylase reactivity and timing of puberty: Vulnerabilities for antisocial behavior in young adolescents. *Psychoneuroendocrinology, 35*, 557–569.

Swanson, H. L. (1999). What develops in working memory? A life span perspective. *Developmental Psychology, 35*, 986–1000.

Vera, J., Ezpeleta, L., Granero, R., & de la Osa, N. (2010). Antisocial behavior, psychopathology and functional impairment: Association with sex and age in clinical children and adolescents. *Child Psychiatry and Human Behavior, 41*, 465–478.

Williams, B. R., Ponesse, J. S., Schachar, R. J., Logan, G. D., & Tannock, R. (1999). Development of inhibitory control across the life span. *Developmental Psychology, 35*, 205–213.

Woodward, L. J., Fergusson, D. M., & Horwood, L. J. (2002). Romantic relationships of young people with childhood and adolescent onset antisocial behavior problems. *Journal of Abnormal Child Psychology, 30*, 231–243.

Yang, Y., & Raine, A. (2009). Prefrontal structural and functional brain imaging findings in antisocial, violent, and psychopathic individuals: A meta analysis. *Psychiatry Research: Neuroimaging, 174*, 81–88.

Zabin, L. S., Emerson, M. R., & Rowland, D. L. (2005). Childhood sexual abuse and early menarche: The direction of their relationship and its implications. *Journal of Adolescent Health, 36*, 393–400.

Personality Disorders in Adolescence

Katherine A. Fowler and Stuart F. White

Personality is intrinsic to our sense of self and each other, and adaptive and maladaptive personality characteristics often help shape the trajectory of personal development. In adolescence, a period fundamentally characterized by rapid and significant emotional, social, and cognitive development, maladaptive changes in personality may be particularly detrimental and hard to understand. This chapter outlines the state of knowledge about personality disorders in adolescence, examines some of the important issues surrounding these disorders, and describes those personality disorders best understood in adolescence.

The most commonly used diagnostic manual for the diagnosis of psychiatric disorders, the DSM-IV-TR (APA, 2000), defines personality disorders broadly. It states: "A Personality Disorder (PD) is an enduring pattern of inner experience and behavior that deviates markedly from the expectations of the individual's culture, is pervasive and inflexible, has an onset in adolescence or early adulthood, is stable over time, and leads to distress or impairment" (p. 629).

This seemingly simple definition is actually quite complex on further inspection, raising both semantic and operational questions. For example, the following terms and phrases, some of which are particularly important when considering the conceptualization and diagnosis of PDs in adolescence, lead to many unanswered questions:

1. *Enduring*: How long must an individual exhibit features of a personality disorder before a diagnosis is applicable? Particularly in the case of diagnosis in adolescence, individuals may have displayed PD features, as they are currently captured by DSM-IV-TR categories, for a very short time.
2. *Pattern*: How consistently over time must an individual exhibit the characteristics in question? Adolescence is a crucial time in identity formation, and behavioral inconsistencies may seem more frequent during this developmental stage than at others.
3. *Deviates markedly*: Whether a deviation is "marked" is clearly subjective. DSM-IV-TR encourages one to consider the individual's context (e.g., family, culture) in making this determination. This is a step in the right direction, as it emphasizes that norms are not universal across all individuals. However, it leads to another question: What constitutes culture? Culture may comprise ethnicity, sexual orientation, socioeconomic status, geographical region, and gender. Can a developmental stage such as adolescence be considered a culture in and of itself, with different norms?
4. *Pervasive and inflexible*: How cross-situationally consistent must personality disorder features be for an individual to meet criteria? For example, can an adolescent meet crite-

K.A. Fowler, Ph.D. • S.F. White, Ph.D. (✉)
National Institute of Mental Health/National Institutes of Health, 9000 Rockville Pike, Building 15K, Bethesda, MD 20892, USA
e-mail: fowlerka@mail.nih.gov; stuart.white@nih.gov

W.T. O'Donohue et al. (eds.), *Handbook of Adolescent Health Psychology*,
DOI 10.1007/978-1-4614-6633-8_29,

ria for a personality disorder if he or she exhibits marked features with peers but not at home?

5. *Onset in adolescence or early adulthood*: How does one discern "onset"? Must the person fully meet criteria, or can some "prodromal" symptoms be included? Particularly in the case of late adolescence and early adulthood, adjusting norms developmentally is a difficult task. How do we find a balance between overpathologizing normal-range teenage behavior and overlooking true pathology? Furthermore, the age limits constituting adolescence and early adulthood are not specified.
6. *Leads to distress/impairment*: What is the threshold for meaningful distress or impairment? And whose distress? Certain personality disorders may be accompanied by a lack of insight and more distress to others than self.

Even beyond these fundamental difficulties in defining personality disorders, several active controversies in the field of personality disorder research are worth mentioning. First, again with respect to defining personality disorders, there is evidence that our current diagnostic categories might be suboptimal. Issues such as high overlap (i.e., comorbidity) among personality disorders call into question their validity and/or existence as independent syndromes. For example, Widiger and Rogers (1989) found that, on average, 85 % of patients who meet criteria for one personality disorder meet criteria for at least one additional personality disorder. Further, the distinction between Axis I and Axis II (where personality disorders fall) psychopathology can be unclear in the case of some PD diagnoses, which some may argue represent subsyndromal variants of Axis I diagnoses.

In both clinical practice and research, there are problems with test-retest reliability (i.e., meeting criteria at different time points within a brief interval) of personality disorder diagnoses (e.g., Loranger, 1988), and the best method for assessing them (e.g., structured or unstructured interviews, self- or other-completed questionnaires, projective techniques) has also been called into question. And to compound all of the issues above (or perhaps in part because of them), the etiology, course, and treatment of most personality disorders is sparsely researched.

Despite all these difficulties, personality disorders are a topic of great interest to researchers, clinicians, and the general public alike. Personality disorder diagnoses frequently bear associations with important social and clinical outcomes (e.g., borderline PD and suicide, schizotypal PD and progression to psychosis). Moreover, when all PDs are taken together, large epidemiological studies have yielded adolescent PD prevalence estimates ranging from 9 to 13 %, higher than many other well-known disorders that impact adolescents, such as eating disorders (Hudson, Hiripi, Pope, & Kessler, 2007), attention-deficit/hyperactivity disorder (ADHD), obsessive-compulsive disorder, and post-traumatic stress disorder (Kessler, Chiu, Demler, & Walters, 2005).

Even within the context of a general paucity of research on most personality disorders, very little research has been done on PDs in adolescence, despite the DSM-IV-TR's suggestion that PDs often emerge during this developmental period. Nonetheless, there are a few PDs that have been the focus of comparatively more research in adolescence. Therefore, despite the fact that the DSM-IV-TR includes ten different PD diagnoses, we will discuss only a subset of these. This chapter will cover the three PDs most researched in adolescent populations: antisocial personality disorder (in this case, its analogue in adolescents, conduct disorder), borderline personality disorder, and schizotypal personality disorder.

For each of these disorders, we will outline the current criteria; describe the disorder in detail; offer a case example; and discuss what is known about the etiology, course, and treatment, all with a particular focus on issues pertaining to adolescent development. Where applicable, we will also discuss what is known about associated social and health (nonmental health) risks. We will conclude by discussing the changing conceptualization of personality disorders, which has arisen as a response to the many difficulties described above, as we move toward DSM-V.

Conduct Disorder

Case Examples

Consider the following three boys, all residing in the same juvenile detention facility. Ryan is a 17-year-old male. He has never known his father and his mother has always worked multiple jobs to support Ryan and his three siblings. Ryan is known as a generally "good kid," but has never been well supervised and has been in trouble for staying out past curfew and throwing parties with alcohol several times. Ryan was convicted of vehicular manslaughter after he was in a serious car accident following an evening of drinking with friends.

Michael is a 13-year-old male. He has an IQ in the "borderline" range and has been diagnosed with several learning disabilities, including ADHD. These impairments are reflected in his very poor educational performance. Michael comes from a dangerous, impoverished neighborhood where drug-related violence is very common. There have been approximately two dozen shootings in his public housing complex in the past 5 years, including several that Michael either witnessed or in which he knew someone involved. Michael was incarcerated after being convicted on assault charges stemming from approximately a dozen fights at school, including one where Michael broke another boy's nose. Michael claims to only fight in self-defense, and states that while he is sorry the other boy's nose was broken, he still feels that the boy should not have threatened him. Teachers indicate that Michael was in fact the one threatening the other student.

John is a 12-year-old male and has been in trouble all his life. John's parents have had him in various treatment programs since he burned his little brother when he was 9 years old "to see what would happen." John's parents have little trouble with their other sons and are well thought of by their community. They indicate that John is not emotionally close to them and they are frightened of him. Recently, John was convicted of murdering an elderly woman that his mother helped care for. When asked about the crime, John indicated that he set the woman on fire after she threatened to report his numerous thefts of her possessions to the police. Laughing, John told a clinician that he had, in fact, been stealing from the woman.

Description and Epidemiology

Antisocial behavior, particularly in adolescence, has a number of implications for adolescent health. Antisocial behavior in the context of conduct disorder, typified by aggressive behaviors, property damage, theft, and serious violations of rules (APA, 2000), is associated with increased risk of physical injury and death, incarceration, substance abuse, sexually transmitted diseases, and teen pregnancy (Moffitt, Caspi, Dickson, Silva, & Stanton, 1996). Antisocial behavior is so common in adolescents that it appears to be a part of the normal teen experience (Elliott, Ageton, Huizinga, Knowles, & Canter, 1983; Moffitt, 1993). Despite the high prevalence of adolescent antisocial behavior, most teens do not suffer lasting health and social problems from these acts; however, for the seriously antisocial and some unlucky few, the impact of delinquent behavior can have serious, long-term consequences (Frick & White, 2008; Moffitt et al., 1996).

Antisocial behavior has several different categorical designations in the current DSM-IV nomenclature, including antisocial personality disorder (APD) and conduct disorder (CD) (APA, 2000). While APD, by definition, cannot be diagnosed before age 18 (APA, 2000), evidence supports a hierarchical relationship between conduct disorder (CD) and APD, in which adults with APD are required to have at least a positive history of CD symptoms and most likely met criteria for CD during adolescence (Burke, Waldman, & Lahey, 2010). This indicates that CD should be viewed as a precursor to the onset of APD in adolescence.

Nevertheless, antisocial youth are a heterogeneous group, as shown in the case examples, with distinct causal mechanisms and correlates (Frick & White, 2008; Moffitt, 1993; 2003). Only some youth diagnosed with CD will go on to develop APD (Burke et al., 2010), with youth from some subgroups of CD much more likely than others to do so (Frick & Dickens, 2006; Moffitt, 2003). The DSM-IV recognizes two subgroups of antisocial behavior, childhood-onset CD and adolescent-onset CD (APA, 2000). Furthermore, research has identified a third subtype, CD with callous-unemotional (CU) traits, which will likely be included in DSM-V (Frick & Moffitt, 2010). The diagnostic criteria for all the subtypes are identical; however, childhood-onset CD requires the presence of symptoms before age 10, and CD with CU traits requires the presence of additional symptoms, namely, a lack of guilt and empathy; a cold, callous interpersonal style; and a willingness to manipulate others for personal gain.

In order to meet overall CD criteria, a youth must display at least three of the following symptoms in the previous 12 months, one of which must have occurred in the previous 6 months: (1) often bullies, threatens, or intimidates others; (2) often initiates physical fights; (3) has used a weapon that can cause serious physical harm to others; (4) has been physically cruel to people; (5) has been physically cruel to animals; (6) has stolen while confronting a victim; (7) has forced someone into sexual activity; (8) has deliberately engaged in fire setting; (9) has deliberately destroyed others' property (other than by fire setting); (10) has broken into someone else's house, building, or car; (11) often lies to obtain goods or favors or to avoid obligations; (12) has stolen items of nontrivial value without confronting a victim; (13) often stays out at night despite parental prohibitions, beginning before age 13 years; (14) has run away from home overnight at least twice while living in parental or parental surrogate home (or once without returning for a lengthy period); or (15) is often truant from school, beginning before age 13 years.

Prevalence of CD has been estimated at between 1 and 10 % of the general population (APA, 2000); however, rates vary widely depending on subtype and age of onset. In a large-scale longitudinal study of the Dunedin, New Zealand, community, Moffitt and colleagues found that approximately 7 % of the sample could be categorized as childhood-onset CD, while 23 % of the sample were categorized as adolescent-onset CD (Moffitt et al., 1996). Furthermore, they found the male to female ratio in the childhood-onset group to be 10:1, while the ratio fell to 1.5:1 in the adolescent-onset CD group (Moffitt & Caspi, 2001). Estimates of the number of youth with CD with CU traits range from 32 to 50 % of those with CD, and most in this subgroup are categorized as childhood-onset (Christian, Frick, Hill, Tyler, & Frazer, 1997; Kahn, Frick, Youngstrom, Findling, & Youngstrom, n.d.; Rowe et al., 2009).

Etiology, Course, and Outcome

Despite being grouped together, the subtypes of conduct disorder differ in etiology, course, and outcome. Adolescent-onset CD is proposed to be a result of failing to meet the demands of adolescence. Moffitt (1993, 2003) suggests that all adolescents show some rebelliousness and seek greater autonomy from their parents to assert their own identity. However, in adolescent-onset CD, this process is exaggerated or becomes extreme and crosses the line into antisocial delinquent behavior (Moffitt, 1993; 2003). Ryan, for example, is likely not a particularly abnormal teenager, but did not receive the necessary supervision. While youth with adolescent-onset CD tend to stop behaving antisocially by early adulthood, there are often long-term consequences to their behaviors, such as poor educational achievement and the stigma of incarceration (Moffitt et al., 1996).

Childhood-onset CD tends to be more severe and chronic relative to adolescent-onset CD (Moffitt, 1993; 2003). It can also be further subdivided into youth with or without callous-unemotional (CU) traits (Frick, 2006; Frick & White, 2008). Even within the childhood-onset CD group, the presence or absence of CU traits has important and unique implications for the severity (Frick & Dickens, 2006), emotional, cognitive (Frick & White, 2008), and neurocognitive correlates of CD (Blair, 2010), as well as unique etiological correlates (Blair, 2010; Frick & White, 2008). While DSM-IV does not currently recognize these distinctions, current DSM-V proposals include a "with CU traits"

(Frick & Moffitt, 2010) specifier to acknowledge the important differences between the two groups of youth.

Most youth with childhood-onset CD do not have CU traits, but do have troubled backgrounds (Frick & Moffitt, 2010). Childhood-onset CD without CU traits is more strongly associated with poor parenting, socioeconomic hardship, and other environmental factors than is CD with CU traits (Hipwell et al., 2007; Oxford, Cavell, & Hughes, 2003; Wootton, Frick, Shelton, & Silverthorn, 1997). CD without CU traits is associated with lower IQ, particularly verbal IQ (Loney, Frick, Ellis, & McCoy, 1998; Salekin, Neumann, Leistico, & Zalot, 2004); psycho-neurological dysfunction (Moffitt, 1993); and increased levels of fear and anxiety (Frick, Lilienfeld, Ellis, Loney, & Silverthorn, 1999). It has been theorized that these types of risk factors combine to create situations that contribute to the development of antisocial behavior. For example, youth may exhibit a "hostile attribution bias," in which the youth incorrectly perceives the actions or intentions of others as hostile even when they are not (Crick & Dodge, 1994) or a situation may arise where increasingly combative and negative interactions between youth and their parents create a dynamic in which children are inconsistently and poorly disciplined and the parent-child relationship becomes cold and distant (Patterson, Reid, & Dishion, 1998). These factors predispose children with childhood-onset CD to increased and inappropriate levels of "reactive aggression," that is, aggression in response to perceived provocation (Berkowitz, 1993). Michael is a good example of this subtype of CD.

Conduct disorder with CU traits appears to have different causal mechanisms. In addition to reactive aggression, youth with CU traits also exhibit goal-oriented aggression (e.g., aggression with a purpose such as stealing) and, as opposed to youth with CD without CU traits, they are much less likely to feel remorse or guilt or to express empathy for their victims (Frick, 2006). As noted above, the genetic influence on antisocial behavior in CD with CU traits appears to be much higher than in CD without CU traits (Viding, Blair, Moffitt, & Plomin, 2005) and several studies show the stability of CU traits from adolescence to adulthood (Blonigen, Hicks, Kruger, Patrick, & Iacono, 2006; Burke, Loeber, & Lahey, 2007; Lynam, Caspi, Moffitt, Loeber, & Stouthamer-Loeber, 2007). Furthermore, youth with CD and CU traits do not have the IQ deficits commonly associated with CD without CU traits (Loney et al., 1998; Salekin et al., 2004) and there is preliminary evidence that the neurobiological impairment associated with CD with CU traits is specific to the amygdala and frontal lobe regions that are highly interconnected with the amygdala, including the orbitofrontal cortex and ventromedial prefrontal cortex (Blair, 2010). An emerging body of evidence suggests that this amgydala dysfunction interferes with the recognition of fear and distress in others (Blair, 2010) and thereby disrupts socialization, possibly by reducing response to punishment and normal socialization techniques (Dadds & Salmon, 2003; White & Frick, 2010) or by interfering with the normal cognitive and emotional processes that keep mammalian aggression within adaptive limits (Blair, Mitchell, & Blair, 2005). Children like John are prototypical examples of youth with CD with CU traits.

Assessment and Treatment

Unlike other disorders, there has not been discussion about large-scale changes to the current CD criteria. Problems of inter-rater reliability and validity that plagued earlier versions of the DSM appear to have been resolved, or are at least not pressing enough to be a major focus of the DSM-V Work Group (Pardini, Frick, & Moffitt, 2010). A wide variety of measures, including the Child Behavior Checklist (Achenbach, 1991) and the Behavior Assessment System for Children (Reynolds & Kamphaus, 2004), among others, have been found to be both reliable and valid for assessing CD across development.

Despite these improvements in assessment, whether to classify broad-based antisocial behavior as a personality disorder remains unclear. As noted previously, personality disorders are defined by DSM-IV as pervasive patterns of inner experience and behavior that *differ substantially from cultural norms* (APA, 2000). In adults, persistent violations of social norms and rules result in a diagnosis of antisocial personality disorder. However, given that the presence of some degree of antisocial behavior in adolescence has been described as normal (Elliot et al., 1983; Moffitt, 1993), making a case for adolescent-onset CD as a personality disorder is difficult as these behaviors are an exaggeration of, not a deviation from, culturally normative behavior. And while many youth may at first appear to meet criteria for childhood-onset CD without CU traits, there is a hurdle: The importance of environmental factors in maintaining CD symptoms and the availability of effective treatments for CD imply childhood-onset CD without CU traits is more similar to other Axis I clinical disorders. In the face of these facts it is difficult to argue that CD without CU traits can be described as a "pervasive pattern of inner experience." Indeed, CD is currently classified as an Axis I disorder and not as a personality disorder.

Childhood-onset CD with CU traits, however, presents much more like a personality disorder. While there do appear to be strong genetic and biological risk factors for CU traits, environmental factors play a role in the etiology of CD with CU traits (White & Frick, 2010). The combination of these genetic/biological and environmental risk factors do appear to produce a pervasive pattern of inner experience (i.e., problems recognizing fear and distress in others) and behavior (i.e., antisocial behavior and violence) that violate cultural norms. Furthermore, while there is some evidence that CU traits do decrease over time and with treatment (Frick, Kimonis, Dandreaux, & Farell, 2003; Lynam et al., 2007; White, Frick, Lawing, & Bauer, 2012), treatment programs with these youth have been much less successful relative to other subtypes of CD. Furthermore, antisocial adults with CU traits commit more crimes, are much more likely to be incarcerated, and are greater institutional management problems than other antisocial adults (Frick & Dickens, 2006).

A number of treatments have been shown to be effective in treating CD. In younger youth with CD (ages 7–13), Parent Management Training, Oregon Model (Patterson, Reid, Jones, & Conger, 1975), which focuses on teaching parents effective parenting strategies and skills, and Problem-Solving Skills Training (Kazdin & Weisz, 2003), which focuses on teaching children more effective problem-solving skills, have substantial evidence to support their use (Eyberg, Nelson, & Boggs, 2008). In adolescents, multisystemic therapy (Henggeler & Lee, 2003) and Multidimensional Treatment Foster Care (Chamberlain & Smith, 2003) have a base of evidence supporting their use (Eyberg et al., 2008). Both of these interventions have an intensive, holistic approach and seek to improve a youth's home life, both interpersonally and economically, and school life and to reduce the influence of deviant peers. However, not all youth appear to respond to treatment equally well. Youth with CD and CU traits in particular have a much poorer record in terms of treatment success than other CD youth (Falkenbach, Poythress, & Heide, 2003; Gretton, McBride, Hare, Shaughnessy, & Kumka, 2001; O'Neill, Lidz, & Heilbrun, 2003; Spain, Douglas, Poythress, & Epstein, 2004). Despite these findings, studies have shown that youth with CD and CU traits can benefit from treatment, though more intensive interventions may be required (Caldwell, Skeem, Salekin, & Van Rybroek, 2006; White, Frick, Lawing, & Bauer, 2012).

Borderline Personality Disorder

Case Example

Jane is a 12-year-old female. She has been referred to an inpatient facility due to aggression toward her foster mother and others, and self-injurious behavior. She has a history of being sexually abused by her mother's boyfriend, starting at approximately age four, and neglect by her mother. Her mother has recently given up custody and parental rights, and is thereby barred from contact with Jane until she turns 18. Jane has been in and out of foster care and inpatient care for several years prior to this hospitalization. At the facility, Jane exhibits sexual behavior that is inappropriate for her age and environment toward male staff and patients. For example, Jane regularly attempts to leave the unit wearing tops many sizes too small and/or without underwear. During her hospitalization, Jane has exhibited extreme emotional volatility. For example, she frequently rapidly goes from physical affection and touching (e.g., hugs, inappropriate touching) to angry outbursts and aggression, often triggered by any kind of redirection. Jane displays several kinds of manipulative behavior, such as offering to perform required tasks (e.g., school work and unit chores) in exchange for special treatment. Also, she attempts to gain extra favors in exchange for de-escalating aggressive behavior. In one instance, Jane threatened to hit staff members with a chair, but said that she would put it down if she were given extra free time that morning.

Description and Epidemiology

Borderline personality disorder (BPD) is described as one of the most "crippling and frequently lethal" psychiatric illnesses (Goodman et al., 2010). It is estimated to affect 2 % of the general population, 20 % of psychiatric inpatients (Goodman et al., 2010), and 30–60 % of psychiatric populations with personality disorders (DSM-IV-TR; APA, 2000). It is much more frequently diagnosed in women (75 % women; however, see Zlotnick, Rothschild, & Zimmerman, 2002, for a review and discussion of possible gender bias in diagnosis of BPD).

According to the criteria outlined in DSM-IV-TR, BPD comprises the following symptoms (five or more are required for diagnosis): (1) frantic efforts to avoid real or imagined abandonment; (2) a pattern of unstable and intense interpersonal relationships characterized by extremes of idealization and devaluation; (3) identity disturbance; (4) impulsivity in at least two areas that are potentially self-damaging; (5) recurrent suicidal behavior, gestures, or threats, or self-mutilating behavior; (6) affective instability due to marked reactivity of mood; (7) chronic feelings of emptiness; (8) inappropriate, intense anger or difficulty controlling anger; or (9) transient, stress-related paranoid ideation or severe dissociative symptoms.

One aspect of BPD that makes it especially troubling (and as referred to above, potentially lethal) is its association with greater risk for suicide. According to DSM-IV-TR, up to 10 % of those meeting BPD criteria eventually commit suicide, a rate 50 times greater than that of the general population (APA, 2000).

Etiology, Course, and Outcome

Identification of BPD and other personality disorders during adolescence is typically discouraged. Unfortunately, this has at least two important implications: (1) important precursors may be missed, and (2) little is known about its developmental antecedents (Goodman et al., 2010).

In fact, there is mounting evidence that BPD may have discernible developmental antecedents, including a childhood onset for some people (Bernstein et al., 1993). Many BPD patients may exhibit early signs: For example, two thirds of BPD patients with a history of deliberate self-harm first started to mutilate themselves as children or adolescents (Zanarini, Frankenburg, Ridolfi et al., 2006), and signs such as abnormal moodiness (Mangelsdorf, Shapiro, & Marzolf, 1995) have been observed even in infancy in patients who later develop BPD (Goodman et al., 2010). Nevertheless, it is very important to likewise note that most children who display features of BPD do not go on to meet criteria for BPD as adults (Lofgren, Bemporad, King, Lindem, & O'Driscoll, 1991).

There is evidence that several integral risk factors for BPD occur in childhood or adolescence, making these developmental periods etiologically important. Family and early experiences appear to be important in the development of BPD in numerous ways. For one, there is some evidence of moderate heritability of BPD symptoms (e.g., Torgerson et al., 2000). Further, parental psychopathology appears to be a risk factor for development of BPD, particularly parental anxiety, substance abuse, depression, and antisocial behavior (Bradley, Jenei, & Westen, 2005; Goldman, D'Angelo, & DeMaso, 1993), which are hypothesized to reflect familial tendencies toward negative affectivity and impulsivity (Bradley et al., 2005).

Moreover, extant empirical evidence indicates that a high percentage of BPD patients report adverse environmental events such as abuse, neglect, trauma, or disturbances in family structure as part of their childhood histories, and that many of these reported events tend to co-occur. There is converging empirical evidence from large-scale epidemiological and clinical samples that the following constitute consistent risk factors for BPD (Zanarini & Frankenburg, 2007):

- Early separations and losses in childhood histories (e.g., Akiskal et al., 1985; Zanarini et al., 1997)
- Disturbed relationships with or absence of one or both parents (e.g., Goldberg, Mann, Wise, & Segall, 1985; Paris & Frank, 1989)
- Verbal and emotional childhood abuse (e.g., Zanarini et al., 1997; Zanarini, Gunderson, Marino, Schwartz, & Frankenburg, 1988)
- Sexual abuse (less frequently present for milder cases, and also more one-time occurrences for milder cases) (e.g., Salzman et al., 1993; Zanarini et al., 1997)
- Emotional neglect (Zanarini et al., 1997)

It is difficult to weight the importance of different types of trauma for the development of BPD; it is likely specific to the individual. Still, it is worth noting that of these factors, emotional neglect particularly distinguishes patients with BPD.

Many contemporary theorists believe that BPD is not appropriately categorized as a personality disorder. Rather, more recent conceptualizations of BPD describe it as an emotion regulation (e.g., Linehan, 1993) or affective spectrum disorder, with concurrent impulse control problems (Links, Heslegrave, & van Reekum, 1999; Zanarini, 1993). Zanarini and Frankenburg (2007) posit that BPD is defined by intense inner pain, maladaptive strategies to cope with that pain, a "hyperbolic temperament" (i.e., one that tends to go to extremes and is very reactive), emotional dysregulation, and disinhibition. They add that the interpersonal difficulties observed in BPD result from this hyperbolic temperament, in that it involves a propensity to take offense, and to insist that others pay attention to the greatness of the person's inner pain. Although it was once thought that a "triggering" event marking symptom onset most often occurred in adolescence, Zanarini et al. add that it can also occur in childhood or young adulthood. They further suggest that the interaction of one or more triggering or "kindling" events and vulnerable or hyperbolic temperament leads to emergence of acute symptoms of BPD. Additionally, temperamental vulnerability (e.g., high neuroticism, low agreeableness, both characteristic of BPD; Clarkin, Hull, Cantor, & Sanderson, 1993; Morey & Zanarini, 2000; Trull, Widiger, Lynam, & Costa, 2003) is likely to interact with childhood adversity. Kindling events, for example, could be more or less normative events viewed through the lens of a hypervigilant child (Zanarini & Frankenburg, 2007).

There is an accumulation of preliminary evidence that suggests biological contributions to this vulnerability, including problems with neurotransmitters such as serotonin, dopamine, acetylcholine, and vasopression; deficits in hypothalamic-pituitary-adrenal (HPA) axis functioning; and dysfunction in frontolimbic brain circuitry (*see* Crowell, Beauchaine, & Linehan, 2009 for a synopsis).

A relatively recent large-sample longitudinal study (McLean Study of Adult Development; Zanarini, Frankenburg, Hennen, Reich, & Silk, 2005) suggests that BPD has a better prognosis than previously thought. Although BPD is a significant risk factor for suicide, suicide in their sample was substantially less common than expected (4 % vs. the predicted 10 %). Furthermore, contrary to what is commonly thought about BPD (and PDs in general), remission of BPD symptoms was common, and recurrences were relatively rare; about two thirds of BPD patients in their sample experienced a remission of symptoms within the 6-year period they were tracked and less than 6 % of those patients met criteria for a recurrence of BPD over that time. This differs from classic conceptualizations of a personality disorder as a fixed part of a person's "character" and is an encouraging finding.

Acute severity of BPD is posited by some (e.g., Zanarini & Frankenburg, 2007) to be determined by severity of temperamental predisposition combined with severity of the kindling event. However, it is important to note that a severe course should not be assumed even given a severe acute presentation. According to Zanarini and Frankenburg, four factors seem to distinguish severity of the course of BPD:

- Number of co-occurring Axis I disorders, in particular, co-occurring anxiety disorders (*see* Zanarini, Frankenburg, & Parachani, 2004)
- Degree of interpersonal impairment
- Strength of patient's will to get better
- Patient's ability to use treatment to help themselves

With respect to other mental health problems, up to 80–90 % of BPD patients meet criteria for a co-occurring mood or anxiety disorder. Additionally, substance abuse and eating disorders frequently co-occur with BPD (Zanarini, Frankenburg, Dubo et al., 1998). With respect to medical comorbidity, BPD bears an association with several other medical problems, including fibromyalgia, chronic fatigue, substance abuse and smoking, and obesity (Frankenburg & Zanarini, 2006).

Assessment and Treatment

There is little work in the domain of adolescent BPD assessment. Systematic assessment with an eye toward developmental norms is just as important for BPD as for other personality disorders. Some BPD criteria may be particularly difficult to disentangle from normative adolescent characteristics. For example, some degree of identity disturbance, unstable relationships, and impulsivity are likely to be observable during some transient period of a young person's life as he or she matures and becomes independent from parents and more peer influenced.

In one promising line of research, however, Crick, Murray-Close, and Woods (2005) demonstrated preliminary evidence that BPD can be meaningfully assessed in childhood. For example, Crick et al. demonstrated that BPD symptoms could be reliably and validly assessed in a large population of preadolescents, and that these features showed moderate stability over a 2-year time period. They administered developmentally appropriate measures of heightened cognitive sensitivity/hostile, paranoid worldview; intense, unstable, inappropriate emotion (i.e., emotional sensitivity); overly close relationships (e.g., exclusivity with a best friend); and impulsivity (in physical and relational aggression) to their sample at several time points. Most of these indicators, excluding emotional sensitivity, predicted overall borderline PD scores even when controlling for depressive symptoms. At this time, however, their measure, the Borderline Personality Features Scale for Children (BPFS-C), is appropriately used in a research context only.

As for treatment, for adult BPD, psychotherapy is designated as the first-line treatment. Three comprehensive psychotherapies for BPD show promising empirical support with adolescent and/or adult patients with BPD: dialectical behavior therapy (DBT; Miller, Rathus, & Linehan, 2007), mentalization-based therapy (MBT; Bateman & Fonagy, 1999), and schema-focused therapy (SFT; Giesen-Bloo et al., 2006). It is noted that "aggressive polypharmacy" is common in the treatment of patients with BPD (Zanarini et al., 2004; Zanarini, Frankenburg, Khera, & Bleichmar, 2001), despite the fact that pharmacological treatment of BPD is currently considered an adjunct to psychotherapy (Zanarini & Frankenburg, 2007), and the fact that there is little empirical evidence supporting its efficacy.

Schizotypal PD

Case Example

Wayne is a 34-year-old Caucasian male who lives in an "apartment" above the garage of his elderly parents' home. As an adolescent, he was considered "strange" by others, but was still accepted by his peers. As he matured, however, he became increasingly withdrawn and no longer maintains friendships. He is currently employed driving an airport taxi shuttle, although he recently transitioned to a more part-time position at the company. Although Wayne had initially coveted the longer shifts, he was finding himself exhausted after each workday. This was largely because Wayne could not shake the feeling that even though the passengers were strangers, they were often taking special notice of him; it sometimes felt like eyes were piercing into the back of his head. After an incident when a passenger complained to Wayne's manager that she felt uncomfortable with the way Wayne was smiling at her in the rear view mirror, management decided it would be best if he took more time off. This news was a relief to Wayne, although he complains of missing his old regular shuttle; Wayne cannot shake the feeling that driving car 131 somehow magically made passengers more generous with tips, even though all the shuttles look the same.

Wayne spends most of his free time on the Internet, actively participating in chat-boards discussing conspiracies about the US Government covering up the existence of ghosts. Wayne is fairly certain that there may be ghost in his neighborhood, as he occasionally sees fleeting shapes, colorful orbs, and shadows flicker out of the corner of his eyes. Although Wayne seems to really enjoy participating in these chat rooms, this often causes him considerable distress afterward, as he feels suspicious that "someone" may be monitoring his Internet activity. Wayne has complained about this to his mother, but when she asks whom, he is unable to say, as this impression is vague. In general, Wayne is not very social, as he feels anxious around others. Wayne's mother feels concerned about her son's isolation; this behavior seems familiar, as her older brother was the same way. When she tries to encourage Wayne to make better friends, he feels incredibly irritated, and explains that his anxiety stays the same no matter how well he knows people. Although Wayne feels his mother is his best friend, Wayne does not feel like she will understand that this anxiety is not associated with poor self-esteem, but rather a feeling that people are out to get him.

Description and Epidemiology

Schizotypal personality disorder (SPD) is summarized in DSM-IV-TR as a "pattern of acute discomfort in close relationships, cognitive or perceptual distortions, and eccentricities of behavior." The following symptoms comprise SPD (five or more are required for diagnosis): (1) ideas of reference (excluding delusions of reference); (2) odd beliefs or magical thinking that influences behavior and is inconsistent with subcultural norms; (3) unusual perceptual experiences, including bodily illusions; (4) odd thinking and speech; (5) suspiciousness or paranoid ideation; (6) inappropriate or constricted affect; (7) behavior or appearance that is odd, eccentric, or peculiar; (8) lack of close friends or confidants other than first-degree relatives; and (9) excessive social anxiety that does not diminish with familiarity and tends to be associated with paranoid fears rather than negative judgments about self.

With respect to differential diagnosis, SPD should not occur exclusively during the course of a disorder involving psychosis, such as schizophrenia or a mood disorder with psychotic features (which could better account for most symptoms), and does not occur within the context of pervasive developmental disorder (which could better account for inappropriate or constricted affect and a lack of relationships, and behavioral eccentricities).

According to DSM-IV-TR (APA, 2000), SPD is estimated to occur in approximately 3 % of the general population. Like schizophrenia, SPD most often emerges in the developmental period ranging from adolescence to young adulthood.

SPD is distinguished from most other personality disorders by a rich history of theory and a strong backbone of empirical evidence. Clinical observations dating back to Kraeplin (1919/1971) and Bleuler (1924) document a syndrome in the biological relatives of schizophrenic patients that appears to comprise attenuated versions of the core symptoms of schizophrenia. Meehl (1962) coined the terms "schizotaxia" to describe a heritable biologically based vulnerability to schizophrenia that either progresses to the full syndrome or to subsyndromal "schizotypy."

Etiology, Course, and Outcome

As noted previously, SPD is estimated to occur in about 3 % of the general population, about three to four times the estimated prevalence rate of schizophrenia (1 %). Large-scale studies such as the Danish Adoption Study (Kety et al., 1968), which included biological relatives of adoptees diagnosed with schizophrenia in young adulthood and normal adoptees, documented that rates of schizophrenia in the relatives of schizophrenic adoptees were significantly higher (5.3 % vs. 1.8 %), strongly suggesting a genetic contribution. Using this same dataset, Kendler, Gruenberg, and Strauss (1981) retrospectively diagnosed SPD in a subset of the biological relatives. In keeping with their predictions, they found higher rates of SPD in relatives of schizophrenic adoptees (10.5 %) than in controls (1.5 %).

This body of literature raises the possibility that schizophrenia and SPD are different phenotypic expressions of a common genetic vulnerability. Several behavioral genetics studies (e.g., Farmer, McGuffin, & Gottesman, 1987; Torgerson & Kringlen, 1991) have shown that monozygotic (MZ; i.e., identical) co-twins of schizophrenic individuals are more likely to meet criteria for SPD than dizygotic (DZ; i.e., fraternal) co-twins, which is interpreted as evidence for shared genetic vulnerability. The way in which this genetic vulnerability is transmitted is still unknown, but assumed to be polygenic, and it is also unknown whether this polygenotype is the same or different for SPD vs. schizophrenia (Bollini & Walker, 2007).

Above and beyond family associations, schizophrenia and SPD share a developmental link: Signs of SPD and/or full-syndrome SPD in adolescence very often predate the onset of schizophrenia. This has raised an important question: Is SPD simply prodromal (i.e., early symptoms indicating the onset of an attack or disease) schizophrenia?

Put succinctly, the answer is no. Nevertheless, SPD certainly indicates a significant risk for schizophrenia: 20–40 % of young adults with SPD develop schizophrenia within 1–5 years (Miller et al., 2002). Miller et al. (2002) found that the single SPD symptom with the best power to predict progression to schizophrenia appears to be social withdrawal: 42 % of patients above their threshold for this symptom developed a psychiatric illness, while 97 % below the threshold did not. The presence vs. absence of a combination of four groups of symptoms (social withdrawal, psychotic-like symptoms, socioemotional dysfunction, and odd behavior) correctly categorized 67 % of later-ill and 99 % of later-well patients.

Despite the utility of SPD as a prospective indicator of schizophrenia, these estimates have a flip side: Taking their inverse, 60–80 % of young adults with SPD do not go on to develop schizophrenia within 1–5 years. Therefore, we must conclude that there is more than one course and outcome for SPD.

Adolescents with SPD show lower-but-present signs of neurological abnormalities experienced by individuals with schizophrenia, including movement anomalies and impaired neurocognitive function (Mittal et al., 2007; Trotman et al., 2006). Additionally, recent unpublished findings suggest that as many as 50 % of patients in a group described as "clinical high risk" on the basis of attenuated psychotic symptoms and/or genetic risk or functional deterioration "progress" to SPD (Schlosser, Jacobson, Niendam, Bearden, & Cannon, 2012). Interestingly, in this sample, the SPD group exhibited lower-level positive symptoms than the group that later converted to psychosis, but was similar in functional impairment, leading Schlosser et al. to conclude that SPD is appropriately characterized as a "persistent functional disability." This suggests that a large subgroup of individuals at high risk for psychosis progress to SPD and stabilize at an impaired but nonpsychotic level of functioning.

Assessment and Treatment

It is particularly important for providers, parents, and educators who interact with adolescents to be aware of the signs and symptoms of SPD and schizophrenia. Signs such as social withdrawal, while highly predictive, must be carefully evaluated against normal teenage behavior as well as the context of the young person's life. For example, is the adolescent withdrawn at home, but maintaining social functioning at school? Have his or her friends noticed any changes? Is this a change from baseline for this particular individual? For example, is this adolescent a shy child who happens to be going through an awkward phase? Is there a possible external reason for withdrawal from friends, such as bullying or exclusion in the adolescent's friend group? Conversely, is this a dramatic and social withdrawal in a formerly gregarious child in all aspects of his or her life?

There are, however, symptoms of SPD that are relatively easier to distinguish from normal development. The "psychotic-like" symptoms referred to by Miler et al. above include particularly odd beliefs such as ideas of reference (i.e., beliefs that innocuous, unrelated phenomena have a personal significance to the individual, or *refer* to them), magical thinking (i.e., evidence of belief in irrational causal associations between the individual's actions or rituals and outcomes in the world), and paranoia (i.e., the irrational belief that others are out to do harm to the person). Additionally, odd behaviors that may be a by-product of these beliefs (e.g., not using e-mail because the FBI might be monitoring one's communications, avoiding contact with former friends because of a suspicion that they are not who they claim to be, etc.) are more easily distinguished from normal development. It is important to note, however, that unusual beliefs associated with SPD should fall below the threshold for a delusion (i.e., the individual should be capable of questioning their validity). Further, it is important to place even seemingly odd beliefs and rituals in the context of a young person's subculture.

This brings up the importance of careful diagnosis. All psychiatric disorders should be carefully diagnosed, of course, but psychotic disorders are unfortunately particularly stigmatized, and misdiagnosis can bear heavy implications, both in the case of false positives (e.g., unfairly restricting a person's opportunities) and false negatives (e.g., foregoing potentially beneficial treatment). Fortunately, there are several well-validated measures for SPD, falling in two basic categories: broad-based structured clinical interviews targeting personality disorders, such as the Structured Clinical Interview for DSM-IV Axis II Personality Disorders (SCID-II; First, Gibbon, Spitzer, Williams, & Benjamin, 1997) and the Structured Interview for DSM-IV Personality (SIDP-IV; Pfohl, Blum, & Zimmerman, 1994), and measures specific to SPD, which include self-report. In the latter category, the revised Structured Interview for Schizotypy (SIS-R; Vollema & Ormel, 2000) comprises both clinician and self-ratings; and the Schizotypal Personality Questionnaire (SPQ; Raine, 1991) and Kings Schizotypy Questionnaire (KSQ; Wiliiams, 1993) employ only self-ratings. All of the above measures exhibit good psychometric properties, including high test-retest reliability and high internal consistency.

Interest in prevention of psychopathology, including psychotic disorders, has increased in the past several decades. Accordingly, there has been a demand for systematic investigation of the best way to intervene during prodromal schizophrenia (which, as mentioned previously, highly overlaps with SPD). As outlined by Larson, Walker, and Compton (2010) in a recent review, the "clinical staging" model of treatment indicates using simpler, safer, less invasive methods (e.g., psychoeducation, omega-3 fatty acids) preceding psychotic onset, then shifting to more aggressive treatment (e.g., antipsychotic medications) post-psychotic onset. It should be noted once again, however, that the choice to pursue preventative treatment for an adolescent with SPD should be balanced against the possibility of stigmatization, adverse events and side effects of medication (including excessive weight gain and associated problems), and importantly, a dearth of evidence for the effectiveness of early intervention. The current status of treatment for SPD, therefore, can be summarized as follows: Research on prodromal intervention is still nascent at this time, and important parameters such as when to start treatment and its duration have not been well established. The primary benefits of early treatment that some patients experience appear to include symptom reduction and delay of psychosis onset while actively engaged in treatment, and intervening at a point when the patient still has insight and may more easily establish trust with mental health professionals (Larson et al., 2010).

Personality Disorders in DSM-V

As can be gathered from the previous sections, personality disorders have long been a topic of great research and clinical interest, and have demonstrated important real-world outcomes. However, as outlined in the introduction and further highlighted by the focus on select PDs in this chapter, there are problems concerning diagnostic specificity and a lack of research with respect to a number of current DSM-IV-TR personality disorders.

In response to these issues, the DSM-V Work Group for Personality Disorders has proposed substantial changes for the new manual, including a completely new approach to defining personality disorders, described as a "hybrid dimensional-categorical" approach (DSM-V PD Work Group, 2010).

Five types of personality disorders, based on DSM-IV PDs with substantial empirical evidence for their validity and clinical utility (Patrick, Fowles, & Krueger, 2009; Skodol et al., 2002), are proposed for DSM-V, including borderline PD, antisocial/psychopathic PD, schizotypal PD, avoidant PD, and obsessive-compulsive PD (DSM-V PD Work Group, 2010). Diverging from the current symptom checklist approach, it is proposed that clinicians rate how well each client matches a diagnostic "prototype" (i.e., a brief text description capturing the essential features) of the given PD. Although the prototype-matching approach is novel, the diagnostic descriptions themselves will likely have a familiar read. Differing more dramatically from the current system, however, a personality trait-based approach will be part of the diagnostic conceptualization. Clinicians will be asked to rate clients on six broad (i.e., "higher order") normal personality trait domains considered useful to case conceptualization: Negative Emotionality, Detachment, Antagonism, Disinhibition, Compulsivity, and Schizotypy (O'Connor, 2005). Each of these traits has a number of facets (*see* http://dsm5.org for details).

Personality disorder diagnoses will be based on these traits and their facets. Each of the five proposed PD types will have as part of its diagnostic description a constellation of facets that should be theoretically elevated or not based on existing research. The diagnostic process is therefore proposed to consist of three major parts: prototype ratings, trait ratings, and impairment ratings. As of now, it is proposed that an individual will be given a PD diagnosis if they attain a rating of a "good match" or "very good match" to the prototype, a rating of "quite a bit" or "extremely" in at least one of the six trait domains, and a rating of at least mild impairment in functioning (self and interpersonal). As of now there are no changes specified for DSM-V that address conceptualization of PDs in a developmental context or directly impact diagnosis of PD in adolescence.

The Work Group has validated this approach and found it superior to using the trait or disorder concepts in isolation (Morey et al., n.d.) (DSM-V PD Work Group, 2010). This new diagnostic system will keep well-established personality disorders with good research bases, but will presumably eliminate several problems with the DSM-IV system. Namely, the Work Group (2010) argues that the use of the six trait dimensional system will eliminate the problems of comorbidities among personality disorders, eliminate the vague "Not Otherwise Specified" category, more clearly identify within-diagnosis heterogeneity, improve diagnostic stability, and improve both convergent and discriminant validity. Furthermore, proponents of the new diagnostic system argue that its greater consistency with existing conceptualizations of normal personality is an asset, as personality disorders would now be acknowledged as configurations of extreme variants of traits and their facets, not categorically different types of personality (O'Connor, 2005). Further, individual deviation from average trait levels in each of these domains could be potentially useful in quantifying the degree of pathology, a clinically relevant but infrequently systematically captured aspect of personality pathology.

Conclusion

Adolescence is a time of rapid and unique developmental change. Few other periods of human development are marked by such sharp, nonlinear cognitive, emotional, and social progress. A chief task of adolescence that reflects some of these changes is the assertion of independence from adult authority figures. Sometimes this task is accomplished partly by behaviors that adults find objectionable or troubling, ranging from relatively benign behaviors such as spending a lot more time with friends to more pernicious, yet still relatively common, activities like experimentation with drugs or alcohol, or other illegal behavior. Of most concern to many adults, adolescence is a time set apart by increased impulsivity and risk-taking, coupled with less-than-fully developed cognitive appreciation of long-term consequences. Still, most adolescent rebelliousness, heightened emotionality, and apparent eccentricities are normal and devoid of serious long-term consequences (though sometimes by sheer luck).

As noted in this chapter, however, adolescence and young adulthood are also extremely common times for the emergence of psychopathology, including personality disorders. When an adolescent is engaging in repeated impulsive risk-taking, is experiencing heightened instability in relationships, is exhibiting signs of harm or potential harm to him- or herself or others, appears to be increasingly withdrawn and odd, or other behaviors highlighted in this chapter, it may be time for parents, educators, or other concerned adults to consider approaching a mental health professional.

We hope that this chapter has served as a useful guide for recognizing the signs of the three most well-researched PDs that may appear in adolescence: borderline PD, schizotypal PD, and antisocial PD/conduct disorder. Moreover, we hope that presenting the current status of research on these disorders has offered insight beyond the common clinical perceptions around each of these disorders. As each of these sections highlights, there are promising evidence-based treatments available for some PDs (i.e., BPD and most subtypes of CD); better rates of remission and relapse than previously thought (once again, for BPD and most subtypes of CD), indicating a hopeful clinical course; and evidence of less progression to feared outcomes than previously thought (e.g., lower rates of suicide in BPD patients than previously estimated, less progression to schizophrenia/psychosis in SPD patients).

It is important to consider these hopeful findings, as they reflect a marked departure from the clinical lore of decades past. All the same, it is also important to keep in mind that while a PD diagnosis is not in and of itself a fixed gateway to a highly predictable course and outcome for a young person, PDs still constitute significant risk factors for a number of negative life outcomes that can be a source of worry even in normally developing adolescents, such as suicide and self-harm, eating disorders, getting in trouble with the legal system, teen pregnancy, and impaired school performance. The more that PDs in adolescence are well researched, accurately assessed, and treated with proven therapies, the more likely it is that these outcomes may be avoided and that the transition to adulthood will be a successful one for these young people. As we move toward DSM-V, hopefully our understanding of PDs and their relation to one other, normal personality, and degree of impairment will improve our ability to conduct rigorous research on the development of these disorders.

Acknowledgements We would like to acknowledge Vijay Mittal for the helpful case example for SPD. We would also like to acknowledge Danielle Schlosser for allowing us access to her recently submitted manuscript.

References

Achenbach, T. M. (1991). *Child behavior checklist/4–18 years (CBCL/4–18)*. Burlington, VT: University of Vermont.

Akiskal, H. S., Chen, S. E., Davis, G. C., Puzantin, V. R., Kashgarian, M., & Bolinger, J. M. (1985). Borderline: An adjective in search of a noun. *Journal of Clinical Psychiatry, 46*, 41–48.

American Psychiatric Association. (2000). Diagnostic and statistical manual of mental disorders (4th ed., Text Revision). Washington, DC: APA.

Bateman, A., & Fonagy, P. (1999). Effectiveness of partial hospitalization in the treatment of borderline personality disorder: A randomized controlled trial. *American Journal of Psychiatry, 156*, 1563–1569.

Berkowitz, L. (1993). *Aggression: Its causes, consequences, and control*. New York: Academic Press.

Bernstein, D. P., Cohen, P., Velez, C. N., Schwab-Stone, M., Siever, L. J., & Shinsato, L. (1993). Prevalence and stability of the DSM-III-R personality disorders in a community-based sample of adolescents. *American Journal of Psychiatry, 150*, 1237–1243.

Blair, R. J. R. (2010). A cognitive neuroscience perspective on child and adolescent psychopathy. In R. T. Salekin & D. R. Lynam (Eds.), *Handbook of child and adolescent psychopathy* (pp. 156–178). New York: Guildford Press.

Blair, R. J. R., Mitchell, D., & Blair, K. (2005). *The psychopath: Emotion and the brain*. Malden, MA, USA: Blackwell Publishing.

Bleuler, E. (1924). *Textbook of psychiatry*. (A. A. Brill, Trans.). New York: Macmillan.

Blonigen, D. M., Hicks, B. M., Kruger, R. F., Patrick, C. P., & Iacono, W. G. (2006). Continuity and change in psychopathic traits as measured via normal-range personality: A longitudinal-biometric study. *Journal of Abnormal Psychology, 115*, 85–95.

Bollini, A. M., & Walker, E. F. (2007). Schizotypal personality disorder. In W. O'Donohue, K. A. Fowler, & S. O. Lilienfeld (Eds.), *Personality disorders: Toward the DSM-V*. Thousand Oaks, CA: Sage.

Bradley, R., Jenei, J., & Westen, D. (2005). Etiology of borderline personality disorder: Disentangling the contributions of intercorrelated antecedents. *Journal of Nervous and Mental Disease, 193*, 24–31.

Burke, J. D., Loeber, R., & Lahey, B. B. (2007). Adolescent conduct disorder and interpersonal callousness as predictors of psychopathy in young adults. *Journal of Clinical Child and Adolescent Psychology, 36*, 334–346.

Burke, J. D., Waldman, I., & Lahey, B. B. (2010, September 20). Predictive validity of childhood oppositional defiant disorder and conduct disorder: Implications for the DSM–V. *Journal of Abnormal Psychology*. 119, 739–751.

Caldwell, M., Skeem, J., Salekin, R., & Van Rybroek, G. (2006). Treatment response of adolescent offenders with psychopathy features. *Criminal Justice and Behavior, 33*(5), 571–596.

Chamberlain, P., & Smith, D. K. (2003). Antisocial behavior in children and adolescents: The Oregon multidimensional treatment foster care model. In A. E. Kazdin & J. R. Weisz (Eds.), *Evidence-based psychotherapies for children and adolescents* (pp. 282–300). New York: Guildford.

Christian, R. E., Frick, P. J., Hill, N. L., Tyler, L., & Frazer, D. (1997). Psychopathy and conduct problems in children: II Implications for subtyping children with conduct problems. *Journal of the American Academy of Child and Adolescent Psychiatry, 36*, 233–241.

Clarkin, J. F., Hull, J. W., Cantor, J., & Sanderson, C. (1993). Borderline personality disorder and personality traits: A comparison of SCID-II BPD and NEO-PI. *Psychological Assessment, 5*, 472–476.

Crick, N. R., & Dodge, K. A. (1994). A review and reformulation of social information processing mechanisms in children's social adjustment. *Psychological Bulletin, 155*, 74–101.

Crick, N., Murray-Close, D., & Woods, K. (2005). Borderline personality features in childhood: A short-term longitudinal study. *Development and Psychopathology, 17*, 1051–1070.

Crowell, S. E., Beauchaine, T. P., & Linehan, M. M. (2009). A biosocial developmental model of borderline personality: Elaborating and extending Linehan's theory. *Psychological Bulletin, 135*, 495–510.

Dadds, M. R., & Salmon, K. (2003). Punishment insensitivity and parenting: Temperament and learning as interacting risks for antisocial behavior. *Clinical Child and Family Psychology Review, 6*, 69–86.

Elliott, D. S., Ageton, S. S., Huizinga, D., Knowles, B. A., & Canter, R. J. (1983). *The prevalence and incidence of delinquent behavior: 1976–1980* (The National Youth Survey Report No. 26). Boulder, CO: Behavioral Research Institute.

Eyberg, S. M., Nelson, M. M., & Boggs, S. R. (2008). Evidence-based psychosocial treatments for children and adolescents with disruptive behavior. *Journal of Clinical Child and Adolescent Psychology, 37*(1), 215–237.

Falkenbach, D., Poythress, N., & Heide, K. (2003). Psychopathic features in a juvenile diverse population: Reliability and predictive validity of two self-report measures. *Behavioral Sciences and the Law, 21*, 787–805.

Farmer, A. E., McGuffin, P., & Gottesman, I. I. (1987). Twin concordance for DSM_III schizophrenia: Scrutinizing the validity of the definition. *Archives of General Psychiatry, 44*, 634–641.

First, M. B., Gibbon, M., Spitzer, R. L., Williams, J. B. W., & Benjamin, L. S. (1997). *Structured clinical interview for DSM-IV axis II personality disorders*. Washington, DC: American Psychiatric Press.

Frankenburg, F. R., & Zanarini, M. C. (2006). Personality disorders and medical comorbidity. *Current Opinions in Psychiatry, 19*, 428–431.

Frick, P. J. (2006). Developmental pathways to conduct disorder. *Child and Adolescent Psychiatric Clinics of North America, 15*, 311–331.

Frick, P. J., & Dickens, C. (2006). Current perspectives on conduct disorder. *Current Psychiatry Reports, 8*, 59–72.

Frick, P. J., Kimonis, E. R., Dandreaux, D. M., & Farrell, J. M. (2003). The 4-year stability of psychopathic traits in non-referred youth. *Behavioral Sciences and the Law, 21*, 713–736.

Frick, P. J., Lilienfeld, S. O., Ellis, M., Loney, B., & Silverthorn, P. (1999). The association between anxiety and psychopathy dimensions in children. *Journal of Abnormal Child Psychology, 27*(5), 383–392.

Frick, P. J., & Moffitt, T. E. (2010). *A proposal to the DSM–V Childhood Disorders and the ADHD and Disruptive Behavior Disorders Work Groups to include a specifier to the diagnosis of conduct disorder based on the presence of callous-unemotional traits*. Retrieved December 8, 2010 from http://www.dsm5.org/Proposed%20Revision%20Attachments/Proposal%20for%20Callous%20and%20Unemotional%20Specifier%20of%20Conduct%20Disorder.pdf.

Frick, P. J., & White, S. F. (2008). The importance of callous-unemotional traits for developmental models of aggressive and antisocial behavior. *Journal of Child Psychology and Psychiatry, 49*(4), 359–375.

Giesen-Bloo, J., van Dyck, R., Spinhoven, P., van Tilburg, W., Dirksen, C., van Asselt, T., et al. (2006). Outpatient psychotherapy for borderline personality disorder. *Archives of General Psychiatry, 63*, 649–658.

Goldberg, R. L., Mann, L. S., Wise, T. N., & Segall, E. A. (1985). Parental qualities as perceived by borderline personality disorders. *Hillside Journal of Clinical Psychiatry, 7*, 134–140.

Goldman, S. J., D'Angelo, E. J., & DeMaso, D. R. (1993). Psychopathology in the families of children and adolescents with borderline personality disorder. *American Journal of Psychiatry, 150*, 1832–1835.

Goodman, M., Patil, U., Triebwasser, J., Diamond, E., Hiller, A., Hoffman, P., et al. (2010). Parental viewpoints of trajectories to borderline personality disorder in female offspring. *Journal of Personality Disorders, 24*, 204–216.

Gretton, H. M., McBride, M., Hare, R. D., Shaughnessy, R., & Kumka, G. (2001). Psychopathy and recidivism in adolescent sex offenders. *Criminal Justice and Behavior, 28*(4), 427–449.

Henggeler, S. W., & Lee, T. (2003). Multisystemic treatment of serious clinical problems. In A. E. Kazdin & J. R. Weisz (Eds.), *Evidence-based psychotherapies for children and adolescents* (pp. 301–322). New York: Guilford Press.

Hipwell, A. E., Pardini, D., Loeber, R., Sembower, M., Keenan, K., & Stouthamer-Loeber, M. (2007). Callous-unemotional behaviors in young girls: Shared and unique effects relative to conduct problems. *Journal of Clinical Child and Adolescent Psychology, 36*, 293–304.

Hudson, J. Hiripi, E. Pope, H. Kessler, R. (2007). The prevalence and correlates of eating disorders in the national comorbidity survey replication. *Biological Psychiatry, 61*, 348–358.

Kahn, R. E., Frick, P. J., Youngstrom, E., Findling, R. L., & Youngstrom, J. K. (2012). The effects of including a callous unemotional specifier for the diagnosis of conduct disorder. *Journal of Child Psychology and Psychiatry, 53*, 271–282.

Kazdin, A. E., & Weisz, J. R. (2003). *Evidence-based psychotherapies for children and adolescents*. New York: Guilford Press.

Kendler, K. S., Gruenberg, A. M., & Strauss, J. S. (1981). An independent analysis of the Copenhagen sample of the Danish Adoption Study of Schizophrenia. *Archives of General Psychiatry, 38*, 982–984.

Kessler, R. C., Chiu, W. T., Demler, O., Merikangas, K. R., & Walters, E. E. (2005). Prevalence, severity, and comorbidity of 12-month DSM-IV disorders in the National Comorbidity Survey replication. *Archives of General Psychiatry, 62*, 617–627.

Kety, S. S., Rosenthal, D., Wender, P. H., & Schulsinger, F. (1968). The types and prevalence of mental illness in the biological and adoptive families of adopted schizophrenics. *Journal of Psychiatry Research, 6*, 345–362.

Kraeplin, E. (1919/1971). *Dementia praecox and paraphrenia* (G. M. Robertson, Ed., R. M. Barclay, Trans.). New York: Krieger.

Larson, M. K., Walker, E. F., & Compton, M. T. (2010). Early signs, diagnosis and therapeutics of the prodromal phase of schizophrenia and related psychotic disorders. *Expert Review of Neurotherapeutics, 10*, 1347–1359.

Linehan, M. (1993). *Cognitive-behavioral treatment of borderline personality disorder*. New York: Guilford Press.

Links, P. S., Heslegrave, R., & van Reekum, R. (1999). Impulsivity: Core aspect of borderline personality disorder. *Journal of Personality Disorders, 13*, 1–9.

Lofgren, D. P., Bemporad, J. R., King, J., Lindem, K., & O'Driscoll, G. (1991). A prospective follow-up study of so-called borderline children. *American Journal of Psychiatry, 148*, 1541–1547.

Loney, B. R., Frick, P. J., Ellis, M. L., & McCoy, M. G. (1998). Intelligence, callous-unemotional traits, and antisocial behavior. *Journal of Psychopathology and Behavioral Assessment, 20*, 231–247.

Loranger, A. W. (1988). *Personality disorders examination (PDE) manual*. Yonkers, NY: DV Communications.

Lynam, D. R., Caspi, A., Moffitt, T. E., Loeber, R., & Stouthamer-Loeber, M. (2007). Longitudinal evidence that psychopathy scores in early adolescence predict adult psychopathy. *Journal of Abnormal Psychology, 116*, 155–165.

Mangelsdorf, S. C., Shapiro, J. R., & Marzolf, D. (1995). Developmental and temperamental differences in emotion regulation in infancy. *Child Development, 66*, 1817–1828.

Meehl, P. E. (1962). Schizotaxia, schizotypy, schizophrenia. *American Psychologist, 17*, 827–838.

Miller, T. J., McGlashan, T. H., Rosen, J. L., Somjee, L., Markovich, P. J., Stein, K., et al. (2002). Prospective diagnosis of the initial prodrome for schizophrenia based on the Structured Interview for Prodromal Syndromes: Preliminary evidence of interrater reliability and predictive validity. *American Journal of Psychiatry, 159*, 863–865.

Miller, A. L., Rathus, J. H., & Linehan, M. (2007). *Dialectical behavior therapy with suicidal adolescents*. New York: Guilford Press.

Mittal, V. A., Tessner, K. D., Trotman, H. D., Esterberg, M., Dhuruv, S. H., Simeonova, D. I., et al. (2007). Movement abnormalities and the progression of prodromal symptomatology in adolescents at risk for psychotic disorders. *Journal of Abnormal Psychology, 116*, 260–267.

Moffitt, T. E. (1993). Adolescence-limited and life-course-persistent antisocial behavior: A developmental taxonomy. *Psychological Review, 100*(4), 674–701.

Moffitt, T. E. (2003). Life-course-persistent and adolescence-limited antisocial behavior: A 10-year research review and a research agenda. In B. B. Lahey, T. E. Moffitt, & A. Caspi (Eds.), *Causes of conduct disorder*

and juvenile delinquency (pp. 49–75). New York: Guilford Press.
Moffitt, T. E., & Caspi, A. (2001). Childhood predictors differentiate life-course persistent and adolescence-limited antisocial pathways among males and females. *Development and Psychopathology, 13*(2), 355–375.
Moffitt, T. E., Caspi, A., Dickson, N., Silva, P. A., & Stanton, W. (1996). Childhood-onset versus adolescent-onset antisocial conduct in males: Natural history from age 3 to 18. *Development and Psychopathology, 8*, 399–424.
Morey, L. C., Hopwood, C, J., Markowitz, J. C., Gunderson, J. G., Grilo, C. M., McGlashan, T. H., et al. (n.d.). Long term predictive validity of diagnostic models for personality disorder: Integrating trait and disorder concepts. Submitted to *American Journal of Psychiatry*.
Morey, L. C., & Zanarini, M. C. (2000). Borderline personality: Traits and disorder. *Journal of Abnormal Psychology, 109*, 733–737.
O'Connor, B. P. (2005). A search for consensus on the dimensional structure of personality disorders. *Journal of Clinical Psychology., 61*, 323–345.
O'Neill, M. L., Lidz, V., & Heilbrun, K. (2003). Adolescent with psychopathic characteristics in a substance abusing cohort: Treatment process and outcomes. *Law and Human Behavior, 27*(3), 299–313.
Oxford, M., Cavell, T. A., & Hughes, J. N. (2003). Callous/unemotional traits moderate the relation between ineffective parenting and child externalizing problems: A partial replication and extension. *Journal of Clinical Child and Adolescent Psychology, 32*, 577–585.
Pardini, D. A., Frick, P. J., & Moffitt, T. E. (2010). Building an evidence base for DSM-5 conceptualizations of Oppositional Defiant Disorder and Conduct Disorder: Introduction to the special edition. *Journal of Abnormal Psychology, 119*(4), 683–688.
Paris, J., & Frank, H. (1989). Perceptions of parental bonding in borderline patients. *American Journal of Psychiatry, 146*, 1498–1499.
Patrick, C. J., Fowles, D. C., & Krueger, R. F. (2009). Triarchic conceptualization of psychopathy: Developmental origins of disinhibition, boldness, and meanness. *Development and Psychopathology, 21*, 913–938.
Patterson, G. R., Reid, J. B., & Dishion, T. J. (1998). *Antisocial boys*. Eugene, OR: Castalia.
Patterson, G. R., Reid, J. B., Jones, R. R., & Conger, R. E. (1975). *A social learning approach to family intervention: Families with aggressive children* (Vol. 1). Eugene, OR: Castalia.
Pfohl, B., Blum, N., & Zimmerman, M. (1994). *Structured interview for DSM-IV personality disorders*. Iowa City: University of Iowa Hospitals and Clinics.
Raine, A. (1991). The SPQ: A scale for the assessment of schizotypal personality based on the DSM-III-R criteria. *Schizophrenia Bulletin, 17*, 555–564.
Reynolds, C. R., & Kamphaus, R. W. (2004). *Behavioral assessment system for children* (2nd ed.). Circle Pines, MN: AGS.
Rowe, R., Maughan, B., Moran, P., Ford, T., Briskman, J., & Goodman, R. (2009). The role of callous and unemotional traits in the diagnosis of conduct disorder. *Journal of Child Psychology and Psychiatry, 51*(6), 688–695.
Salekin, R. T., Neumann, C. S., Leistico, A. R., & Zalot, A. A. (2004). Psychopathy in youth and intelligence: An investigation of Cleckley's hypothesis. *Journal of Clinical Child and Adolescent Psychology, 33*, 731–742.
Salzman, J. P., Salzman, C., Wolfson, A. N., Albanese, M., Looper, J., Ostacher, M., et al. (1993). Association between borderline personality structure and history of childhood abuse in adult volunteers. *Comprehensive Psychiatry, 34*, 254–257.
Schlosser, D. A., Jacobson, S., Chen, Q., Sugar, C. A., Niendam, T. A., Li, G., Bearden, C. E., Cannon, T. D. (2012). Recovery from an at-risk state: clinical and functional outcomes of putatively prodromal youth who do not develop psychosis. *Schizophrenia Bulletin, 3*,1225–1233.
Skodol, A. E., Gunderson, J. G., McGlashan, T. H., Dyck, I. R., Stout, R. L., Bender, D. S., et al. (2002). Functional impairment in patients with schizotypal, borderline, avoidant, or obsessive-compulsive personality disorder. *American Journal of Psychiatry, 159*, 276–283.
Spain, S. E., Douglas, K. S., Poythress, N. G., & Epstein, M. (2004). The relationship between psychopathic features, violence and treatment outcome: The comparison of three youth measures of psychopathic features. *Behavioral Sciences and the Law, 22*, 88–102.
Torgerson, S., & Kringlen, E. (1991). Twin concordance for DSM-III-R schizophrenia. *Acta Psychiatrica Scandinavica, 83*, 395–401.
Torgerson, S., Lygren, S., Oien, P. A., Skre, I., Onstad, S., Edvardsen, J., et al. (2000). A twin study of personality disorders. *Comprehensive Psychiatry, 41*, 416–425.
Trotman, H., McMillan, A., & Walker, E. F. (2006). Cognitive function and symptoms in adolescents with schizotypal personality disorder. *Schizophrenia Bulletin, 32*, 489–497.
Trull, T. J., Widiger, T. A., Lynam, D. R., & Costa, P. T. (2003). Borderline personality disorder from the perspective of general personality functioning. *Journal of Abnormal Psychology, 112*, 193–202.
Viding, E., Blair, R. J. R., Moffitt, T. E., & Plomin, R. (2005). Evidence for substantial genetic risk for psychopathy in 7-year-olds. *Journal of Child Psychology and Psychiatry, 46*, 1–6.
Vollema, M. G., & Ormel, J. (2000). The reliability of the structured interview for Schizotypy-revised. *Schizophrenia Bulletin, 26*, 619–629.
White, S. F., & Frick, P. J. (2010). Callous-unemotional traits and their importance to causal models of severe antisocial behavior in youth. In R. T. Salekin & D. R. Lynam (Eds.), *Handbook of child and adolescent psychopathy* (pp. 135–155). New York: Guildford Press.
White, S. F., Frick, P. J., Lawing, K. and Bauer, D. (2012). Callous–Unemotional traits and response to functional

family therapy in adolescent offenders. *Behavioral Sciences and the Law*. Published online Nov 2012.

Widiger, T. A., & Rogers, J. H. (1989). Prevalence and comorbidity of personality disorders. *Psychiatric Annals, 19*, 132–136.

Williams, M. (1993). *The psychometric assessment of schizotypal personality*. Unpublished doctoral dissertation, London, UK: University of London

Wootton, J. M., Frick, P. J., Shelton, K. K., & Silverthorn, P. (1997). Ineffective parenting and childhood conduct problems: The moderating role of callous-unemotional traits. *Journal of Consulting and Clinical Psychology, 65*, 301–308.

Zanarini, M. C. (1993). BPD as an impulse spectrum disorder. In J. Paris (Ed.), *Borderline personality disorder: Etiology and treatment* (pp. 67–85). Washington, DC: American Psychiatric Press.

Zanarini, M. C., & Frankenburg, F. R. (2007). The essential nature of borderline psychopathology. *Journal of Personality Disorders, 21*, 518–535.

Zanarini, M. C., Frankenburg, F. R., Dubo, E. D., Sickel, A. E., Trikha, A., Levin, A., et al. (1998). Axis I comorbidity of borderline personality disorder. *American Journal of Psychiatry, 155*, 1733–1739.

Zanarini, M. C., Frankenburg, F. R., Hennen, J., Reich, D. B., & Silk, K. R. (2005). The McLean Study of Adult Development (MSAD): Overview and implications of the first six years of prospective follow-up. *Journal of Personality Disorders, 19*, 505–523.

Zanarini, M. C., Frankenburg, F. R., Khera, G. S., & Bleichmar, J. (2001). Treatment histories of borderline inpatients. *Comprehensive Psychiatry, 42*, 144–150.

Zanarini, M. C., Frankenburg, F. R., & Parachani, E. A. (2004). A preliminary trial of fluoxetine, olanzepine, and the olanzepine-fluoxetine combination in women with borderline personality disorder. *Journal of Clinical Psychiatry, 65*, 903–907.

Zanarini, M. C., Frankenburg, F. R., Ridolfi, M. E., Jager-Hyman, S., Hennen, J., & Gunderson, J. G. (2006). Reported childhood onset of self-mutilation among borderline patients. *Journal of Personality Disorders, 20*, 9–15.

Zanarini, M. C., Gunderson, J. G., Marino, M. F., Schwartz, E. O., & Frankenburg, F. R. (1988). DSM-III disorders in the families of borderline outpatients. *Journal of Personality Disorders, 2*, 292–302.

Zanarini, M. C., Williams, A. A., Lewis, R. E., Reich, D. B., Vera, S. C., Marino, M. F., et al. (1997). Reported pathological childhood experiences associated with the development of borderline personality disorder. *American Journal of Psychiatry, 154*, 1101–1106.

Zlotnick, C., Rothschild, L., & Zimmerman, M. (2002). The role of gender in the clinical presentation of patients with borderline personality disorder. *Journal of Personality Disorders, 16*, 277–282.

Deliberate Self-Harm in Adolescents

Catherine Miller and Christian Pariseau

Thin white scars crisscross her left forearm, hidden by a collection of bracelets. He has round burn marks across his shoulders and chest. It is hard to miss the open wounds in various stages of healing, spelling "FAT," etched deep into the skin of her upper thigh. These young people have cut, burned, and carved their skin. Such occurrences of self-injury are commonly encountered when working with adolescents in any healthcare setting, and are extremely common in the mental healthcare setting. Most people go to great lengths to avoid injury and pain, which can make this behavior difficult to understand.

Some evidence suggests an increasing prevalence of self-harm behavior in youth; because these behaviors can be associated with severe psychopathology and suicidality, this trend is alarming. This chapter covers how self-harm is defined and the epidemiology of this behavior. Theories of the psychological function and the currently understood pathophysiology, along with recommended clinical approaches, assessment, and treatment strategies, are discussed.

C. Miller, M.D. (✉)
Center for Adolescent Health, Lucile Packard Children's Hospital at Stanford University, 1174 Castro St. Suite 250, Mountain View, CA 94040, USA
e-mail: camiller@stanford.edu

C. Pariseau, M.D.
Pediatric, Adolescent and Young Adult Medicine, University of Michigan Pediatrics, 1931 Taubman Center, 1500 E. Hospital Dr., Ann Arbor, MI 48109, USA
e-mail: pariseac@umich.edu

Definition

Deliberate self-harm (DSH) is defined as the intentional damage of body tissues in the absence of suicidal intent (Klonsky, 2007a, 2007b). There are multiple terms used to describe this same behavior including non-suicidal self-injury, self-injury, deliberate self-injury, and self-mutilation (Klonsky, 2007a, 2007b). Forms of DSH can include cutting, scratching, carving, burning, hitting, banging, and interfering with wound healing, but generally exclude socially sanctioned forms of tissue injury such as piercing and tattooing (Ballard, Bosk, & Pao, 2010). Also typically excluded from DSH are behaviors such as drug use, restrictive eating, and purging—as the damage done is usually a side effect rather than the primary intent of the behavior (Klonsky, 2007a, 2007b). However, the boundaries around this DSH term can be hazy, as some behaviors not typically thought of as DSH may be included if the primary intent in certain instances is the deliberate damage of body tissues.

Historically, DSH was thought of as a severe expression of a mental disorder, and many clinicians advocated for inpatient treatment approaches (Graff & Mallin, 1967). During the 1960s and 1970s efforts were made to further describe the epidemiology and clinical characteristics of DSH, leading to DSH being officially included as a symptom of borderline personality disorder (BPD) in 1980 in the Diagnostic and Statistical Manual of Mental Disorders (DSM-III-R, 3rd

W.T. O'Donohue et al. (eds.), *Handbook of Adolescent Health Psychology*,
DOI 10.1007/978-1-4614-6633-8_30, © Springer Science+Business Media New York 2013

Edition; Lester, 1972). Currently, although DSH continues to be regarded as a symptom of BPD in DSM-IV-TR, there is extensive research documenting DSH occurring in conjunction with many other diagnoses including depression, anxiety, eating disorders, substance use disorders, and posttraumatic stress disorder (DSM-III-R, 4th Edition). Furthermore, it is now evident that DSH even takes place in nonclinical, high-functioning populations (Klonsky, Oltmanns, & Turkheimer, 2003; Whitlock, Eckenrode, & Silverman, 2006).

Epidemiology

Among the adolescent and young adult age group the prevalence of DSH varies widely depending on the population studied. In nonclinical samples of young adults, lifetime prevalence rates of DSH vary from 4 % in military recruits to 14–38 % in college students (Gratz, Conrad, & Roemer, 2002; Klonsky, 2007a, 2007b; Klonsky et al., 2003). In nonclinical samples of adolescents in the United States and Canada, lifetime prevalence of DSH ranged between 14 and 16 % in three different community high school samples and much higher, 46.5 %, in another recent study from five high schools in the United States (Laye-Gindhu & Schonert-Reichl, 2005; Lloyd-Richardson, Perrine, Dierker, & Kelley, 2007; Muehlenkamp & Gutierrez, 2004; Ross & Heath, 2002). By far, the population with the highest prevalence of DSH is adolescents in psychiatric inpatient settings, with a 12-month prevalence of DSH in this group as high as 80 % (Nock & Prinstein, 2004). Several studies have shown lower lifetime prevalence of DSH in older populations, suggesting an increase in DSH in recent years (Klonsky, 2007a, 2007b).

Age of onset of DSH behavior is typically in the early to middle adolescent years (Klonsky & Muehlenkamp, 2007). In studies examining race and the occurrence of DSH, most have shown Caucasians to have higher rates than non-Caucasian groups, while a few studies have shown similar rates across racial/ethnic groups (Klonsky et al., 2003; Lloyd-Richardson, 2008). Females are commonly perceived to engage in DSH more than males, which is supported by some studies (Ross & Health, 2002). However, more recent studies show no gender difference (Klonsky et al., 2003; Lloyd-Richardson et al., 2007). The main gender difference appears to be the form of injury; females seem more likely to cut themselves while males seem more likely to hit or burn themselves (Klonsky et al., 2003). Overall, skin-cutting or scratching is the most common form of DSH, occurring in 70–97 % of people engaging in DSH (Klonsky, 2007a, 2007b). Banging or hitting (21–44 %) is the next most common form of DSH, followed by burning (15–35 %) (Klonsky, 2007a, 2007b). Most individuals that engage in DSH have used more than one method (Klonsky et al., 2003). The most common body areas injured are the arms, followed by the hands, wrists, thighs, and stomach (Whitlock et al., 2006). Also notable when looking at community samples is that the majority of individuals reporting DSH have only engaged in the behavior once to a few times, and it is the minority of individuals that have chronic, repeated DSH (Whitlock et al., 2006).

Psychological Characteristics

Youth who self-injure are more likely than youth that do not self-injure to share some specific psychological characteristics, including negative emotionality, deficits in emotion skills, and self-derogation (Klonsky et al., 2003). Negative emotionality refers to individuals who experience more intense, frequent negative emotions. People with DSH behaviors have been found to score higher on negative temperament, anxiety, and depression measures. Additionally, DSH is associated with deficits in skills related to experiencing emotions—having more feelings of numbness and dissociation, and difficulty identifying, understanding, and expressing emotions. Also notable is the increase in self-derogation, or self-directed dislike and anger, in people who engage in DSH. In a recent study of 150 high school students, those students with DSH rated themselves lower on academic intelligence, emotional stability, attractiveness, and social skills and had more

Table 1 Functions of DSH

Psychological function	Examples
Affect regulation	"To manage stress," "to stop bad feelings"
Self-punishment	"To punish myself," "to express anger at myself"
Anti-dissociation	"To stop feeling numb," "to feel real and alive"
Anti-suicide	"To prevent me from acting on suicidal thoughts"
Interpersonal influence	"To get help," "to get my parents to stop fighting," "to get people to leave me alone"
Sensation-seeking	"To get a rush," "thought it would be fun"
Interpersonal boundaries	"It's something that only I have control of"

friends with DSH than their peers without DSH (Claes, Houben, Vadereycken, Bijttebier, & Muehlenkamp, 2010).

An association between childhood sexual abuse and DSH has long been noted (Klonsky & Moyer, 2008). However, a 2008 meta-analysis of studies that included measures of self-injury and childhood sexual abuse concluded that the results did not support childhood sexual abuse as having a causal or central role in the development of self-injury behaviors. Rather the meta-analysis showed a modest relationship between DSH and childhood sexual abuse as they tend to be correlated with the same psychological risk factors (Klonsky & Moyer, 2008).

Psychological Function of DSH

Klonsky (2007a, 2007b) found: The most common reported function of DSH is affect regulation. That is, DSH relieves negative emotions or the intensity of negative feelings. Anger, anxiety, or sadness are often present prior to DSH, and DSH seems to bring about feelings of calm or relief. Another reason endorsed by individuals engaging in DSH is self-punishment. Self-punishment is the second most prevalent reason cited in studies for DSH after affect regulation (Klonsky et al., 2003). Anti-dissociation is another reported function of DSH, with individuals seeking to "feel something" to alleviate feelings of numbness and dissociation. In addition, DSH can function as an anti-suicide measure, when adolescents use DSH as a coping mechanism to avoid suicide attempt, or as a distraction or a compromise when dealing with suicidal ideation. Some people also report engaging in DSH in order to influence other people's behavior, actions, or attention, which is referred to as interpersonal influence. Others endorse sensation-seeking as a reason for DSH, finding that inflicting injuries provides excitement or pleasurable stimulation. And finally, DSH has been thought of as a way to indicate interpersonal boundaries, when a person tries to mark or define themselves as different from others, or exert their independence or authority (Table 1).

For many individuals with DSH behaviors, the behaviors may have different functions over time and in different circumstances (Lloyd-Richardson, 2008). Another important part of DSH for some people can be seeing blood, which may help to achieve the desired effect such as relieving tension. In a study of college students, 51.6 % of the students, all with DSH behaviors, reported that it was important to see blood with DSH (Glenn & Klonsky, 2010). The study results also supported that in general those that felt it was important to see blood represented a clinically more severe group.

Pathophysiology of DSH

Looking at the brain processing of pain and emotional distress, and considering the neurodevelopmental changes happening in adolescence, may help clinicians better understand DSH.

Overlap of Physical and Social Pain

Pain sensation is an incredibly complex process that includes sensory and emotional components, with major overlap in brain areas that process physical and emotional/social pain (Ballard et al., 2010). Functional imaging studies comparing healthy adolescents and adults show differential activation of brain areas involved in the experience of social pain. It is possible that adolescents experience social pain differently and perhaps more severely than adults.

The Role of Neurodevelopment

Neuroanatomical brain changes continue throughout adolescence into young adulthood and possibly contribute to increased vulnerability of adolescents to DSH. One of the best characterized changes continuing throughout adolescence is the volume of gray matter over time (Ballard et al., 2010). Gray matter volume (density of neurons) increases until age 11–12 and then declines until young adulthood. This change proceeds in back-to-front direction, with the prefrontal cortex (reasoning, modulating emotional urges) being the last anatomic region of the brain to reach an "adult" pattern of gray matter changes. This maturation correlates with improved impulse control, planning, and emotional regulation.

Many other changes occur during adolescence outside of the brain that directly influence behavior. The hypothalamic-pituitary-adrenal (HPA) axis, a system that is key to the body's response to stress, appears to be more "sensitive" in adolescents (Ballard et al., 2010). Stressors cause a greater release of stress hormones (particularly cortisol) via the HPA system in younger people. Cortisol has effects throughout the body and brain.

The Opioid-Deficit Model

Opioids are naturally occurring (endorphins) and man-made chemicals (e.g., morphine) that have been primarily studied for the treatment of pain. However, growing evidence shows an important role of endogenous opioids in emotion regulation and social behavior. The "opioid-deficit model" is an explanatory hypothesis for DSH in BPD (Fikke, Melinder & Landrø, 2011; Stanley et al., 2010).

The opioid-deficit model has various supporting evidence. Self-harming patients often report self-cutting as a non-painful, non-suicidal act accompanied by a sense of relief or well-being. The opioid-deficit model postulates that people engaging in repeated DSH have abnormally low opioid effect and cutting causes release of endogenous opioids bringing the patient to a "normal" level. DSH could be seen in this light as self-medication. It has long been noted that among adults with BPD, there is a high rate of exogenous opioid abuse and reports of BPD patients who take opiates report feeling "normal" rather than "high."

A study by Prossin et al. examined opioid receptor activity in the cerebral cortex of patients during various moods using positron emission tomography (PET) scanning (Prossin, Love, Koeppe, Zubieta, & Silk, 2010). Unmedicated female BPD patients were studied versus matched healthy controls during both a "neutral" mood and "induced sadness." During the neutral mood, there was greater baseline opioid receptor availability in BPD patients relative to comparison subjects. They hypothesize that greater receptor availability may occur because of lower baseline endogenous opioid neurotransmitter activity in BPD patients. During induced sadness, BPD patients showed greater activation of the endogenous opioid system in many parts of the brain compared to controls. These imaging findings correlate with the clinical findings that BPD patients have a low threshold for becoming emotionally dysregulated, followed by a rise to high levels of emotional arousal.

Stanley et al. researched levels of endogenous neurotransmitters and endogenous opioids in the cerebral spinal fluid (CSF) in adult patients with repetitive DSH versus controls. All study participants were diagnosed with a cluster B personality disorder (all but three had BPD) and had a history of at least one suicide attempt. Of the 29 total patients, 14 had a history of repeated DSH and 25 did not. CSF was collected from all participants via lumbar puncture in the morning after a night of at least 8 h of strict bedrest. The following were measured in all patients: three types of endogenous opioids, the serotonin metabolite 5-hydroxyindoleacetic acid (5-HIAA), and the dopamine metabolite homovanillic acid (HVA). The DSH group had significantly lower levels of two of the three measured opioids. There were no differences in CSF dynorphin, 5-HIAA, and HVA levels between the groups. Also worth noting is that the DSH group reported a higher level of depression and hopelessness.

Extrapolating from both the Prossin and Stanley studies to adolescents has many limitations as the study participants were older in age, had longer lasting illness, mainly included women, and used BPD as a model for studying DSH. However these studies combined with others support opioid system abnormalities in DSH. Further research focusing specifically on adolescents is much needed.

Executive Brain Function

There has been some investigation into whether executive brain functioning differs in adolescents with DSH behaviors. One study looked at 97 high school students, divided into three groups: low-severity DSH, high-severity DSH, and healthy controls (Fikke et al., 2011). The main areas of executive functioning were tested and some differences between the DSH subgroups and controls were found. Overall, there were working memory deficits noted in the high-severity DSH group, and impaired inhibitory control in the low-severity DSH group.

Association Between SI and Suicide

Suicidality and DSH are both common and overlap; DSH is a marker of increased risk of future suicide attempts. Andover et al. studied DSH and suicidality among 117 psychiatric inpatients (Andover & Gibb, 2010). Two-thirds of the patients reported a history of suicide attempt(s) and 45 % reported a history of DSH, with cutting being the most common method. Patients with a history of DSH were more likely to report a history of attempted suicide, and frequency of DSH was correlated with the number of suicide attempts. Interestingly, after controlling for depressive symptoms, hopelessness, current suicidal ideation, and symptoms of BPD, a history of DSH still remained significantly correlated with a presence/absence of suicide attempts. Also, reported DSH frequency positively correlated with patient perceptions of lethality of suicide attempts.

Another study, by Nock et al., looked at the relationship between DSH and suicide attempts (Nock, Joiner, Gordon, Lloyd-Richardson, & Prinstein, 2006). Data was collected from 89 young adults who were admitted to a psychiatric inpatient unit and had engaged in DSH in the previous 12 months. DSH was associated with suicidality in patients with a longer history of DSH, multiple methods of DSH, and absence of physical pain during DSH.

Similar findings were noted by Whitlock, Muehlenkamp, and Eckenrode (2008). They surveyed college students with the goal of determining possible subtypes of DSH. Based on a survey of 2,101 students, those who reported 11 or more incidents of DSH using three or more forms of self-injury were the most likely to report suicidality. Also of note, almost half of the students with the most frequent and varied DSH reported that DSH was not/is not a problem in their life.

A study of 373 high school students looked for differences between adolescents that self-harm versus those who have a history of both DSH and suicidality (Brausch & Gutierrez, 2010). Students were divided into three groups: no history of DSH, a history of DSH but no suicide attempts, and history of both DSH and suicide attempts. Unsurprisingly, the no-self-harm group reported the lowest level of hopelessness and highest levels of self-esteem. Comparing the two groups with a history of DSH, the no-suicide-attempts group reported lower depression scores, less suicidal ideation, greater parental support, and greater self-esteem than the suicide-plus-DSH group.

Clinical Assessment/Approach

A thorough assessment of DSH behavior is imperative in guiding care and treatment approaches. There are multiple formal assessment tools available including questionnaires such as the

Functional Assessment of Self-Mutilation, the Self-Harm Behavior Questionnaire, the Inventory of Statements About Self-Injury, and formal interview tools such as the Self-Injurious Thoughts and Behaviors Interview, and the Suicide Attempt Self-Injury Interview (Gutierrez, Osmann, Barrios, & Kopper, 2001; Klonsky & Glenn, 2009; Linehan, Comtois, Brown, Heard, & Wagner, 2006; Lloyd-Richardson et al., 2007; Nock, Elizabeth, Photos, & Michel, 2007). These tools were largely developed for research purposes and, though not widely used in the clinical setting, can be used clinically and provide guidance on the important elements of a detailed assessment. Below is advice for the initial approach to DSH and an overview of important areas to cover in assessing the behavior.

The initial reaction of a care provider is important. Reactions of shock, disgust, or other intense negative judgments make it less likely that the person engaging in DSH will bring up the behavior in the future and be forthcoming with further details about the behavior. It is recommended that caregivers respond in a low-key, respectful manner (Walsh, 2007). Initial questions such as "What does self-injury do for you?" can help to communicate that you are interested and wanting to gain a better understanding. Attempts to forbid the behavior or quickly "contract for safety" are not helpful. It is not realistic to think that a person who has developed a coping technique can quickly abandon it, without time to work on establishing other coping skills. So the goal will be to establish a long-term therapeutic relationship, in which DSH can be assessed over time and other coping skills can be learned.

Important areas of assessment include a detailed history of DSH, information about recent DSH behaviors, functions of DSH, triggers and consequences of DSH, and screening for suicidality. When taking a detailed history of DSH, it is helpful to explore the age of onset of the behavior, types of injuries, and frequency of DSH, along with the number of wounds typically inflicted, location of the wounds, experience of pain, and the severity of tissue damage. A longer duration of DSH generally portends a more challenging path to alleviating the behavior. And as discussed above, in at least one sample of young adults, greater risk of suicide attempts was associated with a longer history of DSH, use of a greater number of methods, and the absence of physical pain during DSH (Nock et al., 2006).

In gathering information about DSH occurring in the last couple of months, assessing the function of DSH for the individual will be helpful in guiding treatment. Details about the recent frequency of DSH, number of wounds, and the level of tissue damage can help to indicate current level of distress. Also keep in mind that it is rare for individuals to inflict tissue damage requiring stitches or other medical intervention, and that individuals inflicting severe tissue damage may require emergency mental health assessment. Looking at the wounds, with an individual's permission, may provide more objective information than a verbal description. If the DSH involves carved words, exploring the selection of the particular words can be helpful therapeutically. The location of injury is also important, as most people will injure extremities or the abdomen. Reports of DSH to the eyes, face, genitals, or breasts are red flags for psychotic or trauma-related behavior (Walsh, 2007).

Many aspects of timing can be helpful to clarify. The duration of time it takes for completion of the injury points to the length of time it takes to relieve distress; therefore longer periods of DSH may be more concerning. Also exploring the time of day of DSH may help in the development of replacement activities or changing usual routines to decrease DSH. Keeping track of the longest time period between DSH can be motivating for some patients, helping them push themselves to achieve longer and longer DSH-free periods. Other key pieces of information to obtain about recent DSH includes where the behavior usually occurs (e.g., bedroom, bathroom), if tools (e.g., nails, razorblades) are used, and whether DSH occurs alone or in the presence of others (may be virtual presence via online chat groups or social networking sites). All of these details are important when trying to work on altering habits and routines to work toward behavior change.

Examining details about the triggers which precede DSH behavior can help to predict the situations in which future DSH will happen. This allows individuals and care provider to recognize specific opportunities to practice other coping/replacement techniques and can guide attempts to interrupt the chain of thoughts and actions that lead up to DSH. These triggers can be environmental, such as discord in relationship or poor performance in school. Some triggers may be biological factors, such as sleep deprivation, illness, or intoxication. Other triggers are psychological in nature, thought and behavior patterns, affective states, and beliefs. The Suicide Attempt Self-Injury Interview provides a detailed assessment of possible triggers, focusing mainly on environmental triggers, and could be useful as part of a clinical evaluation (Linehan et al., 2006).

In addition, information about the consequences of DSH can help guide treatment. Similar to the assessment of triggers, environmental, biological, and psychological consequences should be examined. An important environmental consequence is the reaction of others to DSH. If the reaction of others reinforces the behavior, it may make sense to try to change that response. Biological consequences include the degree of physical pain experienced, and whether actions are taken to promote wound healing. Important psychological consequences are an individual's emotional state after DSH, their thoughts regarding the DSH (shame, guilt, pride), and the sequence of behaviors afterward. These details may help to inform treatment approaches, for example, working on self-soothing techniques might be helpful for a patient who experiences relief from anxiety and a calm sensation after DSH, but may be less effective for a patient who feels invigorated and energized after DSH.

Though the intent of DSH in most individuals is not suicide, it is very important for care providers to monitor on an ongoing basis suicidal thinking, plans, and attempts, as many of the psychological characteristics of individuals engaging in DSH put them at a high risk of suicide (Nafisi & Stanley, 2007).

Treatment

Treating self-injuring patients can be challenging, as it is usually a slow process of change, and patients using DSH as a coping mechanism often have difficult personality characteristics. These are often patients that are surrounded by negative judgments, from their families, friends, society, and most importantly, themselves. Even after gaining insight into the reasons for their DSH behaviors, individuals may find it very difficult to change. Some of the methods for maintaining a therapeutic relationship with individuals with DSH behaviors are reviewed here, followed by identification of specific therapies that have demonstrated effectiveness in treating DSH (Gratz, 2007; Klonsky et al., 2003).

One important aspect of care is validation of the patients' feelings through listening, reflecting, and understanding. Acknowledging that a patient's emotional pain is real and that you understand DSH provides relief helps a patient feel validated and can facilitate further work on the DSH behavior. This should be validating the effect, not validating DSH as the best means. Also important is for a care provider to firmly support patient self-care and the cessation of DSH behavior. Eliciting the patient's thoughts about the negative consequences of DSH may be helpful as many people are distressed by the behavior. Being able to present additional concerns if patients are unable to come up with adverse consequences can also help to facilitate contemplation about cessation of DSH. Provider concerns might include that DSH can result in infection, pain, and unintentional severe injury or death. It can lead to social embarrassment and shame because it is not a socially acceptable behavior, and most importantly it does not resolve the patient's underlying problems. DSH ends up being a cycle of destructive behavior, which the patient relies upon instead of developing healthier coping strategies.

A pitfall to avoid is that overconcern and effusive compassion in response to DSH may inadvertently reinforce the behavior. On the other hand, DSH often elicits strong negative emotions in care providers, causing providers to reprimand patients, ignore or minimize the DSH behavior, or withdraw from the alliance. The most effective approach is to maintain a dispassionate, nonjudgmental demeanor in discussing DSH. It also may be useful when experiencing intense frustration and negative judgments about an individual with DSH to remember that the behavior is functional instead of labeling the individual as manipulative.

In managing the frustration that can occur during the slow course of treatment, it is important to have realistic expectations—that patients with DSH may take longer to progress with therapy than other patient populations, that there will be relapses of the behavior, that you will need to pay close attention to detect small improvements, and that it is common for patients with DSH to resist the introduction of other coping mechanisms either verbally or through noncompliance. Getting support and outside perspective from colleagues to avoid burnout can also be very useful.

Many types of treatment have been utilized for DSH. Please see Table 2 for a summary of the level of evidence for some of the recognized interventions (Karr, Muehlenkamp, & Turner, 2010). Below is a review of pharmacotherapy and cognitive-behavioral and psychodynamic therapy interventions.

Pharmacotherapy

No medication currently has Food and Drug Administration approval for the treatment of DSH. The existing evidence for medication effectiveness in the treatment of DSH is very preliminary, based on case reports and small non-randomized trials. There are two published reports on naltrexone, an opiate antagonist, showing a decrease in DSH after starting the medication (Griengl, Sendera, & Dantendorfer, 2001; Roth, Ostroff, & Hoffman, 1996). There is also some case-based support for the use of clozapine for treatment of DSH in two published reports (Chengappa, Ebeling, Kang, Levine, & Parepally, 1999; Ferrerri, Loze, Rouillon, & Limosin, 2004). Additionally, there have been two reports on topiramate as helpful in the treatment of DSH (Cassano et al., 2001; Chengappa et al., 1999).

Cognitive-Behavioral Therapies

This general category includes psychotherapies that share the underlying idea that thoughts, rather than external factors like people and events, form our emotions and behaviors. There is a large body of research supporting CBT for mood disorders and substance abuse, and increasing evidence for CBT effectiveness in decreasing DSH. The focus in the literature for DSH intervention has been on a few types of therapy, problem-solving therapy, manual assisted cognitive-behavioral therapy (MACT) and dialectical behavioral therapy (DBT). These types of therapies share some common techniques including recognizing and changing maladaptive thought patterns, teaching skills in problem-solving, effective communication and tolerating distress, and practical behavior intervention (Klonsky et al., 2003). It is not clear which components or combination of techniques are most helpful in treating DSH.

The 1999 Cochrane Review of the available randomized controlled trials looking at effectiveness of treatments in patients with DSH showed a promising trend toward reduction of repeat DSH for problem-solving therapy compared with standard treatment (Hawton et al., 1999). However, the pooled odds ratio was not significant, likely due to the small numbers in these trials. With MACT, a brief, manualized, cost-effective version of CBT, a decrease in DSH behaviors over the course of treatment and post treatment has been demonstrated (Evans et al., 1999; Tyrer et al., 2003). However, additional research is needed to provide support for the superiority of this therapy over other therapeutic approaches, as there was no significant difference between MACT and treatment as usual groups for repeated DSH in the 12-month study of 480 patients (Tyrer et al., 2003).

DBT is the most studied treatment for DSH. DBT was developed for treatment of individuals with BPD, and this is the population included in randomized trials to date. There is evidence for the effectiveness of DBT in reducing DSH during the course of treatment and up to 6–12 months post treatment depending on therapeutic contact (Koons et al., 2001; Linehan, Armstrong, Suarez,

Table 2 Summary of published self-injury interventions and respective levels of evidence

Intervention	Level of evidence	SORT rating	RCTs	Treatment description	Patients treated in published reports or RCTs (*n*)	Effect on self-injury
Topiramate	3	C	N/A	200 mg/day	3	Cessation of self-injury
Clozapine	3	C	N/A	300–550 mg/day for 4–12 months	8	Cessation of self-injury
Naltrexone	3	C	N/A	50 mg/day	8	Cessation of self-injury
Dialectical behavior therapy	1	B	3	12-month outpatient program; weekly individual modified cognitive-behavioral therapy; weekly skills training; ongoing skills coaching between sessions	188	Significant reduction of self-injury in 2/3 RCTs compared with TAU group
Manual assisted cognitive-behavioral therapy	3	C	2	2–7 individual cognitive therapy-oriented sessions; 70-page self-help book	512	No effect on self-injury
Transference-focused psychotherapy	2	C	2	12-month outpatient program; weekly individual psychodynamic therapy	23	No effect on self-injury
Mentalization-based therapy	2	C	0	18-month inpatient program; weekly individual psychodynamic therapy; weekly group psychodynamic therapy (3×); weekly individual psychodrama session	19	Significantly lower proportion of self-injurers compared with TAU group

The number of patients is from randomized controlled trials only when available or from available, published, nonrandomized studies if no randomized controlled trials have been conducted. *SORT* strength of recommendation taxonomy, *RCTs* randomized placebo-controlled trials, *TAU* treatment as usual

Reprinted with permission: Karr et al. (2010). Nonsuicidal self-injury: A review of current research for family medicine and primary care physicians. *The Journal of the American Board of Family Medicine*, 23(2): 240–259

& Allmon, 1991; Linehan, Heardm, & Armstrong, 1994; Linehan et al., 2006). The results about whether DBT is more effective than treatment as usual groups in these studies are mixed. In several earlier studies there were significant differences between treatment groups supporting DBT as more effective than usual treatment in reducing DSH (Koons et al., 2001; Linehan et al., 1991, 1994). However, the most recent randomized controlled trial which had a DBT group and another group treated by community experts using psychodynamic or nonbehavioral approaches showed both groups to be equally effective in decreasing DSH (both groups did have significant decreases in DSH with treatment) (Linehan et al., 2006). But over the 2-year study period, subjects in the DBT group had significantly fewer suicide attempts, fewer hospitalizations for suicidal ideation, and significantly less medical risk with DSH, compared to subjects in the other treatment group (Linehan et al., 2006).

Psychodynamic Therapies

Psychodynamic therapies share a similar approach which emphasizes the importance of the relationship between the patient and therapist in facilitating self-reflection and examination of problematic relationship patterns. Published studies of psychodynamic therapy effectiveness in the treatment of DSH focus on patients with BPD (Levy, Yeomans, & Diamond, 2007). Transference-focused psychotherapy (TFP) was developed specifically for treatment of BPD. A preliminary study did show effectiveness of TFP in reducing suicide attempts, hospitalizations, and the medical risk of DSH episodes; however the therapy did not significantly reduce the overall number of DSH episodes (Clarkin et al., 2001). Later studies of TFP looked at other outcomes in treating BPD, but did not report on DSH (Clarkin, Levy, Lenzenweger, & Kernberg, 2007; Levy, Kelly, & Meehan, 2006).

Another form of psychotherapy, mentalization-based treatment (MBT), was developed for the treatment of patients with severe BPD engaging in an intensive partial hospitalization program for a maximum of 18 months (Bateman & Fonagy, 1999). Results from the 18-month study of 38 patients randomized to the partial hospitalization group or standard psychiatric care showed that the MBT group had a significant decrease in DSH maintained over the course of the 18-month study (Bateman & Fonagy, 1999). The control group did not show a decrease in DSH. Unfortunately, in the 8-year follow-up study DSH was not reported on, though the MBT group continued to show significantly better outcomes than the control group on a number of important measures including suicidality, global functioning, vocational status, and use of medication (Bateman & Fonagy, 2008).

DSH and the Internet

It seems that the incidence of DSH has increased in recent decades and media "conversations" certainly have (Klonsky, 2007a, 2007b; Whitlock, Lader, & Conterio, 2007). During the 1990s, DSH gained significant media exposure in the tabloids, movies, and music. Since that time DSH has found a home on the Internet (Whitlock et al., 2007).

Eighty-seven percent of youth are online regularly and Whitlock et al. have noted a rapid growth of self-injury message boards, blogs, and videos (Whitlock et al., 2007). The dilemma regarding the Internet and DSH for clinicians is: Are these Web sites, blogs, and videos helpful or harmful? In a place of minimal regulation and monitoring, with the chance to be anonymous, the need for self-regulation is paramount. But as discussed earlier in this chapter, self-regulation is often underdeveloped in adolescents who engage in DSH.

Since Internet use is difficult to regulate or control, we agree with Whitlock et al. that the best approach is to discuss Internet use with patients and to specifically ask about the sites devoted to the topic of DSH (Whitlock et al., 2007). Some recommended questions include the following: What sites do you visit? How often? Do you post or just look around? What is the name of your favorite site? Have you shared your own story? If so, how did it feel?

Prevention

Studies of prevention of DSH are severely lacking. One interesting research article looked at a possible school-based prevention program (Muehlenkamp, Walsh, & McDade, 2010). The Signs of Self-Injury (SOSI) program was tested at five schools totaling 274 students. Twenty-six percent (ranging from 10 to 40 % across the five schools) of students reported at least one lifetime act of DSH, with 10 % (range 3–20 % across schools) reporting DSH in the past month. No control group was included.

The researchers found no evidence of iatrogenic harm (i.e., asking students about DSH caused no statistical increase in the risk of youth trying DSH) but students did show improved knowledge about DSH and help-seeking attitudes and intentions. Unfortunately, there was no measurable increase in self-reported help-seeking actions. More work is needed in the area of DSH prevention. Helping adolescents develop more effective coping strategies and a better understanding of DSH may prevent DSH altogether or lead to earlier intervention and better psychological functioning.

Summary

DSH is the intentional damage of body tissues without suicidal intent. The behavior is officially included as a symptom of BPD, but DSH also occurs in the setting of other mental health conditions and in nonclinical, high-functioning populations. The lifetime prevalence of DSH in adolescent and young adults varies depending on the population studied, from a low of 4 % reported by military recruits to 46 % in some high school populations and as high as 80 % in psychiatric inpatient populations. Some evidence suggests an increase in DSH in recent years. Caucasians seem to have higher rates of DSH than non-Caucasian groups, while females and males seem to have similar rates. The most common reported function of DSH is to alleviate negative emotions such as anger, sadness, or anxiety. People often report that DSH brings a feeling of calm or relief. Neurodevelopmental changes happening in adolescence may play a role in DSH, and there are several theories including the opioid-deficit model and differences in executive brain function that may help to explain the pathophysiology of DSH.

DSH is a marker of increased risk of future suicide attempts, and suicidality should be monitored on an ongoing basis. Thorough assessment of the behavior will guide care and treatment approaches. A detailed history should be obtained in a nonjudgmental, respectful manner. For treatment of DSH, there are no medications with Food and Drug Administration approval. Treatment with cognitive-behavioral or psychodynamic therapeutic approaches can help to decrease DSH behaviors, but the process of change is generally slow. More studies regarding preventive interventions in adolescents are needed.

References

Andover, M. S., & Gibb, B. E. (2010). Non-suicidal self-injury, attempted suicide, and suicidal intent among psychiatric inpatients. *Psychiatry Research, 178*(1), 101–105. doi:10.1016/j.psychres.2010.03.019.

Ballard, E., Bosk, A., & Pao, M. (2010). Invited commentary: Understanding brain mechanisms of pain processing in adolescents' non-suicidal self-injury. *Journal of Youth and Adolescence, 39*(4), 327–334. doi:10.1007/s10964-009-9457-1.

Bateman, A., & Fonagy, P. (1999). Effectiveness of partial hospitalization in the treatment of borderline personality disorder: A randomized controlled trial. *The American Journal of Psychiatry, 156*(10), 1563–1569. Retrieved from EBSCO*host*.

Bateman, A., & Fonagy, P. (2008). 8-year follow-up of patients treated for borderline personality disorder: Mentalization-based treatment versus treatment as usual. *The American Journal of Psychiatry, 165*(5), 631–638. doi:10.1176/appi.ajp.2007.07040636.

Brausch, A. M., & Gutierrez, P. M. (2010). Differences in non-suicidal self-injury and suicide attempts in adolescents. *Journal of Youth and Adolescence, 39*(3), 233–242. doi:10.1007/s10964-009-9482-0.

Cassano, P., Lattanzi, L., Pini, S., Dell'Osso, L., Battistini, G., & Cassano, G. B. (2001). Topiramate for self-mutilation in a patient with borderline personality disorder. *Bipolar Disorders, 3*(3), doi:10.1034/j.1399-5618.2001.030306.x.

Chengappa, K., Ebeling, T., Kang, J. S., Levine, J., & Parepally, H. (1999). Clozapine reduces severe self-mutilation and aggression in psychotic patients with borderline personality disorder. *The Journal of Clinical Psychiatry, 60*(7), 477–484. Retrieved from EBSCO*host*.

Chengappa, K. R., Rathore, D., Levine, J., Atzert, R., Solai, L., Parepally, H., et al. (1999). Topiramate as add-on treatment for patients with bipolar mania. *Bipolar Disorders, 1*(1), 42–53. Retrieved April 20, 2011.

Claes, L., Houben, A., Vadereycken, W., Bijttebier, P., & Muehlenkamp, J. (2010). Brief report: The association between non-suicidal self-injury self-concept and acquaintance with self- injurious peers in a sample of adolescents. *Journal of Adolescent Health, 33*(5), 775–778.

Clarkin, J. F., Foelsch, P. A., Levy, K. N., Hull, J. W., Delaney, J. C., & Kernberg, O. F. (2001). The development of a psychodynamic treatment for patients with borderline personality disorder: A preliminary study of behavioral change. *Journal of Personality Disorders, 15*(6), 487–495. doi:10.1521/pedi.15.6.487.19190.

Clarkin, J. F., Levy, K. N., Lenzenweger, M. F., & Kernberg, O. F. (2007). Evaluating three treatments for borderline personality disorder: A multiwave study. *The American Journal of Psychiatry, 164*(6), 922–928. doi:10.1176/appi.ajp.164.6.922.

DSM-III-R. (2000). American Psychiatric Association's diagnostic and statistical manual of mental disorders (3rd ed.). *PsycCRITIQUES, 35*(3), doi:10.1037/028425.

DSM-III-R. (1990). American Psychiatric Association's diagnostic and statistical manual of mental disorders (4th ed.). *PsycCRITIQUES, 35*(3), doi: 10.1037/028425.

Evans, K., Tyrer, P., Catalan, J., Schmidt, U., Davidson, K., Dent, J., et al. (1999). Manual-assisted cognitive-behavior therapy (MACT): A randomized controlled trial of a brief intervention with bibliotherapy in the treatment of recurrent deliberate self-harm. *Psychological Medicine, 29*(1), 19–25.

Ferrerri, M. M., Loze, J., Rouillon, F., & Limosin, F. (2004). Clozapine treatment of a borderline personality disorder with severe self-mutilating behaviours. *European Psychiatry, 19*(3), 177–178. doi:10.1016/j.eurpsy.2003.11.004.

Fikke, L. T., Melinder, A. A., & Landrø, N. I. (2011). Executive functions are impaired in adolescents engaging in non-suicidal self-injury. *Psychological Medicine: A Journal of Research in Psychiatry and the Allied Sciences, 41*(3), 601–610. doi:10.1017/S0033291710001030.

Glenn, C. R., & Klonsky, E. (2010). The role of seeing blood in non-suicidal self-injury. *Journal of Clinical Psychology, 66*(4), 466–473. Retrieved from EBSCO*host*.

Graff, H., & Mallin, R. (1967). The syndrome of the wrist cutter. *The American Journal of Psychiatry, 124*(1), 36–42. Retrieved from EBSCO*host*.

Gratz, K. L. (2007). Targeting emotion dysregulation in the treatment of self-injury. *Journal of Clinical Psychology, 63*(11), 1091–1103. doi:10.1002/jclp.20417.

Gratz, K. L., Conrad, S., & Roemer, L. (2002). Risk factors for deliberate self-harm among college students. *The American Journal of Orthopsychiatry, 72*(1), 128–140. doi:10.1037/0002-9432.72.1.128.

Griengl, H., Sendera, A. A., & Dantendorfer, K. K. (2001). Naltrexone as a treatment of self- injurious behavior: A case report. *Acta Psychiatrica Scandinavica, 103*(3), 234–236. doi:10.1034/j.1600-0447.2001.00087.x.

Gutierrez, P., Osmann, A., Barrios, F., & Kopper, B. (2001). Development and initial validation of the self-harm behavior questionnaire. *Journal of Personality Assessment, 77*, 475–490.

Hawton, K., Townsen, E., Arensman, E., Gunnell, D., Hazell, P., House, A., et al. (1999). Psychosocial and pharmacological treatments for deliberate self harm. *Cochrane Database of Systematic Reviews, 3*. Retrieved April 20, 2011.

Karr, P. L., Muehlenkamp, J. J., & Turner, J. M. (2010). Nonsuicidal self-injury: A review of current research for family medicine and primary care physicians. *Journal of the American Board of Family Medicine, 23*(2), 240–259.

Klonsky, E. (2007a). Non-suicidal self-injury: An introduction. *Journal of Clinical Psychology, 63*(11), 1039–1043. doi:10.1002/jclp.20411.

Klonsky, E. (2007b). The functions of deliberate self-injury: A review of the evidence. *Clinical Psychology Review, 27*(2), 226–239. doi:10.1016/j.cpr.2006.08.002.

Klonsky, E., & Glenn, C. R. (2009). Assessing the functions of non-suicidal self-injury: Psychometric properties of the inventory of statements about self-injury (ISAS). *Journal of Psychopathology and Behavioral Assessment, 31*(3), 215–219. doi:10.1007/s10862-008-9107-z.

Klonsky, E., & Moyer, A. (2008). Childhood sexual abuse and non-suicidal self-injury: Meta analysis. *The British Journal of Psychiatry, 192*(3), 166–170. doi:10.1192/bjp.bp.106.030650.

Klonsky, E., & Muehlenkamp, J. J. (2007). Self-injury: A research review for the practitioner. *Journal of Clinical Psychology, 63*(11), 1045–1056. doi:10.1002/jclp.20412.

Klonsky, E., Oltmanns, T. F., & Turkheimer, E. (2003). Deliberate self-harm in a nonclinical population: Prevalence and psychological correlates. *The American Journal of Psychiatry, 160*(8), 1501–1508. doi:10.1176/appi.ajp.160.8.1501.

Koons, C. R., Robins, C. J., Tweed, J., Lynch, T. R., Gonzalez, A. M., Morse, J. Q., et al. (2001). Efficacy of dialectical behavior therapy in women veterans with borderline personality disorder. *Behavior Therapy, 32*(2), 371–390. doi:10.1016/S0005-7894(01)80009-5.

Laye-Gindhu, A., & Schonert-Reichl, K. A. (2005). Nonsuicidal self-harm among community adolescents: Understanding the 'Whats' and 'Whys' of self-harm. *Journal of Youth and Adolescence, 34*(5), 447–457. doi:10.1007/s10964-005-7262-z.

Lester, D. (1972). Self-mutilating behavior. *Psychological Bulletin, 78*(2), 119–128. doi:10.1037/h0033066.

Levy, K. N., Kelly, K. M., & Meehan, K. B. (2006). Change in attachment patterns and reflective function in a randomized control trial of transference focused psychotherapy for borderline personality disorder. *Journal of Consulting and Clinical Psychology, 74*, 1027–1040.

Levy, K. N., Yeomans, F. E., & Diamond, D. (2007). Psychodynamic treatments of self-injury. *Journal of Clinical Psychology, 63*(11), 1105–1120.

Linehan, M. M., Armstrong, H. E., Suarez, A., & Allmon, D. (1991). Cognitive–behavioral treatment of chronically parasuicidal borderline patients. *Archives of General Psychiatry, 48*(12), 1060–1064. Retrieved from EBSCO*host*.

Linehan, M. M., Comtois, K., Brown, M. Z., Heard, H. L., & Wagner, A. (2006). Suicide attempt self-injury interview (SASII): Development, reliability, and validity of a scale to assess suicide attempts and intentional self-injury. *Psychological Assessment, 18*(3), 303–312. doi:10.1037/1040-3590.18.3.303.

Linehan, M. M., Comtois, K., Murray, A. M., Brown, M. Z., Gallop, R. J., Heard, H. L., et al. (2006). Two-year randomized controlled trial and follow-up of dialectical behavior therapy vs. therapy by experts for suicidal behaviors and borderline personality disorder. *Archives of General Psychiatry, 63*(7), 757–766. doi:10.1001/archpsyc.63.7.757.

Linehan, M. M., Heard, H. L., & Armstrong, H. E. (1994). 'Naturalistic follow-up of a behavioral treatment for chronically parasuicidal borderline patients': Erratum. *Archives of General Psychiatry, 51*(5), 422. Retrieved from EBSCO*host*.

Lloyd-Richardson, E. E. (2008). Adolescent nonsuicidal self-injury: who is doing it and why? *Journal of Developmental and Behavioral Pediatrics, 29*(3), 216–218.

Lloyd-Richardson, E. E., Perrine, N., Dierker, L., & Kelley, M. L. (2007). Characteristic and functions on non-suicidal self-injury in a community sample of adolescents. *Psychological Medicine: A Journal of Research in Psychiatry and the Allied Sciences, 37*(8), 1183–1192. doi:10.1017/S003329170700027X.

Muehlenkamp, J. J., & Gutierrez, P. M. (2004). An investigation of differences between self- injurious behavior and suicide attempts in a sample of adolescents. *Suicide and Life-Threatening Behavior, 34*(1), 12–23. doi:10.1521/suli.34.1.12.27769.

Muehlenkamp, J. J., Walsh, B. W., & McDade, M. (2010). Preventing non-suicidal self-injury in adolescents: The signs of self-injury program. *Journal of Youth and Adolescence, 39*(3), 306–314. doi:10.1007/s10964-009-9450-8.

Nafisi, N., & Stanley, B. (2007). Developing and maintaining the therapeutic alliance with self-injuring patients. *Journal of Clinical Psychology, 63*(11), 1069–1079. doi:10.1002/jclp.20414.

Nock, M. K., Elizabeth, E. B., Photos, V. I., & Michel, B. D. (2007). Self-injurious thoughts and behaviors interview: Development, reliability, and validity in an adolescent sample. *Psychological Assessment, 19*(3), 309–317.

Nock, M. K., Joiner, T. R., Gordon, K. H., Lloyd-Richardson, E., & Prinstein, M. J. (2006). Non- suicidal self-injury among adolescents: Diagnostic correlates and relation to suicide attempts. *Psychiatry Research, 144*(1), 65–72. doi:10.1016/j.psychres.2006.05.010.

Nock, M. K., & Prinstein, M. J. (2004). A functional approach to the assessment of self-mutilative behavior. *Journal of Consulting and Clinical Psychology, 72*(5), 885–890. doi:10.1037/0022-006X.72.5.885.

Prossin, A. R., Love, T. M., Koeppe, R. A., Zubieta, J., & Silk, K. R. (2010). Dysregulation of regional endogenous opioid function in borderline personality disorder: Correction. *The American Journal of Psychiatry, 167*(8), 925–933. Retrieved from EBSCOhost.

Ross, S., & Heath, N. (2002). A study of the frequency of self-mutilation in a community sample of adolescents. *Journal of Youth and Adolescence, 31*(1), 67–77. doi:10.1023/A:1014089117419.

Roth, A. S., Ostroff, R. B., & Hoffman, R. E. (1996). Naltrexone as a treatment for repetitive self-injurious behavior: An open-label trial. *The Journal of Clinical Psychiatry, 57*(6), 233–237.

Stanley, B., Sher, L., Wilson, S., Ekman, R., Huang, Y., & Mann, J. (2010). Non-suicidal self- injurious behavior, endogenous opioids and monoamine neurotransmitters. *Journal of Affective Disorders, 124*(1–2), 134–140. doi:10.1016/j.jad.2009.10.028.

Tyrer, P., Thompson, S., Schmidt, U., Jones, V., Knapp, M., Davidson, K., et al. (2003). Randomized controlled trial of brief cognitive behaviour therapy versus treatment as usual in recurrent deliberate self-harm: The POPMACT study. *Psychological Medicine, 33*(6), 977–986. ISSN 0033-2917.

Walsh, B. (2007). Clinical assessment of self-injury: A practical guide. *Journal of Clinical Psychology, 63*(11), 1057–1068. doi:10.1002/jclp.20413.

Whitlock, J., Eckenrode, J., & Silverman, D. (2006). Self-injurious behaviors in a college population. *Pediatrics, 117*, 1939–1948.

Whitlock, J., Lader, W., & Conterio, K. (2007). The Internet and self-injury: What psychotherapists should know. *Journal of Clinical Psychology, 63*(11), 1135–1143. doi:10.1002/jclp.20420.

Whitlock, J., Muehlenkamp, J., & Eckenrode, J. (2008). Variation in nonsuicidal self-injury: Identification and features of latent classes in a college population of emerging adults. *Journal of Clinical Child and Adolescent Psychology, 37*(4), 725–735. doi:10.1080/15374410802359734.

Eating Disorders in Adolescence

Renee Rienecke Hoste and Daniel Le Grange

Introduction

Eating disorders are psychiatric illnesses that are often associated with significant medical complications, psychiatric comorbidity, and impaired quality of life (APA, 2000; Jenkins, Hoste, Meyer, & Blissett, 2011). These disorders typically begin during adolescence and can potentially result in long-term damage to brain and bone health, fertility, and growth (Golden et al., 2003; Rome & Ammerman, 2003). Anorexia nervosa has the highest rate of mortality of any psychiatric illness (Powers & Bannon, 2004) and has been shown to reduce life expectancy by up to 25 years (Harbottle, Birmingham, & Sayani, 2008), pointing to the need for early and aggressive forms of treatment. Eating disorders are the third most common chronic condition among adolescent females, with a lifetime prevalence rate of 0.5–1 % for anorexia nervosa (AN) and 1–3 % for bulimia nervosa (BN). Among males, prevalence rates are approximately .05 % for AN and 0.1 % for BN (APA, 2000; Hoek & van Hoeken, 2003). However, when subthreshold eating disordered behavior is included, these estimates are much higher. In a longitudinal study of community adolescent girls, Stice, Marti, Shaw, and Jaconis (2009) found that 12 % of their sample engaged in some form of disordered eating.

This chapter will review the diagnostic criteria for eating disorders, risk factors for the development of eating disorders, assessment, and empirically supported forms of treatment.

R.R. Hoste, Ph.D. (✉) • D. Le Grange, Ph.D.
The University of Chicago, 1212 East 59th Street, Chicago, IL 60637, USA
e-mail: rhoste@yoda.bsd.uchicago.edu; legrange@uchicago.edu

Diagnostic Criteria and Clinical Presentation

Anorexia Nervosa

AN is characterized by refusal to maintain weight at or above 85 % of expected weight for age and height, or failure to gain expected weight during a period of growth. This is accompanied by an intense fear of weight gain as well as an overvaluation of the importance of shape and weight, denial of the severity of the illness, or body image distortion. In postmenarcheal females, amenorrhea (the loss of three consecutive menstrual periods) must also be present. Two subtypes of AN are recognized: the restricting subtype, in which individuals lose weight primarily by restricting their food intake, and the binge/purge subtype, in which individuals engage in regular binge eating or purging (APA, 2000).

Individuals with AN often present with perfectionistic or obsessional features, which are often premorbid but seem to be exacerbated by the state of starvation (Pollice, Kaye, Greeno, & Weltzin, 1997). Eating disordered behaviors may include

W.T. O'Donohue et al. (eds.), *Handbook of Adolescent Health Psychology*,
DOI 10.1007/978-1-4614-6633-8_31,

cutting food into very small portions, eating slowly, the excessive use of condiments, an increased interest in recipes or cookbooks, or counting calories (see Beumont, 2002). Physical activity may become compulsive in nature, in that the individual feels driven to exercise and may do so at the expense of other previously enjoyed activities, such as spending time with friends. As the eating disorder worsens, patients often become depressed, irritable, and socially withdrawn. Children and adolescents with AN are often good students and may continue to achieve good grades for some time after the onset of the illness, but concentration is often impaired and it may require more effort to achieve at the same level. In addition to denying or failing to appreciate the severity of their emaciated state, individuals with AN often experience the illness as ego-syntonic and may take pride in their ability to restrict their food intake. This can make treatment challenging, as individuals with AN can be very resistant to therapy.

Bulimia Nervosa

BN is characterized by episodes of binge eating, which are defined as eating an objectively large amount of food and experiencing a loss of control during the eating episode. Some individuals also engage in "subjective" binges, during which they do not eat an objectively large amount of food, but experience a loss of control. Binges are followed by compensatory behavior, such as self-induced vomiting, laxative use, fasting, or excessive exercise. These behaviors must occur at a frequency of at least twice a week for 3 months. As with AN, there is an overemphasis on the importance of body shape and weight when evaluating self-esteem or self-worth. These symptoms cannot occur during an episode of AN, as a diagnosis of AN "trumps" a diagnosis of BN due to the medical severity of the illness. There are two subtypes of BN: the purging type, in which the individual regularly engages in purging as compensatory behavior (e.g., self-induced vomiting, misuse of laxatives or diuretics), and the nonpurging type, in which the individual engages in inappropriate compensatory behavior such as fasting or excessive exercise, but does not purge (APA, 2000).

Although the eating habits of individuals with BN can vary widely, binge episodes are often preceded by periods of restriction during which patients limit their food intake in an effort to lose weight or change their body shape. Restriction may involve not eating for long periods of time, limiting overall caloric intake, or avoiding certain foods such as high-fat or high-carbohydrate foods. Binges are often triggered by negative affective states, including stress or boredom. As opposed to the pride often associated with AN, those with BN are often ashamed of their binge eating and compensatory behaviors and may attempt to hide these behaviors from their parents.

Although patients with BN may be ambivalent about treatment, the ego-dystonic nature of the illness can make it easier to engage these patients in therapy when compared to individuals with AN. Because individuals with BN are usually at a normal weight, they may be able to hide their eating disorder for longer than an individual with AN, whose continued weight loss eventually becomes noticeable to others.

Eating Disorder Not Otherwise Specified

A diagnosis of eating disorder not otherwise specified (EDNOS) is given to those individuals who do not meet full criteria for AN or BN but who experience clinically significant eating-related behaviors or cognitions. The DSM-IV-TR offers examples of symptom profiles that would qualify for a diagnosis of EDNOS, such as an individual who meets all criteria for AN except that she is not amenorrheic. Binge eating disorder (BED), a disorder characterized by recurrent binge episodes but no compensatory behavior, is currently diagnosed as EDNOS. Research has found few differences between individuals with EDNOS and those with full threshold AN or BN, both in terms of psychopathology and medical complications (Fairburn et al., 2007; Moor, Vartanian, Touyz, & Beumont, 2004; Peebles, Hardy, Wilson, & Lock, 2010). This suggests that EDNOS is not a "less serious" disorder, and children and adolescents who display disordered eating but do not meet full criteria for AN or BN should still receive treatment right away. This is particularly important because most children and adolescents who receive a diagnosis of an eating disorder will be given a diagnosis of EDNOS.

Diagnostic Considerations in Children and Adolescents

Although "not otherwise specified" diagnoses in the DSM-IV are meant to be residual categories, studies have found that approximately 60% of adults and adolescents in outpatient treatment receive a diagnosis of EDNOS (Eddy, Doyle, Hoste, Herzog, & Le Grange, 2008; Fairburn et al., 2007; Turner & Bryant-Waugh, 2004). It has been suggested that age-adjusted criteria be used in the diagnosis of eating disorders in children and adolescents, as the current criteria do not seem to be adequate for this age group (Workgroup, 2007).

The variability in the rate and timing of height and weight gain during puberty limits the applicability of the 85% weight criterion for AN. The amenorrhea criterion is also problematic because some individuals with AN will lose their menses prior to losing a significant amount of weight, and others will continue to menstruate at low weights (see Attia & Roberto, 2009). The irregularity of menses after puberty also makes it difficult to determine whether an individual has in fact missed three menstrual cycles, and the criterion cannot be applied to premenstrual females or females who are on birth control, and there is no equivalent criterion for males.

In addition, depending on their level of development, adolescents may have little insight and limited capacity for abstract reasoning, and therefore may not endorse the cognitive symptoms of AN and BN, such as fear of weight gain, overvaluation of shape and weight, or body image distortion, and may be unable to explain the rationale for their behavior.

Risk Factors

Eating disorders are complex illnesses involving biological, psychological, and sociocultural factors. It has been suggested that certain environmental stressors (e.g., familial or sociocultural), combined with certain biological vulnerabilities (e.g., high negative emotionality), can lead to the development of an eating disorder (Steiner et al., 2003). Some influences, such as pubertal timing, self-esteem, and social pressures to be thin, may be particularly salient during adolescence, explaining why eating disorders usually onset during this developmental period.

Many studies have identified correlates of eating disorder symptoms, but fewer studies have determined whether a factor preceded the onset of the eating disorder; only then can the factor be referred to as a "risk factor." In addition, many studies that do assess the temporal sequence of events do so retrospectively, as longitudinal studies, although preferable, are expensive and time-consuming to conduct. However, cross-sectional studies provide important information that can further our understanding of eating disorders and inform the design of later investigations of causal risk factors. The following review includes findings from both cross-sectional and longitudinal studies.

Weight Concerns and Dieting

Negative body image, concerns about weight, and dieting behavior are considered robust predictors of later eating disordered behavior, particularly for BN and AN-binge/purge subtype, and have been found to predict the development of disordered eating in several longitudinal studies (see Jacobi, Morris, & de Zwaan, 2004).

Concerns about weight and an exaggerated focus on appearance are not uncommon among adolescents, and can begin at an early age (Hill, Draper, & Stack, 1994; Maloney, McGuire, Daniels, & Specker, 1989). Weight concerns can lead to experimentation with weight control strategies, which in turn can increase risk for developing an eating disorder. In a cohort study of 888 adolescent females and 811 adolescent males, Patton, Selzer, Coffey, Carlin, and Wolfe (1999) found that 60% of the female sample were moderate dieters, and another 8% dieted at a severe level. Compared to females who did not diet, moderate dieters and severe dieters were, respectively, five and 18 times more likely to develop an eating disorder in the next 6 months. It is believed that continuous efforts to restrict one's eating eventually lead to a breakdown in dietary restraint, as the individual can no longer follow rigid dietary rules. This results in binge eating, often followed by compensatory behavior (Beumont, 2002). Particularly concerning are findings that approximately 60 % of adolescent girls and 30 % of adolescent boys use unhealthy weight control behaviors, such as smoking cigarettes or fasting (Neumark-Sztainer, Story, Hannan, Perry, & Irving, 2002).

Psychiatric Comorbidity and Negative Emotionality

Rates of lifetime anxiety disorders are high among individuals with AN and BN, and Bulik, Sullivan, Fear, and Joyce (1997) found that anxiety disorders preceded the onset of the eating disorder in 90 % of women with AN and 94 % of women with BN. However, 71 % of women with major depression also reported that their anxiety disorder predated the depression. The authors concluded that certain anxiety disorders, such as childhood overanxious disorder and social phobia, may be nonspecific factors that increase risk for later psychopathology in general, but that obsessive-compulsive disorder (OCD) is a specific risk factor for the later development of AN. Many studies have documented high rates of comorbidity among eating disorders and OCD (see Lilenfeld, 2004), and obsessional behaviors are often seen among individuals with AN. Råstam (1992) found that 35 % of their AN sample reported premorbid obsessive-compulsive personality disorder (OCPD), compared to 4 % in the control group.

Perfectionism and negative self-evaluation have been found to be specific correlates of AN (Fairburn, Cooper, Doll, & Welch, 1999), and longitudinal studies have found that low self-esteem predicts the later onset of an eating disorder (Button, Sonuga-Barke, Davies, & Thompson, 1996; Ghaderi & Scott, 2001), although it is unclear to what extent low self-esteem is a specific risk factor for eating disorders as opposed to the development of more general psychopathology.

Childhood Eating

A cross-sectional study found that early feeding and digestive problems were almost twice as common among AN patients than controls (Råstam & Gillberg, 1992), and longitudinal studies have found that early digestive problems, picky eating, eating conflicts, struggles with food, and unpleasant meals during childhood predicted the later onset of an eating disorder (Kotler, Cohen, Davis, Pine, & Walsh, 2001; Marchi & Cohen, 1990).

Puberty

Pubertal changes also seem to coincide with the onset of disordered eating (Attie & Brooks-Gunn, 1989). At particular risk are early-maturing females, who have higher rates of several psychiatric disorders, including eating disorders, than on-time maturers (Graber, Lewinsohn, Seeley, & Brooks-Gunn, 1997), suggesting that this group warrants particular attention from healthcare providers, teachers, and parents.

Family Functioning

Families have historically often been blamed for causing eating disorders (see Hoste, Doyle, & Le Grange, 2012), and several studies have found that eating disorder patients describe their families as more conflictual than do normal controls (e.g., Vidovic, Juresa, Begovac, Mahnik, & Tocilj, 2005). However, the presence of an eating disorder can cause conflict in a family (Nielsen & Barà-Carril, 2003), so it is important to examine family functioning prior to the onset of the eating disorder. Shoebridge and Gowers (2000) found that a history of high-concern parenting and maternal anxiety were more common among mothers of AN adolescents than controls. In a community study comparing individuals with BN, individuals with other psychiatric disorders, and healthy controls, Fairburn, Welch, Doll, Davies, and O'Connor (1997) found that high parental expectations, low contact with parents, and parental critical comments about weight and shape were more common among the BN group than the other two groups, suggesting that these parental characteristics are not related just to general psychopathology but to BN symptoms specifically.

Genetics

Rates of eating disorders are higher among first-degree relatives than among healthy controls for both AN and BN (Strober, Freeman, Lampert, Diamond, & Kaye, 2000), and twin studies have estimated that additive genetic effects account for 28–88 % of the risk for developing an eating disorder (see Jacobi et al., 2004). The first adoption study to examine the impact of genes and environment on disordered eating supported previous studies' findings of high rates of heritability, and found no significant impact of shared environmental factors on disordered eating (Klump, Suisman, Burt, McGue, & Iacono, 2009).

Sociocultural Influences

Adolescents are flooded with images of society's thin ideal, and the increase in concerns about same-sex and opposite-sex relationships during this developmental period may make adolescents particularly sensitive to society's messages about physical beauty. Anne Becker's well-known work with adolescent girls in Fiji found a significant increase in eating disordered attitudes and behaviors following the introduction of television and Western programming (Becker, Burwell, Herzog, Hamburg, & Gilman, 2002). Other studies have found that exposure to thin-ideal images increases body dissatisfaction and negative affect (Groesz, Levine, & Murnen, 2002), particularly among adolescent females who are already dissatisfied with their bodies and who have internalized society's thinness ideal (Heinberg & Thompson, 1995; Stice, Spangler, & Agras, 2001). In a study of adolescents in 7th and 9th grades, McCabe, Ricciardelli, and Finemore (2002) found that females reported pressure from the media to lose weight, while males felt pressure to increase weight and muscle tone, suggesting that although males are receiving different messages from the media, the pressure to change one's body weight or shape to fit the cultural ideal is relevant for most adolescents.

Assessment of Adolescent Eating Disorders

The range of presentations exhibited by adolescents at the assessment is quite varied. Some are angry about being brought to the appointment by their parents, either because they believe that they are not suffering from a disorder or because they are not interested in treatment. These individuals may be reluctant to discuss their symptoms and will attempt to minimize the severity of their illness. Others will be reluctant to discuss their symptoms because they are embarrassed by their behavior. Some adolescents, particularly younger ones, may be willing to discuss their disorder but lack the cognitive capacity to describe the reasons behind their behavior. Still others are quite cooperative, accurate, and insightful in their descriptions of the illness. Regardless of the presentation of the adolescent, it is necessary for the assessor to always meet with the adolescent's parents as well.

Meeting with the adolescent before meeting with the parents is often preferable, as it shows respect for the patient's developing autonomy. Information to obtain during this first meeting will include the onset and course of the eating disorder; the patient's current eating and exercise habits, dieting, weight, and menstrual history; the patient's and family's views of food and weight; the patient's level of body, weight, or shape dissatisfaction; family functioning; other psychiatric diagnoses; suicidal ideation; and the patient's functioning at home, in school, and with friends. The assessor should be familiar with adolescent development and be able to alter his or her questioning style as needed; for example, adolescents who are less developed cognitively may become confused or overwhelmed by open-ended questioning and may prefer a more structured, concrete approach.

After the interview with the adolescent is complete, the assessor should meet with his or her parents separately. If it is a two-parent family, it is preferable to meet with both parents. In addition to confirming the information gathered from the patient, the parents can often provide a broader view of the onset and course of the disorder, including the influence of difficulties that may not be directly related to the eating disorder. For example, parents may notice that their child's eating difficulties began around the same time that he or she started a new school, and that their child has always struggled with transitions. Parents can also provide more general information about the patient's developmental history, temperament, and personality.

In order to accurately assess and diagnose eating disordered symptoms, standardized assessment instruments can be used. The "gold standard" of eating disorder assessment is the Eating Disorder Examination (EDE) (Cooper & Fairburn, 1987), a semi-structured interview that assesses the cognitive and behavioral symptoms of AN, BN, and BED. However, it can be lengthy to administer and requires trained interviewers. The Eating Disorders Examination Questionnaire (EDE-Q; Fairburn & Beglin, 1994) is a self-report version of the EDE. However, adolescents sometimes struggle with accurately identifying instances of somewhat complex concepts such as "loss of control" and may need some guidance when answering these questions. The Eating Attitudes Test (EAT) (Garner & Garfinkel, 1979; Garner, Olmsted, Bohr, & Garfinkel, 1982) is a widely used self-report questionnaire designed to be used as a screening measure.

Because of the medical complications that can accompany eating disorders, it is essential that the patient be assessed for medical stability by a physician before he or she begins outpatient treatment. Medical assessment should include checking the adolescent's vital signs, including blood pressure, orthostatic heart rate and pulse, and temperature, as these can all be affected by malnutrition. Height and weight should be measured during the initial assessment, preferably while the patient is wearing a gown. When weighing a patient, treatment providers should be aware of some patients' attempts to make their weight appear heavier than it actually is, by drinking excessive amounts of fluid (water-loading) before their appointment, placing weights or heavy objects in their pockets, or wearing weights under their clothing. See Katzman, Kanbur, and Steinegger (2010) for a more detailed overview of the information to be gathered during the initial assessment and the challenges that arise when interviewing adolescents.

Treatment for Adolescent Eating Disorders

Eating disorders can be difficult to treat, as eating disordered individuals are often quite ambivalent about recovery and may not readily engage in treatment. However, the potentially serious medical and psychosocial consequences of eating disorders require an assertive team approach, with a mental health expert to address the patient's psychotherapeutic needs, a physician to monitor the patient's physical health, and, if necessary, a psychiatrist to manage comorbid psychiatric concerns. The treatment providers should specialize in the treatment of eating disorders and should have experience working with adolescents (Rome et al., 2003).

Within these suggestions, however, there have been few guidelines for treating eating disorders until 2004, when the UK's National Institute for Clinical Excellence issued clinical guidelines on the treatment of eating disorders (NICE, 2004; Wilson & Shafran, 2005). The Guideline Development Group included professionals from many disciplines, academic experts in psychiatry and psychology, and international experts in eating disorders research. The group met 23 times and employed rigorous methodology to analyze the highest-quality treatment outcome research. Treatment approaches were given grades of A, B, or C. Treatments that had strong empirical support from well-conducted randomized controlled trials (RCTs) were given a grade of A, treatments that had empirical support from well-conducted clinical studies but had not been assessed in an RCT were given a grade of B, and treatment approaches whose support was based on the consensus of experts but did not have strong empirical support were given a grade of C. Over 100 recommendations were made for the treatment of adult and adolescent AN, BN, and EDNOS. With only two exceptions, all treatment approaches were given a grade of C, indicating that there is a great need for more RCTs in the field as a whole. Cognitive-behavioral therapy for adults with BN was given a grade of A, and family-based treatment for adolescents with AN was given a grade of B. These treatment approaches will be reviewed next.

Cognitive-Behavioral Therapy for Bulimia Nervosa

Cognitive-behavioral therapy has a large evidence base to support it as the treatment of choice for adults with BN. However, despite the fact that binge eating and purging behaviors often begin in adolescence (Stice & Agras, 1998), only two RCTs have been conducted with adolescents with BN (Le Grange, Crosby, Rathouz, & Leventhal, 2007; Schmidt et al., 2007). Although CBT has not been widely studied among adolescents with BN, findings suggest that adapting CBT for use with adolescents may have promising results (Schapman, Lock, & Couturier, 2006; Schmidt et al., 2007).

Cognitive-behavioral therapy (CBT) is based on the premise that overconcern with body shape and weight leads to dietary restriction. Dietary restriction in turn leads to hunger, resulting in the temporary lifting of rigid rules around food and consequent binge eating. Binge eating is then followed by some form of compensatory behavior, such as self-induced vomiting, in an attempt to avoid weight gain that may result from the binge (Fairburn, Marcus, & Wilson, 1993).

The first of the three treatment phases focuses on psychoeducation and helping patients change their pattern of eating. The therapist educates the patient about the cognitive-behavioral model of BN and provides information on the adverse effects of dieting, binge eating, and compensatory behavior. Patients are then encouraged to reduce periods of restriction and gradually lessen rigid dietary rules, with the goal of eating meals and snacks regularly throughout the day. In the second phase, patients continue to develop regular patterns of eating and gradually reintroduce "forbidden foods" back into their diet. In addition, patient's overconcern with body weight and shape is addressed. Through cognitive restructuring, patients are taught to challenge their negative thoughts and develop more balanced ways of thinking, and are taught problem-solving techniques to cope with triggers to engage in disordered eating. The third phase focuses on maintaining progress made up to that point in treatment, and addresses relapse prevention.

Although CBT has been found to be quite useful for adults, the developmental level of adolescents necessitates making adjustments to the therapeutic approach (see Lock, 2005, for a more detailed discussion). CBT is a treatment that requires active participation and effort on the part of the patient, including regular homework. For example, self-monitoring is a cornerstone of treatment: patients are asked to keep track of everything they eat and drink, when and where they ate, if they binged or purged, and the circumstances surrounding eating episodes. As described above, adolescents are often unhappy about being brought to treatment by their parents, so therapists can expect a level of motivation that is likely to be much lower than one would expect for a self-referred adult, particularly for a form of treatment that requires work outside of therapy sessions. In addition, adolescents' efforts to establish autonomy from their parents can generalize to other adults, such as the therapist (Lock, 2005), and may take the form of resistance to therapeutic suggestions. Adolescents may take longer to "warm up" to the therapist. Thus, the therapist may need to allow extra time to focus on developing rapport with the patient. The therapist can facilitate this by showing an interest in the adolescent's experiences and allowing for some discussion of issues other than eating that are important to the patient (e.g., problems with peers, romantic relationships). For patients with low motivation, it is important for therapists to "meet them where they're at" to avoid power struggles and show respect for the patient's developing autonomy.

Self-monitoring can also be a challenge when working with adolescents. They are often resistant to keeping food logs because they find them to be too time-consuming, they are embarrassed to write down what they ate, they are worried about others finding the food logs, or they simply forgot. The therapist may need to be more flexible than he or she would need to be with an adult, and brainstorm solutions with the patient in an effort to make it easier to complete the food logs. For example, instead of filling out food logs or writing in a notebook during lunch at school, some patients are more likely to record what they ate if they can keep track of it on their cell phones, making them feel less conspicuous. If patients repeatedly forget, asking parents to remind them can be helpful.

Parental involvement is another way that CBT has been adapted for adolescents. The extent to which parents are involved varies from patient to patient, but usually parents are at least responsible for ensuring that the patient attends sessions regularly. Parents can also assist patients in eating regularly throughout the day, staying with them after meals to prevent purging, and altering shopping habits so that binge foods are not in the house. In addition, parents are often aware of changes in their child's mood that might trigger a binge, and can encourage them to use alternative forms of coping.

In addition to working with parents, therapists may need to intervene in certain school settings. For example, some patients eat lunch quite late in the day, leaving a long gap between breakfast and lunch and inviting the possibility of binge eating in the afternoon. Therapists may need to work with schools to change a patient's lunch period, if necessary, or ask for permission for the patient to eat snacks during class if this is normally forbidden.

Throughout treatment therapists should be careful to use language that is understandable to the patient. While some adolescents may be quite advanced cognitively, others may have limited capacity for abstract reasoning or self-observation, and the therapist will need to adjust his or her approach accordingly. For example, some patients will respond better to concrete, straightforward questions, or may require guidance from the therapist when discussing what triggered a binge episode. Some adolescents struggle with identifying reasons for behaving in a certain manner. If the therapist asks, "What do you think triggered the binge?" the patient may legitimately be unable to answer the question. In these cases, the therapist may need to offer several options: "Your food log says that you didn't have a snack when you got home from school. Do you think you were hungry? You also mentioned earlier that you were feeling stressed that day after the fight you had with your friend. Do you think that had anything to do with it?" In this way the therapist will need to offer a great deal of structure to these patients, and may also need to offer this level of structure when teaching patients cognitive restructuring.

Similarly, when providing psychoeducation to patients, therapists should check to be sure they understand what is being discussed. It can be helpful to ask patients to summarize what the therapist has said in their own words to determine their level of understanding. In addition, therapists should not assume an understanding of eating disorder constructs such as binge eating. The way an eating disorder treatment provider would describe a binge may be very different from the way a patient would describe it, so it is necessary to discuss these issues early on in treatment to ensure that the therapist and patient are on the same page.

Family-Based Treatment for Anorexia Nervosa

A growing body of research is available to suggest that family-based treatment is the treatment of choice for adolescents with an early age of onset (before age 18) and a short duration of illness (less than 3 years) (Le Grange, Lock, Loeb, & Nicholls, 2010; Lock et al., 2010; Russell, Szmukler, Dare, & Eisler, 1987). In addition, follow-up studies have found that patients' weight gain is maintained 5 years later (Eisler et al., 1997).

Family-based treatment (FBT) (also often referred to as the "Maudsley method" or the "Maudsley approach") was developed at the Maudsley Hospital in London, England, in the 1980s. It differs from many traditional forms of psychotherapy in that it takes an agnostic view of the cause of the illness and puts parents in charge of the patient's recovery (Lock, Le Grange, Agras, & Dare, 2001). Because of the severity of AN and the potential long-term medical consequences associated with it, the emphasis in FBT is on a rapid return to health and an assertive approach to weight restoration. Ambivalence about recovery is to be expected with many adolescents and adults with eating disorders, but those with AN seem to be particularly resistant to treatment. This resistance, coupled with the fact that the illness can be fatal and the treatment team therefore cannot afford to wait for the adolescent to be motivated to engage in therapy, necessitates the prominent role of the parents in the treatment approach. Parents are viewed as a crucial resource in the adolescent's recovery, and indeed do the large majority of the therapeutic work. In addition to viewing the family as a resource, another critical tenet of FBT is the separation of the disorder from the patient. Parents are provided with psychoeducation about the nature of AN, particularly about the profound fear of weight gain experienced by the patient and the ways in which this fear can manifest itself at mealtimes, which can vary from quiet, sullen resistance to angry, violent outbursts. Parents are encouraged to remember that this behavior is being driven by the eating disorder rather than their child, which can help parents direct their frustration toward the illness while remaining supportive of the patient.

In the first of three treatment phases, control over the patient's eating is temporarily put in the hands of the parents, who are asked to decide what, when, and how much their child should eat. They are asked to monitor meals and snacks and to curtail physical activity. Parents are encouraged to draw on the knowledge they have about nutrition and adequate food intake to prepare meals and snacks that will reverse their child's state of self-starvation and result in appropriate weight gain and a return to health. The task given to parents is considerable; AN is a powerful illness that does not allow sufferers to easily make decisions that will lead to recovery. Parents often meet great resistance from the eating disorder and it is vitally important that they feel empowered to take on the challenge facing them. Thus, the therapist does not specifically instruct parents as to how to go about feeding their child; parents are regarded as the experts on their own family and are encouraged to approach the refeeding process in the way most fitting for their family, while the therapist is a consultant who provides guidance and expertise on eating disorders. Although families may want to discuss other problems, such as a child's anxiety or increased social withdrawal, other topics are generally not addressed in FBT until the patient is gaining weight and the medical dangers associated with the illness have diminished.

Families begin the second phase of treatment when the patient is approaching his or her ideal body weight and is eating more easily and willingly. The parents gradually return control over eating back to the adolescent. The extent to which the adolescent is given responsibility over food choices will depend greatly on the age of the adolescent. For example, the second phase of treatment for a 10-year-old may look very much like the first phase of treatment, as parents are generally still very much in charge of a 10-year-old's diet. An 18-year-old patient, however, will be given much more responsibility over his or her food choices.

The third phase of treatment can begin when the adolescent is weight-restored and difficulties related to eating have generally diminished. During this phase, issues that may have been set aside earlier in treatment can be addressed. There is a discussion of general adolescent development, upcoming developmental challenges, and how parents can help their children face these challenges without reverting to the eating disorder as a way to cope.

A common criticism of FBT is that it is developmentally inappropriate, and that parents should not be taking control of their adolescent's eating at an age when the adolescent should be developing increased personal autonomy and separating from his or her family of origin. There is no doubt that it would be developmentally inappropriate for parents to take complete control over a healthy adolescent's eating habits. However, as previously noted, the nature of AN is such that the patient is unable to make the decisions necessary to maintain good health, even at times to the point of causing death. As the adolescent is clearly not in control of his or her behavior, FBT temporarily gives this control to the parents, with the goal of restoring the adolescent's weight quickly so that parents can relinquish this control and the patient can return to normal adolescent activities and the normal developmental tasks of separation and individuation.

Other Treatment Approaches

Inpatient treatment is necessary at times, and Golden et al. (2003) have outlined the criteria for admission to an inpatient program. Pharmacotherapy studies with children and adolescents are limited, but there is some evidence for the efficacy of antipsychotics (e.g., olanzapine) (Boachie, Goldfield, & Spettigue, 2003) in the treatment of AN, and fluoxetine in the treatment of BN (Kotler, Devlin, Davies, & Walsh, 2003). In addition, FBT has been shown to be useful in the treatment of adolescents with BN (Le Grange et al., 2007). For adolescents with AN, a form of treatment originally called ego-oriented individual therapy (EOIT) (Robin et al., 1999) and later referred to as adolescent-focused psychotherapy (AFP) (Fitzpatrick, Moye, Hoste, Lock, & Le Grange, 2010) has been found to be helpful.

Conclusion

Eating disorders are serious illnesses that can have a long-term impact on adolescents' health and development. Certain environmental stressors and biological vulnerabilities may be particularly relevant during adolescence, causing these disorders to begin during this stage of development. Early intervention is crucial to minimize the potential damage, even for adolescents who do not meet full criteria for AN or BN. Randomized controlled trials with adolescents with eating disorders are few, but CBT for adolescents with BN may be promising, while FBT for adolescents with AN has been shown to be effective. Regardless of the treatment approach utilized, parental involvement is critical for adolescents with eating disorders.

References

American Psychiatric Association. (2000). *Diagnostic and statistical manual of mental disorders* (4th ed.). Washington, DC: American Psychiatric Association.

Attia, E., & Roberto, C. A. (2009). Should amenorrhea be a diagnostic criterion for anorexia nervosa? *International Journal of Eating Disorders, 42*, 581–589.

Attie, I., & Brooks-Gunn, J. (1989). Development of eating problems in adolescent girls: A longitudinal study. *Developmental Psychology, 25*, 70–79.

Becker, A. E., Burwell, R. A., Herzog, D. B., Hamburg, P., & Gilman, S. E. (2002). Eating behaviours and attitudes following prolonged exposure to television among ethnic Fijian adolescent girls. *The British Journal of Psychiatry, 180*, 509–514.

Beumont, P. J. V. (2002). Clinical presentation of anorexia nervosa and bulimia nervosa. In C. G. Fairburn & K. D. Brownell (Eds.), *Eating disorders and obesity: A comprehensive handbook* (2nd ed., pp. 162–170). New York: Guilford Press.

Boachie, A., Goldfield, G. S., & Spettigue, W. (2003). Olanzapine use as an adjunctive treatment for hospitalized children with anorexia nervosa: Case reports. *International Journal of Eating Disorders, 33*, 98–103.

Bulik, C. M., Sullivan, P. F., Fear, J. L., & Joyce, P. R. (1997). Eating disorders and antecedent anxiety disorders: A controlled study. *Acta Psychiatrica Scandinavica, 96*, 101–107.

Button, E. J., Sonuga-Barke, E. J. S., Davies, J., & Thompson, M. (1996). A prospective study of self-esteem in the prediction of eating problems in adolescent schoolgirls: Questionnaire findings. *British Journal of Clinical Psychology, 35*, 193–203.

Cooper, Z., & Fairburn, C. G. (1987). The eating disorder examination: A semi-structured interview for the assessment of the specific psychopathology of eating disorders. *International Journal of Eating Disorders, 6*, 1–8.

Eddy, K. T., Doyle, A. C., Hoste, R. R., Herzog, D. B., & Le Grange, D. (2008). Eating disorder not otherwise specified in adolescents. *Journal of the American Academy of Child and Adolescent Psychiatry, 47*, 156–164.

Eisler, I., Dare, C., Russell, G. F. M., Szmukler, G. I., Le Grange, D., & Dodge, E. (1997). Family and individual therapy in anorexia nervosa: A five-year follow-up. *Archives of General Psychiatry, 54*, 1025–1030.

Fairburn, C. G., & Beglin, S. J. (1994). Assessment of eating disorders: Interview or self-report questionnaire? *International Journal of Eating Disorders, 16*, 363–370.

Fairburn, C. G., Cooper, Z., Bohn, K., O'Connor, M. E., Doll, H. A., & Palmer, R. L. (2007). The severity and status of eating disorder NOS: Implications for DSM-V. *Behavior Research and Therapy, 45*, 1705–1715.

Fairburn, C. G., Cooper, Z., Doll, H. A., & Welch, S. L. (1999). Risk factors for anorexia nervosa: Three integrated case–control comparisons. *Archives of General Psychiatry, 56*, 468–476.

Fairburn, C. G., Marcus, M. D., & Wilson, G. T. (1993). Cognitive behavioral therapy for binge eating and bulimia nervosa: A comprehensive treatment manual. In C. G. Fairburn & G. T. Wilson (Eds.), *Binge eating: Nature, assessment, and treatment* (pp. 361–404). New York: Guilford Press.

Fairburn, C. G., Welch, S. L., Doll, H. A., Davies, B. A., & O'Connor, M. E. (1997). Risk factors for bulimia nervosa: A community-based case–control study. *Archives of General Psychiatry, 54*, 509–517.

Fitzpatrick, K., Moye, A., Hoste, R., Lock, J., & Le Grange, D. (2010). Adolescent focused psychotherapy for adolescents with anorexia nervosa. *Journal of Contemporary Psychotherapy, 40*, 31–39.

Garner, D. M., & Garfinkel, P. E. (1979). The eating attitudes test: An index of the symptoms of anorexia nervosa. *Psychological Medicine, 9*, 273–279.

Garner, D. M., Olmstead, M. P., Bohr, Y., & Garfinkel, P. E. (1982). The eating attitudes test: Psychometric features and clinical correlates. *Psychological Medicine, 12*, 871–878.

Ghaderi, A., & Scott, B. (2001). Prevalence, incidence, and prospective risk factors for eating disorders. *Acta Psychiatrica Scandinavica, 104*, 122–130.

Golden, N. H., Katzman, D. K., Kreipe, R. E., Stevens, S. L., Sawyer, S. M., Rees, J., et al. (2003). Eating disorders in adolescents: Position paper of the Society for Adolescent Medicine. *Journal of Adolescent Health, 33*, 496–503.

Graber, J. A., Lewinsohn, P. M., Seeley, J. R., & Brooks-Gunn, J. (1997). Is psychopathology associated with the timing of pubertal development? *Journal of the American Academy of Child and Adolescent Psychiatry, 36*, 1768–1776.

Groesz, L. M., Levine, M. P., & Murnen, S. K. (2002). The effect of experimental presentation of thin media images on body satisfaction: A meta-analytic review. *International Journal of Eating Disorders, 31*, 1–16.

Harbottle, E. J., Birmingham, C. L., & Sayani, F. (2008). Anorexia nervosa: A survival analysis. *Eating and Weight Disorders, 13*, e32–e34.

Heinberg, L. J., & Thompson, J. K. (1995). Body image and televised images of thinness and attractiveness: A controlled laboratory investigation. *Journal of Social and Clinical Psychology, 14*, 325–338.

Hill, A. J., Draper, E., & Stack, J. (1994). A weight on children's minds: Body shape dissatisfactions at 9-years old. *International Journal of Obesity and Related Metabolic Disorders, 18*, 383–389.

Hoek, H. W., & van Hoeken, D. (2003). Review of the prevalence and incidence of eating disorders. *International Journal of Eating Disorders, 34*, 383–396.

Hoste, R. R., Doyle, A. C., & Le Grange, D. (2012). Families as an integral part of the treatment team: Treatment culture and standard of care challenges. In J. Alexander & J. Treasure (Eds.), *A Collaborative Approach to Eating Disorders* (pp. 136–143). London: Routledge.

Jacobi, C., Morris, L., & de Zwaan, M. (2004). An overview of risk factors for anorexia nervosa, bulimia nervosa, and binge eating disorder. In T. D. Brewerton (Ed.), *Clinical handbook of eating disorders: An integrated approach* (pp. 117–163). New York: Marcel Dekker.

Jenkins, P., Hoste, R. R., Meyer, C., & Blissett, J. (2011). Eating disorders and quality of life: A review of the literature. *Clinical Psychology Review, 31*, 113–121.

Katzman, D. K., Kanbur, N. O., & Steinegger, C. M. (2010). Medical screening and management of eating disorders in adolescents. In W. S. Agras (Ed.), *The Oxford handbook of eating disorders* (pp. 267–291). New York: Oxford University Press.

Klump, K. L., Suisman, J. L., Burt, S. A., McGue, M., & Iacono, W. G. (2009). Genetic and environmental influences on disordered eating: An adoption study. *Journal of Abnormal Psychology, 118*, 797–805.

Kotler, L. A., Cohen, P., Davis, M., Pine, D. S., & Walsh, B. T. (2001). Longitudinal relationships between childhood, adolescent, and adult eating disorders. *Journal of the American Academy of Child and Adolescent Psychiatry, 40*, 1424–1440.

Kotler, L. A., Devlin, M. J., Davies, M., & Walsh, B. T. (2003). An open trial of fluoxetine for adolescents with bulimia nervosa. *Journal of Child and Adolescent Psychopharmacology, 13*, 329–335.

Le Grange, D., Crosby, R. D., Rathouz, P. J., & Leventhal, B. L. (2007). A randomized controlled comparison of family-based treatment and supportive psychotherapy for adolescent bulimia nervosa. *Archives of General Psychiatry, 64*, 1049–1056.

Le Grange, D., Lock, J., Loeb, K., & Nicholls, D. (2010). Academy for eating disorders position paper: The role of the family in eating disorders. *International Journal of Eating Disorders, 43*, 1–5.

Lilenfeld, L. R. R. (2004). Psychiatric comorbidity associated with anorexia nervosa, bulimia nervosa, and binge eating disorder. In T. D. Brewerton (Ed.), *Clinical handbook of eating disorders: An integrated approach* (pp. 183–207). New York: Marcel Dekker.

Lock, J. (2005). Adjusting cognitive behavior therapy for adolescents with bulimia nervosa: Results of case series. *American Journal of Psychotherapy, 59*, 267–281.

Lock, J., Le Grange, D., Agras, W. S., & Dare, C. (2001). *Treatment manual for anorexia nervosa: A family-based approach*. New York: Guilford Press.

Lock, J., Le Grange, D., Agras, W. S., Moye, A., Bryson, S. W., & Jo, B. (2010). Randomized clinical trial comparing family-based treatment with adolescent-focused individual therapy for adolescents with anorexia nervosa. *Archives of General Psychiatry, 67*, 1025–1032.

Maloney, M. J., McGuire, J., Daniels, S. R., & Specker, B. (1989). Dieting behavior and eating attitudes in children. *Pediatrics, 84*, 482–489.

Marchi, M., & Cohen, P. (1990). Early childhood eating behaviors and adolescent eating disorders. *Journal of the American Academy of Child and Adolescent Psychiatry, 29*, 112–117.

McCabe, M., Ricciardelli, L., & Finemore, J. (2002). The role of puberty, media and popularity with peers on strategies to increase weight, decrease weight and increase muscle tone among adolescent boys and girls. *Journal of Psychosomatic Research, 52*, 145–153.

Moor, S., Vartanian, L. R., Touyz, S. W., & Beumont, P. J. V. (2004). Psychopathology of EDNOS patients: To whom do they compare? *Clinical Psychologist, 8*, 70–75.

Neumark-Sztainer, D., Story, M., Hannan, P. J., Perry, C. L., & Irving, L. M. (2002). Weight-related concerns and behaviors among overweight and nonoverweight adolescents: Implications for preventing weight-related disorders. *Archives of Pediatric and Adolescent Medicine, 156*, 171–178.

NICE. (2004). *Eating disorders: Core interventions in the treatment and management of anorexia nervosa, bulimia nervosa, and related eating disorders*. NICE Clinical Guideline no. 9. Retrieved September 2, 2010, from http://www.nice.org.uk.

Nielsen, S., & Bará-Carril, N. (2003). Family, burden of care and social consequences. In J. Treasure, U. Schmidt, & E. van Furth (Eds.), *Handbook of eating disorders* (2nd ed., pp. 191–206). Chichester, UK: Wiley.

Patton, G. C., Selzer, R., Coffey, C., Carlin, J. B., & Wolfe, R. (1999). Onset of adolescent eating disorders: Population based cohort study over 3 years. *British Medical Journal, 318*, 765–768.

Peebles, R., Hardy, K. K., Wilson, J. L., & Lock, J. D. (2010). Are diagnostic criteria for eating disorders markers of medical severity? *Pediatrics, 125*, e1193–e1201.

Pollice, C. P., Kaye, W. H., Greeno, C. G., & Weltzin, T. E. (1997). Relationship of depression, anxiety, and obsessionality to state of illness in anorexia nervosa. *International Journal of Eating Disorders, 21*, 367–376.

Powers, P. S., & Bannon, Y. (2004). Medical Comorbidity of anorexia nervosa, bulimia nervosa, and binge eating disorder. In T. D. Brewerton (Ed.), *Clinical handbook of eating disorders: An integrated approach* (pp. 231–255). New York: Marcel Dekker.

Råstam, M. (1992). Anorexia nervosa in 51 Swedish adolescents: Premorbid problems and comorbidity. *Journal of the American Academy of Child and Adolescent Psychiatry, 31*, 819–829.

Råstam, M., & Gillberg, C. (1992). Background factors in anorexia nervosa. A controlled study of 51 teenage cases including a population sample. *European Child & Adolescent Psychiatry, 1*, 54–65.

Robin, A. L., Siegel, P. T., Moye, A. W., Gilroy, M., Dennis, A. B., & Sikand, A. (1999). A controlled comparison of family versus individual therapy for adolescents with anorexia nervosa. *Journal of the American Academy of Child and Adolescent Psychiatry, 38*, 1482–1489.

Rome, E. S., & Ammerman, S. (2003). Medical complications of eating disorders: An update. *Journal of Adolescent Health, 33*, 418–426.

Rome, E. S., Ammerman, S., Rosen, D. S., Keller, R. J., Lock, J., Mammel, K. A., et al. (2003). Children and adolescents with eating disorders: The state of the art. *Pediatrics, 111*, e98–e108.

Russell, G. F., Szmukler, G. I., Dare, C., & Eisler, I. (1987). An evaluation of family therapy in anorexia nervosa and bulimia nervosa. *Archives of General Psychiatry, 44*, 1047–1056.

Schapman, A. M., Lock, J., & Couturier, J. (2006). Cognitive-behavioral therapy for adolescents with binge eating syndromes: A case series. *International Journal of Eating Disorders, 39*, 252–255.

Schmidt, U., Lee, S., Beecham, J., Perkins, S., Treasure, J., Yi, I., et al. (2007). A randomized controlled trial of family therapy and cognitive behavior therapy guided self-care for adolescents with bulimia nervosa and related disorders. *The American Journal of Psychiatry, 164*, 591–598.

Shoebridge, P. J., & Gowers, S. G. (2000). Parental high concern and adolescent-onset anorexia nervosa: A case–control study to investigate direction of causality. *The British Journal of Psychiatry, 176*, 132–137.

Steiner, H., Kwan, W., Shaffer, T. G., Walker, S., Miller, S., Sagar, A., et al. (2003). Risk and protective factors for juvenile eating disorders. *European Child & Adolescent Psychiatry, 12*(Suppl 1), 38–46.

Stice, E., & Agras, W. (1998). Predicting onset and cessation of bulimic behaviors during adolescence: A longitudinal grouping analysis. *Behavior Therapy, 29*, 257–276.

Stice, E., Marti, C. N., Shaw, H., & Jaconis, M. (2009). An 8-year longitudinal study of the natural history of threshold, subthreshold, and partial eating disorders from a community sample of adolescents. *Journal of Abnormal Psychology, 118*, 587–597.

Stice, E., Spangler, D., & Agras, W. S. (2001). Exposure to media-portrayed thin-ideal images adversely affects vulnerable girls: A longitudinal experiment. *Journal of Social and Clinical Psychology, 20*, 270–288.

Strober, M., Freeman, R., Lampert, C., Diamond, J., & Kaye, W. (2000). Controlled family study of anorexia nervosa and bulimia nervosa: Evidence of shared liability and transmission of partial syndromes. *The American Journal of Psychiatry, 157*, 393–401.

Turner, H., & Bryant-Waugh, R. (2004). Eating disorder not otherwise specified (EDNOS): Profiles of clients presenting at a community eating disorder service. *European Eating Disorders Review, 12*, 18–26.

Vidovic, V., Juresa, V., Begovac, I., Mahnik, M., & Tocilj, G. (2005). Perceived family cohesion, adaptability and communication in eating disorders. *European Eating Disorders Review, 13*, 19–28.

Wilson, G., & Shafran, R. (2005). Eating disorders guidelines from NICE. *The Lancet, 365*, 79–81.

Workgroup for Classification of Eating Disorders in Children and Adolescents (WCEDCA). (2007). Classification of child and adolescent eating disturbances. *International Journal of Eating Disorders, 40*, S117–S122.

Anxiety in Adolescence

DeMond M. Grant

Introduction

Adolescence is a time of substantial change both physiologically and psychologically. It also is a period of time when individuals are particularly vulnerable to developing symptoms of anxiety disorders (Costello & Angold, 1995). This increased risk for the development of anxiety is likely due in part to the numerous transitions during this period. As a result, adolescence is a particularly important time regarding the development of psychopathology. This period often sets the stage for future beliefs about the self and others, developmental concerns, and interpersonal relationships, which all are factors that are important to the development of anxiety. Therefore, an accurate understanding of the vulnerability factors and the features of anxiety disorders is important for mental health professionals. The goal of this chapter is to review important areas associated with the epidemiology, etiology, assessment, descriptive psychopathology, and treatment of anxiety disorders. This chapter will review these disorders briefly with a focus on adolescence, and will conclude with comments for future research with individuals and adolescents suffering from anxiety disorders.

D.M. Grant, Ph.D. (✉)
Department of Psychology, Oklahoma State University, 107 Whitehurst, Stillwater, OK 74078, USA
e-mail: demond.grant@okstate.edu

Description

Anxiety disorders are one of the most prevalent psychiatric disorders, with lifetime prevalence rates of up to 31 % in the population (Kessler, 1995). The main anxiety disorders that could be the focus of attention for clinicians and researchers include panic disorder (PD), agoraphobia, social anxiety disorder (SAD), generalized anxiety disorder (GAD), obsessive-compulsive disorder (OCD), posttraumatic stress disorder (PTSD), acute stress disorder (ASD), and specific phobias (SP). PD is the fear of experiencing out of the blue physical sensations of anxiety (known as panic attacks). Agoraphobia is characterized by anxiety of places where escape may be difficult in the event that an individual has a panic attack. SAD is an excessive fear of being negatively evaluated in social or performance situations. GAD is characterized by excessive and uncontrollable worry that leads to somatic and cognitive symptoms of anxiety. OCD is characterized by obsessions, which are intrusive and distressing thoughts and images that cause anxiety, and compulsions, which are thoughts or behaviors designed to reduce this anxiety. PTSD is characterized by intrusive thoughts about a past trauma, avoidance of such thoughts, emotional numbing, and physical sensations of anxiety. ASD also involves anxiety about a trauma, although can only be diagnosed within the first month following the event. Specific phobias are excessive fears of particular objects or situations.

W.T. O'Donohue et al. (eds.), *Handbook of Adolescent Health Psychology*,
DOI 10.1007/978-1-4614-6633-8_32, © Springer Science+Business Media New York 2013

Diagnosing the anxiety disorders during adolescence is particularly difficult. The Diagnostic and Statistical Manual (DSM) places the eight above mentioned disorders in their own section, adding anxiety disorders due to a medical condition or a substance, and a Not Otherwise Specified category for clinically impairing symptoms that do not meet full criteria for any of the other disorders (American Psychiatric Association, 2000). This presumes that most of the anxiety disorders develop during adulthood, as there is a separate section in the DSM for disorders that are usually diagnosed during childhood. One of these disorders, separation anxiety disorder, is rarely diagnosed during adolescence (Wicks-Nelson & Israel, 2009). In fact, it is often difficult to determine whether one should draw on what we know about adults with anxiety disorders, or what we know about childhood anxiety among this population. Indeed, it is important to note that not very much research has focused on anxiety during adolescence, and much of the literature that does combines the functioning of adolescents with children. This is surprising, as several studies suggest that anxiety disorders are the most common disorder diagnosed during adolescence (Anderson, 1994; Kim-Cohen et al., 2003). Additionally, there are marked developmental differences between even young and older adolescents, and thus more research is needed to examine how anxiety and its related disorders present during this period.

Etiological Factors

Adolescence represents a period of significant change in several domains that result in the individual increasing their independence from their parents and building their sense of self and way of relating to others. These changes, however, can result in high levels of stress for the adolescent, which in turn can set the stage for psychopathology. How these changes relate to the development of anxiety among adolescents will be discussed in the following section.

Biological Factors

There are extensive biological changes that occur during puberty, mostly involving increased hormone levels via the hypothalamus and the pituitary gland. These hormones result in increased height and weight, changes in the body's composition of fat and muscle, and maturation of the reproductive organs. Some studies indicate that the timing of puberty can increase risk of developing anxiety disorders. Specifically, research has suggested that individuals who experience puberty earlier than their peers are more likely to experience symptomatology compared to peers who develop "on time" or later, particularly among girls (Reardon, Leen-Feldner, & Hayward, 2009). Moreover, the physical changes associated with puberty also may increase risk for anxiety. Females tend to experience increases in the amount of fat compared to males (who experience increases in muscle growth), in addition to growth of the hips and breasts. As a result, body image becomes particularly important for girls, and can result in increased stress and lower self-esteem.

A few studies have begun to examine the effects of pubertal hormones on the development of internalizing disorders. There is some evidence that the hormones that result in puberty may have a relationship with the development of anxiety disorders. For example, one study suggested that hormones released by the adrenal and gonadal systems (which are related to puberty) may increase risk for anxiety among boys, but not girls (Susman et al., 1991). Additionally, cortisol, a hormone that is produced in response to stress and arousal, and is released from the adrenal glands, is increasingly being studied in its relationship with psychopathology. Although it is clear that cortisol is a biological marker of the stress response, its relationship with psychopathology may depend on a number of factors, including the severity and duration of the symptoms. Within the anxiety disorders, some evidence suggests that cortisol is related to PTSD, although the data are equivocal regarding its relation to the other anxiety conditions (Reardon et al., 2009). Given the relatively small number of studies examining this issue, more research is needed in order to draw strong conclusions within this area.

Interpersonal Stress

One robust predictor of the development of anxiety disorders has been the relationship functioning of parents and children. Specifically, several studies suggest that the children of anxious parents are at a greater risk for developing an anxiety disorder compared to those whose parents do not meet criteria for an anxiety diagnosis (Beidel & Turner, 1997; Kearney, Sims, Pursell, & Tillotson, 2003). Other studies have found evidence that attachment patterns during early childhood are predictive of the development of anxiety disorders during adolescence (Muris, Mayer, & Meesters, 2000; Warren, Huston, Egeland, & Sroufe, 1997). Parenting behaviors that are risk factors for anxiety disorders include overprotection, control, rejection, and lack of warmth (McLeod et al., 2007). Thus, parenting behavior that interferes with adolescents' attempts to develop into relatively independent young adults increases risk for the development of anxiety (Davila, La Greca, Starr, & Landoll, 2010).

Moreover, during adolescence peer relationships become more important to an individual's functioning than parental relationships (Larson, 1983). Difficulties in the development of close relationships can lead to chronic stress, which leaves the individual vulnerable to the developmentt of psychopathology. How adolescents function within these relationships can not only affect their future relationship development but also can impact the development of their anxious symptoms (Davila et al., 2010). Thus, positive peer relationships can protect adolescents against the development of anxiety disorders, whereas problematic relationships can increase risk for the development of anxiety (La Greca & Harrison, 2005).

It is important to note that adolescence is a period of time where many sex differences emerge in risks for psychological disorders. With most of the anxiety disorders, females have higher prevalence rates and tend to report more impairment as a result of their symptoms (Chapman, Mannuzza, & Fyer, 1995). One reason why girls are more at risk for the development of anxiety (and depressive) disorders is due to their vulnerability to stress. Particularly, several studies have suggested that girls are more focused on their relationship functioning, and thus are more vulnerable to experiencing stress within these relationships (e.g., Rudolph, 2002). This increased stress results in problematic ways of relating to others, leading to internalizing symptoms characterized by anxiety and depression (Rose & Rudolph, 2006; Rudolph, 2002). Thus, relationship stress is an important vulnerability factor to consider when working with adolescents, particularly for girls.

Cognitive Factors

Cognitive vulnerabilities include ways the individual thinks about themselves and about their world. Specific cognitive vulnerabilities include biases in attention (how one views the world and reacts to threat), interpretation of events, and memory processes. Attentional biases are characterized by excessive focus on perceived threatening or anxiety-provoking stimuli. These biases result in individuals focusing on anxiety-provoking stimuli over neutral or positive stimuli, which serve to maintain their anxious symptoms. Interpretation biases result in the individual inferring negative meanings from ambiguous events. Finally, memory biases involve excessive recall of perceived negative past events. There is considerable evidence of anxiety being associated with biases of attention and interpretation (e.g., Schultz & Heimberg, 2008), although whether anxiety is associated with biases of memory may depend on the specific disorder (Coles & Heimberg, 2002).

Another cognitive factor that has been found to be important to the development of anxiety disorders is anxiety sensitivity. Anxiety sensitivity represents a fear of consequences of experiencing anxiety, such as fear of panic symptoms, mental incapacitation, and others noticing one's anxiety (Reiss, 1991). Studies have suggested that high levels of anxiety sensitivity predict the development of panic attacks and anxiety symptoms prospectively, even when controlling for baseline anxiety symptoms (Hayward, Killen, Kraemer, & Taylor, 2000; Schmidt et al., 2010). Studies also have found evidence of anxiety sensitivity representing a risk factor for anxiety disorders among adolescents (e.g., Anderson & Hope, 2009).

Comorbidity

Among most DSM diagnoses, comorbidity (i.e., where an individual meets criteria for two or more disorders at the same time) is the rule rather than the exception. Thus, when seeing an adolescent with symptoms resembling anxiety, it is important to consider other possible diagnoses. First, individuals who meet DSM criteria for one anxiety disorder are more likely to also meet criteria for another anxiety disorder. Second, depression also exhibits high comorbidity levels with the anxiety disorders. Several studies have suggested a strong relationship between being diagnosed with an anxiety disorder and major depressive disorder (Kessler et al., 1994). Third, anxiety also has been shown to increase risk for substance use disorders. For example, research suggests that individuals often use substances to cope with their anxious symptoms (e.g., Kushner, Sher, & Beitman, 2004). Finally, anxiety disorders also are associated with increased risk for developing eating disorders, particularly among adolescent females (Babio, Canals, Pietrobelli, Perez, & Arija, 2009). Because individuals with eating disorders are less likely to seek treatment, a careful assessment procedure including a physical examination may be useful in distinguishing between anxiety and eating pathology.

As a result of the high levels of comorbidity, it is recommended that clinicians conduct a thorough assessment with adolescents seeking treatment for anxiety. In some cases, approaches effective in treating anxiety also have been useful in treating comorbid cases, although at times comorbidity can negatively impact treatment outcome (e.g., Heimberg & Becker, 2002). Therefore it is important to have a broad understanding of the specific features associated with the anxiety disorders.

Assessment

Assessment of anxiety disorders (and other psychological disorders) is a complex process. The major concerns include focusing on nomothetic assessments with documented psychometric properties, while considering idiographic aspects of the individual patient. In terms of anxiety disorders, examination of an individual's behavior without considering their specific fears can lead to an inaccurate diagnosis. For example, during the assessment phase a clinician may learn that a patient avoids social situations because they make them anxious. However, determining whether this patient is avoiding this situation because they will be negatively evaluated (and thus are experiencing symptoms of SAD) or because they are scared they might have a panic attack (and thus are experiencing symptoms of PD) is an important distinction. Among adolescents, another consideration includes the relationship the adolescent has with his/her parents. Although it is very important for clinicians to focus on the needs of his/her patients, adolescents still are too young to consent to treatment without their parents. Therefore, including the parents during the assessment phase, and determining before treatment the extent that parents will be involved, is essential, regardless of the individual's diagnosis.

The assessment phase ideally would include clinical interviews, self-report measures, and behavioral assessments across multiple sources (i.e., adolescent, parent, teacher). Among adults, one widely used semi-structured interview for assessment of the anxiety disorders is the Anxiety Disorders Interview Schedule for DSM-IV (ADIS-IV; Brown, DiNardo, & Barlow, 1994). The ADIS-IV has been developed for use with children and adolescents, and includes interviews for both the child and the parent (ADIS-C/P; Silverman & Albano, 1996). The ADIS-C/P also includes questions to diagnose related disorders including depression and attention deficit/hyperactivity disorder. Its psychometric properties have been well documented, and it has been used in numerous studies. The full interview takes approximately 2 h, and provides the interviewer with probe questions to differentiate between comorbid conditions. Due to its length, completing the full ADIS can be time consuming, despite its usefulness in differentiating between the different anxiety disorders. Thus, it may be useful to include self-report measures to help determine the specific nature of an individual's fears.

Each anxiety disorder is characterized by a core fear which leads to some form of avoidance or is endured with considerable distress. This fear guides individuals' behavior, typically resulting in avoidance of any situation where they may have to experience or approach the feared object/situation. Thus, understanding anxiety disorders revolves around differentiating between the main fear that characterizes each. A brief review of these disorders will follow, with an eye toward identifying the features of each that are characteristic of adolescents.

Panic Disorder and Agoraphobia

The core fear of panic disorder (PD) involves experiencing a panic attack, a discrete period of intense anxiety typically characterized by increased heart rate, chest pressure, difficulty breathing, and other physiological symptoms of anxiety (American Psychiatric Association, 2000). Panic attacks generally only last a few minutes, and typically observers are not aware of the symptoms that the patient is experiencing. However, from the patient's perspective, these acute anxiety attacks are associated with severe physical and cognitive symptoms of anxiety. Individuals experiencing a panic attack often have catastrophic thoughts about their symptoms. As a result of these fears, individuals with PD have excessive concerns about experiencing future attacks, worry about what these attacks mean about them (e.g., "am I going crazy?"), or change their behavior to avoid having future attacks (e.g., they will avoid exercise or caffeinated drinks; APA, 2000).

A diagnosis of PD can occur either with or without agoraphobia. Agoraphobia involves anxiety about being in a situation where one may not be able to escape in the event that they experience a panic attack (APA, 2000). The additional fears associated with agoraphobia often result in increased avoidance of several situations, including malls, grocery stores, and other situations with large groups of people. Therefore, the symptoms of PD with agoraphobia can result in impairment across a wide variety of situations. Many patients with PD (with or without agoraphobia) will often carry a particular object (e.g., an inhaler, a bottle of pills) around with them to serve as a "safety signal." A safety signal is something that individuals believe will help them cope with anxiety, and is characteristic of all anxiety disorders. Individuals also can rely on close friends, family, and romantic partners. Thus, these individuals can enter their feared situations as long as they have their "safety person" with them. Although these safety signals can help them to enter situations which they normally would fear, use of safety signals can often interfere with treatment.

PD typically has an age of onset around mid to late adolescence. This disorder occurs in about 1 % of adolescents in the community, and as high as 15 % of adolescents seeking treatment, with at least half percent also meeting criteria for agoraphobia (Essau, Conradt, & Petermann, 1999; Last & Strauss, 1989). Research has suggested that the cognitions experienced by adolescents while panicking are similar to those of adults (Nelles & Barlow, 1988). However, data also suggests that many adolescents with PD either are diagnosed with a different disorder (e.g., depression), or are referred for treatment due to comorbid diagnosis (Doerfler, Connor, Volungis, & Toscano, 2007) such as ADHD and mood disorders.

Social Anxiety Disorder

Social anxiety disorder (SAD) is characterized by excessive fears of being negatively evaluated in social situations (APA, 2000). Most individuals with this disorder will avoid social situations with any chance of ambiguity, or hover on the periphery in order to avoid possible embarrassment. Individuals with SAD frequently use close friends, romantic partners, or family members as safety signals. Therefore, the socially anxious individual can attend parties and other evaluative situations as long as their safety person attends with them (and stays by their side). SAD has a fairly early age of onset with many individuals first experiencing clinically significant symptoms during early to mid adolescence (Mannuzza, Fyer, Liebowitz, & Klein, 1990). Therefore, considering the increasing social pressures faced by adolescents, the early teen years are likely a difficult time for individuals with high levels of social fears.

SAD appears to be a relatively common fear among treatment-seeking adolescents. Research suggests that the period of adolescence is one of the highest risks for the development of social anxiety, particularly for girls (e.g., Wittchen, Stein, & Kessler, 1999). Possible reasons include difficulties with body satisfaction, gender role stressors, or changes in physical development (Nolen-Hoeksema & Girgus, 1994). For example, one study suggested that the onset of puberty predicted increased risk for the development of social anxiety among females, but not males during adolescence (Deardorff et al., 2007). Studies have suggested that social fears can decrease the development of appropriate social skills, friendships, and romantic relationships (Johnson & Glass, 1989; Rubin, LeMare, & Lollis, 1990). In fact, socially anxious adolescents experience rejection by peers, fewer friendships, and poor quality friendships (Inderbitzen, Walters, & Bukowski, 1997; La Greca & Lopez, 1998). Social fears also can impact academics, and future occupational functioning. For example, it is not uncommon for socially anxious adolescents to choose a less prestigious career path just because it will allow them to avoid public speaking or interacting with others.

Generalized Anxiety Disorder

Generalized anxiety disorder (GAD) is characterized by excessive and uncontrollable worries about a number of topics within one's life (APA, 2000). As a result of these worries, patients will experience several somatic symptoms including muscle tension, restlessness, and difficulty falling asleep. Among adolescents with this disorder, worries typically focus on the future, school and classwork, family relationships, and friend and romantic relationships (Albano & Hack, 2004). Epidemiological studies suggest that GAD typically has an age of onset during late adolescence (Kendler, Neale, Kessler, Heath, & Eaves, 1992). Previous versions of the DSM have diagnosed children and adolescents with excessive worries with overanxious disorder. However, as of DSM-IV, overanxious disorder has been subsumed under the category of GAD.

Based on available data, the features that characterize adolescents with GAD appear to be similar to adults with the disorder. Typical adolescents with GAD will set high achievement goals for their academics, and will frequently worry about not making these achievements. These perfectionistic tendencies can carry over into other areas, such as being on time for appointments and within their friendships. GAD also is associated with difficulties within close relationships. Studies indicate that GAD is associated with a range of problematic interpersonal behaviors, from excessive dependency to cold and hostile personality traits (e.g., Newman & Erickson, 2010). Finally, due to the nature of the disorder, individuals with GAD frequently engage in checking behavior. For example, these individuals might call a close friend just to "check that they are ok." Therefore, the chronic worry leads to impairment across several domains.

Studies have suggested that similar to adults, adolescents with GAD often experience high levels of comorbid depression (Masi, Favilla, Mucci, & Millipiedi, 2000). Additionally, studies have suggested that adolescents with comorbid GAD and depression are at higher risk for developing suicidal ideation compared to those with either disorder alone (Pawlak, Pascual-Sanchez, Rae, Fischer, & Ladame, 1999; Strauss, Last, Hersen, & Kazdin, 1988). Other studies have suggested that adolescents with GAD may initiate use of alcohol at a lower age compared to their nonanxious peers, perhaps as a self-medication strategy (Clark, Parker, & Lynch, 1999; Kaplow, Curran, Angold, & Costello, 2001).

Obsessive-Compulsive Disorder

The characteristic symptoms of obsessive-compulsive disorder (OCD) are made up of obsessions, or intrusive thoughts or images that cause anxiety or distress, and compulsions, or repetitive behaviors used to reduce anxiety or distress (APA, 2000). Although the focus of the obsessions (to increase anxiety) and the compulsions (to decrease anxiety) remain rather constant, the specific rituals and symptoms vary greatly for each patient. Indeed, there are several areas of obsessions and compulsions that are only somewhat functionally related. For example, upon experiencing an obsession that one's hand is contaminated or dirty, a typical response is to excessively wash one's hand. Alternatively, it is not at all uncommon for a patient with OCD to experience obsessions related to a close friend or family member being hurt which leads to a compulsion to count objects in the environment. Although DSM criteria do not require both obsessions and compulsions for a diagnosis, individuals experiencing only one type of symptom are rare (Swedo et al., 1989). In trying to diagnose this disorder, it is important to keep in mind the function of the thoughts and behaviors.

Research indicates that OCD often develops during childhood or adolescence, with prevalence rates at this time being around 1–2 % (Rasmussen & Eisen, 1990). Although some studies suggest that among children boys tend to develop OCD earlier than girls (Swedo et al., 1989), during adolescence prevalence rates appear to be equal among the sexes (Flament et al., 1988). Despite these data, not much research has examined the particular impairments associated with OCD during adolescence. It appears that OCD presents similarly across adults and adolescents, with both being characterized by difficulties across interpersonal, academic, and home environments. Common difficulties associated with adolescent OCD include difficulties completing homework, difficulties grooming, and other situations where the obsessions and compulsions interfere with concentration. There is evidence that parents are more likely to notice the problems associated with OCD compared to their adolescent children, although a multi-informant assessment procedure may still be important for these patients (Piacentini, Bergman, Keller, & McCracken, 2003). One important aspect to note is that although adolescents with OCD often seek treatment for their symptoms, many are often diagnosed incorrectly or do not receive an empirically supported treatment (Flament et al., 1988).

Posttraumatic Stress Disorder and Acute Stress Disorder

Posttraumatic stress disorder (PTSD) is relatively well known amongst the general population, yet the specific features and symptoms of this disorder are not. PTSD is an anxiety disorder that develops following a particularly frightening or traumatic event that was either experienced or witnessed directly (APA, 2000). Although traumatic events can lead to the development of a variety of psychological disorders (e.g., Grant, Beck, Marques, Palyo, & Clapp, 2008), PTSD is made up of a particular constellation of symptoms, grouped into "clusters" by our current diagnostic system. The first cluster is known as "Reexperiencing" symptoms because individuals repeatedly think of their trauma. Symptoms of reexperiencing include intrusive thoughts and dreams of the event, and flashbacks during which individuals feel as if the event is actually recurring. The second cluster of symptoms is known as the "Avoidance and Numbing" cluster, which consists of avoiding thoughts and activities that remind one of the event and symptoms in which people's emotions and ways of relating to others are reduced. The third cluster is called "Hyperarousal," and consists of typical symptoms of excessive anxiety, including difficulty sleeping, hypervigilance (being on alert for danger), and an exaggerated startle response. Importantly, PTSD can only be diagnosed if the symptoms persist for longer than 1 month after the trauma.

PTSD can develop from a wide variety of traumas, including natural disasters, motor vehicle accidents, sexual abuse, and sexual and physical assault. Despite these differences, the presentation of this disorder across different traumas is highly similar. Adolescents appear to experience similar symptoms and presentations as adults. When discussing their trauma, typical PTSD patients will only describe the basic details, avoiding any negative thoughts or emotions experienced during the event. Many patients have not told anyone about the event, and thus it may take several sessions to build a rapport with the patient before they discuss the details of the event. A thorough PTSD assessment would also include the details of the trauma. Although a multi-informant perspective is useful for diagnosing PTSD, adolescents may be less likely to divulge to their parents that they experienced a trauma. This is an important consideration both for parents and clinicians. Adolescent PTSD appears to be relatively common, with prevalence rates reported as high as 16 % and 19 % for boys and girls, respectively (Kilpatrick et al., 2003). The development of PTSD during adolescence is associated with similar risk factors as adults, including difficulties in social functioning, anxiety and depression, difficulty remembering the trauma, and negative feelings about the trauma (Udwin, Boyle, Yule, Bolton, & O'Ryan, 2000).

Acute stress disorder (ASD) is characterized by excessive anxiety and dissociative symptoms following a trauma (APA, 2000). ASD can only be diagnosed within 1 month of the trauma. ASD shares several symptoms of PTSD, including intrusive thoughts or images, avoidance of trauma-related stimuli, and increased arousal. However, ASD also is characterized by dissociative symptoms that are not part of a PTSD diagnosis, such as a subjective sense of numbing or detachment, derealization, and depersonalization. The rationale for including dissociation as a symptom of ASD is that use of such coping in the early aftermath of trauma is predictive of later PTSD (Harvey & Bryant, 2002).

Not much is known about the presentation of ASD among adolescents. Studies indicate that as many as 28 % of adolescents experiencing trauma may experience ASD (e.g., Meiser-Stedman et al., 2005). Although there is evidence of ASD predicting later PTSD status (Brewin, Andrews, Rose, & Kirk, 1999), other data suggests little predictive utility of the dissociative symptoms of ASD, even among adolescents. This has led some to question the utility of the ASD diagnosis (e.g., Dalgleish et al., 2008).

Specific Phobias

Specific phobias (SP) are characterized by excessive anxiety about a number of discrete events. Based on DSM criteria, these fears are divided into five types: animal type, natural environment type, situational type, blood/injection/injury type, and "other" for fears that cannot be included in the previous categories (APA, 2000). Adolescent samples appear to be characterized by similar subtypes (Muris, Schmidt, & Merckelbach, 1999). Although there is considerable heterogeneity in the specific fears associated with SP, individuals who meet criteria for this disorder tend to avoid the situations that elicit their anxiety. Diagnosing individuals with a specific phobia is contingent on these fears not being accounted for by another disorder. For example, a patient who fears driving, but whose fear is related to a past accident that also results in reexperiencing symptoms, avoidance, and excessive arousal, would be diagnosed with PTSD rather than a specific phobia of driving. In diagnosing SP, it is important to consider the impairment that results from the individual's fears. In addition, the specific fears that result in a diagnosis of SP must be excessive to a fear reaction that is normal to the situation, and must lead to excessive avoidance.

Related Disorders

Body dysmorphic disorder (BDD) is characterized by excessive concern that a specific aspect of one's appearance is flawed in the absence of any real deformity (APA, 2000). As a result, individuals with BDD experience negative thoughts about their perceived deformity, and excessively engage in behaviors focused on checking or hiding this deformity. Given the importance of body image during adolescence, this developmental period is particularly vulnerable for the development of BDD. Among adolescents with BDD, typical areas of the body which may be of concern include the skin, hair, or muscle shape and size (APA, 2000). These thoughts can become so distressing that they interfere with school, homework, and socializing with peers (Hadley,

Greenberg, & Hollander, 2002). Although this disorder was originally thought to be a somatoform disorder, more recent evidence suggests that it may be more closely related to the anxiety disorders. In particular, research has suggested that BDD is highly related to SAD, with BDD being the fourth most common comorbid disorder associated with SAD (Hollander & Aronowitz, 1999). In support of this, a recent review paper suggested that these two disorders are highly similar with respect to age of onset, trajectory, and cognitive biases (Fang & Hofmann, 2010). Further research is needed to examine the similarity of BDD with SAD, and whether BDD may be better conceptualized as an anxiety disorder.

Another disorder related to anxiety concerns is trichotillomania (TTM), which is characterized by an excessive urge to pull one's hair (APA, 2000). Research suggests that between 1 and 3.5 % of adolescents will experience this disorder (Christenson, Pyle, & Mitchell, 1991). Onset during adolescence appears to be common (Christenson & MacKenzie, 1995). However, few studies have examined the presentation of TTM among adolescents. Research suggests that across developmental age, the scalp appears to be the most common area of pulling hair (e.g., Tolin, Franklin, Diefenbach, Anderson, & Meunier, 2007). Although both OCD and TTM are characterized by repetitive behaviors, the former is generally focused on a variety of compulsive behaviors, whereas the latter is focused exclusively on hair pulling. In addition, whereas some evidence suggests that hair pulling at times may be automatic, at other times hair pulling may be preceded by anxiety (e.g., Woods, Piacentini, Himle, & Chang, 2005).

Treatment

In general, treatment of anxiety disorders among adolescents can be exceedingly complex. First, because of the changes and adjustments that occur during adolescence, a major consideration involves considering where the adolescent falls developmentally. That is, some adolescents may be more likely to respond to treatments that involve the parent, whereas in other cases including the parent may actually hinder rapport building or treatment adherence. Inclusion of developmental processes and idiographic differences is important when treating adolescents. Therefore, as part of the assessment process, clinicians also should consider the adolescent's environment, forms of social support, and the close relationships identified by the patient.

There have been several empirically supported treatments developed for the anxiety disorders. These treatments tend to have several similar elements, including psychoeducation, relaxation skills, cognitive restructuring (i.e., changing anxiety-related thought patterns into more balanced or neutral thoughts), and exposure. Exposure therapy involves having a patient experience the negative thoughts and feelings associated with their anxiety disorder in a controlled environment. The rationale is that repeated exposure to the anxiety-provoking stimuli will result in habituation or a reduced anxiety response to subsequent exposures to the stimuli. Cognitive-behavioral treatments (CBT) for anxiety disorders, which focus on reducing problematic thoughts and behaviors, all involve some type of exposure therapy. CBT also includes a substantial homework component, in which the patient applies the skills they learned during sessions to real-world applications.

Only recently have these therapies been adapted for use with adolescent samples. Although the core components of CBT (psychoeducation, cognitive therapy, relaxation training, and exposure) are kept, two major facets are added to make these treatments more applicable to adolescents. First, the language and examples are simplified to help younger populations understand the rationale and procedures of the treatment. Second, components are included to help parents and their children during treatment. This can include educating the parent about the nature of anxiety disorders, including parents in part of the sessions, and having parents help the adolescent with homework. Downward extensions of adult CBT treatments are now being developed for all of the anxiety disorders (e.g., Foa, Chrestman, & Gilboa-Schechtman, 2009; Hoffman & Mattis, 2000; Pincus, May, Whitton, Mattis, & Barlow, 2010). However, it is important to note that some disorders have only limited evidence of effectiveness in reducing symptoms among adolescents.

There also is a considerable literature examining the use of psychotropic medications for the treatment of anxiety disorders. There are several different drug classes that have demonstrated effectiveness in reducing symptoms of anxiety, particularly the antidepressants (e.g., Rockhill et al., 2010). Selective serotonin reuptake inhibitors (SSRIs), a particular type of antidepressant, have been shown to decrease anxiety symptoms in adolescents across several of the main anxiety disorders. OCD likely has the strongest support for pharmacological treatments reducing symptomatology (Rockhill et al., 2010). Less research has examined psychotropic medications among the other anxiety disorders in adolescent samples, although there is some evidence for their efficacy. For example, one study compared CBT, a commonly used SSRI (sertraline), and combined CBT and SSRI to placebo among a sample of children and adolescents diagnosed with SAD, GAD, and separation anxiety disorder. Results suggested that all three treatments evidenced higher reductions in anxiety symptoms compared to placebo, supporting their efficacy (Walkup et al., 2008). Additionally, the combined treatment resulted in the highest reductions in symptoms, suggesting that a combination of medication and CBT may be the most effective in reducing symptoms of anxiety among adolescents (similar to adults).

It is salient to note that all medications will have side effects, which should be carefully considered with a medical professional before starting an adolescent on any medications. For SSRIs, side effects can range from headaches and nausea to increased risk for suicidal ideation or attempts. Thus, it is important for parents to carefully monitor their child when starting a new medication regimen.

Conclusions

Overall, there are several conclusions that can be drawn with respect to anxiety disorders among adolescents. First, based on the literature, there is evidence that the presentations of anxiety symptoms during adolescence are similar to that of adults. This is important, as developmental processes can impact both our assessment procedures and treatments for these impairing psychological conditions. However, further research is needed to examine the similarities and differences of the anxiety disorders among adolescents and adults. Second, anxiety symptomatology is highly prevalent among this population. In fact, adolescence appears to be the most vulnerable time for the development of significant symptoms of all or almost all of the anxiety disorders. Third, there is evidence that many of the anxiety disorders may be either misdiagnosed or left untreated until a comorbid disorder develops. This is highly unfortunate, as anxiety disorders tend to be chronic conditions that are unlikely to remit without treatment.

Therefore, there are several considerations to be kept in mind whether treating or researching anxiety among adolescents. Most youth are less likely to seek treatment for their concerns until their parents become aware of their difficulties. As a result, externalizing disorders (e.g., attention deficit/hyperactivity disorder) are more likely to be noticed than internalizing disorders such as anxiety and depression. Assessing a wide range of symptomatology may be important in order to obtain an accurate diagnosis. Additionally, consideration of the developmental age of the adolescent is crucial in order to obtain an accurate and thorough assessment. Although some patients may feel comfortable discussing their difficulties with parents, as adolescents become older they are less likely to do so. Keeping this in mind during the assessment and adjusting one's procedures accordingly is crucial in this population.

Finally, the literature examining anxiety among adolescents is still in its infancy. This is unfortunate, because the study of psychopathology during adolescence can help inform both how subclinical symptoms become diagnosable conditions and ways to decrease those at risk for significant psychopathology. Presently, although there are some general guidelines for assessing and treating adolescents with anxiety, most studies lump adolescents with children samples. Although these studies are highly informative, they limit the type of conclusions that can be drawn regarding the specific aspects of anxiety during this developmental period. Moreover, examining anxiety and its related disorders during adolescence can increase our understanding of the etiologies associated with these disorders, and inform our knowledge of ways to reduce risk for these chronic, debilitating conditions.

References

Albano, A. M., & Hack, S. (2004). Children and adolescents. In R. G. Heimberg, C. L. Turk, & D. S. Mennin (Eds.), *Generalized anxiety disorder: Advances in research and practice* (pp. 383–408). New York: The Guilford Press.

American Psychiatric Association. (2000). *The diagnostic and statistical manual of mental disorders* (4th ed.). Washington, DC: American Psychiatric Association.

Anderson, J. C. (1994). Epidemiological issues. In T. H. Ollendick, N. J. King, & W. Yule (Eds.), *International handbook of phobic and anxiety disorders in children and adolescents* (pp. 43–66). New York: Plenum Press.

Anderson, E. R., & Hope, D. A. (2009). The relationship among social phobia, objective and perceived physiological reactivity, and anxiety sensitivity in an adolescent population. *Journal of Anxiety Disorders, 23*, 18–26.

Babio, N., Canals, J., Pietrobelli, A., Perez, S., & Arija, V. A. (2009). A two-phase population study: Relationships between overweight body composition, and risk of eating disorders. *Nutricion Hospitalaria, 24*, 485–491.

Beidel, D. C., & Turner, S. M. (1997). At risk for anxiety: I. Psychopathology in the offspring of anxious parents. *Journal of the American Academy of Child and Adolescent Psychiatry, 36*, 918–924.

Brewin, C. R., Andrews, B., Rose, S., & Kirk, M. (1999). Acute stress disorder and posttraumatic stress disorder in victims of violent crime. *The American Journal of Psychiatry, 156*, 360–366.

Brown, T. A., DiNardo, P. A., & Barlow, D. H. (1994). *Anxiety disorders interview schedule for DSM-IV (ADIS-IV)*. Albany, NY: Graywind.

Chapman, T. F., Mannuzza, S., & Fyer, A. J. (1995). Epidemiology and family studies of social phobia. In R. G. Heimberg, M. R. Liebowitz, D. A. Hope, & F. R. Schneier (Eds.), *Social phobia: Diagnosis, assessment, and treatment* (pp. 21–40). New York: Guilford Press.

Christenson, G. A., & MacKenzie, T. B. (1995). Trichotillomania, body dysmorphic disorder, and obsessive-compulsive disorder. *The Journal of Clinical Psychiatry, 56*, 211–212.

Christenson, G. A., Pyle, R. L., & Mitchell, J. E. (1991). Estimated lifetime prevalence of trichotillomania in college students. *The Journal of Clinical Psychiatry, 52*, 415–417.

Clark, D. B., Parker, A. M., & Lynch, K. G. (1999). Psychopathology and substance-related problems during early adolescence: A survival analysis. *Journal of Clinical Child Psychology, 28*, 333–341.

Coles, M. E., & Heimberg, R. G. (2002). Memory biases in the anxiety disorders: Current status. *Clinical Psychology Review, 22*, 587–627.

Costello, E. J., & Angold, A. (1995). Epidemiology. In J. S. March (Ed.), *Anxiety disorders in children and adolescents* (pp. 109–124). New York: Guilford Press.

Dalgleish, T., Meiser-Stedman, R., Kassam-Adams, N., Ehlers, A., Winston, F., Smith, P., et al. (2008). Predictive validity of acute stress disorder in children and adolescents. *The British Journal of Psychiatry, 192*, 392–393.

Davila, J., La Greca, A. M., Starr, L. R., & Landoll, R. R. (2010). Anxiety disorders in adolescence. In J. G. Beck (Ed.), *Interpersonal processes in the anxiety disorders: Implications for understanding psychopathology and treatment*. Washington, DC: American Psychological Association.

Deardorff, J., Hayward, C., Wilson, K. A., Bryson, S., Hammer, L. D., & Agras, S. (2007). Puberty and gender interact to predict social anxiety symptoms in early adolescence. *Journal of Adolescent Health, 41*, 102–104.

Doerfler, L. A., Connor, D. F., Volungis, A. M., & Toscano, P. F. (2007). Panic disorder in clinically referred children and adolescents. *Children Psychiatry and Human Development, 38*, 57–71.

Essau, C. A., Conradt, J., & Petermann, F. (1999). Frequency of panic attacks and panic disorder in adolescents. *Depression and Anxiety, 9*, 19–26.

Fang, A., & Hofmann, S. G. (2010). Relationship between social anxiety disorder and body dysmorphic disorder. *Clinical Psychology Review, 30*, 1040–1048.

Flament, M. F., Whitaker, A., Rapoport, J. L., & Davies, M. (1988). Obsessive compulsive disorder in adolescence: An epidemiological study. *Journal of the American Academy of Child and Adolescent Psychiatry, 27*, 764–771.

Foa, E. B., Chrestman, K. R., & Gilboa-Schechtman, E. (2009). *Prolonged exposure therapy for adolescents with PTSD: Emotional processing of traumatic experiences: Therapist guide*. New York: Oxford University Press.

Grant, D. M., Beck, J. G., Marques, L., Palyo, S. A., & Clapp, J. D. (2008). The structure of distress following trauma: Posttraumatic stress disorder, major depressive disorder, and generalized anxiety disorder. *Journal of Abnormal Psychology, 117*, 662–672.

Hadley, S. J., Greenberg, J., & Hollander, E. (2002). Diagnosing and treatment of body dysmorphic disorder in adolescents. *Current Psychiatry Reports, 4*, 108–113.

Harvey, A. G., & Bryant, R. A. (2002). Acute stress disorder: A synthesis and critique. *Psychological Bulletin, 128*, 886–902.

Hayward, C., Killen, J. D., Kraemer, H. C., & Taylor, C. B. (2000). Predictors of panic attacks in adolescents. *Journal of the American Academy of Child and Adolescent Psychiatry, 39*, 207–214.

Heimberg, R. G., & Becker, R. E. (2002). *Cognitive-behavioral group therapy for social phobia: Basic mechanisms and clinical strategies*. New York: Guilford Press.

Hoffman, E. C., & Mattis, S. G. (2000). A developmental adaptation of panic control treatment for panic disorder in adolescence. *Cognitive and Behavioral Practice, 7*, 253–261.

Hollander, E., & Aronowitz, B. R. (1999). Comorbid social anxiety and body dysmorphic disorder: Managing the complicated patient. *The Journal of Clinical Psychiatry, 60*, 27–31.

Inderbitzen, H. M., Walters, K. S., & Bukowski, A. L. (1997). The role of social anxiety in adolescent peer relations: Differences among sociometric status groups and rejected groups. *Journal of Clinical Child Psychology, 26*, 338–348.

Johnson, R. L., & Glass, C. R. (1989). Heterosocial anxiety and direction of attention in high school boys. *Cognitive Therapy and Research, 13*, 509–526.

Kaplow, J. B., Curran, P. J., Angold, A., & Costello, E. J. (2001). The prospective relation between dimensions of anxiety and the initiation of adolescent alcohol abuse. *Journal of Clinical Child Psychology, 30*, 316–326.

Kearney, C. A., Sims, K. E., Pursell, C. R., & Tillotson, C. A. (2003). Separation anxiety disorder in young children: A longitudinal and family analysis. *Journal of Clinical Child and Adolescent Psychology, 32*, 593–598.

Kendler, K. S., Neale, M. C., Kessler, R. C., Heath, A. C., & Eaves, L. J. (1992). Generalized anxiety disorder in women: A population based twin study. *Archives of General Psychiatry, 49*, 267–272.

Kessler, R. C. (1995). The national comorbidity survey: Preliminary results and future directions. *International Journal of Methods in Psychiatric Research, 5*, 139–151.

Kessler, R. C., McGonagle, K., Zhao, S., Nelson, C., Hughes, M., Eshleman, S., et al. (1994). Lifetime and 12-month prevalence of DSM-III-R psychiatric disorders in the United States. *Archives of General Psychiatry, 51*, 8–19.

Kilpatrick, D. G., Ruggiero, K. J., Acierno, R., Saunders, B. E., Resnick, H. S., & Best, C. L. (2003). Violence and risk of PTSD, major depression, substance abuse/dependence, and comorbidity: Results from the national survey of adolescents. *Journal of Consulting and Clinical Psychology, 71*, 692–700.

Kim-Cohen, J., Caspi, A., Moffitt, T. E., Harrington, H., Milne, B. J., & Poulton, R. (2003). Prior juvenile diagnoses in adults with mental disorder: Developmental follow-back of a prospective-longitudinal cohort. *Archives of General Psychiatry, 60*, 709–717.

Kushner, M. G., Sher, K. J., & Beitman, B. D. (2004). The relationship between alcohol problems and the anxiety disorders. *The American Journal of Psychiatry, 147*, 685–695.

La Greca, A. M., & Harrison, H. M. (2005). Adolescent peer relations, friendships, and romantic relationships: Do they predict social anxiety and depression? *Journal of Clinical Child and Adolescent Psychology, 34*, 49–61.

La Greca, A. M., & Lopez, N. (1998). Social anxiety among adolescents: Linkages with peer relations and friendships. *Journal of Abnormal Child Psychology, 26*, 83–94.

Larson, R. W. (1983). Adolescents' daily experience with family and friends: Contrasting opportunity systems. *Journal of Marriage and the Family, 45*, 739–750.

Last, C. G., & Strauss, C. C. (1989). Panic disorder in children and adolescents. *Journal of Anxiety Disorders, 3*, 87–95.

Mannuzza, S., Fyer, A. J., Liebowitz, M. R., & Klein, D. F. (1990). Delineating the boundaries of social phobia: Its relationship to panic disorder and agoraphobia. *Journal of Anxiety Disorders, 4*, 41–59.

Masi, G., Favilla, L., Mucci, M., & Millepiedi, S. (2000). Depressive comorbidity in children and adolescents with generalized anxiety disorder. *Child Psychiatry and Human Development, 30*, 205–215.

McLeod, B. D., Wood, J. J., & Weisz, J. R. (2007). Examining the association between parenting and childhood anxiety: A meta-analysis. *Clinical Psychology Review, 27*, 155–172.

Meiser-Stedman, R., Yule, W., Smith, P., Glucksman, E., & Dalgleish, T. (2005). Acute stress disorder and post-traumatic stress disorder in children and adolescents involved in assaults or motor vehicle accidents. *The American Journal of Psychiatry, 162*, 1381–1383.

Muris, P., Mayer, B., & Meesters, C. (2000). Self-reported attachment style, anxiety, and depression in children. *Social Behavior and Personality, 28*, 157–162.

Muris, P., Schmidt, H., & Merckelbach, H. (1999). The structure of specific phobia symptoms among children and adolescents. *Behaviour Research and Therapy, 37*, 863–868.

Nelles, W. B., & Barlow, D. H. (1988). Do children panic? *Clinical Psychology Review, 8*, 359–372.

Newman, M. G., & Erickson, T. M. (2010). Generalized anxiety disorder. In J. G. Beck (Ed.), *Interpersonal processes in the anxiety disorders: Implications for understanding psychopathology and treatment* (pp. 125–152). Washington, DC: American Psychological Association.

Nolen-Hoeksema, S., & Girgus, J. S. (1994). The emergence of gender differences in depression during adolescence. *Psychological Bulletin, 115*, 424–443.

Pawlak, C., Pascual-Sanchez, T., Rae, P., Fischer, W., & Ladame, F. (1999). Anxiety disorders, comorbidity, and suicide attempts in adolescence: A preliminary investigation. *European Psychiatry, 14*, 132–136.

Piacentini, J., Bergman, L., Keller, M., & McCracken, J. (2003). Functional impairment in children and adolescents with obsessive-compulsive disorder. *Journal of Child and Adolescent Psychopharmacology, 13*(Supp 1), S61–S69.

Pincus, D. B., May, J. E., Whitton, S. W., Mattis, S. G., & Barlow, D. H. (2010). Cognitive-behavioral treatment of panic disorder in adolescence. *Journal of Clinical Child and Adolescent Psychology, 39*, 638–649.

Rasmussen, S. A., & Eisen, J. L. (1990). Epidemiology of obsessive compulsive disorder. *The Journal of Clinical Psychiatry, 56*, 11–16.

Reardon, L. E., Leen-Feldner, E. W., & Hayward, C. (2009). A critical review of the empirical literature on the relation between anxiety and puberty. *Clinical Psychology Review, 29*, 1–23.

Reiss, S. (1991). Expectancy model of fear, anxiety, and panic. *Clinical Psychology Review, 11*, 141–474.

Rockhill, C., Kodish, I., DiBattisto, C., Macias, M., Varley, C., & Ryan, S. (2010). Anxiety disorders in children and adolescents. *Current Problems in Pediatric and Adolescent Health Care, 40*, 66–99.

Rose, A. J., & Rudolph, K. D. (2006). A review of sex differences in peer relationship processes: Potential trade-offs for the emotional and behavioral development of girls and boys. *Psychological Bulletin, 132*, 98–131.

Rubin, K. H., LeMare, L. J., & Lollis, S. (1990). Social withdrawal in childhood: Developmental pathways to peer rejection. In S. R. Asher & J. D. Coie (Eds.), *Peer rejection in childhood* (pp. 217–249). Cambridge, UK: Cambridge University Press.

Rudolph, K. D. (2002). Gender differences in emotional responses to interpersonal stress during adolescence. *Journal of Adolescent Health, 30*, 3–13.

Schmidt, N. B., Keough, M. E., Mitchell, M. A., Reynolds, E. K., MacPherson, L., Zvolensky, M. J., et al. (2010). Anxiety sensitivity: Prospective prediction of anxiety among early adolescents. *Journal of Anxiety Disorders, 24*, 503–508.

Schultz, L. T., & Heimberg, R. G. (2008). Attentional focus in social anxiety disorder: Potential for interactive processes. *Clinical Psychology Review, 28*, 1206–1221.

Silverman, W. K., & Albano, A. M. (1996). *The anxiety disorders interview schedule for children for DSM-IV: Child and parent versions*. San Antonio, TX: Psychological Corporation.

Strauss, C. C., Last, C. G., Hersen, M., & Kazdin, A. E. (1988). Association between anxiety and depression in children and adolescents with anxiety disorders. *Journal of Abnormal Child Psychology, 16*, 57–68.

Susman, E. J., Dorn, L. D., & Chrousos, G. P. (1991). Negative affect and hormone levels in young adolescents: Concurrent and predictive perspectives. *Journal of Youth and Adolescence, 20*, 167–190.

Swedo, S. E., Rapoport, J. L., Leonard, H., Lenane, M., & Cheslow, D. (1989). Obsessive-compulsive disorder in children and adolescents: Clinical phenomenology of 70 consecutive cases. *Archives of General Psychiatry, 46*, 335–341.

Tolin, D. F., Franklin, M. E., Diefenbach, G. J., Anderson, E., & Meunier, S. A. (2007). Pediatric trichotillomania: Descriptive psychopathology and an open trial of cognitive-behavioral therapy. *Cognitive Behaviour Therapy, 36*, 129–144.

Udwin, O., Boyle, S., Yule, W., Bolton, D., & O'Ryan, D. (2000). Risk factors for long-term psychological effects of a disaster experienced in adolescence: Predictors of post traumatic stress disorder. *Journal of Child Psychology and Psychiatry, 41*, 969–979.

Walkup, J. T., Albano, A. M., Piacentini, J., Birmaher, B., Compton, S. N., Sherrill, J. T., et al. (2008). Cognitive behavioral therapy, sertraline, or a combination in childhood anxiety. *The New England Journal of Medicine, 359*, 2753–2766.

Warren, S. L., Huston, L., Egeland, B., & Sroufe, L. A. (1997). Child and adolescent anxiety disorders and early attachment. *Journal of the American Academy of Child and Adolescent Psychiatry, 36*, 637–644.

Wicks-Nelson, R., & Israel, A. C. (2009). *Abnormal child and adolescent psychology* (7th ed.). Upper Saddle River, NJ: Pearson Prentice Hall.

Wittchen, H. U., Stein, M. B., & Kessler, R. C. (1999). Social fears and social phobia in a community sample of adolescents and young adults: Prevalence, risk factors, and co-morbidity. *Psychological Medicine, 29*, 309–323.

Woods, D. W., Piacentini, J., Himle, M. B., & Chang, S. (2005). Premonitory Urge for Tics Scale (PUTS): Initial psychometric results and examination of the premonitory urge phenomenon in youths with Tic disorders. *Journal of Development and Behavioral Pediatrics, 26*, 397–403.

Depression and Suicide-Related Behaviors in Adolescence

Roisin M. O'Mara, Adabel Lee, and Cheryl A. King

Introduction

Depressive disorders become increasingly prevalent during adolescence and are associated with significant psychosocial impairment. Because suicidal thoughts and behaviors are symptoms of a depressive disorder and because adolescents with depressive disorders are at elevated risk for suicide, depressive disorders and suicide risk are often considered together. This chapter provides an overview of these two public health concerns, addressing etiology and risk factors, course and outcome, assessment, and treatment.

Sources of support: Funding was provided by a National Institute of Mental Health Career Development Award to Dr. Cheryl King (K24 MH077705).

R.M. O'Mara, Ph.D.
Bradley Hospital, 1011 Veterans Memorial Parkway, Riverside, RI 02915, USA
e-mail: Lifespan.org

A. Lee, Ph.D.
Global Center for Children and Families, University of California Los Angeles Semel Institute, 10920 Wilshire Boulevard, Suite 350, Los Angeles, CA 90024, USA
e-mail: adabellee@mednet.ucla.edu

C.A. King, Ph.D. (✉)
Division of Child and Adolescent Psychiatry, Department of Psychiatry, University of Michigan, 4250 Plymouth Road, Ann Arbor, MI 48109-2700, USA

Department of Psychology, University of Michigan, Institute for Human Adjustment, 530 Church, Ann Arbor, MI 48109, USA
e-mail: kingca@med.umich.edu

Depression in Adolescence

Definition of Terms

Depression is a mood disorder that is characterized by low mood, irritability, less interest in engaging in pleasurable activities, changes in appetite or weight, significant changes in sleep, restlessness or slowing down of cognitive processes or behaviors, excessive tiredness, change in self-esteem, feelings of worthlessness, poor concentration, and suicidal thoughts or recurrent thoughts of death and dying (American Psychiatric Association, 2000). In order to receive a diagnosis of major depressive episode, a subset of these symptoms must be present for 2 or more weeks and must cause significant distress or functional impairment in the person's everyday life. Once an individual has experienced 2 or more major depressive episodes, they are said to have a recurrent major depressive disorder. A diagnosis of dysthymic disorder is defined primarily by a significant level of depressed or irritable mood for at least 1 year that is present in combination with at least two other depressive symptoms. Adolescents with either of these

W.T. O'Donohue et al. (eds.), *Handbook of Adolescent Health Psychology*,
DOI 10.1007/978-1-4614-6633-8_33, © Springer Science+Business Media New York 2013

disorders are generally considered to be clinically depressed.

Epidemiology of Adolescent Depression

Depression is one of the most common mental health disorders, with point prevalence (i.e., proportion of adolescents who experience depression at any given time) rates for adolescent depression ranging between 2 % and 5 % (see Lewinsohn, Rohde, Klein, & Seeley, 1999 for review) and 12-month prevalence rates ranging from 2 % (McGee et al., 1990) to 13 % (Feehan, McGee, Raja, & Williams, 1994). Findings from the National Comorbidity Survey—Adolescent Supplement (NCS-A; Merikangas et al., 2010) describe significantly higher rates of depression in older adolescents, with lifetime prevalence rates doubling from 8.4 % (at ages 13–14) to 15.4 % (at ages 17–18), with some evidence of up to a 25 % lifetime prevalence by the end of adolescence (Lewinsohn, Rohde, & Seeley, 1998). Significantly more adolescent girls report depression than adolescent boys (15.9 % vs. 7.7 %) (Merikangas et al., 2010). This gender difference first appears between the ages of 13 and 15 years, and then becomes more pronounced between the ages of 15 and 18 years (Hankin et al., 1998). There is some variability in the prevalence rates reported in different studies, as these rates are dependent to a certain degree on the threshold criteria and methodology used by researchers (Boyle et al., 1996; Roberts, Attkisson, & Rosenblatt, 1998).

Etiology and Risk Factors for Adolescent Depression

It is helpful to conceptualize the development of psychopathology within a diathesis–stress model (Abramson, Alloy, & Metalsky, 1988). In this model, an individual has some degree of vulnerability to developing depression (e.g., genetic predisposition, psychological vulnerabilities). This vulnerability, or diathesis, is triggered by stress (either an acute stressor or accumulation of stressors). Each individual's vulnerability varies, such that a person with a high level of vulnerability may need only a relatively minor stressor to trigger a depressive episode, whereas a person with a low level of vulnerability may need a higher level of stress, or multiple stressors, to trigger a depressive episode. Stressors may include trauma and abuse, academic challenges, interpersonal conflicts, and lack of social support. It is noteworthy that stressors at one point in time may become diatheses at a later point in time. For example, an adolescent may initially experience some form of abuse as a stressor, and over time, this experience may increase that adolescent's vulnerability by lowering the amount of stress needed to exacerbate depressive symptoms at a later point in time.

Evidence suggests that there may be genetic or biological risk factors for depressive symptoms in adolescents. For example, Van den Bergh and Van Calster (2009) found that adolescents with high levels of depressive symptoms had cortisol profiles that differed from those who had low or moderate levels of depressive symptoms. There is also evidence to suggest that there are significant genetic influences on adolescent mood, which may change over time from childhood to young adulthood (Kendler, Gardner, & Lichtenstein, 2008). Related to this and reflecting possible genetic and environment influences, adolescents who have a family history of depression are at an increased risk for depression (e.g., Silberg, Maes, & Eaves, 2010). Cognitive vulnerability, a consistent pattern of negative thinking or distortions, may also function as a diathesis that increases an individual's likelihood of experiencing depression (e.g., Abela & Hankin, 2008). Although negative thought patterns are believed to develop over time as a result of interactions with important others (e.g., caregivers), over time they may begin to function as a preexisting vulnerability that is triggered by stress(ors).

Stressors that may trigger a depressive episode, or exacerbate depressed mood, include a history of trauma and abuse (Harkness, Lumley, & Truss, 2008; Suliman et al., 2009). Individuals who have a history of trauma or abuse are at increased risk for developing later depressive symptoms, and evidence suggests that chronicity (or greater number) of abuse or trauma confers even greater risk for poor outcomes (Suliman et al., 2009). Stressors for adolescents may also be school related. This may be either academic stress or difficulties with teachers or classmates. Even when adolescents do not have specific difficulties with academics or peers, they often experience stress during transitions, such as the change from middle school to high school; academic demands increase and changes in peer groups may occur. Finally, depression may be triggered or exacerbated by interpersonal problems, such as conflicts and arguments with parents or peers, being excluded or ostracized from one's peer group (relational aggression; e.g., Crick, Ostrov, & Werner, 2006), or a lack of social support (Rao, Hammen, & Poland, 2010).

Course and Outcome of Adolescent Depression

The recurrence rates for depression are relatively high and depression is often cyclical in nature, with episodes frequently triggered by stress(ors). Rates of recurrence during adolescence are approximately 40 % within 2 years (Birmaher et al., 2004) and 70 % within 5 years (Birmaher et al., 1996). Further, there is an increased likelihood of recurrence with each additional episode, as previous depressive episodes confer greater risk for subsequent episodes. There is also evidence that adolescents who experience depression have an increased likelihood of experiencing depressive episodes during adulthood (e.g., Costello, Angold, & Keeler, 1999; Kessler, Avenevoli, & Merikangas, 2001). More recent research suggests that earlier age of onset and recurrence are associated with particularly poor outcomes (Hammen, Brennan, Keenan-Miller, & Herr, 2008).

Additionally, depression in adolescents is often comorbid with other diagnoses. Costello, Mustillo, Erkanli, Keeler, and Angold (2003) found that depressed adolescent girls were 28 times more likely to report an anxiety disorder, ten times more likely to report conduct disorder, seven times more likely to report oppositional defiant disorder, and three times more likely to report substance use. Depressed adolescent boys were 28 times more likely to report anxiety, ten times more likely to report substance use, twice as likely to report attention-deficit/hyperactivity disorder, and 17 times more likely to report oppositional defiant disorder. Compared to other adolescent mental health disorders, depression has the highest comorbidity rate, and this comorbidity appears to affect risk and course of depression, as well as treatment outcomes (see Birmaher et al., 1996 for review).

Assessment of Adolescent Depression

The two major diagnostic classification systems used to diagnose depression are the *International Statistical Classification of Diseases and Related Health Problems* (*ICD-10*; World Health Organization, 1992), which is used internationally, and the *Diagnostic and Statistical Manual of Mental Disorders* (DSM-IV-TR; American Psychiatric Association, 2000), which is used predominantly in the United States. With either diagnostic system, a thorough assessment needs to be conducted before diagnosing an adolescent with depression.

An evaluation of depressive symptoms in adolescents generally requires a clinical interview with the adolescent (perhaps with a semi-structured diagnostic instrument), a clinical interview with the parent(s), and behavioral observations of the adolescents. It may also include adolescent self-report questionnaires, parent report questionnaires, and teacher report questionnaires (with parent and adolescent consent) (Klein, Dougherty, & Olino, 2005).

The clinical interview with the adolescent is generally considered to be the most important method of assessing depressive symptoms due to the need to understand the adolescents' level of subjective distress. Parents, however, can provide important information about significant changes in observable behavior, such as sleep, appetite, irritability, and loss of pleasure, as well as about significant life events, transitions, and stressors. Supplemental information about the adolescent's depressive symptoms and co-occurring conditions, and about the adolescent's psychosocial strengths, may also be obtained using self-report questionnaires. Finally, behavioral observations of the adolescent during the session, as well as of the adolescent's interactions with parents or caregivers, can provide valuable information about the adolescent's depressive affect, level of behavioral activation, and communication patterns. It is important to gather information about the presence of symptoms, as well as their severity (e.g., mild, moderate, severe), duration (i.e., history of length illness and amount of time per day), and frequency (e.g., weekly or daily basis). Given that depression can develop from many different pathways and is often accompanied by co-occurring disorders, collecting broader information such as developmental and social history, family psychiatric history, symptoms of co-occurring disorders, and psychosocial stressors is also an essential part of a thorough assessment of depression.

Finally, typically via the clinical interview, the level of impairment in functioning should be assessed in the domains of school, family, friends, and activities. Although many of the symptoms that are used to assess for depression are internal states, there are several behavioral indicators that may indicate that an adolescent is experiencing depressed mood. These behaviors may include a decline in grades or school performance, changes in peer relationships, behavior problems at home or school, attention difficulties, loss of interest in engaging in regular activities, or withdrawing from family and friends.

It is important to note that depressed mood often manifests as irritability in children and adolescents, as noted in the *DSM-IV-TR* (American Psychiatric Association, 2000); thus, it is important to carefully discern between depressed mood manifesting as irritability from the presence of both depressed mood and oppositional behaviors. Also, it should be noted that it can be difficult to distinguish between normative adolescent development (e.g., greater independence, less time spent with family) and some depressive symptoms, such as withdrawal and isolative behaviors. It may also be difficult to differentiate some of the symptoms of depressive disorders and alcohol or substance abuse, such as an altered sleep pattern, change in sleeping habits, or declining academic achievement.

When depressive symptoms co-occur with another mental health disorder, such as attention-deficit/hyperactivity disorder, this may result in a more complicated clinical picture. For example, in some instances, the presence of both major depressive disorder and attention-deficit/hyperactivity disorder may resemble bipolar disorder symptoms with depressed mood, irritability, and impulsive emotional reactions. As well, depressive symptoms may be secondary to a medical condition (e.g., depressed mood in reaction to a cancer diagnosis) or to substance use. In these situations, it is important to clarify the timing of the onset of symptoms to determine whether the depression is secondary to another issue.

Treatment of Adolescent Depression

There is evidence for the efficacy of both cognitive behavioral therapy (CBT; Beck, Rush, Shaw, & Emery, 1979) and interpersonal therapy for adolescents (IPT-A) (Mufson et al., 2004) for treating adolescent depression. Additionally, family therapy may be particularly helpful when conflictual family relationships are closely linked to the adolescent's mood (Diamond & Josephson, 2005). Finally, there is significant evidence for pharmacological treatment of depressive symptoms, particularly with the use of SSRIs (Cohen, Gerardin, Mazet, Purper-Ouakil, & Flament, 2004). Other treatments, such as electroconvulsive therapy and light therapy, are currently being studied in adolescents. A review of these treatments is as follows:

1. *Cognitive Behavioral Therapy* (CBT; Beck et al., 1979): CBT is based on the conceptualization that cognitions, behaviors, and emotions are interrelated, and focuses on modifying an individual's cognitions and behaviors to improve mood. *Negative core beliefs* are pervasive beliefs

about the self at a very fundamental level. These negative core beliefs are theorized to manifest in the form of *automatic thoughts*. The goal of CBT is to modify or counteract these negative core beliefs; these changes then lead to improved mood. CBT also targets changing behaviors. This may include "behavioral activation" which targets avoidant behaviors or amotivation; the individual is encouraged to increase his or her activity level by engaging in pleasurable activities. Common examples of this include taking a walk, exercising, and spending time with friends. Behavior change may also include changing a maladaptive behavior, such as decreasing fighting with a sibling, which would then presumably lead to lower levels of distress.

Within CBT, family psychoeducation plays an important role in helping the family understand the extent to which depression may be impacting an adolescent's mood, behavior, and functioning. It is often helpful to provide parents with information about depressive symptoms, particularly regarding the fact that depression in adolescents may manifest as irritability. Oftentimes, oppositional behaviors are an indication of depressed mood. It is also important to emphasize to parents some of the adolescent's functional limitations as the adolescent is working towards feeling better and improving his or her mood. CBT has been adapted for use with adolescents and there is good evidence that supports both the efficacy (e.g., Clarke, Rohde, Lewinsohn, Hops, & Seeley, 1999; David-Ferdon & Kaslow, 2008) and effectiveness (Klein, Jacobs, & Reinecke, 2007) to treat depression in adolescents.

2. *Interpersonal Therapy for Adolescents* (IPT-A; Mufson, Moreau, Weissman, & Klerman, 1993): IPT-A focuses on examining how interpersonal relationships and dynamics relate to mood. The adolescent works with the therapist to identify a "problem area" relating to unresolved grief, role disputes, role transitions, interpersonal deficits, or living situations with a single parent. Identification of the "problem area" is determined after completing an interpersonal inventory, in which the adolescent is asked to describe the nature of his or her important relationships (both positive and negative). Once identified, the therapist and adolescent work together to examine the impact of mood on the relationship, and vice versa, and begin to develop skills and strategies to address conflicts, transitions, or losses. Evidence supports the efficacy and David-Ferdon and Kaslow (2008) have reviewed studies demonstrating the effectiveness of IPT in treating depression in adolescence.
3. *Family Therapy*: Family therapy can also be effective in treating depression in adolescents (Diamond & Josephson, 2005; Larner, 2009), particularly if family relationships (e.g., parent–child conflicts) are a significant source of stress and conflict for the adolescent.

   The term "family therapy" is often used loosely, so it is important to differentiate specific forms of family therapy that emphasize the parent–adolescent relationship from therapies that involve parents more generally (e.g., generic psychoeducation about depressive symptoms). For example, evidence from a randomized controlled trial suggests that attachment-based family therapy (ABFT), which focuses on improving parent–adolescent relationships by addressing communication skills and patterns, increasing awareness of negative relationship dynamics, and decreasing conflict, for example, may be an efficacious treatment for adolescent depression and suicidal ideation (Diamond et al., 2010; Diamond, Siqueland, & Diamond, 2003).
4. *Psychopharmacology*: Antidepressants are often prescribed to treat moderate to severe depression and reduce the severity of depressive symptoms by regulating the levels of neurotransmitters in the brain. There are various types of antidepressants: monoamine oxidase inhibitors (MAOIs), tricyclic and tetracyclic antidepressants, selective serotonin reuptake inhibitors (SSRIs), serotonin and norepinephrine reuptake inhibitors (SNRIs), and atypical antidepressants. MAOIs and tricyclics are not typically used as a first line due to the number and/or severity of possible side effects. SSRIs

are prescribed more frequently as these are considered to be safer than the older antidepressants. In particular, there is good evidence to support the efficacy of fluoxetine in treating adolescent depression (Kratochvil et al., 2006).

Antidepressants have been associated with an increase in the broad category of suicidal ideation and/or attempts (4% among youth taking antidepressants vs. 2% among youth taking a placebo), which prompted the Food and Drug Administration to impose a "black box" warning on antidepressant medications for this age group. It is important to note that no increase in suicide deaths have been reported with antidepressant use (Posner et al., 2007). The warning states that there may be an increased risk in suicidality (i.e., suicidal thoughts and behaviors) in youth, particularly during the first 1–2 months of treatment, and that frequent monitoring during this time is recommended.

5. *Combination Therapy*: The combination of both psychopharmacology and psychotherapy is typically recommended as the most effective treatment for moderate to severe depression (March et al., 2004; Vitiello, 2008). The use of antidepressants may help to alleviate some of the vegetative symptoms (i.e., psychomotor retardation, hypersomnia) that are more physiologically based, while the use of psychotherapy targets any maladaptive thought or behavior patterns. Results from the Treatment of SSRI-Resistant Depression in Adolescents (TORDIA) study found that if adolescents did not obtain significant relief from depressive symptoms from an initial SSRI trial, a switch to another antidepressant in combination with cognitive behavioral therapy was more effective than a change in medication alone (Brent et al., 2008). The TORDIA study also found that combination therapy was most effective for adolescents who have depression comorbid with another disorder (Asarnow et al., 2009).
6. *Electroconvulsive Therapy* (ECT): At this time, there is limited evidence available (i.e., case studies or small samples) about the effectiveness of electroconvulsive therapy (ECT) for depressed adolescents. Evidence suggests that ECT is effective for severe and persistent, treatment-resistant depression (i.e., depression that has not responded to psychotherapy, multiple medication trials) in adults. There are strict practice guidelines for the use of ECT in adolescents (Ghaziuddin et al., 2004). Additional research on these treatments is needed to determine the effectiveness and long-term outcomes of this treatment in the adolescent population.

Suicide-Related Behaviors in Adolescence

Definition of Terms

In this section we use the nomenclature originally developed by O'Carroll et al. (1996) and further revised by Silverman et al. (2007) for defining suicidal ideation and suicide attempt. Accordingly, *suicidal ideation* is defined as thoughts of killing oneself without regard to intention to act on the thoughts. A *suicide attempt* is a self-inflicted, potentially injurious behavior with a nonfatal outcome, for which there is evidence (either explicit or implicit) of intent to die. *Death by suicide* refers to a self-inflicted death with either explicit or implicit evidence of intent to die. Taken together, suicidal ideation, suicide attempt, and/or suicide death will be referred to as *suicide-related behaviors*.

Epidemiology of Adolescent Suicide-Related Behaviors

Adolescent death by suicide is a tragedy of substantial public health significance, both in the United States and throughout the world. Suicide is the third leading cause of death among adolescents and young adults in the United States and the rate of suicide deaths in the United States from 2000 to 2007 (the most recent data available) among adolescents (13–19 years old) was

6.03 per 100,000 (Centers for Disease Control and Prevention, 2010a). In addition to suicide death, suicidal ideation, planning, and attempting are significant public health problems. When asked about suicide-related behaviors in the past year, 13.8 % of high school students report seriously having considered attempting suicide in the past year, 10.9 % made a plan for how they would attempt suicide, 6.3 % attempted suicide, and 1.9 % made a suicide attempt that required medical attention (Centers for Disease Control and Prevention, 2010b).

Etiology and Risk Factors for Adolescent Suicide-Related Behaviors

Although the etiology of suicide-related behaviors is not fully understood, there are multiple risk factors that have been identified for suicide-related behaviors. These risk factors can be organized into the following categories:

1. *Demographic Factors*: In the United States, adolescent boys are approximately three times more likely to die by suicide than girls (Centers for Disease Control and Prevention, 2010a). However, high school-aged females are significantly more likely than males to have seriously considered attempting suicide (17.5 % vs. 10.5 %), made a specific plan (13.2 % vs. 8.6 %), attempted suicide (8.1 % vs. 4.6 %), and made a suicide attempt that required medical attention (2.3 % vs. 1.6 %) in the previous year (Centers for Disease Control and Prevention, 2010b). Some have proposed that the means that adolescent males and females choose in attempting suicide drive the gender difference in suicide death, with girls predominantly using less lethal means thus leading to lower death rates (Beautrais, 2003). Others have offered alternative explanations, such as differences in rates of reporting between male and female suicide attempts and suicide deaths, differing socialization patterns between males and females towards suicidal behavior, and cultural differences (Canetto & Sakinofsky, 1998; Moscicki, 1994). Recent years have seen an increase in adolescent females using hanging/suffocation as a method of suicide (Centers for Disease Control and Prevention, 2010a). During the years 1999–2007, 50 % of adolescent males died by firearm, 41 % died by suffocation, and 4 % died by poisoning. Among adolescent females, 52 % died by suffocation, 29 % died by firearms, and 21 % died by poisoning.

   Suicide-related behaviors also vary with race and ethnicity. From 2000 to 2007, the racial/ethnic rates of suicide deaths among adolescents aged 13–19 years were as follows: African American: 3.58 per 100,000; Asian/Pacific Islander: 4.09 per 100,000; Hispanic: 4.49 per 100,000; Caucasian: 6.48 per 100,000; and American Indian/Native Alaskan: 14.53 per 100,000 (Centers for Disease Control and Prevention, 2010a). The significantly higher rate of suicide deaths among American Indian/Native Alaskan adolescents may be related to high rates of alcohol abuse and dependence and limited employment opportunities (Goldston et al., 2008).
2. *Mental Health Disorders*: Mental health disorders are extremely common among adolescents with suicide-related behaviors. Between 80 and 90 % of adolescents who die by suicide suffer from significant psychopathology such as mood disorders, anxiety disorders, conduct disorders, and substance abuse (e.g., Brent et al., 1994; Shaffer et al., 1996; Shafii et al., 1988). Studies investigating risk factors for suicide ideation and attempt (as opposed to suicide death) are much more prevalent in the research literature. Among a nationally representative sample, adolescents with depression plus anxiety or depression plus a disruptive disorder were at the highest risk for suicide ideation and attempt. Anxiety and substance use disorders were only associated with suicide-related behaviors if they were comorbid with other disorders (Foley et al., 2006). Among a clinical sample of youth who were experiencing suicidal ideation or had attempted suicide, Gould et al. (1998) reported that mood, anxiety, and substance use disorders significantly increased the risk of suicide-related behaviors. Disruptive disorders did not increase the risk for suicide attempt, but were

significantly associated with suicide ideation. Furthermore, substance abuse differentiated suicide ideators from attempters, suggesting it plays an important role in escalating from suicidal thoughts to actions.

3. *Prior Suicide Attempt*: A prior suicide attempt is one of the strongest predictors of a future suicide attempt and death by suicide. Shaffer et al. (1996) found that a previous suicide attempt conferred a 30-fold increase in death by suicide among boys, and a threefold increase among girls. Groholt et al. (1997) reported that between one quarter and one-third of adolescents who die by suicide have made a prior attempt. Adolescents with multiple suicide attempts are at an even greater risk of future suicide attempts (Miranda et al., 2008) and ultimately of dying by suicide (Hultén et al. 2001). Adolescents with a history of multiple suicide attempts versus single suicide attempters display higher levels of psychiatric severity and comorbidity, and higher levels of levels of intent, planning, and perceived lethality related to their suicide attempts (e.g., Forman et al., 2004; Rosenberg et al., 2005).
4. *Psychological Factors*: Certain psychological factors, such as hopelessness (e.g., Beck et al., 1990), and aggression and impulsivity (e.g., Giegling et al., 2009) can increase the risk for suicide-related behaviors in adolescents, especially when combined with mental health or substance abuse disorders.
5. *Social and Interpersonal Factors*: In order to understand suicide risk in adolescents, we must consider the social context in which they are living and environmental stressors to which they are exposed. Experiencing a trauma, such as sexual or physical abuse (e.g., Ystgaard et al., 2004), being either the victim or the perpetrator of bullying (e.g., Kaltiala-Heino et al., 1999), low levels of social support (Winfree & Jiang, 2010), being gay or bisexual (Foley et al., 2006; Gould et al., 1998), and exposure to a peer suicide (Gould et al., 1994), are all important social factors that are associated with an increased risk in adolescents for suicide-related behaviors. Stressful life events such as interpersonal conflict or loss and legal and disciplinary problems are common precipitants for suicide-related behaviors (e.g., Brent et al., 1999). For a full review of social and interpersonal risk factors relating to adolescent suicide-related behaviors, see King and Merchant (2008).

Course and Outcome of Adolescent Suicide-Related Behaviors

Suicide-related behaviors appear to be a chronic problem for a significant number of adolescents. In a 10-year follow-up study of adolescents with suicide-related behavior, suicide ideation persisted for over one-third of participants, suicide planning persisted for 21 %, and suicide attempts persisted for 15 % of those who reported these suicide-related behaviors at baseline (Borges et al., 2008). Other studies have shown a higher long-term rate of suicide attempting among adolescents, whereby 44 % of adolescents hospitalized for a suicide attempt had made at least one more attempt during the following 9 years (Groholt & Ekeberg, 2009).

In one of the few studies to report suicide deaths as an outcome, Kotila (1992) conducted a 5-year follow-up of 422 adolescent suicide attempters who were admitted to a hospital in Helsinki. Of the suicide attempts, 120 were made by boys (5 of which were repetitions) and 302 were made by girls (55 of which were repetitions). At the end of the follow-up period, 5 of the males (4.2 %) and 3 of the females (0.99 %) had died by suicide. The mean annual mortality rate among these adolescent suicide attempters was 723 per 100,000, which was 20 times the average mortality for suicide and violent death among individuals of the same age in Finland during the same time period.

An important area of research involves studying the outcomes of adolescents who have been psychiatrically hospitalized (both for suicide-related behavior and for other mental health disorders) in order to identify the prevalence and predictors of suicide-related behaviors post-discharge. Various studies have shown that between 7 % and 18 % of psychiatrically hospitalized adolescents made a suicide attempt within 6 months of discharge, and 25 % made an attempt within 5 years of discharge (Brent et al., 1993; Goldston et al., 1999; King et al., 1995; Prinstein et al., 2008). Factors across these studies that increased the risk of a post-discharge suicide attempt included a history of a previous suicide attempt, perceived high levels of family discord, not living with a parent, a diagnosis of dysthymia (fewer symptoms, less severe, but more chronic type of depression), high levels of suicidal ideation during hospitalization, an affective disorder, conflict with a peer, and death of a non-parental relative.

Assessment of Adolescent Suicide-Related Behaviors

Given the multiple risk factors and pathways to suicide-related behavior, taking a broad and comprehensive approach to assessment is critical. Conducting a thorough suicide risk assessment and developing a comprehensive and accurate formulation guide effective treatment planning and care management, thereby also helping to protect the adolescent at risk for suicide. A careful clinical evaluation and documentation of the evaluation also provide some degree of legal protection for the mental health provider. It is very important to utilize multiple methods and sources in order to assess an adolescent's risk of suicide-related behavior. In addition to interviewing the adolescent individually, providing them with self-report measures of suicide-related behaviors, mental health disorders, traumatic experiences, and drug and alcohol use may provide important additional information that the adolescent would not necessarily share in person. It is also important to collect collaborative information from the parents/guardians of the adolescent and previous treatment providers. Assessment should be an ongoing part of treatment, as the risk for suicide-related behavior is not static over time.

In collaboration with the Suicide Prevention Resource Center, the Substance Abuse and Mental Health Services Administration (2009) developed a five-step method of evaluating for suicide risk, which is an extremely useful guide for clinicians working with this population. The five steps are as follows:

1. Identify risk factors such as previous suicide-related behaviors, current/past suicide attempts, key symptoms (e.g., hopelessness, anxiety/panic, impulsivity).
2. Identify protective factors which may mitigate the risk of suicide, such as internal factors (e.g., ability to cope with stress, religious beliefs) and external factors (e.g., family and social supports).
3. Conduct a systematic inquiry about suicide ideation (frequency, duration, intensity), plans (timing, location, lethality, availability, preparatory acts), behaviors (past attempts, aborted attempts, rehearsals), and intent (extent to which individual expects to carry out the plan and believes that the plan/act will be lethal, explore reasons to die vs. reasons to live). In the case of youths, ask parent/guardian about evidence of suicidal thoughts, plans, or behaviors, and changes in mood, behaviors, or disposition.
4. Determine risk level and intervention based on clinical judgment, after completing steps 1–3. Risk levels may be described as high (suicidal intent or preparatory behavior for suicide attempt, protective factors not relevant), moderate (multiple risk factors, few protective factors), or low (few or low level risk factors, strong protective factors).
5. Document the individual's risk level, treatment plan, means restriction plan if applicable, and follow-up plan.

Treatment of Adolescent Suicide-Related Behaviors

Once a thorough assessment has been completed, the next step is to develop and implement a treatment plan. Treatment of adolescents with suicide-related behaviors should be rooted in empirically supported interventions while also tailoring the treatment for the individual adolescent and their specific diagnoses, risk and protective factors, and social and cultural contexts.

There are only a limited number of interventions that have been specifically developed for and tested among adolescents with suicidal behavior. Many large-scale treatment studies for depression, anxiety, conduct problems, and drug and alcohol use exclude adolescents who are determined to be at risk for suicide, resulting in them being a much-neglected population in clinical research. The difficulties of studying adolescents with suicide-related behavior include the high level of risk management, the challenge of addressing the clinical needs of a group characterized by diagnostic heterogeneity and frequent comorbid conditions, and ethical considerations in conducting randomized controlled treatments and therefore withholding potentially beneficial treatments from adolescents who are at high risk of dying by suicide.

Multisystemic therapy (MST; Henggeler et al., 2002) is an intensive home- and community-based approach whereby a team of professionals work with adolescents and also target the multiple systems within which adolescents are imbedded. In a study of MST's effectiveness with youth who were experiencing a psychiatric emergency, participants were randomized to receive treatment as usual (i.e., psychiatric hospitalization) or to receive MST (Huey et al., 2004). After a 1-year follow-up period, the authors reported that MST was more effective than psychiatric hospitalization in reducing adolescent-reported (but not parent-reported) suicide attempts. However, it was not shown to improve depression, hopelessness, or suicide ideation.

Originally developed by Linehan (1993) for adults with borderline personality disorder and self-harming behaviors, dialectical behavior therapy (DBT) is currently being studied for its use with suicidal adolescents. Briefly, DBT focuses on the balance of acceptance and change, validation strategies, case management, and teaching emotion regulation, effective communication, and problem solving strategies. In a quasi-experimental study, Rathus and Miller (2002) reported that suicidal adolescents in an outpatient setting had fewer psychiatric hospitalizations during treatment and a higher rate of treatment completion than those in the treatment as usual group. In a feasibility study, Katz, Cox, Gunasekara, and Miller (2004) found that when a child/adolescent psychiatric unit adopted a DBT protocol, there was a significant reduction in behavioral incidents during psychiatric admission than the treatment as usual group. There were no significant differences in the reduction of self-harming behavior, depression, or suicidal ideation after 1 year. Both of these studies suggest that DBT is a promising treatment for suicide-related behaviors among adolescents, but further research is necessary.

The Youth-Nominated Support Team (YST), developed by King et al. (2006, 2009), is a psychoeducational social support intervention that was designed to help adolescents during the period of time immediately following psychiatric hospitalization for acute suicide risk. Adolescents were invited to nominate adults who could serve as a "support team," and these adults were then provided with psychoeducation concerning the adolescent's treatment plan, effective strategies for communicating with adolescents, and crisis management. The results of the first study indicated a significant reduction in suicidal ideation for female participants, but not for males. The results of the second larger and more rigorous randomized controlled trial showed that YST was associated with a more rapid decrease in suicidal ideation for multiple suicide attempters during the initial weeks after hospitalization (small to moderate effect size). There was no effect on suicide attempt rates in either study.

The Treatment of Adolescent Suicide Attempters Study (TASA; Brent et al., 2009) sought to compare the effects of psychotherapy (either supportive or a cognitive behavioral therapy specifically designed to target suicide-related behaviors), medication, and a combination of both psychotherapy and medication, among adolescents with depression and a recent suicide attempt. Due to the open nature of this trial, the authors were not able to comment on the efficacy of the different treatments. However, when they compared the 6-month outcomes of their participants to a similar sample of suicidal youths who were followed naturalistically, the risk of suicide attempt among participants in their sample (regardless of what treatment group they were in) was lower.

As part of the TASA study, Stanley et al. (2009) developed cognitive behavioral therapy for suicide prevention (CBT-SP), a specific therapy for adolescents who have made a suicide attempt. CBT-SP is theoretically grounded in cognitive behavioral therapy, dialectical behavioral therapy, and targeted therapies for suicidal youths with depression. CBT-SP includes conducting a chain analysis of the suicide attempt, safety plan development, skill building, psychoeducation, family intervention, and relapse prevention. In a recently published feasibility and acceptability study, the Treatment of Adolescent Suicide Attempters (TASA) authors reported high retention rates of participants with 100 % of patients reporting that CBT-SP was helpful (Stanley et al., 2009).

While still widely used in some mental health treatment settings, the effectiveness of "no suicide contracts" has not been studied empirically and is frequently debated in the literature (e.g., Busch et al., 2003). Some of the concerns with such "contracts" are that they represent verbal agreements that may have little or no meaning or impact when working with an adolescent who may be under the influence of alcohol or other drugs when acutely suicidal, may struggle with interpersonal relationships and agreements, or may have a history of impulsivity (an absence of thinking about what one has "agreed" to). Furthermore, Rudd et al. (2006) argue that the use of the word "contract" implies that the patient gives away their autonomy at a time when their sense of control is often minimal, and asks them not to harm themselves without necessarily giving them any tools to actually follow through on this contract to stay alive. Rudd and colleagues (2006) suggest using a "commitment to treatment" agreement, in place of a "no suicide contract," whereby the patient and the clinician (1) come to an agreement each of their roles, obligations, and expectations in treatment; (2) communicate openly and honestly about all aspects of treatment including suicide; and (3) access identified emergency resources outlined in the patient's "crisis response plan" when necessary. Rather than a "no suicide contract," we recommend that a crisis response plan be developed early in treatment in order to come up with various strategies for how to deal with an increase in suicidal thoughts (e.g., engaging in self-soothing behaviors, calling a supportive person, or going to the emergency room).

To date, specific pharmacotherapies have not been developed for suicide-related behavior among adolescents. Instead, the common practice is to utilize medication(s) to treat the underlying mental health disorder(s) when appropriate in order to provide symptom relief that may reduce suicide-related behaviors.

In summary, treatment recommendations for this population include a comprehensive assessment and thoughtful formulation which guides the selection of appropriate and evidence-based treatments, developing a crisis plan, ensuring close monitoring and supervision of the youth during and after the suicidal crisis, providing intensive mental health services and case management in the aftermath of suicide-related behavior, treating the underlying mental health disorder if applicable, helping the youth to develop more adaptive coping skills to manage suicidal urges, providing psychoeducation and support to family members, increasing social support for the youth, and providing ongoing assessment of suicide-related behavior risk.

Conclusion

Depressive disorders are relatively common among adolescents, and adolescents with depressive disorders frequently experience suicidal thoughts and sometimes engage in suicidal behavior. Other types of psychopathology, in addition to a wide range of psychosocial factors, are also associated with elevated risk for suicidal thoughts and behaviors among adolescents. A substantial evidence base is available to guide the mental health provider's evaluation and treatment of these adolescents. Continued research on the causes and risk factors, course and outcome, assessment, and treatment of both depression and suicide-related behaviors is extremely important so that we may continue to improve our management of these serious public health concerns.

References

Abela, J. Z., & Hankin, B. L. (2008). Cognitive vulnerability to depression in children and adolescents: A developmental psychopathology perspective. In J. Z. Abela, B. L. Hankin, J. Z. Abela, & B. L. Hankin (Eds.), *Handbook of depression in children and adolescents* (pp. 35–78). New York: Guilford Press.

Abramson, L. Y., Alloy, L. B., & Metalsky, G. I. (1988). The cognitive diathesis-stress theories of depression: Toward an adequate evaluation of the theories' validities. In L. B. Alloy (Ed.), *Cognitive processes in depression*. New York: Guilford Press.

American Psychiatric Association. (2000). *Diagnostic and statistical manual of mental disorders* (4th ed.). Washington, DC: Author. Text Rev.

Angst, J., & Merikangas, K. (2001). Multi-dimensional criteria for the diagnosis of depression. *Journal of Affective Disorders, 62*, 7–15.

Asarnow, J., Emslie, G., Clarke, G., Wagner, K., Spirito, A., Vitiello, B., et al. (2009). Treatment of selective serotonin reuptake inhibitor-resistant depression in adolescents: Predictors and moderators of treatment response. *Journal of the American Academy of Child and Adolescent Psychiatry, 48*(3), 330–339.

Beautrais, A. L. (2003). Suicide and serious suicide attempts in youth: A multiple-group comparison study. *The American Journal of Psychiatry, 160*(6), 1093–1099.

Beck, A. T., Brown, G., Berchick, R. J., Stewart, B. L., & Steer, R. A. (1990). Relationship between hopelessness and ultimate suicide: A replication with psychiatric outpatients. *The American Journal of Psychiatry, 147*, 190–195.

Beck, A. T., Rush, J., Shaw, B. F., & Emery, G. (1979). *Cognitive therapy of depression*. New York: Guilford Press.

Birmaher, B., Ryan, N. D., Williamson, D. E., Brent, D. A., et al. (1996). Childhood and adolescent depression: A review of the past 10 years, Part I. *Journal of the American Academy of Child and Adolescent Psychiatry, 35*, 1427–1439.

Birmaher, B., Williamson, D. E., Dahl, R. E., Axelson, D. A., Kaufman, J., Dorn, L. D., et al. (2004). Clinical presentation and course of depression in youth: Does onset in childhood differ from onset in adolescence? *Journal of the American Academy of Child and Adolescent Psychiatry, 43*, 63–70.

Borges, G., Angst, J., Nock, M. K., Ruscio, A. M., & Kessler, R. C. (2008). Risk factors for the incidence and persistence of suicide-related outcomes: A 10-year follow-up study using the National Comorbidity Surveys. *Journal of Affective Disorders, 105*(1–3), 25–33.

Boyle, M. H., Offord, D. R., Racine, Y., Szatmari, P., et al. (1996). Identifying thresholds for classifying childhood psychiatric disorder: Issues and prospects. *Journal of the American Academy of Child and Adolescent Psychiatry, 35*, 1440–1448.

Brent, D., Emslie, G., Clarke, G., Wagner, K., Asarnow, J., Keller, M., et al. (2008). Switching to another SSRI or to venlafaxine with or without cognitive behavioral therapy for adolescents with SSRI-resistant depression: The TORDIA randomized controlled trial. *Journal of the American Medical Association, 299*(8), 901–913.

Brent, D. A., Greenhill, L. L., Compton, S., Emslie, G., Wells, K., Walkup, J. T., et al. (2009). The treatment of Adolescent Suicide Attempters Study (TASA): Predictors of suicidal events in an open treatment trial. *Journal of the American Academy of Child and Adolescent Psychiatry, 48*(10), 987–996.

Brent, D. A., Kolko, D. J., Wartella, M. E., & Boylan, M. B. (1993). Adolescent psychiatric inpatients' risk of suicide attempt at 6-month follow-up. *Journal of the American Academy of Child and Adolescent Psychiatry, 32*(1), 95–105.

Brent, D. A., Perper, J. A., Moritz, G., Allman, C., Friend, A., Roth, C., et al. (1999). Age- and sex-related risk factors for adolescent suicide. *Journal of the American Academy of Child and Adolescent Psychiatry, 38*(12), 1497–1505.

Brent, D. A., Perper, J. A., Moritz, G., & Liotus, L. (1994). Familial risk factors for adolescent suicide: A case–control study. *Acta Psychiatrica Scandinavica, 89*(1), 52–58.

Busch, K. A., Fawcett, J., & Jacobs, D. G. (2003). Clinical correlates of inpatient suicide. *The Journal of Clinical Psychiatry, 64*(1), 14–19.

Canetto, S., & Sakinofsky, I. (1998). The gender paradox in suicide. *Suicide & Life-Threatening Behavior, 28*(1), 1–23.

Centers for Disease Control and Prevention. (2010a). *Web-based injury statistics query and reporting system (WISQARS)*. Retrieved January 10, 2011, from http://www.cdc.gov/ncipc/wisqars.

Centers for Disease Control and Prevention. (2010b). Youth risk behavior surveillance—United States. *Morbidity and Mortality Weekly Report, 59*, SS-5.

Clarke, G. N., Rohde, P., Lewinsohn, P. M., Hops, H., & Seeley, J. R. (1999). Cognitive-behavioral treatment of adolescent depression: Efficacy of acute group treatment and booster sessions. *Journal of the American Academy of Child and Adolescent Psychiatry, 38*(3), 272–279.

Cohen, D., Gerardin, P., Mazet, P., Purper-Ouakil, D., & Flament, M. F. (2004). Pharmacological treatment of adolescent major depression. *Journal of Child and Adolescent Psychopharmacology, 14*(1), 19–31.

Costello, E., Angold, A., & Keeler, G. P. (1999). Adolescent outcomes of childhood disorders: The consequences of severity and impairment. *Journal of the American Academy of Child and Adolescent Psychiatry, 38*(2), 121–128.

Costello, E., Mustillo, S., Erkanli, A., Keeler, G., & Angold, A. (2003). Prevalence and development of psychiatric disorders in childhood and adolescence. *Archives of General Psychiatry, 60*(8), 837–844.

Crick, N. R., Ostrov, J. M., & Werner, N. E. (2006). A longitudinal study of relational aggression, physical aggression, and children's social-psychological adjustment. *Journal of Abnormal Child Psychology, 34*, 131–142.

David-Ferdon, C., & Kaslow, N. J. (2008). Evidence-based psychosocial treatments for child and adolescent depression. *Journal of Clinical Child and Adolescent Psychology, 37*(1), 62–104.

Diamond, G., & Josephson, A. (2005). Family-based treatment research: A 10-year update. *Journal of the American Academy of Child and Adolescent Psychiatry, 44*, 872–887.

Diamond, G. S., Siqueland, L., & Diamond, G. M. (2003). Attachment-based family therapy for depressed adolescents: Programmatic treatment development. *Clinical Child and Family Psychology Review, 6*(2), 107–127.

Diamond, G. S., Wintersteen, M. B., Brown, G. K., Diamond, G. M., Gallop, R., Shelef, K., et al. (2010). Attachment-based family therapy for adolescents with suicidal ideation: A randomized controlled trial. *Journal of the American Academy of Child and Adolescent Psychiatry, 49*(2), 122–131.

Feehan, M., McGee, R., Raja, S. N., & Williams, S. M. (1994). DSM-III-R disorders in New Zealand 18 year-olds. *The Australian and New Zealand Journal of Psychiatry, 28*, 87–99.

Foley, D. L., Goldston, D. B., Costello, E. J., & Angold, A. A. (2006). Proximal psychiatric risk factors for suicidality in youth: The Great Smoky Mountains study. *Archives of General Psychiatry, 63*, 1017–1024.

Forman, E. M., Berk, M. S., Henriques, G. R., Brown, G. K., & Beck, A. T. (2004). History of multiple suicide attempts as a behavioral marker of severe psychopathology. *The American Journal of Psychiatry, 161*(3), 437–443.

Ghaziuddin, N., Kutcher, S. P., Knapp, P., Bernet, W., Arnold, V., Beitchman, J., et al. (2004). Practice parameter for use of electroconvulsive therapy with adolescents. *Journal of the American Academy of Child and Adolescent Psychiatry, 43*(12), 1521–1539.

Giegling, I., Olgiati, P., Hartmann, A. M., Calati, R., Möller, H., Rujescu, D., et al. (2009). Personality and attempted suicide. Analysis of anger, aggression and impulsivity. *Journal of Psychiatric Research, 43*(16), 1262–1271.

Goldston, D. B., Daniel, S. S., Reboussin, D. M., Reboussin, B. A., Frazier, P. H., & Kelley, A. E. (1999). Suicide attempts among formerly hospitalized adolescents: A prospective naturalistic study of risk during the first 5 years after discharge. *Journal of the American Academy of Child and Adolescent Psychiatry, 38*(6), 660–671.

Goldston, D. B., Molock, S. D., Whitbeck, L. B., Murakami, J. L., Zayas, L. H., & Hall, G. C. N. (2008). Cultural considerations in adolescent suicide prevention and psychosocial treatment. *American Psychologist, 63*, 14–31.

Gould, M. S., King, R. A., Greenwald, S., Fisher, P., Schwab-Stone, M., Kramer, R., et al. (1998). Psychopathology associated with suicidal ideation and attempts among children and adolescents. *Journal of the American Academy of Child and Adolescent Psychiatry, 37*(9), 915–923.

Gould, M. S., Petrie, K., Kleinman, M. H., & Wallenstein, S. (1994). Clustering of attempted suicide: New Zealand national data. *International Journal of Epidemiology, 23*(6), 1185–1189.

Groholt, B., & Ekeberg, Ø. (2009). Prognosis after adolescent suicide attempt: Mental health, psychiatric treatment, and suicide attempts in a nine-year follow-up study. *Suicide & Life-Threatening Behavior, 39*(2), 125–136.

Groholt, B., Ekeberg, Ø., Wichstrøm, L., & Haldorsen, T. (1997). Youth suicide in Norway, 1990–1992: A comparison between children and adolescents completing suicide and age- and gender-matched controls. *Suicide & Life-Threatening Behavior, 27*(3), 250–263.

Hammen, C., Brennan, P. A., Keenan-Miller, D., & Herr, N. R. (2008). Early onset recurrent subtype of adolescent depression: Clinical and psychosocial correlates. *Journal of Child Psychology and Psychiatry, 49*(4), 433–440.

Hankin, B. L., Abramson, L. Y., Moffitt, T. E., Silva, P. A., McGee, R., & Angell, K. E. (1998). Development of depression from preadolescence to young adulthood: Emerging gender differences in a 10-year longitudinal study. *Journal of Abnormal Psychology, 107*(1), 128–140.

Harkness, K. L., Lumley, M. N., & Truss, A. E. (2008). Stress generation in adolescent depression: The moderating role of child abuse and neglect. *Journal of Abnormal Child Psychology, 36*(3), 421–432.

Henggeler, S. W., Schoenwald, S. K., Rowland, M. D., & Cunningham, P. B. (2002). *Serious emotional disturbance in children and adolescents: Multisystemic therapy*. New York: Guilford Press.

Huey, J. S., Henggeler, S. W., Rowland, M. D., Halliday-Boykins, C. A., Cunningham, P. B., Pickrel, S. G., et al. (2004). Multisystemic therapy effects on attempted suicide by youths presenting psychiatric emergencies. *Journal of the American Academy of Child and Adolescent Psychiatry, 43*(2), 183–190.

Hultén, A., Jiang, G. X., Wasserman, D., Hawton, K., Hjelmeland, H., De Leo, D., et al. (2001). Repetition of attempted suicide among teenagers in Europe: Frequency timing, and risk factors. *European Child & Adolescent Psychiatry, 10*(3), 161–169.

Kaltiala-Heino, R., Rimpelä, M., Marttunen, M. J., Rimpelä, A., & Rantanen, P. (1999). Bullying, depression, and suicidal ideation in Finnish adolescents: School survey. *British Medical Journal, 319*(7206), 348–351.

Katz, L. Y., Cox, B. J., Gunasekara, S., & Miller, A. L. (2004). Feasibility of dialectical behavior therapy for suicidal adolescent inpatients. *Journal of the American Academy of Child and Adolescent Psychiatry, 43*(3), 276–282.

Kendler, K. S., Gardner, C. O., & Lichtenstein, P. P. (2008). A developmental twin study of symptoms of anxiety and depression: Evidence for genetic innovation and attenuation. *Psychological Medicine, 38*(11), 1567–1575.

Kessler, R., Avenevoli, S., & Merikangas, K. (2001). Mood disorders in children and adolescents: An epidemiologic perspective. *Biological Psychiatry, 49*, 1002–1014.

King, C. A., Klaus, N., Kramer, A., Venkataraman, S., Quinlan, P., & Gillespie, B. (2009). The Youth-Nominated Support Team–Version II for suicidal adolescents: A randomized controlled intervention trial.

Journal of Consulting and Clinical Psychology, 77(5), 880–893.

King, C. A., Kramer, A., Preuss, L., Kerr, D. R., Weisse, L., & Venkataraman, S. (2006). Youth-Nominated Support Team for suicidal adolescents (Version 1): A randomized controlled trial. *Journal of Consulting and Clinical Psychology, 74*(1), 199–206.

King, C. A., & Merchant, C. R. (2008). Social and interpersonal factors relating to adolescent suicidality: A review of the literature. *Archives of Suicide Research, 12*(3), 181–196.

King, C. A., Segal, H. G., Kaminski, K., & Naylor, M. W. (1995). A prospective study of adolescent suicidal behavior following hospitalization. *Suicide & Life-Threatening Behavior, 25*(3), 327–338.

Klein, D. N., Dougherty, L. R., & Olino, T. M. (2005). Toward guidelines for evidence-based assessment of depression in children and adolescents. *Journal of Clinical Child and Adolescent Psychology, 34*(3), 412–432.

Klein, J. B., Jacobs, R. H., & Reinecke, M. A. (2007). Cognitive-behavioral therapy for adolescent depression: A meta-analytic investigation of changes in effect-size estimates. *Journal of the American Academy of Child and Adolescent Psychiatry, 46*(11), 1403–1413.

Kotila, L. (1992). The outcome of attempted suicide in adolescence. *Journal of Adolescent Health, 13*(5), 415–417.

Kratochvil, C. J., Vitiello, B., Brent, D., Bostic, J. Q., Naylor, M. W., & Kratochvil, C. (2006). Selecting an antidepressant for the treatment of pediatric depression. *Journal of the American Academy of Child and Adolescent Psychiatry, 45*(3), 371–373.

Larner, G. (2009). Integrating family therapy in adolescent depression: An ethical stance. *Journal of Family Therapy, 31*(3), 213–232.

Lewinsohn, P. M., Rohde, P., Klein, D. N., & Seeley, J. R. (1999). Natural course of adolescent major depressive disorder: I. Continuity into young adulthood. *Journal of the American Academy of Child & Adolescent Psychiatry, 38*, 56–63.

Lewinsohn, P. M., Rohde, P., & Seeley, J. R. (1998). Major depressive disorder in older adolescents: Prevalence, risk factors, and clinical implications. *Clinical Psychology Review, 18*, 765–794.

Linehan, M. M. (1993). *Skills training manual for treating borderline personality disorder*. New York: Guilford Press.

March, J., Silva, S., Petrycki, S., Curry, J., Wells, K., Fairbank, J., et al. (2004). Fluoxetine, cognitive-behavioral therapy, and their combination for adolescents with depression: Treatment for adolescents with depression study (TADS) randomized controlled trial. *Journal of the American Medical Association, 292*(7), 807–820.

McGee, R., Feehan, M., Williams, S., Partridge, F., et al. (1990). DSM-III disorders in a large sample of adolescents. *Journal of the American Academy of Child and Adolescent Psychiatry, 29*, 611–619.

Merikangas, K., He, J., Burstein, M., Swanson, S., Avenevoli, S., Cui, L., et al. (2010). Lifetime prevalence of mental disorders in U.S. adolescents: Results from the National Comorbidity Survey Replication-Adolescent Supplement (NCS-A). *Journal of the American Academy of Child and Adolescent Psychiatry, 49*, 980–989.

Miranda, R., Scott, M., Hicks, R., Wilcox, H., Munfakh, J., & Shaffer, D. (2008). Suicide attempt characteristics, diagnoses, and future attempts: Comparing multiple attempters to single attempters and ideators. *Journal of the American Academy of Child and Adolescent Psychiatry, 47*(1), 32–40.

Moscicki, E. K. (1994). Gender differences in completed and attempted suicides. *Annals of Epidemiology, 4*, 152–158.

Mufson, L., Dorta, K., Wickramaratne, P., Nomura, Y., Olfson, M., & Weissman, M. M. (2004). A randomized effectiveness trial of interpersonal psychotherapy for depressed adolescents. *Archives of General Psychiatry, 61*(6), 577–584.

Mufson, L., Moreau, D., Weissman, M. M., & Klerman, G. (1993). *Interpersonal psychotherapy for depressed adolescents*. New York: Guilford Press.

O'Carroll, P. W., Berman, A., Maris, R. W., & Moscicki, E. K. (1996). Beyond the tower of Babel: A nomenclature for suicidology. *Suicide & Life-Threatening Behavior, 26*(3), 237–252.

Posner, K., Oquendo, M. A., Gould, M., Stanley, B., & Davies, M. (2007). Columbia Classification Algorithm of Suicide Assessment (C-CASA): Classification of suicidal events in the FDA's pediatric suicidal risk analysis of antidepressants. *The American Journal of Psychiatry, 164*(7), 1035–1043.

Prinstein, M. J., Nock, M. K., Simon, V., Cheah, C. S. L., Spirito, A., & Aikins, J. W. (2008). Longitudinal trajectories and predictors of adolescent suicidal ideation and attempts following inpatient hospitalization. *Journal of Consulting and Clinical Psychology, 76*(1), 92–103.

Rao, U., Hammen, C. L., & Poland, R. E. (2010). Longitudinal course of adolescent depression: Neuroendocrine and psychosocial predictors. *Journal of the American Academy of Child and Adolescent Psychiatry, 49*(2), 141–151.

Rathus, J. H., & Miller, A. L. (2002). Dialectical behavior therapy adapted for suicidal adolescents. *Suicide & Life-Threatening Behavior, 32*(2), 146–157.

Roberts, R. E., Attkisson, C. C., & Rosenblatt, A. (1998). Prevalence of psychopathology among children and adolescents. *The American Journal of Psychiatry, 155*, 715–725.

Rosenberg, H. J., Jankowski, M. K., Sengupta, A., Wolfe, R. S., Wolford, G. L., & Rosenberg, S. D. (2005). Single and multiple suicide attempts and associated health risk factors in New Hampshire adolescents. *Suicide & Life-Threatening Behavior, 35*(5), 547–557.

Rudd, M., Mandrusiak, M., & Joiner, T. E., Jr. (2006). The case against no-suicide contracts: The commitment to

treatment statement as a practice alternative. *Journal of Clinical Psychology, 62*(2), 243–251.
Shaffer, D., Gould, M. S., Fisher, P., & Trautman, P. (1996). Psychiatric diagnosis in child and adolescent suicide. *Archives of General Psychiatry, 53*(4), 339–348.
Shafii, M., Steltz-Lenarsky, J., Derrick, A. M., & Beckner, C. (1988). Comorbidity of mental disorders in the post-mortem diagnosis of completed suicide in children and adolescents. *Journal of Affective Disorders, 15*(3), 227–233.
Silberg, J. L., Maes, H., & Eaves, L. J. (2010). Genetic and environmental influences on the transmission of parental depression to children's depression and conduct disturbance: An extended children of twins study. *Journal of Child Psychology and Psychiatry, 51*(6), 734–744.
Silverman, M., Berman, A. L., Sanddal, N. D., O'Carroll, P. W., & Joiner, T. E., Jr. (2007). Rebuilding the Tower of Babel: A revised nomenclature for the study of suicide and suicidal behaviors: Part 2: Suicide-related ideations, communications, and behaviors. *Suicide & Life-Threatening Behavior, 37*(3), 264–277.
Stanley, B., Brown, G., Brent, D. A., Wells, K., Poling, K., & Curry, J. (2009). Cognitive-behavioral therapy for suicide prevention (CBT-SP): Treatment model, feasibility, and acceptability. *Journal of the American Academy of Child and Adolescent Psychiatry, 48*(10), 1005–1013.
Substance Abuse and Mental Health Services Administration. (2009). Retrieved February 4, 2011, from http://store.samhsa.gov/shin/content//SMA09-4432/SMA09-4432.pdf.
Suliman, S., Mkabile, S. G., Fincham, D. S., Ahmed, R., Stein, D. J., & Seedat, S. (2009). Cumulative effect of multiple trauma on symptoms of posttraumatic stress disorder, anxiety, and depression in adolescents. *Comprehensive Psychiatry, 50*(2), 121–127.
Van den Bergh, B. H., & Van Calster, B. B. (2009). Diurnal cortisol profiles and evening cortisol in post-pubertal adolescents scoring high on the Children's Depression Inventory. *Psychoneuroendocrinology, 34*(5), 791–794.
Vitiello, B. (2008). Recent NIMH clinical trials and implications for practice. *Journal of the American Academy of Child and Adolescent Psychiatry, 47*(12), 1369–1373.
Winfree, L. T., & Jiang, S. (2010). Youthful suicide and social support: Exploring the social dynamics of suicide-related behavior and attitudes within a national sample of US adolescents. *Youth Violence and Juvenile Justice, 8*(1), 19–37.
World Health Organization. (1992). *The ICD-10 classification of mental and behavioural disorders*. Geneva: WHO.
Ystgaard, M., Hestetun, I., Loeb, M., & Mehlum, L. (2004). Is there a specific relationship between childhood sexual and physical abuse and repeated suicidal behavior? *Child Abuse & Neglect, 28*(8), 863–875.

Adolescents with Intellectual Disabilities

Megan M. Griffin, Marisa H. Fisher, Elisabeth M. Dykens, and Robert M. Hodapp

By definition, adolescence is a time of change, marking the transition from childhood to adulthood. During this period, the hormonal and physical changes of puberty are accompanied by concurrent transitions related to social relationships, family dynamics, and engagement in school and the community. Also during this period, adolescents navigate new social roles, develop a social identity, and explore romantic relationships. Adolescents also typically take on new roles and responsibilities within the family, producing a shift in the family dynamic. Finally, similar changes in roles are often evident in community contexts, with adolescents meeting greater challenges at school and in their communities—from taking more advanced classes to entering the workforce.

Though their experiences often differ from those of typically developing adolescents, adolescents with intellectual and developmental disabilities also experience changes in most aspects of their lives. Some attain the typical milestones of adolescence, such as getting a driver's license or going to college. For many youth with intellectual and developmental disabilities, however, these milestones are delayed, modified, or do not occur at all. At the same time, a host of unique issues, challenges, and systems arise for these individuals.

This chapter addresses the experiences of adolescents with intellectual and developmental disabilities. Our focus throughout will be on youth with intellectual disabilities (ID). These adolescents encounter similar transitions and challenges as the larger group of individuals with various developmental disabilities; all such individuals (regardless of type of disability) need similar considerations, accommodations, and supports during adolescence. In addressing the needs of adolescents with ID, we first present the definition and classification of ID, its varied causes, and specific manifestations among individuals with certain genetic disorders. We then address issues related to the physical and mental health of individuals with ID, before discussing other transitions experienced by adolescents with ID—in terms of education, socialization, and post-school engagement. Finally, we conclude by considering the experiences of adolescents with ID in the context of the family.

M.M. Griffin, Ph.D. (✉) • M.H. Fisher, Ph.D.
R.M. Hodapp, Ph.D.
University of New Mexico, MSC05 3040,
1 University of New Mexico, Albuquerque,
NM, 87131-0001, USA
e-mail: griffinm@unm.edu; marisa.fisher@vanderbilt.edu; robert.hodapp@vanderbilt.edu

E.M. Dykens, Ph.D.
Vanderbilt University, 230 Appleton Place,
Peabody Box 40, Nashville, TN 37203, USA
e-mail: elisabeth.dykens@vanderbilt.edu

W.T. O'Donohue et al. (eds.), *Handbook of Adolescent Health Psychology*,
DOI 10.1007/978-1-4614-6633-8_34, © Springer Science+Business Media New York 2013

Intellectual Disabilities

Definition and Classification

The current edition of the *Diagnostic and Statistical Manual of Mental Disorders* characterizes ID with a three-factor definition (American Psychiatric Association [*DSM-IV-TR*], 2000). First, individuals with ID have subaverage intellectual functioning, as evidenced by an intelligence quotient (IQ) score of 70 or below on an individually administered test. Second, this subaverage intellectual functioning must be associated with or result in impairments in adaptive behavior. Finally, to be considered an intellectual disability, these characteristics begin during childhood or adolescence, before the individual is 18 years of age.

Though the general components of this three-factor definition are mostly accepted, the ways in which these components are defined and emphasized remain open to debate (Hodapp, Griffin, Burke, & Fisher, 2011). For example, the validity of the IQ criterion has been questioned, as the intellectual ability of an individual with an IQ slightly above 70 and an individual with an IQ slightly below 70 are not readily apparent. Because of this and other issues related to reliable measurement, the most recent definition of ID suggested by the field's main professional group, the American Association on Intellectual and Developmental Disabilities (AAIDD, 2011), emphasizes the need for clinical judgment related to the assessment of IQ. Similarly, much debate relates to the criterion of impaired adaptive behavior—including the ways in which adaptive behavior is measured and categorized, as well as its importance in relation to the IQ criterion.

Among individuals with ID, great variation exists in levels of functioning. Traditionally, professionals have categorized people with ID according to their level of intellectual impairment (Hodapp et al., 2011). These categories are associated with a range of IQ scores: mild (IQ = 55–70), moderate (40–54), severe (20–25—40), and profound (below 20–25) intellectual disabilities. More recently, a different system of classification has emerged based on the intensity of support needed by individuals, rather than their levels of intellectual functioning (AAIDD, 2011).

Etiology and Behavioral Phenotypes

Just as variation exists in their levels of functioning, individuals with ID also vary in the causes of their disabilities (Zigler & Hodapp, 1991). Traditionally, professionals have categorized the causes of ID into two groups, undifferentiated and organic. The term "undifferentiated" refers to unknown causes of ID, and may include such factors as polygenic inheritance, environmental deprivation, or undetected organic causes (Hodapp, 1994). The term "organic" refers to identified origins of ID, including hundreds of causes that can occur before, during, or after birth. Prenatal causes encompass over 1,000 genetic disorders, fetal alcohol syndrome, and accidents in utero. Other causes include such birth-related complications as prematurity and anoxia. Finally, postnatal causes encompass both illness and accidents resulting in subaverage intellectual functioning and impairments in adaptive behavior.

Among individuals with certain types of organic ID—particularly those with certain genetic disorders—specific behavioral phenotypes, or profiles, have been identified (Dykens, Hodapp, & Finucane, 2000). These profiles denote the greater likelihood for individuals with a given disorder to manifest certain cognitive, linguistic, or adaptive strengths and weaknesses or periods of faster or slower development. In addition, even compared to adolescents with ID more generally, adolescents with several of these genetic conditions show increased risks for specific psychiatric disorders, maladaptive behaviors, or physical health problems.

Two genetic conditions can serve as examples. In the first condition, Williams syndrome, many individuals demonstrate relative strengths in expressive language and relative weaknesses in visuospatial skills. Many individuals with Williams syndrome are also hypersensitive to sound and demonstrate musicality in various ways (e.g., interest in or talent for music). In addition, people with Williams syndrome are often described as hyper-social and friendly; at the same time, compared with the typically developing population, these individuals more often experience numerous anxieties and fears (Dykens, 2003).

Adolescents with another genetic condition, Prader–Willi syndrome, also show a distinct profile (Dykens et al., 2000). Though most such individuals have mild to moderate ID, children and adolescents with Prader–Willi syndrome excel in tasks that involve visual organization and perception (e.g., completing jigsaw puzzles; Dykens, 2002). In contrast, individuals with Prader–Willi syndrome typically do not perform well on tasks that involve sequential processing. Additionally, a hallmark behavior of people diagnosed with Prader–Willi is hyperphagia, or compulsive overeating. If unchecked, hyperphagia can result in morbid obesity, other related health problems, and even death. In addition to compulsive eating, people with Prader–Willi often engage in other repetitive, obsessive-compulsive behaviors (Dykens, Leckman, & Cassidy, 1996; Dykens & Roof, 2008).

This brief consideration of behavioral phenotypes highlights the variability that exists among individuals with ID. Ultimately, behavioral phenotypes may help identify the most effective interventions for a certain individual or group (Hodapp & Fidler, 1999). These examples also offer a more nuanced view of the characteristics of individuals with ID—too often defined negatively—by including their positive characteristics and strengths. Differences related to etiology are revisited throughout the chapter.

Health of Adolescents with ID

In considering the health of adolescents with ID, we begin by discussing issues related to physical health, including adverse health conditions, pubertal development, and health literacy. Next, we address the many issues related to mental health, before examining health care for adolescents with ID.

Physical Health

Associated Health Conditions and Secondary Conditions

Adolescents with ID experience higher rates of a variety of "secondary conditions" (Krahn, Hammond, & Turner, 2006). These conditions are health problems that are not directly related to ID per se, but that nonetheless affect individuals with ID disproportionately. For example, individuals with ID, including teens, are much more likely than those in the general population to experience obesity, poor oral health, pressure ulcers, and various other health problems. With improvements in health literacy and access to health care, such secondary conditions are preventable. Though preventable, individuals with ID nonetheless experience these secondary health problems at disproportionately high rates.

Various other associated health problems are also related specifically to certain conditions or etiologies of ID. Consider, for example, Down syndrome and cerebral palsy. Summarizing health concerns among children and adolescents with Down syndrome, Roizen (2010) noted that children with Down syndrome are especially prone to congenital heart disease, respiratory issues, gastrointestinal problems, celiac disease, thyroid problems, leukemia, obesity, and visual and hearing problems (see also, Schieve, Boulet, Boyle, Rasmussen, & Schendel, 2009). Likewise, individuals with cerebral palsy may experience a whole host of co-occurring conditions related to their disability. Such children and adolescents more often experience motor impairment, sensory loss, epilepsy, and other impairments (Rosenbaum, Paneth, Leviton, Goldstein, & Bax, 2007). Great variation exists in both the types and levels of health problems experienced among individuals with cerebral palsy.

Development During Puberty

Compared with the general population, people with developmental disabilities are prone to differences in pubertal development. For example, one study estimated that youth with neurodevelopmental disabilities are about 20 times more likely to experience early pubertal development

(Siddiqi, Van Dyke, Donohue, & McBrien, 1999). Within specific genetic disorders, adolescents with Williams syndrome typically begin puberty earlier than adolescents in the general population, though pubertal development otherwise proceeds normally (Wang & Blum, 2003). In contrast, teens with Prader–Willi experience many issues related to puberty, including genital abnormalities and incomplete maturation (Crinò et al., 2003).

Partly because pubertal development may be atypical, teens with ID need to be educated about pubertal changes. Just like their peers without disabilities, adolescents with disabilities have sex drives and sexual interests, and are just as likely to experiment with sexuality (Murphy & Elias, 2006). Consequently, adolescents with ID need to learn about appropriate sexual behavior, including the appropriateness of behaviors in certain situations. Unfortunately, many adolescents with ID are not provided with appropriate sex education. Programs need to be tailored to meet the comprehension levels of these adolescents, starting with basic information about the physical changes experienced during adolescence. These courses should also extend to comprehensive sexual health education, including information about contraception, sexually transmitted diseases, and pregnancy. In addition to appropriate sex education, a broader knowledge of health and self-care needs should be fostered among adolescents with ID.

Knowledge of Health and Self-Care Needs

Multiple factors have been identified that influence the health of individuals with ID (Walsh & McConkey, 2009). These include genetic factors, social circumstances, environmental factors, and inadequate health care (Krahn et al., 2006). In addition to these influences on the health of individuals with ID, Krahn et al. (2006) note the influence of individual behaviors that precipitate or exacerbate secondary conditions. Inadequate knowledge of healthy lifestyle choices puts many individuals with ID at additional risk of poor health outcomes—outcomes that are largely preventable by adopting healthy habits.

Low health literacy has been linked with a variety of negative outcomes (Marks, Sisirak, & Hsieh, 2008). For example, people with low health literacy are more likely to be hospitalized or need emergency services, and less likely to utilize preventive services. People with poor health literacy might not understand the importance of healthy behaviors (e.g., nutritious diet, regular exercise). Additionally, some individuals might lack basic safety knowledge related to exercise (e.g., the importance of warming up; ways to safely use equipment). To address these issues, curricula are available to educate individuals with ID about the importance of cultivating healthy habits (e.g., *Health Matters*; Marks, Sisirak, & Heller, 2010).

In addition to addressing topics related to diet and exercise, curricula are available that include information about other health-related topics. For example, *My Health, My Choice, My Responsibility* (Vitale, Levitz, & Crimmins, 2007) includes lessons on preparing for medical appointments, self-advocacy in health care, and personal hygiene. Written at a reading level appropriate for adolescents and young adults with ID, these curricula also include age-appropriate examples and activities. Parents, educators, and other professionals can use these curricula to teach health literacy skills to individuals with ID.

Beyond promoting knowledge about the importance of a healthy lifestyle, adolescents with ID must also have opportunities to apply this knowledge. Many individuals with ID have a troubling combination of high body fat, poor strength, and low cardiovascular endurance (Rimmer, 2000). The importance of an active lifestyle is therefore critical to these adolescents, who as a group have generally poor physical fitness. Recognizing this issue, Special Olympics International, in addition to its "Healthy Athletes" screening program, provides opportunities for individuals with ID to participate in athletic training and competition (Horwitz, Kerker, Owens, & Zigler, 2000; Special Olympics, 2005). Such participation in Special Olympics has been linked to greater social competence and more positive self-perceptions (Dykens & Cohen, 1996).

Mental Health

Adolescents with ID also have unique needs related to mental health. Like their typically developing peers, individuals with ID experience great changes during puberty related to brain development and hormonal levels. These changes are often accompanied by intense emotions and changes in mood, and may make individuals more susceptible to various mental health problems. In addition, compared to individuals with typical intellectual functioning, individuals with ID are at a heightened risk for psychiatric disorders (Dykens, 2000). Thus, adolescence is a particularly sensitive time for individuals with ID.

People with ID who also have a diagnosis of a psychiatric disorder are considered to have a "dual diagnosis" (Jopp & Keys, 2001). Because psychiatric conditions among those with ID are often difficult to diagnose or remain undiagnosed, prevalence estimates of dual diagnosis range from 10 to 70 % of individuals with ID (Dykens, 2000). Due to misidentification and misdiagnosis of psychiatric disorders, individuals with dual diagnoses are less likely to receive appropriate treatment, supports, and services. Misidentification of mental health conditions may occur for several reasons, which include diagnostic overshadowing, atypical manifestation of the mental illness, and unavailability of appropriate assessments to measure symptoms among individuals with ID.

Misidentification and Misdiagnosis

"Diagnostic overshadowing" refers to instances when the mental health problems of an individual with ID are attributed to impairments in adaptive behavior related to ID rather than to a concurrent psychiatric disorder (Jopp & Keys, 2001). For example, if an individual with ID displays behaviors symptomatic of depression or anxiety, a professional might attribute these to the person's level of intellectual functioning, rather than considering the possible need for psychiatric diagnosis and treatment. In general, the more severe the individual's symptoms, the more likely a clinician will be to consider the possibility of dual diagnosis.

Another issue concerns atypical manifestations of psychiatric disorders. Specifically, many individuals with ID display atypical symptoms, behaviors that do not generally denote a particular psychiatric disorder among typically developing adolescents (Antonacci & Attiah, 2008). For example, obsessive-compulsive disorder (OCD) is associated with a variety of "classic" compulsions (e.g., repetitively washing hands); among individuals with ID, however, these compulsions may not occur (King, Stavrakaki, & Gedye, 2007). Compulsions that require abstract thinking or counting skills may be rare or absent among individuals with ID, as well. Additionally, individuals who have limitations in expressive language are less able to report their experience of obsessive thoughts. Finally, individuals with ID might not meet the typical criteria for OCD involving awareness that their compulsions are excessive, or that compulsions are causing them distress.

Assessment

Issues such as diagnostic overshadowing and atypical manifestation are problems involving the assessment of individuals with ID. As noted above, appropriate assessment is difficult when individuals with ID have limited expressive language. In a psychiatric interview, limitations in language may result in the inability to communicate information concerning the nature, onset, duration, frequency, and severity of symptoms. In addition, limitations in language and intellectual ability may prohibit individuals with ID from expressing abstract thoughts or feelings that relate to their experience of a psychiatric condition.

To provide appropriate psychiatric assessments for individuals with ID, several groups have developed alternatives to typical psychiatric interviews (e.g., Psychiatric Assessment Schedule for Adults with Developmental Disability). An alternative set of diagnostic criteria have also been developed, with criteria based on DSM-IV-TR but adapted for use among individuals with ID. The *Diagnostic Manual-Intellectual Disability: A Textbook of Diagnoses of Mental Disorders in Persons with Intellectual Disability*

(DM-ID; Fletcher, Loschen, Stavrakaki, & First, 2007) provides adaptations of the diagnostic criteria to be applied for persons with ID, and provides alternative assessment methods for providing a diagnosis. In addition to providing adaptations to specific diagnostic criteria, the DM-ID provides information about common behaviors of individuals with ID and how to differentiate these from the behavioral manifestations of psychiatric disorders.

Beyond assessments related to a formal diagnosis, other tools have been developed to assess maladaptive behavior of individuals with ID. These measures—including the Reiss Screen for Maladaptive Behavior, the Aberrant Behavior Checklist, and the Developmental Behaviour Checklist—are all normed on children and adolescents with ID and are summarized in the DM-ID (Hurley, Levitas, Lecavalier, & Pary, 2007). In addition, the field of applied behavior analysis has developed an approach to obtain information about an individual's specific problem behaviors. By conducting a functional behavioral assessment (FBA), professionals can identify what purpose the behavior serves for the individual (Cooper, Heron, & Heward, 2007). This information is then used to develop effective interventions to decrease the rate of problem behaviors and increase the rate of appropriate replacement behaviors.

Correlates of Maladaptive Behavior

Various factors correlate with maladaptive behavior in individuals with ID. As noted earlier, one such factor concerns the individual's specific genetic disorder. Compared to the general population (or even to the population of persons with ID), for example, children and adolescents with Williams syndrome are more prone to anxiety disorders (Dykens, 2003). Likewise, individuals with Prader–Willi syndrome are much more likely to engage in overeating and compulsive food-related behaviors, as well as other compulsions that are unrelated to food (Dykens et al., 1996).

Persons with certain genetic syndromes may also experience developmental changes in their maladaptive behavior with age. For example, compared to younger children with Prader–Willi syndrome, adolescents and adults with Prader–Willi syndrome more often display withdrawal, isolation, and depression (Dykens & Cassidy, 1995). A similar age-related pattern of behavior has been identified among individuals with Down syndrome (Dykens, Shah, Sagun, Beck, & King, 2002). Specifically, lower level aggressive behaviors—such as being argumentative and swearing—are more prevalent among younger adolescents with Down syndrome, while internalizing behaviors associated with depression (e.g., being withdrawn) are more common among older adolescents (Dykens, 2007). In a few cases, adolescents with Down syndrome have been reported to show extreme, rapid regressions in adaptive and cognitive-linguistic skills, as well as sudden-onset, severe psychiatric symptoms (Devenny & Matthews, 2011; Dykens, Shah, Davis, & Fitzpatrick, 2011). Although the characteristics, prevalence, and reasons underlying any such age-related changes remain unknown, etiology and age are clearly correlates of psychopathology among individuals with ID.

Health Care

Related to the physical and mental health of adolescents with ID are the systems and services available to provide them appropriate health care. Krahn et al. (2006) have described a "cascade" of disparities among individuals with ID related to the prevalence of adverse health conditions, access to health care services, and availability of appropriately trained health care professionals. For example, few health care professionals are appropriately trained in disabilities (Voelker, 2002), and similarly there are few health care professionals who are willing to accept these adolescents as patients (Surgeon General, 2002). Professionals who have training in and experience with patients with ID are thus in short supply, even as these patients experience disproportionate needs in the areas of health and mental health.

This problem is compounded during adolescence, when individuals face transitions on multiple fronts. Many individuals with ID and their families, for example, need to transition from the care of a pediatrician to that of a primary care doctor. This change can be difficult, especially as many individuals and families have long-standing relationships with their pediatricians, and may encounter barriers to finding a primary care physician. To address this transition as well as other health-related issues, young adults with ID can access a curriculum called *Being a Healthy Adult: How to Advocate for Your Health and Health Care* (Roberson, 2010). This curriculum includes lessons and activities related to health and health care, understanding disabilities, and self-advocacy. It is written at a reading level and includes content appropriate for adolescents and young adults with ID.

In addition to the transition from one health care provider to another, adolescents with ID and their families face a second important health care transition. Specifically, Medicaid recipients have reported how difficult it is to transition from the more expansive benefits available under pediatric coverage to less available benefits as an adult (Surgeon General, 2002). To access more flexible benefits, many individuals with ID and their families sign up for the waiting list to receive Medicaid waivers. Due to limited funding in most states, however, waiting lists are exceptionally long, with many individuals never receiving these benefits.

Transitions from Adolescence to Adulthood

To this point, we have discussed changes related to health and mental health. These changes occur alongside transitions in various other areas, such as schooling, socialization, and family dynamics. We now describe issues arising for adolescents with ID in these areas.

Educational Issues

Like most adolescents, high school is a big part of the lives of adolescents with ID. However, these students may have very different high school experiences than their typically developing peers. The Individuals with Disabilities Education Improvement Act (IDEIA, 2004) is a key determinant of the school experiences of students with ID. Under this legislation, students with disabilities are entitled to a free appropriate public education. IDEIA includes regulations regarding the education of students with disabilities until the age of 21. In order to receive an appropriate education, students may need a variety of supports and services provided by the school.

For each school-age student with a disability, a plan is developed that documents the needed supports and services. Such plans are called Individualized Education Programs (IEPs). The team that develops this plan is composed of general education and special education teachers, service providers, parents, and students (as appropriate). An IEP should include the student's present level of performance, measurable goals, and a specific plan to meet those goals—including the supports and services which the student will receive. IDEIA also includes regulations that apply only to adolescents aged 16 and older. The purpose of these regulations is to help the student transition smoothly from the school years to adult life.

Unfortunately, such regulations are necessary because, compared to their typically developing peers, students with disabilities more often experience poor outcomes (Newman, Wagner, Cameto, & Knokey, 2009). Compared with 66 % of their peers without disabilities, only 57 % of youth with disabilities were employed after high school. Similarly, compared with 53 % of their same-age peers, only 45 % of students with disabilities attended postsecondary schooling. Of students with any disability during the post-high school years, those with ID are the least likely to be involved in education, training, or paid employment (Wagner, Newman, Cameto, Garza, & Levine, 2005).

Thus, transition services are particularly important to support teenage students with ID. As mandated by IDEIA, transition services involve a coordinated set of activities that focus on improving the student's academic and functional skills and facilitate the transition to post-school activities (e.g., work or postsecondary education, PSE). Similar to the instruction and services identified in the student's IEP, transition services should be individualized to each student's particular strengths, needs, and preferences.

IDEIA requires that each student's IEP must include a transition plan before the student turns 16 years old. The plan should include measurable goals related to various areas of adult life (e.g., employment), as well as the services needed to support the student in meeting these goals (e.g., vocational training). Additionally, when transition services are discussed, students with disabilities should be invited to attend their IEP meetings. In this way, students can become involved in decisions related to their own lives, both during and after high school.

In contrast with the experiences of their typically developing peers, students with ID are influenced greatly by provisions in IDEIA. First, their instruction and classroom placement is guided by their IEPs. Such placements can range from instruction in a segregated setting to inclusion in a general education classroom. Second, their schooling can extend through age 21. Thus, while their peers often graduate from high school at age 18 or 19, students with ID may continue to receive educational services for several additional years. Students with ID who attend high school past age 18 may continue to learn in a traditional classroom setting in the high school; however, for some, community-based classrooms are an option. These community-based classrooms are located throughout the local community, and are age-appropriate settings in which students can learn functional skills needed for employment and independent living.

Finally, students with ID may also differ from their typically developing peers in what they are taught. Whereas most high school students receive academic instruction for the majority of the day, students with ID also often receive training in other areas. Students with ID may receive training in functional skills necessary for employment and independent living (e.g., using money). Students may also receive training in appropriate social skills, as well as self-determination skills (e.g., goal-setting, choice-making, self-advocacy; Wehmeyer et al., 2007).

Social Issues

Adolescents with ID also experience transitions related to their social lives. Like other teenagers, individuals with ID are more prone to take risks, seek novelty, and value the company of their same-age peers during adolescence. Despite these similarities, individuals with ID also experience some differences in socialization during adolescence. Many do not enjoy an active social life, and may rarely interact with typically developing peers. Such limitations often continue after high school, as many young adults with ID experience segregation and isolation (Chambers, Hughes, & Carter, 2004).

Limited friendships and social experiences may stem from a variety of causes. Adolescents with ID may lack appropriate social skills, including skills such as initiating a conversation or understanding nonverbal social cues. These deficits may occur for many reasons, including limited cognitive abilities, limited receptive or expressive communication, and engaging in maladaptive behaviors. It should be noted that competency with social skills can vary widely among individuals with ID—some individuals may have few impairments, whereas others may be highly affected by such deficits. For example, impairments in communication and social interaction typical of individuals with autism spectrum disorders make the social aspects of transitioning to adulthood very challenging for these adolescents (Taylor, 2009).

Socialization differences also relate to the inadequate opportunities that many adolescents with ID have to interact with typically developing peers. Especially for students who are placed in segregated classrooms, the opportunities for interaction with same-age typically developing peers may be rare. Unfortunately, segregated educational settings do not include typically developing peers who can model appropriate social behaviors. To address this problem, some schools have established "peer buddy" programs in which general education students and special education students are encouraged to interact (Hughes & Carter, 2000). Additionally, Best Buddies is an organization that enhances the lives of people with intellectual and developmental disabilities by pairing them in one-to-one friendships with individuals without disabilities (Hardman, Clark, & Kliewer, 2006). Best Buddies can foster social inclusion of adolescents with ID both within and outside of the school setting.

Social Vulnerability

Because some adolescents with ID lack social skills and support systems (e.g., communication skills, large network of friends), they are more vulnerable to teasing, bullying, and other mistreatment. Other factors that heighten the risk for such mistreatment include low self-esteem, a tendency to look toward others for guidance, and co-occurring physical impairments. Unfortunately, due to such risk factors, individuals with ID are more likely to experience minor abuses such as being teased or cheated out of money (Halpern, Close, & Nelson, 1986). They are also more likely to be the victims of more serious crimes and abuse (Sullivan & Knutson, 2000; Wilson & Brewer, 1992).

Risks of experiencing exploitation and abuse also relate to other individual factors (Fisher, Hodapp, & Dykens, 2008). Though somewhat counterintuitive, higher rates of abuse occur among adolescents with lesser degrees of disability (Petersilia, 2001). Likewise, males with disabilities are more likely to experience physical abuse or neglect (Sobsey et al., 1997), whereas females are more likely to experience sexual abuse. Vulnerability to such mistreatment or abuse greatly concerns parents of adolescents with ID, even affecting their decisions related to the postsecondary activities of their children (Griffin, McMillan, & Hodapp, 2010).

Transition to Postsecondary Options and Services

Although youth with ID are among the least likely to be engaged in education, training, or employment after exiting high school (Wagner et al., 2005), more transition options have become available in recent years. Notably, opportunities for individuals with ID to participate in inclusive PSE have recently expanded. Historically, receiving an inclusive education after high school has not been an option for students with ID; however, this has changed in recent years. Currently, 150 PSE programs in the United States offer adolescents and young adults with ID the opportunity to go to college alongside their typically developing peers (Grigal & Hart, 2010). Such PSE programs are as diverse as the colleges and universities in which they are housed, but most include opportunities for students with ID to expand their social circles, continue learning academics, and gain employment skills.

In addition to PSE, employment remains a primary goal for young adults with ID. Schooling at both the secondary and postsecondary levels can focus on employment skills and experiences, and adolescents with ID can also gain work experience through job-shadowing, volunteering, or interning (Luecking, 2009). For those adolescents needing significant support in these activities or in competitive employment, service agencies can provide assistance from job coaches. If adolescents with ID require lower levels of support, then parents, social-service personnel, and others can identify those "natural supports" (e.g., coworkers) within the workplace who can help. Other types of accommodations can also foster the success of employees with ID.

Families of Adolescents with ID

The transitions of adolescence can be accompanied by stress among parents of individuals with ID, in much the same way that parental stress accompanies the transitions of adolescents without disabilities. Though the nature and timing of these transitions may differ, adolescence is nonetheless a period of adjustment for all individuals and their families. Like the parents of most typically developing children, parents of children with ID provide primary support through childhood. Though this support typically wanes as adolescents and young adults become more independent, parents of adolescents with ID may continue to provide high levels of support.

This greater need for support among adolescents with ID relates, in part, to a difficulty or a delay in reaching typical milestones. For example, among typically developing adolescents in the United States, obtaining a driver's license is a rite of passage. However, many young adults with ID do not achieve this milestone due to challenges with passing the required tests. In some cases, parents of adolescents with ID may support them in receiving training to obtain a driver's license; alternatively, parents may assist their son or daughter in accessing other forms of transportation (e.g., biking, public transportation). However, in general, the independent travel of adolescents with ID is much more restricted than that of their typically developing peers. This, in itself, is a support that many families of individuals with ID continue to provide well into adulthood.

Also, as previously discussed, many adolescents with ID remain in high school longer than their typically developing peers. This delay in exiting high school is also often accompanied by delays in other areas. For example, many young adults with ID continue to depend on their parents for support in terms of education, employment, and needed services. As many as 60 % or more of these young adults also continue to live in their parents' home (National Center for Family Support, 2000), and depend on them financially.

Parents may assume the responsibilities for caregiving independently, or may share some of these responsibilities with siblings, grandparents, and other extended family members. Especially given that individuals with ID are living longer lives and may outlive their parents, it is important to consider the future support needs of individuals with ID. Because the siblings of individuals with ID may take on primary caregiving responsibilities as parents become less able to do so, these siblings play an important role in the lives of individuals with ID.

To that end, several studies have focused on the experiences of the siblings of people with disabilities. In one study, most of the adult siblings reported having close, positive relationships with their siblings with disabilities (Hodapp, Urbano, & Burke, 2010). Indeed, researchers have begun to focus on the uniquely positive aspects of having a family member with ID, recognizing the effects this can have on individual family members and on the family system as a whole (Dykens, 2005). Due to close relationships with a sibling with disabilities, many adult siblings have reported considering their sibling when making major life choices such as marriage, and transitions, such as relocating for work. Many also anticipate taking on future caregiving for their sibling with a disability, with female siblings more likely to anticipate adopting caregiving roles in the future (Krauss, Seltzer, Gordon, & Friedman, 1996).

Conclusion

Thus, adolescence is a critical time for individuals with ID and their families. These adolescents encounter a variety of health and mental health disparities, school and work challenges, and ongoing needs for support. Throughout this chapter, we have addressed how the experiences of adolescents with ID are both similar to and different from the experiences of their typically developing peers. Like all young adults, individuals with ID experience physical and mental changes during adolescence. These changes develop alongside extra challenges that they face in terms of health problems, health care, dual diagnosis, schooling, and socialization. Though these teens and their families often face unique challenges, adolescence remains an exciting time filled with new experiences as individuals with ID transition to adulthood.

References

American Association on Intellectual and Developmental Disability (AAIDD). (2011). *Intellectual disability: Definition, classification, and systems of supports* (11th ed.). Washington, DC: American Association on Intellectual and Developmental Disability.

American Psychiatric Association. (2000). *Diagnostic and statistical manual of mental disorders* (4th ed.). Washington, DC: American Psychiatric Association. Text revised.

Antonacci, D. J., & Attiah, N. (2008). Diagnosis and treatment of mood disorders in adults with developmental disabilities. *Psychiatric Quarterly, 79*, 171–192.

Chambers, C. R., Hughes, C., & Carter, E. W. (2004). Parent and sibling perspectives on the transition to adulthood. *Education and Training in Developmental Disabilities, 39*, 79–94.

Cooper, J. O., Heron, T. E., & Heward, W. L. (2007). *Applied behavior analysis* (2nd ed.). Upper Saddle River, NJ: Pearson Education Inc.

Crinò, A., Schiaffini, R., Ciampalini, P., Spera, S., Beccaria, L., Benzi, F., et al. (2003). Hypogonadism and pubertal development in Prader-Willi syndrome. *European Journal of Pediatrics, 162*, 327–333.

Devenny, D., & Mathews, A. (2011). Regression: Atypical loss of attained functioning in children and adolescents with Down syndrome. *International Review of Research in Developmental Disabilities, 41*, 233–264.

Dykens, E. M. (2000). Annotation: Psychopathology in children with intellectual disability. *Child Psychopathology and Psychiatry, 41*, 407–418.

Dykens, E. M. (2002). Are jigsaw puzzle skills 'spared' in persons with Prader-Willi syndrome? *Journal of Child Psychology & Psychiatry, 43*, 343–352.

Dykens, E. M. (2003). Anxiety, fears, and phobias in persons with Williams syndrome. *Developmental Neuropsychology, 23*, 291–316.

Dykens, E. M. (2005). Happiness, well-being, and character strengths: Outcomes for families and siblings of persons with mental retardation. *Mental Retardation, 43*, 360–364.

Dykens, E. M. (2007). Psychiatric and behavioral disorders in persons with Down syndrome. *Mental Retardation and Developmental Disabilities Research Reviews, 13*, 272–278.

Dykens, E. M., & Cassidy, S. B. (1995). Correlates of maladaptive behavior in children and adults with Prader-Willi syndrome. *American Journal of Medical Genetics, 60*, 546–549.

Dykens, E. M., & Cohen, D. J. (1996). Effects of Special Olympics International on social competence in persons with mental retardation. *Journal of the American Academy of Child and Adolescent Psychiatry, 35*, 223–229.

Dykens, E. M., Hodapp, R. M., & Finucane, B. (2000). *Genetics and mental retardation syndromes: A new look at behavior and treatments*. Baltimore: Paul H. Brookes Publishing Company.

Dykens, E. M., Leckman, J. F., & Cassidy, S. B. (1996). Obsessions and compulsions in Prader-Willi syndrome. *Journal of Child Psychology and Psychiatry, 37*, 995–1002.

Dykens, E. M., & Roof, E. (2008). Behavior in Prader-Willi syndrome: Relationship to genetic subtypes and age. *Journal of Child Psychology and Psychiatry, 49*, 1001–1008.

Dykens, E. M., Shah, B., Davis, B., & Fitzpatrick, J. (2011). Psychiatric complexities of clinic-referred adolescents and young adults with Down syndrome. *Journal of Intellectual Disability Research*.

Dykens, E. M., Shah, B., Sagun, J., Beck, T., & King, B. H. (2002). Maladaptive behaviour in children and adolescents with Down's syndrome. *Journal of Intellectual Disability Research, 46*, 484–492.

Fisher, M. H., Hodapp, R. M., & Dykens, E. M. (2008). Child abuse among children with disabilities: What we know and what we need to know. *International Review of Research in Mental Retardation, 35*, 251–289.

Fletcher, R., Loschen, E., Stavrakaki, C., & First, M. (Eds.). (2007). *Diagnostic manual-intellectual disability (DM-ID): A textbook of diagnosis of mental disorders in persons with intellectual disability*. Kingston, NY: NADD Press.

Griffin, M. M., McMillan, E. D., & Hodapp, R. M. (2010). Family perspectives on post-secondary education for students with intellectual disabilities. *Education and Training in Autism and Developmental Disabilities, 45*, 339–346.

Grigal, M., & Hart, D. (2010). *Think college*. Baltimore: Brookes.

Halpern, A., Close, D. W., & Nelson, D. J. (1986). *On my own: The impact of semi-independent living programs for adults with mental retardation*. Baltimore: Brookes.

Hardman, M. L., Clark, C., & Kliewer, C. (2006). Promoting friendship through Best Buddies: A national survey of college program participants. *Mental Retardation, 44*, 56–63.

Hodapp, R. M. (1994). Cultural-familial mental retardation. In R. Sternberg (Ed.), *Encyclopedia of intelligence* (pp. 711–717). New York: Macmillan.

Hodapp, R. M., & Fidler, D. J. (1999). Special education and genetics: Connections for the 21st century. *Journal of Special Education, 33*, 130–137.

Hodapp, R. M., Griffin, M. M., Burke, M. M., & Fisher, M. H. (2011). Intellectual disabilities. In R. J. Sternberg & S. B. Kaufman (Eds.), *Cambridge handbook of intelligence* (pp. 193–209). Cambridge, UK: Cambridge University Press.

Hodapp, R. M., Urbano, R. C., & Burke, M. M. (2010). Adult female and male siblings of persons with disabilities: Findings from a national survey. *Intellectual and Developmental Disabilities, 48*, 52–62.

Horwitz, S. M., Kerker, B. D., Owens, P. L., & Zigler, E. (2000). *The health status and needs of individuals with mental retardation*. New Haven, CT: Yale University.

Hughes, C., & Carter, E. W. (2000). *The transition handbook: Strategies high school teachers use that work!* Baltimore: Brookes.

Hurley, A. D., Levitas, A., Lecavalier, L., & Pary, R. J. (2007). Assessment and diagnostic procedures. In R. Fletcher, E. Loschen, C. Stavrakaki, & M. First (Eds.), *Diagnostic manual—intellectual disability: A clinical guide for diagnosis of mental disorders in persons with intellectual disability*. Kingston, NY: NADD Press.

Individuals with Disabilities Education Improvement Act of 2004, 20 U.S.C. 1400 et seq.

Jopp, D. A., & Keys, C. B. (2001). Diagnostic overshadowing reviewed and reconsidered. *American Journal on Mental Retardation, 106*, 416–433.

King, R., Stavrakaki, C., & Gedye, A. (2007). Obsessive-compulsive disorder. In R. Fletcher, E. Loschen, C. Stavrakaki, & M. First (Eds.), *Diagnostic manual-intellectual disability (DM-ID): A textbook of diagnosis of mental disorders in persons with intellectual disability*. Kingston, NY: NADD Press.

Krahn, G. L., Hammond, L., & Turner, A. (2006). A cascade of disparities: Health and health care access for people with intellectual disabilities. *Mental Retardation and Developmental Disabilities Research Reviews, 12*, 70–82.

Krauss, M. W., Seltzer, M. M., Gordon, R., & Friedman, D. H. (1996). Binding ties: The roles of adult siblings of persons with mental retardation. *Mental Retardation, 34*, 83–93.

Luecking, R. G. (2009). *The way to work: How to facilitate work experiences for youth in transition*. Baltimore: Brookes.

Marks, B., Sisirak, J., & Heller, T. (2010). *Health matters: The exercise and nutrition health education curriculum for people with developmental disabilities*. Baltimore: Brookes.

Marks, B., Sisirak, J., & Hsieh, K. (2008). Health services, health promotion, and health literacy: Report from the State of the Science in Aging with Developmental Disabilities Conference. *Disability and Health Journal, 1*, 136–142.

Murphy, N. A., & Elias, E. R. (2006). Sexuality of children and adolescents with developmental disabilities. *Pediatrics, 18*, 398–403.

National Center for Family Support. (2000). Aging family caregivers: Needs and policy concerns. Family support policy brief #3. National Center for Family Support @ HSRI. Winter.

Newman, L., Wagner, M., Cameto, R., & Knokey, A. M. (2009). *The post-high school outcomes of youth with disabilities up to 4 years after high school*. Menlo Park, CA: SRI International.

Petersilia, J. R. (2001). Crime victims with developmental disabilities. *Criminal Justice and Behavior, 28*, 655–694.

Rimmer, J. H. (2000). Physical fitness in people with mental retardation. The Arc of the United States.

Roberson, K. (2010). *Being a healthy adult: How to advocate for your health and health care*. New Brunswick, NJ: The Elizabeth M. Boggs Center on Developmental Disabilities.

Roizen, N. (2010). Overview of health issues among persons with Down syndrome. *International Review of Research in Mental Retardation, 39*, 3–33.

Rosenbaum, P., Paneth, N., Leviton, A., Goldstein, M., & Bax, M. (2007). Definition and classification of cerebral palsy. *Developmental Medicine & Child Neurology, 49*, 8–14.

Schieve, L. A., Boulet, S. L., Boyle, C., Rasmussen, S. A., & Schendel, D. (2009). Health of children 3 to 17 years of age with Down syndrome in the 1997–2005 National Health Interview Survey. *Pediatrics, 123*, e253–e260.

Siddiqi, S. U., Van Dyke, D. C., Donohoue, P., & McBrien, D. M. (1999). Premature sexual development in individuals with neurodevelopmental disabilities. *Developmental Medicine and Child Neurology, 41*, 392–395.

Sobsey, D., Randall, W., & Parrila, R. K. (1997). Gender differences in abused children with and without disabilities. *Child Abuse and Neglect, 21*, 707–720.

Special Olympics. (2005). *Changing attitudes, changing the world: The health and health care of people with intellectual disabilities*. Washington, DC: Special Olympics.

Sullivan, P. M., & Knutson, J. F. (2000). Maltreatment and disabilities: A population-based epidemiological study. *Child Abuse & Neglect, 24*, 1257–1273.

Surgeon General. (2002). *Closing the gap: A national blueprint to improve the health of persons with mental retardation*. Washington, DC: US Department of Health and Human Services.

Taylor, J. L. (2009). The transition out of high school and into adulthood for individuals with autism and their families. *International Review of Research in Mental Retardation, 38*, 1–32.

Vitale, M., Levitz, M., & Crimmins, D. (2007). *My health, my choice, my responsibility: A training program on health self-advocacy*. Valhalla, NY: Westchester Institute for Human Development.

Voelker, R. (2002). Improved care for neglected population must be the rule rather than the exception. *Journal of the American Medical Association, 288*(3), 299–301.

Wagner, M., Newman, L., Cameto, R., & Levine, P. (2005). *Changes over time in the early post-secondary outcomes of youth with disabilities*. Menlo Park, CA: SRI International.

Walsh, P. N., & McConkey, R. (2009). Inclusive health and people with intellectual disabilities. *International Review of Research in Mental Retardation, 38*, 1–32.

Wang, P., & Blum, N. (2003). Williams syndrome. In M. Wolraich (Ed.), *Disorders of development and learning* (pp. 283–298). Hamilton, Ontario, CA: BC Decker.

Wehmeyer, M. L., Agran, M., Hughes, C., Martin, J. E., Mithaug, D., & Palmer, S. (2007). *Promoting self-determination for students with developmental disabilities*. New York: Guilford.

Wilson, C., & Brewer, N. (1992). The incidence of criminal victimization of individuals with an intellectual disability. *Australian Psychologist, 27*, 114–117.

Zigler, E., & Hodapp, R. M. (1991). Behavioral functioning in individuals with mental retardation. *Annual Review of Psychology, 42*, 29–50.

Part V

Physical Health in Adolescent Health Psychology

Pregnancy in Adolescence

Mary M. Aruda and P. Burke

Introduction

Pregnancy during the adolescent years has long been an area of controversy and interest. Adolescent pregnancy is a complex experience because of its effects on the youth and their families, as well as their infant offspring. Additionally, the occurrence of pregnancy during the adolescent developmental period has economic and societal level impacts (Holcombe, Peterson, & Manlove, 2009). Teen childbearing in the United States cost taxpayers (federal, state, and local) at least $10.9 billion in 2008, according to an updated analysis by The National Campaign to Prevent Teen and Unplanned Pregnancy (2011). Most of the costs of teen childbearing are associated with negative consequences for the children of teen mothers, including increased costs for health care, foster care, incarceration, and lost tax revenue. Within the United States, there are multiple stakeholders including large government agencies and organizations that compile and analyze data and produce voluminous reports on the topic. In clinical practice, the complexity of dealing with pregnant teens and their significant others often taxes even the most empathetic of health care professionals. This chapter reviews teen pregnancy statistics, and explores the phenomenon of teenage pregnancy from a developmental perspective as well as in the context of social, health, and cultural influences. Interventions for working with pregnant teens and promising prevention strategies are also discussed.

M.M. Aruda, Ph.D., P.N.P., F.N.P., F.A.A.N.P. (✉)
College of Nursing and Health Sciences,
University of Massachusetts Boston, 100 Morrissey Boulevard, Boston, MA 02125, USA
e-mail: mary.aruda@umb.edu; mary.aruda@gmail.com

P. Burke, Ph.D., F.N.P., P.N.P., F.S.A.H.M.
Bouve' College of Health Sciences,
Northeastern University, 360 Huntington Avenue, Boston, MA 02115, USA
e-mail: pj.burke@neu.edu

Current Statistics

The birthrate for teenagers aged 15–17 has fallen since 1991 for all racial and ethnic groups (Ventura & Hamilton, 2011). The US birthrate for teenagers in 2009 was the lowest it has ever been in nearly 70 years for which national data are available; the rate was 39.1 births per 1,000 females aged 15–19 years (Ventura & Hamilton, 2011). Three in ten girls become pregnant at least once by age 20. One in five pregnancies is to a teen mother. The majority of pregnancies among 15–19-year-olds (82 %) are unplanned (Mathews, Sutton, Hamilton, & Ventura, 2010). Large disparities persist in race and ethnicity. Hispanic and black women, especially under age 25, have higher birth and pregnancy rates than non-Hispanic white women (Kaye, Suellentrop, & Sloup, 2009). Black and Hispanic youth comprised nearly 60 % of the US teen births in 2009, although

W.T. O'Donohue et al. (eds.), *Handbook of Adolescent Health Psychology*,
DOI 10.1007/978-1-4614-6633-8_35, © Springer Science+Business Media New York 2013

they represent only 35 % of the total population of 15–19-year-old females (Hamilton, Martin, & Ventura, 2010). Unprotected sex, contraceptive failure, and inconsistent or incorrect use of contraceptives are among the reasons for unplanned pregnancy. Despite many efforts to increase access to confidential clinical services, many adolescents continue to experience unwanted, mistimed, or unintended pregnancies.

There are some promising trends indicating that teen sexual activity declined or leveled off in the 1990s through the mid-2000s, and that contraceptive use increased or stabilized (Aba, Martin, & Copez, 2010). According to the latest 2009 Youth Risk Behavior Surveillance System, slightly less than half of all adolescents (46 %) have had sexual intercourse by high school graduation. Many sexually active teens (61 %) report using a condom at last intercourse, but only 23 % report use of more effective birth control, including birth control pills or depo provera (CDC, 2011c). Mosher and Jones (2010) found that lack of knowledge and ambivalence were the top two rated reasons for not using contraception reported by women (N=842) who had experienced a recent unintended birth. When presented with a list of possible reasons for not using contraception, their rank-ordered responses were as follows: *Did not think you could get pregnant* (43.9 %); *Did not really mind if you got pregnant* (22.8 %); *Worried about side effects of birth control* (16.2 %); *Did not expect to have sex* (14.1 %); *Male partner did not want to use birth control* (9.6 %); *and Male partner did not want female to use birth control* (7.3 %). The newer contraceptives on the market, implants, and intrauterine devices, also known as long-acting reversible contraceptives, LARC, which are now approved for adolescents, hold promise as a more reliable and less effort-dependent form of birth control.

The recent dramatic headlines reporting a decline in the adolescent birthrate (Ventura & Hamilton, 2011) may be falsely reassuring to those who are under the impression that the teen pregnancy problem has been resolved. Clinicians who are at the front lines working with large number of pregnant teens are not encouraged by such reports. Pregnancy rates are an estimate, based on the actual countable births and sophisticated estimates of planned terminations (abortions) and spontaneous terminations (miscarriages). A helpful module for calculating pregnancy rates is found on the Center for Disease Control and Prevention (CDC) Web site (CDC, 1999). Because half of all adolescent pregnancies end in either abortion or miscarriage, the number of teen pregnancies is often estimated by doubling the actual number of adolescent births. Consistent with national estimates, in a review of 6 years of clinical quality improvement data for pregnant adolescent patients (N=601), 48.2 % continued their pregnancy, 45.8 % terminated their pregnancy, and 6 % had a miscarriage (Aruda, McCabe, Litty, & Burke, 2008). Table 1 summarizes adolescent birth data for the United States for the last 10 years. Doubling the total number of teen birth will yield an estimate of the annual number of adolescent pregnancies. For this past decade, due to the decline in birthrates, the annual estimate is below the previously popular number quoted of *one million adolescent pregnancies*.

Table 1 Total number of live births to adolescents in the United States

Year	Under 15	15–19	Total teen births	Birthrate (15–19)
2000	8,219	369,456	377,675	47.7
2001	7,510	352,953	360,463	45.3
2002	7,315	425,493	432,493	43.0
2003	6,661	414,580	421,241	41.6
2004	6,781	415,262	422,043	41.1
2005	6,722	414,593	421,315	40.5
2006	6,396	435,436	441,832	41.9
2007	6,218	445,045	451,263	42.5
2008	5,764	434,758	440,522	41.5
2009	5,030	409,840	414,870	39.1

The United States continues to have one of the highest rates of adolescent pregnancy among the world's developed nations (Santelli, Linberg, Finer, & Singh, 2007). Quite simply, adolescent pregnancy is the result of unprotected sexual intercourse, which also places the teen at risk for sexually transmitted infections (STIs), including HIV/AIDS. Youth aged 15–24 years account for nearly half of all new STIs each year (Finer &

Henshaw, 2006). In their classic study, Darroch and colleagues (2001) found adolescent sexual behavior similar across developed nations for initiation and frequency of intercourse; however, the US teens were less likely to use or consistently use contraception compared to teens in the other developed nations. The US teens were also more likely to desire motherhood than teens in other countries. One possible explanation that has been offered is that European teenagers have universal sexuality education as well as greater access to and acceptance of contraception (Klein, 2005). When an underlying behavior like adolescent sexual activity exists across cultures, yet with vastly different outcomes, it becomes a prime target for public health intervention. Indeed, adolescent pregnancy prevention, using a broad perspective to reduce high-risk sexual behavior including the reduction of STIs, is one of CDC's top six priorities, because it is a "winnable battle" in public health and of paramount importance to health and quality of life for youth (CDC, 2011b).

Consequences of Pregnancy in Adolescence

Research has demonstrated the impact of teen pregnancy on adolescents as well as their offspring. Children born to teenage mothers are more likely to be of low birth weight and to be born prematurely (Martin et al., 2010). The incidence of having a low-birth-weight infant (<2,500 g) among adolescents is more than double the rate for adults, and the neonatal death rate (within 28 days of birth) is almost three times higher (Klein, 2005; Cox, 2008). Children of teen mothers are at higher risk of lower cognitive attainment and lower academic achievement, and also exhibit greater behavioral problems (Hoffman & Maynard, 2008). Long term, the sons of teen mothers are significantly more likely to be incarcerated and the daughters of teen mothers are significantly more likely to become teen mothers (Farber, 2009).

Teen mothers are more likely to interrupt their education or drop out of high school, leading to limited vocational opportunities (Hoffman & Maynard, 2008). Often however, pregnancy in adolescence places mothers at greater risk of poverty (Meade, Kershaw, & Ickovics, 2008).

Repeat births before 18 years of age have an even stronger negative effect on high school completion. Factors associated with increased high school completion for pregnant teenagers include race (black teenagers fare better than do white teenagers), being raised in a smaller family, presence of reading materials in the home, employment of the teenager's mother, and having parents with higher educational levels (Klein, 2005).

Teens face physical challenges during pregnancy due to immature development and inadequate nutritional intake. Biological factors that have been consistently associated with negative pregnancy outcomes are poor nutritional status, low prepregnancy weight and height, poor pregnancy weight gain, and parity. In addition, adolescent pregnancy has been associated with medical problems including pregnancy-induced hypertension, anemia, and STDs. The mortality rate for adolescent mothers, although low, is twice that for adult pregnant women (Klein, 2005). Lack of or late entry to prenatal care is a contributing factor to prenatal morbidity and mortality. As the authors found from their own clinical practice and research, despite intense case management and outreach, almost half (45 %) of the pregnant teens seen in an urban adolescent clinic did not begin prenatal care until the end of the first trimester at 12 weeks or later (Aruda et al., 2008). Some teens deny or ignore their pregnancy and avoid prenatal care despite being eligible for medical coverage.

Historical Influences on Adolescent Pregnancy

Teenage pregnancy is not a new phenomenon; however, over the years the sociocultural context has varied along with changing societal attitudes toward women, marriage, and adolescence (Best Start: Ontario's Maternal, Newborn and Early Child Development Resource Center). Their publication, *Teen pregnancy prevention: Exploring out-of-school approaches*, provides a summary of the historical trends in teenage pregnancy.

In the late nineteenth and early twentieth centuries, society focused on the unmarried condition of pregnant women, rather than on age. Unwed mothers were characterized as immoral. Numbers increased with industrialization and the movement of young women from rural areas to cities, where they were beyond family control. In 1904, the concept of adolescence as a distinct time of transition was introduced by G. Stanley Hall. The early to mid twentieth century was influenced by the eugenics movement which was based on the beliefs that the wrong people were having children. Unmarried, sexually active young women were seen as unfit. The concept of prevention was introduced in the social work field, to try to ensure that poverty and delinquency were not passed from one generation to another. Post World War I focused more on the "unwed mothers" and "illegitimate children" versus the age of the mother. Post World War II, unmarried teenagers who became pregnant were classified as delinquents or having emotional or psychological problems. Prior to the 1960s, most teenage pregnancies led to marriage—hence the term *shotgun marriage*—and thus the pregnancy was a societal nonissue. This subtle societal shift is documented even through literature searches in databases such as PsychInfo, where "UNWED MOTHERS" became a search term in1973, followed in 1985 by the search term "ADOLESCENT MOTHERS."

During the 1960s and early 1970s, more women decided not to get married and public concern rose; teen pregnancy was presented as a medical problem requiring increased access to clinics, birth control and abortion. There was a shift from viewing "teen pregnancy" as a moral problem to viewing it as a psychological or a health problem, with estimates of the economic costs to society. The 1970s and 1980s saw a dramatic increase in research of the causes and consequences of teen pregnancy, emphasizing the negative outcomes for teen mothers and their children, without considering preexisting socioeconomic factors. The teen parent was depicted as "perpetrator of poverty" (Furstenberg, 2003), and a social problem requiring government intervention. From 1990 to present, teen pregnancy is still stigmatized as a social problem, and yet the media's focus on individual teen parents may actually glamorize the role. Adolescent pregnancy research and prevention efforts broaden beyond individual behavior to explore the link between socioeconomic factors and disadvantage, the social determinants of health.

Developmental Influences on Adolescent Pregnancy

Consistent with current health guidelines, such as Bright Futures (Hagan et al., 2008), clinicians often find it helpful to view adolescence in stages: early adolescence (11–14 years), middle adolescence (15–17 years), and late adolescence (18–21 years). The period of early adolescence is marked by the physical transformations of puberty along with a shift from dependence on parents to increased independence. Appearance and feeling "normal" become vitally important.

Of particular importance for young adolescents has been the trend toward earlier entry into puberty. In the nineteenth century when data were first recorded, the average age of first period or menarche was 16 or 17. Since then, the age of menarche has decreased by 3 months for every decade and now appears to be leveling off at age 12, with earlier menarche noted in black and Hispanic youth (Cox, 2008). The age range and pattern for the development of secondary sex characteristics in girls are breast buds (8–12); pubic hair (11–14); and menarche (9–16). Male pubertal development typically begins about 2 years later than females. The pattern for male puberty is as follows: testicles enlarge (as early as 9-1/2); pubic hair (10–15); onset of spermarche; and lengthening of genitals (11–14) (McNeeley & Blanchard, 2009). While the development of secondary sex characteristics gives young adolescents the appearance of being more mature, their brain development, in particular their prefrontal cortex, is still maturing. The prefrontal cortex is responsible for advanced reasoning, including the ability to plan, understand cause and effect, think through scenarios, and manage impulses. From a developmental perspective, it is not surprising that curious, socially driven teens, who are in the process of forming their personal identity, might engage in sexual relations as a means for meeting their basic needs for belonging, intimacy, and mastery (Weinberger, Elvevag, & Giedd, 2005; NIMH, 2011).

Early puberty has been linked to earlier romantic expectations and experiences. A recent, nationwide multiyear survey found that girls who experience menarche before age 12 were more likely to live with or marry someone at an earlier age (Cavanagh, 2011). Teens who mature earlier and initiate intercourse at younger ages have been found to have a greater number of sexual partners (Abma, Martinez, Mosher, & Dawson, 2004).

Pregnancy in an early adolescent is vastly different from pregnancy in an older adolescent. Health care for early adolescents requires comprehensive support to maximize nutritional intake and growth for both the pregnant teen and her fetus (Cox, 2008). For teens younger than 15 years, there are increased risks for prematurity, low birth weight, and mortality. While survey reports indicate a decline, 6 % of youth reported initiating sexual intercourse before age 13, and 13 % of youth reported having had intercourse by 15 years of age (Abma, Martinez, & Coben, 2010). Younger teenagers are especially vulnerable to coercive and nonconsensual sex. A 2002 study of girls who were age 14 or younger when they first had sex found that 18 % characterized their first sexual experience as involuntary, and 27 % indicated it was unwanted (Kirby, 2007). One of the caveats of identifying pregnancy in a young adolescent is to be alert for the risk of incest or sexual assault.

One of the hallmarks of middle adolescence (high school years) is intense interest in peer activities. Indeed, as peer group values become more important, so too the potential for conflicts with parents increases. Likewise a sense of omnipotence and immortality may lead to adolescent risk-taking behavior. At this stage there is usually an increase in dating activity or involvement in partnering relationships, and as such more opportunity for sexual experimentation and intercourse (Radzic, Sherer, & Neinstein, 2008). It is not surprising that most young people have sex for the first time at about age 17 (Guttmacher, 2011).

Half (46 %) of all adolescents have had sexual intercourse by graduation from high school, with only slightly more than a third (39 %) using a condom at last intercourse (CDC, 2011c). Teens having sex tend to do so sporadically, as suggested by the report that only 34 % of sexually active youth had had sex in the prior 3 months. Because of the sporadic nature of teen sexual activity, adolescents often do not plan to have sex on a particular occasion, but sometimes do so anyway, and this unprotected intercourse places them at risk for pregnancy. Age of sexual partner is another risk factor. Research indicates that when adolescent females have sex at a young age with much older partners, there is a greater chance that their first sexual experience was involuntary or unwanted and that they can become pregnant because under these circumstances intercourse is more likely to be unprotected (Kirby, 2007).

In late adolescence, there is the potential for greater independence and movement toward adult roles and responsibilities; however, there is significant variation, depending upon what developmental tasks they have managed to accomplish up to that point, in the context of both their assets or protective factors and stressors or risk factors. The term "emerging adults" that was coined for 18–25-year-olds connotes the complex developmental process that older adolescents experience (Arnett, 2000). Birthrates overall by race and ethnicity are consistently higher for ages 18–19 than for 15–17. Although downward trends for both age groups have been similar, long-term declines were smaller for older teens (Ventura & Hamilton, 2011). A decrease in the median age of menarche, coupled with an increase in the median age of marriage for females to 25.3 years, results in a protracted period of time—nearly a decade—during which youth are at risk for unprotected intercourse and the consequences of an unintended pregnancy and STIs (Guttmacher, 2011).

New research on adolescent brain development provides an understanding of cognitive differences. It is important to remember that adolescents think differently than adults do (Weinberger et al., 2005). Immature cognitive processing and egocentric thinking can lead to distortions in judgment and the belief that a pregnancy could not possibly happen to them, often leading to delays in pregnancy diagnosis. Emotional factors, such as fear or shame, can perpetuate denial. For some adolescents, finding out that they are pregnant initially can be immobilizing, leading them to simply ignore it and hope that things will work out. Under stress, an adolescent may revert to concrete thinking and focus on daily routines, which can subvert abstract decision making and planning for the future. Due to immature cognitive development, becoming a parent during early or middle adolescence has limitations because a teen parent may not accurately perceive and/or respond to her child's intentions or needs (Farber, 2009).

Social Influences on Teen Pregnancy

Adolescent development and behavior take place in a social context—home, school, and community. While family relationships are transformed over the course of adolescence and young adulthood, parental influences remain important. Parents of adolescents are typically in the midst of their own midlife crisis, which in turn can affect their ability or desire to monitor their teen's behavior. Adolescents raised in single-parent households are at increased risk for teenage pregnancy (Salazar, Santelli, Crosby, & Diclemente, 2009). The National Institute on Drug Abuse (2003) described the following family protective factors: a strong bond between children and their families; parental involvement in a child's life; supportive parenting; and clear limits and consistent enforcement of discipline. One of the largest research studies on teens in the United States is the National Longitudinal Study of Adolescent Health (Add Health), a longitudinal study of a nationally representative sample of the US adolescents who were in grades 7–12 during the 1994–1995 school year. The Add Health cohort has been followed into young adulthood with four in-home interviews, the most recent of which was conducted in 2008. One of the key early findings of the Add Health study was the power of family connectedness as a potential protective factor across all risks in adolescence, including early pregnancy (http://www.cpc.unc.edu/projects/addhealth).

Teenage pregnancy may be both an antecedent as well as a consequence of poor academic performance and poverty. High expectations from parents, school officials, and the community at large provide extrinsic motivating factors for success. Adolescents need to feel hopeful, optimistic, and confident in their ability to achieve. Resources, opportunities, and nurturing environments are critical adjuncts to their preventing an early or unintended pregnancy. Similarly, when a pregnant teenager opts to become a parent, she needs the support of her family and school system, as well as access to essential health care and social service programs. Researchers have demonstrated an increased risk of becoming an adolescent parent if other family members have been teen parents (Furstenberg, 2003). Teen parents often have mothers, sisters, or brothers who were themselves teen parents (East & Jacobson, 2001).

The influence of male partners on teen pregnancy is important but until recently has been overlooked by researchers, funders, or policy makers. According to the Office of Adolescent Health (OAH), of the approximately ten million adolescent males who were aged 12–16 in 1996, almost one in ten became a father before their 20th birthday (OAH, 2011). Teen fathers were more likely to report that they did not want the pregnancy and were less likely than older fathers to report that the pregnancy occurred at or about the right time. Younger fathers (<24 years) were more likely to report having wanted the pregnancy later (32 %) than were fathers aged 25–34 and 35 and older (19 and 13 %, respectively) (Bronte-Tinkew, Horowitz, Kennedy, & Perper, 2007). Eight of ten teen fathers do not marry their first child's mother. These absent fathers pay less than $800 annually for child support, often because they are quite poor themselves (National Campaign for Teen Pregnancy Prevention). Male involvement in contraception has been gaining increased focus and integration into federal Title X family planning efforts.

Working with Pregnant Teens

The initial challenge in working with pregnant adolescents is identification of the pregnancy. Adolescents present for pregnancy testing under a variety of circumstances. While most women have pregnancy concerns with delayed or missing periods, many adolescents may ordinarily have irregular periods for a number of medical reasons, and thus they may not be concerned by amenorrhea (missed menstrual periods). Similarly, many teens mistake early pregnancy implantation bleeding/staining for a light period. When scheduling a medical appointment or walking in for an urgent care visit, an adolescent may be hesitant to divulge sensitive information. This reluctance to disclose sexual history underscores the importance of confidentiality for adolescent reproductive health visits, which is supported by law in all 50 states (English, Bass, Boyle & Eshragh, 2010).

Health professionals need to be prepared to ascertain an adolescent's "hidden agenda." As we know from YRBSS data, approximately half of all teens are sexually active and thus it is recommended that all adolescents be screened for sexual risk behaviors. Many young women may be unaware of the possibility of being pregnant or reluctant to raise the question until a health care provider inquires about their sexual activity. Despite the availability of home pregnancy test kits, research has demonstrated that only approximately one-third of adolescents presenting to clinics have already conducted a pregnancy test at home and thus were seeking confirmation and referral (Shew, Hellerstedt, Sieving, Smith, & Fee, 2000). For many adolescents, the cost of a home pregnancy test kit may be prohibitive or they may be reluctant to purchase a pregnancy test from their neighborhood pharmacy because of privacy concerns. Adolescents are selective regarding to whom they disclose information and may refrain from disclosing their concern about a pregnancy unless they feel comfortable. Health professionals are encouraged to create welcoming, adolescent-friendly environments.

Estimates are that one-third of the population of children has special health care needs. Adolescents with chronic health conditions often underestimate their ability to become pregnant or may engage in unprotected intercourse, in an attempt to test their fertility status. Sexual risk assessments are especially important for adolescents with chronic medical conditions, such as cystic fibrosis, diabetes, renal disease, and cancer. One cannot assume that an adolescent is abstinent or using protection, even if she has a serious medical condition or is on medication that has known teratogenic effects. The authors have worked with many teens whose desire to become or remain pregnant outweighed what was in their own best interest from a medical perspective, including patients who were post-transplant or on chemotherapy. Likewise, teens with complex mental health issues, such as depression, anxiety, or substance abuse, are at risk for engaging in unprotected sexual activity (Aruda, Waddicor, Frese, Cole, & Burke, 2010).

All teens, regardless of any preexisting health issues, should be counseled about their potential reproductive capacity (i.e., fecundity) and the risks of unprotected intercourse. "In normally fertile couples, cycle fecundity averages 20 % and does not exceed approximately 35 % even when coitus is carefully timed" (Fritz & Speroff, 2011, p. 1,155). After 3, 6, or 12 months of exposure, approximately 57, 72, and 85 % of sexually active couples will attain a pregnancy (Fritz & Speroff, 2011). Adolescents who have never been pregnant and therefore begin to doubt that they can ever become pregnant need to understand their future risk for pregnancy and what they can do to protect their reproductive health status, such as ensuring adequate intake of folic acid (http://www.womenshealth.gov/publications/our-publications/fact-sheet/folic-acid.cfm#b).

Once a pregnancy is confirmed, it is important to assess the adolescent's emotional response, coping skills, and social support resources. Options counseling is one of the most important aspects of early pregnancy management. It is imperative for clinicians to utilize neutral, factual information and nondirective statements when discussing options. For example, the following script was previously developed for a multidisciplinary adolescent practice (Aruda, 2007). "*You have a decision to make about your pregnancy. Any pregnant adolescent has three options. Alphabetically, these options are: (a) abortion or pregnancy termination; (b) continuing the pregnancy and arranging for an adoption, infant care, or foster care; and (c) continuing the pregnancy, entering prenatal care, and becoming a parent. At this point, which option do you think you will choose?*"

Choosing what to do about a pregnancy may be the biggest decision that an adolescent has ever had to make in her life. The clinician's words are very powerful and must be chosen with care. Adolescent ambivalence is normal. A teen will need time and energy to thoughtfully consider all of the options, along with their potential impact. For some teens, the choice may seem clear-cut, and they reach a decision quickly. Others need more time to talk with people in their personal support network as they carefully weigh each option. They may vacillate between continuing and terminating the pregnancy. Adolescents who have cognitive limitations or are emotionally fragile will need extensive support and counseling, and will benefit from mental health services. In some cases, the pregnant adolescent may feel pressured by her partner or a parent to choose a certain option and this situation requires careful exploration. Such pressure, at a time when the teen is already feeling vulnerable, can be volatile and requires careful exploration. If the pregnant teen is interested, arranging a family or a couple's meeting can help to diffuse some of the angst while providing a safe environment and support. Ultimately it is the pregnant teen's right and responsibility to choose her option for abortion, adoption, or parenting. Anecdotally, the authors have found that adolescents who felt forced into a decision to terminate their pregnancy were more likely to experience an early repeat pregnancy. There are no available statistics for repeat adolescent pregnancy post abortion, and thus more research is needed in this area. Similarly, prematurely choosing to continue a pregnancy without careful consideration of all the ramifications can have a great impact on the adolescent, her family, as well as her partner and his family. Although very few adolescents choose adoption, a variety of relatively new options are now available, including temporary infant care placements, foster care, and placements with extended family. It is helpful to have written materials available (Aruda et al., 2010). Once a decision is made, prompt referral for prenatal or termination services is important. Providers should follow up by confirming that the adolescent has kept her first prenatal appointment or arrange for a postabortion follow-up visit (Aruda et al., 2010).

Professionals working with newly pregnant teens need to have knowledge of options for pregnancy termination, including medical and aspiration abortion as well as reputable referral sites within their communities. Abortion rules and regulations are subject to continuing evolution in different states and updates are posted by organizations such as Planned Parenthood. A comprehensive review of medical care for pregnant teens can be found in the Teenage Pregnancy chapter by Cox (2008).

Motivations for Unprotected Sexual Intercourse

The area of adolescent sexuality has generated tremendous research over the years and investigators have examined a large number of variables to explain adolescent sexual behavior. In a meta-analysis, Kirby (2007) found that over 500 factors have been identified that affect one or more sexual behaviors (e.g., the initiation of sex, frequency of sex, number of sexual partners, use of condoms, and use of other contraceptives) or consequences of those behaviors (i.e., pregnancy, childbearing, or STD). Important risk and protective factors include characteristics of the teens as well as their communities, families, and relationships with friends, peers, and partners. Sexual partners may be a casual or a romantic partner. Furthermore, sexual behavior should not be confused with sexual identity.

Kirby (2007) has organized risk and protective factors for teen pregnancy into four key themes:

1. Individual biological factors (e.g., age, physical maturity, and gender)
2. Disadvantage, disorganization, and dysfunction in the lives of the teens themselves and their environments (e.g., rates of substance abuse, violence, and divorce; also levels of education)
3. Sexual values, attitudes, and modeled behavior (e.g., teens' own values about sexual behavior as well as those expressed by parents, peers, and romantic partners)
4. Connection to adults and organizations that discourage sex, unprotected sex, or early childbearing (e.g., attachment to parents and other adults in their schools and places of worship)

Blum et al. (2000) confirmed the importance of connections as a foundation for building resiliency in youth development. Home and community environments, as well as connections to family and school, were found to influence adolescent behavior. Understanding the complex web of influences leading adolescents to engage in unprotected intercourse is critically important to the design and implementation of risk reduction interventions and public health and prevention education policies, as well as informing clinical practice and counseling guidelines (Bearinger et al., 2007; DiClemente et al., 2007).

The interactions between affect, thought, and behavior are powerful. Indeed adolescents' motivations for sexual activity and pregnancy prevention need to be understood in the context of normal human development (Burke, 1987). In their 1995 landmark report, *The Best Intentions*, Brown and Eisenberg (1995) noted that there is persuasive evidence that unprotected sexual activity is influenced not only by knowledge and access but also by personal and emotional factors. Kirby (2007) stated that among the known risk and protective factors, adolescents' own sexual beliefs, values, attitudes, and intentions are the most strongly related to sexual behavior. Personal attitudes and feelings, as both an individual and as one connected to another through sexual relations, exert a major influence on sexual behavior and the decision (implicit or explicit) about whether or not to use protection during sexual intercourse.

Concerns about fertility or in adolescent terms, "just checking" to see if they could get pregnant, have been identified as possible motivator for adolescents to engage in intercourse. It is not surprising then that adolescent females become curious about their fertility while at the same time trying to make sense of their environmental norms (Burke, Tonelli, & Chalfin, 2011). Rainey, Stevens-Simon, and Kaplan (1993) first described female adolescents' potentially problematic self-perception of fertility fears. In a sample of 200 urban females aged 14–18 years, 21.5 % were concerned about their ability to conceive and were 45 % less likely to use contraception. Other researchers have noted "urban lore" associated with adolescents' fertility concerns related to the use of specific contraceptive methods (Clark, 2001). Wimberly et al. (2003), using focus groups, reported an extensive range of adolescent beliefs about the causes of infertility. Trent, Millstein, and Ellen (2006) found that 72 % of adolescent girls surveyed from a high-STI-prevalence community thought there was some chance they would have future fertility problems and 58 % thought they would have little or no control over developing fertility problems in the future. White, Rosengard, Weitzen, Meers, and Phipps (2006) documented that 42 % of newly pregnant adolescents expressed fears about their ability to conceive when surveyed at a first prenatal visit.

Aruda (2011) found in a survey that of 305 adolescents requesting pregnancy testing in a clinic, 51 % ($n=153$) expressed worries (fertility fears) about their ability to become pregnant. This is an interesting finding considering that nearly half, 45 % ($n=137$), reported a prior pregnancy. Most teens (75 %) had been exposed to discussions of fertility concerns in the media and 10 % had been told that they could not get pregnant. Most (79 %) responded that they were trying to prevent pregnancy; 72 % ($n=213$) hoped that their pregnancy test was negative, 12 % ($n=35$) hoped for a positive test, and 17 % ($n=50$) were not sure what they wanted for a test result.

The majority (81 %, $n=241$) of the pregnancy tests were negative at the time of the visit, making these adolescents prime candidates for further preventative interventions targeted at reducing unprotected intercourse.

Worries about the ability to become pregnant (fertility fears) have emerged as a predictor for unprotected sexual intercourse for certain groups of adolescents (Aruda, 2011). In a national survey, 59 % of women and 47 % of men say that it is at least slightly likely they are infertile (19 % of women and 14 % of men describe it as quite or extremely likely) (Kay, Suellentrop, & Slop, 2009). Assisted reproductive technologies have dramatically changed reproductive health care in the past decades, and marketing efforts have heightened women's concerns about their reproductive capacity. Adolescents, described as the "sponges" of cultural influence, often take in these messages and internalize them (Brown & Gilligan, 1992). With record high rates of STIs in the United States, and globally, some of these adolescents' fertility fears may indeed be warranted.

Future Directions to Prevent Adolescent Pregnancy

A body of research is emerging on programs that have proven effective and many which have been retested through replication, to prevent adolescent pregnancy. Comprehensive research reviews have been commissioned both privately and by the US Government. The OAH, under Health and Humans Services (HHS) commissioned a review of the evidence by Mathematica and recommended 28 programs to be used for funding requests. The programs reflected a range of program models and target populations; 20 had evidence of impacts on sexual activity (sexual initiation, number of partners, or frequency of sexual activity), 9 on contraceptive use, 4 on STIs, and 5 on pregnancy or births (OAH, 2011). The National Campaign for Teen Pregnancy Prevention, *Emerging Answers 2007*, reviewed 115 studies, but also acknowledged that many creative community programs may not have the resources for evaluation and publication. Kirby (2007) has stated that because teen pregnancy has many causes, and because even effective programs do not eliminate the problem—it is unreasonable to expect any single curriculum or community program to make a serious dent in the problem of teen pregnancy on its own. Making true and lasting progress in preventing teen pregnancy requires a combination of community programs and broader efforts to influence values and popular culture, to engage parents and schools, to change the economic incentives that face teens, and more (Kirby 2007). Current, evidence-based information is crucial for professionals working to prevent adolescent pregnancy.

In our experience and recent updated review of the literature, there are several areas to be highlighted that hold great promise for prevention of teen pregnancy. First is the identification and targeting of resources toward high-risk groups. The Teen Pregnancy Prevention Initiative (TPPI), the CDC funding initiative for 2010–2015, has targeted nine communities nationally with high teen pregnancy rates and is looking for a 10 % decrease through four key components: implementation of evidence-based programs, quality community linkages, education, and sustainability (CDC, 2011b). Comprehensive youth development interventions hold great promise in reducing pregnancy risk among high-risk groups. A recent report of a 12-month, randomized clinical trail showed increased condom use, increased hormonal and dual contraceptive use, as well as greater stress management and higher levels of prosocial connectedness at school and with family (Sieving et al., 2011).

Researchers have focused attention on adolescents who present for pregnancy testing and identified them as a potential group to target for prevention. As discussed earlier, the majority of pregnancy tests done in clinical practice settings are negative, and research surrounding this testing time is developing. A longitudinal study by Zabin, Sedivy, & Emerson (1994) revealed that 58 % of teens with an initial negative pregnancy test become pregnant within 18 months of that index test. A subsequent cross-sectional study of 2,926 young women aged 17 or younger who presented to clinics for pregnancy testing revealed that 62.3 % of the tests were negative and 36.4 % were positive (Zabin, Emerson, Ringers, & Sedivy, 1996). Recent research indicates 77 % negative pregnancy test results within an urban setting and further reinforced pregnancy testing as an important and often missed opportunity for clinicians (Daley, Sadler, Leventhal, Cromwell, & Reynolds, 2005). They suggested that identifying and intervening with adolescents seeking pregnancy testing could potentially reduce early childbearing and other consequences of unprotected intercourse. Unfortunately, clinical sites, under pressure to generate volume and meet productivity demands, often have difficulty accommodating the counseling and health education needs of adolescents presenting for pregnancy testing, which means a missed opportunity for prevention.

For those youth who decide to be engaged in sexual intercourse, contraceptives have entered a new era. A comprehensive analysis of contraceptives by Jaccard (2009) broadens our prior perspective. The term contraceptive behavior is ambiguous and can be thought of as having four facets: *contraceptive choice*, which refers to choosing a major method of contraception and acquiring it; *accuracy of use*, which refers to whether the contraceptive is used correctly; *consistency of use*, which refers to whether the contraceptive is used at each instance of intercourse; and *contraceptive switching*, which refers to changing from one method of contraception to another. All four facets are important to unplanned pregnancy. Choice of a less effective method increases the risk of an unplanned pregnancy, as does using a method incorrectly or inconsistently. Switching methods often results in gaps in protection, higher failure rates as individuals learn a new method, and, if the new method is less effective, increased risk of unplanned pregnancy.

New contraceptive methods now available to adolescents hold great promise regarding increased choice, accuracy, consistency, and decreased switching to prevent pregnancy. The older hormonal contraceptives (pill, patch, and vaginal ring) are readily available but depend on the correct use. Depo provera can be given every 3 months but patients need to come to clinic to receive the injection. The new options, LARC, including intrauterine devices such as the Mirena, which releases a hormone (levonorgestrel) or the Copper T, and subdermal implants (Implanon). LARC is encouraged by the American College of Obstetricians and Gynecologists for most women, including adolescents (ACOG, 2009). Despite this encouragement, use of LARC remains quite low among American women. Only 1.3 % of American women of any age relies on an intrauterine contraception and less than 1 % relies on a contraceptive implant (Mosher & Jones, 2010). Although overall use is low, the IUD appears to be a well-accepted contraceptive among adolescents (Yen, Saah, & Hillard, 2010). Multiple studies of adolescents using IUDs have shown high rates of continuation, ranging from 45 to 83 % at 6 months, 48–88 % at 12 months, and 60–73 % at 24 months (Godfrey et al., 2010). Few studies have examined the use of implants in the adolescent population, though one study determining which components of a maternity program helped teenage mothers delay subsequent pregnancies found that failure to have Norplant inserted during the puerperium was the strongest predictor of repeat pregnancy during the first 2 postpartum years (Stevens-Simon, Kelly, & Kulick, 2001).

It is clear that the voice and emotional responses of youth need to be acknowledged to increase contraceptive use. Recent national survey demonstrates that many unmarried young women fear the side effects of contraception and these fears reduce their likelihood of using the more effective methods of birth control. Many unmarried young adults, both men and women, simply do not believe that contraception is very effective. And many unmarried young adults believe they are infertile (Kaye et al., 2009). This confusion, and the misinformation often found in media, points to the need for clear, organized, direct sex education for adolescents. The education needs to present clear, balanced information about the basics—anatomy, reproduction, fertility, pregnancy, STIs, sexuality, and related issues. In addition, education programs need to include full and accurate information about contraception, including the types of methods available, how to use them correctly, and their benefits as well as their risks. Programs need to allow adolescents to voice their fears and concerns and counteract and correct specific myths and misinformation about contraception. In addition, educational programs for youth build skills for healthy and respectful relationships (Kaye et al., 2009). The public debate over "abstinence-only" education has been at times contentious. However, in their position paper on abstinence-only education policies and programs issued by the Society for Adolescent Health and Medicine (Santelli, Ott, Lyon, Rogers, & Summers, 2006), the organization "supports a comprehensive approach to sexual risk reduction including abstinence as well as correct and consistent use of condoms and contraception among teens who choose to be sexually active" (p. 86).

More challenging are attempts to change social environments and to tackle the social determinants of health which lead to adolescent pregnancy. We are all influenced by the larger social environment around us. Parents and other caring adults need to communicate with their teens and young adults about the importance of pregnancy planning—when, with whom, and under what circumstances it might be best to start a family. They should also acknowledge the desire that so many unmarried young adults express for children and family life, and how such feelings relate to longer term goals. Parents, other caring adults, and larger social systems need to encourage unmarried young adults to *align* their plans for pregnancy and family with their sexual and contraceptive behavior—for example, using protection "most of the time" is not a reliable way to prevent pregnancy; it must be used "all the time" (Kaye et al., 2009).

In summary, adolescent pregnancy continues to be a major issue and challenge within the United States. Adolescent childbearing has a negative impact on three dimensions: health of the adolescents and their infants; individual social and economic effects; and societal level impacts (WHO, 2008). Much research and many promising interventions are in process. Funding needs to be sustained for program development and evaluation, as well as for intervention research. Adolescent pregnancy prevention demands continued diligent efforts by adults who care for and about teens.

References

Abma, J. C., Martinez, G. M., & Copen, C. E. (2010). Teenagers in the United States: Sexual activity, contraceptive use, and childbearing, National Survey of Family Growth 2006–2008. National Center for Health Statistics. *Vital and Health Statistics, 23*(30).

American College of Obstetricians and Gynecologists (ACOG). (2009). Opinion no 450: Increasing use of contraceptive implants and intrauterine devices to reduce unintended pregnancy. *Obstetrics and Gynecology, 114*, 1434–1438.

Arnett, J. J. (2000). Emerging adulthood, a theory of development from the late teens through the twenties. *American Psychologist, 55*(5), 469–480.

Aruda, M. (2007). Diagnosing and tracking pregnant teens: Development of a quality improvement project. *Women's Health Care, 6*(9), 25–33.

Aruda, M. M. (2011). Predictors of unprotected intercourse for female adolescents measured at their request for a pregnancy test. *Journal of Pediatric Nursing, 26*, 216–223.

Aruda, M. M., McCabe, M., Litty, C., & Burke, P. (2008). Adolescent pregnancy diagnosis and outcomes: A six year clinical sample. *Journal of Pediatric and Adolescent Gynecology, 21*, 17–19.

Aruda, M. M., Waddicor, K., Frese, L., Cole, J., & Burke, P. (2010). Early pregnancy in adolescents: Diagnosis, assessment, options counseling, and referral. *Journal of Pediatric Health Care, 24*(1), 4–13.

Bearinger, L. H., Sieving, R. E., Ferguson, J., & Sharma, V. (2007). Global perspectives on the sexual and reproductive health of adolescents: Patterns, prevention, and potential. *The Lancet, 369*, 1220–1231.

Blum, R. W., Beuhring, T., Shew, M. L., Bearinger, L. H., Sieving, R. E., & Resnick, M. D. (2000). The effects of race/ethnicity, income, and family structure on adolescent risk behaviors. *American Journal of Public Health, 90*(12), 1879–1884.

Best start: Ontario's Maternal, Newborn and Early Child Development Resource Center. *Teen pregnancy prevention: Exploring out-of-school approaches.* Retrieved August 10, 2011, from http://www.beststart.org/resources/rep_health/pdf/teen_pregnancy_08_5.pdf.

Bronte-Tinkew, J., Horowitz, A., Kennedy, E., & Perper, K. (2007). *Men's pregnancy intentions and prenatal behaviors: What they mean for fathers' involvement with their children. Child trends research brief #2007: 18.* Retrieved August 22, 2011, from http://www.childtrends.org/files/Child_Trends-2007_06_11_RB_Prenatal.pdf.

Brown, S. S., & Eisenberg, L. (Eds.). (1995). *The best intentions: Unintended pregnancy and the well-being of children and families..* Institute of Medicine, Washington, DC: National Academy Press.

Brown, L., & Gilligan, C. (1992). *Meeting at the crossroads.* New York: Ballantine Books.

Burke, P. (1987). Adolescents' motivation for sexual activity and pregnancy prevention. *Issues in Comprehensive Pediatric Nursing, 10*(3), 161–171.

Burke, P., Tonelli, M., & Chalfin, S. (2011). Adolescents' fertility concerns: "I'm not trying to get pregnant but if I did..." *Journal of Pediatric and Adolescent Gynecology, 24*(6), 413–414.

Cavanagh, S. (2011). Early pubertal timing and the union formation behaviors of young women. *Social Forces*.

Centers for Disease Control and Prevention (CDC). (2011a). *Teenage pregnancy prevention: Integrating services, programs, and strategies through community-wide initiatives*. Retrieved August 22, 2010, from http://www.cdc.gov/TeenPregnancy/PreventTeenPreg.htm.

Centers for Disease Control and Prevention (CDC). (2011b). *Teen pregnancy: Improving the lives of young people and strengthening communities by reducing teen pregnancy at a glance 2011*. Retrieved August 7, 2011, from http://www.cdc.gov/chronicdisease/resources/publications/aag/teen-preg.htm.

Centers for Disease Control and Prevention (CDC). (2011c). *Youth Risk Behavior Surveillance System (YRBSS) fact sheet 2009*. Retrieved August 7, 2011, from http://www.cdc.gov/healthyyouth/yrbs/factsheets/index.htm#sexual.

Centers for Disease Control and Prevention (CDC). (1999). *Public health data module 2: Calculating teen birth and pregnancy rates*. Retrieved August 20, 2011, from http://www.cdc.gov/nchs/data/training/module2.pdf.

Clark, L. (2001). Will the pill make me sterile? Addressing reproductive health concerns and strategies to improve adherence to hormonal contraceptive regimens in adolescent girls. *Journal of Pediatric and Adolescent Gynecology, 14*, 153–162.

Cox, J. E. (2008). Teenage pregnancy. In L. S. Neinstein, C. M. Gordon, D. K. Katzman, D. S. Rosen, & E. R. Woods (Eds.), *Adolescent health care: A practical guide* (5th ed., pp. 565–580). Philadelphia: Lippincott Williams & Wilkins.

Daley, A. M., Sadler, L. S., Leventhal, J. M., Cromwell, P. F., & Reynolds, H. D. (2005). Negative pregnancy tests in urban adolescents: An important and often missed opportunity for clinicians. *Pediatric Nursing, 31*, 87–89.

Darroch, J. E., Singh, S., Frost, J. J., & The Study Team. (2001). Differences in teen pregnancy rates among five developed countries: The role of sexual activity and contraceptive use. *Family Planning Perspectives, 33*, 244–250.

DiClemente, R. J., Salazar, L. F., & Crosby, R. A. (2007). A review of STD/HIV preventative interventions for adolescents: Sustaining effects using an ecological approach. *Journal of Pediatric Psychology, 32*, 888–906.

East, P. L., & Jacobson, L. J. (2001). The younger siblings of teenage mothers: A follow-up of their pregnancy risk. *Developmental Psychology, 37*, 254–264.

English, A., Bass, L., Boyle, A. D., & Eshragh, F. (2010). *State minor consent laws: A summary* (3rd ed.). Chapel Hill, NC: Center for Adolescent Health & the Law.

Farber, N. (2009). *Adolescent pregnancy, 2nd ed.: Policy and prevention services*. New York: Springer.

Finer, L. B., & Henshaw, S. K. (2006). Disparities in rates of unintended pregnancy in the United States, 1994 and 2001. *Perspectives on Sexual and Reproductive Health, 38*(2), 90–96.

Fritz, M. A., & Speroff, L. (2011). *Clinical gynecologic endocrinology and infertility*. Philadelphia: Wolters Kluwer-Lippincott-Williams & Wilkins.

Furstenberg, F. (2003). Teenage childbearing as a public issue and private concern. *Annual Review of Sociology, 29*, 23–39.

Godfrey, E. M., Memmel, L. M., Neustadt, A., et al. (2010). Intrauterine contraception for adolescents aged 14–18 years: A multicenter randomized pilot study of levonorgestrel-releasing intrauterine system compared to the Copper T 380A. *Contraception, 81*, 123–127.

Guttmacher Institute. (2011). *Facts on American teens sexual and reproductive health*. Retrieved August 15, 2011, from http://www.guttmacher.org/pubs/FB-ATSRH.pdf.

Hagan, J. F., Shaw, J. S., & Duncan, P. M. (2008a). *Bright futures: Guidelines for health supervision of infants, children and adolescents* (3rd ed.). Elk Grove Village, IL: American Academy of Pediatrics.

Hamilton, B. E., Martin, J. A., & Ventura, S. J. (2010). Births: Preliminary data for 2009. *National Vital Statistics Reports, 59*(3):Table 2.

Hoffman, S., & Maynard, R. (2008). *Kids having kids*. Washington, D.C.: The Urban Institute Press.

Holcombe, E., Peterson, K., & Manlove, J. (2009). *Ten reasons to still keep the focus on teen childbearing. Child trends research brief publication #2009–10*. Retrieved August 7, 2011, from http://www.childtrends.org/Files//Child_Trends-2009_04_01_RB_KeepingFocus.pdf.

Jaccard, J. (2009). *Unlocking the contraceptive conundrum*. Washington, DC: The National Campaign to Prevent Teen and Unplanned Pregnancy.

Kaye, K., Suellentrop, K., & Corinna Sloup, C. (2009). *The fog zone: Misperceptions, magical thinking, and ambivalence put young adults at risk for unplanned pregnancy. Washington, DC: National Campaign to Prevent Teen and Unplanned Pregnancy*. Retrieved August 20, 2011, from http://www.thenationalcampaign.org/fogzone/PDF/FogZone.pdf.

Kirby, D. (2007). *Emerging answers: Research findings on programs to reduce teen pregnancy and sexually transmitted diseases*. Washington, DC: National Campaign to Prevent Teen and Unplanned Pregnancy.

Klein, J. D., & The Committee on Adolescence, American Academy of Pediatrics. (2005). Adolescent pregnancy: Current trends and issues. *Pediatrics, 116*, 281–286.

Martin, J. A., Hamilton, B. E., Sutton, P. D., et al. (2010). *Births: Final data for 2008. National vital statistics reports; vol 59 no 1*. Hyattsville, MD: National Center for Health Statistics.

Mathews, T. J., Sutton, P. D., Hamilton, B. E., & Ventura, S. J. (2010). *State disparities in teenage birth rates in the United States. NCHS data brief, no 46*. Hyattsville, MD: National Center for Health Statistics.

McNeeley, C. & Blanchard, J. (2009). Explaining the teen years: A guide to healthy adolescence. Center for adolescent health, John Hopkins, Bloomberg School of Public Health. http://www.jhsph.edu/bin/s/e/Interactive%20Guide.pdf.

Meade, C. S., Kershaw, T. S., & Ickovics, J. R. (2008). The intergenerational cycle of teenage motherhood: An ecological approach. *Health Psychology, 27*(4), 419–429.

Mosher, W. D., & Jones, J. (2010). Use of contraception in the United States: 1982–2008. National Center for Health Statistics. *Vital and Health Statistics, 23*(29).

National Campaign for Teen Pregnancy Prevention. *Teen pregnancy and responsible fatherhood.* Retrieved August 22, 2011, from http://www.thenationalcampaign.org/why-it-matters/pdf/fatherhood.pdf.

National Institute on Drug Abuse (2003). Preventing drug use among children and adolescents: A research-based guide for parents, educators and community leaders. (2nd edition). Bethesda, MD: US DHHS, NIH, NIDA.

National Institute of Mental Health (NIMH). (2011). *The teen brain: Still under construction.* Retrieved from http://www.nimh.nih.gov/health/publications/the-teen-brain-still-under-construction/teen-brain.pdf.

Office of Adolescent Health (OAH). (2011). Retrieved August 22, 2011, from http://www.hhs.gov/ash/oah/index.html.

Rainey, D. Y., Stevens-Simon, C., & Kaplan, D. W. (1993). Self-perception of infertility among female adolescents. *American Journal of Disease in Children, 147*, 1053–1057.

Radzik, M., Sherer, S., & Neinstein, L. (2008). Psychosocial development in adolescents. In L. S. Neinstein, C. M. Gordon, D. K. Katzman, D. S. Rosen, & E. R. Woods (Eds.), *Adolescent health care: A practical guide* (5th ed., pp. 27–31). Philadelphia: Lippincott Williams & Wilkins.

Salazar, L. F., Santelli, J. S., Crosby, R. A., & Diclemente, R. J. (2009). Sexually transmitted disease transmission and pregnancy among adolescents. In R. J. DiClemente, J. S. Santelli, & R. A. Crosby (Eds.), *Adolescent health: Understanding and preventing risk behaviors* (pp. 275–302). San Francisco: Jossey-Bass.

Santelli, J., Ott, M. A., Lyon, M., Rogers, J., & Summers, D. (2006). Abstinence-only education policies and programs: A position paper of the Society for Adolescent Medicine. *Journal of Adolescent Health, 38*, 83–87.

Santelli, J., Lindberg, L. D., Finer, L. B., & Singh, S. (2007). Explaining recent declines in adolescent pregnancy in the United States: The contribution of abstinence and improved contraceptive use. *American Journal of Public Health, 97*(1), 150–156.

Shew, M. L., Hellerstedt, W. L., Sieving, R. E., Smith, A. E., & Fee, R. M. (2000). Prevalence of home pregnancy testing among adolescents. *American Journal of Public Health, 90*, 9746.

Sieving, R. E., McMorris, B. J., Beckman, K. J., Pettingell, S. L., Secor-Turner, M., Kugler, K., et al. (2011). Prime time: 12-month sexual health outcomes of a clinic-based intervention to prevent pregnancy risk behaviors. *Journal of Adolescent Health, 49*(2), 172–179.

Stevens-Simon, C., Kelly, L., & Kulick, R. (2001). A village would be nice but…it takes a long-acting contraceptive to prevent repeat adolescent pregnancies. *American Journal of Preventive Medicine, 21*, 60–65.

The National Campaign on Teen and Unplanned Pregnancy. (2011). *National cost of teen childbearing.* Retrieved August 20, 2011, from http://www.thenationalcampaign.org/costs/default.aspx.

Trent, M., Millstein, S. G., & Ellen, J. E. (2006). Gender-based differences in fertility beliefs and knowledge among adolescents from high sexually transmitted disease-prevalence communities. *Journal of Adolescent Health, 38*, 282–287.

Ventura, S. J., & Hamilton, B. E. (2011). *U.S. teenage birth rate resumes decline. NCHS data brief, no 58.* Hyattsville, MD: National Center for Health Statistics.

Weinberger, D. R., Elvegag, B., & Giedd, J. N., (2005). The adolescent brain: A work in progress. The National Campaign to Prevent Teen Pregnancy. http://www.thenationalcampaign.org/resources/pdf/BRAIN.pdf.

White, E., Rosengard, C., Weitzen, S., Meers, A., & Phipps, M. (2006). Fear of inability to conceive in pregnant adolescents. *Obstetrics and Gynecology, 108*, 1411–1416.

Wimberly, Y. H., Kahn, J. A., Kollar, L. M., & Slap, G. B. (2003). Adolescent beliefs about infertility. *Contraception*, Vol. 68(5), pp. 385–391.

World Health Organization. (October 2008). Adolescent pregnancy. *MPS Notes*, Geneva, Switzerland. http://www.who.int/maternal_child_adolescent/documents/mpsnnotes_2_lr.pdf.

Yen, S., Saah, T., & Hillard, P. J. A. (2010). IUDs and adolescents—An under-utilized opportunity for pregnancy prevention. *Journal of Pediatric and Adolescent Gynecology, 23*(3), 123–128.

Zabin, L. S., Emerson, M. R., Ringers, P. A., & Sedivy, V. (1996). Adolescents with negative pregnancy test results: An accessible at- risk group. *JAMA, 275*(2), 113–117.

Zabin, L. S., Sedivy, V., & Emerson, M. R. (1994). Subsequent risk of childbearing among adolescents with a negative pregnancy test. *Family Planning Perspectives, 26*(5), 212–217.

Sexually Transmitted Infections (STIs) and the Developing Adolescent: Influences of and Strategies to Reduce STI Acquisition

Beth A. Auslander, Marina Catallozzi, and Susan L. Rosenthal

Sexually transmitted infections (STIs) among adolescents continue to be a major public health concern. Among the estimated 19 million STI cases reported each year, approximately half of the cases were among adolescents. This is particularly concerning when considering that only 25 % of the sexually experienced population is adolescents (Weinstock, Berman, & Cates, 2004). Racial/ethnic and gender disparities exist with higher rates of STIs being noted among minority youth compared to white youth and females compared to males (Centers for Disease Control and Prevention, 2010b). In 2009, the highest rates of chlamydia (3,329.3 cases per 100,000 females) and gonorrhea (568.8 per 100,000 females) were seen among 15–19-year-old females (Centers for Disease Control and Prevention, 2010b).

Given these rates, we begin with a brief overview of STIs, and then discuss factors that influence adolescents' risk of acquisition and strategies designed to prevent STI transmission and acquisition among adolescents.

Overview of STIs

Common STIs in adolescents are trichomonas, chlamydia, gonorrhea, human papillomavirus (HPV), and herpes simplex virus (HSV). Additional STIs which adolescents may experience include syphilis and pubic lice. Human immunodeficiency virus (HIV) may be transmitted sexually, as well as other infections including bacterial vaginosis and hepatitis B. STIs that are reported to the Centers for Disease Control include chlamydia, gonorrhea, and syphilis.

STIs are frequently asymptomatic or unrecognizable to the individual. When there are symptoms, there is overlap in symptoms across STIs, but certain symptoms are associated with particular STIs. Below, we describe examples of typical symptoms associated with some of the common STIS; however, it is important to remember that STIs can present in a variety of ways and that it is also best to confirm the diagnosis with laboratory testing. For example, chlamydia, gonorrhea, and trichomonas infection can be associated with

B.A. Auslander, Ph.D. (✉)
Division of Adolescent and Behavioral Health, Department of Pediatrics and Sealy Center for Vaccine Development, University of Texas Medical Branch, 301 University Boulevard, Galveston, TX 77555-0319, USA
e-mail: baauslan@utmb.edu

M. Catallozzi, M.D.
Department of Pediatrics & Population and Family Health, Columbia University Medical Center-College of Physicians and Surgeons, New York, NY, USA

S.L. Rosenthal, Ph.D., A.B.P.P.
Department of Pediatrics, Columbia University Medical Center-College of Physicians & Surgeons, New York, NY, USA

W.T. O'Donohue et al. (eds.), *Handbook of Adolescent Health Psychology*,
DOI 10.1007/978-1-4614-6633-8_36, © Springer Science+Business Media New York 2013

discharge from the penis or vagina, burning sensation during urination, and vaginal bleeding (Centers for Disease Control and Prevention, 2011a, 2011c, 2011f). Chlamydia and gonorrhea infections can be associated with pelvic inflammatory disease or prostatitis, which can cause severe abdominal pain, rectal pain, and even fever (Centers for Disease Control and Prevention, 2011a, 2011c). For women, long-term consequences of untreated or pelvic inflammatory disease and/or tubo-ovarian abscesses can lead to scarring and infertility later in life (Centers for Disease Control and Prevention, 2011a, 2011c). Neonatal exposure to chlamydia can result in neonatal conjunctivitis or pneumonia (Centers for Disease Control and Prevention, 2011a). In the short term, syphilis can cause genital lesions and rash. In the long term, untreated and unrecognized syphilis can lead to serious cardiovascular and neurologic problems (Centers for Disease Control and Prevention, 2011e). HSV can either be symptomatic or cause painful genital lesions and pain on urination. Neonatal infection with HSV can result in severe complications, and even death (Centers for Disease Control and Prevention, 2011d). Depending on the HPV strain causing infection, HPV can cause genital warts or cervical or penile changes leading to cancer (Centers for Disease Control and Prevention, 2011a, 2011b, 2011c). Regardless of whether the individual experiences symptoms or recognizes symptoms, infections can be transmitted to another partner who may or may not experience symptoms and significant consequences (Leone, 2005). Another biological consequence of STIs is that having an STI increases the risk of HIV transmission and acquisition (Fleming & Wasserheit, 1999; Gupta, Warren, & Wald, 2007).

Psychosocial Impact

Individuals can experience a variety of psychological sequelae to an STI diagnosis. For instance, 28 % of adolescent females and 31 % of adolescents diagnosed with an STI subsequently reported high levels of depressive symptoms (Shrier, Harris, & Beardslee, 2002). High levels of shame (i.e., blaming oneself for failing to live up to certain societal expectations; Corrigan & Penn, 1999; Tangney, 1996) have also been reported by some adolescents in relation to possible diagnosis or diagnosis of an STI (Cunningham, Kerrigan, Jennings, & Ellen, 2009; Sales et al., 2007). Adult research indicates that about 32 % of individuals diagnosed with herpes experience moderate to severe anxiety at the time of diagnosis (Bickford, Barton, & Madalia, 2007). Unfortunately, it is not uncommon for a person to be concerned about stigma or fear of being rejected from others because of his/her STI diagnosis (Fortenberry, 2004; Scrambler & Hopkins, 1986).

A person's response to an STI can be moderated by both physical aspects associated with an STI and psychosocial factors. For example, severity and frequency of reoccurrences of genital herpes have been found to influence an individual's quality of life (Patel et al., 2001). Psychosocial factors influencing response to an STI include social support and coping mechanisms. For example, adolescents/young adults who perceived more social support from religious/spiritual figures reported more positive psychological adjustment to genital herpes than individuals who perceived less support (Barnack-Tavlaris, Reddy, & Ports, 2011). Further, use of more effective coping mechanisms, problem solving and acceptance coping, is associated with positive psychological adjustment to STIs among both adolescents and young adults (Barnack-Tavlaris et al., 2011; Manne & Sandler, 1984) while use of ineffective coping techniques, including wishful thinking and self-blame, was associated with poor psychological adjustment (Manne & Sandler, 1984).

Detection of STIs and Care-Seeking Behavior

Annual routine screening for chlamydia and gonorrhea in any sexually experienced adolescent female is recommended and can be done through urine testing. Currently there are no recommendations for screening males. HIV screening through serological testing or oral mucosa is recommended for both sexually active males and females, and is typically done based on the background prevalence in the local community. HPV screening is done through pap smears and is recommended for girls after age 21. HSV is not typically part of screening, but can be detected by serological testing (Centers for Disease Control and Prevention, 2010c). It is important to note that many adolescents incorrectly believe that they have been screened for HSV when having been "checked for STIs." Symptomatic testing is available for all STIs and should be done, although sometimes in low-resource settings, syndromic or presumptive treatment occurs (i.e., treatment based on the presentation of typical symptoms and a consistent history; World Health Organization, 1991). There are medications or treatments available for STIs that can treat the infection, reduce the likelihood of transmission, manage or treat the symptoms, and/or minimize the sequelae (Centers for Disease Control and Prevention, 2010c). This underscores the importance of adolescents to have adequate access to sexual and reproductive health care. Yet despite the availability of screening and treatment and its importance, studies indicate that 39–44 % of adolescents report not seeking treatment for an STI until 7 or more days after recognizing symptoms (Fortenberry, 1997; Meyer-Weitz, Reddy, Van Den Borne, Kok, & Pietersen, 2000). Multiple factors are associated with delays in STI care seeking. Among adolescents, perceived stigma related to STIs (Cunningham, Tschann, Gurvey, Fortenberry, & Ellen, 2002) has been found to be associated with delayed care seeking while belief in the effectiveness of treatment and social support from peers for STI care is associated with early care seeking (Godin et al., 1993). Perceiving that an STI is serious is helpful in motivating an adolescent for care seeking to a point. However, if the adolescent views the STI as too serious, he/she may become fearful and be less likely to seek care (Cunningham, Kerrigan, Pillay, & Ellen, 2005). For a detailed review of the screening and treatment of STIs, the reader is referred to the Sexually Transmitted Diseases Treatment Guidelines (Centers for Disease Control and Prevention, 2010c).

Contextual Factors Influencing Adolescents' Risk of STI Exposure/Acquisition

Behavioral factors that place both male and female adolescents at increased risk for being exposed to an STI include (1) sexual risk behaviors and (2) exposure from infected partners. In addition, the immature gynecological tract of a young adolescent female may place her at further biological vulnerability.

Sexual Risk Behaviors

Sexual risk behaviors that have consistently been found to be associated with higher STI rates include initiating sex at an early age (Kaestle, Halpern, Miller, & Ford, 2005; Kahn, Rosenthal, Succop, Ho, & Burk, 2002), having multiple partners (Fatusi & Wang, 2009; Woodhead, Chung, & Joffe, 2009), and not using condoms (Warner, Stone, Macaluso, Buehler, & Austin, 2006). Concerning are reports from a 2009 national survey (Centers for Disease Control and Prevention, 2010d) which indicated that approximately 6 % of adolescents reported having sex before the age of 13 years, 14 % reported having four or more sexual partners, and 39 % of sexually active adolescents reported not using a condom at last intercourse. These percentages are even higher among minority youth which may partly explain their higher rates of STIs compared to whites (Centers for Disease Control and Prevention, 2010d).

The likelihood that an adolescent will engage in these risk behaviors is related to the timing of their physical maturity, their underlying psychological health, and their sociocultural context. It is important to keep in mind that these factors do not act independently but rather interact in a complex manner to influence adolescent sexual behavior.

Physical maturity takes place as a result of pubertal/hormonal changes and brain structural changes that occur during adolescence. The hormonal changes are associated with physical changes, including body size and secondary characteristics, and sexual motivation (Buck Louis et al., 2008; Wallen & Zehr, 2004). The brain structural changes which recently have been thought to be connected to the hormonal changes (Blakemore, Burnett, & Dahl, 2010; Sisk & Foster, 2004) have been linked with cognitive and affective changes (Steinberg, 2004, 2010a). Interestingly the parts of the brain that are associated with reward sensitivity, preference for immediate rewards, and sensation seeking have been shown to develop much faster (Wahlstrom, Collins, White, & Luciana, 2010) than the parts of the brain believed to be responsible for self-regulation and impulse control (Gogtay & Thompson, 2010; Schmithorst & Yuan, 2010). This temporal disconnect places the individual vulnerable to engaging in risk-taking behavior, including sexual risk-taking behavior (Steinberg, 2010b).

When pubertal timing/developmental changes occur early, the adolescent has a greater likelihood of engaging in sexual risk taking. That is, for both males and females, early maturity is linked with early sexual initiation (Copeland et al., 2010; Downing & Bellis, 2009) and frequency of sexual behavior (Michaud, Suris, & Deppen, 2006). Researchers have hypothesized that early bodily changes can have a negative effect on the adolescent self-image, making the adolescent more self-conscious of their bodies and thus more prone to engaging in sexually risk behaviors. Another proposed explanation for the relationship between early pubertal timing and sexual risk behavior is that the adolescent experiences pressure from peers and adults to act older than he/she truly is or engage in behaviors (i.e., sexual behavior) for which they are not ready (Michaud et al., 2006).

Psychological comorbidities, such as depression, anxiety, and conduct problems, also influence sexual risk behavior which in turn increases STI exposure. Both internalizing (e.g., depression) (Brown et al., 2010; Rubin, Gold, & Primack, 2009; Seth, Raiji, DiClemente, Wingood, & Rose, 2009; Wilson, Asbridge, Kisely, & Langille, 2010) and externalizing behaviors (e.g., antisocial behaviors, substance use, manic behaviors); (Brown et al., 2010; Cavazos-Rehg et al., 2011; Schofield, Bierman, Heinrichs, Nix, & Conduct Problems Prevention Research Group, 2008) have been found to predict sexual risk taking and STIs among adolescents. However, when considering both internalizing and externalizing problems in a model to predict sexual initiation, only externalizing problems remained significant (McLeod & Knight, 2010). In sum, it appears that psychopathology characterized by a lack of self-control is the type of psychopathology most associated with sexual risk behaviors.

Sociocultural context (i.e., parents, peers, community/society, partners) is another important determinant of adolescent sexual risk behavior. Parents can provide a protective effect on adolescent sexual risk taking through their parenting style and their communication with the adolescent about sexuality. An authoritative parenting style (i.e., sets firm limits but yet is warm and nurturing) and/or parent communication are associated with delayed age of sexual initiation, greater condom use, fewer partners among adolescents (DiClemente et al., 2001; Feldman & Brown, 1993; Gillmore, Chen, Haas, Kopak, & Robillard, 2011; Hadley et al., 2008; Lammers, Ireland, Resnick, & Blum, 2000; Luster & Small, 1994; Parkes, Henderson, Wight, & Nixon, 2011; Wight, Williamson, & Henderson, 2006), and lower likelihood of acquiring STIs (Bettinger et al., 2004; Crosby, DiCllemente, Wingood, Lang, & Harrington, 2003; Ford et al., 2005).

Peers, race/ethnicity, communities, and the media may influence adolescents by establishing the social norms for sexual behavior (Boyer et al., 2000; Brown, Halpern, & L'Engle, 2005; Wilson & Kelling, 1982). Having friends who engage in sexually risky behaviors (Boyer et al., 2000), living in high-risk neighborhoods (Cubbin, Brindis, Jain, Santelli, & Braveman, 2010; Lang et al., 2010), being of minority race (Centers for Disease Control and Prevention, 2010d), and viewing sexual media material (Collins et al., 2004; L'Engle, Brown, & Kenneavy, 2006) are associated with increased likelihood of engaging in sexual risk-taking behaviors (e.g., having had sex, engaging in frequent sex, having casual partners, not using condoms/contraception). On a positive note, parents can help buffer these effects through parent responsiveness in parent–adolescent sex discussions (Fasula & Miller, 2006).

Adolescent partner characteristics as well as relationship characteristics have been shown to be related to sexual risk-taking behavior, thereby increasing their risk for STIs. For example, adolescents who have older partners are more likely to engage in sex at an early age (Pettifor, O'Brien, Macphail, Miller, & Ress, 2009) and to not use condoms than adolescents with similar-age partners (Ford, Sohn, & Lepkowski, 2001). It could be that when adolescents have older partners, the power in the relationship is not equally distributed, thereby limiting the younger adolescent from negotiating abstinence and condom use (Ford et al., 2001). In terms of the relationship context, adolescents who have been in relationships longer have been shown to use condoms more inconsistently (Brady, Tschann, Ellen, & Flores, 2009; Ellen, Cahn, Eyre, & Boyer, 1996) than adolescents in relationship of shorter duration. Interestingly, both positive qualities of the adolescent relationship, such as trust and feelings of love, intimacy, and enmeshment within the relationship (Brady et al., 2009; Foulkes, Pettigrew, Livingston, & Niccolai, 2009; Manning, Flanigan, Giordano, & Longmore, 2009), and negative qualities, such as relationship conflict and mistrust, have been associated with less consistent condom use (Manning et al., 2009).

Exposure to STIs

There is no perfect association between engaging in sexual risk behaviors and acquiring an STI, since one has to have sex with an infected partner for acquisition to occur. The risk of being exposed to an infected partner is partly determined by the adolescent's social network. That is, in social networks where the STI rates are high, e.g., black youth (Forhan et al., 2009), incarcerated youth (Joesoef, Kahn, & Weinstock, 2006), and homeless youth (Haley et al., 2002; Tyler, Whitbeck, Chen, & Johnson, 2007), the risk of exposure to an infected partner is high. Consequently, an individual in a high-STI-prevalence social network does not have to engage in much sexual risk taking to acquire an STI. For example, one study found that among African-American college women, the risk of acquiring HSV-2 was substantial even among those who reported having only one partner during their lifetime (Lewis, Bernstein, Rosenthal, & Stanberry, 1999). Having sex with a partner outside of one's social network (i.e., sexual mixing) has also been thought to increase STI risk in some cases, particularly when the selected partner is from a high-STI-prevalence social network (Aral et al., 1999; Begley, Corsby, Diclemengte, Wingood, & Rose, 2003; Ford & Lepkowski, 2004). Adolescents also may be exposed to infected partners when their partners delay seeking care as research with adults suggests that symptomatic individuals report continuing to have sex while waiting for treatment (Mercer et al., 2007). In addition, adolescents can be reinfected by partners who are not notified of possible infection and provided the necessary treatment. In a recent study, 74 % of the adolescent women treated for an STI at baseline experienced 1 or more repeat infections. Analysis of these infections indicated that most of those (84 %) were likely due to reinfections from partners as opposed to treatment failures (Batteiger et al., 2010).

Strategies to Reduce Adolescent STI Exposure/Acquisition

Reducing the STI epidemic among adolescents requires routine screening and partner notification, interventions to delay sexual initiation and promote condom use in those choosing to have intercourse, and uptake of other biomedical strategies, including vaccines and microbicides.

Routine Screening and Partner Notification

Given that STIs are often asymptomatic, routine screening is a critical component of strategies to reduce the spread. Though STI screening among adolescents has risen since 2000 (Centers for

Disease Control and Prevention, 2009), the current STI screening rates are still well below what is recommended. For instance, chlamydia screening rates ranged from 26 to 42 % in women aged 15–25 years (Centers for Disease Control and Prevention, 2009; Wiehe, Rosenman, Wang, & Fortenberry, 2010). Disparities in STI testing exist. For example, in a sample of 14–25-year-old women, 14- and 15-year-olds were the least likely of all the ages to be tested. Also, white women compared to minority women, and women with private insurance versus public insurance/self-pay, were less likely to have been tested for chlamydia. The disparities in testing were thought to reflect physician stereotyping as opposed to purposeful physician risk evaluation (Wiehe et al., 2010).

Adolescents report barriers to routine STI screening including difficulties accessing and negotiating the health care system, limited information about STI testing, negative reactions and interactions with providers, concerns about confidentiality, and stigmatizing social norms associated with getting STI testing (Balfe, Brugha, DO'Donovan, O'Connell, & Vaughan, 2010; Goldenberg, Shoveller, Koehoorn, & Ostry, 2008). Providers note that lack of time, lack of training on sexual history taking, limited knowledge regarding screening guidelines and STI prevalence rates, and lack of clinic reminders for testing prevent them from offering STI testing (Cook et al., 2001; Hocking, Parker, Pavlin, Fairley, & Gunn, 2008). On a positive note, interventions aimed at reducing some of these barriers (e.g., by providing physician training on sexual history taking, increasing physician knowledge about STI risk among sexually active adolescents) have been found to increase STI screening rates (Ginige, Fairley, Hocking, Bowden, & Chen, 2007). Thus more efforts should be made to implement and further design programs to increase STI screening.

Another strategy to reduce infection rates is partner notification, which has been shown to be successful in getting partners treated. For example, in one study, 66 % of the adolescents informed their partners, and 82 % of the notified male partners received treatment (James, Hughes, Ahmed-Jushuf, & Slack, 1999). Partner notification can be done by the adolescent alone, the adolescent with assistance from a health professional, and the provider alone (Mathews & Coetzee, 2007). However, not all partners of adolescents get notified. Individual and relationship factors have been shown to influence partner notification. For instance, having greater self-efficacy in notifying a partner and being in a higher quality relationship have been shown to predict greater likelihood of notifying a partner (Fortenberry, Brizendine, Katz, & Orr, 2002). These results suggests that adolescents may require special skills training for notifying partners and perhaps extra assistance notifying partners in lower quality relationships.

To further increase likelihood of partners being treated, expedited partner therapy (EPT) has been implemented in some areas. EPT is a strategy wherein the partners of the infected person presenting for treatment are provided STI treatment without medical evaluation. The most frequent method for delivering medication is through the infected partner. However, health care personnel have also delivered the medication directly to partners of infected individuals. A review of clinical trials with adolescents infected with chlamydia and/or gonorrhea found that partner-delivered partner therapy (PDPT) led to significantly reduced or trends of reduced infection rates of the original partner presenting for treatment compared to partner notification alone (Hogben & Burstein, 2006).

Despite this effectiveness and the acceptability of this approach to patients, this option remains underutilized. Barriers to this approach include provider or physician concerns regarding the legality of dispensing medication to individuals without medical evaluation, providing treatment to minors without parental consent despite the fact that minors are able to consent for STI-related care, confidentiality issues related to mandated reporting of sexual activity of minors related to billing, costs of providing medication, and documentation of medication dispensing (Hogben & Burstein, 2006).

Delaying Sexual Activity and Condom Use Among Adolescents

In effort to reduce adolescents' engagement in sexually risky behaviors, comprehensive sex education programs have been developed. In these programs, adolescents are encouraged to delay sexual activity until an older age and to use condoms in the event that they engage in sexual behavior. The most effective programs address social influences, are grounded within social learning theory (Kirby, 1992), and have three components: information about STIs, motivational training, and behavior skills for negotiation of abstinence and condoms (Johnson, Scott-Sheldon, Huedo-Medina, & Carey, 2011). These programs tend to be in community or school settings. The material and content are usually provided in group settings over multiple sessions for a median number of 10.5 h (Underhill, Operario, & Montgomery, 2007b). Evaluations of comprehensive education programs indicate that they are successful at delaying sexual initiation, increasing condom use, and reducing unprotected intercourse. At the same time, they have not been found to increase sexual behavior as critics have suggested (Kirby, Laris, & Rolleri, 2007; Underhill et al., 2007b). Further, the results from one program indicated that incorporation of a parental monitoring intervention enhanced the effects (Stanton et al., 2004).

A few brief one-session programs have been designed for primary care settings (Boekeloo et al., 1999; Jemmott, Jemmott III, & O'Leary, 2007). In "Sister to Sister! Respect Yourself! Protect Yourself! Because You are Worth It!," African-American adolescent girls were administered a 20-min cognitive-behavioral skill-building intervention by a nurse in the clinic. The single session focused on increasing condom use skills. Participants read about condom use, viewed a video demonstrating proper way to use a condom, practiced applying a condom to an anatomical model, and role-played ways to negotiate condom use with their partner. The results indicated that participating in this brief skill-based intervention increased condom use up to 12 months later and reduced rate of STI acquisition at 12 months (Jemmott et al., 2007).

In contrast to comprehensive sex education programs, abstinence-only programs which teach that abstinence until marriage is the only method to be used by adolescents have not been shown to be effective at reducing adolescents' sexual risk behaviors (Trenholm et al., 2007; Underhill, Operario, & Montgomery, 2007a) and in fact have been criticized for their medical inaccuracies. While abstaining from sex certainly reduces one's exposure to STIs, the actual failure rate of practicing abstinence until marriage is high among adolescents with 88 % of adolescents reporting having sex before marriage (Fortenberry, 2005).

Vaccines

Vaccines are currently available for the prevention of hepatitis B and the human papilloma virus and vaccines for other STIs are in development (Food and Drug Administration; Mast et al., 2005; Stanberry et al., 2002). However, much of the marketing of the hepatitis B vaccine failed to acknowledge that it was sexually transmitted as it is currently given as a routine infant vaccine (Mast et al., 2005). There are two HPV vaccines, a bivalent one which protects against HPV 16 and 18 (HPV2), (Food and Drug Administration, 2009) and a quadrivalent (HPV4) one that also protects against types 6 and 11. (Food and Drug Administration, 2006) HPV 16 and 18 are two of the most common types causing cervical cancer (Tota et al., 2011) and HPV 6 and 11 cause genital warts (Lacey et al., 2006). The current Advisory Committee on Immunization Practices (ACIP; Centers for Disease Control and Prevention, 2010a) recommendation for the HPV vaccination is for it to be routinely administered for males and females aged 11–12 and catch up vaccination for those aged 13–26 years (Centers for Disease Control and Prevention, 2007, 2011g). According to the 2009 National Immunization Survey, 44 % of adolescent females aged 13–17 years have had one or more doses of the HPV vaccine and only 26.7 % have had all three doses (Centers for Disease Control and Prevention, 2010a). These numbers suggest that despite the effectiveness of these vaccines and the recommendations, many adolescent females still remain unvaccinated or under-vaccinated.

There are many reasons for the current rates of HPV vaccine uptake. First, we do not have high rates of vaccine uptake for non-mandated vaccines, and many parents continue to have concerns about side effects despite the clear evidence of its safety. Second, particularly at the initial availability of the vaccine, there was limited knowledge by both parents and providers regarding HPV (Bendik, Mayo, & Parker, 2011; Esposito et al., 2007; Slonim et al., 2005; Zimet, Shew, & Kahn, 2008). Less provider knowledge of HPV is associated with less provider intent to recommend the vaccine (Riedesel et al., 2005) and less adolescent knowledge is associated with less intent to get the vaccine (Jones & Cook, 2008) as well as less likelihood of adolescents having received the vaccine (Bendik et al., 2011; Read, Joseph, Polishchuk, & Suss, 2010). Providers and parents consistently have been shown to prefer vaccinating mid-adolescents (those 14–16 years) as opposed to the recommended age of 11–12 years (Kahn et al., 2005; Kahn et al., 2007; Raley, Followwill, Zimet, & Ault, 2004; Riedesel et al., 2005). In general, factors associated with increased parents' and/or adolescents' acceptance of the vaccine are perceived greater susceptibility (Forster, Marlow, Wardle, Stephenson, & Waller, 2010); perceived risk (Dempsey, Ziment, Davis, & Koutsky, 2006; Olshen, Woods, Austin, Luskin, & Bauchner, 2005; Woodhall et al., 2007); perceived seriousness of the STI/HPV like cervical cancer (Allen et al., 2009; Bendik et al., 2011; Constantine & Jerman, 2007; Zimet et al., 2005); belief that the vaccine is effective at preventing an STI, like HPV (Davis, Dickman, Ferris, & Dias, 2004; Ogilvie et al., 2010); perception of fewer barriers to getting the vaccine (e.g., cost; Reiter, McRee, Gottlieb, & Brewer, 2010); and perception of support for the vaccine (e.g., physicians, parents; Allen et al., 2009; Bendik et al., 2011; Guerry et al., 2011). Although mode of transmission is not a factor in the decision-making for most parents, parents who oppose STI vaccination may describe concerns about the potential for adolescent sexual disinhibition (Zimet et al., 2008).

For those adolescents who are unvaccinated (i.e., cases wherein parents refused the vaccine) interventions need to focus on changing attitudes (Davis et al., 2004; Dempsey et al., 2006). Recent research suggests that persuasive theory-based interventions targeted at certain health beliefs (e.g., perceived susceptibility) could serve to be an effective and easily implemented method to promote uptake (Cox, Cox, Sturm, & Zimet, 2010). For those that are under-vaccinated, that is, adolescents who failed to complete the three dose series, the focus may need to be on structural interventions such as reminder/recall programs. One novel approach that has been successful is the use of text messaging (Kharbanda et al., 2011).

Microbicides

Scientists have been working on developing products, called microbicides, that could be inserted into the vagina or rectum to prevent STIs/HIV and possibly pregnancy. Though more clinical trials of microbicides have been conducted with gels, other dosage forms include vaginal tablets and films are in development (Garg et al., 2010). These products would be female initiated and hence are thought to potentially give women more control over STI/HIV protection than the male condom which requires negotiation with the male partner (Cutler & Justman, 2008).

A report from AVAC: Global Advocacy for HIV Prevention dated May 2011 indicated that there are 15 ongoing microbicide clinical trials (AVAC: Global Advocacy for HIV Prevention, 2011; Cutler & Justman, 2008). To date, only one product (tenofovir, a reverse transcriptase inhibitor) has been shown to be safe and effective in preventing HIV and HSV-2. However, the effectiveness was directly related to consistency of use; those women who used the gel during 80 % of their sexual acts reduced their risk by 54 %, whereas those who used the gel in less than 50 % of the sexual acts only reduced their risk of HIV acquisition by 28 % (Abdool Karim et al., 2010). This trial included women aged 18–40 and thus it is not known whether these results would generalize to younger adolescents. A study is planned to assess the safety of the tenofovir gel among younger adolescents (AVAC: Global Advocacy for HIV Prevention, 2011).

As noted, by the tenofovir trial results, using a microbicide consistently will be critical for effectiveness. Thus, a few studies have been conducted with hypothetical products and microbicide surrogates (e.g., vaginal products without the active ingredient of a microbicide) to examine acceptability among adolescents. This research suggests that adolescents may prefer a gel over a suppository (Zubowicz et al., 2006). Physical characteristics, such as messiness of the product, leakage, and clumping, have been reported as concerns of female adolescents. In contrast, the lubricating quality of microbicide surrogates has been viewed in a positive manner by adolescent girls, most likely because of its effect on sexual pleasure (Zubowicz et al., 2006). Female adolescents may also be most concerned about side effects and more interested in products that prevent problems (i.e., pregnancy or non-HIV STIs) for which they view themselves at high risk (Tanner et al., 2008).

Relationship context and partners could be influential in the acceptability of these products. Adolescents have been found to be more likely to use a microbicide surrogate in more established, mutual, and satisfying relationships that are monogamous (Short, Rosenthal, Auslander, & Succop, 2009). Communication with partners about using these products may be difficult for some adolescents; some have reported that they do not know how to initiate the conversation and/or how to handle their partners' reactions and questions regarding the product (Zubowicz et al., 2006). Adolescents also report that they may not talk with partners about using the product, because they believed an explanation was not needed within the relationship context and because they did not even think to communicate about the product (Short, Ramos, Oakes, & Rosenthal, 2007). Thus adolescents likely will require education about the product itself as well as education and skills training about how to communicate with partners about using these products.

Parental figures may be influential in the acceptance of these products. A recent study found that 50 % of the adolescent girls participating in a microbicide acceptability study spoke with their mothers about using the microbicide surrogate (Sunder, Ramos, Short, & Rosenthal, 2006). Further, adolescents who talked with their mothers about using these products were more likely to talk to their partners about microbicide use (Short et al., 2007). Thus, when microbicides become available to the public, parents could be in a position to promote the use of this new method and perhaps encourage adolescents to communicate with partners about microbicides.

Conclusions

STIs are prevalent among adolescents and can cause significant physical and psychological sequelae. Though screening and treatment are available, many adolescents may not be getting adequate routine reproductive and sexual health care, and may delay seeking care when faced with symptoms. Their increased risk for STIs is due to their developing bodies, sexual risk behaviors, and exposure to infected partners. Multiple strategies are needed to reduce the STI epidemic among adolescents, including routine screening, partner notification, comprehensive sex education, and new biomedical approaches, such as vaccines and microbicides. Challenges and barriers to the implementation of each of these STI prevention strategies exist and will need to be addressed in order for them to be effective. To conclude, STIs are a significant problem among adolescents with multiple factors influencing acquisition, thereby requiring a complex interplay of prevention strategies.

References

Abdool Karim, Q., Abdool Karim, S., Frohlich, J., Grobler, A., Baxter, C., Mansoor, L., et al. (2010). Effectiveness and safety of tenofovir gel, an antiretroviral microbicide, for the prevention of HIV infection in women. *Science, 329*, 1168–1174.

Allen, J. D., Mohllajee, A. P., Shelton, R. C., Othus, M. K. D., Fontenot, H. B., & Hanna, R. (2009). Stage of adoption of the human papillomavirus vaccine among college women. *Preventive Medicine, 48*, 420–425.

Aral, S. O., Hughes, J. P., Stoner, B. S., Whittington, W. L. H., Handsfield, H. H., Anderson, R. M., et al. (1999). Sexual mixing patterns in the spread of gonococcal and chlamydian infections. *American Journal of Public Health, 89*, 825–833.

AVAC: Global Advocacy for HIV Prevention. (2011, May). *Ongoing Trials of Topical Microbicide Candidates*. Retrieved from http://www.avac.org/ht/d/sp/i/3512/pid/3512.

Balfe, M., Brugha, R., DO'Donovan, D., O'Connell, E., & Vaughan, D. (2010). Young women's decisions to accept chlamydia screening: Influences of stigma and doctor-patient interactions. *BMC Public Health, 10*, 425.

Barnack-Tavlaris, J., Reddy, D., & Ports, K. (2011). Psychological adjustment among women living with genital herpes. *Journal of Health Psychology, 16*, 12–21.

Batteiger, B., Tu, W., Ofner, S., Van Der Pol, B., Stothard, D., Orr, D., et al. (2010). Repeated Chlamydia trachomatis genital infections in adolescent women. *Journal of Infectious Diseases, 201*, 42–51.

Begley, E., Crosby, R. A., Diclemente, D., Wingood, G. M., & Rose, E. (2003). Older partners and STD prevelance among pregnant African American teens. *Sexually Transmitted Diseases, 30*, 211–213.

Bendik, M. K., Mayo, R. M., & Parker, V. G. (2011). Knowledge, perceptions, and motivations related to HPV vaccination among college women. *Journal of Cancer Education, 26*, 459–464.

Bettinger, J. A., Celentano, D. D., Curriero, F. C., Adler, N. E., Millstein, S. G., & Ellen, J. M. (2004). Does parental involvement predict new sexually transmitted diseases in female adolescents? *Archives in Pediatric and Adolescent Medicine, 158*, 666–670.

Bickford, J., Barton, S. E., & Madalia, S. (2007). Chronic genital herpes and disclosure. The influence of stigma. *International Journal of STD and AIDS, 18*, 589–592.

Blakemore, S.-J., Burnett, S., & Dahl, R. E. (2010). The role of puberty in the developing adolescent brain. *Human Brain Mapping, 31*, 921–933.

Boekeloo, B. O., Schamus, L. A., Simmens, S. J., Cheng, T. L., O'Connor, K., & D'Angelo, L. J. (1999). A STD/HIV prevention trial among adolescents in managed care. *Pediatrics, 103*, 107–115.

Boyer, C. B., Shafer, M., Wibbelsman, C. J., Seeberg, D., Teitle, E., & Lovell, N. (2000). Associations of sociodemographic, psychosocial, and behavioral factors with sexual risk and sexually transmitted diseases in teen clinic patients. *Journal of Adolescent Health, 27*, 102–111.

Brady, S. S., Tschann, J. M., Ellen, J. M., & Flores, E. (2009). Infidelity, trust, and condom use among Latino youth in dating relationships. *Sexually Transmitted Diseases, 36*, 227–331.

Brown, L., Hadley, W., Stewart, A., Lescano, C., Whiteley, L., Donenberg, G., et al. (2010). Psychiatric disorders and sexual risk among adolescents in mental health treatment. *Journal of Consulting and Clinical Psychology, 78*, 590–597.

Brown, J., Halpern, C., & L'Engle, K. (2005). Mass media as a sexual super peer for early maturing girls. *Journal of Adolescent Health, 36*, 420–427.

Buck Louis, G. M., Gray, E., Marcus, M., Ojeda, S. R., Pescovitz, O. H., Witchel, S. F., et al. (2008). Environmental factors and puberty timing: Expert panel research needs. *Pediatrics, 121*, S192–S207.

Cavazos-Rehg, P., Krauss, M., Spitznagel, E., Schootman, M., Cottler, L., & Bierut, L. (2011). Substance use and the risk for sexual intercourse with and without a history of teenage pregnancy among adolescent females. *Journal of Studies on Alcohol and Drugs, 72*, 194–198.

Centers for Disease Control and Prevention. (2007). Quadrivalent human papillomavirus vaccine: Recommendations of the Advisory Committee on Immunization Practices (ACIP). *Morbidity and Mortality Weekly Report, 56*, 1–24.

Centers for Disease Control and Prevention. (2009). Chlamydia screening among sexually active young female enrollees of health plans—United States, 2000–2007. *Morbidity and Mortality Weekly Report, 58*, 362–365.

Centers for Disease Control and Prevention. (2010a). National, state, and local area vaccination coverage among adolescents aged 13–17 years—United States, 2009. *Morbidity and Mortality Weekly Report, 59*, 1018–1023.

Centers for Disease Control and Prevention. (2010b). *Sexually transmitted disease surveillance, 2009*. Atlanta, Georgia: National Center for HIV/AIDS, Viral Hepatitis, STD, and TB Prevention.

Centers for Disease Control and Prevention. (2010c). Sexually transmitted disease treatment guidelines, 2010. *Morbidity and Mortality Weekly Report, 59*, 1–110.

Centers for Disease Control and Prevention. (2010d). Youth risk behavior surveillance—United States. Surveillance summaries 2009. *Morbidity and Mortality Weekly Report, 59*, SS-5.

Centers for Disease Control and Prevention. (2011a). *Fact sheet for chlamydia*. Atlanta, Georgia.

Centers for Disease Control and Prevention. (2011b). *Fact sheet for genital herpes*. Atlanta, Georgia.

Centers for Disease Control and Prevention. (2011c). *Fact sheet for gonorrhea*. Atlanta.

Centers for Disease Control and Prevention. (2011d). *Fact sheet for herpes*. Atlanta, Georgia

Centers for Disease Control and Prevention. (2011e). *Fact sheet for syphilis*. Atlanta, Georgia

Centers for Disease Control and Prevention. (2011f). *Fact sheet for Trichomoniasis*. Atlanta, Georgia.

Centers for Disease Control anad Prevention. (2011g). Recommendations on the use of the quadrivalent human papilloma virus vaccine in males – Advisory Committee on Immunization Practices (ACIP), 2011. *Morbidity and Mortality Weekly Report, 60*, 1705–1708.

Collins, R. L., Elliott, M. N., Berry, S., Kanouse, D. E., Kunkel, D., Hunter, S. B., et al. (2004). Watching sex on television predicts adolescent initiation of sexual behavior. *Pediatrics, 114*, e280–e289.

Constantine, N. A., & Jerman, P. (2007). Acceptance of human papillomavirus vaccination among Californian parents of daughters: A representative statewide analysis. *Journal of Adolescent Health, 40*, 108–115.

Cook, R., Wiesenfeld, H., Ashton, M., Krohn, M., Zamborsky, T., & Scholle, S. (2001). Barriers to screening sexually active adolescent women for chlamydia: A survey of primary care physicians. *Journal of Adolescent Health, 28*, 204–210.

Copeland, W., Shanahan, L., Miller, S., Costello, E., Angold, A., & Maughan, B. (2010). Outcomes of early pubertal timing in young women: A prospective population-based study. *American Journal of Psychiatry, 167*, 1218–1225.

Corrigan, P. W., & Penn, D. L. (1999). Lessons from social psychology on discrediting psychiatric stigma. *American Psychologist, 54*, 765–766.

Cox, D. S., Cox, A. D., Sturm, L. A., & Zimet, G. D. (2010). Behavioral interventions to increase HPV vaccination acceptability among mothers of young girls. *Health Psychology, 29*, 29–39.

Crosby, R. A., DiCllemente, R. J., Wingood, G. M., Lang, D. L., & Harrington, K. (2003). Infrequent parental monitoring predicts sexually transmitted infections among low-income African American female adolescents. *Archives of Pediatrics and Adolescent Medicine, 157*, 169–173.

Cubbin, C., Brindis, C., Jain, S., Santelli, J., & Braveman, P. (2010). Neighborhood poverty, aspirations and expectations, and initiation of sex. *Journal of Adolescent Health, 47*, 399–406.

Cunningham, S., Kerrigan, D., Jennings, J., & Ellen, J. (2009). Relationships between perceived STD-related stigma, STD-related shame and STD screening among a household sample of adolescents. *Perspectives on Sexual and Reproductive Health, 41*, 225–230.

Cunningham, S. D., Kerrigan, D., Pillay, K. B., & Ellen, J. M. (2005). Understanding the role of perceived severity in STD-related care-seeking delays. *Journal of Adolescent Health, 37*, 69–74.

Cunningham, S., Tschann, J., Gurvey, J., Fortenberry, J., & Ellen, J. M. (2002). Attitudes about sexual disclosure and perceptions of stigma and shame. *Sexually Transmitted Infections, 78*, 334–338.

Cutler, B., & Justman, J. (2008). Vaginal microbicides and the prevention of HIV transmission. *Lancet Infection Diseases, 8*, 685–697.

Davis, K., Dickman, E. D., Ferris, D., & Dias, J. K. (2004). Human papillomavirus vaccine acceptability among parents of 10–15 year-old adolescents. *Journal of Lower Genital Tract Disease, 8*, 188–194.

Dempsey, A. F., Zimet, G. D., Davis, R. L., & Koutsky, L. A. (2006). Factors that are associated with parental acceptance of human papillomavirus vaccines: A randomized intervention study of written information about HPV. *Pediatrics, 117*, 1486–1493.

DiClemente, R. J., Wingood, G. M., Crosby, R., Cobb, B. K., Harrington, K., & Davies, S. L. (2001). Parent-adolescent communication and sexual risk behaviors among African American adolescent females. *Journal of Pediatrics, 139*, 407–412.

Downing, J., & Bellis, M. (2009). Early pubertal onset and its relationship with sexual risk taking, substance use, and anti-social behaviour: A preliminary cross-sectional study. *BMC Public Health, 9*, 446.

Ellen, J. M., Cahn, S., Eyre, S. L., & Boyer, C. B. (1996). Types of adolescent sexual relationships and associated perceptions about condom use. *Journal of Adolescent Health, 18*, 417–421.

Esposito, S., Bosis, S., Pelucchi, C., Begliatti, E., Rognoni, A., Bellasio, M., et al. (2007). Pediatrician knowledge and attitudes regarding human papillomavirus disease and its prevention. *Vaccine, 25*, 6437–6446.

Fasula, A., & Miller, K. (2006). African-American and Hispanic adolescents' intentions to delay first intercourse: Parental communication as a buffer for sexually active peers. *Journal of Adolescent Health, 38*, 193–200.

Fatusi, A., & Wang, W. (2009). Multiple sexual partnership mediates the association between early sexual debut and sexually transmitted infection among adolescent and young adult males in Nigeria. *European Journal of Contraception and Reproductive Health Care, 14*, 134–143.

Feldman, S. S., & Brown, N. (1993). Family influences on adolescent male sexuality: The mediation role of self-restraint. *Social Development, 2*, 15–35.

Fleming, D., & Wasserheit, J. (1999). From epidemiological synergy to public health policy and practice: The contribution of other sexually transmitted diseases to sexual transmission of HIV infection. *Sexually Transmitted Infections, 75*, 3–17.

Food and Drug Administration. (2006). Approval letter – Gardisil. Retrieved February 24, 2013. http://www.fda.gov/BiologicsBloodVaccines/Vaccines/ApprovedProducts/ucm111283.htm.

Food and Drug Administration. (2009). Approval Letter – Cervarix. Retrieved February 24, 2013. http://www.fda.gov/BiologicsBloodVaccines/Vaccines/ApprovedProducts/ucm186959.htm.

Ford, K., & Lepkowski, J. (2004). Characteristics of sexual partners and STD infection among American adolescents. *International Journal of STD and AIDS, 15*, 260–265.

Ford, C., Pence, B., Miller, W., Resnick, M., Bearinger, L., Pettingell, S., et al. (2005). Predicting adolescents' longitudinal risk for sexually transmitted infection: Results from the National Longitudinal Study of Adolescent Health. *Archives of Pediatric and Adolescent Medicine, 159*, 657–664.

Ford, K., Sohn, W., & Lepkowski, J. (2001). Characteristics of adolescents' sexual partners and their association with use of condoms and other contraceptive methods. *Family Planning Perspectives, 33*(100–105), 132.

Forhan, S., Gottlieb, S., Sternberg, M., Xu, F., Datta, S., McQuillan, G., et al. (2009). Prevalence of sexually transmitted infections among female adolescents aged 14 to 19 in the United States. *Pediatrics, 124*, 1505–1512.

Forster, A. S., Marlow, L. A. V., Wardle, J., Stephenson, J., & Waller, J. (2010). Understanding adolescents' intentions to have the HPV vaccine. *Vaccine, 28*, 1673–1676.

Fortenberry, J. D. (1997). Health care seeking behaviors related to sexually transmitted diseases among adolescents. *American Journal of Public Health, 87*, 417–420.

Fortenberry, J. D. (2004). The effects of stigma on genital herpes care-seeking behaviours. *Herpes, 11*, 8–11.

Fortenberry, D. (2005). The limits of abstinence-only in preventing sexually transmitted infections. *Journal of Adolescent Health, 36*, 269–270.

Fortenberry, J. D., Brizendine, E. J., Katz, B. P., & Orr, D. P. (2002). The role of self-efficacy and relationship quality in partner notification by adolescents with sexually transmitted infections. *Archives of Pediatrics and Adolescent Medicine, 156*, 1133–1137.

Foulkes, H. B. S., Pettigrew, M. M., Livingston, K. A., & Niccolai, L. M. (2009). Comparison of sexual partnership characteristics and associations with inconsistent condom use among a sample of adolescents and adult women diagnosed with chlamydia trachomatis. *Journal of Women's Health, 18*, 393–399.

Garg, S., Goldman, D., Krumme, M., Rohan, L. C., Smoot, S., & Friend, D. R. (2010). Advances in development, scale-up, and manufacturing of microbicide gels, films, and tablets. *Antiviral Research, 885*, 519–529.

Gillmore, M. R., Chen, A. C., Haas, S. A., Kopak, A. M., & Robillard, A. G. (2011). Do family and parent factors in adolescence influence condom use in early adulthood in a multiethnic sample of young adults? *Journal of Youth and Adolescence, 40*, 1503–1518.

Ginige, S., Fairley, C., Hocking, J., Bowden, F., & Chen, M. Y. (2007). Interventions for increasing chlamydia screening in primary care: A review. *BMC Public Health, 9*, 95.

Godin, G., Fortin, C., Mahnès, G., Boyer, R., Nadeau, D., Duval, B., et al. (1993). University students' intention to seek medical care promptly if symptoms of sexually transmitted diseases were suspected. *Sexually Transmitted Diseases, 20*, 100–104.

Gogtay, N., & Thompson, P. M. (2010). Mapping gray matter development: Implications for typical development and vulnerability to psychopathology. *Brain and Cognition, 72*, 6–15.

Goldenberg, S., Shoveller, J., Koehoorn, M., & Ostry, A. (2008). Barriers to STI testing among youth in a Canadian oil and gas community. *Health Place, 14*, 718–729.

Guerry, S., De Rosa, C., Markowitz, L., Walker, S., Liddon, N., Kerndt, P., et al. (2011). Human papillomavirus vaccine initiation among adolescent girls in high-risk communities. *Vaccine, 29*, 2235–2241.

Gupta, R., Warren, T., & Wald, A. (2007). Genital herpes. *Lancet, 370*, 2127–2137.

Hadley, W., Brown, L., Lescano, C., Kell, H., Spalding, K., Diclemente, R., et al. (2008). Parent-adolescent sexual communication: Associations of condom use with condom discussions. *AIDS Behavior, 13*, 997–1004.

Haley, N., Roy, E., Leclerc, P., Lambert, G., Boivin, J., Cédras, L., et al. (2002). Risk behaviours and prevalence of chlamydia trachomatis and neisseria gonorrhoeae genital infections among Montreal street youth. *International Journal of STD and AIDS., 13*, 238–245.

Hocking, J., Parker, R., Pavlin, N., Fairley, C., & Gunn, J. M. (2008). What needs to change to increase chlamydia screening in general practice in Australia? The views of general practitioners. *BMC Public Health, 8*, 425.

Hogben, M., & Burstein, G. (2006). Expedited partner therapy for adolescents diagnosed with gonorrhea or chlamydia: A review and commentary. *Adolescent Medicine Clinics, 17*, 687–695.

James, N., Hughes, S., Ahmed-Jushuf, I., & Slack, R. (1999). A collaborative approach to management of chlamydial infection among teenagers seeking contraceptive care in a community setting. *Sexually Transmitted Infections, 75*, 156–161.

Jemmott, L. S., Jemmott, J. B., III, & O'Leary, A. (2007). Effects on sexual risk behavior and STD rate of brief HIV/STD prevention interventions for African American women in primary care settings. *American Journal of Public Health, 97*, 1034–1040.

Joesoef, M., Kahn, R., & Weinstock, H. (2006). Sexually transmitted diseases in incarcerated adolescents. *Current Opinion in Infectious Disease, 19*, 44–48.

Johnson, B. T., Scott-Sheldon, L. A. J., Huedo-Medina, T. B., & Carey, M. P. (2011). Interventions to reduce sexual risk for human immunodeficiency virus in adolescents: A meta-analysis of trials, 1985-2008. *Archives of Pediatric and Adolescent Medicine, 165*, 77–84.

Jones, M., & Cook, R. L. (2008). Intent to receive an HPV vaccine among university men and women and implications for vaccine administration. *Journal of American College Health, 57*, 23–31.

Kaestle, C., Halpern, C., Miller, W., & Ford, C. (2005). Young age at first sexual intercourse and sexually transmitted infections in adolescents and young adults. *American Journal of Epidemiology, 161*, 774–780.

Kahn, J., Rosenthal, S., Succop, P., Ho, G., & Burk, R. (2002). The interval between menarche and age of first sexual intercourse as a risk factor for subsequent HPV infection in adolescent and young adult women. *Journal of Pediatrics, 141*, 718–723.

Kahn, J., Rosenthal, S., Tissot, A., Bernstein, D., Wetzel, C., & Zimet, G. (2007). Factors influencing pediatricians' intention to recommend human papillomavirus vaccines. *Ambulatory Pediatrics, 7*, 367–373.

Kahn, J., Zimet, G., Bernstein, D., Riedesel, J., Lan, D., Huang, B., et al. (2005). Pediatricians' intention to administer human papillomavirus vaccine: The role of practice characteristics, knowledge, and attitudes. *Journal of Adolescent Health, 37*, 502–510.

Kharbanda, E., Stockwell, M., Fox, H., Andres, R., Lara, M., & Rickert, V. (2011). Text message reminders to promote human papillomavirus vaccination. *Vaccine, 29*, 2537–2541.

Kirby, D. (1992). School-based programs to reduce sexual risk-taking behaviors. *Journal of School Health, 62*, 280–287.

Kirby, D., Laris, B. A., & Rolleri, L. A. (2007). Sex and HIV education programs: Their impact on sexual behavior of young people throughout the world. *Journal of Adolescent Health, 40*, 206–217.

Lacey, C. J., Lowndes, C. M., & Shah, K. V. (2006). Chapter 4: Burden and management of non-cancerous HPV-related conditions: HPV-6/11 disease. *Vaccine, 24*(Suppl 3), S3/35–41.

L'Engle, K. L., Brown, J. D., & Kenneavy, K. (2006). The mass media are an important context for adolescents' sexual behavior. *Journal of Adolescent Health, 38*, 186–192.

Lammers, C., Ireland, M., Resnick, M., & Blum, R. (2000). Influences on adolescents' decision to postpone onset of sexual intercourse: A survival analysis of virginity among youths aged 13 to 18 years. *Journal of Adolescent Health, 26*, 42–48.

Lang, D., Salazar, L., Crosby, R., DiClemente, R., Brown, L., & Donenberg, G. (2010). Neighborhood environment, sexual risk behaviors and acquisition of sexually transmitted infections among adolescents diagnosed with psychological disorders. *American Journal of Community Psychology, 46*, 303–311.

Leone, P. (2005). Reducing the risk of transmitting genital herpes: Advances in understanding and therapy. *Current Medical Research and Opinion, 21*, 1577–1582.

Lewis, L. M., Bernstein, D. I., Rosenthal, S. L., & Stanberry, L. R. (1999). Seroprevalence of herpes simplex virus type 2 in African-American college women. *Journal of the National Medical Association, 91*, 210–212.

Luster, T., & Small, S. A. (1994). Factors associated with sexual risk-taking behaviors among adolescents. *Journal of Marriage and the Family, 56*, 622–632.

Manne, S., & Sandler, I. (1984). Coping and adjustment to genital herpes. *Journal of Behavioral Medicine, 7*, 391–410.

Manning, W., Flanigan, C., Giordano, P., & Longmore, M. (2009). Relationship dynamics and consistency of condom use among adolescents. *Perspectives on Sexual and Reproductive Health, 41*, 181–190.

Mast, E., Weinbaum, C., Fiore, A., Alter, M., Bell, B., Finelli, L., et al. (2005). A comprehensive immunization strategy to eliminate transmission of hepatitis B virus infection in the United States: Recommendations of the Advisory Committee on Immunization Practices (ACIP) Part 1: Immunization of Infants, Children, and Adolescents. *Morbidity and Mortality Weekly Report, 54*(16), 1–23.

Mathews, C., & Coetzee, N. (2007). Partner notification. *Clinical Evidence* (*Online*), 1605.

McLeod, J. D., & Knight, S. (2010). The association of socioemotional problems with early sexual initiation. *Perspectives on Sexual and Reproductive Health, 42*, 93–101.

Mercer, C., Sutcliffe, L., Johnson, A., White, P., Brook, G., Ross, J., et al. (2007). How much do delayed healthcare seeking, delayed care provision, and diversion from primary care contribute to the transmission of STIs? *Sexually Transmitted Infections, 83*, 400–405.

Meyer-Weitz, A., Reddy, P., Van Den Borne, H., Kok, G., & Pietersen, J. (2000). The determinants of health care seeking behaviour of adolescents attending STD clinics in South Africa. *Journal of Adolescence, 23*, 741–752.

Michaud, P.-A., Suris, J.-C., & Deppen, A. (2006). Gender-related psychological and behavioral correlates of pubertal timing in a national sample of Swiss adolescents. *Molecular and Cellular Endocrinology, 254–255*, 172–178.

Ogilvie, G. S., Anderson, M., Marra, F., McNeil, S. A., Pielak, K., Dawar, M., et al. (2010). A population-based evaluation of a publicly funded, school-based HPV vaccine program in British Columbia, Canada: Parental factors associated with HPV vaccine receipt. *PLoS Medicine, 7*, e1000270.

Olshen, E., Woods, E. R., Austin, B., Luskin, M., & Bauchner, H. (2005). Parental acceptance of the human papillomavirus vaccine. *Journal of Adolescent Health, 37*, 248–251.

Parkes, A., Henderson, M., Wight, D., & Nixon, C. (2011). Is parenting associated with teenagers' early sexual risk-taking, sexual autonomy, and relationship with sexual partners. *Perspectives on Sexual and Reproductive Health, 43*, 30–40.

Patel, R., Boselli, F., Cairo, I., Barnett, G., Price, M., & Wulf, H. (2001). Patients' perspectives on the burden of recurrent genital herpes. *International Journal of STD and AIDS, 12*, 640–645.

Pettifor, A., O'Brien, K., Macphail, C., Miller, W., & Rees, H. (2009). Early coital debut and associated HIV risk factors among young women and men in South Africa. *International Perspectives on Sexual and Reproductive Health, 35*, 82–90.

Raley, J. C., Followwill, K. A., Zimet, G. D., & Ault, K. A. (2004). Gynecologists' attitudes regarding human papilloma virus vaccination: A survey of fellows of the American college of obstetricians and gynecologists. *Infecious Diseases in Obstetrics and Gynecology, 12*, 127–133.

Read, D. S., Joseph, M. A., Polishchuk, V., & Suss, A. L. (2010). Attitudes and perceptions of the HPV vaccine in Caribbean and African-American adolescent girls and their parents. *Journal of Pediatric and Adolescent Gynecology, 23*, 242–245.

Reiter, P. L., McRee, A.-L., Gottlieb, S. L., & Brewer, N. T. (2010). HPV vaccine for adolescent males: Acceptability to parents post-vaccine licensure. *Vaccine, 28*, 6292–6297.

Riedesel, J., Rosenthal, S., Zimet, G., Bernstein, D., Huang, B., Lan, D., et al. (2005). Attitudes about human papillomavirus vaccine among family physicians. *Journal of Pediatric and Adolescent Gynecology, 18*, 391–398.

Rubin, A., Gold, M., & Primack, B. (2009). Associations between depressive symptoms and sexual risk behavior in a diverse sample of female adolescents. *Journal of Pediatric and Adolescent Gynecology, 22*, 306–312.

Sales, J., DiClemente, R., Rose, E., Wingood, G., Klein, J., & Woods, E. (2007). Relationship of STD-related shame and stigma to female adolescents' condom-protected intercourse. *Journal of Adolescent Health, 40*, 573.e571–573.e576.

Schmithorst, V. J., & Yuan, W. (2010). White matter development during adolescence as shown by diffusion MRI. *Brain and Cognition, 72*, 16–25.

Schofield, H., Bierman, K., Heinrichs, B., Nix, R., & Conduct Problems Prevention Research Group. (2008). Predicting early sexual activity with behavior problems exhibited at school entry and in early adolescence. *Journal of Abnormal Child Psychology, 36*, 1175–1188.

Scrambler, G., & Hopkins, A. (1986). Being epileptic, coming to terms with stigma. *Sociology of Health and Illness, 8*, 26–43.

Seth, P., Raiji, P., DiClemente, R., Wingood, G., & Rose, E. (2009). Psychological distress as a correlate of a biologically confirmed STI, risky sexual practices, self-efficacy and communication with male sex partners in African-American female adolescents. *Psychology, Health, and Medicine, 14*, 291–300.

Short, M., Ramos, S., Oakes, J., & Rosenthal, S. (2007). Adolescent girls' communication with partners about microbicide use. *Sexual Health, 4*, 243–248.

Short, M., Rosenthal, S., Auslander, B., & Succop, P. (2009). Relationship context associated with microbicide-like product use. *Journal of Pediatric and Adolescent Gynecology, 22*, 313–317.

Shrier, L. A., Harris, S. K., & Beardslee, W. R. (2002). Temporal associations between depressive symptoms and self-reported sexually transmitted disease among adolescents. *Archives in Pediatric and Adolescent Medicine, 156*, 599–606.

Sisk, C., & Foster, D. (2004). The neural basis of puberty and adolescence. *Nature and Neuroscience, 7*, 1040–1047.

Slonim, A., Roberto, A., Downing, C., Adams, I., Fasano, N., Davis-Satterla, L., et al. (2005). Adolescents' knowledge, beliefs, and behaviors regarding hepatitis B: Insights and implications for programs targeting vaccine-preventable diseases. *Journal of Adolescent Health, 36*, 178–186.

Stanberry, L. R., Spruance, S. L., Cunningham, A. L., Bernstein, D. I., Mindel, A., Sacks, S., et al. (2002). Glycoprotein-D-adjuvant vaccine to prevent genital herpes. *New England Journal of Medicine, 347*, 1652–1661.

Stanton, B., Cole, M., Galbraith, J., Li, X., Pendleton, S., Cottrell, L., et al. (2004). Randomized trial of a parent intervention: Parents can make a difference in long-term adolescent risk behaviors, perceptions, and knowledge. *Archives in Pediatric and Adolescent Medicine, 158*, 947–955.

Steinberg, L. (2004). Risk taking in adolescence: What changes and why? *Annals of New York Academy of Sciences, 1021*, 51–58.

Steinberg, L. (2010a). A behavioral scientist looks at the science of adolescent brain development. *Brain and Cognition, 72*, 160–164.

Steinberg, L. (2010b). A dual systems model of adolescent risk-taking. *Developmental Psychobiology, 52*, 216–224.

Sunder, P. K., Ramos, S., Short, M. B., & Rosenthal, S. L. (2006). Adolescent girls' communication with "mothers" about topical microbicides. *Journal of Pediatric and Adolescent Gynecology, 19*, 373–379.

Tangney, J. (1996). Conceptual and methodological issues in the assessment of shame and guilt. *Behavior Research and Therapy, 34*, 741–754.

Tanner, A. E., Katzenstein, J. M., Zimet, G. D., Cox, D. S., Cox, A. D., & Fortenberry, D. (2008). Vaginal microbicide preferences among midwestern urban adolescent women. *Journal of Adolescent Health, 43*, 349–356.

Tota, J. E., Chevarie-Davis, M., Richardson, L. A., Devries, M., & Franco, E. L. (2011). Epidemiology and burden of HPV infection and related diseases: implications for prevention strategies. *Preventative Medicinem, 53*(Suppl 1), S12–21.

Trenholm, C., Devaney, B., Fortson, K., Quay, L., Wheeler, J., & Clark, M. (2007). *Impacts of four title V, section 510 abstinence education programs, final report.* Princeton, NJ: Matematica Policy Research.

Tyler, K. A., Whitbeck, L. B., Chen, X., & Johnson, K. (2007). Sexual health of homeless youth: Prevalence and correlates of sexually transmissible infections. *Sexual Health, 4*, 57–61.

Underhill, K., Operario, D., & Montgomery, P. (2007a). Abstinence-only programs for HIV infection prevention in high-income countries (Review). *Cochrane Database System Review, 4*, CD005421.

Underhill, K., Operario, D., & Montgomery, P. (2007b). Systematic review of abstinence-plus HIV prevention programs in high-income countries. *PLoS Medicine, 4*, 1471–1485.

Wahlstrom, D., Collins, P., White, T., & Luciana, M. (2010). Developmental changes in dopamine neurotransmission in adolescence: Behavioral implications and issues in assessment. *Brain and Cognition, 72*, 146–159.

Wallen, K., & Zehr, J. (2004). Hormones and history: The evolution and development of primate female sexuality. *Journal of Sex Research, 41*, 101–112.

Warner, L., Stone, K., Macaluso, M., Buehler, J., & Austin, H. (2006). Condom use and risk of gonorrhea and chlamydia: A systematic review of design and measurement factors assessed in epidemiologic studies. *Sexually Transmitted Diseases, 33*, 36–51.

Weinstock, H., Berman, S., & Cates, W. (2004). Sexually transmitted diseases among American youth: Incidence and prevalence estimates, 2000. *Perspectives on Sexual and Reproductive Health, 36*, 6–10.

Wiehe, S., Rosenman, M., Wang, J., & Fortenberry, J. (2010). Disparities in chlamydia testing among young women with sexually transmitted infection symptoms. *Sexually Transmitted Diseases, 37*, 751–755.

Wight, D., Williamson, L., & Henderson, M. (2006). Parental influences on young people's sexual behaviour: A longitudinal analysis. *Journal of Adolescence, 29*, 473–494.

Wilson, K., Asbridge, M., Kisely, S., & Langille, D. (2010). Associations of risk of depression with sexual risk taking among adolescents in Nova Scotia high schools. *Canadian Journal of Psychiatry, 55*, 577–585.

Wilson, J. Q., & Kelling, G. L. (1982). The police and neighborhood safety: Broken windows. *Atlantic Monthly, 127*, 29–38.

Woodhall, S. C., Lehtinen, M., Verho, T., Huhtala, H., Hokkanen, M., & Kosunen, E. (2007). Anticipated acceptance of HPV vaccination at the baseline of implementation: A survey of parental and adolescent knowledge and attitudes in Finland. *Journal of Adolescent Health, 40*, 466–469.

Woodhead, N., Chung, S., & Joffe, A. (2009). Protective and risk factors for sexually transmitted infections in middle school students. *Sexually Transmitted Diseases, 36*, 280–283.

World Health Organization. (1991). *Management of patients with sexually transmitted diseases: WHO technical report series 810*. Geneva: WHO.

Zimet, G. D., Perkins, S. M., Sturm, L. A., Bair, R. M., Juliar, B. E., & Mays, R. M. (2005). Predictors of STI vaccine acceptability among parents and their adolescent children. *Journal of Adolescent Health, 37*, 179–186.

Zimet, G. D., Shew, M. L., & Kahn, J. A. (2008). Appropriate use of cervical cancer vaccine. *Annual Review of Medicine*, 223–236.

Zubowicz, E. A., Oakes, J. K., Short, M. B., Perfect, M. M., Succop, P. A., & Rosenthal, S. L. (2006). Adolescents' descriptions of the physical characteristics of microbicide surrogates and experiences of use. *Journal of Women's Health, 15*, 952–961.

HIV Among Adolescents in the United States in the Twenty-First Century: Learning to Manage a Chronic Illness

Maureen E. Lyon

One of the most tragic aspects of HIV diagnosis is that adolescents often do not get the support from their family, classmates, and friends that another illness might elicit so easily, because of the secrecy social stigma sustains. Since the time of the ancient Greeks certain illnesses have been perceived as a punishment from the gods. As discussed in Susan Sontag's book *Illness as Metaphor and AIDS and Its Metaphors* (Sontag, 1989), this belief is social death. Furthermore, HIV-infected persons who believe their HIV is a punishment from god are more likely to reject life-prolonging treatments and less likely to adhere to medication regimens (Kaldjian, Jekel, & Friedland, 1998; Lyon et al., 2011). This metaphor may be a major obstacle to self-care and care by loved ones and the community.

Social isolation for adolescents with HIV has high costs especially with respect to mental health (Abramowitz et al., 2009). Krauss, Godfrey, O'Day, Freidin, and Kaplan (2006) have done outstanding work successfully implementing a program in public housing projects and hospitals in New York City to decrease the stigma associated with HIV. As they note, all emerging illnesses in which there is a fear of transmission are accompanied by stigma with its associated social isolation for the victim of the disease. As they so wisely point out, the virus does not do an interview to figure out what group an individual belongs to before infecting someone. Stigma decreases with increasing awareness of cross-categories, for example that a person with HIV is also a sibling, a friend, and a respected teacher. Social isolation may have an even greater impact on the families and caregivers, who often do not have the benefit of participating in summer camps or supportive programs provided by hospital-based clinics funded through Ryan White or philanthropic foundations. So targeting a decrease in social isolation is an important goal for therapists working with HIV-positive children, adolescents, and their families.

Epidemiology

Unfortunately, adolescents, ages 13–19 years old, account for more than a third of new HIV infections each year in the USA (CDC, 2008). African-American adolescents (ages 13–19) are disproportionately represented, as they are only 17 % of the US teenagers, but account for 75 % of new HIV diagnoses. African-American females have nearly 20 times the HIV rate compared to white females. Among 13–24-year-olds, the estimated percentage of diagnosed HIV infections attributed to male-to-male sexual (MSM) contact increased from 57 % in 2005 to 68 % in 2008, the

M.E. Lyon, Ph.D., A.B.P.P. (✉)
Division of Adolescent and Young Adult Medicine, Center for Translational Science, Children's National Medical Center, Children's Research Institute, 111 Michigan Avenue, NW, Washington, DC 20010-2970, USA
e-mail: mlyon@childrensnational.org

W.T. O'Donohue et al. (eds.), *Handbook of Adolescent Health Psychology*,
DOI 10.1007/978-1-4614-6633-8_37, © Springer Science+Business Media New York 2013

last year that data are available (CDC Fact Sheet, 2008). The percentage of diagnosed HIV infections attributed to heterosexual contact decreased from 32 % to 25 % during this time. Among young MSM 26–50 % reported recent unprotected anal intercourse, and much of this unprotected sex occurred with a partner of unknown or different HIV status. These data suggest that the new cohort of young MSM need programs specifically targeted to their generation (Garofalo et al., 2008).

Health psychologists play an important role as members of multidisciplinary teams, advocates for youth, and psychotherapists in establishing safe and supportive environments, especially for sexual minority youth, who disproportionately are experiencing the burden of HIV. These youth are often victimized at school, which is, in turn, associated with HIV risk behaviors and may interfere with the efforts of HIV-positive youth to treat themselves and others with care. Health psychologists can act as advocates for programs for professional development for school staff, such as the American Psychological Association (APA) Healthy Lesbian, Gay, and Bisexual Students Project to help schools and youth-serving organizations improve health and mental health outcomes for sexual minority youth. For more information, visit www.apa.org/pi/lgbc/hlgbsp. Finally, health psychologists can advocate for the implementation of evidence-based effective policies, practices, and interventions. CDC's Division of HIV/AIDS Prevention funds health departments and community organizations to promote the use of evidence-based HIV interventions, many of which are geared toward young men who have sex with men and young people of color. Information about these interventions is available at www.cdc.gov/hiv/topics/research/prs/evidence-based-interventions.htm.

With respect to children with perinatal HIV, the Pediatric HIV/AIDS Cohort Study (Van Dyke et al., 2011) found that US children born with HIV are doing fairly well as adolescents, and with a mean age of 12 years, 68 % had suppressed viral load. Independent predictors of a suppressed viral load were male gender, recent birth cohort (1994–2002), antiretroviral therapy (ART) use at entry into care, and fewer prior ART treatments. Most children with perinatal HIV maintained virologic suppression and good CD4 values, a measure of immune outcome.

In the seventeenth annual British HIV Association conference Dr. Tania Wan (2011) presented data on young adults who were infected at birth, being transitioned to adult care in Britain. One-fifth had CDR cell count below 200 cells/mm (the old CDC criteria for defining AIDS). Some of those with undetectable viral load had failed to fully restore their immune function. One in eight had severe lipodystrophy, and over half were identified as having clinically significant psychological issues.

As HIV-positive adolescents emerge into adulthood there will be more concern with heart disease and other illnesses associated with the side effects of ART (Leyden et al., 2010), than death from opportunistic infections, caused by a compromised immune system (Brady et al., 2010). Perinatal transmission of the virus had been reduced from 40 % to 1–2 % by a combined use of ART for pregnant women, ART prophylaxis in the newborn, and refraining from breast feeding (Buchholz, Hien, Weichert, & Tenenbaum, 2010).

HIV/AIDS is no longer a death sentence. Adolescents infected in their teens and 20s have the potential to live into their 50s (Harrison, Song, & Zhang, 2010; van Sighem, Gras, Reiss, Brinkman, & de Wolf, 2010) and not transmit the virus sexually, as long as they can maintain an undetectable viral load (Vernazza et al., 2008) through sustained adherence to ART.

Disclosure of HIV Status

HIV disclosure is one of the most salient psychosocial challenges facing people living with HIV/AIDS. For most adolescents with chronic illnesses, disclosure elicits support from others. But because HIV is a sexually transmitted disease, related to behavior and has no cure, HIV often elicits fear and aversion (Krauss et al., 2006). Among adults 65 % stated that they had not disclosed their HIV status because they feared discrimination (Kalichman et al., 2011). Such concerns are particularly salient for adolescents, who are normatively sensitive to peer evaluation and motivated by a strong desire to fit in. For most patients society is on the side of protecting private health information, but for HIV patients society has made it a crime to not disclose one's HIV status to sexual partners in some states.

Complex levels of disclosure exist—starting within the family. Should adolescents tell siblings, school personnel or the school nurse, their religious leader, boyfriends/girlfriends, or sexual partners? Although there are protocols developed to help parents/legal guardians tell their children their HIV diagnosis (Wiener & Lyon, 2006), standardized protocols have not yet been adapted for HIV-positive adolescents to disclose to others. Families are often counseled to disclose to school nurses on a need-to-know basis. This is especially important if a child is on a medical regimen that requires more than twice a day dosing or liquid medications that need to be refrigerated. Yet, many adolescents decide to break school rules, hiding their meds and self-administering during the school day, rather than trust a school nurse to keep their confidence.

Failure to disclose can negatively impact health, either impeding adherence to care or medications or hindering reduction of sexual risk behavior (Crepaz & Marks, 2003). Barriers to disclosure have been reported for HIV-positive adolescents (D'Angelo et al., 2001), similar to those found in adults (Chandra et al., 2003). These barriers include fear of discrimination, rejection in relationships, and a desire to protect oneself and others emotionally and physically from abuse or violence. Among HIV-positive adolescents diagnosis disclosure varies by gender, ethnicity, sexual orientation, and age (see review for adolescents in Wiener & Lyon, 2006). Perinatally infected adolescents' families usually know their diagnosis, but their friends and sexual partners may not know. In contrast behaviorally infected adolescents are more likely to tell a friend or sexual partner, especially if they are lesbian, gay, bisexual, transgendered, or questioning (LGBTQ). In each instance there is tension between the potential of social and instrumental support and fear of discrimination and rejection. For LGBTQ this may also mean coming out about their sexual orientation.

All HIV-positive adolescents have to weigh the meaning of HIV disclosure for their ability to form and maintain romantic relationships, as well as the possibility of sexual transmission. High rates of nondisclosure to sexual partners (Koenig et al., 2006) are consistently found among adolescents, ranging from 68 % who had disclosed to their main sex partner to 27 % who had never disclosed to any sex partners. Although most adolescents described supportive responses to disclosure over time, Koenig found that negative experiences were reported by 35 %. These included judgmental comments, contagion fear, relationship deterioration, physical assault, actual/threatened disclosure to others, and housing discrimination.

On the other hand, individuals who fail to disclose miss the potential positive effects that post-disclosure support has on health and well-being (Wiener & Lyon, 2006). Furthermore, research suggests that among adolescents living with HIV who are in care, those who disclose to others have better immune function, psychosocial adjustment, and social support (Wiener, 2004). Shellmer et al. (2005) found that younger adolescents felt more ready to disclose than older adolescents, suggesting that this may be an opportune time to target an intervention.

Adolescence is a time of moral questioning and deciding on a set of principles to guide one's life. This developmental period affords an opportunity to approach the disclosure process from an ethical perspective, as well as a health perspective. Many adolescents have not had training in a systematic method of ethical decision-making. O'Leary and Wolitski of the CDC (2009) proposed reducing transmission risk behavior through fostering values clarification and learning an ethical decision-making process, so that individuals' self-standards become more salient to them and resistant to change. This is similar to the process of focusing on altruism and personal responsibility by encouraging adolescents living with HIV to "express [their] higher selves" in the only program to date for adolescents living with HIV (Rotheram-Borus et al., 2004).

A disclosure process model has been proposed (Chaudoir, Fisher, & Simoni, 2011) to provide a theoretical framework with which to study how HIV-positive individuals make decisions about disclosing their serostatus and how these decisions affect them, which should guide future research and program development. Evidence-based protocols have been developed for adults to help with disclosure to sexual partners and to decrease unprotected sex acts which may be useful for adolescents (Kalichman et al., 2001). Disclosure to HIV status was found to reduce HIV transmission risks in HIV-positive adults (Crepaz & Marks, 2003; Kalichman et al., 2001; Parsons et al., 2005), and to improve mental health (Lam et al., 2007; Lee & Rotheram-Borus, 2002).

Within the CDC's Diffusion of Effective Behavioral Interventions Project (DEBI) programs, only one had modules which focused on disclosure of seropositive status to sex partners. Kalichman et al.'s (2001) *Healthy Relationships* is a five-session, small group intervention for adults living with HIV/AIDS. The intervention has been demonstrated to be effective with adults (Lyles et al., 2007). It teaches decision-making skills about disclosure of HIV status through the use of role plays and observation of video clips. To our knowledge no similar program exists for HIV-positive adolescents. Mary Jane Rotheram-Borus (personal communication, October 30, 2008) and her team have developed an intervention to help African-American women disclose their HIV status.

We do not know if HIV-positive adolescents are using Internet partner notification for HIV disclosure or exposure, but such web sites are active (Hogben & Kachur, 2008; Mimiaga et al., 2008). Health psychologists have an important role in adapting existing evidence-based strategies to be sensitive to the complexity of the disclosure process which requires information, skills, and support so that we can help adolescents make informed choices about how to disclose safely and sensitively.

Health psychologists can help guide adolescents as they make informed choices about who to tell, depending on the unique circumstances of the adolescent. It is also critical that treatment teams honestly inform adolescents of the decreased likelihood of transmitting HIV if they can maintain an undetectable viral load and good immune functioning, as well as its benefit for their own health.

Treatment Adherence as Prevention

ART is a comprehensive HIV prevention strategy. The HIV Prevention Trials Network (HPTN 052, Press release May 12, 2011) demonstrated a 96 % reduction in HIV transmission among serodiscordant heterosexual couples who initiated ART early, rather than following current CDC guidelines. Furthermore, European data suggest that maintaining an undetectable viral load also prevents transmission of the virus to sexual partners (Vernazza et al., 2008) and concerns about telling patients this, such as the potential for transmission during acute HIV infection, behavioral disinhibition, or resistance have not materialized (Hull & Montaner, 2011; Johnstone-Robertson et al., 2011; Kalichman et al., 2011).

As a consequence the Joint United Nations AIDS (UNAIDS) program has called for the inclusion of antiretroviral treatment as a key pillar in the global strategy to control the spread of HIV and others have discussed the ethical challenges of providing oral preexposure prophylaxis (PrEP) for uninfected MSM (Leibowitz, Parker, & Rotheram-Borus, 2011). Thus, maximizing adherence to treatment is not only fundamental to the well-being of adolescents with HIV but is also important for public health (Simoni et al., 2007; HTPN 052, 2011).

There is no gold standard for treating problems with medication adherence (Chesney, 2006). The World Health Organization (2003) has estimated that if all individuals living with a chronic illness were adherent with their medication regimens, the results would be equal to curing cancer. WHO warns against blaming the patient for failures in adherence to medication regimens. There are many systems issues that pose barriers to adherence, such as lack of access to care or distrust of the doctor or medical establishment. Adhering to ART regimens is even more challenging than that found with other illnesses, as HIV regimens are often complex and always lifelong.

The rapid and continual replication of HIV in the infected host makes development of mutant strains of HIV likely. This in turn can cause resistance to the medications a patient is taking (D'Angelo, 2006). The best way to avoid this is to completely suppress (to the degree possible) replication of the virus. This is the major reason to insist on high levels of patient adherence, so that medication levels remain high enough to stop replication. The emergence of resistance can signal a major change in the illness and make therapy quite challenging. It usually means that some or all of medications in use with this patient need to be switched and can ultimately lead to the inability to stop the progression of HIV replication and further suppression of the immune system.

Side effects from ART include but are not limited to depression, nausea, diarrhea, and malaise or a general run down feeling. Side effects may mimic depressive symptomatology (e.g., fatigue, sleep disturbance, and weight loss) and may interfere with adherence. There are also more serious toxicities associated with ART medications, which require monitoring with routine lab testing. Patients need to be educated about when to speak with their practitioner about side effects. Psychotropic treatment of psychiatric symptoms improves the overall care and functioning of youth with HIV and is generally safe (Cohen et al., 2010). Behavioral manifestations of the disease process may also remit with effective adherence to ART.

New research suggests that the old belief that effective treatment requires 90–95 % adherence is incorrect. Rather the *effectiveness of viral suppression interacts with adherence* and the nature of the ART regimen and whether or not it is a boosted regimen (Bangsberg, 2008). With the introduction of once a day dosing adherence rates are expected to improve. Stigma, lack of disclosure, and secrecy are additional barriers to adherence to medication. There are also cultural barriers to ability and willingness to take medication. In Thailand, for example, adherence rates for adolescents are close to the ideal of 95 % (Rongkavilit et al., 2007), whereas in the United States (Flynn et al., 2007) the majority of adolescents started on ART stopped treatment (63 %) within the 3-year period of observation. Only 24 % of behaviorally infected adolescents (29/120) who were started on an ART regimen achieved and maintained undetectable viral loads over 3 years. Importantly, adherence during the first 16 weeks on medication appeared to be critical for achieving undetectable viral loads, confirming results those from the Reaching for Excellence in Adolescent Care and Health (REACH) study in which only 28.3 % of HIV-positive adolescents ($N=161$) reported having missed no doses in the previous month (Murphy et al., 2005). For a review of barriers to adherence among adolescents, see Koenig and Bachanas (2006). Therefore, health psychologists and treatment teams should endeavor to provide maximal support during this initial critical period of first starting ART.

How can we improve adherence? Going beyond the context of institutional and community variables, there are very few published interventions aimed at increasing adherence to medication in adolescents living with HIV (Reisner et al., 2009). One of the first (Lyon et al., 2003) found that self-reported adherence and satisfaction with treatment increased in a 12-session pilot study of a multifamily "HAART" Group ($N=46$; 23 families). The intervention alternated six "family group" psychoeducational sessions with six "adolescent only" support sessions for a total of 12 sessions for adolescents living with HIV and 6 sessions for the family at the hospital where they received treatment. Participants discussed the dynamics of HIV, why they should take therapy, how to manage side effects, and how to communicate with doctors. Of the 46 participants, 78 % completed the intervention; and 91 % of the adolescents reported increased adherence. Four adolescents experienced a one-log reduction in viral load to undetectable levels at the end of the 12-week intervention. At 6-month evaluation two of four participants who had not been taking any medication started ART. Two adolescents continued to decline antiretroviral medications. One lesson learned was that in future studies family members should receive reimbursement and incentives, as well as adolescents.

Participants reported what they gained most from the group were connectedness and decreased isolation. Family/treatment buddies rated the overall program as highly helpful, citing social support as most valuable. An unanticipated benefit was an increase in other health behaviors, including medical and dental appointments, hepatitis B and influenza immunizations, and referrals to mental health and substance abuse treatment. Games and prizes were used to review the content of the six educational/skill sessions, making the time together fun. Adolescents rated a multiple alarm watch as the best aid to medication adherence.

The Therapeutic Regimens Enhancing Adherence in Teens (TREAT) program (Rogers, Miller, Murphy, Tanney, & Fortune, 2001) was an 8-week intervention. It was designed to prepare adolescents who had never taken HAART by providing them with education through written materials and a video. Contrary to the hypothesis, 40 % of the 79 participants were found to be at stages of readiness that did not match with their treatment stage, nor their actual adherence behavior. The lesson learned from this trial was not to use stage of readiness as a reason to deny access to medication. Understandably, many physicians want patients to at least begin to accept and deal with and process their psychological and emotional feelings about being positive, before making a lifetime commitment to taking medications daily, because lapses in therapy or subtherapeutic regimens may result in viral resistance and therapy failure.

Depression is consistently associated with nonadherence to HIV medications (Hosek, Harper, & Domanico, 2005; Murphy, Wilson, Durako, Muenz, & Belzer, 2001). Chronic substance use and mental health issues have been shown to make it hard for HIV-infected adolescents and adults to maintain treatment adherence. For example, for REACH participants, depression and substance use were significantly associated with decreased adherence, both during the time period in which the participant was depressed and using substances, as well as later (Murphy et al., 2001, 2005). These findings highlight the importance of standardizing assessments of adolescents' emotional functioning and substance abuse when making a treatment plan. When caregivers have primary responsibility for calling to obtain refills adolescents were more likely to adhere (Marhefka et al., 2008).

Teens Linked to Care (TLC) is the only adherence intervention to be evaluated in a clinical trial (Rotheram-Borus et al., 2001). Because of poor attendance, it was modified to be delivered as one-to-one counseling, offered either in person or by phone. Unfortunately, despite decreases in risk behavior, the intervention did not significantly improve medication use or adherence. A randomized clinical trial funded by the CDC to improve adherence to treatment and to reduce risk behaviors for adolescents living with HIV, Adolescent IMPACT, is currently in the data analytic phase with dissemination of results expected soon (Lyon, Marhefka, Abramowitz, & Koenig, 2008).

A surprising number of adolescents have ongoing difficulty in swallowing pills. Specialized training on pill swallowing and the use of liquid formulations is often necessary to ensure adherence (Garvie, Lensing, & Rai, 2007). Directly observed therapy has also been found to be helpful for adolescents (Garvie et al., 2011). Clearly, multiple strategies to overcome barriers to adherence, rather than any one strategy, are necessary.

One explanatory model to help persons with HIV to start care and maintain it consistently is the situated Information, Motivation, Behavioral Skills model of Care Initiation and Maintenance (sIMB-CIM) (Amico, 2011). Other approaches have involved the use of technology, such as LifeWindows, which is a computer-based intervention in HIV clinical care settings that demonstrated improved antiretroviral adherence in patients who persisted in care at the clinical care sites (Fisher et al., 2011). Another brief intervention developed by Kalichman et al. (2011) focuses on behavioral self-regulation counseling delivered by cell phone to increase HIV treatment adherence. They demonstrated a clinically significant increase in ART adherence from baseline, compared to the standard of care control, which was found at 4 months post baseline. Behavioral interventions for adults such as the Healthy Living Project show promise for being adapted with adolescents (Johnson et al., 2007). Recent research also suggests that effective interventions should include a focus on promoting patients' autonomy and religious/spiritual beliefs regarding ART adherence (Finocchario-Kessler et al., 2011a, 2011b). Spiritual and mind-body beliefs and religious practices can be either barriers or motivators to HIV-treatment decision making and medication adherence (Finocchario-Kessler et al., 2011a, 2011b; Lyon et al., 2011).

Transition to Adult Health Care

The nature of the United States health care system poses special challenges for HIV-positive youth transitioning to adult health care. Insurance and privacy regulations make the study of existing transition programs' effectiveness difficult to evaluate. Nevertheless, a few small studies exist. Donohoe, Allison, Garvie, and Knapp (2004) found that HIV-positive youth with a history of neglect or foster care were less likely to successfully make the transition to an adult health care facility. Although the reasons were not elucidated, institutional barriers, such as the loss of insurance when reaching age 21 or 18, depending on the state, likely accounted for part of this. In an unpublished study at Children's National Medical Center patients who did not make a successful transition to adult health care were likely to die in their 20s. The psychiatrist, Harry Stack Sullivan, suggested long ago that we treat ourselves as others have treated us. So it is not surprising that youth who have a history of neglect by caregivers are more likely to neglect their own health than those who were not neglected. Adolescents with a history of neglect will need additional support as they make the transition to adult health care.

Research (Valenzuela et al., 2011; Wiener et al., 2011) supports the need for a clear and structured transition process. In one study of 59 youth, with a mean age of 22 years, living with HIV, 45 % reported transition to adult health care to be more difficult than expected, and 32 % reported they could not find emotional supports (Wiener et al., 2011). Our Canadian colleague, Dr. Miriam Kaufman, has developed an effective program to help all adolescents with a chronic illness transition to adult health care and provides free tools for this purpose on the web site http://www.sickkids.ca/Go-Positive/index.html.

HIV-Associated Neurological Disorders

Unfortunately, HIV-associated neurological disorders (HAND) persist in the ART era. The HIV Neuroimaging Consortium (Harezlak et al., 2011), using proton magnetic resonance spectroscopy (MRS) ($N=268$ patients: $n=28$ control HIV-negative; $n=124$ neuroasymptomatic individuals; $n=50$ AIDS dementia complex), found cognitive impairment in 48 % of HIV-infected individuals. Brain inflammatory changes were ubiquitous among HIV-infected individuals, whereas neuronal injury occurred predominantly in those with cognitive impairment. In a new mouse model, Dash et al. (2011) demonstrated that HIV infection of the nervous system leads to inflammatory responses, changes in brain cells, and damage to neurons. This is the first study to show neuronal loss during the initial stages of HIV infection in an animal model. These findings have implications for decision-making and risk behavior in individuals with HIV and contribute to the ongoing debate on whether or not to start ART earlier. For the interested reader an excellent review of the cognitive neuropsychology of HAND is provided by Woods et al. (2009), as well as Cohen and colleagues' *Handbook of AIDS Psychiatry* (2010).

Assessment of HAND has been studied in adolescents with HIV. Lyon et al. (2009) examined the ability of the HIV-Dementia Scale (HDS; Power, Selnes, Grim, & McArthur, 1995) and the mini-mental state examination (MMSE) in screening for HAND in adolescents ($N=76$). Six patients (13 %) (all males, all perinatally infected, all CDC categories B and C) had a clinical HAND diagnosis, confirmed by a neurologist blind to the study. Perceptual organization, working memory, and processing speed on intelligence testing were significantly correlated with HDS scores.

Depression and age were not correlated with HAND. When the HDS cut point was lowered to less than 8, sensitivity was 83.33 % and specificity was 87.14 % (87 % correct classification). The HDS is a valid 10-min, well-tolerated, screening tool for HAND in adolescents. This measure is free, readily available, and used internationally.

Reproductive Decision-Making: Desire for a Child

Planning for pregnancy for HIV-positive adolescents and youth is critical to prevention of transmission to their babies and to uninfected sexual partners who desire children. This is because most mothers and their babies benefit from ART, particularly when it is started prior to pregnancy (United States Department of Health and Human Services, 2010). Caesarean section further reduces the risk of transmission of HIV to a child through pregnancy (perinatal transmission rate) which overall has been reduced to a rate of 0.99 % in 2001–2002 from a rate of 5.1 % in 1997–1998 (Bartlett, 2005) from the highest rate of 78 % in 1993 (Lindegren et al., 1999). The International AIDS Society (ISA-USA) guidelines recommend ART in all HIV+ women who are considering pregnancy to decrease the chances of transmission to unborn children (Waldura, 2011).

Health care providers in the United States may be reluctant to give medical advice on reproduction to HIV-positive adolescents (Panozzo et al., 2003; Sherr & Barry, 2004), even though a significant proportion of HIV-infected persons express a wish for parenthood. In Europe fertility clinics have experience in providing both intrauterine inseminations and in vitro fertilization to couples to achieve pregnancy where the male is HIV infected and the female is uninfected, without HIV transmission to the uninfected female partner (Bendikson, Anderson, & Hornstein, 2002).

Adolescents with HIV are more likely to become pregnant than their noninfected peers (Agwu, Jang, Korthuis, Araneta, & Gebo, 2011). Compared to perinatally infected adolescents, behaviorally infected adolescents are five times more likely to become pregnant and get pregnant more than once (36.8 % vs. 14.3 %) (Agwu et al., 2011). The median age at pregnancy was 18 years. Transmission occurred in one birth (1/61) despite prenatal ART. In another study, among 75 perinatally infected young women, six females became pregnant and of those, three individuals had more than one pregnancy (Bernstein, Trexler, & D'Angelo, 2006). The average age of first conception was 17.2 years. Compared to their community peers, adolescents infected at birth with HIV were more likely to have become pregnant (14 % vs. 11.8 %). A recent study found that if the HIV-positive adolescents perceived that their parent and partner had the desire for a child, the adolescent was more likely to have the intention to become pregnant and was significantly more likely not to be using condoms (Krupincza, LaGrange, & Vyas, 2011). These data suggest an opportunity to intervene to support planned pregnancies by informing patients that maintaining an undetectable viral load and good immune functioning through adherence to ART will likely prevent the transmission of HIV to their baby or their uninfected partner.

Adolescents and youth have a basic human right to all information and services related to their reproductive health (United Nations; Gruskin, Ferguson, & O'Malley, 2007). The primary ethical concern should be for the autonomy of the HIV-positive adolescent to make decisions about having a child and that, for this reason, fertility services should never be denied to adolescents with HIV/AIDS, particularly given that techniques and treatments are available to minimize harm to the uninfected partner and unborn child (United States Department of Health, 2010). Empowering young people to promote and safeguard their rights may enable them to act on their own behalf to gain access to the information and services they need to make an informed choice. Otherwise, HIV-positive adolescents may avoid contact with the health care system, endangering not only their lives but also the lives of their uninfected partner and unborn children. For these reasons, health psychologists should make a point to inquire about the desire of their HIV-positive patients for children.

Family Centered Advance Care Planning/Palliative Care

Despite our best efforts, HIV/AIDS remains a disease without a cure. HIV/AIDS has a disproportionate adverse impact on adolescents and minorities, although most youth with HIV are now expected to live well into adulthood (Justice et al., 2009; McConnell et al., 2005). In 2006, in a perinatally infected cohort, mean age at death was 18 years (Brady et al., 2010). Once the immune system is compromised, a patient with AIDS can die suddenly from an overwhelming infection or following a long period of chronic illness (Brady et al., 2010; Nachman et al., 2000; van Rossum, Fraaij, & de Groot, 2002). Consequently, prognosis is difficult and time of death uncertain, underscoring the importance of ACP. Declining death rates can lead to a false belief that, once people have access to ART, end-of-life (EOL) issues cease to be of great concern (McConnell, 2006). Instead, medical breakthroughs have expanded the timeframe for palliative care and blurred the definition of EOL (Grady, Knebel, & Draper, 2001). Adolescents at risk of dying cannot wait until their mental abilities are blunted or incapacitated by HAND (Allison, Wolters, & Brouwers, 2009; Lyon, McCarter, & D'Angelo, 2009; Wood, Shah, Steenhoff, & Rutstein, 2009) to participate in decision-making about their own EOL care.

Children who die of AIDS rarely have do not resuscitate (DNR) orders or hospice enrollment (Lyon, Williams et al., 2008). National guidelines recommend that quality palliative care be integrated routinely with HIV care. Thus, incorporating ACP into the care and treatment of HIV-positive adolescents is critical in preparing for the EOL.

EOL decisions are emotional and challenging for adults. For adolescents and their families, EOL decisions are even more complex, emotionally charged, and potentially overwhelming. Left unprepared for EOL decisions, miscommunication and disagreements may result in families being charged with neglect (Mercurio, 2007), court battles, and even legislative intervention (Fins & Schiff, 2005). Families may be torn apart (Wijngaards-de Meij et al., 2005) rather than strengthened (Chandan & Richter, 2009). Standardized protocols for ACP may prevent such adverse outcomes.

Respect for adolescent autonomy supports including adolescents in ACP, defined as a process for preparing for EOL, including discussion of death (Grady, 2005; Johnstone & Kanitsaki, 2009). Cognitive capacities required for "informed consent" for medical treatment develop in early adolescence (Badzek & Kanosky, 2002). Interviews with terminally ill adolescents indicate they are capable of participating in and understanding the consequences of their decision(s) (Hinds et al., 2005). Interviews with parents of terminally ill children show they found an ACP interview helpful (Hammes et al., 2005). Parents find talking to their children about death acceptable, and those who talked to their child about death did not regret it after their child died (Kreicbergs et al., 2004). Adolescents are capable of using an advance directive (Wiener et al., 2008).

Nevertheless, the structure of the adolescent brain is not fully formed, particularly the prefrontal cortex, which is involved in understanding the consequences of decisions (Weinberger, Elvevag, & Giedd, 2005). Thus, the wisdom of having families is involved in EOL decision-making for 18–24-year-olds who are legally able to do so, on their own. Studies suggest talking about death and dying and decision-making with adolescents benefits them and their families (Field & Behrman, 2002; Lyon et al., 2009; Lyon et al., 2009a, 2009b; Lyon et al., 2010). Furthermore, adolescents want involvement in their own EOL decisions (Lyon et al., 2004).

Currently, the only structured, developmentally appropriate, culturally sensitive, and family-centered program which exists to help the families of children or adolescents with HIV/AIDS or other life-threatening conditions to speak directly and honestly about EOL care is the Family Centered (FACE) ACP protocol. FACE, developed and pilot tested by Lyon and colleagues (Lyon et al., 2010; Lyon et al., 2009a, 2009b), demonstrated the feasibility, acceptability, safety, and efficacy in a randomized controlled clinical trial.

FACE is a 3-session (60 min, 1 week apart) intervention that integrates five of the eight domains of variables relevant to EOL care from the 2004 National Consensus Project for Quality Palliative Care (National Consensus Project: Clinical Practice Guidelines for palliative Care, 2004): (1) psychological, (2) social (family), (3) spiritual, (4) cultural, and (5) ethical/legal aspects of care with respect to patient goals, preferences, and choices. FACE is implemented in hospital-based clinics supported by the Ryan White CARE Act which provides comprehensive interdisciplinary assessment and care, providing the context for the other three domains: (6) structure and processes of care, (7) physical aspects of care, and (8) care of the imminently dying patient.

FACE provides the adolescent and family with the opportunity to have a facilitated discussion of their hopes, needs, and goals in an honest conversation about preferences for end-of-life care. This process can increase trust within the family and with the multidisciplinary team. FACE demonstrated that making ACP explicit increased congruence in treatment preferences between the adolescent and family and decreased decisional conflict for the adolescent without any adverse outcomes. FACE is now being studied longitudinally to determine if the increased congruence in treatment preferences between adolescents and their families can be maintained over time as well as the impact of spiritual struggle (http://projectreporter.nih.gov/project_info_description.cfm?aid=8076110&icde=7530683).

A Tool for Engagement

In June 2009, Wiener and her colleague at the National Cancer Institute published a board game, *Shop Talk*, to use with patients living with cancer or HIV. The object of the game is to have a fun time "shopping" while talking about the child/adolescents' life, interests, illness, and feelings; the game can be "played" with one or more people at a time. The therapist can use the player's response as a point of departure for further discussion or exploration. *Shop Talk* is designed for children ages 7–16 years. Because critical information can be revealed through the course of play—suicidal feelings, for example, or non-adherence to medication regimens—the game should only be used with the supervision of a trained therapist so that opportunities for intervention aren't missed. *Shop Talk* is available in two versions, one for HIV patients and one for their siblings. Spanish and English versions are also available free of charge by contacting Dr. Wiener at wienerl@mail.nih.gov.

Living Well

Adolescents living with any chronic illness, including HIV, should be encouraged to consider, with their families when possible, the following: "What does living well mean to you?" "What gives your life meaning?" "What do you hope for from your future medical plan of care?" "What other hopes do you have, if your first hope is not possible?" In this way the health psychologist can enhance motivation and facilitate growth along the path the adolescent has chosen to reach their goals for a life well lived, considering their values and lived experience.

References

Abramowitz, S., Koenig, L. J., Chandwani, S., Orban, L., Stein, R., LaGrange, R., et al. (2009). Characterizing social support: Global and specific social support experiences of HIV-infected youth. *AIDS Patient Care and STDs, 23*, 323–330.

Agwu, A. L., Jang, S. S., Korthuis, P. T., Araneta, M. R. G., & Gebo, K. A. (2011). Pregnancy incidence and outcomes in vertically and behaviorally HIV-infected youth. *Journal of the American Medical Association, 305*, 468–470.

Allison, S., Wolters, P. L., & Brouwers, P. (2009). Youth with HIV/AIDS: Neurobehavioral consequences. In R. H. Paul et al. (Eds.), *HIV and the brain. Current clinical neurology* (pp. 187–211). New York: Humana Press.

Amico, K. R. (2011). A situated-Information Motivation Behavioral Skills Model of Care Initiation and Maintenance (sIMB-CIM): An IMB model based approach to understanding and intervening in engagement in care for chronic medical conditions. *Journal of Health Psychology, 16*(7), 1071–1081.

Badzek, L., & Kanosky, S. (2002). Mature minors and end-of-life decision making: A new development in their legal right to participation. *Journal of Nursing Law, 8*(3), 8223–8229.

Bangsberg, D. (2008). The importance of adherence: Resistance, viral fitness, and adherence patterns in determining outcomes. Grand rounds, George Washington University HIV/AIDS Institute.

Bartlett, J. G. (2005). Mother-to-child transmission of HIV infection in the era of highly active antiretroviral therapy. *Clinical Infectious Disease, 40*(3), 458–465.

Bendikson, K. A., Anderson, D., & Hornstein, M. D. (2002). Fertility options for HIV patients. *Current Opinion in Obstetrics and Gynecology, 14*(5), 453–457.

Bernstein, K., Trexler, C., & D'Angelo, L. (2006). "I'm just like anyone else": Risk behaviors and health consequences in perinatally infected HIV-positive adolescents. Annual Meeting of the Society of Adolescent Medicine, Boston, MA.

Brady, M. T., Oleske, J. M., Williams, P. L., Elgie, C., Mofenson, L. M., Dankner, W. M., et al. (2010). Declines in mortality rates and changes in causes of death in HIV-1 infected children during the HAART era. *Journal of Acquired Immune Deficiency Syndrome, 53*(1), 86–94.

Buchholz, B., Hien, S., Weichert, S., & Tenenbaum, T. (2010). Pediatric aspects of HIV1-infection—an overview. *Minerva Pediatrics, 62*, 371–387.

Centers for Disease Control and Prevention. (2008). HIV/AIDS Surveillance Rep Diagnoses of HIV infection and AIDS in the United States and Dependent Areas (Vol. 20). Retrieved from www.cdc.gov/hiv/surveillance/resources/reports/2008report/pdf /2008SurveillanceReport.pdf.

Centers for Disease Control and Prevention Fact Sheet (2008). *HIV Fact Sheet*. Retrieved from www.cdc.gov/HealthyYouth/sexualbehaviors/pdf/hiv_factsheet_ymsm.pdf.

Chandan, U., & Richter, L. (2009). Strengthening families through early intervention in high HIV prevalence countries. *AIDS Care, 21*, 76–82.

Chandra, P. S., Deepthivarma, S., & Manjula, V. (2003). Disclosure of HIV infection in South India: Patterns, reasons, and reactions. *AIDS Care, 15*, 207–215.

Chaudoir, S. R., Fisher, J. D., & Simoni, J. M. (2011). Understanding HIV disclosure: A review and application of the Disclosure Processes Model. *Social Science and Medicine, 72*, 1618–1629.

Chesney, M. A. (2006). The elusive gold standard. *Future perspectives for HIV adherence assessment and intervention. Journal of Acquired Immune Deficiency Syndrome., 43*(Suppl 1), S149–S155.

Cohen, M. A., Goforth, H., Lux, J., Batista, S., Khalife, S., Cozza, K., et al. (2010). *Handbook of AIDS psychiatry*. New York: Oxford University Press.

Crepaz, N., & Marks, G. (2003). Serostatus disclosure, sexual communication and safer sex in HIV positive men. *AIDS Care: Psychological Socio-Medical Aspects of AIDS/HIV, 15*(3), 379–387.

D'Angelo, L. J. (2006). Caring for HIV-infected teens. In M. E. Lyon & L. J. D'Angelo (Eds.), *Teenagers, HIV, and AIDS: Insights from youths living with the virus* (pp. 29–43). Westport, CT: Praeger Press.

D'Angelo, L., Abdalian, S. E., Sarr, M., Hoffman, N., & Belzer, M. (2001). Disclosure of serostatus by HIV infected youth: The experience of the REACH study. *Journal of Adolescent Health, 29*(Suppl 3), 72–79.

Dash, P. K., Gorantla, S., Gendelman, H. E., Knibbe, J., Casale, G. P., Makarov, E., et al. (2011). Loss of neuronal integrity during progressive HIV-1 infection of humanized mice. *Journal of Neuroscience, 31*(9), 3148. doi:10.1523/JNEUROSCI.5473-10.2011.

Donohoe, M., Allison, K., Garvie, P. A., & Knapp K. M. (2004, July). Needs and barriers of youth infected with HIV when transitioning from pediatric to adult health care settings. Presented at the Annual NIMH Conference on the Role of Families in Preventing and Adapting to HIV/AIDS, Atlanta, GA.

Field, M. J., & Behrman, R. E. (2002). *When children die: Improving palliative and end-of-life care for children and their families*. Washington, DC: Institute of Medicine, National Academy Press.

Finocchario-Kessler, S., Catley, D., Berkley-Patton, J., Gerkovich, M., Williams, K., Banderas, J., et al. (2011). Baseline predictors of ninety percent or higher antiretroviral therapy adherence in a diverse urban sample: The role of patient autonomy and fatalistic religious beliefs. *AIDS Patient Care and STDs, 25*, 103–111.

Finocchario-Kessler, S., Catley, D., Berkley-Patton, J., Gerkovich, M., Willimas, K., Banderas, J., et al. (2011). Computer-based intervention in HIV clinical care setting improves antiretroviral adherence: The LifeWindows Project. *AIDS Behavior, 15*(8), 1635–1646.

Fins, J., & Schiff, N. (2005). In brief: The afterlife of terri schiavo. *The Hastings Center Report., 35*(4), 8. http://www.medscape.com/viewarticle/511647.

Fisher, J. D., Amico, K. R., Fisher, W. A., Corman, D. H., Shuper, P. A., et al. for the Life Windows Team. (2011). Computer based intervention in HIV clinical care setting improves antiretroviral adherence: The Life Windows Project. *AIDS Behavior, 15*(8), 1635–1646.

Flynn, P. M., Rudy, B. J., Lindsey, J. C., et al. (2007). Long-term observation of adolescents initiating HAART therapy: Three-year follow-up. *AIDS Research and Human Retroviruses, 23*(10), 1208–1214.

Garofalo, R., Mustanski, B., & Donenberg, G. (2008). Parents know and parents matter; Is it time to develop family-based HIV prevention programs for young men who have sex with men? *Journal of Adolescent Health, 43*, 201–204.

Garvie, P. A., Flynn, P. M., Belzer, M., Britto, P., Hu, C., For Pediatric AIDS Clinical Trials Group (PACTG) P1036B Team, et al. (2011). Psychological factors, beliefs about medication, and adherence of youth with human immunodeficiency virus in a multisite directly observed therapy pilot study. *Journal of Adolescent Health, 48*(6), 637–640.

Garvie, P. A., Lensing, S., & Rai, S. N. (2007). Efficacy of a pill-swallowing training intervention to improve antiretroviral medication adherence in pediatric patients with HIV/AIDS. *Pediatrics, 119*(4), e893–e899.

Grady, P. A. (2005). Introduction: Papers from the National Institutes of Health State-of-the-Science Conference on improving end-of-life care. *Journal of Palliative Medicine, 8*(Suppl 1), S1–S3.

Grady, P. A., Knebel, A. R., & Draper, A. (2001). End-of-life issues in AIDS: The research perspective. *Journal of the Royal Society of Medicine, 94*, 479–482. discussion 84–85.

Gruskin, S., Ferguson, L., & O'Malley, J. (2007). Ensuring sexual and reproductive health for people living with HIV: An overview of key human rights, policy and health systems issues. *Reprod Health Matters, 15*(Suppl 29), 4–26.

Hammes, B. J., et al. (2005). Pediatric advance care planning. *Journal of Palliative Medicine, 8*(4), 766–773.

Harezlak, J., Buchthal, S., Taylor, M., Schifitt, G., Zhong, J., Daar, E., et al. (2011). The HIV Neuroimaging Consortium. Persistence of HIV-associated cognitive impairment, inflammation, and neuronal injury in era of highly active antiretroviral treatment. *AIDS, 25*, 625–633.

Harrison, K. M. C. D., Song, R., & Zhang, X. (2010). Life expectancy after HIV diagnosis based on national HIV surveillance data from 25 states, United States. *Journal of Acquired Immune Deficiency Syndromes, 53*(1), 124–130.

Hinds, P. S., Drew, D., Oakes, L. L., Fouladi, M., Spunt, S. L., Church, C., et al. (2005). End-of-life care preferences of pediatric patients with cancer. *Journal of Clinical Oncology, 23*(36), 9055–9057.

Hogben, M., & Kachur, R. (2008). Internet partner notification: Another arrow in the quiver. (Editorial). *Sexually Transmitted Diseases, 35*, 117–118.

Hosek, S. G., Harper, G. W., & Domanico, R. (2005). Predictors of medication adherence among HIV-infected youth. *Psychological Health Medicine, 10*, 166–179.

Hull, M. W., & Montaner, J. (2011). Antiretroviral therapy: A key component of a comprehensive HIV prevention strategy. *Current HIV/AIDS Report, 8*(2), 85–93.

Johnson, M. O., Charlebois, E., Morin, S. F., Remien, R. H., Chesney, M. A., & NIMH Healthy Living Project Team. (2007). Effects of a behavioral intervention on antiretroviral medication adherence among people living with HIV: The Healthy Living Project randomized controlled study. *Journal of Acquired Immune Deficiency Syndrome, 42*, 574–580.

Johnstone, M. J., & Kanitsaki, O. (2009). Ethics and advance care planning in a culturally diverse society. *Journal of Transcultural Nursing, 20*, 405–415. http://tcn.sagepub.com/cgi/content/abstract/20/4/405.

Johnstone-Robertson, S. P., Hargrove, J., & Williams, B. G. (2011). Antiretroviral therapy initiated soon after HIV diagnosis as standard care: Potential to save lives? *HIV/AIDS: Research and Palliative Care, 3*, 9–17.

Justice, A. C., McGinnis, K. A., Skanderson, M., Chang, C. C., Gibert, C. C., For the VACS Project Team, et al. (2009). Towards a combined prognostic index for survival in HIV infection: The role of "no-HIV" biomarkers. *HIV Medicine, 11*(2), 143–151. 10.1111/j.1468-1293.2009.00757.x.

Kaldjian, L. C., Jekel, J. F., & Friedland, G. (1998). End-of-life decisions in HIV-positive patients: The role of spiritual beliefs. *AIDS, 12*(1), 103–107.

Kalichman, S. C., Cherry, C., Kalichman, M. O., Amaral, C. M., White, D., et al. (2011). Integrated behavioral intervention to improve HIV/AIDS treatment adherence and reduce HIV transmission. *American Journal of Public Health, 101*(3), 531–538.

Kalichman, S. C., Rompa, D., Cage, M., DiFonzo, K., Simpson, D., Austin, J., et al. (2001). Effectiveness of an intervention to reduce HIV transmission risks in HIV-positive people. *American Journal of Preventive Medicine, 21*, 84–92.

Koenig, L. J., & Bachanas, P. J. (2006). Adherence to medications for HIV: Teens say, "Too many, too big, too often". In M. E. Lyon & L. J. D'Angelo (Eds.), *Teenagers, HIV and AIDS: Insights from youths living with the virus* (pp. 45–65). Westport, CT: Praeger Publishers.

Koenig, L. J., Demas, P., Bachanas, P., Morris, M., Ferndon, C. D., Bell, A., & Wiener, J. (2006, August). *Keeping secrets: Disclosure experiences of youth with HIV/AIDS*. Paper presented at the annual meeting of the American Psychological Association, New Orleans, LA.

Krauss, B. J., Godfrey, C., O'Day, J., Freidin, E., & Kaplan, R. (2006). Learning to live with an epidemic: Reducing stigma and increasing safe and sensitive socializing with persons with HIV. In M. E. Lyon & L. J. D'Angelo (Eds.), *Teenagers HIV and AIDS: Insights from youths living with the virus* (pp. 83–103). Westport, CT: Praeger.

Kreicbergs, U., et al. (2004). Talking about death with children who have severe malignant disease. *New England Journal of Medicine, 351*(12), 1175–1186.

Krupincza, K., LaGrange, R., Vyas, A. (2011, April). Pregnancy wantedness among HIV positive adolescents and young adults. Poster session presented at the annual Medical Center Research Week 2011, Washington, DC.

Lam, P. K., Naar-King, S., & Wright, K. (2007). Social support and disclosure as predictors of mental health in HIV-positive youth. *AIDS Patient Care and STDS, 21*, 20–29.

Lee, M. B., & Rotheram-Borus, M. J. (2002). Parents' disclosure of HIV to their children. *AIDS, 16*, 2201–2207.

Leibowitz, A. A., Parker, K. B., & Rotheram-Borus, M. J. (2011). A US policy perspective on oral preexposure prophylaxis for HIV. *American Journal of Public Health, 101*(6), 982–985.

Leyden, W. A., Xu, L., Chao, C. R., Horberg, M. A., Towner, W. J., Hurley, L. B., Quesenberry, C. P., Silverberg, M. J., & Klein, D. (2010). Contribution of

Immunodeficiency to Coronary Heart Disease: Cohort Study of HIV-infected and HIV-uninfected Kaiser Permanente Members. Retrieved from www.retroconference.org/2011/PDFs/810.pdf.

Lindegren, M. L., Byers, R. H., Jr., Thomas, P., Davis, S. F., Caldwell, B., Rogers, M., et al. (1999). Trends in perinatal transmission of HIV/AIDS in the United States. *Journal of the American Medical Association, 282*(6), 531–538.

Lyles, C. M., Kay, L. S., Crepaz, N., Herbst, J. H., Passin, W. F., Kim, A. F., et al. (2007). Best-evidence interventions: Findings from a systematic review of HIV behavioral interventions for US populations at high risk, 2000–2004. *American Journal of Public Health, 97*, 133–143.

Lyon, M. E., Garvie, P. A., Briggs, L., He, J., D'Angelo, L., & McCarter, R. (2009a). Development, feasibility and acceptability of the family-centered (FACE) advance care planning intervention for adolescents with HIV. *Journal of Palliative Medicine, 12*(4), 363–372.

Lyon, M. E., Garvie, P. A., Briggs, L., He, J., Malow, R., D'Angelo, L. J., et al. (2010). Is it safe? Talking to teens with HIV/AIDS about death and dying: A 3-month evaluation of family centered (FACE) advance care planning—anxiety, depression quality of life. *HIV/AIDS: Research and Palliative Care, 2*, 1–11.

Lyon, M. E., Garvie, P. A., Kao, E., Briggs, L., He, J., Malow, R., et al. (2011). An exploratory study of spirituality in HIV infected adolescents and their families: Family Centered advance care planning and medication adherence. *Journal of Adolescent Health, 48*(6), 633–636.

Lyon, M. E., Garvie, P. A., McCarter, R., Briggs, L., He, J., & D'Angelo, L. (2009b). Who will speak for me? Improving end-of-life decision-making for adolescents with HIV and their families. *Pediatrics, 123*(2), e199–e206.

Lyon, M. E., Marhefka, S. L., Abramowitz, S., & Koenig, L. J. (2008, August). ADIMPACT Team. Psychosocial issues of adolescents with HIV infection acquired at birth and later in life. Symposium. Annual Meeting of the American Psychological Association, Boston, MA.

Lyon, M. E., McCarter, R., & D'Angelo, L. (2009). Detecting HIV associated neurocognitive disorders in adolescents: What is the best screening tool? *Journal Adolescent Health, 44*(2), 133–135. doi:10.1016/j.jadohealth.2008.06.023.

Lyon, M. E., Trexler, C., Akpan-Townsend, C., et al. (2003). A family group approach to increasing adherence to therapy in HIV infected youth: Results of a pilot project. *AIDS Patient Care and STDs, 17*(6), 299–308.

Lyon, M. E., Williams, P. L., Woods, E. R., Hutton, N., Butler, A. M., Sibinga, E., et al. (2008). Do not resuscitate orders and/or hospice care, psychological health and quality of life among children/adolescents with AIDS. *Journal of Palliative Medicine, 11*, 459–469.

Lyon, M. E., et al. (2004). What do adolescents want? An exploratory study regarding end-of-life decision-making. *Journal of Adolescent Health, 35*(6), 529.e1–529.e6.

Lyon, M. E., et al. (2009). Development, feasibility and acceptability of the Family-Centered (FACE) Advance Care Planning Intervention for adolescents with HIV. *Journal of Palliative Medicine, 12*(4), 363–372.

Marhefka, S. L., Koenig, L. J., Allison, S., et al. (2008). Family experiences with pediatric antiretroviral therapy: Responsibilities, barriers, and strategies for remembering medications. *AIDS Patient Care STDS, 22*(8), 637–647.

McConnell, M. (2006). Trends in antiretroviral therapy use and survival rates for a cohort of HIV-infected children and adolescents in the United States, 1989–2001. *Journal of Acquired Immune Deficiency Syndrome, 38*, 488–494.

McConnell, M. S., Byers, R. H., Frederick, T., Peters, V. B., Dominguez, K. L., For the Pediatric Spectrum of HIV Disease Consortium, et al. (2005). Trends in antiretroviral therapy use and survival rates for a large cohort of HIV-infected children and adolescents in the United States, 1989–2001. *Epidemiology and social Science, 38*(4), 488–494.

Mercurio, M. R. (2007). An adolescent's refusal of medical treatment: Implications of the Abraham Cheerix case. *Pediatrics, 120*(6), 1357–1358.

Mimiaga, M. J., Tetu, A. M., Gortmaker, S., Koenen, K. C., Fair, A. D., et al. (2008). HIV and STD status among MSM and attitudes about internet partner notification for STD exposure. *Sexually Transmitted Diseases, 35*, 111–116.

Murphy, D. A., Belzer, M., Durako, S. J., Sarr, M., Wilson, C. M., & Muenz, L. R. (2005). Longitudinal antiretroviral adherence among adolescents infected with human immunodeficiency virus. *Archives of Pediatric and Adolescent Medicine, 159*(8), 764–770.

Murphy, D. A., Wilson, C. M., Durako, S. J., Muenz, L. R., & Belzer, M. (2001). Antiretroviral medication adherence among the REACH HIV-infected adolescent cohort in the USA. *AIDS Care, 13*(1), 27–40.

Nachman, S. A., et al. (2000). Nucleoside analogs plus ritonavir in stable antiretroviral therapy-experienced HIV-infected children: A randomized controlled trial. Pediatric AIDS Clinical Trials Group 338 Study Team. *Journal of the American Medical Association, 283*(4), 492–498.

National Consensus Project: Clinical Practice Guidelines for Palliative Care. (2004). Retrieved from www.nationalconsensusproject.org.

O'Leary, A., & Wolitski, R. J. (2009). Moral agency and the sexual transmission of HIV. *Psychological Bulletin, 135*(3), 478–494.

Panozzo, L., Battegay, M., Friedl, A., & Vernazza, P. L. (2003). High risk behaviour and fertility desires among heterosexual HIV-positive patients with a serodiscordant partner—two challenging issues. *Swiss Medical Weekly, 133*(7–8), 124–127.

Parsons, J. T., Scrimshaw, E. W., Bimbi, D. S., Wolitski, R. J., Gomez, C. A., & Halkitis, P. N. (2005).

Consistent, inconsistent, and non-disclosure to casual sexual partners among HIV-seropositive gay and bisexual men. *AIDS, 19*(Suppl), S87–S97.

Power, C., Selnes, O. A., Grim, J. A., & McArthur, J. C. (1995). HIV-D scale: A rapid screening test. *Journal of AIDS and Human Retrovirology, 8*, 273–278.

Reisner, S. L., Mimiaga, M. J., Skeer, M., Perkovich, B., Johnson, C. V., & Safren, S. A. (2009). A review of HIV antiretroviral adherence and intervention studies among HIV-infected youth. *Topics in HIV Medicine, 17*(1), 14–25.

Rogers, A. S., Miller, S., Murphy, D. A., Tanney, M., & Fortune, T. (2001). The TREAT (therapeutic regimens enhancing adherence in teens) program: Theory and preliminary results. *Journal of Adolescent Health, 29*(Suppl 3), 30–38.

Rongkavilit, C., Naar-King, S., Chuenyam, T., Wang, B., Wright, K., & Phanuphak, P. (2007). Health risk behaviors among HIV-infected youth in Bangkok, Thailand. *Journal of Adolescent Health, 40*(4), 358.e1–358.e8.

Rotheram-Borus, M. J., Lee, M. B., Murphy, D. A., et al. (2001). Efficacy of a preventive intervention for youths living with HIV. *American Journal of Public Health, 91*(3), 400–405.

Rotheram-Borus, M. J., Swendeman, D., Comulada, S., Weiss, R. E., Lee, M., & Lightfoot, M. (2004). Prevention for substance-using HIV-positive young people: Telephone and in-person delivery. *Journal of Acquired Immune Deficiency Syndrome, 37*, S68–S77.

Shellmer, D. A., Lyon, M. E., Zea, M. C., Radcliffe, J., D'Angelo, L. D., & Rutstein, R. (2005, August). Pediatric HIV: Effects of adjustment, social support, and disclosure on cognitive and psychosocial functioning. Poster presented at the 113th Annual American Psychological Association Annual Convention, Washington, DC.

Sherr, L., & Barry, N. (2004). Fatherhood and HIV-positive heterosexual men. *Journal of HIV Medicine, 5*(4), 258–263.

Simoni, J. M., Montgomery, A., Martin, E., New, M., Demas, P. A., & Rana, S. (2007). Adherence to antiretroviral therapy for pediatric HIV infection: A qualitative systematic review with recommendations for research and clinical management. *Pediatrics, 119*(6), e1371–e1383.

Sontag, S. (1989). *Illness as metaphor and AIDS and its metaphors*. New York: Picador.

United States Department of Health and Human Services. (December, 2010. updated April 2011). Fact sheet: AIDS info HIV and pregnancy health information for patients. Retrieved from http://www.aidsinfo.nih.gov.

United Nations Population Fund. *Supporting Adolescents and Youth*. Retrieved from http://www.unfpa.org/about/index/htm.

Valenzuela, J., Buchanan, C., Radcliffe, J., Ambrose, C., Hawkins, L., & Tanney, M. (2011). Transition to adult services among behaviorally infected adolescents with HIV—a qualitative study. *Journal of Pediatric Psychology, 36*(2), 134–140.

Van Dyke, R. B., Patel, K., Siberry, G. K., Burchett, S. K., Spector, S. A., For the Pediatric HIV/AIDS Cohort Study, et al. (2011). Antiretroviral treatment of U.S. children with perinatally-acquired HIV infection: Temporal changes in therapy between 1991 and 2009 and predictors of immunologic and virologic outcomes. *Journal of Acquired Immune Deficiency Syndromes, 57*(2), 165–173.

Van Rossum, A. M., Fraaij, P. L., & de Groot, R. (2002). Efficacy of highly active antiretroviral therapy in HIV-1 infected children. *The Lancet Infectious Disease, 2*(2), 93–102.

Van Sighem, A. I., Gras, L., Reiss, P., Brinkman, K., de Wolf, F., & ATHENA National Observational Cohort Study. (2010). Life expectancy of recently diagnosed asymptomatic HIV-infected patients approaches that of uninfected individuals. *AIDS, 24*, 1527–1535.

Vernazza, P., Hirschel, B., Bernasconi, E., & Flepp, M. (2008). Les personnes séropositives ne souffrant d'aucune autre MST et suivant un traitment antirétroviral efficace ne transmettent pas le VIH par voie sexuelle. *Bulletin des médecins suisses* 89(5). Link to English translation of the report *HIV-positive individuals without additional sexually transmissible diseases (STD) and on effective anti-retroviral therapy are sexually noninfectious*. Retrieved from http://www.ternyata.org/books/wisdom/swiss_english.pdf.

Waldura, J. F. (2011). Perspective: Prevention of perinatal HIV transmission: The perinatal HIV hotline perspective. *Prevention of Perinatal HIV Transmission, 19*, 23–26.

Wan, T. et al. (2011). Health outcomes for young adults with perinatally acquired HIV-1 infection following transfer to adult services. 17th annual British HIV Association conference, Bournemouth, abstract 031.

Weinberger, D. R., Elvevag, B., & Giedd, J. N. (2005). The adolescent brain: A work in progress. Monograph published by The National Campaign to Prevent Teen Pregnancy. See also "Inside the Teenage Brain." Retrieved from www.frontline.org.

Wiener, L. S. (2004). Disclosure. In S. L. Zeichner & J. S. Read (Eds.), *Textbook of pediatric HIV care* (pp. 667–671). Cambridge: Cambridge University Press.

Wiener, L., Ballard, E., Brennan, T., Battles, H., Martinez, P., & Pao, M. (2008). How I wish to be remembered: The use of an advance care planning document in adolescent and young adult populations. *Journal of Palliative Medicine, 11*, 1309–1313.

Wiener, L., Kohrt, B., Battles, H., & Pao, M. (2011). The HIV experience: Youth identified barriers for transitioning from pediatric to adult care. *Journal of Pediatric Psychology, 36*(2), 141–154.

Wiener, L. S., & Lyon, M. E. (2006). HIV disclosure: Who knows? Who needs to know? Clinical and ethical considerations. In M. E. Lyon & L. J. D'Angelo (Eds.), *Teenagers, HIV, AIDS: Insights from adolescents living with the virus* (pp. 105–126). Westport, CT: Praeger Publishers/Division of Greenwood Press.

Wijngaards-de Meij, L., Stroebe, M., Schut, H., Stroebe, W., Van den Bout, J., Van der Jeijden, P., et al. (2005).

Couples at risk following the death of their child: Predictors of grief versus depression. *Journal of Consulting and Clinical Psychology, 76*, 617–623.

Wood, S. M., Shah, S. S., Steenhoff, A. P., & Rutstein, R. M. (2009). The impact of AIDS diagnoses on long-term neurocognitive and psychiatric outcomes of surviving adolescents with perinatally acquired HIV. *AIDS, 23*(14), 1859–1865.

Woods, S. P., Moore, D. J., Weber, E., & Grant, I. (2009, May, Published on line). Cognitive neuropsychology of HIV-associated neurocognitive disorders. *Neuropsychological Review* DOI 10.1007/s11065-009-9102-5.

World Health Organization. (2003). *Adherence to long-term therapies*. Retrieved from www.who.int/chronic_conditions/adherencereport/en/.

Obesity in Adolescence

Alan M. Delamater, Elizabeth R. Pulgaron, and Amber Daigre

Obesity has increased dramatically in American youth over the past several decades. Given the fact that obesity increases health risks, decreases quality of life, and is a chronic condition and difficult to treat, it constitutes a significant public health issue. The objective of this chapter is to review research concerning the epidemiology and prognosis of obesity in adolescents, etiologic factors, as well as physical health and psychosocial correlates, and approaches to intervention.

Epidemiology and Prognosis

Being overweight is defined as being heavier than is healthy given a person's height. This includes having more body fat than is desired. Typically being classified as an overweight adult consists of having a body mass index (BMI) between 25 and 29.9. An adult is considered obese once his/her BMI is 30 or higher. BMI is calculated by taking a person's weight in kilograms and dividing it by the square of the person's height in meters (CDC, 2009a). A similar calculation is computed to determine a child's BMI; however, gender and age are also added into the equation to account for differences in expected body fat at different developmental levels according to gender. A child or adolescent's BMI which is at or above the 95 percentile compared to same aged and gender peers is considered obese (CDC, 2011); a BMI between the 85th and 95th percentile would be considered in the overweight range.

Although BMI is a generally accepted measure for obesity, it is not diagnostic since it is not a direct measure of body fat. Other measures of body fat distribution include skinfold thickness tests, waist circumference, calculation of waist-to-hip circumference ratios, ultrasound, computed tomography, and magnetic resonance imaging (MRI; CDC, 2009a).

Data from the United States National Health and Nutrition Examination Survey (NHANES) from 2007 to 2008 indicated that 17 % of children aged 2–19 years old met criteria for being obese according to BMI (Ogden, Carroll, Curtin, Lamb, & Flegal, 2010). For the 12–19-year-old group, the overall rate of obesity across ethnic groups and gender was 18 %, with 12 % of the sample having a BMI at or above the 97th percentile. When adolescents were divided into ethnic groups, the data indicated that 24 % of non-Hispanic Black adolescents, 22 % of Hispanic adolescents, and 16 % of non-Hispanic Caucasians met criteria for obesity according to BMI. Using logistic regression models, significant differences in the prevalence of obesity among ethnic groups were evident for adolescents. Specifically, Hispanic males had significantly higher odds of having a high BMI compared with non-Hispanic Caucasian males, and non-Hispanic Black

A.M. Delamater, Ph.D. (✉) • E.R. Pulgaron, Ph.D.
A. Daigre, Ph.D.
University of Miami Miller School of Medicine,
1601 Northwest 12th Avenue, Miami, FL 33136, USA
e-mail: adelamater@med.miami.edu

W.T. O'Donohue et al. (eds.), *Handbook of Adolescent Health Psychology*,
DOI 10.1007/978-1-4614-6633-8_38,

females were significantly more likely than non-Hispanic Caucasian females to have a high BMI.

In addition to the data available from NHANES, there is another national study focused specifically on adolescents and their weight trajectories over time. The US National Longitudinal Study of Adolescent Health began in 1994 and initially recruited over 20,000 adolescents across the country in order to follow this nationally representative cohort into adulthood. Recent reports from this study indicate that obesity prevalence doubled from adolescent years to when the sample entered their early 1920s and then doubled again by the time the sample was in their late 1920s to early 1930s (Gordon-Larsen, The, & Adair, 2010). By 2008, obesity prevalence increased to 36.1 %, and was highest among non-Hispanic Black females. Obesity in adolescence has been associated with continued obesity in young adulthood, especially for non-Hispanic Black females, while across all ethnic and racial groups and for both men and women, only 5 % of normal-weight adolescents become severely obese (BMI > 40) in adulthood (The, Suchindran, North, Popkin, & Gordon-Larsen, 2010).

Etiologic Factors

Being obese is generally thought to be the result of a chronic caloric imbalance, with more calories being consumed than expended each day. History of obesity, hereditary factors, environment, metabolism, behavior, culture, and socioeconomic status all play a role in obesity.

Hereditary Factors and Early Growth

Most obese adolescents were overweight and/or obese as children. In fact, the origins of obesity are being traced to early childhood development. Adiposity rebound is a relatively new construct studied in the pediatric obesity literature. This refers to the time at which young children's BMI begins to increase after a nadir. Children who experience early adiposity rebound (before the age of 5 years) have increases in mean BMI from age three to adolescence while those that experience late adiposity rebound have decreases in BMI from age three to adolescence. Early rebound has also been associated with increased depositions of fat in middle childhood. Data indicate that these differences are maintained into adulthood (Rolland-Cachera, Deheeger, Maillot, & Bellisle, 2006; Williams & Goulding, 2009).

There is also evidence to support a genetic component to obesity. For example, Whitaker, Wright, Pepe, Seidel, and Dietz (1997) found that parental obesity significantly increased the risk of obesity in adulthood for both children that were obese and those who were not, especially when children were under the age of 10 years old. Among those who were obese during childhood, 79 % in the 10–14-year-old group had at least one parent who met criteria for obesity.

Although some of the increased risk for obesity may be attributed to genetics, it is difficult to distinguish the genetic from the environmental component. Historically, high drives for storing fat were followed by periods of stress or high energy use resulting in decreases in body fat. Babies became thinner once they started growing and walking. However, the current environment consists of an excessive availability of high-fat and energy-dense foods combined with an increase in sedentary activities. This combination results in a disconnect between our biology and environment. While there is some inconsistency in the literature, there is evidence to support that both under- and overnutrition while a child is in utero can be related to obesity development (Adair, 2008).

Environmental Factors

The significant rise of obesity rates, specifically within adolescents, may be attributed to several multidimensional environmental changes that have impacted adolescents' perceptions and value of nutritional intake, physical activity, and cognitions about maintaining a healthy lifestyle. While research has implicated the role of genetics and metabolism (Allison, Matz, Pietrobelli, Zannolli, & Faith, 1999; Meyer & Stunkard, 1993) in determining adolescents' weight, the significant rise in adolescent obesity suggests that environmental factors (e.g., changes in nutrition, physical activity, and family environmental factors) are influential.

Dietary Factors

One important environmental factor is the current degree and type of food available to adolescents. Changes in dietary intake among adolescents have been linked to higher daily total energy intake. The consumption of food and beverages with higher levels of fat and sugar has increased substantially (Kantor, 1999; Putnam & Gerrior, 1999; Tippett & Cleveland, 1999). For example, data from the 2007 Youth Risk Behavior Survey indicated that in the past week 79 % of high school students had not eaten fruits and vegetables five or more times per day and 34 % had consumed soda at least one time per day (Eaton et al., 2008). Similar findings regarding factors related to fatty food consumption across countries have been documented (Gerrits et al., 2010), with self-control, concern about diet, and unhealthy eater prototype being related to the amount of fatty foods consumed.

Adolescents' access and frequency of visits to fast-food restaurants, where food is higher in fat and energy relative to food served at home, has increased substantially with over 30 % of youth eating at least one fast-food meal a day and 75 % reporting eating fast food at least once a week (Bowman, Gortmaker, Ebbeling, Pereira, & Ludwig, 2004; French, Story, Neumark-Sztainer, Faulkerson, & Hannan, 2001; Lin, Guthrie, & Blaylock, 1996; Lin, Guthrie, & Frazao, 1999a, 1999b). Further, the frequency of fast-food restaurant use by adolescents has been linked to increased intake of total calories, percent of calories from fat, daily servings of soft drinks, cheeseburgers, french fries, and pizza. An inverse relationship between fast-food restaurant usage and daily servings of fruit, vegetables, and milk has also been documented (French, Story, Neumark-Sztainer, Faulkerson, & Hannan, 2001). In addition to nutritional associations, fast-food restaurant use has also been associated with other behaviors including increased rates of student employment, more time spent watching television, greater availability of "junk food" in the home, and more perceived barriers to healthy eating (French et al., 2001).

Not all unhealthy eating habits can be attributed to the fast-food industry. Even at school, adolescents are frequently limited to school lunches consisting of high calorie foods such as pizza or hamburgers (Miller, Gold, & Silverstein, 2003). In addition, school-wide food practices such as allowing students to have food in the classroom and hallways and using food as a reward are linked to increased BMI in middle school students (Kubik, Lytle, & Story, 2005). Further, the cost of healthy food relative to foods with higher fat and sugar content appears to affect adolescents' food choice. That is, there is some support to suggest that reducing the price of fruit and vegetables within high schools results in a substantial increase in fresh fruit and vegetable sales (French, 2003). There is even evidence to support that adolescents would prefer to have healthier options offered at school. Goslinger, Madsen, Woodward-Lopez, and Crawford (2011) conducted a study with a sample of over 5,000 youth in low-income areas across California which found that most students reported that it was important to have access to purchase fruit at school, more so than they valued the availability of chips, candy, or soda. Although students report wanting healthier choices, there is also evidence to support that the actual behavior of students may differ depending on the availability of unhealthy foods and snacks at school. For example, nearly 20 % of middle school students reported buying snacks from a vending machine at least 2 out of 5 days in the past school week instead of purchasing school lunch (Parks, Sappenfield, Huang, Sherry, & Bensyl, 2010). In general, the choices available from school vending machines include sodas and calorie-dense snacks. Therefore, many researchers and obesity activists promote making environmental changes, especially in the school setting, to assist students in making better nutritional choices.

Physical Activity

In addition to caloric intake, lack of energy expenditure (typically as a result of physical activity) is also a major contributor to adolescent obesity. Sallis, Prochaska, and Taylor (2000) conducted a comprehensive review of the literature on variables that are potentially related to physical activity in youth. Results indicated that adolescents who were males, white, and younger; perceived themselves as competent athletically; previously engaged in physical activity; had support from parents and others; and had opportunities to exercise were more likely to engage in physical activity than those who did not have these attributes.

Several studies have shown that physical activity levels decrease significantly from childhood to adolescence (Heath, Pratt, Warren, & Kann, 1994), particularly among black girls (Kimm et al., 2002). While it is generally believed that the current generation of adolescents is far less active than past generations, an examination of physical activity of high school students between 1993 and 2003 using the Youth Risk Behavior Survey (YRBS) demonstrated that while there were statistically significant decreases in physical activity by high school boys and adolescents in grades nine and ten, decreases over time were generally small (Adams, 2006). That is, children decrease physical activity as they enter adolescence, but the overall trend in decreased physical activity among adolescents from 1993 to 2003 was minimal. However, results from the 2007 national YRBS indicated that among high school students nationwide, 35 % had watched television 3 or more hours per day on an average school day during the past month and 65 % had not met recommended levels of physical activity during the past week (Eaton et al., 2008). Specific traits associated with declines in physical activity in adolescence have been examined. For example, higher perceived behavioral control, support for physical activity, and self-efficacy have been associated with smaller declines in physical activity in a review of the available literature on longitudinal patterns of physical activity in adolescents (Craggs, Corder, Van Sluijs, & Griffin, 2011).

Adolescents' access to physical activity facilities (e.g., parks, public facilities, YMCAs, and schools) within their neighborhood is related to their engagement in exercise and risk of being overweight (Gordon-Larsen, Nelson, Page, & Popkin, 2006). That is, the risk of being an overweight adolescent decreases with increasing number of physical activity facilities available to adolescents within their neighborhood. However, adolescents who live in neighborhoods with a high proportion of ethnic minorities and those with a lower education are at a higher risk for lack of physical activity facilities.

Family Factors

It also appears that the family environment impacts adolescent overweight. Family influence on eating habits begins at a young age and continues into adulthood. One important factor in influencing young children's energy intake is maternal behavior or style related to children's eating. There is substantial research documenting the significant role of maternal behavior in affecting young children's eating behavior. For example, research shows that stringent parental controls over children's food intake can result in preferences for high-fat, energy-dense foods; negatively affect the variety of food children are willing to eat; and alter children's responsiveness to internal cues of hunger and satiety (Birch & Fisher, 1998). Modeling of eating behaviors is another way parents influence childhood obesity. Breakfast consumption in adolescents (which has been identified as having multiple health benefits) has been associated with parental breakfast eating and living in two-parent families (Pearson, Biddle, & Gorely, 2009). In addition to parental modeling of positive eating habits, other aspects of parent involvement have been found to positively influence physical activity in adolescents. Family cohesion, effective parent-child communication and parental engagement have been found to positively predict bouts of moderate to vigorous physical activity per week in both adolescent males and females (Ornelas, Perreira, & Ayala, 2007).

There are also various negative parental influences on obesity rates that have been identified in the literature. Even after controlling for sociodemographic variables, adolescents with an overweight mother or father were at an increased likelihood of being overweight or obese as a young adult based on the US National Longitudinal Study of Adolescent Health (Crossman, Sullivan, & Benin, 2006). Lower parental education and a weaker perception that parents care during adolescence were related to a higher risk for being overweight as an adult female, whereas being African American or Native American reduced the risk for being overweight (Crossman, Sullivan, & Benin, 2006). Adolescent males were at increased risk for becoming overweight as adults when they perceived a close relationship with their parents and when their parents were viewed as trying to control their eating behaviors. Further, the amount of television viewing within the home by adolescents was positively related to an increased BMI in young adulthood (Hancox, Milne, & Poulton, 2004).

Health and Psychological Correlates of Obesity in Adolescence

With increasing rates of obesity among youth populations, it is also important to consider the physical health and psychological correlates and consequences of this condition. The consequences of childhood and adolescent obesity are far reaching, not only including health-related physical outcomes but also psychological, social, and behavioral consequences. The consequences of being overweight may be severe, including higher risk for cardiovascular diseases, type 2 diabetes, cancer, hypertension, dyslipidemia, stroke, orthopedic problems, and sleep apnea (CDC, 2009b). In addition to health consequences, there are also significant psychological and psychosocial consequences of being overweight, including psychological distress, discrimination, and medical treatment expenses for various health problems.

Health Correlates

With increasing rates of obesity among youth, it is important to consider the potential adverse health effects of this condition. The toll of obesity on adolescents' health is well documented. Today adolescents exhibit a higher frequency of health difficulties that were once only seen in adults. Such conditions include high blood pressure, type 2 diabetes, metabolic syndrome, polycystic ovary disease, fatty liver disease, sleep apnea, and orthopedic complications (Daniels, 2006; Dietz, 1998; Reilly, 2005).

Reilly et al. (2003) compiled empirical data which described the health consequences of obesity in youth. Among these health problems were associations between obesity (as measured by BMI and central obesity/waist circumference) and cardiovascular risk factors such as high blood pressure, dyslipidemia, abnormal left ventricular mass, and insulin resistance. The prevalence of cardiovascular risk factors among obese youth is high and has been estimated at 58 % with one risk factor and 25 % with two or more (Freedman, Dietz, Srinivasan, & Berenson, 1999).

Related to increased cardiovascular risk is the risk for metabolic syndrome among obese children and adolescents. This condition refers to the clustering of metabolic and cardiovascular risk factors (i.e., large waist circumference, high triglycerides, low levels of HDL cholesterol, high blood pressure, and high fasting blood glucose or insulin resistance) and is associated with increased risk for type 2 diabetes. Estimates of the prevalence of metabolic syndrome among obese youth range from 6.8 to 28.7 %, though it is speculated that these may underestimate the true extent of the problem (Cook, Weitzman, Auinger, Nguyen, & Dietz, 2003; Weiss et al., 2004). Weiss et al. (2004) found that the prevalence of metabolic syndrome increased with the severity of obesity, reaching as much as 50 % in extremely obese children. Nathan and Moran (2008) recently estimated that half of obese adolescents have metabolic syndrome.

Asthma also represents a common and prevalent complication associated with obesity in youth. Previously, researchers were unclear about the association between asthma and obesity, but recent studies illustrate a significant relationship between these conditions (Gennuso, Epstein, Paluch, & Cerny, 1998; Reilly, 2005). Visness et al. (2010) reported results on the relationship between asthma and obesity based on data collected in a 7-year NHANES. Results of the survey, which reflected data on 16,000 children and adolescents, showed significant relationships between obesity and a diagnosis of asthma, with non-atopic asthma showing a greater correlation. This relationship was previously demonstrated in a study of 300 Israeli youth, where obesity was associated with more wheezing, more frequent physician-diagnosed asthma, and more prevalent inhaler use than in non-obese youth (Bibi et al., 2004).

The long-term health consequences of obesity in youth are also important to consider. Several researchers have reported the long-term continuation of cardiovascular risk from childhood into adulthood (Freedman et al., 1999; Reilly, 2005) and have cited a significant relationship between obesity in adolescence with premature mortality (Daniels, 2006; Must, Jacques, Dallal, Bajema, & Dietz, 1992). Such studies are difficult to conduct given their longitudinal design; however, there is evidence to support the lifetime trajectory of obesity and related health complications.

Psychological and Psychosocial Correlates

In addition to the health consequences of obesity, psychological and psychosocial functioning are also areas of concern for obese adolescents. Body image difficulties represent one area where obese adolescents may struggle with psychological challenges. Researchers have noted adolescence as a time of particular vulnerability to body image concerns (Wardle & Cooke, 2005). There is an established relationship between weight issues and body dissatisfaction, most notably in girls (Davidson & Birch, 2002; Davidson, Markey, & Birch, 2003; Ricciardelli & McCabe, 2001). Among adolescent boys, findings show body dissatisfaction among overweight as well as underweight boys (Presnell, Bearman, & Stice, 2004). These findings suggest that body dissatisfaction is certainly a prevalent concern among obese adolescents; however, it is not a concern that is specific only to the overweight adolescent population.

Obese and overweight adolescents exhibit psychological difficulties beyond those related to dissatisfaction with body image. The effects may extend into other parts of their lives such as perceptions of competence with physical activity, school, as well as in social settings. For example, obese girls are more likely to be victims of bullying, while obese boys are more likely to be victims of bullying as well as perpetrators of bullying (Griffiths, Wolke, Page & Horwood, 2006). The social effects of obesity were described in an investigation of the relationship between overweight and social marginalization (Strauss & Pollack, 2003). Results showed that overweight adolescents were rated as less popular than their normal-weight peers and were less likely to be selected as friends by their peers, a social stigmatization trend that has also been shown among preschool-aged children (Musher-Eizenman, Holub, Barnhart Miller, Goldstein, & Edwards-Leeper, 2004). Overweight adolescents have been described as being "more isolated and more peripheral to social networks" and reported to have lower rates of best friend reciprocity (Strauss, Smith, Frame, & Forehand, 1985).

The social correlates of obesity may be largely explained by the societal stigma related to obesity that is well documented in the literature. Obese individuals are frequently stereotyped as ugly, mean, stupid, and lazy (Faulkner et al., 2001; Latner & Stunkard, 2003; Wardle, Volz, & Golding, 1995). Similar descriptions have been given in studies with young children presented with pictures of children of varying physical characteristics. Young children consistently rated overweight children as least liked and least likely to be a playmate (Richardson, 1971). Given the association between adolescent friendships and self-esteem, it is hypothesized that social marginalization contributes to reduced self-esteem and increased rates of depression among overweight teens (Caskey & Felker, 1971; Strauss et al., 1985).

Of the many psychological consequences of obesity, the prevalence of depression among overweight and obese adolescents is a topic of considerable debate. Some studies found no association between depressive symptoms and BMI (e.g., Friedman & Brownell, 1995; Vila et al., 2004). Stice and Bearman (2001) found that higher body mass in adolescent girls did not predict depression 20 months and 4 years after enrollment.

Similar results were described by Goodman and Whitaker (2002), showing no association between obesity at the time of enrollment and depression at a 1-year follow-up visit.

However, other researchers have found a significant relationship between obesity and depression among teens. In a study of Chinese adolescents, Xie et al. (2005) reported a significant relationship between high BMI and higher self-reported depressive symptoms among girls, mediated by perceived peer isolation. When compared to normal-weight peers, obese adolescents had significantly more depressive symptoms, and this difference persisted when comparing obese adolescents to those who were in the overweight range (Sjoberg, Nilsson, & Leppert, 2005). In a study by Stice, Hayward, Cameron, Killen, and Barr (2000), body dissatisfaction and dietary restraint were shown to be significant risk factors for depression among adolescent girls and in a study of seventh, ninth, and eleventh graders, Faulkner et al. (2001) found more and stronger associations for obese adolescent girls than for obese boys. These associations included greater likelihood of social isolation, feelings of hopelessness, as well as greater likelihood for past suicide attempts. Together these results indicate an inconsistent relationship between obesity and depression in adolescents.

In addition to the psychological and psychosocial consequences of obesity, there has also been research addressing the prevalence of psychiatric disorders among obese adolescents. Lamertz, Jacobi, Yassouridis, Arnold, and Henkel (2002) investigated this issue in their community survey study of German youth ranging in age from 14 to 24 years. Results indicated no significant relationships between BMI and mental disorders or psychopathology (i.e., anxiety, substance abuse, mood disorders, somatoform disorders). In another community-based study, researchers found clinical diagnoses of anxiety and depression to be associated with higher weight status and higher BMI (Anderson, Cohen, Naumova, & Must, 2006), which they suggested may support anxiety and depression as precursors to obesity later in life. When the rates of psychopathology were investigated among a population of extremely obese adolescents (BMI>40), significant differences emerged between the extremely obese group and the obese population-based controls, with the extremely obese teens having higher rates of mood, anxiety, somatoform, and eating disorders (Britz et al., 2000).

Overall, the research findings indicate that obese adolescents are at increased risk for psychological and psychosocial difficulties which are more likely the consequence of obesity rather than causal factors. Quality of life has been shown to be significantly lower in obese youth and at a level comparable to youth with cancer (Schwimmer, Burnwinkle, & Varni, 2003). A study conducted by Gortmaker, Must, Perrin, Sobol, and Dietz (1993) followed obese adolescents for 7 years. Results indicated that young obese women completed less years of school, had lower household incomes, experienced higher rates of poverty, and were less likely to be married than women who had not been obese. Obese men were less likely to be married. This study demonstrated the socioeconomic discrimination that many obese individuals may experience.

Obesity Interventions

Given the increasing rates and persistence of obesity in youth as well as the many adverse consequences, researchers have focused their efforts on developing interventions to treat obesity in adolescents and prevent its persistence into adulthood. Interventions have targeted increasing physical activity and improving dietary behavior through several approaches (Kamath et al., 2008), including schools, clinics, community-based programs, and eHealth programs delivered over the Internet or with mobile technology. Medical interventions including various medications and bariatric surgery have also been studied.

School-Based Interventions

Parents identify schools as having a great responsibility in reducing obesity in youth (Kropski, Keckley, & Jensen, 2008). Furthermore, recent trends in national legislation identify school-based intervention programs as preferable methods for reducing rates of obesity (Foster et al., 2008). Several approaches have been used in school-based obesity programs, including nutritional interventions (e.g., James, Thomas, Cavan, & Kerr, 2004), physical activity interventions (e.g., Sallis et al., 1993), and combinations of both intervention strategies (e.g., Coleman et al., 2005). The objective in these programs is generally preventive in focus, with an attempt to change behavioral patterns in all youth rather than selecting only overweight youth.

School-based health education programs have been somewhat successful in reducing dietary fat intake, increasing fruit and vegetable consumption, and increasing physical activity in children (Kelder, Perry, Lytle, & Klepp, 1994; Killen et al., 1988; Luepker et al., 1996; Perry et al., 1998; Sallis et al., 1997). These school-based programs have had several components, including a health education curriculum, as well as making changes in the school food service and physical education (PE) curriculum. Newer school-based programs have emphasized changing the school environment through social marketing approaches (Walsh, Rudd, Moeykens, & Maloney, 1993) so that health promotion attains a higher priority for children, teachers, school administrators, food service personnel, as well as parents.

In school-based obesity intervention programs focused on physical activity, researchers have geared programs toward increased duration of aerobic exercise during PE times (e.g., Sallis et al., 1993, 1997). The Eat Well and Keep Moving classroom-based intervention program focused on increasing fruit and vegetable consumption, limiting television viewing, and increasing physical activity (Lin et al., 1999a). The intervention was delivered by classroom teachers who integrated the intervention into their typical classroom curriculum. Similarly, Project SPARK included a physical activity curriculum whereby students participated in a "recommended schedule" of three 30-min classes per week, divided into three segments (i.e., warm up, cardiovascular, cool down/stretch) (Sallis et al., 1993, 1997).

Newer school-based health promotion programs have focused specifically on reducing obesity and several have been shown to be effective (Davis, Davis, Northington, Moll, & Kolar, 2002; Doak, Visscher, Renders, & Seideil, 2006). For example, Planet Health (Gortmaker et al., 1999) focused specifically on reducing obesity and added intervention components that targeted reducing time spent viewing television and playing video games. This intervention was successful at reducing obesity in girls, and decreasing television influenced the reduction in obesity. Another school-based study focused only on reducing television viewing and demonstrated a reduction in obesity (Robinson, 1999). The reduction of sedentary behavior is clearly an integral component of weight loss programs (Epstein et al., 1995) and has become a more prominent focus of treatment of obese youth in recent years (Leung, Agaronov, Grytsenko, & Yeh, 2011; Wahi, Parkin, Beyene, Uleryk, & Birken, 2011).

This focus on nutrition and physical activity is common among school-based intervention programs. Physical activity is often measured via minutes of participation in a PE classroom protocol. For example, participants in the Healthy Study Group diabetes risk reduction project participated in a minimum of 150 min of moderate to vigorous activity over 2 weeks during the required minimum of 225 min of PE class time (The Healthy Study Group, 2010). This multisite national study evaluated the effects of a comprehensive multicomponent school-based program to reduce obesity and risk of type 2 diabetes in 6th grade children followed until the end of 8th grade. Besides increasing physical activity, the program emphasized healthy nutrition, behavioral knowledge and skills, and communication strategies and social marketing to support the intervention. Results showed the intervention schools had greater reductions in BMI, prevalence of obesity, and fasting insulin (indicating reduced risk for type 2 diabetes).

Clinic-Based Interventions

Dietary Approaches

Several clinic-based studies have compared the effects of different dietary interventions with overweight adolescents, and preliminary findings suggest that type of nutritional intake may affect weight loss. In a 12-week randomized controlled trial comparing the effects of a low-carbohydrate diet with those of a low-fat diet on weight loss and serum lipids in overweight adolescents, those in the low-carbohydrate group displayed significantly greater reductions in their BMI and improvements in non-HDL cholesterol levels relative to adolescents in the low-fat group (Sondike, Copperman, & Jacobson, 2003). Adolescents in the low-fat group displayed improvements in LDL cholesterol level, but those in the low-carbohydrate group did not show these improvements. Less than half of treatment participants returned for a 1-year follow-up assessment, but none of them returned to their baseline BMI. In another trial with overweight adolescents comparing reduced carbohydrate and fat diets, the reduced carbohydrate treatment group displayed greater reductions in BMI and fat mass at 6- and 12-month follow-up (Ebbeling, Leidig, Sinclair, Hangen, & Ludwig, 2003).

Another approach to obesity intervention involves hospitalization or residential treatment to implement specific dietary interventions. One comparative study of dietary restrictions was conducted in a residential setting over 9 months. In this study, 121 extremely overweight adolescents were randomized into either an increased protein dietary intake or decreased carbohydrate intake group. Participants significantly reduced their weight, but there were no differences between dietary groups in weight loss (Rolland-Cachera et al., 2004). At 2-year follow-up, adolescents regained a significant portion of their weight due to increased energy intake (particularly snacking) and sedentary behaviors after returning home. However, it is important to note that recent research with obese adults indicates that reduced calorie diets result in weight loss regardless of which macronutrients are emphasized (Sacks et al., 2009).

Seventeen obese adolescents were admitted into a hospital for 1 month and then followed in an outpatient setting for a total of 12 months to implement a protein-sparing modified fast diet (a high-protein, low-calorie diet). Results indicated that nearly half displayed significant decreases in body weight after 1 year (Stallings, Archibald, Pencharz, Harrison, & Bell, 1988). In another report involving inpatient treatment, 122 obese youth participated in a 10-month comprehensive program with dietary restriction with a 14-month follow-up. Results from this non-randomized study indicated that these youth lost 49 % of their weight after 10 months, and at follow-up they maintained a 32 % weight loss; they also reported improved dietary habits and psychological well-being (Braet, Tanghe, Decaluwé, Moens, & Rosseel, 2004).

In another non-randomized study, 56 obese adolescents participated in a comprehensive 1-year outpatient program consisting of an acute phase with a very low-calorie diet (800 calories per day) followed by a less restrictive hypocaloric diet, moderate-intensity physical exercise, and behavior modification with parental involvement to reinforce behavioral changes (Sothern, Udall, Suskind, Vargas, & Blecker, 2000). Most youth (93 %) completed the acute phase with a mean weight loss of 9.4 kg; 63 % completed the 1-year program. The results at 1 year indicated that significant reductions in BMI occurred, particularly for the most obese adolescents. This study provides preliminary support for very low-calorie dietary approaches, but it is difficult to evaluate the unique effects of parent participation, exercise, and diet on treatment outcome. More controlled work using this approach is needed.

Multicomponent Family Approaches

Family-based behavioral interventions targeting both dietary intake and physical activity have been shown to be efficacious in overweight children, with significant weight loss maintained even 10 years after treatment (Epstein, Valoski, Wing, & McCurley, 1994, 1998), but fewer family-based studies have been conducted with overweight adolescents. In an early study of multicomponent family intervention, overweight adolescents (ages 13–17) were randomly assigned to either a mother and adolescent seen separately condition or adolescent seen alone condition (Coates, Killen, & Slinkard, 1982). Treatment included 14 weekly, 90-min group sessions, two-parent sessions, on-site exercise, and leader-facilitated interactions about weight control behaviors. At posttreatment, both treatment groups exhibited decreases in percentage overweight (8.6 % and 5.1 %, respectively, for adolescent-mother and adolescent alone). At 18-month follow-up, both groups continued to show decreases in percentage overweight from baseline (8.4 % adolescent-mother, 8.2 % child alone).

In a study with a predominately Caucasian sample of 12–16-year-old adolescents that were randomly assigned to three treatment formats (i.e., mothers and adolescents seen separately, mothers and adolescents seen together, adolescents seen alone), treatment type affected outcomes (Brownell, Kelman, & Stunkard, 1983). Treatment included 45–60-min group sessions for 1 year (16 weekly sessions then 1 session every 2 months) and participants were provided with nutrition and exercise education, rewards for attendance and weight loss, stimulus control, and behavior modification. At posttreatment, the mothers and adolescents that were seen separately displayed better outcomes (17.1 % decrease in percent overweight) than when mothers and adolescents were seen together (7.0 % decrease in percent overweight) or when adolescents were seen alone (6.8 % decrease in percent overweight). However, a study that sought to replicate these findings in a predominately African American adolescent sample was unsuccessful (Wadden et al., 1990). That is, treating the adolescent and the mother separately did not have a differential impact on treatment outcomes, although weight loss was positively correlated to the number of sessions attended by the parent.

In a randomized controlled trial of a family-based intervention conducted in Israel, 46 6–16-year-old overweight youth were randomly assigned to a multicomponent 3-month treatment group or a control group (Nemet et al., 2005). Youth were first invited to a session with their parents and a dietitian, and then youth meetings alternated with parent meetings, for a total of six meetings in the 3-month program. Participants followed a balanced hypocaloric diet, with a deficit of 30 % from reported intake or intake 15 % less than daily required intake, and also participated in an hour-long physical training program twice weekly; they were also encouraged to complete 30–45 min of walking or weight-bearing sport activities at least once per week. At posttreatment, youths in the multicomponent intervention group achieved significant reductions in body weight, BMI, and body fat percentage and significant increases in physical activity compared to participants in the control group. Long-term effects were positive with maintenance of body weight and a reduction in BMI and body fat percentages of the intervention group.

One promising intervention for adolescent obesity is the ShapeDown program (Mellin, Slunkard, & Irwin, 1987). In this non-randomized study, adolescents (ages 12–18) attended 14 weekly, 90-min group sessions. Sessions included nutrition education, on-site exercise, two parent sessions, and discussions about weight control behaviors. At posttreatment, adolescents who participated in the program demonstrated a significant decrease in their percentage overweight (5.9 %) and at a 15-month follow-up, program participants displayed further decreases in the percentage overweight (9.9 %).

A randomized controlled trial was conducted to evaluate the effects of an exercise program on BMI and psychological outcomes in 81 overweight adolescents (Daley, Copeland, Wright, Roalfe, & Wales, 2006). Overweight youth (ages 11–16 years) were randomly assigned to receive exercise therapy, an equal contact exercise placebo, or usual care. The exercise therapy group engaged in aerobic exercise activities for 30 min three times weekly for eight weeks (24 sessions). During the first 12 sessions, participants were also introduced to cognitive-behavioral strategies consistent with the transtheoretical model. During the last 12 sessions, behavioral interventions including goal setting, self-monitoring, and increasing social support were utilized. The results did not show significant reductions in BMI; however, the exercise therapy group and exercise contact group displayed significant improvements in physical self-worth compared to the usual care group which persisted 14- and 28-week follow-ups.

A recent trial examined the effects of a multicomponent family-based behavioral outpatient program, relative to a brief family intervention in overweight children and adolescents (Steele et al., 2012). Significant reductions in BMI and improved quality of life occurred for both treatment groups at posttreatment and maintained at 1-year follow-up. However, these effects were noted for children; neither intervention approach was effective at reducing BMI of adolescents.

Primary Care Interventions

Besides the outpatient specialty clinic setting and residential treatment facilities, clinical interventions for overweight adolescents have been implemented in the primary care setting. Pediatricians have an excellent opportunity to screen adolescents for weight status at regular office visits. However, a national survey of pediatrician's practices indicated that adolescent overweight is diagnosed significantly less by pediatricians than the national prevalence of adolescent overweight (Cook, Weitzman, Auinger, & Barlow, 2005). This indicates that many overweight adolescents go undiagnosed and untreated. Despite this, innovative attempts are being made to develop feasible interventions for overweight adolescents that can be conducted in primary care settings.

For example, a multicomponent treatment called Patient-Centered Assessment and Counseling for Exercise Plus Nutrition (PACE+) was developed for use in a primary care setting (Patrick et al., 2001). In this study of 117 youth ages 11–18 years, participants completed an interactive computer program designed to increase their moderate physical activity to vigorous physical activity, reduce fat intake, and increase fruit and vegetable intake. PACE+ components were based on the trans-theoretical model and guided participants to set specific goals for one nutrition and one physical activity behavior they were most ready to change. After completing the computer program, participants received physical activity and nutrition counseling from a health care provider, and then were randomly assigned to a no-contact control group, frequent mail group, infrequent mail and telephone group, or frequent mail and telephone group to evaluate a low-cost follow-up strategy over a 4-month trial. All groups exhibited significant improvements in healthy dietary intake and in moderate physical activity.

In another multicomponent behavioral weight control intervention implemented in a primary care office, 43 overweight adolescents were randomly assigned to a Healthy Habits program group or a traditional single session of physician weight counseling group (Saelens et al., 2002). Youth in the Healthy Habits group completed a computer program adapted from the PACE+ specifically designed for overweight adolescents that developed an individualized action plan. The action plan was then discussed with their physician, who tailored their counseling to the specific action plans. Participants then received weekly follow-up phone counseling calls for eight weeks and then biweekly calls for an additional 6–8 weeks. Phone counseling included teaching adolescents about weight change and dietary and physical activity behaviors, goals, and self-monitoring to facilitate goal achievement. Manuals were provided to assist in acquiring behavioral skills related to weight change, and parents were sent information sheets highlighting how to reinforce their child and assist their child with structuring the environment to promote healthy lifestyle habits. The results indicated that the intervention resulted in modest decreases in BMI; the intervention group did not return to their baseline weight at follow-up, but the control group's BMI increased at posttreatment and follow-up. These results suggest that the Healthy Habits program at least helps overweight adolescents maintain their BMI, whereas those who did not receive the intervention continued to gain weight.

In a recent large randomized trial including 878 young overweight adolescents, a primary care-delivered behavioral intervention was compared with a sun exposure intervention (Patrick et al., 2006). The intervention consisted of office-based, computer-assisted diet and physical activity assessment and stage-based goal setting followed by brief health care provider counseling and 12 months of monthly mail and telephone counseling. Although there were no reductions in BMI over 1 year, youth in the behavioral intervention did show significant improvements in several health behaviors, including reduced time spent in sedentary behavior; girls in the intervention group exhibited reduction in saturated fat consumption, and boys showed increases in physical activity. Overall, these findings suggest that brief computer-assisted behavioral interventions delivered in the primary care setting with follow-up can improve health behaviors of overweight adolescents.

Community-Based Interventions

Given the large numbers of overweight adolescents, and the challenges of providing treatment to them through clinic-based programs, researchers have examined the effects of delivering programs based in various community settings. For example, programs for overweight adolescents have been delivered in churches, schools, and other programs available in the community.

Churches may be a particularly effective setting to deliver weight loss interventions for adolescents because they are located in convenient locations close to home, and many families attend church regularly. In a multicomponent intervention for overweight African American girls ages 12–16 years, 10 churches were randomly assigned to either a high-intensity or moderate-intensity intervention (Resnicow, Taylor, Baskin, & McCarty, 2005). The high-intensity intervention included 24–26 sessions and girls participated in every session with parents attending every other session. Each session included information about dietary intervention and 30 min of physical exercise. In addition, girls were provided two-way paging devices so that they could receive messages throughout the day about dietary intake and physical exercise. Participants also received four to six motivational interviewing telephone calls over the course of treatment. Motivational interviewing for the treatment of obesity in adolescents has received increasing research attention in recent years (Resnicow, Davis, & Rollnick, 2006). The moderate-intensity intervention included six sessions and topics addressed included fat, fad diets, barriers to physical activity, and the benefits of physical activity. The results showed no significant differences in BMI over time or between groups over the 6-month intervention period. However, girls who attended greater than 75 % of sessions showed a small decrease in BMI (0.8 units), suggesting that adherence to treatment has an impact on adolescent treatment outcomes.

In another community application, "adventure therapy" was combined with cognitive-behavioral treatment for overweight adolescents in a randomized trial comparing the peer-enhanced adventure therapy with a standard cognitive-behavioral weight loss intervention involving parents and structured exercise activities held at the clinic (Jelalian, Mehlenbeck, Lloyd-Richardson, Birmaher, & Wing, 2005). The peer group adventure activities occurred in various community settings. Participants in both groups demonstrated significant reductions in weight over time, 4 months after treatment and also at follow-up 6 months later. More youth in the adventure therapy group maintained a significant weight loss at follow-up than those in standard treatment, and older adolescents in the adventure group had greater weight loss than older adolescents in the standard group. These findings suggest the benefits of adding peer group fun activities as an adjunct to more traditionally delivered outpatient family programs.

Providing effective treatment is especially challenging for the population of ethnic minority youth who have greater obesity rates and are more likely to be of lower income status. Delivering treatment programs using neighborhood schools may be a more effective way to reach many overweight youth than asking families to take their children to specialty outpatient programs at tertiary care medical centers, particularly because of the limited transportation options of many lower income families. This method was used in a recent study that compared delivery of a family program held at schools compared with a control group in which youth visited the outpatient clinic every 6 months for medical monitoring by physicians along with brief counseling by dietitians and social workers (Savoye et al., 2011). The healthy lifestyle program delivered at schools included an intensive phase of two meetings each week for 6 months followed by a less intensive phase of meetings held every 2 weeks for an additional 6 months. Youth participated in exercise activities and nutrition behavior modification, while parents attended nutrition-related meetings that emphasized the importance of them modeling healthy behavior change for their children.

In this study, 209 obese 6–16-year-old children of mixed ethnic minority and low-income backgrounds participated and were randomized to receive either the program held at schools or the standard clinical follow-up program. After the 12-month treatment program, follow-up measures were obtained 12 months later, allowing for determination of effects over a 2-year period. Although there was considerable attrition over time, the results demonstrated significant reductions in BMI for the school group relative to the control group which were maintained at 2-year follow-up. In addition, these youth had significant improvements in their metabolic risk profile, including reductions in cholesterol and insulin resistance (Savoye et al., 2011).

A community site was also utilized in a study designed to examine the effects of exercise intensity on cardiovascular fitness and insulin resistance in overweight adolescents over an 8-month treatment program. Eighty participants were randomly assigned to one of three groups: lifestyle education (LSE), LSE and moderate-intensity physical training, or LSE and high-intensity physical training (Gutin et al., 2002; Kang et al., 2002). Most youth (69 %) were African American and were provided transportation to the community-based program after school. During LSE, adolescents received information about nutrition, physical activity, psychosocial factors associated with obesity, coping skills, and behavior modification. While no groups displayed changes in BMI, the combined physical training (high-intensity and moderate-intensity groups) and LSE group displayed significant improvements in cardiovascular fitness and the high-intensity group displayed improvements in insulin resistance compared to the LSE alone group.

Medical Interventions

Pharmacological Therapies

Three of the most common drugs in recent adolescent obesity treatment research include sibutramine, orlistat, and metformin. In two randomized controlled trials, the efficacy of combined sibutramine and behavior treatment on reducing weight in overweight adolescents was evaluated (Berkowitz, Wadden, Tershakovec, & Cronquist, 2003; Berkowitz et al., 2006). The first study with 82 overweight adolescents demonstrated the short-term efficacy of the addition of sibutramine to a 6-month family-based behavioral weight loss program in reducing weight compared to the behavioral therapy and placebo control group (Berkowitz et al., 2003). However, medication dose had to be reduced or discontinued in many participants to manage the increases in blood pressure, heart rate, and other symptoms.

In a larger multicenter double-blind trial of the efficacy of a 1-year sibutramine and behavior intervention, the behavior therapy plus sibutramine treatment group resulted in significantly greater improvements in overweight adolescents' (ages 12–16) BMI, body weight, triglyceride levels, high-density lipoprotein cholesterol levels, insulin levels, and insulin sensitivity relative to the behavior therapy plus placebo group (Berkowitz et al., 2006). Overall, adverse events led to 23 sibutramine participants (6.3 %) being removed from the medication. In much smaller trials examining the efficacy of sibutramine with Brazilian and Mexican overweight adolescents, significant reductions in BMI were also found (Garcia-Morales et al., 2006; Godoy-Matos et al., 2005). However, because of the risk of adverse cardiovascular side effects, sibutramine is no longer being considered a front-line medical approach to treatment of obesity in youth.

In a study that employed similar multicenter randomized controlled trial methodology, the efficacy of a 1-year trial of an orlistat plus diet, exercise, and family-based behavioral intervention was evaluated with overweight adolescents ages 12–16 years (Chanoine, Hampl, Jensen, Boldrin, & Hauptman, 2005). There was a significant decrease in BMI in both treatment groups until week 12. The BMI of participants in the orlistat treatment group stabilized from 12 weeks to 1 year, whereas the control group's BMI increased slightly over time. A smaller randomized trial also supported the use of orlistat in reducing overweight adolescents' weight, BMI, total cholesterol, low-density lipoprotein-cholesterol, fasting insulin, and fasting glucose (Ozkan, Bereket, Turan, & Keskin, 2004). However, there are significant gastrointestinal side effects with this medication that may not be acceptable to most adolescents.

Metformin has also been evaluated for the treatment of adolescent obesity. Three randomized trials with relatively small sample sizes provided preliminary support for the use of metformin in treating obese adolescents. Specifically, metformin treatment (from 8 weeks to 6 months in length) resulted in greater weight loss, reductions in BMI, and fasting insulin compared to control groups (Freemark & Bursey, 2001; Kay et al., 2001; Srinivasan et al., 2006). However, the long-term effect of metformin on adolescent overweight is unknown. Larger multisite trials of this medication are needed to gain a better understanding of its long-term effectiveness for weight control in adolescents as well as their potential side effects.

Bariatric Surgery

Bariatric surgery for morbidly obese adolescents is being increasingly used and generating considerable controversy. The development of effective weight management surgery is leading to a decrease in postoperative complications associated with surgery in adolescents (Inge et al., 2004). Decreased complications and increased safety of bariatric surgery are providing severely obese adolescents who have a history of failing at other organized weight loss interventions an alternative intervention for weight control.

Research indicates that bariatric gastric bypass surgery is efficacious for treating severely overweight adolescents and related health comorbidities (Garcia, Langford, & Inge, 2003). Research has shown that bariatric surgery has larger improvements in short-term and long-term follow-up BMIs compared with other weight loss interventions (Inge, Xanthakos, & Zeller, 2007; Rand & MacGregor, 1994). However, the effectiveness of bariatric surgery in reducing weight should be viewed with caution as adolescents who receive the surgery are morbidly obese with BMIs greater than 40. As a result, they have more weight to lose than moderately or mildly overweight adolescents. Besides significant weight loss, other positive results reported include excellent psychosocial adjustment (i.e., improved self-esteem, social relationships, and appearance) up to 6 years after surgery (Rand & MacGregor, 1994).

Adjustable banding is increasingly being used with adolescent patients because the adjustability in the gastric band can better accommodate the needs of a physically developing individual. This can allow for a progression of weight loss and degree of restriction most appropriate over time, avoiding potential problems with nutritional deficiencies (Garcia et al., 2003). If there are complications, the gastric band can be surgically removed. Preliminary studies have demonstrated that laparoscopic adjustable gastric banding in severely overweight adolescents results in significant reductions in weight at short-term follow-up (as early as 6 months) and at long-term follow-up (up to 6 years postoperative) (Angrisani et al., 2005; Fielding & Duncombe, 2005; Nadler, Youn, Ginsburg, Ren, & Fielding, 2007). However, more well-controlled larger studies of adolescent bariatric surgery are needed to demonstrate the potential benefits and risks associated with bariatric surgery before surgery is integrated as a standard treatment for extreme adolescent overweight. In addition, more studies concerning the psychosocial outcomes for adolescents after bariatric surgery are needed.

eHealth Interventions

The Internet is considered by many to be "next transformation in the delivery of health care" (Kassirer, 1995). The use of the Internet and other digital technologies such as smart cell phones and text messaging for the delivery of behavioral health interventions has been termed eHealth. Over 75 % of Americans are estimated to have Internet access (Bell, Redd, & Rainie, 2004) and studies show that about 80 % of adult Internet users in the USA seek health-related information (Fox, 2005). Parents of children with a chronic health condition are more likely to use the Internet for health information than parents of healthy children (Tuffrey & Finlay, 2002). Research has generally shown that Internet health interventions have favorable treatment outcomes (Murray, Burns, See Tai, Lai, & Nazareth, 2009).

Several studies have demonstrated the efficacy of Internet-based approaches for weight control (Fontaine & Allison, 2002). Favorable results were obtained in several Internet behavioral weight loss programs for adults (McCoy, Couch, Duncan, & Lynch, 2005; Rothert et al., 2006; Tate, Jackvony, & Wing, 2003). A recent review of weight loss programs delivered over the Internet concludes that this approach may be an alternative to face-to-face weight loss programs (Saperstein, Atkinson, & Gold, 2007) with tailored social cognitive theory-based interventions associated with lifestyle behaviors and weight loss for up to a year (Winett, Tate, Anderson, Wojcik, & Winett, 2005). A recent weight loss study conducted in primary care settings with adults showed that a remotely delivered behavioral intervention (i.e., study-specific web site, email, and telephone support) was as effective as the same intervention delivered in person for achieving weight loss over 2 years (Appel et al., 2011).

A recent meta-analytic review of eHealth interventions for various pediatric health conditions demonstrated that eHealth programs that incorporated behavioral methods such as self-monitoring, feedback, and contingency management had larger effect sizes than those that were didactic and educational (Cushing & Steele, 2010). Several reports suggest the efficacy of web-based interventions for use with adolescents, particularly for improving lifestyle health behaviors related to weight loss (Winett et al., 1999), with better results among youth utilizing the web site more frequently (Frenn et al., 2005; Williamson et al., 2005). However, decreased web use occurred over time and weight loss was not maintained at 2 years (Williamson et al., 2006). Other studies have demonstrated the efficacy of web interventions for improving dietary (Long et al., 2006) and physical activity (Jago et al., 2006) habits of young adolescents. An Internet program was also successful in increasing fruit and vegetable intake and physical activity in 8–10-year-old African American girls at risk for obesity (Thompson, Baranowski, Cullen, & Baranowski, 2007). Text messaging was positively received by adolescents participating in a weight loss program (Woolford et al., 2011).

Summary and Conclusions

Epidemiologic studies indicate that there is an epidemic of obesity among adolescents in the United States, with about one-third of all adolescents being classified as overweight and approximately 17 % being considered obese. Studies indicate that adolescents from lower income and ethnic minority backgrounds have greater rates of obesity. Because most overweight adolescents were overweight during their childhood, the prevention of adolescent overweight and obesity must begin with prevention of childhood obesity. Overweight adolescents are at increased risk for various health-related and psychosocial co-morbidities, both now and in the future. The likelihood is very high that overweight adolescents will remain overweight as adults, increasing their risks for developing various health problems, including cardiovascular disease and type 2 diabetes. Therefore, identifying and implementing effective treatments for overweight adolescents is an urgent issue of great public health significance.

While hereditary and early growth factors are significant influences, it is clear that environmental factors, including family behaviors such as parental modeling and feeding styles, play a major role in the etiology of adolescent obesity. Research findings indicate that adolescents who engage in unhealthy dietary behaviors such as frequent consumption of fast food, sweetened beverages, and high-fat foods, and in combination with reduced levels of physical activity and increased sedentary behaviors, achieve a positive energy balance over time which results in increased fat storage and excess body weight. Overweight adolescents are likely to experience psychological distress, depression, and reduced quality of life, particularly if they are teased by others about their weight.

Review of intervention studies provides some support for the efficacy of multicomponent family-based behavioral interventions delivered in outpatient clinical programs that address weight loss through modification of dietary and physical activity lifestyle behaviors. Such interventions that include parental involvement and support, as well as the involvement of peers, appear to hold promise for sustained weight loss, but more research is needed to achieve greater weight loss that can be maintained over time, particularly for severely obese adolescents. However, given the large numbers of overweight adolescents needing treatment, researchers must focus on ways to reach and deliver effective interventions, considering the fact that most families will likely not seek out specialty outpatient programs located in tertiary medical centers. More research is therefore needed to evaluate the efficacy and costs of interventions delivered in community settings such as schools, churches, and primary care clinics, as well as over the Internet, in order to provide treatment to more adolescents.

More work is also needed on methods to motivate, engage, and sustain adolescents and their families in treatment, as research indicates better outcomes with increased program participation and longer duration of treatment. Motivational interviewing appears to be a useful therapeutic strategy, but more studies demonstrating its effectiveness with weight control in adolescents are needed. While residential programs may be another treatment option for extremely overweight adolescents, there are currently no controlled studies with long-term follow-up to support their use. Medical interventions including pharmacological and surgical approaches have shown some efficacy, but more research is needed to demonstrate their safety and acceptability, as well as long-term effects.

Given the tremendous challenge in successfully treating adolescent obesity, and the costs of its continuation into adulthood, a public health approach is needed to address the environmental factors that are responsible for the increased incidence of obesity in youth over the past few decades. Prevention of obesity should begin early in life, and there is a need for more work in this area. A societal response including intervention at many levels may be needed to achieve a reduction in adolescent obesity rates. Besides intervention at the level of individual adolescents and their families, social marketing, legislation related to food marketing and production, school health policy changes, and changes in the built environment are all needed in this effort. Health care providers, schools, communities, and families must all work together to support the behavioral health of adolescents in order to reduce the epidemic of child and adolescent obesity.

References

Adair, L. S. (2008). Child and adolescent obesity: Epidemiology and developmental perspectives. *Physiology and Behavior, 94*, 8–16.

Adams, J. (2006). Trends in physical activity and inactivity amongst US 14–18 year olds by gender, school grade and race, 1993–2003: Evidence from the youth risk behavior survey. *BioMed Central Public Health, 6*, 57–63.

Allison, D. B., Matz, P. E., Pietrobelli, A., Zannolli, R., & Faith, M. S. (1999). Genetic and environmental influences on obesity. In A. Bendich & R. J. Deckelbaum (Eds.), *Primary and secondary preventive nutrition* (pp. 147–164). Totowa, NJ: Humana Press.

Anderson, S. E., Cohen, P., Naumova, E. N., & Must, A. (2006). Association of depression and anxiety disorders with weight change in a prospective community based study of children followed up into adulthood. *Archives of Pediatric Adolescent Medicine, 160*, 285–291.

Angrisani, L., Favretti, F., Furbetta, F., Paganelli, M., Basso, N., Soldi, S. B., et al. (2005). Obese teenagers treated by lap-band system: The Italian experience. *Surgery, 138*, 877–881.

Appel, L. J., Clark, J. M., Yeh, H. C., et al. (2011). Comparative effectiveness of weight-loss interventions in clinical practice. *New England Journal of Medicine, 365*(21), 1959–1968.

Bell, P., Redd, P., & Rainie, L. (2004). *Rural areas and the internet*. Washington, DC: Pew Internet and American Life Project.

Berkowitz, R., Fujioka, K., Daniels, S., et al. (2006). Effects of sibutramine treatment in obese adolescents: A randomized trial. *Annals of Internal Medicine, 145*, 81–90.

Berkowitz, R., Wadden, T. A., Tershakovec, A. M., & Cronquist, J. L. (2003). Behavior therapy and sibutramine for the treatment of adolescent obesity. *Journal of the American Medical Association, 289*, 1805–1812.

Bibi, H., Shoseyov, D., Feigenbaum, D., et al. (2004). The relationship between asthma and obesity: Is it real or a case of over diagnosis. *Journal of Asthma, 41*, 403–410.

Birch, L. L., & Fisher, J. O. (1998). Development of eating behaviors among children and adolescents. *Pediatrics, 101*(3), 539–549.

Bowman, S., Gortmaker, S., Ebbeling, C., Pereira, M., & Ludwig, D. (2004). Effects of fast food consumption on energy intake and diet quality among children in a national household survey. *Journal of Pediatrics, 113*(1), 112–118.

Braet, C., Tanghe, A., Decaluwé, V., Moens, E., & Rosseel, Y. (2004). Inpatient treatment for children with obesity: Weight loss, psychological well-being, and eating behavior. *Journal of Pediatric Psychology, 29*(7), 519–529.

Britz, B., Siegfried, W., Ziegler, A., Lamertz, C., Herpertz-Dahlmann, B. M., Remschmidt, H., et al. (2000). Rates of psychiatric disorders in a clinical study group of adolescents with extreme obesity and in obese adolescents ascertained via a population based study. *International Journal of Obesity, 24*, 1707–1714.

Brownell, K. D., Kelman, S. H., & Stunkard, A. J. (1983). Treatment of obese children with and without their mothers: Changes in weight and blood pressure. *Pediatrics, 71*, 515–523.

Caskey, S. R., & Felker, D. W. (1971). Social stereotyping of female body image by elementary school age girls. *Research Quarterly, 42*, 251–255.

CDC. (2009a). *Overweight and obesity*. Retrieved January 31, 2011, from http://www.cdc.gov/obesity/defining.html.

CDC. (2009b). *Overweight and obesity*. Retrieved January 31, 2011, from http://www.cdc.gov/obesity/causes/health.html.

CDC. (2011). *Basics about childhood obesity*. Retrieved from http://www.cdc.gov/obesity/childhood/basics.html.

Chanoine, J., Hampl, S., Jensen, C., Boldrin, M., & Hauptman, J. (2005). Effect of orlistat on weight and body composition in obese adolescents. *Journal of American Medical Association, 293*, 2873–2883.

Coates, T. J., Killen, J. D., & Slinkard, L. A. (1982). Parent participation in a treatment program for overweight adolescents. *International Journal of Eating Disorders, 1*, 37–48.

Coleman, K. J., Tiller, C. L., Sanchez, J., Heath, E. M., Sy, O., Milliken, G., et al. (2005). Prevention of epidemic increase in child risk of overweight in low-income schools. *Archives of Pediatrics and Adolescent Medicine, 159*, 217–224.

Cook, S., Weitzman, M., Auinger, P., & Barlow, S. (2005). Screening and counseling associated with obesity diagnosis in a national survey of ambulatory pediatric visits. *Pediatrics, 116*, 112–116.

Cook, S., Weitzman, M., Auinger, P., Nguyen, M., & Dietz, W. H. (2003). Prevalence of a metabolic syndrome phenotype in adolescents. *Archives of Pediatrics and Adolescent Medicine, 157*, 821–827.

Craggs, C., Corder, K., Van Sluijs, E., & Griffin, S. (2011). Determinants of change in physical activity in children and adolescents: A systematic review. *American Journal of Preventive Medicine, 40*(6), 645–658.

Crossman, A., Sullivan, D. A., & Benin, M. (2006). The family environment and American adolescents' risk of obesity as young adults. *Social Sciences and Medicine, 63*(9), 2255–2267.

Cushing, C., & Steele, R. (2010). A meta-analytic review of eHealth interventions for pediatric health promoting and maintaining behaviors. *Journal of Pediatric Psychology, 35*, 937–949.

Daley, A. J., Copeland, R. J., Wright, N. P., Roalfe, A., & Wales, J. K. (2006). Exercise therapy as a treatment for psychopathologic conditions in obese and morbidly obese adolescents: A randomized controlled trial. *Pediatrics, 118*, 2126–2134.

Daniels, S. (2006). The consequences of childhood overweight and obesity. *The Future of Children, 16*, 47–67.

Davidson, K. K., & Birch, L. L. (2002). Processes linking weight status and self concept among girls from ages 5 to 7 years. *Developmental Psychology, 38*, 735–748.

Davidson, K. K., Markey, C. N., & Birch, L. L. (2003). A longitudinal examination of patterns in girls' weight concerns and body dissatisfaction from ages 5 to 9 years. *International Journal of Eating Disorders, 33*, 320–332.

Davis, S., Davis, M., Northington, L., Moll, G., & Kolar, K. (2002). Childhood obesity reduction by school based programs. *ABNF Journal, 13*(6), 145–149.

Dietz, W. H. (1998). Health consequences of obesity in youth: Childhood predictors of adult disease. *Pediatrics, 101*, 518–525.

Doak, C. M., Visscher, T. L., Renders, C. M., & Seideil, J. C. (2006). The prevention of overweight and obesity in children and adolescents: A review of interventions and programmes. *International Life Sciences Institute Obesity Reviews, 7*(111–136), 2006.

Eaton, D., Kann, L., Kinchen, S., Shanklin, S., Ross, J., Hawkins, J., et al. (2008). Youth risk behavior surveillance—United States, 2007. *MMWR Surveillance Summaries, 57*(4), 1–131.

Ebbeling, C. B., Leidig, M. M., Sinclair, K. B., Hangen, J. P., & Ludwig, D. S. (2003). A reduced-glycemic load diet in the treatment of adolescent obesity. *Archives of Pediatric Adolescent Medicine, 157*, 773–779.

Epstein, L. H., Myers, M., Raynor, H., & Saelens, B. (1998). Treatment of pediatric obesity. *Pediatrics, 101*, 554–570.

Epstein, L. H., Valoski, A. M., Vara, L. S., et al. (1995). Effects of decreasing sedentary behavior and increasing activity on weight change in obese children. *Health Psychology, 14*, 109–115.

Epstein, L. H., Valoski, A., Wing, R. R., & McCurley, J. (1994). Ten-year outcomes of behavioral family-based treatment for childhood obesity. *Health Psychology, 13*, 373–383.

Faulkner, N. H., Neumark-Sztainer, D., Story, M., Jeffery, R. W., Beuring, T., & Resnic, M. D. (2001). Social, educational, and psychological correlates of weight status in adolescents. *Obesity Research, 9*, 32–42.

Fielding, G. A., & Duncombe, J. E. (2005). Laparoscopic adjustable banding in severely obese adolescents. *Surgery for Obesity and Related Diseases, 1*, 399–407.

Fontaine, K. R., & Allison, D. B. (2002). Obesity and the internet. In C. Gairburn & K. Brownell (Eds.), *Eating disorders and obesity* (2nd ed.). New York: Guilford Press.

Foster, G. D., Sherman, S., Borradaile, K. E., Grundy, K. M., Vander Veur, S. S., Nachmani, J., et al. (2008). A policy-based school intervention to prevent overweight and obesity. *Pediatrics, 121*, 794–802.

Fox S. (2005). *Digital divisions*. Washington, DC: Pew Internet, October 5.

Freedman, D. S., Dietz, W. H., Srinivasan, S. R., & Berenson, G. R. (1999). The relation of overweight to cardiovascular risk factors among children and adolescents: The Bogalusa heart study. *Pediatrics, 103*, 1175–1182.

Freemark, M., & Bursey, D. (2001). The effects of metformin on body mass index and glucose tolerance in obese adolescents with fasting hyperinsulinemia and a family history of type 2 diabetes. *Pediatrics, 107*, E55.

French, S. A. (2003). Pricing effects on food choices. *The Journal of Nutrition, 133*, 841S–843S.

French, S. A., Story, M., Neumark-Sztainer, D., Faulkerson, J. A., & Hannan, P. (2001). Fast food restaurant use among adolescents: Associations with nutrient intake, food choices and behavioral and psychosocial variables. *Division of Epidemiology, 25*, 1823–1833.

Frenn, M., Malin, S., Brown, R. L., Greer, Y., Fox, J., Greer, J., et al. (2005). Changing the tide: An internet/video exercise and low-fat intervention with middle-school students. *Applied Nursing Research, 18*, 13–21.

Friedman, M. A., & Brownell, K. D. (1995). Psychological correlates of obesity: Moving to the next research generation. *Psychological Bulletin, 117*, 3–20.

Garcia, V. F., Langford, L., & Inge, T. H. (2003). Application of laparoscopy for bariatric surgery in adolescents. *Current Opinion in Pediatrics, 15*, 248–255.

Garcia-Morales, L. M., Berber, A., Macias-Lara, C. C., Lucio-Ortiz, C., Del Rio-Navarro, B. E., & Dorantes-Alvarez, L. M. (2006). Use of sibutramine in obese Mexican adolescents: A 6-month, randomized, double-blind, placebo-controlled, parallel-group trial. *Clinical Therapeutics, 28*, 770–782.

Gennuso, J., Epstein, L., Paluch, R., & Cerny, F. (1998). The relationship between asthma and obesity in urban minority children and adolescents. *Archives of Pediatric and Adolescent Medicine, 152*, 1197–1200.

Gerrits, J. H., O'Hara, R. E., Bettina, P. F., Gibbons, F. X., Ridder, D., Keresztes, N., et al. (2010). Self-control, diet concerns and eater prototypes influence fatty foods consumption of adolescents in three countries. *Health Education Research, 25*(6), 1031–1041.

Godoy-Matos, A., Carraro, L., Vieira, A., et al. (2005). Treatment of obese adolescents with sibutramine: A randomized, double-blind, controlled study. *The Journal of Clinical Endocrinology and Metabolism, 90*, 1460–1465.

Goodman, E., & Whitaker, R. C. (2002). A prospective study of the role of depression in the development and persistence of adolescent obesity. *Pediatrics, 110*, 497–504.

Gordon-Larsen, P., Nelson, M. C., Page, P., & Popkin, B. M. (2006). Inequality in the built environment underlies key health disparities in physical activity and obesity. *Pediatrics, 117*, 417–424.

Gordon-Larsen, P., The, N. S., & Adair, L. S. (2010). Longitudinal trends in obesity in the United States from adolescents to the third decade of life. *Obesity, 18*, 1801–1804.

Gortmaker, S. L., Cheung, L. W. Y., Peterson, K. E., et al. (1999). Impact of a school-based interdisciplinary intervention on diet and physical activity among urban primary school children. *Archives of Pediatrics and Adolescent Medicine, 153*, 975–983.

Gortmaker, S. L., Must, A., Perrin, J. M., Sobol, A. M., & Dietz, W. H. (1993). Social and economic consequences of overweight in adolescence and young adulthood. *New England Journal of Medicine, 32*, 1008–1012.

Gortmaker, S., Peterson, K., Wiecha, J., Sobol, A., Dixit, S., Fox, M., et al. (1999). Reducing obesity via a school-based interdisciplinary intervention among youth. *Archives of Pediatric and Adolescent Medicine, 153*, 409–418.

Goslinger, W., Madsen, K., Woodward-Lopez, G., & Crawford, P. (2011). Would students prefer to eat healthier foods at school? *Journal of School Health, 81*(3), 146–151.

Griffiths, L. J., Wolke, D., Page, A. S., & Horwood, J. P. (2006). Obesity and bullying: Different effects for boys and girls. *Archives of Disease in Childhood, 91*, 121–125.

Gutin, B., Barbeau, P., Owens, S., Lemmon, C. R., Bauman, M., Allison, J., et al. (2002). Effects of exercise intensity on cardiovascular fitness, total body composition, and the visceral adiposity of obese adolescents. *American Journal of Clinical Nutrition, 75*, 818–826.

Hancox, R. J., Milne, B. J., & Poulton, R. (2004). Associations between child and adolescent television viewing and adult health: A longitudinal birth cohort study. *Lancet, 364*(9430), 257–262.

Heath, G. W., Pratt, M., Warren, C. W., & Kann, L. (1994). Physical activity patterns in American high-school-student-results from the 1990 youth risk behavior survey. *Archives of Pediatric and Adolescent Medicine, 148*(11), 1131–1136.

Inge, T. H., Krebs, N. F., Garcia, V. F., Skelton, J. A., Guice, K. S., Strauss, R. S., et al. (2004). Bariatric surgery for severely overweight adolescents: Concerns and recommendations. *Pediatrics, 114*, 217–223.

Inge, T. H., Xanthakos, S. A., & Zeller, M. H. (2007). Bariatric surgery for pediatric obesity: Now or later? *International Journal of Obesity, 31*, 1–14.

Jago, R., Baranowski, T., Baranowski, J., Thompson, D., Cullen, K., Watson, K., et al. (2006). Fit for life Boy Scout badge: Outcome evaluation of a troop and internet intervention. *Preventive Medicine, 42*, 181–187.

James, J., Thomas, P., Cavan, D., & Kerr, D. (2004). Preventing childhood obesity by reducing consumption of carbonated drinks: Cluster randomized controlled trial. *British Medical Journal, 328*, 1237.

Jelalian, K., Mehlenbeck, R., Lloyd-Richardson, E. E., Birmaher, V., & Wing, R. R. (2005). "Adventure therapy" combined with cognitive-behavioral treatment for overweight adolescents. *International Journal of Obesity, 30*, 31–39.

Kamath, C. C., Vickers, K. S., Ehrlich, A., McGovern, L., Johnson, J., Singhal, V., et al. (2008). Behavioral Interventions to prevent childhood obesity: A systematic review and meta-analyses of randomized trials. *The Journal of Clinical Endocrinology and Metabolism, 93*, 4606–4615.

Kang, H. S., Gutin, B., Barbeau, P., Owens, S., Lemmon, C. R., Allison, J., et al. (2002). Physical training improves insulin resistance syndrome markers in obese adolescents. *Medicine and Science in Sports and Exercise, 34*, 1920–1927.

Kantor, L. S. (1999). A comparison of the US food supply with the Food Guide Pyramid recommendations. In E. Frazo (Ed.), *America's eating habits: Changes and consequences* (pp. 71–95). Washington, DC: USDA/Economic Research Division.

Kassirer, J. P. (1995). The next transformation in the delivery of health care. *New England Journal of Medicine, 332*, 52–54.

Kay, J. P., Alemzadeh, R., Langley, G., D'Angelo, L., Smith, P., & Holshouser, S. (2001). Beneficial effects of metformin in normoglycemic morbidly obese adolescents. *Metabolism, 50*, 1457–1461.

Kelder, S., Perry, C., Lytle, L., & Klepp, K. (1994). Community-wide youth nutrition education: Long-term outcomes of the Minnesota Heart Health Program. *Health Education Research, 9*, 119–131.

Killen, J., Telch, M., Robinson, T., Maccoby, N., Taylor, C., & Farquhar, J. (1988). Cardiovascular disease risk reduction for tenth graders: A multiple-factor school-based approach. *Journal of the American Medical Association, 260*, 1728–1733.

Kimm, S. Y. S., Glynn, N. W., Kriska, A. M., Barton, B. A., Kronsberg, S. S., Daniels, S. R., et al. (2002). Decline in physical activity in black girls and white girls during adolescence. *The New England Journal of Medicine, 347*, 709–715.

Kropski, J. A., Keckley, P. H., & Jensen, G. L. (2008). School-based obesity prevention programs: An evidence-based review. *Obesity, 16*, 1009–1018.

Kubik, M. Y., Lytle, L. A., & Story, M. (2005). Schoolwide food practices are associated with body mass index in middle school students. *Archives of Pediatrics and Adolescent Medicine, 159*, 1111–1114.

Lamertz, C. M., Jacobi, C., Yassouridis, A., Arnold, K., & Henkel, A. W. (2002). Are obese adolescents and young adults at higher risk for mental disorder? A community survey. *Obesity, 10*, 1152–1160.

Latner, J. D., & Stunkard, A. J. (2003). Getting worse: The stigmatization of obese children. *Obesity Research, 11*, 452–456.

Leung, M. M., Agaronov, A., Grytsenko, K., & Yeh, M. C. (2011). Intervening to reduce sedentary behaviors and childhood obesity among school-age youth: A systematic review of randomized trials. *Journal of Obesity, 2012*, 1–14.

Lin, B. H., Guthrie, J., & Blaylock, J. R. (1996). *The diets of America's children: Influence of dining out, household characteristics, and nutrition knowledge.* Washington, DC: U.S. Department of Agriculture, Economic Research Service, No. AER746.

Lin, B. H., Guthrie, J., & Frazao, E. (1999a). *Away-from-home foods increasingly important to quality of American diet.* Washington, DC: U.S. Department of Agriculture, Economic Research Service, Agricultural Bulletin No. 791.

Lin, B. H., Guthrie, J., & Frazao, E. (1999b). *Nutrient contribution of food away from home.* Washington, DC: U.S. Department of Agriculture, Economic Research Service, Agricultural Bulletin Number 750.

Long, J. D., Armstron, M. I., Amos, E., Shriver, B., et al. (2006). Pilot using World Wide Web to prevent diabetes in adolescents. *Clinical Nursing Research, 15*, 67–79.

Luepker, R., et al. (1996). Outcomes of a field trial to improve children's dietary patterns and physical activity: The Child and Adolescent Trial for Cardiovascular Health (CATCH). *Journal of the American Medical Association, 275*, 768–776.

McCoy, M. R., Couch, D., Duncan, N. D., & Lynch, G. S. (2005). Evaluating an internet weight loss program for diabetes prevention. *Health Promotion International, 20*, 221–228.

Mellin, L. M., Slunkard, L. A., & Irwin, C. E. (1987). Adolescent obesity intervention: Validation of the SHAPEDOWN program. *Journal of the American Dietetic Association, 87*, 333–338.

Meyer, J. M., & Stunkard, A. J. (1993). Genetics and human obesity. In A. J. Stunkard & T. A. Wadden (Eds.), *Obesity: Theory and therapy* (2nd ed., pp. 137–149). New York: Raven Press.

Miller, J., Gold, M. S., & Silverstein, J. (2003). Pediatric overeating and obesity: An epidemic. *Psychiatric Annals, 33*(2), 94–103.

Murray, E., Burns, J., See Tai, S., Lai, R., & Nazareth, I. (2009). Interactive health communication applications for people with chronic disease. *The Cochrane Library, 1.* http://www.thecochranelibrary.com.

Musher-Eizenman, D. R., Holub, S. C., Barnhart Miller, A., Goldstein, S. E., & Edwards-Leeper, L. (2004). Body size stigmatization in preschool children: The role of control attributions. *Journal of Pediatric Psychology, 29*, 613–620.

Must, A., Jacques, P. F., Dallal, G. E., Bajema, C. J., & Dietz, W. J. (1992). Long-term morbidity and mortality of overweight adolescents: A follow-up of the Harvard Growth Study of 1922 to 1935. *New England Journal of Medicine, 327*, 1350–1355.

Nadler, E. P., Youn, H. A., Ginsburg, H. B., Ren, C. J., & Fielding, G. A. (2007). Short-term results in 53 US obese pediatric patients with laparoscopic adjustable gastric banding. *Journal of Pediatric Surgery, 42*, 137–142.

Nathan, B. M., & Moran, A. (2008). Metabolic complications of obesity in childhood and adolescence: More than just diabetes. *Current Opinion in Endocrinology, Diabetes, and Obesity, 15*(1), 21–29.

Nemet, D., Barkan, S., Epstein, Y., Friedland, O., Kowen, G., & Eliakim, A. (2005). Short- and long-term beneficial effects of a combined dietary-behavioral-physical activity intervention for the treatment of childhood obesity. *Pediatrics, 115*, 443–449.

Ogden, C. L., Carroll, M. D., Curtin, L. R., Lamb, M. M., & Flegal, K. M. (2010). Prevalence of high body mass index in US children and adolescents, 2007–2008. *Journal of the American Medical Association, 303*(3), 242–249.

Ornelas, I. J., Perreira, K., & Ayala, G. X. (2007). Parental influences on adolescent physical activity: A longitudinal study. *International Journal of Behavioral Nutrition and Physical Activity, 4*(3).

Ozkan, B., Bereket, A., Turan, S., & Keskin, S. (2004). Addition of orlistat to conventional treatment in adolescents with severe obesity. *European Journal of Pediatrics, 163*, 738–741.

Parks, S., Sappenfield, W., Huang, Y., Sherry, B., & Bensyl, D. (2010). The impact of the availability of school vending machines on eating behavior during lunch: The youth physical activity and nutrition survey. *American Dietetic Association, 110*, 1532–1536.

Patrick, K., Calfas, K. J., Norman, G. J., et al. (2006). Randomized controlled trial of a primary care and home-based intervention for physical activity and nutrition behaviors. *Archives of Pediatrics and Adolescent Medicine, 160*, 128–136.

Patrick, K., Sallis, J. F., Prochaska, J. J., Lydston, D. D., Calfas, K. J., Zabinski, M. F., et al. (2001). A multicomponent program for nutrition and physical activity change in primary care. *Pediatric and Adolescent Medicine, 155*, 940–946.

Pearson, N., Biddle, S., & Gorely, T. (2009). Family correlates of breakfast consumption among children and adolescents: A systematic review. *Appetite, 52*(1), 1–7.

Perry, C., Bishop, D., Taylor, G., et al. (1998). Changing fruit and vegetable consumption among children: The 5-a-Day Power Plus Program in St. Paul, Minnesota. *American Journal of Public Health, 88*, 603–609.

Presnell, K., Bearman, S. K., & Stice, E. (2004). Risk factors for body dissatisfaction in adolescent boys and girls: A prospective study. *International Journal of Eating Disorders, 36*, 389–401.

Putnam, J., & Gerrior, S. (1999). Trends in the US food supply, 1970–1997. In E. Frazo (Ed.), *America's eating habits: Changes and consequences* (pp. 133–160). Washington, DC: USDA/Economic Research Division.

Rand, C. S., & MacGregor, A. M. (1994). Adolescents having obesity surgery: A six year follow-up. *Southern Medical Journal, 87*, 1208–1213.

Reilly, J. J. (2005). Descriptive epidemiology and health consequences of childhood obesity. *Best Practice and Research Clinical Endocrinology and Metabolism, 19*(3), 327–341.

Reilly, J. J., Methven, E., McDowell, Z. C., et al. (2003). Health consequences of obesity. *Archives of Disease of Childhood, 88*, 748–752.

Resnicow, K., Davis, R., & Rollnick, S. (2006). Motivational interviewing for pediatric obesity: Conceptual issues and evidence review. *Journal of the American Dietetic Association, 106*(12), 2024–2033.

Resnicow, K., Taylor, R., Baskin, M., & McCarty, F. (2005). Results of go girls: A weight control program for overweight African-American adolescent females. *Obesity Research, 13*(10), 1739–1748.

Ricciardelli, L. A., & McCabe, M. P. (2001). Children's body image concerns and eating disturbance: A review of the literature. *Clinical Psychological Review, 21*, 325–344.

Richardson, S. A. (1971). Handicap, appearance and stigma. *Social Science and Medicine, 5*, 621–628.

Robinson, T. (1999). Reducing children's television viewing to prevent obesity: A randomized trial. *Journal of the American Medical Association, 282*, 1561–1567.

Rolland-Cachera, M. F., Deheeger, M., Maillot, M., & Bellisle, F. (2006). Early adiposity rebound: Causes and consequences for obesity in children and adults. *International Journal of Obesity, 30*, S11–S17.

Rolland-Cachera, M. F., et al. (2004). Massive obesity in adolescents: Dietary interventions and behaviors associated with weight regain at 2 year follow-up. *International Journal of Obesity, 28*, 514–519.

Rothert, K., Strecher, V. J., Doyle, L. A., et al. (2006). Web-based weight management programs in an integrated health care setting: A randomized, controlled trial. *Obesity, 14*, 266–272.

Sacks, R. M., Bray, G. A., Carey, V. J., et al. (2009). Comparison of weight-loss diets with different compositions of fat, protein, and carbohydrates. *New England Journal of Medicine, 360*(9), 859–873.

Saelens, B. E., Sallis, J. F., Wilfley, D. E., Patrick, K., Cella, J. A., & Buchta, R. (2002). Behavioral weight control for overweight adolescents initiated in primary care. *Obesity Research, 10*(1), 22–32.

Sallis, J. F., McKenzie, T. L., Alcaraz, J. E., Kolody, B., Faucette, N., & Hovell, M. F. (1997). The effects of a 2-year physical education program (SPARK) on physical activity and fitness in elementary school students. *American Journal of Public Health, 87*, 1328–1334.

Sallis, J. F., McKenzie, T. L., Alcaraz, J. E., Kolody, B., Hovell, M. F., & Nader, P. R. (1993). Project SPARK: Effects of physical education on adiposity in children.

Annals of the New York Academy of Sciences, 699, 127–136.

Sallis, J. F., Prochaska, J. J., & Taylor, W. C. (2000). A review of correlates of physical activity of children and adolescents. *Medicine and Science in Sports and Exercise, 32*(5), 963–975.

Saperstein, S. L., Atkinson, N. L., & Gold, R. S. (2007). The impact of Internet use for weight loss. *Obesity Research, 8*(459–465), 2007.

Savoye, M., Nowicka, P., Shaw, M., et al. (2011). Long-term results of an obesity program in an ethnically diverse pediatric population. *Pediatrics, 127*(3), 401–410.

Schwimmer, J. B., Burnwinkle, T. M., & Varni, J. W. (2003). Health related quality of life of severely obese children and adolescents. *Journal of the American Medical Association, 289*(14), 1813–1819.

Sjoberg, R. L., Nilsson, K. W., & Leppert, J. (2005). Obesity, shame, and depression in school aged children: A population based study. *Pediatrics, 116*, 389–392.

Sondike, S. B., Copperman, N., & Jacobson, M. S. (2003). Effects of a low-carbohydrate diet on weight loss and cardiovascular risk factors in overweight adolescents. *Journal of Pediatric Psychology, 142*, 253–258.

Sothern, M. S., Udall, J. N., Suskind, R. M., Vargas, A., & Blecker, U. (2000). Weight loss and growth velocity in obese children after very low calorie diet, exercise, and behavior modification. *Acta Paediatrica, 89*, 1036–1043.

Srinivasan, S., Ambler, G. R., Baur, L. A., Garnett, S. P., Tepsa, M., Yap, F., et al. (2006). Randomized, controlled trial of metformin for obesity and insulin resistance in children and adolescents: Improvement in body composition and fasting insulin. *The Journal of Clinical Endocrinology and Metabolism, 91*, 2074–2080.

Stallings, V. A., Archibald, E. H., Pencharz, P. B., Harrison, J. E., & Bell, L. E. (1988). One-year follow-up of weight, total body potassium, and total body nitrogen in overweight adolescents treated with the protein-sparing modified fast. *The American Journal of Clinical Nutrition, 48*, 91–94.

Steele, R. G., Aylward, B., Jensen, C. D., Cushing, C. C., Davis, A. M., & Bovaird, J. A. (2012). Comparison of a family-based group intervention for youths with obesity to a brief individual family intervention: a practical clinical trial of Positively Fit. *Journal of Pediatric Psychology, 37*, 53–63.

Stice, E., & Bearman, S. K. (2001). Body-image and eating disturbances prospectively predict increases in depressive symptoms in adolescent girls: A growth curve analysis. *Developmental Psychology, 37*, 597–607.

Stice, E., Hayward, C., Cameron, R. P., Killen, J. D., & Barr, T. C. (2000). Body-image and eating disturbances predict onset of depression among female adolescents: A longitudinal study. *Journal of Abnormal Psychology, 109*, 438–444.

Strauss, R. S., & Pollack, H. A. (2003). Social marginalization of overweight children. *Archives of Pediatric and Adolescent Medicine, 157*, 746–752.

Strauss, C. C., Smith, K., Frame, C., & Forehand, R. (1985). Personal and interpersonal characteristics associated with childhood obesity. *Journal of Pediatric Psychology, 10*, 337–343.

Tate, D. F., Jackvony, E. H., & Wing, R. R. (2003). Effects of internet behavioral counseling on weight loss in adults at risk for type 2 diabetes: A randomized trial. *Journal of the American Medical Association, 289*, 1833–1836.

The Healthy Study Group. (2010). A school-based intervention for diabetes risk reduction. *The New England Journal of Medicine, 363*, 443–453.

The, N. S., Suchindran, C., North, K. E., Popkin, B. M., & Gordon-Larsen, P. (2010). Association of adolescent obesity with risk of severe obesity in adulthood. *Journal of the American Medical Association, 304*(18), 2042–2047.

Thompson, D., Baranowski, J., Cullen, K., & Baranowski, T. (2007). Development of a theory-based internet program promoting maintenance of diet and physical activity change to 8-year-old African American girls. *Computers and Education, 48*, 446–459.

Tippett, K. S. & Cleveland, L. E. (1999). How current diets stack up: Comparison with dietary guidelines. In E. Frazao (Eds.), *America's Eating Habits: Changes and Consequences* (pp. 51–70). *ERS Agriculture Information Bulletin No. 750*. Washington, DC: US Department of Agriculture.

Tuffrey, C., & Finlay, F. (2002). Use of the internet by parents of paediatric outpatients. *Archives Disease Children, 87*(534–536), 2002.

Vila, G., Zipper, E., Dabbas, M., Bertrand, C., Robert, J. J., Ricour, C., et al. (2004). Mental disorders in obese children and adolescents. *Psychosomatic Medicine, 66*, 387–394.

Visness, C., London, S., Daniels, J., et al. (2010). Association of childhood obesity with atopic and non-atopic asthma: Results from the National Health and Nutrition Examination Survey 1999–2000. *Journal of Asthma, 47*, 822–829.

Wadden, T. A., Stunkard, A. J., Rich, L., Rubin, C. J., Sweidel, G., & McKinney, S. (1990). Obesity in black adolescent girls: A controlled clinical trial of treatment by diet, behavior modification, and parental Support. *Pediatrics, 85*, 345–352.

Wahi, G., Parkin, P. C., Beyene, J., Uleryk, E. M., & Birken, C. S. (2011). Effectiveness of interventions aimed at reducing screen time in children. *Archives of Pediatric and Adolescent Medicine, 165*(11), 979–986.

Walsh, D., Rudd, R., Moeykens, B., & Maloney, T. (1993). Social marketing for public health. *Health Affairs, 12*, 104–119.

Wardle, J., & Cooke, L. (2005). The impact of obesity on psychological well-being. *Best Practice and Research Clinical Endocrinology and Metabolism, 19*, 421–440.

Wardle, J., Volz, C., & Golding, C. (1995). Social variation in attitudes to obesity in children. *International Journal of Obesity Related Metabolism Disorders, 19*, 562–569.

Weiss, R., Dziura, J., Burgert, T. S., Tamborlane, W. V., Taksali, S. E., Yeckel, C. W., et al. (2004). Obesity and the metabolic syndrome in children and adolescents. *The New England Journal of Medicine, 350*, 2362–2374.

Whitaker, R. C., Wright, J. A., Pepe, M. S., Seidel, K. D., & Dietz, W. H. (1997). Predicting obesity in young adulthood from childhood and parental obesity. *The New England Journal of Medicine, 337*(13), 869–873.

Williams, S. M., & Goulding, A. (2009). Patterns of growth associated with the timing of adiposity rebound. *Obesity, 17*, 335–341.

Williamson, D. A., Martin, P. D., White, M. A., Newton, R., Walden, H., York-Crowe, E., et al. (2005). Efficacy of an internet-based behavioral weight loss program for overweight adolescent African-American girls. *Eating and Weight Disorders, 10*, 193–203.

Williamson, D., Walden, H., White, M., York-Crowe, E., Newton, R., Alfonso, A., et al. (2006). Two-year Internet-based randomized controlled trial for weight loss in African-American girls. *Obesity, 14*, 1231–1243.

Winett, R. A., Roodman, A. A., Winett, S. G., Bajzek, W., Rovniak, L. S., & Whiteley, J. A. (1999). The effects of Eat4Life internet-based health behavior program on the nutrition and activity practices of high school girls. *Journal of Gender, Culture, & Health, 4*, 239–254.

Winett, R. A., Tate, D. F., Anderson, E. S., Wojcik, J. R., & Winett, S. G. (2005). Long-term weight gain prevention: A theoretically based Internet approach. *Preventive Medicine, 41*, 629–641.

Woolford, S. J., Barr, K. L. C., Derry, H. A., et al. (2011). OMG do not say LOL: Obese adolescents' perspectives on the content of text messages to enhance weight loss efforts. *Obesity, 19*, 2382–2387.

Xie, B., Chou, C. P., Spruijt-Metz, D., Liu, C., Xia, J., Gong, J., et al. (2005). Effects of perceived peer isolation and social support availability on the relationship between body mass index and depressive symptoms. *International Journal of Obesity, 29*, 1137–1143.

Cardiovascular Complaints in Adolescence: Clinical Considerations

Melissa Horn, Jessica Ford, David Fairbrother, and Samuel F. Sears

Introduction

Cardiac conditions that appear in childhood and adolescence are rare, leaving the general population less knowledgeable about the symptoms and effects of such diseases. When hearing the term "heart disease," it brings to mind ischemic disease processes, such as coronary artery disease and heart attack. However, ischemic cardiac issues tend to develop many years before symptoms surface, making them anomalies in the pediatric population. Several less known, non-ischemic cardiac conditions are either present at birth, or they are newly diagnosed in the teenage years. This chapter will focus on the following forms of heart disease that plague children and adolescents: congenital heart defects, electrophysiological disorders, and cardiomyopathy.

The aforementioned diseases present adolescents with a plethora of physical, psychosocial, familial, and, in some cases, neurological difficulties. While teens without chronic diseases are acquiring independence, exploring new roles, and excitedly looking toward their future, those with cardiac conditions often face the barriers of existential uncertainty, physical restrictions, and parental overprotection. As such, development is undoubtedly impacted by the presence of heart disease.

While this chapter does not include all forms of pediatric cardiac conditions, it focuses on some of the most common complaints. For each disease state, discussion will center on etiology, treatment, and the adolescent's experience of the condition, including physical, psychosocial, familial, and neurological components. Further, special focus will be given to teens whose conditions are treated with implantable cardioverter defibrillators, medical devices that pose recipients with unique adjustment challenges. The chapter will close with discussion of measures that can be used in the psychosocial assessment of teens with cardiac conditions, as well as forms of intervention that may aide adjustment and

M. Horn (✉)
Department of Veterans Affairs,
510 West Union Street, Athens, OH, USA
e-mail: Melissa.Horn@va.gov

J. Ford
Department of Psychology, East Carolina University,
East Fifth Street, Greenville, NC 27858, USA
e-mail: haufj07@students.ecu.edu

D. Fairbrother
Department of Pediatrics, Division of Pediatric Cardiology, East Carolina University, East Carolina Heart Institute, 115 Heart Drive, Greenville, NC 27834, USA
e-mail: fairbrotherd@ecu.edu

S.F. Sears
Department of Psychology, East Carolina University,
115 Heart Drive, Greenville, NC 27834, USA

Department of Cardiovascular Sciences,
East Carolina University, 115 Heart Drive,
Greenville, NC 27834, USA
e-mail: searss@ecu.edu

W.T. O'Donohue et al. (eds.), *Handbook of Adolescent Health Psychology*,
DOI 10.1007/978-1-4614-6633-8_39, © Springer Science+Business Media New York 2013

development. It is hoped that this information will serve as a guide to increase knowledge about cardiac conditions in teens, as well as provide a resource for treating this population with high-quality, whole-person interventions.

Congenital Heart Defects

Etiology

The term congenital heart defects (CHD) refers to a variety of structural defects in the heart. Typically discovered in neonates and infants, CHD occur in approximately one in 100–150 live births and are the most common birth defect (Liebson, 2010). There are a large number of different CHD, which vary in severity (Hoffman, Kaplan, & Liberthson, 2004). These defects can be considered either acyanotic or cyanotic, with the latter group being more severe (Miyagul et al., 2003). A cyanotic defect is the result of bidirectional or right to left shunting in which some blood bypasses the lungs and enters circulation without being oxygenated. Acyanotic lesions tend to result in fewer complications and do not prevent blood from being oxygenated properly. The most common cyanotic lesion is tetralogy of Fallot and the most common acyanotic lesion is ventricular septal defect (Miyagul et al., 2003). For a more detailed review of each defect and specific surgical interventions, please see Hoffman and associates (2004). Table 1 contains some of the common CHD, as well as typical symptoms and physical limitations of each category of CHD. As the majority of these are diagnosed and have surgical repair or palliation early in life, symptoms and limitations in the adolescent are often related to both the type of surgical intervention and any residual defect.

Treatment

If a lesion is considered of sufficient severity or risk, surgical repair is the most common treatment for CHD (Hoffman et al., 2004). In 2000, 80 % of those who underwent surgery survived to adulthood. This dramatic increase in survival rates has resulted in increased need for care of adolescents and adults with CHD. In fact, in 2000, nearly half of those alive with CHD were adults (Marelli, Mackie, Ionescu-Ihu, Rahme, & Pilote, 2007). Unfortunately, although mortality rates are substantially lower following surgical intervention, one out of every five CHD survivors will need an additional operation. Arrhythmias resulting in hospitalization are also experienced by adolescents and adults with CHD. Somerville (1997) reported on common nonmedical reasons adolescents and adults with CHD contact their cardiologist, including such psychological difficulties as anxiety and suicidal ideation.

In addition to surgical correction, some adolescents and teens with CHD take medication to improve or maintain optimal heart functioning. Adolescents may be prescribed none or several medications listed below to help palliate the effects of CHD (The Task Force on the Management of Grown-up Congenital Heart Disease of the European Society of Cardiology, 2003). Angiotensin-converting enzyme (ACE) inhibitors may be prescribed to induce relaxation of blood vessels and thus decrease the vascular resistance that the heart pumps against (i.e., afterload reduction). Other medications to reduce the effort the heart muscle include beta-adrenergic blocking agents (beta-blockers), calcium channel blockers, and vasodilators. Antiarrhythmics are often prescribed to regulate the rhythm of the heart and prevent potentially lethal ventricular arrhythmias. Another medication that helps regulate rate and rhythm and that also improves the strength of the heart muscle is digitalis. Anticoagulants or blood thinners keep the blood from clotting and thus prevent blood clots which may travel and result in heart attack or stroke. These are sometimes used in patients with man-made shunts or that have low-velocity blood flow. Diuretics may be used to reduce swelling or edema due to excess pulmonary blood flow or poor cardiac function. Finally, antibiotics are regularly prescribed to prevent infection (specifically endocarditis).

Table 1 Common congenital heart defects and associated physical symptoms and limitations

	Cyanotic	Acyanotic
Type	• Tetralogy of Fallot • Transposition of great arteries • Total anomalous pulmonary venous return • Truncus arteriosus • Tricuspid atresia • Hypoplastic left heart syndrome	• Patent ductus arteriosus • Coarctation of the aorta • Atrial septal defects • Ventricular septal defects • Aortic stenosis • Pulmonary stenosis
Physical symptoms	• Bluish discoloration of the lips, fingers, and toes • Breathing problems (e.g., dyspnea/hyperventilation) • Anxiety • Syncope • Chest pain • Reduced appetite • Puffy eyes or face • Fatigue • Delay in physical growth	• Clinical signs are not always apparent • Increased pulmonary blood flow • Increased cardiac workload • Fatigue • Chest pain • Shortness of breath upon exertion
Limitations	• Physical limitations depend on severity of the defect and clinical presentation of the adolescent with CHD and will vary from teen to teen, but are more likely in those with cyanotic lesions	

Physical Experience of Disease

When asked about his experience with CHD, the 116-year-old said, "When I was younger I guess I thought it didn't really make a difference because no one cared—I didn't bother to tell them. But no I mean, it's a big factor because everyone is so critical and judgmental. Having a heart problem makes me more of a loner and unpopular because I'm not physical and stuff like that" (Tong et al., 1998, p. 306). His experience was marked by the physical limitations of his heart defect. This physical limitation resulted in social exclusion. This evaluation of the effects of CHD is not an isolated experience, but a shared experience of many with CHD. In fact, in a qualitative study of the challenges teens face coping with CHD, illness management (via medication adherence or limiting physical activity) and social integration were among the six most frequently mentioned challenges of living with CHD (Tong et al., 1998). Other challenges included seeking independence, developing strategies for coping with uncertainty, determining to whom and when to disclose medical status, and seeking normality. In empirical quantitative research, physical capacity is a predictor of psychosocial functioning among adolescents with CHD (Spurkland, Bjornstad, Lindberg, & Seem, 1993).

Physical activity may negatively affect someone with CHD through hemodynamic effects, fluid depletion, blood pressure disturbance, tachycardia, hypertrophy of the cardiac muscle, and arrhythmias which may result in sudden death. Physical limitations depend on severity of CHD, the type of defect, the surgical repair, and the impact of the activity on cardiac hemodynamics. According to the task force on the management of grown-up CHD of the European Society of Cardiology, those with Marfan's syndrome, with aortic anomalies, taking oral anticoagulants, or with pacemakers are asked not to participate in impact sports (2003). In addition, many persons with CHD are encouraged to participate in social/leisure exercise, but not competitive or impact sports.

Psychosocial Functioning

Having CHD undoubtedly has the potential to affect the psychosocial functioning of adolescents. Foster et al. (2001) developed a long list of the tasks these teens face, including coping with body image and physical activity limitations, seeking peer acceptance, dealing with stigma, managing anxiety about medical procedures, learning to manage intellectual or learning difficulties, becoming more independent and responsible for their health care, and forming appropriate educational and vocational goals. These challenges are likely contributors to the reduced functioning in a variety of domains found in adolescents with CHD.

Poor emotional functioning has been found in many studies of those with CHD (Alpern, Uzark, & Dick, 1989; Aurer, Senturia, Shopper, & Biddy, 1971; Barrett, Van der Feen, Spieth, Berul, & DeMaso, 2001; DeMaso, Twente, Spratt, & O'Brien, 1995; 2000; Fricchione & Vlay, 1986; Green & Levitt, 1962; Kovacs et al., 2009; Linde, Rasof, & Dunn, 1966; Spurkland et al., 1993; Todaro, Fennell, Sears, Rodrigue, & Roche, 2000). Behavioral difficulties (especially internalizing problems) have been noted in 27 % of children with surgical repair of CHD at birth (Majnemer et al., 2008). Among teens with CHD there were a significantly greater number of patients who report anxiety and depression on the Child Behavior Check List than the reference group (Utens, Verhulst, Meijboom, Duivenvoorden, & Hess, 1993). In one sample of young adults with CHD, the prevalence of those with clinically significant depression or anxiety was 36.4 %. A significant minority had clinically significant depression (27.3 %) and a smaller, but still significant, group had clinically significant anxiety (9.1 %; Bromberg, Beasley, D'Angelo, Landzberg, & DeMaso, 2003). Adjustment difficulties have also been noted in these children (DeMaso et al., 1991; DeMaso, Beardslee, Silbert, & Fyler, 1990; 1991). Finally, health-related quality of life (QoL) has also been found to be significantly lower in children and adolescents with CHD according to patient and parent report on both generic and disease-specific indices of QoL (Kamphuis et al., 2004; Spijkerboer et al., 2006). Some of the key risk factors for poor emotional adjustment include CNS impairment, poor family functioning, more complex lesions (DeMaso, 2004), and older age (Kardsorp, Evaraerd, Kindt, & Mulder, 2007). Unfortunately, despite the large quantity of research studies on emotional difficulties in children and adolescents with CHD, these studies suffer from problems such as small sample size, heterogeneity of measures, and little consistency regarding type of lesion or age (DeMaso, 2004).

In addition to emotional issues, children and adolescents may also experience difficulties relating with peers. Majnemer and associates (2008) noted significantly lower than normative socialization in 13.3 % of children with CHD. Children and adolescents with CHD are rated as more withdrawn than their same-aged peers by teachers. Among adolescents and adults (aged 15–30) with CHD surveyed, social impairment was found in many domains including school functioning (19 %) and during free time activities (15 %). In addition, adolescents with CHD reported expectations of social impairment in sports (26 %), future career (11 %), and family planning (10 %) (Fekkes et al., 2001). Level of family strain related to the illness appears to be an important factor that impacts social functioning (Casey, Sykes, Craig, Power, & Mulholland, 1996). Other risk factors include low self-esteem, high levels of depression, lower IQ or cognitive impairment (DeMaso, 2004; Youssef, 1988), physical limitations, and altered physical appearance (DeMaso, 2004). Altered physical appearance may include blue lips, clubbed fingers and toes, or moon face (DeMaso, 2004).

Family Functioning

Having a child with a chronic illness like CHD can change family functioning, which may also impact the child's ability to cope with and manage chronic disease. This is especially true during the transition to adolescence, which causes strain even in families that do not have a chronically ill member. Overall, families of children and adolescents with CHD report concerns about normality, when to disclose information about CHD to others, how to manage a chronic illness, social integration, and the impact of CHD on family coping (Sparacino et al., 1997). These concerns have been found to negatively impact family functioning in families coping with a CHD diagnosis (Peterson & Harbaugh, 1995; Van Horn, DeMaso, Gonzalez-Heydrich, & Dahlmeier Erickson, 2001). Mothers are especially distressed, with studies showing difficulties with adjustment, anxiety, and depression (DeMaso et al., 1990, 1991, 1995; Thompson, Gustafson, George, & Spock, 1994). Mothers report additional concerns about medical prognosis, QoL, psychosocial functioning, effects on the family, and impact on finances (Van Horn et al., 2001). Maternal adjustment to these additional stressors has been linked with child adjustment, mother-reported child behavior problems, and child-reported physical symptoms (DeMaso et al., 1990, 1991, 1995; Thompson et al., 1994). Other studies have also found maternal adjustment to be negatively correlated with increased daily stressors and increased palliative coping (e.g., self-blame, avoidance, emotion-focused, and wishful thinking; Davis, Brown, Bakeman, & Campbell, 1998). Risk factors for reduced parental QoL include child posttraumatic stress, high impact of CHD on family life, lower socioeconomic status, and foreign nationality (Landolt, 2011). Fathers tend to be less studied, so conclusions about the relative impact on mothers vs. fathers should be considered tentatively.

Neurological Functioning

In a meta-analysis of the neurocognitive consequences of CHD, Miatton and associates (2006) noted that the majority of children and adolescents with CHD do not have significantly lower IQ scores than healthy controls. However, certain groups have been found to have significantly lowered IQ scores, specifically those with hypoplastic left heart syndrome or who have had surgery for CHD, which are also likely markers of relative disease severity. In school functioning, those with cyanotic lesions, especially transposition of the great arteries, have more difficulties in arithmetic, spelling, and reading (Linde et al., 1966; Silbert, Wolff, Mayer, Rosenthal, & Nadas, 1969). Additional meta-analyses revealed attentional difficulties in children and adolescents with transposition of the great arteries, tetralogy of Fallot, or ventricular septal defects (Miatton, DeWolf, Francois, & Thiery, 2006). Most adolescents with CHD have normative memory functioning. On the other hand, those with single ventricle defects have significantly lowered abilities on learning and memory tasks. Meta-analysis also examined language development studies and found that children and adolescents with transposition of the great arteries, staged palliation survivors, and ventricular septal defects exhibit a language delay of 2–4 months (Miatton et al., 2006; Majnemer et al., 2008). Overall, in tests of linguistic skills, these groups also perform below average. Finally, tests of motor functioning reveal that those with transposition of the great arteries experience fine motor disturbance, those with hypoplastic left heart syndrome have weaker visual-motor integration, and those who have had surgery for CHD exhibit poor locomotor skills compared to same-aged peers. These findings highlight the importance of understanding the specific disease state children and adolescents with CHD suffer from, as well as the interventions they have undergone as a result.

Additionally, some preoperative factors are noted to contribute to increased risk for neurocognitive deficits (Miatton et al., 2006). Malformations and deletions of the 22q11.2 chromosome, polymorphisms of the apolipoprotein E, and Down syndrome have all been shown as risk factors for worse neurological outcomes following surgery. Additionally, among persons with CHD, there is a greater prevalence of structural brain abnormalities, for example ventriculomegaly, cerebral atrophy, periventricular leukomalacia, poor brain growth due to hemodynamic disturbance, embolic infarction, cerebrovascular thrombosis, and abscess formation. New lesions and worsening of preexisting lesions is a significant risk for children and adolescents with complex congenital heart disease following surgical intervention. There is also a negative correlation between age at time of surgery and IQ scores (O'Dougherty, Wright, Garmezy, Loewenson, & Torres, 1983; O'Dougherty, Wright, Loewenson, & Torres, 1985). Further, specific surgical techniques such as use of deep hypothermic circulatory arrest and hemodilution have been shown to result in lowered cognitive abilities (Majnemer et al., 2008). Finally, there are several other postoperative factors to consider when determining risk for neurocognitive deficits in those who have had surgery for CHD. Having a greater number of operations, a longer stay in the intensive care unit, and being older at age of testing have all been shown to be correlated with greater neurocognitive dysfunction (Majnemer et al., 2008).

Arrhythmias and Electrophysiological Disorders of the Heart

Etiology

Although rare, a variety of arrhythmias of the heart may surface and persist in adolescence. The American Heart Association (AHA, 2011) describes an arrhythmia as any change in the normal sequence of electrical impulses of the heart. Arrhythmias can fall into two categories: bradycardia, a rhythm that is too slow, and tachycardia, a rhythm that is too fast (above 100 beats per minute). Arrhythmias can be described as benign or life-threatening, and individuals who experience them may be symptomatic or asymptomatic. Further, arrhythmias can be secondary to structural problems of the heart or they can be primary, deriving from a faulty cardiac electrical system.

Quite often, arrhythmias occur in the context of those who have had repairs of CHD, wherein the altered structure of the heart interferes with the electrical impulses and pathways. It is estimated that more than 50 % of pediatric patients who experience symptomatic ventricular arrhythmias have proof of organic heart disease (Davis, Gow, McCrindle, & Hamilton, 1996; Paul, Marchal, & Garson, 1990). Thus, these individuals are at risk for tachycardia, leading to palpitations, fainting, or sudden cardiac death.

Alternatively, those with no structural damage or repair of the heart can experience problems with the electrical system thereof. For clarity, these primary electrical conditions will be referred to in this chapter as "electrophysiological disorders." Disorders in which ventricular arrhythmias are the hallmark complication in a structurally normal heart include long QT syndrome (LQTS; Moss & Robinson, 1992), Brugada syndrome (Antzelevitch et al., 2002), catecholaminergic polymorphic ventricular tachycardia (CPVT; Francis, Sankar, Nair, & Priori, 2005), and Wolff–Parkinson–White syndrome (WPW; Gallagher, Gilbert, Svenson, Sealy, Kasell, Wallace, 1975). The exact prevalence of these disorders in the overall population is unknown, but overall, they are rare. For instance, LQTS is one of the more well known of these diseases, and its estimated prevalence is approximately 1 in 5,000 (Tester, Will, Haglund, & Ackerman, 2006).

To understand the etiology of electrophysiological disorders, one must first understand the electrical impulses of the heart. An action potential creates the electrical impulse of the heart, and this impulse is influenced by the opening and closing of the calcium, potassium, and sodium channels. DNA variations in these ion channels are most commonly implicated in arrhythmias in structurally normal hearts (Noseworthy & Newton-Cheh, 2008). In most cases, the aforementioned electrophysiological disorders are hereditary in nature, and within the affected family, each child has a 50 % chance of inheriting the disorder (Schimpf, Veltmann, Wolpert, & Borggrefe, 2009). To complicate matters, these disorders can exist in silent carriers of the DNA mutation, and further, affected individuals may or may not be symptomatic (Schimpf, Veltmann, Wolpert, & Borggrefe, 2009). Therefore genetic testing is often encouraged when electrophysiological disorders are suspected.

The most significant implication of arrhythmia is the potential for sudden cardiac arrest (SCA), leading to sudden cardiac death. SCA is the sudden, unexpected death from a cardiac cause, which occurs in a short period of time (minutes to 1 h) after the onset of symptoms (Zipes & Wellens, 1998). In the United States, it is estimated that 300,000 lives are lost due to SCA every year (Zheng, Croft, Giles, & Mensah, 2001). The majority of cases, 80 % of SCAs, are related to underlying coronary heart disease, while fewer, 10–15 %, are accounted for by non-ischemic processes, such as cardiomyopathy. Only 5 % of SCA cases are thought to be due to primary electrophysiological disorders existing in a structurally normal heart (Huikuri, Castellanos, & Myerburg, 2001). Unfortunately, in this minority of diseases, SCA may be the first and only manifestation of the disease, resulting in death.

Fatal arrhythmias may make their first appearance during strenuous physical activity. This is particularly troubling for adolescence because demanding exercise is often prevalent in the form of competitive sports (Schimpf, Veltmann, Wolpert, & Borggrefe, 2009). This is not to say that sports are the cause of increased rates of SCA; rather research has demonstrated that sports have elicited sudden death in those young persons who were predisposed to life-threatening ventricular arrhythmias during physical exercise (Corrado, Basso, Rizzolo, Schiavon, & Thiene, 2003). Screening through use of a 12-lead EKG is beneficial for athletes who may be at risk of SCA; however, there is a great deal of heterogeneity in screening practices, lending to continued fatalities (Corrado et al., 2005).

Treatment

Electrophysiological disorders often cannot be cured, rather managed through medication, ablation, and therapy from an implantable cardioverter defibrillator. Medications for persons with electrophysiological disorders and those prone to arrhythmias include beta-blockade and other antiarrhythmic medications, which are designed respectively to slow the rate of the heart and to prevent arrhythmias (Aleong, Milan, & Ellinor, 2007). While beta-blockade has mild risk, antiarrhythmic medications can elicit serious side effects, such as exacerbation of ventricular tachycardia, which is known as a pro-arrhythmic effect (Ali, 2008). Consequently, in some cases, the treatment of the underlying disease can increase risk of SCA.

Radiofrequency catheter ablation is another treatment option for those with some types of life-threatening arrhythmias. This is a procedure in which a catheter tip is positioned over the area of the heart that is responsible for triggering the tachycardia. The tissue is then heated with the catheter, thereby burning the myocardium and creating a scar, to prevent an electrical current from passing through or originating from this tissue (AHA, 2011a). This approach provides more permanent protection from arrhythmias. When there is a discrete arrhythmogenic focus, a recent meta-analysis demonstrated that ablation is feasible and safe in pediatric patients, and the success and low recurrence rates of tachycardia were encouraging after this procedure (Tomaske, Candina, Weiss, & Bauersfeld, 2011). However, for some of the arrhythmias which are known as channelopathies, such as LQTS or Brugada syndrome, catheter ablation is ineffective because all the ventricular myocardium is involved, rather than a small defined area. However, ongoing evaluation of the effectiveness of ablation procedures is ongoing in adults and children.

Those with risk of arrhythmias or primary electrophysiological disorders are often treated with an implantable cardioverter defibrillator (ICD) for either prophylactic or secondary prevention of SCA. The ICD is a device that operates by monitoring potentially lethal electrical rhythms of the heart and terminating them with an immediate high-voltage shock. Several large-scale clinical trials have demonstrated the mortality benefit of the ICD over antiarrhythmic medication. All-cause mortality has been reduced by 23–30 % in patients who are treated with the ICD in addition to antiarrhythmic medication (Bardy et al., 2005; Moss et al., 2002). Criteria for implantation often include survival of SCA, syncope, significant family history of sudden death, and/or diminished ejection fraction (Aleong et al., 2007).

Physical Experience of the Disease

Individuals with electrophysiological disorders may present with or without symptoms. When the heart beats too slow (bradycardia), the affected individual is prone to fatigue, loss of oxygen to the body and the brain, and syncope (near and actual fainting). In the case of tachycardia, which is the hallmark symptom of electrophysiological disorders, the most common warning signs are palpitations, light-headedness, dizziness, dyspnea (shortness of breath), and syncope, possibly leading to SCA and death (Schimpf, Veltmann, Wolpert, & Borggrefe, 2009). Those who are asymptomatic experience the same underlying pathology, but have no awareness of such, presenting the possibility of syncope and SCA, seemingly without forewarning. In these individuals, their first symptom may be their last.

In those with electrophysiological disorders, symptoms can be triggered by a plethora of stimuli. They include, but are not limited to, the following: strenuous exercise, auditory stimuli, sudden bursts of activity, swimming, sudden changes in temperature, caffeine, certain medications, and/or during sleep patterns (Schimpf et al., 2009). Not only do these triggers vary by disorder but also by genetic variation of each disorder. The complexity of the disorders and their variants can make it difficult for adolescents and their parents to know which triggers to avoid, and may lead some parents to take measures to overprotect their child from such stimuli.

The most significant limitation that those with electrophysiological disorders face is restraint from sports activity. Risk stratification for sports participation is complex and depends on the child's disorder and presentation (Schimpf et al., 2009). It is difficult for medical providers themselves to know how to make the most accurate recommendations regarding sports (Heidbuchel et al., 2006). Several studies have demonstrated accord that those with LQTS, Brugada syndrome, and CPVT should not perform competitive sports (Heidbuchel et al., 2006). There is much more variation in medical providers' approach toward acceptable leisure-time activities, lending to more uncertainty about limitations and the possibility of overprotection, which may or may not be necessary for the adolescent.

Psychosocial Adjustment

Children and adolescents with arrhythmias often face psychosocial struggles to adjust to their disease and treatment. These adjustment difficulties are made complex not only by the child's reactions to his/her limitations but also by the parental reactions of overprotection and anxiety. Due to the low incidence of electrophysiological disorders, there is a paucity of research in the coping processes of these individuals, especially adolescents. This section will primarily focus on studies regarding the adjustment of individuals with one of the most common electrophysiological diseases, which is LQTS.

Due to the threat of sudden death, those with or at risk for arrhythmias often struggle with anxiety. Few studies actually focus on the psychosocial adjustment of the child with the arrhythmias; however, one study compared the adjustment of children with LQTS (mean age 13) and children with asthma (mean age = 11; Giuffre, Gupta, Crawford, & Leung, 2008). With use of standardized measures of anxiety and behaviors, these researchers illustrated that children with both asthma and LQTS had extensive fears, yet the fears varied between the medical conditions. The fears of children with asthma were the following: medical fears, fear of danger/death, and fear of minor injury, whereas those with LQTS experienced fear of failure and criticism, and they tended to keep feelings in while minimizing their true feelings of anxiety. Also, children with LQTS showed more internalizing problems than their counterparts with asthma. This suggests that adolescents with LQTS may experience fears related to their disorder, but find difficulty in sharing their anxiety openly.

A qualitative study that included adults with LQTS likewise demonstrated that anxiety and worry often surface in the psychosocial adjustment of this population (Anderson, Oyen, Bjorvatn, & Gjengedal, 2008). Through interviews, these researchers found that anxiety can be related to the high level of uncertainty about when/why symptoms surface and the relatively little known about LQTS by medical providers. In those who have experienced and survived manifestations of their illness, anxiety seems related to those specific cardiac events that threatened their lives. For instance, the youngest person in the study at hand, a 23-year-old female, made the following statement related to her worry, "It comes when I'm about to go to rest, then… Well, it's not every night, but quite a few nights of the week that I go to bed at night thinking: What was it like that night? What was it like when I passed out?" (Anderson et al., 2008, p. 492).

Next, treatments for electrophysiological disorders can be equally as distressing as the cardiac condition itself. Often a medication regimen is required, which can unfortunately cause side effects including fatigue, depression, or even exacerbation of ventricular tachycardia. Further, electrophysiological disorders are often treated with the ICD, and while it is a life-saving device, coping with the possibility of intense electrical shock to the body can cause anxiety. This will be addressed in the section titled *Special Consideration: The Experience of Adolescents with Implantable Cardioverter Defibrillators*.

Family Functioning

A broader set of research studies have been conducted on parents' adjustment to having a child with an electrophysiological disorder. Naturally, having a child or adolescent with a disorder that could suddenly claim his or her life with little warning due to SCA increases the anxiety of parents and family members. Researchers found a significant fear of their child's death in parents of children with LQTS (Farnsworth, Fosyth, Haglund, & Ackerman, 2006). One parent made the comment, "When I walk into their rooms in the morning to wake them, I am always aware in the back of my mind… will they be cold?" (Farnsworth et al., 2006, p.287).

Family function is often consequently centered on reducing the risk of sudden death of a child. Parents find themselves taking on the role of educator since these conditions are rare and relatively new to the scientific community. In one qualitative study of parents with a child with LQTS, a parent reported, "I educated the doctor; I talk to the older doctors who have never heard of it [LQTS]" and "I went to the school and talked to the teachers and told them if he passes out to call 911" (Farnsworth et al., 2006, p. 287).

Families often use avoidance as a coping mechanism when a family member suffers from an electrophysiological disorder. Certain electrophysiological problems can be triggered by arousal and strenuous activity; henceforth, parents attempt to reduce exposure to such stimuli (Farnsworth et al., 2006). This may be especially difficult when diagnosis presents in the adolescent time period, as it often does, since a child must suddenly stop physical activities that he or she had engaged in most of his or her young life. Parents may become overprotective, limiting activities that may not be necessary to stop. This overprotection may be allayed by treatment with the implantable cardioverter defibrillator, to be discussed later in this chapter.

Cardiomyopathy

Etiology

Cardiomyopathy is a term for a diseased state of the heart, in which there is a structural abnormality in the ventricular muscle fibers. There are four main forms of the disease, including dilated and hypertrophic cardiomyopathy, the most common forms, and restrictive and arrhythmogenic right ventricular cardiomyopathy, which occur less frequently in children. For relevance to adolescents, the focus in this chapter will be on dilated and hypertrophic cardiomyopathy. In their vital facts resource, the Children's Cardiomyopathy Foundation (2008) has compiled research on statistics of the disease. The prevalence of cardiomyopathy is estimated at one in every 100,000 children under the age of 18 in the United States, yet this is thought to be an underestimation since many undiagnosed children can die suddenly with SCA. The majority of the time, the disease is detected when children are under the age of 12 months; however, the second largest age range of detection is adolescents aged 12–18 years. Cardiomyopathy can be a primary inherited problem, or it can be acquired from secondary causes, such as infections, cancer chemotherapy, low blood flow to the heart, oxygen, or high blood pressure. However, in 75 % of cases of the disease, the cause is unknown.

Those with cardiomyopathy are highly susceptible to life-threatening arrhythmias and heart failure. Cardiomyopathy is the most common cause of sudden cardiac death (including trained athletes; Maron, 2003). Also, cardiomyopathy can lead to heart failure, a state in which the heart is unable to pump blood in a substantial enough way to meet the body's needs for oxygen and nutrients. Heart failure is a progressive disease, meaning that once symptoms thereof present, they must be actively monitored and managed to prevent further episodes of decline.

Treatment

There is no cure for cardiomyopathy; rather treatment is aimed at the management of symptoms. Treatment varies dependent upon the type of cardiomyopathy. In general, however, disease management often involves medications, including diuretics, inotropic agents, afterload-reducing agents, and beta-blockers (AHA, 2011b). Respectively, these medications serve to decrease excess fluid in the lungs or other organs, to help the heart contract more effectively, to relax the arteries and allow the blood to flow with more ease to the body, and to slow the heartbeat and decrease the effort needed for contraction of the heart muscle. Also, depending on the subtype and severity, medication management may include anticoagulation therapy to reduce the risk of blood clots and antiarrhythmic medications to reduce episodes of tachycardia, which can lead to SCA.

When individuals with hypertrophic cardiomyopathy develop symptoms of heart failure, alcohol septal ablation (ASA) and septal myomectomy may be recommended. Both procedures are designed to reduce the impact of heart failure symptoms by decreasing obstruction to blood flow out of the heart; however, they are not cures for cardiomyopathy or heart failure. Recent research was conducted with a patient sample with hypertrophic cardiomyopathy and concurrent significant psychological distress and compromised well-being. Participants were evaluated pre- and post-ASA, and post-scores demonstrated reductions in distress, and improvement in well-being and disease severity (Serber, Sears, & Nielsen, 2007).

Other forms of cardiomyopathy management include pacemaker implantation and ICD technology. Because individuals with cardiomyopathy are prone to life-threatening arrhythmias, ICD therapy is beneficial for protection against SCA and sudden death. Further, recent pacemaker technology has been updated with the biventricular pacing function. Biventricular pacing is used often in cases of dilated cardiomyopathy and when cardiomyopathy has progressed to heart failure. The biventricular pacemaker involves pacing in both the right and left ventricles to allow them to contract together and improve synchrony. Biventricular pacing has shown promising long-term benefits in those implanted with this form of pacemaker (Linde et al., 2002).

In the most severe forms of cardiomyopathy, heart transplantation is necessary to improve survival and QoL. Cardiomyopathy is one of the leading causes of heart transplantation in youth (AHA, 2011b). Survival rates are promising. When pediatric age groups and diagnoses are combined in analysis, the 1-year survival rate is 75–85 %. At 5 years, the survival rate is 65–75 %, while long-term survival rates continue to be monitored and are forecast to improve with better rejection surveillance and medications (Morrow, 2000). Despite the promise of heart transplantation, the procedure is related to its own complications, such as infection, organ rejection, coronary artery disease, and the side effects of medications, thereby creating its own unique disease state.

If a heart transplant is not available in adequate timing for the adolescent, ventricular assist devices may be helpful. Ventricular assist devices are mechanical devices that assist in the pumping of the heart for short periods of time. However, these devices are not intended for long-term use, and they prove beneficial primarily in those cases wherein the device is used as a bridge to actual heart transplantation (Sharma et al., 2006).

Physical Experience of the Disease

Adolescents with cardiomyopathy can vary in presentation from having no or mild symptoms to the more severe state, wherein cardiomyopathy has caused congestive heart failure and the symptoms thereof. In some cases, an adolescent may have no evident symptoms of cardiomyopathy and suddenly develop a life-threatening arrhythmia, prompting abrupt and immediate diagnosis and intervention. In other cases, the affected individual may have the mild symptoms of decreased exercise capacity or becoming easily fatigued. In the more severe state, such as when cardiomyopathy becomes suddenly and rapidly evident as the result of a viral infection, heart failure develops. The symptoms of heart failure include difficulty breathing, fatigue with non-strenuous activities, coughing, swelling, pale color, decreased urine output, and excessive sweating; unfortunately, if not promptly diagnosed, some of these symptoms may be mistaken as asthma (AHA, 2011b) and effective treatment may be delayed.

Medications used to manage cardiomyopathy often result in multiple side effects. Depending on the type of medication, the following are some of the complaints that may arise: dizziness, fatigue, excessive bruising or bleeding from minor injury, and lowered blood pressure/heart rate (AHA, 2011b). Medication management is more intense if heart failure occurs or transplantation is needed, resulting in more doctors' appointments and, possibly, dietary restrictions.

Unfortunately, those with cardiomyopathy have many physical restrictions. Due to the risk of SCA/death and increased heart failure, adolescents with both hypertrophic and dilated cardiomyopathy are not permitted to play competitive sports, as defined as organized team activity involving training (AHA, 2011b). Leisure-time and less strenuous activity restrictions should be tailored by the treating cardiologist due to varying degrees of cardiomyopathy.

Psychosocial Functioning

Adolescents with cardiomyopathy are prone to layers of psychosocial difficulties. First, since these adolescents are prone to arrhythmias and SCA, they are susceptible to the psychosocial problems that were discussed in previous section regarding adjustment to electrophysiological disorders. Refer to that section for more information. Second, since cardiomyopathy is a lifelong disease that cannot be "cured," it results in episodes of decompensation that can incur the acute stressors of symptom flare-ups and increased need for medical attention. This aspect of the disease envelops uncertainty about prognosis and need for strict adherence to one's medical regimen.

Few studies have been conducted on the psychosocial adjustment of adolescents with cardiomyopathy; thus, studies of adults will be used in this section. One study systematically explored the impact of dilated cardiomyopathy on QoL and well-being (Steptoe, Mohabir, Mahon, & McKenna, 2000). The mean age of participants was 47.6, with the youngest person at the age of 16. When compared to the normative population, results illustrated a significant decrement in those with cardiomyopathy in the domains of activities of daily living, emotional functioning, social functioning, vitality, general perceptions of health, and sleep. These results were similar to those found in a closely related study of participants with hypertrophic cardiomyopathy by the same investigators. Further, participants with dilated cardiomyopathy experienced more depression and anxiety than the normative population. These results were only partially accounted for by symptoms and the severity of the underlying disease, indicating that simply being diagnosed with such a condition incurs a substantial level of ongoing stress.

For those with cardiomyopathy that advances to heart failure, more psychosocial decrements are expected. In adults, depression in patients with heart failure is more common than in the normative population (Johansson, Dahlstrom, & Brostrom, 2006). Further, heart failure is related to decrements in health status and an increased risk of hospitalization (Havranek, Ware, & Lowes, 1999).

Since cardiomyopathy is a leading cause for heart transplantation, it is necessary to discuss coping with this significant form of medical intervention. Coping with transplantation entails many facets including awaiting an appropriate and timely donor, concerns related to rejection of the donated heart, concerns related to the surgery, and the rigorous medical regimen that follows transplantation. Very little has been researched on the coping of the adolescent who undergoes heart transplantation, but some research suggests that those who survive fare quite well. One small-scale study demonstrated positive outcomes in QoL, function, and psychological well-being in adolescents who survived successful transplantation when compared to healthy populations (Pollock-BarZiv, Anthony, Niedra, Dipchand, & West, 1997). In terms of adult psychological functioning, an extensive study detailed the 5-year adjustment rates of individuals who survived a cardiac transplant (Rybarczyk et al., 2007). Participants were a minimum age of 21, indicating that some were adolescent-age at time of transplant. The results indicated normal long-term adjustment of transplanted patients when compared to the normative population. Depression scores were lower in transplanted patients than in those counterparts who had heart failure, but no transplantation. Also, negative affect ratings in transplanted individuals were similar to those seen in the normative population. These are promising results; however they highlight the risk to the adolescent; the best predictors of depression were younger age, lower recreational functioning, neurological problems, and lower satisfaction with emotional support.

Finally, due to the limited research on youth coping with cardiomyopathy, there is also a lack of research on the familial adjustment to the disorder. The ever-present risk of SCA leads to the postulation that families presented with cardiomyopathy struggle with the same fears and avoidant behaviors as those families affected by electrophysiological disorders. Further, families in which a child is diagnosed with cardiomyopathy or heart transplant often have a taxing medical regimen that can create stress on the dynamics of the entire family.

Special Consideration: The Experience of Adolescents Treated with Implantable Cardioverter Defibrillators

As previously mentioned, the implantable cardioverter defibrillator (ICD) is a medical device that has dramatically decreased the incidence of sudden cardiac death. Both youth and adults with CHDs, electrophysiological disorders of the heart, and cardiomyopathy (among other cardiac conditions) are prone to life-threatening arrhythmias that lead to SCA and death. The ICD is a medical device that monitors the heart to detect and treat potentially lethal electrical rhythms with an immediate high-voltage shock.

Although the ICD was initially designed for adults, clinical research and modifications have extended the use of the device to children and teens. Researchers have demonstrated excellent survival rates of children with ICDs and congenital heart disease of 95.8 % at 4 years (Gradaus et al., 2004) and 89 % at 5 years (Sreeram, Trieschmann, & de Haan, 2008). Consistent rates of appropriate, life-saving shock therapy in young patients have been documented at 28 % (Alexander et al., 2004) and 26 % (Berul et al., 2008), demonstrating high utility of the device in young patients who are at risk for SCA. However, while survival rates are impressive, existing research suggests that pediatric ICD recipients are at greater risks for device and health-related complications when compared to adult recipients. Growth, as measured by change in height, weight, or body surface area, may be a strong predictor of lead failure in pediatric patients, which may result in lead extractions and replacements, as well as inappropriate multiple shocks and psychological distress (Alexander et al., 2004; Korte, Koditz, Niehaus, & Tebbenjohanns, 2004).

Knowledge of the psychosocial experiences of pediatric ICD patients is limited compared to the extensive research that has been documented for adult patients. In adult ICD recipients, the prevalence of anxiety is 13–38 % (Burke, Hallas, Clark-Carter, & Connelly, 2003; Camm et al., 1999;

Sears & Conti, 2002) while 24–46 % of patients are affected by depression (Bilge et al., 2006; Camm et al., 1999). Further, a recent meta-analysis suggested that QoL remained the same or improved in the majority of adult ICD patients who received the device (Francis, Johnson, & Niehaus, 2006); however, this did not hold true for patients who received multiple ICD shocks. The majority of these studies evidenced that patients receiving shocks experienced worsening QoL. Passmann et al. (2007) demonstrated that the experience of one shock is associated with a decrement in QoL, but clinically significant deficits do not appear to occur until a patient experiences 5 or more device discharges.

Shock has been described as a "6" on a pain scale of 1–10 (Ahmad, Bloomstein, Roelke, Bernstein, & Parsonnet, 2000; Pelletier, Gallagher, Mitten-Lewis, McKinley, & Squire, 2002) and in adults, it is the feature of the ICD most associated with decrements in QoL (Passman et al., 2007). The unpredictable and uncomfortable ICD shock serves as a potential aversive stimulus in patients' everyday lives, which may activate a host of maladaptive feelings and cognitions. Cognitive reactions include making faulty conclusions that the ICD is actually harmful, instead of life-saving, and that physical functioning will "cause" the ICD to discharge, leading to an attitude of learned helplessness (Goodman & Hess, 1999). Further, patients who have experienced shock may make flawed associations between shock and activities during shock when in most cases, arrhythmias occur without regard to activity. These feelings and cognitions often lead patients to avoid situations and people due to fear of being shocked and fear of embarrassment.

A recent study shed light on the psychosocial adjustment specific to children and adolescents with ICDs. Sears et al. (2011) explored the perceptions of youth with ICDs ($n=65$; ages 8–18) and their parents. Participants reported both lower physical and psychological QoL scores when compared with scores of healthy youth in the normative population. When compared with chronically ill youth, ICD recipients had lower physical QoL scores. When parents of ICD recipients rated their perception of their child's physical and psychological QoL, their ratings were significantly lower than those of parent-perceived scores of children in the normative and chronically ill populations. Surprisingly, there were no differences in the perceived QoL of ICD recipients in terms of ICD shocks and medical severity. One of the most significant findings of the study was that 87 % of the participants reported avoidance behaviors since ICD implantation, especially in females.

One final aspect of ICD therapy is device maintenance. Patients can expect device generator replacement every 5–7 years, as well as lead extraction/replacement every 10–15 years. Device maintenance requires patients to attend regular device interrogation appointments with their electrophysiologists every 3–6 months whereby information is obtained from the device to assess the presence of arrhythmias, device therapy, and device malfunctioning. As they transition to young adulthood, younger ICD patients must learn to stay abreast on recall notices and ways of managing distressful reactions to the possibility of recall (Sears & Conti, 2006; Stutts et al., 2007).

Assessment

Due to the nature of cardiac disease and its incompatibility with normal development, adolescents with such cardiac conditions often benefit from comprehensive assessment, which can guide appropriate intervention. As already mentioned, teens with cardiac conditions face substantial barriers to maintaining adequate QoL and developing independence. These issues also lend to decrements in mental health as evidenced in psychological and social domains. Utilizing appropriate standardized instruments not only provides clinicians with a better understanding of the adolescent experience of heart disease but also allows for a comparison to a healthy peer sample. Members of an interdisciplinary team who may administer these tools vary, but often include nurses and psychologists. However, a general rule of thumb is to seek supervision in the case that the administrator has limited experience

Table 2 Assessment tools utilized in studies of children and adolescents with heart disease

Measurement tool	Reference	Disease specific
Severity		
Cardiologist's Perception of Medical Severity Scale (CSEV)	DeMaso et al. (1991)	Yes
Family functioning		
Parental HRQoL	Landolt (2011)	No
Maternal Cognitive Processes	Moos and Tsu (1977)	No
Hassles and Uplifts Scale	DeLongis, Folkman, and Lazarus (1988)	No
Multidimensional Health Locus of Control Scales	Wallston, Wallston, and Lazarus (1978)	No
Ways of Coping Questionnaire	Folkman and Lazarus (1980)	No
Family Environment Scale	Moos and Moos (1981)	No
Brief Symptom Inventory	Derogatis (1975)	No
Parenting Stress Index	Abidin (1990)	No
Emotional functioning		
TNO-AZL Child Quality of Life Questionnaire (TACQOL)	Vogels et al. (2000)	No
Cardiac-Specific Module (CHD-TAAQOL)	Kamphuis et al. (2004)	Yes
Pediatric Cardiac Quality of Life Inventory (PCQLI)	Marino et al. (2008)	Yes
Social functioning		
Child Behavior Checklist (CBCL)	Achenbach (1991)	No
Vineland Adaptive Behavior Scale (VABS)	Sparrow, Balla, and Cicchetti (1984)	No
Functional Independence Measure for Children (WeeFIM)	Uniform Data System for Medical Rehabilitation (1998)	No
Functioning related to implantable cardioverter defibrillators (ICDs)		
Avoidance Measure	Lemon, Edelman, and Kirkness (2004)	Yes
Cognitive Coping with ICD Shock	Godemann et al. (2004)	Yes
Florida Patient Acceptance Survey (FPAS)	Burns, Serber, Keim, and Sears (2005)	Yes

giving an assessment. Table 2 provides assessment tools which have been used with children and teens with heart disease.

Neuro-cognitive assessment tools, often applicable to the pediatric population with CHD, are not included in this table. This is because a full neuropsychological battery for children displaying symptoms of neurological deficits is required for appropriate intervention. In the case that neuropsychological assessment is needed, adolescents and teens may be referred to a school psychologist and/or a neuropsychology practice.

Psychosocial Interventions

Despite a great deal of evidence that adolescents with cardiac conditions face many challenges, at the present time there are few empirical interventions designed specifically for children and adolescents with CHD, electrophysiological disorders, or cardiomyopathy. In the case that a child or adolescent requires psychosocial intervention, an appropriate referral would be to a pediatric, school, or health psychologist. For the teen or adolescent facing cognitive or neuropsychological impairments, some behavioral interventions delivered by a neuropsychologist may improve functioning.

One hypothesis regarding psychosocial interventions for youth with cardiac conditions is that they should focus on the child's coping with limitations with physical activities, and on reducing parental overprotective behaviors. According to a prominent developmental psychologist, Erik Erikson (1968), early stages of development involve a certain degree of exploration, mastery over skills, and investigation of roles (athlete, student, worker, etc.). If these critical activities are limited or halted (i.e., when an adolescent is newly diagnosed, and physical activity must be stopped), stages of development may not be mastered in a linear fashion. See Diagram 1 for an illustration of the possible effects of heart disease on pediatric development through adolescence.

With guidance from Diagram 1 and other treatment models, psychosocial interventions may include the elements of education, parent–child communication, acceptance, and identity exploration. Both the adolescent and parent should be encouraged to obtain a clear understanding of the child's disease state, as well as accurate recommendations for restrictions, rather than assuming what activities are on or off-limits. Consequently, communication on these issues should be facilitated between the child and parent. Interventions likely to benefit adolescents are those that promote acceptance of physical limitations and exploration of alternative skills and roles within the constraints of their restrictions. While there is a lack of empirical evidence regarding this matter, psychosocial interventions that involve acceptance and commitment therapy (ACT; Greco & Hayes, 2008) and cognitive-behavioral therapy (CBT; Friedburg & McClure, 2002) may be helpful in achieving the aforementioned goals.

Treatments that address anxiety may be paramount for adolescents with heart disease and their parents. As previously mentioned in each of the three sections on heart disease, anxiety surfaces due to uncertainty about one's future, fears about which triggers will cause arrhythmias or further decline, and fears about how a child will be perceived by peers due to his/her heart condition, among many others. Again, CBT and ACT may be helpful to both the child and parents. The family will need to understand and gain awareness of their fears to address them through cognitive restructuring or acceptance. Further, the application of relaxation strategies and deep breathing techniques may assist the child and parent to ease the strain of anxiety on the body.

Teens with heart disease often have a medical regimen to follow; therefore interventions that promote adherence are encouraged. Adolescents with heart disease are likely to be gaining independence and increasing their responsibilities for managing their diseases. They contend with responsibilities to medication, physical restrictions, and attendance of doctor's appointments, among others. Often seen with cardiomyopathy, those who develop heart failure and/or require a heart transplant face a strict, life-threatening need for adherence (McAllister, Buckner, & White-Williams, 2006). Again, the literature is sparse on empirical psychosocial treatment approaches specific to adherence in adolescents with heart disease. Some qualitative studies stress that adherence in adolescents with cardiac conditions can be enhanced through a supportive environment, knowledge of their medications and disease, a positive self-concept, and doctor–patient communication (Ittenbach, Cassedy, Marino, Spicer, & Drotar, 2009).

Some intervention models for teens with specific cardiac conditions involve interdisciplinary collaboration and physical components. Fredriksen et al. (2000) created an intervention protocol for adolescents with CHD. The intervention itself consisted of either a 2-week sports rehabilitation center training or 5 months of home-based training. Physical activities were chosen to increase strength, flexibility, stamina, balance, and coordination. In addition to supervised physical training, intervention groups were provided information about CHD and physical activity. Ultimately, the rehab center group was not different from the home-based training group. When compared to controls that were only provided assessment and information about CHD and physical activity, the intervention group had significantly lowered internalizing behavior. In fact, decreased withdrawal and somatic complaints scales of the Child Behavior Checklist had the greatest improvement following physical activity intervention. Physical activity intervention also resulted in increased oxygen uptake and greater physical activity. On the contrary, this intervention was not sufficient to reduce externalizing behavioral problems or anxiety and depression scores.

There is a paucity of research targeting psychosocial interventions for both teens and adults

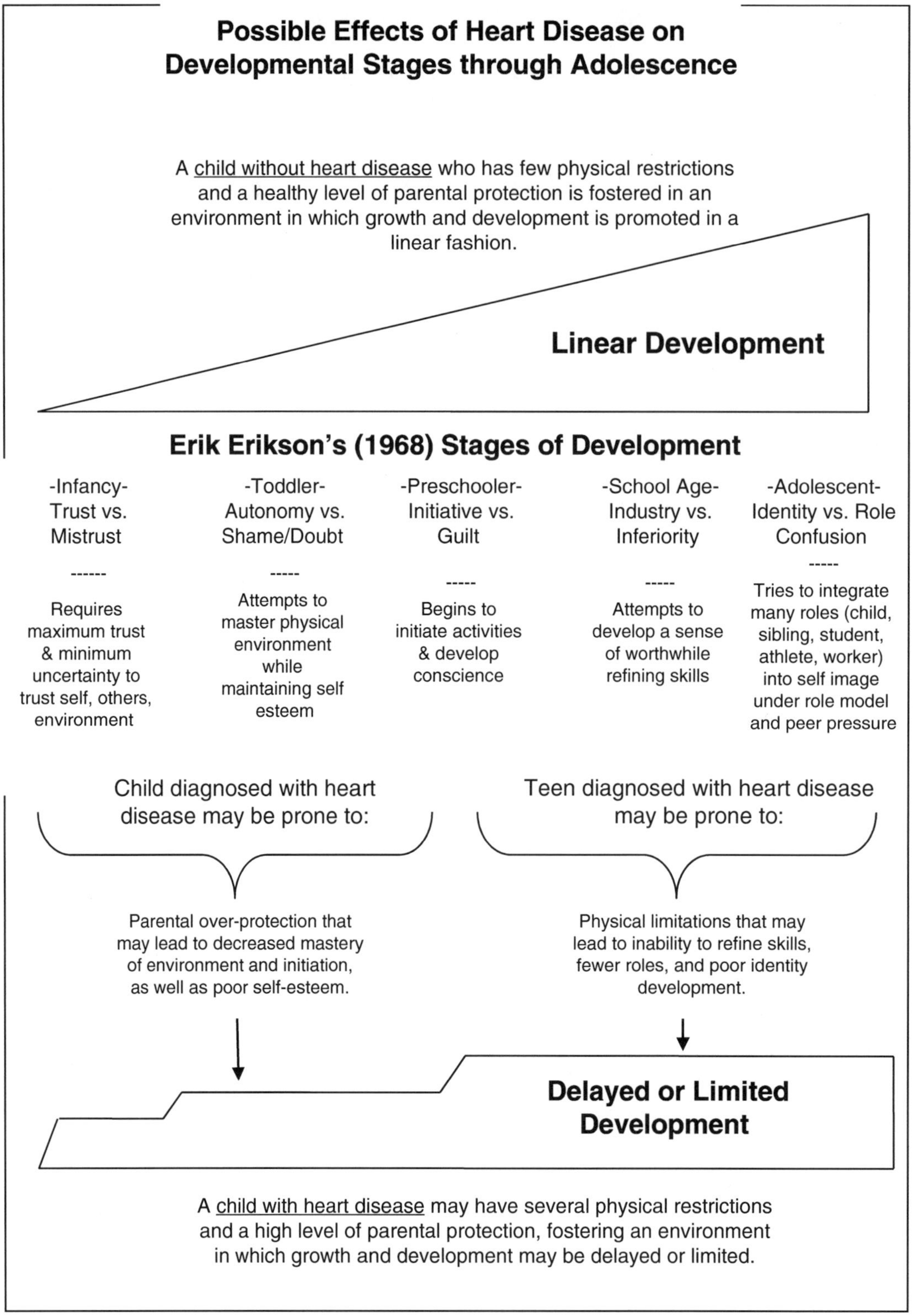

Diagram 1 Possible effects of heart disease on developmental stages through adolescence

alike with electrophysiological disorders and cardiomyopathy. However, there are interventions designed for individuals with ICDs, many of whom are diagnosed with the two aforementioned cardiac conditions to treat or prevent life-threatening arrhythmias. All of these interventions are designed for adults, yet they are worthy of mention as they shed light on treatment components that may be helpful for adolescents coping with the threat of SCA and ICDs.

A recent review of intervention trials has demonstrated that psychosocial interventions are indeed worthwhile for the adult ICD patient population (Pedersen, Van Den Broek, & Sears, 2007). This meta-analysis revealed that several interventions demonstrated a reduction in depressive symptoms and gains in QoL. The most prominent effects in the included studies demonstrated improved exercise capacity and decrements in anxiety in ICD patients. Further, Sears et al. (2007) introduced the shock and stress management program, which included a combination of ICD-specific education, relaxation/stress management, CBT techniques, and group discussion/social support. Special attention was paid to assist participants to cope with shock, to separate faulty associations between shock and certain activities, and to engage in important life's pleasurable activities without preoccupation and fear of shock. This comprehensive treatment package resulted in a significant reduction of anxiety and salivary cortisol, as well as a significant increase in patient acceptance of ICD technology. It is likely that this treatment protocol would be quite helpful to the pediatric population, and empirical research is encouraged to fill this gap in the literature.

Finally, high-quality interdisciplinary interventions should assist adolescents in transitioning from pediatric care to adult care. In 2011 the AHA published guidelines intended to assist pediatric and adult cardiologists during the transition to receiving adult care (Sable et al., 2011). The guidelines suggest that the goal for optimal transition is to provide uninterrupted, patient-centered, age and developmentally appropriate, flexible, and comprehensive care during transition. Specific to adolescents with CHD, Reid and associates (2004) found that correlates of successful transition to adult cardiology include older age at last pediatric cardiology appointment, previous independence during pediatric cardiology appointments, CHD-specific health beliefs (e.g., perceived risk of not attending appointments), higher frequency of pediatric cardiology appointments, health status, substance use, and distance to the nearest health care center. The AHA suggests that parents be included in the transition, that transition be considered a process rather than a discreet event, that developmental and medical needs be considered, and that the adult and pediatric cardiologist collaborate with the adolescent's primary care physician. The following are some specific guidelines delineated by age group:

1. Childhood: begin informing child about condition in developmentally appropriate language.
2. Early adolescence: begin foreshadowing with parents and adolescents about the imminent transfer to adult care and engage adolescents in transition planning; have discussion about the risks of smoking, alcohol use, and illicit drug use; ask adolescent about their understanding of their condition, physical activity limitations, and future goals.
3. Middle to late adolescence: begin conversations about vocational and employment advice, birth control, pregnancy, genetic counseling, and long-term prognosis; ensure all medical and surgical needs are satisfied prior to transfer; create a portable and accessible medical history; write a transfer of care letter; and provide the adolescent with a health-care transition resource binder.

During each of these points, it is suggested that providers address concerns with a nonjudgmental and empathetic nature and that emotional maturity be considered so that each adolescents' transition is appropriately tailored.

Conclusion

Modern medicine has succeeded in preventing mortality in many manifestations of cardiovascular disease in children and adolescents. With increased longevity, comprehensive management and adjustment to cardiovascular disease warrants attention to both psychosocial assessment and treatment interventions addressing specific patient and family needs. The current review highlighted the heterogeneity of common disease states and presentations as well as their broad impact on major areas of life functioning. The review brings attention to the clearly indicated need for multidisciplinary care in order to achieve the desired broad-based health outcomes, beyond simply mortality. Attention to the psychosocial functioning of young patients with cardiovascular disease makes good sense but requires a greater degree of medical team building and interdisciplinary dialogue and availability. The goal remains clear: help patients achieve optimal quality of life and daily functioning, despite their disease state. Innovation in disease-specific, tailored service delivery and health policy is ongoing and needed to achieve these ambitious goals.

References

Abidin, R. R. (1990). *Parenting stress index (PSI)*. Odess, FL: Psychological Assessment Resources.

Achenbach, T. M. (1991). *Manual for the CBCL/4–18 and 1991 profile*. Burlington, VT: University of Vermont, Department of Psychiatry.

Ahmad, M., Bloomstein, L., Roelke, M., Bernstein, A. D., & Parsonnet, V. (2000). Patients' attitudes toward implanted defibrillator shocks. *Pacing and Clinical Electrophysiology, 23*(6), 934–938.

Aleong, R. G., Milan, D. J., & Ellinor, P. T. (2007). The diagnosis and treatment of cardiac ion channelopathies: Congenital long QT syndrome and Brugada Syndrome. *Current Treatment Options in Cardiovascular Medicine, 9*(5), 364–371.

Alexander, M. E., Cecchin, F., Walsh, E. P., Triedman, J. K., Bevilacqua, L. M., & Berul, C. I. (2004). Implications of implantable cardioverter defibrillator therapy in congenital heart disease and pediatrics. *Journal of Cardiovascular Electrophysiology, 15*(1), 72–76.

Ali, K. M. S. (2008). Collateral effects of antiarrhythmics in pediatric age. *Current Pharmaceutical Design, 14*(8), 782–787.

Alpern, D., Uzark, K., & II Dick, M. (1989). Psychosocial responses of children to cardiac pacemakers. *Journal of Pediatrics, 114*, 494–501.

American Heart Association. (2011). *Children and Arrhythmia*. Retrieved July 30, 2011, from http://www.heart.org/HEARTORG/Conditions/Arrhythmia/AboutArrhythmia/Types-of-Arrhythmia-in-Children_UCM_302023_Article.jsp.

Anderson, J., Oyen, N., Bjorvatn, C., & Gjengedal, E. (2008). Living with Long-QT Syndrome: A qualitative study of coping with increased risk of sudden cardiac death. *Journal of Genetic Counseling, 17*, 489–498.

Antzelevitch, C., Brugada, P., Brugada, J., Brugada, R., Shimizu, W., Gussak, I., et al. (2002). Brugada syndrome: A decade of progress. *Circulation Research, 91*(12), 1114–1118.

Aurer, E. T., Senturia, A. G., Shopper, M., & Biddy, R. (1971). Congenital heart disease and child adjustment. *Psychiatric Medicine, 2*, 210–219.

Bardy, G. H., Lee, K. L., Mark, D. B., Poole, J. E., Packer, D. L., Boineau, R., et al. (2005). Amiodarone or an implanted cardioverter defibrillator for congestive heart failure. *The New England Journal of Medicine, 352*, 225–237.

Barrett, K., Van der Feen, J. R., Spieth, L., Berul, C., & DeMaso, D. R. (2001) *Worries in adolescents with implantable cardioverter defibrillators: A pilot study*. Poster session presented at the annual meeting of the North American Society of Pacing and Electrophysiology, Boston, MA.

Berul, C. I., Van Hare, G. F., Kertesz, N. J., Dubin, A. M., Cecchin, F., Collins, K. K., et al. (2008). Results of a multicenter retrospective implantable cardioverter-defibrillator registry of pediatric and congenital heart disease patients. *Journal of the American College of Cardiology, 51*(17), 1685–1691.

Bilge, A. K., Ozben, B., Demircan, S., Cinar, M., Yilmaz, E., & Abelet, K. (2006). Depression and anxiety status of patients with implantable cardioverter defibrillator and precipitating factors. *Pacing and Clinical Electrophysiology, 29*(6), 619–626.

Bromberg, J. I., Beasley, P. J., D'Angelo, E. J., Landzberg, M., & DeMaso, D. R. (2003). Depression and anxiety in adults with congenital heart defects: A pilot study. *Heart & Lung, 32*, 105–110.

Burke, J. L., Hallas, C. N., Clark-Carter, D., & Connelly, W. D. (2003). The psychosocial impact of the implantable cardioverter defibrillator: A meta-analytic review. *British Journal of Health Psychology, 8*(Pt 2), 165–178.

Burns, J. L., Serber, E. R., Keim, S., & Sears, S. F. (2005). Measuring patient acceptance of implantable cardiac device therapy: Initial psychometric investigation of the Florida patient acceptance survey. *Journal of Cardiovascular Electrophysiology, 16*(4), 384–390.

Camm, A. J., Sears, S. F., Jr., Todaro, J. F., Lewis, T. S., Sotile, W., & Conti, J. B. (1999). Examining the psychosocial impact of implantable cardioverter defibrillators: A literature review. *Clinical Cardiology, 22*(7), 481–489.

Casey, F. A., Sykes, D. H., Craig, B. G., Power, R., & Mulholland, H. C. (1996). Behavioral adjustment of children with surgically palliated complex congenital heart disease. *Journal of Pediatric Psychology, 21*, 335–352.

Children's Cardiomyopathy Foundation. (2008). *Vital facts*. Retrieved July 29, 2011, from http://www.childrenscardiomyopathy.org/site/vital.php.

Corrado, D., Basso, C., Rizzolo, G., Schiavon, M., & Thiene, G. (2003). Does sports activity enhance the risk of sudden death in adolescents and young adults? *Journal of the American College of Cardiology, 42*, 1959–1963.

Corrado, D., Pelliccia, A., Bjornstad, H. H., Vanhees, L., Biffi, A., Borjesson, M., et al. (2005). Cardiovascular pre-participation screening of young competitive athletes for prevention of sudden death: Proposal for a common European protocol. *European Heart Journal, 26*(5), 516–528.

Davis, C. C., Brown, R. T., Bakeman, R., & Campbell, R. (1998). Psychological adaptation of mother of children with congenital heart disease: Stress, coping, and family functioning. *Journal of Pediatric Psychology, 23*, 219–228.

Davis, A. M., Gow, R. M., McCrindle, B. W., & Hamilton, R. M. (1996). Clinical spectrum, therapeutic management, and follow-up of ventricular tachycardia in infants and young children. *American Heart Journal, 131*, 186–191.

DeLongis, A., Folkman, S., & Lazarus, R. S. (1988). The impact of daily stress on health and mood: Psychological and social resources as mediators. *Journal of Personality and Social Psychology, 54*, 486–495.

DeMaso, D. R. (2004). Pediatric Heart Disease. In R. T. Brown (Ed.), *Handbook of pediatric psychology in school settings* (pp. 283–298). Mahwah, NJ: Lawrence Erlbaum Associates.

DeMaso, D. R., Beardslee, W. R., Silbert, A. R., & Fyler, D. C. (1990). Psychological functioning in children with cyanotic heart defects. *Journal of Developmental and Behavioral Pediatrics, 11*, 289–293.

DeMaso, D. R., Camis, L. K., Wypij, D., Bertram, S., Lipshitz, M., & Freed, M. (1991). The impact of maternal perceptions and medical severity on the adjustment of children with congenital heart disease. *Journal of Pediatric Psychology, 16*, 137–149.

DeMaso, D. R., Spratt, E. G., Vaughan, B. L., D'Angelo, E. J., Van der Feen, J. R., & Walsh, E. (2000). Psychological functioning in children and adolescents undergoing radiofrequency catheter ablation. *Psychosomatics, 41*, 134–139.

DeMaso, D. R., Twente, A. W., Spratt, E. G., & O'Brien, P. (1995). The impact of psychological functioning, medical severity, and family functioning in pediatric heart transplantation. *The Journal of Heart and Lung Transplantation, 14*, 1102–1108.

Derogatis, L. R. (1975). *Brief Symptom Inventory*. Baltimore, ML: Clinical Psychometric Research.

Erikson, E. H. (1968). *Identity: Youth and crisis*. New York, NY: Norton.

Farnsworth, M. M., Fosyth, D., Haglund, C., & Ackerman, M. J. (2006). When I go in to wake them … I wonder: Parental perceptions about congenital long QT syndrome. *Journal of the American Academy of Nurse Practitioners, 18*, 284–290.

Fekkes, M., Kamphuis, R. P., Ottenkamp, J., Verrips, E., Vogels, T., Kamphuis, M., et al. (2001). Health-related quality of life in young adults with minor congenital heart defects. *Psychology and Health, 16*, 239–250.

Folkman, S., & Lazarus, R. S. (1980). An analysis of coping in a middle-aged community sample. *Journal of Pediatric Psychology, 15*, 347–358.

Foster, E., Graham, T. P., Driscoll, D. J., Reid, G. J., Reiss, J. G., Russell, I. A., et al. (2001). Task force 2: Special healthcare needs of adults with congenital heart disease. *Journal of the American College of Cardiology, 37*, 1183–1187.

Francis, J., Johnson, B., & Niehaus, M. (2006). Quality of life in patients with implantable cardioverter defibrillators. *Indian Pacing Electrophysiology Journal, 6*(3), 173–181.

Francis, J., Sankar, V., Nair, V. K., & Priori, S. G. (2005). Catecholaminergic polymorphic ventricular tachycardia. *Heart Rhythm, 2*(5), 550–554.

Fredriksen, P. M., Kahrs, N., Braasvaer, S., Sigurdsen, E., Gundersen, O., Roeksund, G., et al. (2000). Effects of physical training in children and adolescents with congenital heart disease. *Cardiology in the Young, 10*, 107–114.

Fricchione, G. L., & Vlay, S. C. (1986). Psychiatric aspects of patients with malignant ventricular arrhythmias. *The American Journal of Psychiatry, 143*, 1518–1526.

Friedburg, R. D., & McClure, J. M. (2002). *Clinical practice of cognitive therapy with children and adolescents: The nuts and bolts*. New York City: The Guilford Press.

Gallagher, J. J., Gilbert, M., Svenson, R. H., Sealy, W. C., Kassell, J., Wallace, A. G. (1975). Wolff-Parkinson-White syndrome. The problem, evaluation, and surgical correction. *Circulation, 51*, 767–785.

Giuffre, M., Gupta, S., Crawford, S. G., & Leung, A. K. C. (2008). Fears and anxiety in children with Long-QT Syndrome compared to children with asthma. *Journal of the National Medical Association, 100*(4), 420–424.

Godemann, F., Butter, C., Lampe, F., Linden, M., Schlegl, M., Schulthess, H. P., et al. (2004). Panic disorders and agoraphobia: Side effects of treatment with an implantable cardioverter defibrillator. *Clinical Cardiology, 27*(6), 321–326.

Goodman, M., & Hess, B. (1999). Could implantable cardioverter defibrillators provide a human model supporting the learned helplessness theory of depression? *General Hospital Psychiatry, 21*(5), 382–385.

Gradaus, R., Wollmann, C., Kobe, J., Hammel, D., Kotthoff, S., Block, M., et al. (2004). Potential benefit from implantable cardioverter-defibrillator therapy in children and young adolescents. *Heart, 90*(3), 328–329.

Greco, L. A., & Hayes, S. C. (Eds.). (2008). *Acceptance and mindfulness treatments for children and adolescents: A practitioner's guide*. Oakland: New Harbinger Publications.

Green, M., & Levitt, E. (1962). Constriction of body image in children with congenital heart disease. *Pediatrics, 29*, 438–443.

Havranek, E., Ware, M., & Lowes, B. (1999). Prevalence of depression in congestive heart failure. *The American Journal of Cardiology, 84*, 348–350.

Heidbuchel, H., Corrado, D., Biffi, A., Hoffmannd, E., Panhuyzen-Goedkoope, N., Hoogstenf, J., et al. (2006). Recommendations for participation in leisure-time physical activity and competitive sports of patients with arrhythmias and potentially arrhythmogenic conditions. Part II: Ventricular arrhythmias, channelopathies and implantable defibrillators. *European Journal of Cardiovascular Preventative Rehabilitation, 13*, 676–686.

Hoffman, J. I. E., Kaplan, S., & Liberthson, R. R. (2004). Prevalence of congenital heart disease. *American Heart Journal, 147*, 425–439.

Huikuri, H. V., Castellanos, A., & Myerburg, R. J. (2001). Sudden death due to cardiac arrhythmias. *The New England Journal of Medicine, 345*, 1473–1482.

Ittenbach, R. F., Cassedy, A. E., Marino, B. S., Spicer, R. L., & Drotar, D. (2009). Adherence to treatment among children with cardiac disease. *Cardiology in the Young, 19*, 545–551.

Johansson, R., Dahlstrom, U., & Brostrom, A. (2006). The measurement and prevalence of depression in patients with chronic heart failure. *Progress in Cardiovascular Nursing, 21*, 28–36.

Kamphuis, M., Zwinderman, K. H., Vogels, T., Vliegen, H. W., Kamphuis, R. P., Ottenkamp, J., et al. (2004). A cardiac-specific health-related quality of life module for young adults with congenital heart disease: Development and validation. *Quality of Life Research, 13*, 735–745.

Kardsorp, P. A., Evaraerd, W., Kindt, M., & Mulder, B. J. (2007). Psychological and cognitive functioning in children and adolescents with congenital heart disease: A meta-analysis. *Journal of Pediatric Psychology, 32*, 527–541.

Korte, T., Koditz, H., Niehaus, M., & Tebbenjohanns, J. (2004). High incidence of appropriate and inappropriate ICD therapies in children and adolescents with implantable cardioverter defibrillator. *Pacing and Clinical Electrophysiology, 27*(7), 924–932.

Kovacs, A. H., Saide, A. S., Kuhl, E. A., Sears, S. F., Silversides, C., Harrison, J. L., et al. (2009). Depression and anxiety in adult congenital heart disease: Predictors and prevalence. *International Journal of Cardiology, 137*, 158–164.

Landolt, M. A. (2011). Predictors of parental quality of life after child open heart surgery: A 6-month prospective study. *Journal of Pediatrics, 158*, 37–43.

Lemon, J., Edelman, S., & Kirkness, A. (2004). Avoidance behaviors in patients with implantable cardioverter defibrillators. *Heart & Lung, 33*(3), 176–182.

Liebson, P. R. (2010). Cardiovascular risk in special populations IV: Congenital heart defects. *Preventative Cardiology, 13*, 49–55.

Linde, C., Leclercq, C., Rex, S., Garrigue, S., Lavergne, T., Cazeau, S., et al. (2002). Long-term benefits of biventricular pacing in congestive heart failure: Results from the MUltisite STimulation in cardiomyopathy (MUSTIC) study. *Journal of the American College of Cardiology, 40*(1), 111–118.

Linde, L. M., Rasof, B., & Dunn, O. J. (1966). Attitudinal factors in congenital heart disease. *Pediatrics, 38*, 92–101.

Majnemer, A., Limperopoulos, C., Shevell, M., Rohlicek, C., Rosenblatt, B., & Tchervenkov, C. (2008). Developmental and functional outcomes at school entry in children with congenital heart defects. *Journal of Pediatrics, 153*, 55–60.

Marelli, A. J., Mackie, A. S., Ionescu-Ihu, R., Rahme, E., & Pilote, L. (2007). Congenital heart disease in the general population changing prevalence and age distribution. *Circulation, 115*, 163–172.

Marino, B. S., Shera, D., Wernovsky, G., Tomlinson, R. S., Aguirre, A., Gallagher, M., et al. (2008). The development of the pediatric cardiac quality of life inventory: A quality of life measure for children and adolescents with heart disease. *Quality of Life Research, 17*, 613–626.

Maron, B. J. (2003). Sudden death in young athletes. *The New England Journal of Medicine, 349*, 1064–1075.

McAllister, S., Buckner, E. B., & White-Williams, C. (2006). Medication adherence after heart transplantation: Adolescents and their issues. *Progress in Transplantation, 16*(4), 317–323.

Miatton, M., DeWolf, D., Francois, K., & Thiery, E. (2006). Neurocognitive consequences of surgically corrected congenital heart defects: A review. *Neuropsychology Review, 16*, 65–85.

Miyagul, N. I., Cardoso, S. M., Meyer, M., Utramari, F. T., Araujo, F. H., Rozkowisk, I., et al. (2003). Epidemiological study of congenital heart defects in children and adolescence: Analysis of 4,538 cases. *Arquivos Brasileiros de Cardiologia, 80*, 274–278.

Moos, R. H., & Moos, B. S. (1981). *Family environmental scale manual*. Palo Alto, CA: Consulting Psychologists Press.

Moos, R. H., & Tsu, V. D. (1977). The crisis of physical illness: An overview. In R. Moos (Ed.), *Coping with physical illness* (pp. 3–21). New York, NY: Plenum Press.

Morrow, W. R. (2000). Cardiomyopathy and heart transplantation in children. *Current Opinion in Cardiology, 15*(4), 216–223.

Moss, A. J., & Robinson, J. (1992). Clinical features of the idiopathic long QT syndrome. *Circulation, 85*((Suppl I)), 140–144.

Moss, A. J., Zareba, W., Hall, W. J., Klein, G., Wilber, D. J., Cannom, D. S., et al. (2002). Prophylactic implantation of a defibrillator in patients with myocardial infarction and reduced ejection fraction. *The New England Journal of Medicine, 346*(12), 877–883.

Noseworthy, P. A., & Newton-Cheh, C. (2008). Genetic Determinants of sudden cardiac arrest. *Circulation, 118*, 1854–1863.

O'Dougherty, M., Wright, F. S., Garmezy, N., Loewenson, R. B., & Torres, R. (1983). Later competence and adaptation in infants who survive severe heart defects. *Child Development, 54*, 1129–1142.

O'Dougherty, M., Wright, F. S., Loewenson, R. B., & Torres, R. (1985). Cerebral dysfunction after chronic hypoxia in children. *Neurology, 35*, 42–46.

Passman, R., Subacius, H., Ruo, B., Schaechter, A., Howard, A., Sears, S. F., et al. (2007). Implantable cardioverter defibrillators and quality of life: Results from the defibrillators in nonischemic cardiomyopathy treatment evaluation study. *Archives of Internal Medicine, 167*(20), 2226–2232.

Paul, T., Marchal, C., & Garson, A., Jr. (1990). Ventricular couplets in the young: Prognosis related to underlying substrate. *American Heart Journal, 119*(Pt. 1), 577–582.

Pedersen, S. S., Van Den Broek, K., & Sears, S. F. (2007). Psychological intervention following implantation of an implantable defibrillator: A review and future recommendations. *PACE, 30*, 1–9.

Pelletier, D., Gallagher, R., Mitten-Lewis, S., McKinley, S., & Squire, J. (2002). Australian implantable cardiac defibrillator recipients: Quality-of-life issues. *International Journal of Nursing Practice, 8*(2), 68–74.

Peterson, C., & Harbaugh, B. L. (1995). Children and adolescent's experiences while undergoing cardiac catheterization. *Maternal–Child. Nursing Journal, 23*, 15–25.

Pollock-BarZiv, S. M., Anthony, S. J., Niedra, R., Dipchand, A. I., & West, L. J. (1997). Quality of life and function following cardiac transplantation in adolescents. *Transplantation Proceedings, 35*(7), 2468–2470.

Reid, G. J., Irvine, M. J., McCrindle, B. W., Sananes, R., Ritvo, P. G., Sui, S. C., et al. (2004). Prevalence and correlates of successful transfer from pediatric to adult health care among a cohort of young adults with complex congenital heart disease. *Pediatrics, 113*, e197–e205.

Rybarczyk, B., Grady, K. L., Naftel, D. C., Kirklin, J. K., White-Williams, C., Kobashigawa, J., et al. (2007). Emotional adjustment 5 years after heart transplant: A multisite study. *Rehabilitation Psychology, 57*(2), 206–214.

Sable, C., Foster, E., Uzark, K., Bjornsen, K., Canobbio, J., Connolly, H. M., et al. (2011). Best practices in managing transition to adulthood for adolescents with congenital heart disease: The transition process and medical and psychosocial issues: A scientific statement from the American heart association. *Circulation, 123*, 1454–1485.

Schimpf, R., Veltmann, C., Wolpert, C., & Borggrefe, M. (2009). Channelopathies: Brugada Syndrome, Long QT Syndrome, Short QT Syndrome, and CPVT. *Herz, 34*, 281–288.

Sears, S. F., Jr., & Conti, J. B. (2002). Quality of life and psychological functioning of ICD patients. *Heart, 87*(5), 488–493.

Sears, S. F., Jr., & Conti, J. B. (2006). Psychological aspects of cardiac devices and recalls in patients with implantable cardioverter defibrillators. *The American Journal of Cardiology, 98*(4), 565–567.

Sears, S. F., Hazelton, A. G., St Amant, J., Matchett, M., Kovacs, A., Vazquez, L. D., et al. (2011). Quality of life in pediatric patients with implantable cardioverter defibrillators. *The American Journal of Cardiology, 107*(7), 1023–1027.

Sears, S. F., Sowell, L. D., Kuhl, E. A., Kovaks, A. H., Serber, E. R., Handburg, E., et al. (2007). The ICD shock and stress management program: A randomized trial of psychosocial treatment to optimize quality of life in ICD patients. *Pacing and Clinical Electrophysiology, 30*(7), 858–864.

Serber, E. R., Sears, S. F., & Nielsen, C. D. (2007). Depression, anxiety, and quality of life in patients with obstructive hypertrophic cardiomyopathy three months after alcohol septal ablation. *The American Journal of Cardiology, 100*(10), 1592–1597.

Sharma, M. S., Webber, S. A., Morell, V. O., Gandhi, S. K., Wearden, P. D., Buchanan, J. R., et al. (2006). Ventricular assist device support in children and adolescents as a bridge to heart transplantation. *The Annals of Thoracic Surgery, 82*(3), 926–932.

Silbert, A., Wolff, P. H., Mayer, B., Rosenthal, A., & Nadas, A. S. (1969). Cyanotic heart disease and psychological development. *Pediatrics, 143*, 192–200.

Somerville, J. (1997). Management of adults with congenital heart disease: An increasing problem. *Annual Review of Medicine, 48*, 283–293.

Sparacino, P. A., Tong, E. M., Messias, D. K., Foote, D., Chesla, C. A., & Gilliss, C. L. (1997). The dilemmas of parents of adolescents and young adults with congenital heart disease. *Heart & Lung, 26*, 187–195.

Sparrow, S., Balla, D. A., & Cicchetti, D. V. (1984). *Vineland adaptive behavior scales, interview edition. Survey form manual: A revision of the vineland social maturity scale by EA Doll.* Circle Pines, MN: American Guidance Service.

Spijkerboer, A. W., Utens, E. M. W. J., Koning, W. B. D., Bogers, A. J. J. C., Helbing, W. A., & Verhulst, F. C. (2006). Health-related quality of life in children and adolescents after invasive treatment for congenital heart disease. *Quality of Life Research, 15*, 663–673.

Spurkland, I., Bjornstad, P. G., Lindberg, H., & Seem, E. (1993). Mental Health Functioning in adolescents with congenital heart disease: A comparison between adolescents born with severe heart defect and atrial septal defect. *Acta Paediatrica, 82*, 71–76.

Sreeram, N., Trieschmann, U., & de Haan, E. (2008). Device therapy in children: Current indications. *Indian Pacing and Electrophysiology Journal, 8*(Suppl. 1), S92–S104.

Steptoe, A., Mohabir, A., Mahon, M. G., & McKenna, M. J. (2000). Health related quality of life and psychological wellbeing in patients with dilated cardiomyopathy. *Heart, 83*, 645–650.

Stutts, L. A., Conti, J. B., Aranda, J. M., Jr., Miles, W. M., Burkart, T. A., & Sears, S. F. (2007). Patient evaluation of ICD recall communication strategies: A vignette study. *Pacing and Clinical Electrophysiology, 30*(9), 1105–1111.

Tester, D. J., Will, M. L., Haglund, C. M., & Ackerman, M. J. (2006). Effect of clinical phenotype on yield of long QT syndrome genetic testing. *Journal of the American College of Cardiology, 47*, 764.

The Task Force on the Management of Grown-Up Congenital Heart Defects of the European Society of Cardiology. (2003). Management of grown-up congenital heart defects. *European Heart Journal, 24*, 1035–1084.

Thompson, R. J., Gustafson, K. E., George, L. K., & Spock, A. (1994). Change over a 12-month period in the psychological adjustment of children and adolescents with cystic fibrosis. *Journal of Pediatric Psychology, 19*, 189–204.

Todaro, J. F., Fennell, E. B., Sears, S. F., Rodrigue, J. R., & Roche, A. K. (2000). Review: Cognitive and psychological outcome of pediatric heart transplantation. *Journal of Pediatric Psychology, 25*, 567–576.

Tomaske, M., Candina, R., Weiss, M., & Bauersfeld, U. (2011). Safety and efficacy of paediatric outpatient radiofrequency catheter ablations. *International Journal of Cardiology, 148*(3), 276–279.

Tong, E. M., Sparacino, P. S. A., Messias, D. K. H., Foote, D., Chesla, C. A., & Gillis, C. L. (1998). Growing up with congenital heart disease: The dilemmas of adolescents and young adults. *Cardiology in the Young, 8*, 303–309.

Uniform Data System for Medical Rehabilitation. (1998). *WeeFIM system clinical guide*. Buffalo, NY: University of Buffalo.

Utens, E. M. W. J., Verhulst, F. C., Meijboom, F. J., Duivenvoorden, H. J., & Hess, J. (1993). Behavioral and emotional problems in children and adolescents. *Psychological Medicine, 23*, 415–424.

Van Horn, M., DeMaso, D. R., Gonzalez-Heydrich, J., & Dahlmeier Erickson, J. (2001). Illness-related concerns of mothers with congenital health disease. *Journal of the American Academy of Child and Adolescent Psychiatry, 40*, 847–854.

Vogels, T., Verrips, G. H. W., Koopman, H. M., Theunissen, N. C. M., Fekkes, M., & Kamphuis, R. P. (2000). *TACQOL Manual. Parent Form and Child Form*. Leiden: Leiden Center for Child Health and Pediatrics LUMC-TNO.

Wallston, K. A., Wallston, T. T., & Lazarus, R. S. (1978). Family support in the black community. *Journal of Clinical Child Psychology, 19*, 347–355.

Youssef, N. M. (1988). School adjustment of children with congenital heart disease. *Maternal–Child Nursing Journal, 17*, 217–302.

Zheng, Z., Croft, J. B., Giles, W. H., & Mensah, G. A. (2001). Sudden cardiac death in the United States, 1989 to 1998. *Circulation, 104*, 2158–2163.

Zipes, D. P., & Wellens, H. J. (1998). Sudden cardiac death. *Circulation, 98*, 2334–2351.

Asthma in Adolescence

Cassandra Snipes

Definitions and Epidemiology

Asthma is the most common adolescent chronic health condition (Goodwin, Fergusson, & Horwood, 2004); nearly 7.1 million children under the age of 17 years in the United States are affected by asthma (Akinbami, Moorman, & Liu, 2011). Unfortunately, the prevalence, morbidity, and mortality associated with pediatric asthma have increased over the recent years and are relatively high among adolescents (Bruzzese et al., 2011; Goodwin, Pine, & Hoven, 2003; Spencer, Serdar, Johnston, & Harrigan, 2000; Thomsen et al., 2011).

Ages 11–17 years have more asthma exacerbation, increased hospitalization as a result of exacerbations, intubation, and higher asthma-related mortality rates than younger children (Bruzzese et al., 2011; Drotar, Witherspoon, Zaebracki, & Peterson, 2006). In a survey conducted by the Center for Disease Control and Prevention (CDC), among high school students with current asthma, 37.9 % reported an asthma episode or attack during the 12 months (Center for Disease Control and Prevention, 2003). Additionally, adolescents, ages 11–17 years, had an annual asthma attack prevalence of 61.5 per 1,000, compared to 57.5 (ages 5–10 years) and 43.5 (ages 0–4 years). Adolescents had an annual mortality rate of 4.4 per 1,000,000, compared to 2.7 (ages 5–10 years) and 2.5 (ages 0–4 years) (Akinbami & Shoendorf, 2002). This may be due to the fact that adolescents are less likely to receive regular medical care compared to younger children. Another possibility for the increased burden on adolescents may be the transfer of responsibility for managing treatment from parent to child, and adolescents may be ill equipped to manage asthma independently (Bruzzese et al., 2011). In addition, more individuals of this age tend to smoke. An additional possible explanation is that deficiency in lung function already present at 9–10 years at least persists until mid-adulthood and may become exacerbated with time (Morgan et al., 2005). Although childhood asthma is more prevalent in boys, in the mid-teenage years the trend reverses with female adolescents having higher rates of asthma (Akinbami et al., 2011; Bruzzese et al., 2011). This prevalence trend may be due to suggested gender-specific reduced adaptive immunity in young boys, changes in baseline lung functioning during puberty, as well as sex-specific hormonal contribution during puberty (Osman, Hansell, Simpson, Hollowell, & Helms, 2007). Ethnic minority youths, children with obesity, adolescents that smoke tobacco, and those with a family history of asthma are at greater risk for developing asthma. Adolescent asthma is a pervasive chronic illness and has significant public health implications.

C. Snipes, B.A. (✉)
Department of Psychology: MS 0296 Reno, University of Nevada, Mail Stop 297, Reno, NV 89512, USA
e-mail: snipes.cassandra@gmail.com

W.T. O'Donohue et al. (eds.), *Handbook of Adolescent Health Psychology*,
DOI 10.1007/978-1-4614-6633-8_40, © Springer Science+Business Media New York 2013

According the American Lung Association (ALA), asthma is a chronic upper respiratory disease that is characterized by intermittent and variable periods of acute reversible airway obstruction (American Lung Association, 2011). Episodic exacerbations that involve symptoms such as shortness of breath, cough, wheezing, and chest tightness can range from mild to life-threatening. An asthma attack is characterized by constriction of the bronchial smooth muscles, swelling of bronchial tissues, and increased mucous secretion that narrow the airways and cause breathing difficulties. If severe this can cause severe shortness of breath and low blood oxygen. Allergen or irritant-induced airway constriction is due to a release of histamine, tryptase, leukotrienes, and prostaglandins from mast cells (The National Institute of Health, 2007). Attacks are often followed by airway swelling that persists after the initial acute episode has resolved and can result in extended periods of impaired functioning. As the disease and inflammation progresses, other factors can also limit airflow. These include edema, inflammation, mucus hypersecretion, and the formation of mucus plugs, as well as structural changes including hypertrophy and hyperplasia of the airway smooth muscle. Airway hyperresponsiveness to wide range of stimuli is also an important feature of asthma. Additionally, permanent structural changes in the airway can take place. These structural changes include thickening of the subbasement membrane, blood vessel proliferation and dilation, and airway smooth muscle hypertrophy (The National Institute of Health, 2007). These complications can result in a significantly reduced quality of life for adolescents suffering from even mild asthma.

Asthma can be trigged by environmental factors such as allergens particularly tobacco smoke, dust mites, furred and feathered animals, certain molds, chemicals, strong odors, and air pollution (Agency for Toxic Substances & Disease Registry, 2010); seasonal factors (e.g., weather change); and genetic factors such as atopy (the tendency to develop allergies) (Goodwin et al., 2003). Additionally, exposure and sensitization to allergens and irritants found in the indoor environment are major factors in the development and exacerbation of asthma. Moisture, dampness, poor ventilation, deteriorated carpeting, and structural deficits such as water intrusion (leading to damp housing), dead spaces in walls that harbor pests, and poorly functioning ventilation appliances are all indoor asthma triggers (Krieger & Higgins, 2002; Takaro, Krieger, Song, Sharify, & Beaudet, 2011; Thomsen et al., 2011). Controlling exposure to asthma triggers is imperative in the management of asthma (American Lung Association, 2011). The ability to achieve control and avoid exacerbations is related to provider knowledge and practices, access to and use of health-care services, asthma education, self-management, and the availability of insurance to pay for care (Ungar et al., 2011).

Asthma, depending on the severity of the disease and level of control of exacerbations, can be associated with functional impairment. Adolescents suffering from asthma experience reductions in functioning in many aspects including school absences, frequent doctor visits, reduced physical activity, and hospitalizations (Wise et al., 2007). Approximately 5.7 per 1,000 adolescents experience limitation of activity due to asthma (National Center for Health Statistics, 2010). In fact, the Center for Disease Control and Prevention (CDC) recently found that asthma is one of the leading causes of school absenteeism (Centers for Disease Control and Prevention, 2007). The economic burden from pediatric-related asthma related to lost school days has been estimated to total $1 billion each year in the United States alone. Asthma can lead to limited function in adolescents and indirect, costly expenditures.

The estimated cost of treating pediatric asthma is $3.2 billion (Spencer et al., 2000), and nearly half of overall asthma-related expenditures are allocated to individuals under 18 years of age (Drotar et al., 2006). Additionally, a majority of the health-care costs devoted to the treatment of asthma are allocated to a relatively small portion of the patient population that experience recurrent, severe symptoms (Drotar et al., 2006; Godard, Chanez, Siraudin, Nicoloyannis, & Duru, 2002). Serra-Bastlles, Plaza, Cornella, and

Brugues (1998) found that the progressive increase in the severity of the disease causes a considerable increase in the total costs of asthma; a small amount (14 %) of all asthmatic patients account for large percentage (47 %) of the overall annual costs. Some estimates have been as high as 20 % of the asthmatic population utilizing 80 % of the resources allocated to asthma (Smith et al., 1997). These high utilizers have increased emergency room visits and hospitalizations due to poorly controlled asthma, and in turn, the consumption of these high-cost health-care options greatly increases health-care expenditures (ten Brinke, Ouwerkerk, Zwinderman, & Spinhoven, 2001). Adolescent asthma is costly and it is imperative that the treatment of asthma focuses on those with uncontrolled asthma exacerbations, in order to reduce overall health-care costs.

It has been shown that multiple health status domains are affected by pediatric asthma, with regard to frequency and severity of recent symptoms. Adolescent asthma causes impairment for individuals and is a significant burden on the health-care system, with those with poorly controlled asthma utilizing the bulk of the allotted health-care resources.

The Role of SES

The relationship between low SES and asthma is well documented. There is some evidence that inadequate access to or use of asthma medications may contribute to this relationship (Bruzzese et al., 2011). It has been shown that children from families without prescription drug insurance have a higher rate of ED visits. However, with government-sponsored drug insurance, children from lower-income families underused corticosteroids (Bruzzese et al., 2011; Ungar et al., 2011). Studies have also shown as much as 40 % of the excess asthma risk in minority children may be attributable to exposure to residential allergens (Takaro et al., 2011). This is supported by findings that urban, minority youth experience greater asthma morbidity even when controlling for ethnicity and race (Bruzzese et al., 2011; Wise et al., 2007). The role of SES in asthma development and maintenance are still relatively unknown, and this area deserves further consideration.

Cultural Considerations

Racial and ethnic disparities in medication adherence and asthma outcomes have been well documented. Multiracial youths have a higher asthma prevalence of asthma (13.6 %) as compared to non-Hispanic Whites (8.2 %) (Moorman, Zahran, Truman, & Molla, 2011). Additionally, African American children with asthma have particularly high disease severity, morbidity, and mortality (Drotar et al., 2006). One study found that Black and Hispanic adolescents were more likely to have poorer adherence as recorded by electronic recording (Bender et al., 2000). Another study showed that Black and Latino children were more likely to underuse asthma preventative medications in comparison to White children after adjusting for sociodemographic variables and asthma status (Lieu et al., 2002). Adolescence, Black race, and living in rural regions independently predicted failure of families to fill oral corticosteroid prescriptions following children's hospitalization or visit to the ED (Kaugars, Klinnert, & Bender, 2004). Among 15–19-year-olds with asthma, Black adolescents have 3 times the amount of emergency department (ED) visits, 4.5 times the hospitalizations, and 5 times the mortality rate of White adolescents (Naimi et al., 2009). However, understanding these racial and ethnic differences is complex. The most frequent reported barriers to the treatment of asthma among parents from urban, minority backgrounds were patient and family characteristics such as behavior problems, family conflict, and distress; environmental factors such as geographic location and transportation; health-care provider factors such as continuity of care and availability of providers; and health-care system factors such as a lack of health insurance (Mansour, Lanphear, & DeWitt, 2000). Evaluating cultural competence of health-care systems may be important in for improving adolescent asthma outcomes (Kaugars et al., 2004).

Additionally, exposure to allergens and environmental tobacco smoke may be related to racial or ethnic group differences. Different patterns of environmental risk factors, such as tobacco smoke and cat and cockroach exposure, were found among European Americans, African Americans, high-acculturated Hispanics, and low-acculturated Hispanics. The low-acculturated Hispanics had no measurable pet dander in the home, since indoor pets are not normative in this ethnic group. Within the African American group, better maternal mental health was associated with cat exposure (Kaugars et al., 2004). These findings suggest that cultural differences may underlie families' efforts and decisions to alter their home environments consistent with treatment recommendations (i.e., removing pets from the home).

A shifting of responsibility from caregiver to children generally occurs as the child grows older. However, racial and ethnic identify may play a role in the relative successfulness of this transition. A significant level of disagreement concerning allocation for family responsibility for asthma management was found in a sample of Black adolescents and their caregivers. Families where caregivers overestimated the level of adolescents' involvement for self-care tasks had adolescents with increased nonadherence and greater functional morbidity (Kaugars et al., 2004). Although the pathways are unclear, race and ethnicity play a role in adolescent asthma.

Despite the fact that the mechanisms by which cultural factors influence adolescent asthma are unknown, there are still steps that can be implemented within the health-care system to better care for these individuals. In order to address the disparities in health status and health provision, providers must be scientifically minded, have skills in "dynamic sizing," and acquire information about different cultural groups (Duckworth, Iezzi, Vijay, & Gerber, 2009). It is important to apply the scientific method to health provision by reserving judgment and not forming false conclusion based on bias. Instead, providers must form hypotheses, develop ways to test these hypotheses, and provide services consistent with the obtained data. Secondly, dynamic sizing involves the ability to know when to generalize and when to individualize. More specifically, this skill helps providers to avoid applying stereotypes to members of a particular cultural group, while still appreciating the importance of the larger cultural group. Next, it is important for providers to seek information on specific cultural groups that they may encounter in practice. Ultimately, providers need to incorporate the patient's cultural history and racial identity when assessing and conceptualizing presenting problems and outlining treatment goals. By reserving judgment, acquiring knowledge regarding specific cultural groups, and conducting culturally sensitive assessment and treatment conceptualization, both primary care and behavioral health providers can create a culturally aware health-care system.

Obesity

Obesity has been shown to contribute to the development and persistence of adolescent asthma. In the United States, adolescents with a body mass index (BMI) above the 85th percentile were at the highest risk for developing asthma (Ho et al., 2010). Several studies have demonstrated that obesity is associated with the prevalence and incidence with asthma both cross-sectionally and longitudinally, especially among female adolescents (Chen, Dales, Tang, & Krewski, 2002; Guerra et al., 2004). Additionally, being overweight or obese at age 11 was associated with a twofold increase risk for persistence of asthma from childhood through adolescence (Guerra et al., 2004). Ho and colleagues (2010) found that increased body mass index (BMI) exaggerates the risk of acquiring asthma in female adolescents, but not in male adolescents; therefore, it appears that gender may be an important moderator of BMI-related asthma risk. It remains unclear if this increased risk for females is due to genetic, psychological, or behavioral factors.

It is possible that those adolescents with asthma are less likely to exercise, due to their disease symptomology, and in turn would be more likely to gain weight and be classified as obese. However, the hypothesis that obesity plays a direct role in the persistence of asthma is supported by the finding that weight reduction in obese patients with asthma improves lung function and symptoms (Guerra et al., 2004). Although the mechanisms through which obesity influences asthma are still unclear, it is important to recognize obesity as a risk factor for asthma in clinical practice.

Smoking

Both active and passive tobacco smoking are risk factors for adolescent asthma. A higher risk of current and lifetime asthma is seen in adolescents exposed to passive smoking of parents or peers. In addition, parental passive smoking is associated with children's frequency of asthma exacerbations, severity of symptoms, number of emergency rooms visits, and length of recovery time following hospitalization (Zbikowski, Klesges, Robinson, & Alfano, 2002). Active smoking has also been clearly linked to the severity of asthma in adolescents due to tobacco's ability to increase inflammation and bronchial and nasal hyperresponsiveness (Annesi-Maesano et al., 2004; Gilliland et al., 2006). There is also evidence that regular active smoking impacts the development of asthma in adolescence after a short period of time (Gilliland et al., 2006). Results consistently show that smoking rates among adolescents with asthma are equivalent or higher than youths without asthma (Zbikowski et al., 2002). Evidence also suggests that once asthmatic youths try smoking tobacco they are more likely to become regular smokers (Van De Ven, Engels, Kerstjens, & Van Den Eijnden, 2007). These smoking trends may be due to the short-term anti-inflammatory effects of cigarette smoke on allergic inflammation or greater susceptibility to nicotine dependence in adolescents with asthma (Van De Ven et al., 2007). Adolescence is a major risk period for becoming a cigarette smoker, due to the developmental changes that occur. Therefore, smoking intervention that educates youth about how smoking can worsen their asthma is extremely important.

Comorbid Psychiatric Symptoms

There is a clear link between psychiatric symptoms such as depression and anxiety and asthma (Goodwin et al., 2003; Kanton, Richardson, Lozano, & McCauley, 2004; Katon, Richardson, Russo, Lozano, & McCauley, 2006; Kaugars et al., 2004; Slattery & Essex, 2010). For example, Katon and colleagues (2006) found that 17 % of youths with asthma enrolled in a large health-maintenance organization (HMO) met diagnostic criteria or a DSM-IV disorder. Some studies show up to one-third of asthmatic youths meet criteria for anxiety disorders (Kanton et al., 2004).

Both community and clinical samples provide evidence of a link between asthma and anxiety disorders, and panic disorder in particular. However, there is some evidence that panic disorder may only be associated with severe asthma (Goodwin et al., 2003). In a recent study by Slattery and Essex (2010), a lifetime history of asthma was associated with anxiety symptoms in an adolescent community sample. An association between asthma and depression has also been shown, although results are mixed (Goodwin et al., 2004; Lavoie et al., 2005; Slattery & Essex, 2010). Comorbid anxiety and depressive disorders in youth with asthma have been shown to be associated with increased asthma symptoms, functional impairment, and higher rates of smoking when compared with youth with asthma alone (Katon et al., 2006).

Asthmatic adolescents are also at an increased risk of suicide. Both epidemiological and prospective studies have shown a significant increase in suicide incidence in adolescents with asthma (Kuo et al., 2010). In fact, Kuo and colleagues found that suicide incidence for asthmatic adolescents was more than twice that of those without asthma. This study also found that higher severity of baseline asthma symptoms was associated with higher suicide mortality (Kuo et al., 2010). In a community youth sample, elevated suicide risk in asthmatic adolescents was found independent of comorbid mental disorders (Goodwin & Marusic, 2004). This increased suicide risk in adolescents suffering from asthma must be addressed through assessment and appropriate mental health referral in primary care settings.

The underlying mechanisms of the association between asthma and psychiatric symptoms remain unclear (Lavoie et al., 2005). A recent meta-analysis demonstrates a bidirectional relationship between mental health symptoms and atopic disorders such as asthma (Slattery & Essex, 2010). Generally accepted theories include that the association may reflect activation of an innate, fear-based neural network to perceived or experienced breathlessness or, alternatively, activation of a suffocation alarm system due to alterations in central mechanisms of carbon dioxide sensitivity. Specifically, asthma may increase the likelihood of panic attacks through increased vulnerability to difficulty breathing and other panic symptoms associated with respiratory abnormalities (Goodwin et al., 2003). It is also possible that the fear induced by asthma attacks, which can be sudden and life-threatening, is associated with the onset of panic. Finally, it is conceivable that a third common factor, either genetic or environmental, is associated with the increased likelihood of the co-occurrence of asthma and psychiatric symptoms (Goodwin et al., 2003, 2004). This association between anxiety disorders and asthma may also be the result of broader issues related to a sense of well-being as individual attempt to cope with an ongoing illness (Slattery & Essex, 2010).

As stated above, psychiatric symptoms as well as behavioral adjustment difficulties may be related at least in part to asthma-related stressors. Take the example of Laura, a 13-year-old female, who experienced several severe attacks over the past year that required hospitalization. Recently, her anxiety has increased, as evidenced by experiencing symptoms of panic at the first sign of asthma symptoms. Laura's anxiety is now significantly interfering with self-management of her asthma. Additionally, her quality of life has been affected by her limited interaction with friends in settings that may exacerbate her asthma symptoms. Adolescents with psychological problems may have less well-controlled asthma, indirectly due to poor adherence or directly due through psychosomatic pathways (Vila et al., 2003). Behavioral and psychiatric problems such as those Laura is experiencing require intervention (Drotar et al., 2006).

Regardless of the underlying mechanisms, assessing for comorbid psychiatric symptomology is important in adolescents presenting to primary care for asthma treatment and must be taken into account when prescribing treatment (Lavoie et al., 2005). There is evidence that rates of recognition of anxiety and depressive disorders in youth with asthma are low and significant deficits remain in quality of mental health treatment these youths receive (Katon et al., 2006). One study showed only 125 of youths with asthma and a DSM-IV diagnosis received 90 days or longer antidepressant medication at minimally effective doses, and only 10.5 % received more than three psychotherapy visits. This is particularly concerning given the elevated suicide risk in asthmatic adolescents. Additionally, it has been demonstrated that psychological dysfunction contributes to morbidity and costs of asthma, independently of asthma severity (ten Brinke et al., 2001). In order to provide proper treatment and reduce health-care costs, psychiatric comorbidity must be taken into account when treating adolescent asthma.

Family Dysfunction

Adolescent asthma can have a significant psychological impact on families. Findings clearly indicate that quality of life for the asthmatic adolescent and their caregivers are significantly influenced by both emotional and behavioral problems of the adolescent. Specifically, the self-esteem and anxiety of adolescents are linked to the impact on themselves and their caregivers (Vila et al., 2003). Interestingly, Vila and colleagues (2003) also showed that quality of life for both adolescents with asthma and their parents does not depend on medical variables such as duration of the disease, its initial severity, or past control by treatment. Families can be significantly influenced by the burden of adolescent asthma, specifically by the psychological distress that can accompany the disease.

In turn, the quality of family resources and relationships may have an impact on the level of control and morbidity in adolescent asthma. There is strong evidence for relationships between caregivers, mental health, and youth's asthma morbidity. The literature consistently shows that poorer caregiver psychological functioning is associated with worse asthma outcomes for children. In an inner-city population, caregivers who reported clinically significant mental health problems had children who were 1.78 times more likely to be hospitalized in the next 9 months, when compared to caregivers with nonclinically significant psychopathology scores (Kaugars et al., 2004). Additionally, the National Cooperative Inner-City Asthma Study (NCICAS) found a relationship between hospitalization rates for children with asthma and caregiver mental health problems.

Psychological and family dysfunction, problematic asthma management, and asthma-related morbidity can be clustered together and result in problematic outcomes (Drotar et al., 2006). For example, family social environments that include conflict, aggression, and deficient nurturing may produce poorer pediatric asthma outcomes (Kaugars et al., 2004). Conflict between children with asthma, their parents, and hospital staff differentiated those children who died of asthma from a control group matched for asthma severity (Kaugars et al., 2004). Parental criticism may also play a role in adolescents' management of asthma. Among adolescents hospitalized for asthma, higher parental criticism was more likely to be associated with greater treatment noncompliance upon admission and with better response to treatment when adolescents were separated from their parents and participating in a structured treatment regimen (Kaugars et al., 2004).

As previously mentioned, the burdens imposed by these asthma symptoms and the necessary treatment may cause additional stresses and burdens for families. It is important to recognize this bidirectional relationship between psychological functioning in the parents and the child's physical symptoms, and the challenge that having a child with asthma presents (and thereby increases the psychological stress of the caregivers) (Kaugars et al., 2004). For this reason, family-centered psychological interventions are important in the promotion of psychological adaptation and illness management in adolescent asthma (Drotar et al., 2006).

A Stepped Care Approach to Medical Intervention

Because of the high prevalence and cost of treating adolescent asthma, enhancing care outcomes in primary care settings is a public health imperative. Effective health-care delivery involves adopting a stepwise approach to treatment (Byrd, Ferguson, Henderson, Oksol, & O'Donohue, 2005). Under stepped care protocols simpler interventions are tried first, with more intensive interventions reserved for when a desired outcome is not achieved (Von Korff & Tiemens, 2000). Progress is monitored and stepped care plans are individualized according to each patient's preference. The levels of stepped care for chronic illness are (1) systematic routine assessment and preventative medicine, (2) self-care with low intensity support, (3) care management in primary care, (4) intensive care management with specialized advice, and (5) specialist care (Von Korff, Glasglow, & Sharpe, 2002). Stepped care based on patient outcomes increases effectiveness and lowers cost.

The least intensive intervention when treating adolescent asthma involves systematic routine assessment and preventative medicine. The National Institute of Health outlines three important functions of asthma assessment: (1) severity, the intrinsic intensity of the disease process; (2) control, the degree to which symptoms, functional impairment, and risk of untoward events are minimized and the goals of therapy are met; and (3) responsiveness, the ease with which control is achieved by medical intervention (The National Institute of Health, 2007). Assessment should be accomplished through careful, directed history and lung function measurement and should accomplish identifying precipitating factors, assessing comorbid conditions that may aggravate asthma, assessing patient's knowledge and skills for self-management, and classifying asthma severity (The National Institute of Health, 2007).

Health-related quality of life (HRQOL) is also an important dimension in the treatment of adolescent asthma. HRQOL refers specifically to the functional effect of an illness and its consequent therapy upon a patient, as perceived by the patient (Rutishauser, Sawyer, Bond, Coffey, & Bowes, 2001). Due to the immense physical, cognitive, social, and emotional changes that occur during adolescence, it is important to utilize only measures that have been validated for this particular age group. The adolescent quality of life questionnaire (AAQOL) is a well-validated self-report measure that assesses six domains: symptoms, medication, physical activities, emotion, social interaction, and positive effects (Rutishauser et al., 2001). The AAQOL is intended for use with ages 12–17 years and requires only 5–7 min to complete. The AAQOL is an age-appropriate and valid asthma-related quality of life measure for use in adolescents with asthma. HRQOL is an important factor in adolescent asthma management.

The second element of the least intrusive intervention for asthma, preventative medicine, can be accomplished by avoiding asthma triggers in the environment. As mentioned previously, triggers that include smoke, pollen, pet dander, dust mites, and poor ventilation can all contribute to asthma exacerbation (American Lung Association, 2011). Avoiding these triggers or eliminating them from the home is a preventative step in the management of asthma.

The next element of stepped care, self-care with low intensity support, can be addressed through self-management and specifically written action plans. Self-management, which is understood as the adolescent's ability to manage his or her own treatment, is an integral part of successful long-term treatment. Effective self-management has been shown to reduce asthma symptoms, health-related morbidity, and social, emotional, and financial burden associated with asthma for the suffering adolescent and his or her family (Zebracki & Drotar, 2004).

It is imperative that the primary care providers practice self-management education, as opposed to traditional patient education, when treating adolescents with asthma. Self-management education teaches problem-solving skills rather than simply disease-specific information and technical skills. Problem-solving skills provide techniques to help the patient make decisions, take appropriate action, and alter these changes as they encounter changes in circumstance or the disease. Self-management includes medical management of the condition, maintaining important life roles, and managing negative emotions that often accompany chronic disease (Lorig, Ritter, Laurent, & Plant, 2006). The forming of the patient/health-care provider relationship should also be a focus of self-management training (Lorig & Holman, 2003). The adolescent and their family are largely responsible for his or her own care on a day-to-day basis over the length of the illness, and therefore, self-management is an integral element of asthma management.

The need for active participation on the part of the parent or adolescent with asthma to prevent exacerbations has led to the universal recommendation by national and international asthma guidelines to provide written action plans (WAP) for home management of asthma (Bhogal, Zemek, & Ducharme, 2009; Guendelman, Meade, Benson, Chen, & Samuels, 2002). WAPs consist of a written set of instructions given to the adolescent with asthma for the management of chronic, ongoing symptoms as well the prevention and management of exacerbations. A WAP serves many functions. First, it serves as a communication tool between the health-care provider and the patient, and second, it serves as a reminder to patients of the treatment plan. WAPs should be tailored to each individual patient's type and severity of asthma, including but not limited to what medications should be used as maintenance therapy; when, how, and for how long to modify medications in case of deterioration; and when to access the medical system during an exacerbation (i.e., contact physician, go to the ED) (Bhogal et al., 2009). Ungar and colleagues (2011) found that those children with an action plan had 28 % few exacerbations. In addition, those who do not have a written action plan are four times more likely to have an asthma attack requiring emergency hospital treatment (Asthma, 2011).

Self-management can be problematic for adolescents for several reasons. Firstly, asthma symptoms are episodic and therefore require frequent monitoring and adjustment of treatment accordingly. Next, asthma management is multidimensional and requires behaviors that accomplish the following objectives: (1) minimize the frequency and severity of asthma episodes, (2) reduce dysfunction caused by asthma, and (3) optimize involvement of daily activities (Zebracki & Drotar, 2004). Self-management can also be difficult to achieve in adolescence due to the unique developmental and behavioral challenges faced by this age group. A wish for independence from parental authority, involvement in risk taking behaviors, and a focus on more immediate consequences rather than long-term outcomes can interfere with successful self-management and treatment adherence (Naimi et al., 2009; Price, 1996; Zebracki & Drotar, 2004). There is evidence to suggest that adolescents' self-efficacy, an individual's expectations about their ability to successfully perform a health-related behavior to manage a chronic condition, may influence adherence to asthma treatment (Zebracki & Drotar, 2004). In light of these findings, interventions designed to increase adolescents' sense of self-efficacy for asthma management may effectively promote treatment adherence. Therefore, it is important that the providers work together with the adolescent to create a written action plan. In order to promote self-efficacy, successful completion of the action plan is more important than the plan itself. The purpose of action plans is to give patients confidence in the management of their disease, that in turn fuels internal motivation (Bodenheime, Lorig, Homan, & Grumbach, 2002).

Action plans must be based on patient perceived problems, in order to promote completion of the plan (Lorig & Holman, 2003). For example, if maintaining regular exercise is important to the adolescent, then self-management skills are taught in the context of exercise (e.g., "If you would like to maintain being active in sports, take regular corticosteroids in order to limit the probability of an asthma exacerbation."). Framing self-management in the context of patient values is imperative.

As noted above, promoting self-efficacy is an important goal of self-management programs. In order to accomplish enhancing self-efficacy, the concept must be translated into tools that providers can utilize. The four key ingredients of promoting self-efficacy are performance mastery, modeling, interpretation of symptoms, and social persuasion (Lorig & Holman, 2003). Performance mastery is addressed by involving the patient in their behavior change by asking them to create manageable, specific weekly goals. In the event that the goal was not accomplished, problem-solving skills are utilized. Next, modeling is accomplished through having peers teach self-management skills (Lorig et al., 2008). A program that utilizes the concept of modeling, the Triple A Program, will be discussed in more detail in the following sections. Reinterpreting physiological symptoms is also important. When symptoms are explained as having multiple causes, this leads to multiple ways of managing the symptoms. Finally, social persuasion is a powerful tool in increasing self-efficacy. If others around you are participating in a behavior, you are more likely to follow. Therefore, if members of self-management group are gaining benefits from a behavior change such as increasing exercise, other members are more likely to engage in the same behavior (Lorig & Holman, 2003). By practicing these four ingredients of promoting self-efficacy, providers can enhance the self-management of teens with asthma.

A large body of empirical evidence supports the efficacy of the self-management approach. Many self-management programs for patients' chronic conditions have demonstrated an increase in the number of minutes exercised per week and an increase in the practice of cognitive symptom management skills such as relaxation (Lorig et al., 2008). Patients have also demonstrated improved communication with their provider and benefited from improved health status (Lorig & Holman, 2003). Self-management is absolutely imperative to address when treating adolescents with asthma due to the strong evidence supporting the success of the approach.

The third level of stepped care medical intervention for asthma, care management in primary care, is accomplished through medication management. Adolescents with persistent forms of asthma characterized by underlying inflammation of the airways generally require both quick-relief medication and long-term control medication for optimal management. Quick-relief medications are used to reduce symptoms associated with bronchoconstriction. In addition, for children with moderate to severe asthma, long-term control medications (e.g., corticosteroids) should be taken on a daily basis to achieve management of persistent asthma symptoms (Kuethe, Vaessen-Verberne, Mulder, Bindles, & van Alderen, 2011). Currently, asthma guidelines recommend a dose of up to 200 μg/day beclomethasone dipropionate (BDP)-hydrofluoroalkane equivalent for adolescents with mild-to-moderate asthma. Maximum effect is achieved with a dose of 500 μg/day. Any dose above that leads to minimal further improvement and may be more likely associated with side effects (Zhang, Axelsson, Chung, & Lau, 2011). However, it should be noted that asthma medications have significant side effects, which may intensify problems with treatment adherence. Side effects of inhaled corticosteroids may include delayed growth acceleration and increased aggressive or oppositional behavior and effects on memory and mood (Zhang et al., 2011). Although these medications are associated with side effects, it has been demonstrated that regular use of low-dose inhaled corticosteroids can prevent a significant proportion of hospital admissions during the course of the disease and these medications continue to be the treatment of choice for asthma (Suissa, Ernst, & Kezouh, 2002).

Regular follow-up is also an important element of adolescent asthma management. The follow-up should include assessment of asthma control status, patient education, prescription of inhaled medication and instructions on use, implementation of a self-management or action plan, and regular medical review (Kuethe et al., 2011).

The fourth element of stepped care for asthma, intensive care management with specialized advice, can involve instituting more frequent follow-ups or an emergency room visit in which the patient receives immediate specialized care. Additionally, in an integrated care milieu the patient may have the opportunity to meet with a behavioral health specialist in order to address any psychiatric concerns that often accompany this disease (Byrd et al., 2005).

The fifth and most intensive step of care involves specialist care. Patients who have poor outcomes in the lower levels of care, are chronically noncompliant, or have complex clinical presentations can be referred to providers that specialize in pulmonary disease. At this level of treatment patients may also be referred to specialty mental health providers such as psychologists and psychiatrists (Byrd et al., 2005). In the context of adolescent asthma this specialized level of care is also understood as hospitalization for asthma exacerbations. Because hospitalization is the most costly and invasive treatment option, it should be reserved for only the most severe cases. All previous treatment steps should be utilized in order to prevent these costly hospitalizations.

Medical treatment for teens with asthma should adhere to the stepped care model in order to provide the least intrusive care to patients and to reduce overall health-care costs.

Interventions for Medical Providers

Medical providers' nonadherence to NHLBI practice guidelines may in part be contributed to adolescent asthma morbidity. Medical providers' nonadherence includes not prescribing controller medication, not recommending daily peak flow monitoring, not screening and counseling patients regarding smoking cessation, and not counseling regarding allergen exposure. Barriers to adherence to NHLBI practice guidelines include a lack of familiarity and agreement with the guideline recommendations, not believing that the recommendations are helpful, limited confidence in their ability to implement the guidelines, and insufficient training (Bruzzese et al., 2011). Interventions with clinicians targeting prescription and communication behaviors have been shown to be effective in improving pediatric outcome as evidenced by reduction in acute medical visits, emergency department visits, and hospitalizations (Bruzzese et al., 2011). Medical provider behavior has a significant impact on adolescent asthma and should be the continued target of intervention.

A Stepped Care Approach to Psychological Intervention

Adolescent asthma has many psychosocial and psychological complications, as evidenced by the high comorbidity of panic disorder, anxiety, and depression. Therefore, the behavioral health specialist is a key addition to a treatment team for adolescent asthma (Cordaro & Wamboldt, 2011). Just as stepped care interventions are the most cost-effective approach to medical interventions for asthma, stepped care is also the most desirable approach to treatment in the case of a referral to a behavioral specialist. The stepwise levels of care for psychological disorders in adolescent asthma are (1) assessment and triage, (2) watchful waiting, (3) psychoeducation, (4) bibliotherapy, (5) computer-based interventions/eHealth, (6) group therapy, (7) individual therapy, (8) medication, and (9) inpatient treatment (Mercer, 2011).

Once the asthmatic patient is referred to a behavioral health specialist, assessment should be focused on several important psychological domains, namely, overall psychological health, self-management, cognitive processing, and emotion regulation (Mercer, 2011). Overall psychological health includes general psychological functioning, DSM-IV diagnosis (or symptoms), and treatment-interfering behaviors. As mentioned previously, anxiety and depression commonly co-occur and must be properly addressed in assessment (Cordaro & Wamboldt, 2011). Self-management assessment includes lifestyle factors (i.e., diet, exercise, substance use), medication use, disease knowledge, problem-solving and goal setting skills, and social support (Mercer, 2011). Specifically, social support has been shown to have a strong influence on symptom reports in adolescence (Kang, Coe, Karaszewski, & McCarthy, 1998). It has been demonstrated that immune changes during times of stress are greatest for teenagers with low social support (Kang et al., 1998). Therefore, this domain is important in assessment of asthmatic adolescents, particularly if their asthma is not well controlled. Next, cognitive processing includes maladaptive and adaptive coping strategies, self-defeating thoughts, and any catastrophic interpretations. Emotion regulation consists of emotional functioning, emotional avoidance, and emotional expression. After a behavioral health assessment is completed, the patient must be triaged to the appropriate level of care based on their level of psychological distress, impact of social and lifestyle factors, motivation, and skills and preferences. Regardless of the level of care that the adolescent is triaged to, a case manager must continually assess patient participation and outcome.

Watchful waiting is the least intrusive behavioral health level of stepped care. This process involves closely monitoring a patient's condition until symptoms appear or change. In the case of an asthmatic adolescent experiencing depression, monitoring symptoms of depression (i.e., low mood, weight gain or loss, difficulty concentrating) before intervention is important due to relatively equal rates of remitting, improving, or declining of depression (Mercer, 2011). In the event that the symptoms of depression do not remit or improve, the patient is referred to the next level of care.

Psychoeducation should focus on stress management, behavior modification, and disease education. Information can be delivered as handouts, DVDs, through the Internet, or verbally (Oser, 2006). This material can serve the function of connecting adolescents to community health resources, can facilitate long-term care planning, and can also be part of prevention tools in community agencies and schools. In fact, psychoeducational school-based interventions have been shown to be successful in managing adolescent asthma. Bruzzese and colleagues (2011) found that asthma self-management for adolescents (ASMA), a school-based intervention that uses both group and individual sessions and provides education for their medical providers, was effective in (1) improving asthma self-management; (2) had better medical management from medical providers; (3) had reductions in night awakenings, days with activity restrictions, and self-reported asthma-related school absences; (4) had improved quality of life; and (5) had reductions in acute care visits, ED visits, and hospitalizations. Although these programs may be difficult to implement due to schools' limited resources, schools may consider partnering with health insurance companies or a university with a medical school with the personnel available to implement these interventions (Bruzzese et al., 2011).

The Triple A Program (Adolescent Asthma Action) is another school-based asthma education program that was developed to raise asthma awareness among adolescents with asthma (Saini et al., 2011). The program utilizes social modeling and supportive environments by recruiting senior students who first learn from trained educators and then teach younger students and has been shown to improve knowledge of students with asthma and their peers (Saini et al., 2011).

Open airways for Schools (OAS) is a similar school-based intervention that has been shown to be effective in increasing successful pediatric asthma management (Saini et al., 2011; Spencer et al., 2000). The program is designed to address children's management of and feeling towards their asthma by covering (1) basic information and feelings about asthma, (2) recognizing and managing asthma symptoms, (3) solving problems with medicine and deciding how bad symptoms are, (4) finding and controlling asthma triggers, (5) getting enough exercise, and (6) doing well in school (Spencer et al., 2000). The OAS program has been shown to produce a significant decrease in health-care utilization through a reduction in emergency room visits, hospital stays, and doctor's visits. School-based interventions are viable options to psychoeducation to reduce asthma-related health-care costs.

Bibliotherapy is a significantly less stigmatizing and costly way to receive professional psychological treatment. This self-help book method of treatment delivery can cover a variety of ailments such as depression, anxiety, coping, and stress management (Mercer, 2011). However, this level of intervention is not appropriate for all patients. Only patients that are motivated, have an appropriate level of literacy, and are willing to participate in their own treatment will experience success with bibliotherapy.

Computer-based interventions and eHealth are similar to bibliotherapy, although delivered through different media. Several eHealth pediatric asthma programs that utilize games, experiential learning, or skill-building exercises have been shown to improve asthma knowledge, self-efficacy, and behavior (Wise et al., 2007).

"Health Buddy" improved the asthma outcomes of inner-city children through enabling children to access and monitor their asthma symptoms and quality of life and send them to health-care providers through a secure Web site (Guendelman et al., 2002). This eHealth intervention also included interactive telephone education; 11 asthma questions (each followed by a short tailored message); a clinic-based, asthma education session with a nurse who reviewed the telephone data; and a physician examination. Compared to children using an asthma diary, those that used Health Buddy reported 48 % lower odds of reporting a limitation in activity, had significantly lower odds of reporting a peak air flow below 80 % of their personal best, and were more likely to improve self-care behaviors and to reduce asthma symptoms, while making fewer urgent calls to the hospital (Guendelman et al., 2002).

There is also evidence that e-mail pharmacy case management, another element of computer-based intervention, has promising results for pediatric asthma behaviors (Wise et al., 2007).

Although these computer-based interventions are not conclusive, the results are promising enough to warrant replication (Drotar et al., 2006; Guendelman et al., 2002). It is also important to note the reduction of the burden of care placed on the health-care system by these relatively cheap, and easy to implement, computer-based and eHealth interventions.

Group therapy is the next level of stepped care for the treatment of adolescent asthma. Psychoeducation and psychosocial groups typically provide cognitive techniques to manage stress, emotion regulation, and self-management (Mercer, 2011). As aforementioned, family conflict is a risk factor for adolescent asthma and can lead to problems with treatment adherence. Therefore, multifamily group discussions that focus on the fact that many families struggling with chronic illness have reduced coping skills because they fear expressing negative emotion about the illness can be helpful (Cordaro & Wamboldt, 2011). These groups can be facilitated by individuals from a range of training backgrounds and are able to treat many patients at one time, making them a very cost-effective approach to psychosocial treatment for adolescents with asthma.

Individual therapy is a viable option for adolescents that do not show symptom improvement with less intrusive interventions (Cordaro & Wamboldt, 2011). Cognitive behavior therapy, problem-solving therapy, prolonged exposure, and other empirically based therapies should be utilized when treating adolescents with asthma (Mercer, 2011).

Next, psychopharmacological management of psychological symptoms can be utilized with adolescents with asthma. While SRRIs have been shown to be relatively effective and safe for treating depression in this population, teens typically have difficulty adhering to these medications because of the side effects (Cordaro & Wamboldt, 2011). The use of antidepressants should be closely monitored in adolescents, and steps should be taken to minimize the chance of causing harm to the patient such as conducting a comprehensive review of the patient's current medication and consulting with a pharmacist to review the safety and risk associated with adding an additional medication. Psychopharmacological treatments should only be utilized when all other levels of stepped care have proved to be ineffective in reducing psychological symptomology.

Inpatient treatment is the highest level of stepped care and involves intensive treatment in a secure and regulated setting for acute and severe psychological distress (Mercer, 2011). In adolescents with asthma inpatient treatment would typically be a response to severe depression or anxiety or a threat to harm self or others. It is imperative that inpatient treatment adheres to empirically supported treatments and focus on disease management, stress inoculation, and relapse prevention (Mercer, 2011). Inpatient treatment is costly and should only be utilized under the direst of circumstances.

Behavioral health treatment for adolescents with asthma should follow the stepped care model. The least intrusive and costly intervention is utilized first, moving to more intensive treatment if symptoms persist. Accurate assessment of teens with asthma is crucial, as anxiety and depression often co-occur with this disease and a behavioral health specialist should absolutely be a part of the treatment team for this population.

Final Considerations

Adolescent asthma is a significant public health concern and is increasing in prevalence. We must identify cost-effective ways to manage asthma in this specific population and the co-occurring psychological disorders that often accompany the disease. Specifically, assessment of anxiety, panic disorder, and depression is imperative in teens with asthma due to the high prevalence of these comorbidities. Assessment of and interventions for active smoking and obesity is crucial in order to effectively manage asthma in this population. Medical intervention, as well as behavioral health care, must be delivered with adherence to guidelines and in a stepped care model. A stepped care approach to treatment reduces costs and the burden of treatment on the individual patient. Special consideration should also be paid to the treatment adherence barriers faced by adolescents with chronic disease. It is only through comprehensive assessment and a stepped care approach to treatment that the burden of adolescent asthma with be reduced.

References

Agency for Toxic Substances & Disease Registry (2010). Retrieved, from http://www.atsdr.cdc.gov/csem/csem.asp?csem=18&po=9.

Akinbami, L., Moorman, J., & Liu, X. (2011). *Asthma prevalence, health care use, and mortality: United States, 2005-2009*. Hyattsville, MD: U.S. Department of Health and Human Services, National Health Statistics Report.

Akinbami, L., & Shoendorf, K. (2002). Trends in childhood asthma: Prevalence, health care utilization, and mortality. *Pediatrics, 101*, 315–322.

American Lung Association (2011). Retrieved, from http://www.lung.org/lung-disease/asthma/learning-more-about-asthma/.

Annesi-Maesano, I., Oryszczyn, M., Raherison, C., Kopferschmitt, C., Pauli, G., Taytard, A., et al. (2004). Increased prevalence of asthma and allied diseases among active adolescent tobacco smokers after controlling for passive smoking exposure. A cause for concern? *Clinical and Experimental Allergy, 34*, 1017–1023.

Asthma, U.K. (2011). Retrieved, from http://www.rcn.org.uk/__data/assets/pdf_file/0004/488371/Asthma_Management_in_the_21st_Century.pdf.

Bender, B., Annett, R., Ikle, D., DuHamel, T., Rand, C., & Strunk, R. (2000). Relationship between disease and psychological adaptation in children in the Childhood Asthma Management Program and their families. *Archives of Pediatrics & Adolescent Medicine, 154*, 706–713.

Bhogal, S., Zemek, R., & Ducharme, F. (2009). Written action plans for asthma in children (review). *The Cochrane Library, 1*, 1–59.

Bodenheime, T., Lorig, K., Homan, H., & Grumbach, K. (2002). Patient self-management of chronic disease in primary care. *Journal of the American Medical Association, 288*, 2469–2475.

Bruzzese, J., Sheares, B., Vincent, E. D., Sadeghi, S., Levinson, M., Mellins, R., et al. (2011). Effects of a school-based intervention for urban adolescents with asthma: A controlled trial. *American Journal of Respiratory and Critical Care Medicine, 183*, 998–1006.

Byrd, M., Ferguson, K., Henderson, D., Oksol, E., & O'Donohue, W. (2005). The integrated management of adult asthma. In W. O'Donohue, M. Byrd, N. Cummings, & D. Henderson (Eds.), *Behavioral integrated care: Treatments that work in the primary care setting* (pp. 367–381). New York: Brunner-Routledge.

Centers for Disease Control and Prevention (2003). Self-reported asthma among high school students–United States 2003. *Mortality and Morbidity Weekly Report, 54*(31), 765–767.

Centers for Disease Control and Prevention (2007). Retrieved, from http://www.cdc.gov/datastatistics/archive/asthma-absences.html.

Chen, Y., Dales, R., Tang, M., & Krewski, D. (2002). Obesity may increase the incidence in asthma in women but not in men: Longitudinal observations from the canadian national population health surveys. *American Journal of Epidemiology, 155*, 191–197.

Cordaro, A., & Wamboldt, M. (2011). Integrated care practice guidelines for adolescents with asthma. In W. O'Donohue & L. Woodward Tolle (Eds.), *Behavioral approaches to chronic disease in adolescence: A guide to integrative care* (pp. 111–128). New York: Springer.

Drotar, D., Witherspoon, D., Zaebracki, K., & Peterson, C. (2006). Psychological interventions: Asthma. In D. Drotar, D. Witherspoon, K. Zaebracki, & C. Peterson (Eds.), *Psychological interventions in childhood chronic illness* (pp. 123–138). Washington, DC: American Psychological Association.

Duckworth, M., Iezzi, T., Vijay, A., & Gerber, E. (2009). Cultural competency in the primary care setting. In L. James & W. O'Donohue (Eds.), *The primary care toolkit: Practical resources for the integrated behavioral care provider* (pp. 63–76). New York: Springer.

Gilliland, F., Islam, T., Berhane, K., Gaunderman, W., McConnell, R., Avol, E., et al. (2006). Regular smoking and asthma incidence in adolescents. *American Journal of Respiratory and Critical Care Medicine, 174*, 1094–1100.

Godard, P., Chanez, P., Siraudin, L., Nicoloyannis, N., & Duru, G. (2002). Costs of asthma are correlated with severity: A 1-yr prospective study. *European Respiratory Journal, 19*, 61–67.

Goodwin, R., Fergusson, D., & Horwood, L. (2004). Asthma and depressive and anxiety disorders among young persons in the community. *Psychological Medicine, 34*, 1465–1474.

Goodwin, R., & Marusic, A. (2004). Asthma and suicidal ideation among youth in the community. *Crisis: The Journal of Crisis Intervention and Suicide Prevention, 25*, 99–102.

Goodwin, R., Pine, D., & Hoven, C. (2003). Asthma and panic attacks among youth in the community. *The Journal of Asthma, 40*, 139–145.

Guendelman, S., Meade, K., Benson, M., Chen, Y., & Samuels, S. (2002). Improving asthma outcomes and self-management behaviors of inner-city children: A randomized trial of the health buddy interactive device and asthma diary. *Archives of Pediatrics & Adolescent Medicine, 156*, 114–120.

Guerra, S., Wright, A., Morgan, W. J., Sherrill, D., Holberg, C., & Martinez, F. (2004). Persistence of asthma symptoms during adolescence. *American Journal of Respiratory and Critical Care Medicine, 170*, 78–85.

Ho, W., Lin, Y., Caffrey, J., Lin, M., Hsu, H., Myers, L., et al. (2010). Higher body mass index may induce asthma among adolescents with pre-asthmatic symptoms: A prospective cohort study. *BMC Public Health, 11*, 542–560.

Kang, D., Coe, C., Karaszewski, J., & McCarthy, D. (1998). Relationship of social support to stress responses and immune function in healthy and asthmatic adults. *Research in Nursing and Health, 21*(2), 117–128.

Kanton, W., Richardson, L., Lozano, P., & McCauley, E. (2004). The relationship of asthma and anxiety disorders. *Psychosomatic Medicine, 66*, 349–355.

Katon, W., Richardson, L., Russo, J., Lozano, P., & McCauley, E. (2006). Quality of mental health care for youth with asthma and comorbid anxiety and depression. *Medical Care, 44*, 1064–1072.

Kaugars, A., Klinnert, M., & Bender, B. (2004). Family influences on pediatric asthma. *Journal of Pediatric Psychology, 29*, 475–491.

Krieger, J., & Higgins, D. (2002). Housing and health: Time again for public health action. *American Journal of Public Health, 92*, 758–768.

Kuethe, M., Vaessen-Verberne, A., Mulder, P., Bindles, P., & van Alderen, W. (2011). Paediatric asthma outpatient care by asthma nurse, paediatrician or general practitioner: Randomised controlled trial with two year follow-up. *Primary Care Respiratory Journal, 20*, 84–91.

Kuo, C., Chen, V., Lee, W., Chen, W., Ferri, C., Stewart, R., et al. (2010). Asthma and suicide mortality in young people: A 12-year follow-up study. *The American Journal of Psychiatry, 167*, 1092–1099.

Lavoie, K., Cartier, A., Labrecque, M., Bacon, S., Lemiere, C., Malo, J., et al. (2005). Are psychiatric disorders associated with worse asthma control and quality of life in asthma patients? *Respiratory Medicine, 99*, 1249–1257.

Lieu, T., Lozano, P., Finkelstien, J., Chi, F., Jensvold, N., & Capra, A. (2002). Racial/ethnic variation in asthma status and management practices among children managed in Medicaid. *Pediatrics, 109*, 857–865.

Lorig, K. R., & Holman, H. (2003). Self-management education: History, definitions, outcomes, and mechanisms. *Annals of Behavioral Medicine, 26*, 1–7.

Lorig, K. R., Ritter, P., Laurent, D., & Plant, K. (2006). Internet-based chronic disease self-management. *Medical Care, 44*, 964–971.

Lorig, K. R., Ritter, P. L., Dost, A., Plant, K., Laurent, D. D., & Mcneil, I. (2008). The expert patients programme online, a 1-year study of an Internet-based self-management programme for people with long-term conditions. *Chronic Illness, 4*(4), 247–256.

Mansour, M., Lanphear, B., & DeWitt, T. (2000). Barriers to asthma care in urban children: Parent perspectives. *Pediatrics, 106*, 512.

Mercer, V. (2011). Chronic disease management. In W. O'Donohue & C. Draper (Eds.), *Stepped care and e-health* (pp. 151–179). New York: Springer.

Moorman, J., Zahran, H., Truman, B., & Molla, M. (2011). Current asthma prevalence—United States, 2006–2008. *Morbidity and Mortality Weekly Report Supplements, 60*, 84–86.

Morgan, W., Stern, D., Sherrill, D., Guerra, S., Holberg, C., Guilbert, T., et al. (2005). Outcome of asthma and wheezing in the first six years of life: Follow-up through adolescence. *American Journal of Respiratory and Critical Care Medicine, 172*, 1253–1258.

Naimi, D., Freedman, T., Ginsberg, K., Bogen, D., Rand, C., & Apter, A. (2009). Adolescents and asthma: Why bother with our meds? *The Journal of Allergy and Clinical Immunology, 123*, 1335–1341.

National Center for Health Statistics. (2010). *Health, United States, 2009: With special feature on medical technology*. Hyattsville, MD: U.S. Department of Health and Human Services.

Oser, M. (2006). Patient education to promote adherence to treatments. In W. O'Donohue & E. Levensky (Eds.), *Promoting treatment adherence: A practical handbook for health care providers* (pp. 85–97). Thousand Oaks: Sage.

Osman, M., Hansell, A., Simpson, C., Hollowell, J., & Helms, P. (2007). Gender-specific presentations for asthma, allergic rhinitis and eczema in primary care. *Primary Care Respiratory Journal, 16*, 28–35.

Price, J. (1996). Issues in adolescent asthma: What are the needs? *Thorax, 51*, 13–17.

Rutishauser, C., Sawyer, S., Bond, L., Coffey, C., & Bowes, G. (2001). Development and validation of the adolescent asthma quality of life questionnaire (AAQOL). *European Respiratory Journal, 17*, 52–58.

Saini, B., Shah, S., Kearey, P., Bosnic-Anticevich, S., Grootjans, J., & Armour, C. (2011). An interprofessional learning module on asthma health promotion. *American Journal of Pharmaceutical Education, 72*, 1–10.

Serra-Bastlles, J., Plaza, V. M., Cornella, A., & Brugues, J. (1998). Cost of asthma according to the degree of severity. *European Respiratory Journal, 12*, 1322–1326.

Slattery, M., & Essex, M. (2010). Specificity in the association of anxiety, depression, and atopic disorders in a community sample of adolescents. *Journal of Psychiatric Research, 45*, 1–8.

Smith, D., Malone, D., Lawson, K., Okamoto, L., Battista, C., & Saunders, W. (1997). A national estimate of the economic costs of asthma. *American Journal of Respiratory and Critical Care Medicine, 156*, 787–793.

Spencer, G., Serdar, A., Johnston, Y., & Harrigan, J. (2000). Managing childhood asthma: The effectiveness of the open airways for schools program. *Family & Community Health, 23*, 20–30.

Suissa, S., Ernst, P., & Kezouh, A. (2002). Regular use of inhaled corticosteroids and the long term prevention of hospitalisation for asthma. *Thorax, 57*, 880–884.

Takaro, T., Krieger, J., Song, L., Sharify, D., & Beaudet, N. (2011). The breathe-easy home: The impact of asthma-friendly home construction on clinical outcomes and trigger exposure. *American Journal of Public Health, 101*, 55–62.

ten Brinke, A., Ouwerkerk, M., Zwinderman, A., & Spinhoven, P. (2001). Psychopathology in patients with severe asthma is associated with increased health care utilization. *American Journal of Respiratory and Critical Care Medicine, 163*, 1093–1096.

The National Institute of Health. (2007). *Expert panel report 3: Guidelines for the diagnosis and management of asthma*. Bethesda, MD: The National Institute of Health, U.S. Department of Health and Human Services.

Thomsen, S., van der Sluis, S., Ohm Kyvik, K., Skytthe, A., Skadhauge, L., & Backer, V. (2011). Increase in the heritability of asthma from 1994 to 2003 in among adolescent twins. *Respiratory Medicine, 105*, 1–6.

Ungar, W., Paterson, M., Gomes, T., Bikangaga, P., Gold, M., To, T., et al. (2011). Relationship of asthma management, socioeconomic status, and medication insurance characteristics to exacerbation frequency in children with asthma. *Annals of Allergy, Asthma & Immunology, 106*, 17–23.

Van De Ven, M., Engels, R., Kerstjens, H., & Van Den Eijnden, R. (2007). Bidirectionality in the relationship between asthma and smoking in adolescents: A population-based cohort study. *Journal of Adolescent Health, 41*, 444–454.

Vila, G., Hayder, R., Bertrand, C., Falissard, B., de Blic, J., Mouren-Simeoni, M., et al. (2003). Psychopathology and quality of life for adolescents with asthma and their parents. *Psychosomatics, 44*, 319–328.

Von Korff, M., Glasglow, R., & Sharpe, M. (2002). Organising care for chronic illness. *British Medical Journal, 325*, 92–94.

Von Korff, M., & Tiemens, B. (2000). Individualized stepped care of chronic illness. *The Western Journal of Medicine, 172*, 133–137.

Wise, M., Gustafson, D., Sorkness, C., Molfenter, T., Staresinic, A., Meis, T., et al. (2007). Internet telehealth of pediatric asthma case management: Integrating computerized and case manager features for tailoring a web-based asthma education program. *Health Promotion Practice, 8*, 282–291.

Zbikowski, S., Klesges, R., Robinson, L., & Alfano, C. (2002). Risk factors for smoking among adolescents. *Journal of Adolescent Health, 30*, 279–287.

Zebracki, K., & Drotar, D. (2004). Outcome expectancy and self-efficacy in adolescent asthma self-management. *Children's Health Care, 33*, 133–149.

Zhang, L., Axelsson, I., Chung, M., & Lau, J. (2011). Dose response of inhaled corticosteroids in children with persistent asthma: A systematic review. *Pediatrics, 127*, 129–138.

Endocrine Disorders in Adolescence

Michael B. Ranke

Introduction

Most endocrine disorders are congenital or have their origin during childhood and are of relevance for the individual during the entire life. Some disorders are specifically related with the transition from childhood to adult life, which are summarised with the term "adolescence" and encompass physical and psychosocial changes, which lead to sexual maturity and the maturation of the individual personality. Other disorders pose specific problems of treatment during this transitional phase due to physical, behavioural and social changes which occur and are experienced in special ways by adolescents. Several chapters in this book are dealing with specific aspects of endocrine changes and disorders during adolescence. In this chapter the specific focus is on disorders treated with steroid hormones and the implications of such treatment on growth. Congenital adrenal hyperplasia and Turner syndrome are two relatively frequent disorders in which the role of sexual development and growth is closely intertwined and therefore serve as models for the discussion of these topics.

M.B. Ranke, M.D., F.R.C.P. (Edin) (✉)
University Children's Hospital, Hoppe Seylerstr.1, 72076 Tübingen, Germany
e-mail: Michael.ranke@gmx.de

Congenital Adrenal Hyperplasia

Pathophysiology

The adrenal cortex is the source of basically three types of steroid hormones which are metabolites of cholesterone: glucocorticoids, androgens and mineralocorticoids (Miller, Achermann, & Flueck, 2008; Speiser et al., 2010). The cells of the adrenal cortex located in different zones of the gland are specialised. The zona glomerulosa (outer) produces mineralocorticoids (mainly aldosterone) which is under the regulation of the renin-angiotensin system, the zona reticularis (inner) produces androgens (mainly dehydroepiandrosterone = DHEA) and the zona fasciculata (middle) produces glucocorticoids (mainly cortisol). The blood levels of cortisol are regulated via a classical endocrine feedback system (hypothalamus-pituitary-adrenal axis) which involves the secretion of a hypothalamic hormone (CRH = corticotrophin-releasing hormone), a pituitary hormone (ACTH = adrenocorticotropic hormone), a signal transduction system at the adrenal cells (involving an ACTH receptor) and a complex pathway of steroidogenesis, which requires the functioning of a multitude of enzymes mostly of the cytochrome P450 (CYP) family. The enzymes and their activity are under genetic control.

Glucocorticoids have essential roles for the metabolic functioning (e.g. glucose homeostasis) and the composition of the body. Aldosterone is prominently involved in the regulation of fluids,

W.T. O'Donohue et al. (eds.), *Handbook of Adolescent Health Psychology*,
DOI 10.1007/978-1-4614-6633-8_41, © Springer Science+Business Media New York 2013

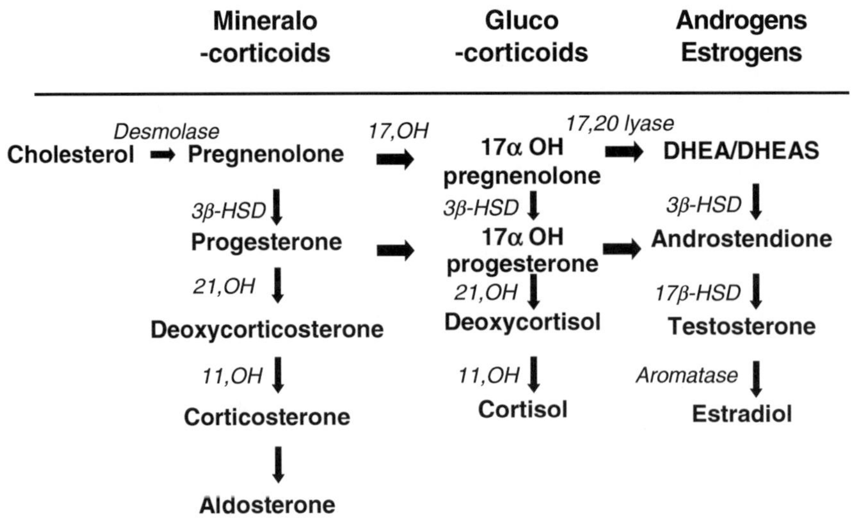

Fig. 1 Simplified diagram of steroid hormone synthesis. (Coursiv letters mark enzymes; - OH = hydroxylase; e.g. 21, OH = 21-hydrohylase, if defect is the key enzyme for CAH)

salts and blood pressure (Miller, 2005; New, 2003). Severe deficiency of both hormones is not compatible with life. Due to a circadian rhythm within the hypothalamus-pituitary unit, cortisol is secreted at higher levels in the morning and lower levels at night. While the secretion per body mass of cortisol and mineralocorticoids is principally constant after early childhood, there is a rise of adrenal androgen production after an age of about 6 years (adrenarche).

Congenital adrenal hyperplasia (CAH) is a term used for a group of inborn errors of the steroidogenic pathway associated with an impairment of cortisol secretion which by a subsequent activation of the hypothalamus-pituitary unit leads to a hyperplasia of the adrenal gland. Depending on the enzyme blockade, the disorders are associated with an excess of adrenal androgens and/or a lack or excess of mineral corticoids. The metabolites after the enzyme blockade are lacking, and the metabolites before the blockade are accumulating and continue to be metabolised into further metabolites with subsequent clinical effects. The most frequent disorder is the 21-hydroxylase (CYP21) [21-OHD] deficiency (see Fig. 1) which is the model disease in the context discussed here. The aetiology is a mutation of the 21-B-gene located on chromosome 6. The incidence varies and is about 1:6,000 newborns. Since the disorder is transmitted in a recessive mode, only children with two defective alleles are affected. The disorder affects both genders with equal frequency. Depending on the remnant enzyme activity, which is correlated with the nature of the gene defect, the hormone deficiencies—deficiency of cortisol and aldosterone, excess of androgens—vary in magnitude. In case cortisol and aldosterone are lacking, the disorder is called salt-wasting ("classical") 21-OHD, and in the case of cortisol deficiency only, it is called simple virilising 21-OHD. Both forms present at birth. There is also a late-onset (nonclassical) form of 21-OHD seen after adolescence (New, 2006). Typically the metabolite 17-OH progesterone (before the enzyme blockade) is elevated. The diagnosis is made by hormone analysis and confirmed by gene analysis. In some countries there is 17-OH progesterone screening for 21-OHD in newborns.

In the case of salt-wasting 21-OHD, newborns develop vomiting, hyponatremia, weight loss, hypotension (salt-losing crisis) and hypoglycaemia and will die if not treated appropriately. While male newborns are clinically usually not conspicuous and may just present with pigmented, slightly enlarged genitalia, newborn females present with ambiguous external genitalia.

The degree of virilisation may range from a mild clitoromegaly to a phallic transformation of the clitoris with varying degrees of fusion of the labia majora, which may give a scrotum-like appearance (classification according to Prader—stages I–V) (Prader, 1954). Urethra and vagina may thus end in a urogenital sinus. The inner part of the vagina as well as uterus and ovaries is however developed as in normal girls. Thus, once the diagnosis is established in these children, there is no doubt of their female gender and the rearing as girls. In cases of late-onset 21-OHD female's tall stature with an advanced bone age, moderate clitoromegaly or hirsutism may lead the differential diagnosis.

Aside from the anatomical aspects in virilised girls with CAH, there is an ongoing discussion about the implications of elevated androgen levels during pre- and postnatal life on the brain and the personality of a female (Meyer-Bahlburg, 2001; Meyer-Bahlburg et al., 2008; Money and Ehrhartdt, 1972). Although there is no dissension that girls with CAH should be reared as girls and will function as females in any aspect, there is ample evidence that affected girls often tend to be attracted to activities previously thought to be more typically associated with boys ("rough and tumble play") and to behave tomboyish. Although these categories are of lesser relevance in our Western societies, the fundamental role of hormonal imprinting on the brain is still not unravelled.

Treatment of CAH

Hormonal Replacement

The aims of treatment in CAH are to enable the affected children a normal development in terms of their metabolism, a normal growth process, a normal timing of puberty which ends in the ability to function sexually according to gender and to be fertile in adult life (Hindmarsh, 2009; Speiser et al., 2010). Under- and overtreatment with glucocorticoids and mineralocorticoids should be avoided at any time during development. Replacement with mineralocorticoids [e.g. fludrocortisone—orally 50–200 μg/day (or 150 μg/m²/day)]—potentially with sodium chloride supplementation—is relatively easy after infancy, when the monitoring of plasma rennin activity (PRA) and blood pressure shows stable results. Treatment with glucocorticoids, however, is difficult and less standardised. The main reason for this is the fact that blood glucocorticoid levels need not only be adequate in terms of mimicking the diurnal needs of the body but need to be given in such a mode that an excessive androgen production is avoided. This means that glucocorticoids need to be available for the feedback to the pituitary when the endogenous activity of the hypothalamus-pituitary is highest. Thus, the therapy can be oriented not only at the total daily cortisol production but also at its circadian distribution. Hydrocortisone is usually given in a daily dose of 10–15 mg/m²/day divided into three doses (morning 50 %, lunchtime and evening 25 % each). Given the fact that hydrocortisone has a biological half-life of only about 6 h, there may be periods of low glucocorticoid exposure. During childhood, this treatment can usually be done without avoiding under-treatment (virilisation, early puberty, loss of growth potential) or overtreatment (obesity, growth impairment, delayed puberty).

During adolescence, the standard therapy which was successful at a younger age is often no longer effective (Bonfig et al., 2009). There are several reasons for this: (1) in adolescent boys and girls, there is less control by parents, and often there is a higher degree of negation of rules. Adolescents find it difficult to adhere to frequent and fixed schedules. There is also the pubertal identity "crisis" which is aggravated by the recognition of the disease. (2) Some problems connected to elevated androgens in childhood such as growth problems or hirsutism are not easily recognisable during puberty. Particularly in boys an inadequate (irregular) replacement of glucocorticoids which may result in smaller testes or testicular adenoma is not obvious to the adolescent alongside normal pubertal development.

Signs of androgen excess such as acne, hirsutism and hair loss of the scull (male-pattern balding) are alarming symptoms for female adolescents. Such a development should be documented systematically with a scoring system (Ferryman-Gallwey Score) (Ferryman & Gallwey, 1961).

In addition to treating the hormonal basis (see below), it may also be required to involve a dermatologist for the treatment of acne (James, 2005) and the optical (bleaching) or physical (epilation) removal of hirsutism (Rosenfield, 2005). Today both aspects of treatment are multifaceted and may require an expertise, which is beyond the paediatric and adult endocrinologist. In adolescent girls, the processes starting and maintaining regular ovulation require a higher degree of optimisation of glucocorticoid replacement. Therefore, adolescents may need a more frequent control by the paediatric endocrinologist and repeated and more personalised information about the nature of the disease. It is inadequate to believe that everything is clear to the adolescent (and its parents) only because the family has been coming to the office for years. In my experience additional interventions by experienced psychologists are however only needed in rare cases.

When impaired adherence to the regimen of hydrocortisone is the cause of an inadequate control of the disease, the use of more potent glucocorticoid derivates ought to be considered, and this will reduce the frequency of medication during the day. Prednisone/prednisolone with a potency about five times higher than hydrocortisone may be given twice daily [total dose 4–5 mg/m^2/day (morning to evening—1/3 to 2/3)]. Dexamethasone is even more potent (30–100 times) and may be given at the end of the growth phase (50–150 μg in the evening). Changes in treatment patterns should always be guided by experienced endocrinologists.

Growth

Already at birth, children with CAH tend to be slightly larger. Children whose disorder is discovered in childhood are tall and have an advanced bone age, which impairs the growth potential. On average the adult height in children treated is impaired compared to the population (Hargitai et al., 2001) by about one standard deviation (about 6–7 cm). A reduction in height is more pronounced in cases with salt wasting, which probably reflects a greater difficulty to control the disorder. It is the rule that any growth impairment is more likely to be the result of insufficient treatment with glucocorticoids rather than its excess. The latter however may occur subtly and slowly and may be accompanied with a gain in weight, which may be misinterpreted as simple obesity in times when this is exploding in incidence particularly among juveniles and adolescents. Any gain in weight (BMI) with a slowing down of the height velocity and a subnormal progression of the bone age should stimulate to search for further signs of hypercortisolism. The potentially positive psychotropic effect of glucocorticoids holds the risk of an addiction with higher than recommended doses in adolescents.

The onset of puberty in children with CAH tends to be in the normal age range, provided that the hormonal treatment has been optimal. In a small number of cases, central puberty may be precocious, which may then require treatment with gonadotropin-releasing hormone analogues for psychological reasons and for the preservation of a normal growth potential (Carel et al., 2009). In cases of a poor adult height, prognosis at puberty onset of treatment with growth hormone is a discussed option.

Genitalia and Sexuality

Issues related to sexuality should, in general, always be addressed openly, sensitively and with competence, since they are an essential element of human life and in particular a major concern of adolescents (Casteras et al., 2009; Frisen et al., 2009; Otten et al., 2005). In girls with virilised genitalia at birth, surgical correction needs to be performed by experienced surgeons after counselling of the parents about all aspects relevant to the disorder. The goals of surgery are (1) genital appearance compatible with gender, (2) unobstructed urinary emptying without incontinence or infection and (3) good adult sexual and reproductive function (Speiser et al., 2010). When there is only minimal virilisation (Prader stage I–II), surgery may not be required at all, since the clitoris will reduce in size relative to the growth of the child's body and with proper medical care.

Clitorectomy should never be performed. Any reduction of clitoral size needs to be performed with the greatest care to preserve its sensitivity. Today the correction of the vaginal opening using up-to-date surgical technology is recommended during the first year of life (2–6–[12] months). Such early procedures are supposed to ensure good sexual functionality. However, experience shows that many girls now in their adolescence have not been treated surgically under optimal conditions in infancy, thus necessitating a second surgery in adolescence. Aside from technical aspects of the procedure, the most important issue is its timing (Vidal et al., 2010).

When puberty has started it must be investigated whether the genital situation is likely to allow a normal intercourse. This investigation should be done after explaining the reasons and potential consequences to the girls with utmost sensitivity. The issue often needs to be put forward by the treating paediatrician. An examination should only be done by the team qualified for the potentially necessary surgery. The procedure should then be done not too early before the first intercourse can be expected. At the same time it should be done at a time point sufficiently before the cohabitarche is imminent in order to provide time for healing and the feeling of normality to the female adolescent. Thus, the timing of genital surgery in adolescence also depends on the personal and social settings. In the author's experience a practical timing is when menarche is imminent. In conflicts between parents and the adolescent, the physician needs to find compromises in the interest of the affected girls and must respect their privacy within the legal frameworks. Manipulations with devices to widen a narrow vaginal introitus by the adolescents themselves, as was recommended previously, are considered obsolete today.

Like any other adolescent girls with CAH also need to be counselled about conception and its prevention. In the case of a pregnant adolescent, monitoring needs to be done in an experienced centre. Treatment with hydrocortisone or prednisone should be guided so that serum testosterone remains in the upper normal range. Dexamethasone treatment should be avoided. The problems of prenatal therapy of CAH in an affected fetus are beyond the scope of this article. If reconstructive surgery has been performed, primary caesarean section should be advised to avoid further damage to the genital tract.

The issues of genital development and sexuality also need to be discussed with adolescent boys. They should be taught that their sexual functioning and fertility is absolutely normal as long as the management of the disorder is appropriate. They should also be advised that non-compliance may result in the development of adrenal and/or testicular adenoma (adrenal rest tumours) (Mouritsen et al., 2010).

Hypogonadism

Hypogonadism is a term describing the inability to develop functioning gonads which leads to normal organic and functional development enabling normal reproduction. Hypogonadism usually becomes apparent when puberty does not occur timely or does not progress according to its natural pattern. In a strict sense disorders of puberty which are of transient nature (*see Chapter of Rogol*) are distinguished from those with permanent hypogonadism. The causes of hypogonadism vary (see Table 1). In principle disorders with the cause located in the gonads (testes, ovaries) are termed "primary or peripheral hypogonadism" (e.g. Turner syndrome, Klinefelter syndrome), and disorders with the cause located in the regulating centres hypothalamus and pituitary are termed "secondary or central hypogonadism" (e.g. gonadotropin deficiency, combined pituitary hormone deficiency). In the case of a delay in the pubertal development, there are several tasks: (1) to establish a diagnosis and to find out whether the condition is transient or permanent, (2) to ensure a normal phenotypical and psychological development of the affected adolescent and (3) to ensure fertility. Since there is a high degree of complexity depending on the cause of hypogonadism, this chapter will only deal with selected aspects of the topic taking specific disorders as models to discuss the relevant issues.

Table 1 Classification of hypogonadism

	Affected area	Example
Impaired hypothalamus-pituitary function		
"*Secondary hypogonadism*"	Congenital anomalies	Septo-optic dysplasia
	CNS tumours	Craniopharyngioma
	CNS irradiation	Post-X-ray
	Trauma/surgery	Head injury
	Defects of GnRH, LH, FSH	Kallman's syndrome
Impaired gonadal function		
"*Primary hypogonadism*"	Loss of the gonads	Torsion on gonads
	Irradiation damage	Post-X-ray
	Chemical damage	Cyclophosphamide
	Syndromes	Prader-Willi S.
	Chromosomal disorders	Turner S. Klinefelter S.

Turner Syndrome

Background

Turner syndrome (TS) or Ullrich-Turner syndrome (UTS) may be defined as the combination of characteristic physical features—short stature, gonadal dysgenesis, typical visible dysmorphic stigmata and abnormalities in organs—which is present in individuals with a female phenotype and is caused by the complete or partial absence of one of the X chromosomes (Bondy, 2007; Ranke and Saenger, 2001). The main topics discussed here will be sexual development and fertility, growth promotion and psychosocial aspects.

Turner syndrome affects approximately 1:2,000 live-born females. In about 50 % of cases, the karyotype analysis of peripheral lymphocytes reveals the complete loss of one X chromosome (karyotype 45, X), while the remaining patients display a multitude of chromosomal abnormalities. The wide range of somatic features in TS indicates that a number of different X-located genes are responsible for the complete phenotype. Short stature in TS has been associated with haploinsufficiency of a critical chromosomal region (distal of Xp22.2), which escapes inactivation (pseudoautosomal region of X and Y) and in which the short stature homeobox (SHOX) gene resides (Xp22.33) (Rao et al., 1997). Skeletal defects in TS include mesomelia, micrognathia, cubitus valgus, high-arched palate, short metacarpals and Madelung deformity. SHOX defects are known to cause mesomelic short stature associated with varied phenotypical features. Thus, haploinsufficiency of SHOX may explain a major part of short stature in TS, but does not entirely clarify this issue. To date, there is neither conclusive genetic data available which would explain the soft tissue and visceral stigmata in TS, such as lymphoedema, webbing of the neck and congenital heart failure, nor a firm knowledge about the genetic basis of the defect of ovarian function (gonadal dysgenesis).

Sexual Development and Fertility in TS

A consistent feature documented in TS is the unambiguous identification with the female gender. The completion of female development may, however, be thwarted by certain factors during adolescence and in adult life: ovarian failure occurs in the majority of patients, and up to 30 % experience late but spontaneous puberty (Pasquino et al., 1997). Puberty and the menstrual cycle will however only continue in a fraction of these patients. We now know that ovarian failure in TS results from premature ovarian senescence which, in several patients, ends during infancy as it progresses at a faster pace than normal. External genitalia, vagina and uterus are normally developed at birth and may grow normally on oestrogens.

Due to their short stature, young as well as adolescent TS patients are likely to be overprotected by adults and possibly rejected by their peers.

Growth-promoting therapy with recombinant human growth hormone (rhGH) is an accepted method for attempting to normalise height during childhood and adult life (see below). Its aims are not only to achieve a normal height during childhood and in adult life but also to assure that measures to induce puberty can be initiated within the normal developmental window for girls. A delay of oestrogen replacement resulting in the postponement of feminisation may affect the process in which the role of the mature female is learned, as primary deficits involving cognition hinder the development of appropriate social relations and interaction with the opposite sex (Burnett et al., 2010; McCauley et al., 1987). However, patients with partners tend to develop normal sexual relationships (Sheaffer et al., 2008).

The ultimate biological goal of women is childbearing. As a rule ovarian failure and infertility are major features of TS. It is extremely rare for a TS patient to experience a spontaneous pregnancy and delivery of a healthy baby. The almost uniform prospect of infertility is by far the most existential threat to patients with TS, particularly during adolescence. In women with TS, like in any other women with ovarian failure, recent endeavours to alleviate this situation include in vitro fertilisation of donated oocytes or embryos. The success of such attempts depends, to a great extent, on the maturity of the uterus. The fact that this approach entails a higher-than-normal risk of spontaneous abortion possibly indicates that an optimal developmental window is required in order to ensure complete anatomical and functional uterine development (Bryman et al., 2011). Cryopreservation of oocytes makes it possible for the patient's own cells to be used at a suitable time point after the technical difficulties of this procedure are completely resolved (Lau et al., 2009). Finally, the maintenance of ovarian function may possibly be a further mean of resolving the problem of infertility in UTS (Simpson and Rajkovic, 1999).

It also needs to be kept in mind that in part of the girls with TS, puberty will start but will progress incompletely due to remnant ovarian function. The fact that spontaneous fertility is reported means that potentially fertile adolescents need to be identified and contraception may be advised in time.

Oestrogen Replacement in TS

In a large study of 566 adults with TS, it was documented that the timely induction of puberty was extremely important for the self-esteem, for the development of social relations to the peers and for the initiation of sexual activities (Carel et al., 2006). Given that the mean onset of puberty in girls visible through breast budding (Tanner stage B2) occurs at about 10 years with a natural variation of about 2 years, the induction of puberty should ideally not be delayed much beyond an age of 12 years. Of course the intentions of the adolescents, their parents and the overall circumstances will eventually decide the time point. The principal problem related to oestrogen replacement during puberty is that oestrogens fasten the tempo of growth but do not augment it and lead to the closure of the epiphyses of the long bones, thus bringing the growth process to an end. Any therapy with oestrogen should therefore be conducted in a way that does not impair the growth potential. At a chronological age of 12 years at which the bone age in TS is about 10 years, it can be expected that an adolescent on GH will still grow—even very conservatively estimated—10 cm (Ranke and Lindberg, 2011). Thus, when a child with TS has reached about 140+ cm at puberty onset, it can be assumed that she is likely to reach an adult height of more than 150 cm. Timely and appropriate oestrogen replacement is also considered important for the lifelong bone health of adult women.

In addition to the timing of the initiation of oestrogens, the choice of the hormone preparation, the dose and the dose progression play a major role. This is relevant in all adolescents irrespective of the cause of hypogonadism. Oral oestrogen preparations which are most convenient in daily life are available as 17ß-estradiol (=E2), estradiol valerate (=E2val), ethinyl estradiol (EE) and conjugated oestrogens. Ethinyl estradiol is no longer recommended for oestrogen replacement. Oestrogen valerate and oestrogen cypionate are given i.m., a mode which is rarely indicated. Transdermal estradiol can be given as an ointment or as matrix patches, which release E2 in a standardised mode. The medicaments and the equivalent therapeutic doses of the different preparations are listed in Table 2. The choice of the oestrogen used obviously also depends on its availability, the experience of the physicians and habits in the medical environment (Drobac et al., 2006; Kiess et al., 2002). The dose increments over time are chosen in such a way that the normal pubertal course (about 3 years from the onset to menarche) is mimicked. Unfortunately oestrogen measurements in blood during replacement cannot be used for the guidance of treatment. Therefore, clinical parameters (e.g. breast staging), sonography of the uterus, body growth and bone age development need to guide treatment. Usually we start with about 1/6 of the adult oestrogen dose and increase the dose by this amount every 6 months. We give oestrogens unopposed with gestagens until the pubertal development (including uterine size) is equivalent to Tanner stage 4. Then derivates of progesterone (progestagens) are added in a cyclic mode (e.g. 10–14 out of 28–30 days) in order to induce a menstruation. The phenotypical feminisation of girls with TS and in other disorders with hypogonadism is usually very satisfying. Unfortunately neither the treatment with oestrogens "for the induction of puberty" nor "treatment of oestrogen deficit in adolescents" is a licensed indication but constitutes formally an "off label use".

Male Hypogonadism

In the male Klinefelter syndrome (karyotype 47,XXY) (Rogol and Tartaglia, 2010; Ryan, 2010) and testicular insufficiency due to the treatment of malignancies (Edgar et al., 2009) are probably the most frequent causes of peripheral hypogonadism, while congenital or acquired pituitary deficits with combined loss of hypothalamus-pituitary hormone secretion are the most frequent causes of central hypogonadism (Table 1). In Klinefelter syndrome boys are tall (they have three active SHOX loci) and have minor intellectual deficits. Since the disorder affects predominantly the Sertoli cells, thus impairing fertility, the Leydig cells, which produce testosterone, are less affected. Therefore, puberty often begins less conspicuous with low-normal testosterone levels and moderate penile growth but smaller testes. With time progressing the testicular abnormality becomes more evident. Treatment for malignancies frequently involves exposure of gonads (in males and females) to chemotherapeutically or X-rays. This leads more often to infertility than to complete loss of sex steroids since Leydig cells are also more resistant to these factors than Sertoli cells. Since during adolescence masculine physical development (growth, muscular development and strength, secondary sex characteristics such as pubic and facial hair growth, deepening of the voice) and penile growth rather than testicular size and fertility are the major concerns for adolescent boys, treatment of hypogonadism in adolescence means basically adequate replacement of testosterone.

Like in females (see above), the timing of therapy and the nature of the medication and its dose are prominent issues of therapy (Drobac et al., 2006; Kiess et al., 2002; Rogol and Tartaglia, 2010; Yin and Swerdloff, 2010). For psychological reasons, the initiation of puberty should not be postponed beyond the age of 14 years. There are a multitude of testosterone (T) preparations available for its replacement (Table 3). However, for the induction and maintenance of puberty, mostly testosterone enanthate alone or in combination with T. propionate or T. cypionate for i.m. injection is used. The starting dose of 50 mg/month is increased by this amount about every 6–9 months, until the adult maintenance dose of about 250 mg per months is reached. In order to ensure moderately constant blood levels of testosterone, injections need to be given every 3 (or 2) weeks. Testosterone undecanoate can be taken orally (capsules per 40 g). The adult replacement dose is 2–6 capsules. Thus, for the induction of puberty for which there is less experience, lower doses need to be given. Clinical features typical for pubertal development (*see Chapter of Rogol*) and the blood levels before the next injection may guide the dosing. Severe acne and priapism are rare indicators of overdosing. It is important to explain the expected changes induced by therapy to the boys and their parents. Preserving fertility in Klinefelter syndrome is an issue of research (Houk et al., 2010).

Table 2 Medication available for oestrogen replacement therapy

Substance	Mode of application	Medicament (availability may vary from country to country)	Dose (daily) for adult women	Use in Europe (%)	Use in the USA (%)
17ß-estradiol	t.d.	25/37.5/50/75/ 100 μg—release/24 h (patches)	50–100 μg	10	5
17ß-estradiol	p.o.	1.0/2.0/4.0 mg (tablets)	1.0–2.0 mg	32	
Estradiol valerate	p.o.	1.0/2.0 mg (tablets)	1.0–2.0 mg	5	
Ethinyl estradiol	p.o.	25 μg (tablets)	25 μg	39	12
Conjugated estrogens	p.o.	0.3/0.6/1.25 mg (tablets)	1.25 mg/day	12	78

Europe = Kiess et al., 2002; USA = Drobac et al., 2006

Table 3 Testosterone substances available for hormone replacement and mode of application

Oral	i.m.	Transdermal
Testosterone (T)	T. propionate	T. gel
T. cyclodextrin	T. enanthate	T. plaster
T. undecanoate	T. undecanoate	
17a-methyl-T.	T. buciclate	
	T. decanoate	DHT gel
Fluoxymesterone	T. microspheres	
	T. pellets	

T testosterone, *DHT* dihydrotestosterone

In the case of hypogonadotropic (secondary) hypogonadism without additional growth impairment, the underlying disorder is usually diagnosed because of an absence of the occurrence of signs of true puberty (oestrogen effects in girls, testicular enlargement in boy—pubic hair development is not an indicator of true puberty). The doubtless diagnosis of hypogonadotropic hypogonadism (GnRh) deficiency (Balasubramanian et al., 2010) or gonadotropin (LH, FSH) deficiency (Walvoord, 2009) is often difficult, and delayed spontaneous puberty may occur after a challenge of the system with external sex steroids. Like in secondary hypogonadism the most important aspect for the child is the induction of puberty and normal growth. Thus, the therapy to induce puberty should be initiated in time (not after age 12 years in girls or 14 years in boys) using the same approach as discussed for children with primary hypogonadism. To assure future fertility is also a goal but of lesser concern for adolescents who primarily want to be fully integrated into their peer group. In boys it is of some relevance to experience testicular growth, which can be achieved by treatment with gonadotropins or gonadotropin-releasing hormone (GnRH). Whether—or when—such a treatment is required to preserve future fertility is an open question.

Growth Promotion in Adolescence

Short stature is a symptom which is exclusively present during childhood development and may have a multitude of causes, most of which are still unknown (Table 4) (Wit et al., 2007). A growth failure may be congenital or acquired. A growth failure is termed primary in case the growing tissue is inherently abnormal, while it is called secondary if the factors regulating the growth process directly (e.g. growth hormone) or indirectly (e.g. nutrition, organ function) are impaired. If the cause or the pathogenesis of a growth disorder is known, specific measures can possibly be taken to correct the symptom. The most prominent secondary growth disorder is growth hormone (GH) deficiency which in its most severe form leads to an adult height of about 130 cm ("dwarfism") if not treated. Growth hormone deficiency is frequently associated with an impaired secretion of other pituitary hormones (TSH, ACTH, LH, FSH). Replacement with recombinant human GH (by injection s.c. once daily) allows children with GH deficiency (GHD) to reach a normal adult height. In addition, GH has also been proven to be effective in treating short stature in a number of disorders with primary growth failure not caused by an impaired

Table 4 Classification of short stature (Wit et al., 2007)

ESPE code	Main category	Second category	Subcategory (examples)
1A	*Primary growth disorders*		
1A.1		Clinically defined syndromes	Turner S., Noonan S., Silver-Russell S.
1A.2		Small for gestational age (SGA)	
1A.3		Skeletal dysplasia	Achondroplasia
1A.4			
1B	*Secondary growth disorders*		
1B.1		Insufficient nutrient intake	
1B.2		Disorders of organ systems	Cardiac, pulmonary, liver, renal
1B.3		Growth hormone deficiency (secondary IGF-I deficiency)	Impaired GH secretion
1B.4		Other disorders of the GH axis	Laron S., IGF-I deficiency
1B.5		Other endocrine disorders	Hypothyroidism, Cushing S.
1B.6		Metabolic disorders	
1B.7		Psychosocial	Anorexia nervosa
1B.8		Iatrogenic	Chemotherapy, corticoids
1C	*Idiopathic short*		
1C.1		Familial	
2C.2		Nonfamilial	

GH secretion (e.g. Turner S., shortness after small size at birth (SGA), Chronic Renal Failure, Idiopathic Short Stature (ISS)). Growth is a complex and long process, and it can be accepted as a principle that any growth disorder should be treated well before the onset of puberty. During normal puberty the total growth remaining to adult height is only 20–40 cm compared to about 80–100 cm from birth to puberty onset. Thus, any gain in height is a smaller fraction of prepubertal growth which is easier to achieve.

In children with secondary hypogonadism and growth hormone deficiency, the issue of an induction of puberty is associated with the question of growth hormone replacement and the preservation of the growth potential (MacGillivray, 2004; Walvoord; 2009). During normal puberty oestrogens in girls and boys (in boys testosterone is converted to estradiol [Fig. 1]) augment GH secretion directly and IGF secretion indirectly. At the same time oestrogens promote ossification at the growth plate. Testosterone and its active derivative dihydrotestosterone (DHT) do not enhance the GH-IGF axis but have a direct growth-promoting effect at the growth plate, which probably explains the greater pubertal growth in boys. Thus, any steroid which can be transformed into oestrogen (aromatisation) also holds the potential to impair growth. The replacement with sex steroids should therefore be considered cautiously and along the lines as described above. Whether or not the dose of GH needs to be increased above the prepubertal level is not clear. Certainly an increase in GH dose is able to augment growth during puberty, but usually in GHD total pubertal growth is in the expected magnitude on prepubertal GH dose levels (Ranke & Lindberg, 2011).

In TS short stature is the most consistent finding. It begins during the prenatal phase and ends with an adult height that is 20 cm below the female average of the corresponding ethnic group (Ranke and Grauer, 1994). The availability of unlimited GH has made it possible to conduct carefully designed studies aimed at evaluating the growth response. In the proof-of-concept study by Rosenfeld et al. (1998), 70 patients with TS were treated with GH—partly in conjunction with the anabolic steroid oxandrolone—from an age of about 9 years onward. While the patients in the control group achieved an adult height of 144 cm, the treated patients grew to a mean of 152 cm. The GH dose was 0.375 mg/kg/week divided into daily injections. This dose is about 50 % higher than the replacement dose given in GH-deficient children. Summarising many studies in which relatively old children with TS were treated with similar GH doses suggest that the following factors are predictive of the degree of height gain during GH treatment: (1) age (the younger, the better), (2) age at onset of puberty (not before 13–14 years of age) and (3) GH dose (the higher, the better). This was confirmed in a Dutch cooperative study in which girls at a median age of 7 years were started on GH therapy in doses of up to 0.5 mg/kg/week and did not begin oestrogen substitution before the patients reached 12 years of age. Almost all of the girls in the study achieved a height within the normal range for adult women. Many of them exceeded 160 cm (van Pareren et al., 2003). Growth promotion therapy in these patients did not elicit any major clinical or metabolic side effects, although the long-term risk of diabetes mellitus and cardiovascular disorders is increased; neither was disproportional growth observed among patients. Based on a large observational cohort of TS girls treated with GH, we observed that the predictors of adult height on GH are chronological age at GH start (the younger, the better), age at puberty start (the later, the better), GH dose (the more, the better), mid-parental height (the taller, the better), height at GH start (the taller, the better) and the responsiveness during the first year on GH (the more, the better) (Ranke et al., 2007). Growth hormone is an approved therapy for the growth promotion of height in TS up to a dose of about 0.35 mg/kg/week. The attainment of normal height already during childhood has wide implications, not the least the induction of puberty at an earlier time point than is the case in current practice, a strategy that will certainly influence the psychosocial integration of TS patients in a positive way (Reiter et al., 2001). Unfortunately even today late diagnosis of the disorder is still the cause of inappropriate growth development and causes a delay in achieving feminisation.

Tall Stature

Like short stature tall stature—a height >97th centile for age—in a child and adolescent is a symptom requiring a diagnosis (Table 5). In particular any height outside the familial target range is suggestive for an abnormality. Tall stature may be only transient during childhood or may be permanent leading to tall stature in adult life (Wit et al., 2007). Aside from familial tall stature and tall stature of unknown cause (idiopathic), chromosomal abnormalities (males: 47, XXY; 47, YYX and females: 47, XXX) and dysmorphic syndromes (e.g. Marfan syndrome, Sotos syndrome) are accompanied with tall stature. Growth hormone-producing tumours during childhood leading to gigantism (after closure of the epiphyses, acromegaly develops) and the lack of an oestrogen receptor are rare causes of excessive growth. Most frequently tall stature is familial or of unknown (idiopathic) origin.

Excessive adult height (>185 cm in girls, >200 cm in boys) is often considered a psychological handicap and practical disadvantage irrespective of its cause. Therefore, parents quite often seek advice about the potential growth of their tall child (Thomsett, 2010). Height prediction methods involving bone age ratings are able to offer moderately accurate information about the expected height, in particular at an age just before puberty onset (Venn et al., 2008). In the case of an excessive height expectation, attempts to reduce the adult height and thereby preventing psychological suffering have been offered for children with tall stature caused by a primary disorder or with normal variant tall stature (see Table 5). The demand for an intervention in such cases is depending on the sex (tall stature is considered more disadvantageous in females) and certainly depending on the social environment. The mechanism of the therapies to diminish excessive adult height is principally the same in boys and girls. High concentrations of oestrogens—given directly to girls (e.g. 7.5 mg conjugates oestrogens [or equivalent] per day p.o. plus cyclic

Table 5 Classification of tall stature (Wit et al., 2007)

ESPE code	Main category	Second category	Subcategory (examples)
2A	*Primary growth disorders*		
2A.1		Clinically defined syndromes with sex chromosome abnormality	47,XXY (Klinefelter S.) 47,XXX S. 47,XYY S.
2A.2		Dysmorphic syndromes due to metabolic/connective tissue abnormality	Marfan S. Homocystinuria
2A.3		Other dysmorphic syndromes with symmetrical overgrowth	Fragile X S. Sotos S. Weaver S.
2A.4		Dysmorphic syndromes with partial/asymmetrical overgrowth	Beckwith-Wiedemann S.
2B	*Secondary growth disorders*		
2B.1		Growth hormone overproduction	GH producing adenoma GHRH excess
2B.2		Hyperinsulinism	
2B.3		Familial glucocorticoid deficiency	
2B.4		Hyperthyroidism	
2B.5		Conditions with tall stature in childhood leading to short/normal adult stature	Precocious puberty CAH
2B.6		Conditions with normal height in childhood leading to tall adult stature	Aromatase deficiency Oestrogen receptor deficiency
2C	*Normal variant tall*		
2C.1		Genetic (familial, constitutional) tall stature	
2C.2		Nonfamilial idiopathic tall stature	

S. = syndromes

gestagens) or given indirectly by high doses of testosterone to boys (about 500 mg per month i.m.)—advance bone maturation, thus shortening the growth process. The effect of such therapies depends on the bone age at its initiation. If a bone age is below 11 years in girls or 13 years in boys, a reduction in expected adult height of about 5 cm and more can be expected (Binder et al., 1997; Drop et al., 1998). Although the therapies appear to be generally safe in the short and the long run, including the prospect of fertility, it is advised to apply such a treatment with utmost restriction.

Psychological and Behavioural Comorbidities

While in the disorders discussed—congenital adrenal hypoplasia (CAH), hypogonadism and growth problems in small or tall stature—the problems are often straightforward and can be resolved by means of standard medical intervention or psychological advice. However, in a segment of patients severe psychological and behavioural problems may arise. The problems may cover a broad range of child/adolescent psychological disorders and behavioural problems. Anxiety, depression, social phobia and dissocial behaviour may be observed. Such situations call for an integrated approach involving experienced psychologists and/or behavioural health professionals. Particularly in CAH and in hypogonadism, a variety of problems may arise at different stages of childhood development. In females with CAH and disorders of sex differentiation, the medical strategies to assure a female phenotype after birth need to be accompanied with support of the family. This may be more difficult today, since there are partly confliction positions as to what determines gender identity of the individual. In case of a conflict between biological (chromosomal, gonadal and genital) female sex and the individually perceived gender during adolescence, guidance needs to be sought with a specialist in the field. In order to avoid mistakes, which are often difficult to compensate, the health specialist should seek advice about the medical facts first and take a cautious attitude before offering advice. The health professional should also know the details of the patient's (families) social and cultural setting, which has a major impact on attitudes in this area. It should also be considered that health professionals must primarily defend/protect the interest of the patient (particularly before full age) over the position and interests of the family. This may often be achieved, if not only problems verbalised directly are dealt with but if known areas of potential conflicts (e.g. gender identity, sexuality, fertility) are approached with the parties prophylactically. This may be done with the parties separately and in a mode appropriate for the development of the child and acceptable for the family. Since completely unresolvable conflicts are rare, caregivers should be generally guided by a positive attitude towards arising problems.

References

Balasubramanian, R., Dwyer, A., Seminara, S. B., Pitteloud, N., Kaiser, U. B., & Crowley, W. F., Jr. (2010). Human GnRH deficiency: A unique disease model to unravel the ontogeny of GnRH neurons. *Neuroendocrinology, 92*, 81–99.

Binder, G., Grauer, M. L., Wehner, A. V., Wehner, F., & Ranke, M. B. (1997). Outcome in tall stature. Final height and psychological aspects in 220 patients with and without treatment. *European Journal of Pediatrics, 156*, 905–910.

Bondy, C. A., & for the Turner Syndrome Consensus Study Group. (2007). Care of girls and women with Turner syndrome: A guideline of the Turner Syndrome Study Group. *Journal of Clinical Endocrinology and Metabolism, 92*, 10–25.

Bonfig, W., Pozza, S. B., Schmidt, H., Pagel, P., Knorr, D., & Schwarz, H. P. (2009). Hydrocortisone dosing during puberty in patients with classical congenital adrenal hyperplasia: An evidence-based recommendation. *Journal of Clinical Endocrinology and Metabolism, 94*, 3882–3888.

Bryman, I., Sylvén, L., Berntorp, K., Innala, E., Bergström, I., Hanson, C., et al. (2011). Pregnancy rate and outcome in Swedish women with Turner syndrome. *Fertility and Sterility, 95*(8), 2507–2510.

Burnett, A. C., Reutens, D. C., & Wood, A. G. (2010). Social cognition in Turner's syndrome. *Journal of Clinical Neuroscience, 17*, 283–286.

Carel, J. C., Eugster, E. A., Rogol, A., Ghizzoni, L., Palmert, M. R., ESPE-LWPES GnRH Analogs Consensus Conference Group, et al. (2009). Consensus statement on the use of gonadotropin-releasing hormone analogs in children. *Pediatrics, 123*, e752–e762.

Casteràs, A., De Silva, P., Rumsby, G., & Conway. (2009). GS.rate. *Clinical Endocrinology, 70*, 833–837.

Drobac, S., Rubin, K., Rogol, A. D., et al. (2006). A workshop on pubertal hormone replacement options in the United States. *Journal of Pediatric Endocrinology & Metabolism, 19*, 55–64.

Drop, S. L., De Waal, W. J., & De Muinck Keizer-Schrama, S. M. (1998). Sex steroid treatment of constitutionally tall stature. *Endocrine Reviews, 19*, 540–558.

Edgar, A. B., Morris, E. M., Kelnar, C. J., & Wallace, W. H. (2009). Long-term follow-up of survivors of childhood cancer. *Endocrine Development, 15*, 159–180.

Ferriman, D., & Gallwey, J. D. (1961). Clinical assessment of body hair growth in women. *Journal of Clinical Endocrinology and Metabolism, 21*, 1440–1447.

Frisén, L., Nordenström, A., Falhammar, H., Filipsson, H., Holmdahl, G., Janson, P. O., et al. (2009). Gender role behavior, sexuality, and psychosocial adaptation in women with congenital adrenal hyperplasia due to CYP21A2 deficiency. *Journal of Clinical Endocrinology and Metabolism, 94*, 3432–3439.

Hargitai, G., Sólyom, J., Battelino, T., Lebl, J., Pribilincová, Z., Hauspie, R., et al. (2001). Growth patterns and final height in congenital adrenal hyperplasia due to classical 21-hydroxylase deficiency. Results of a multicenter study. *Hormone Research, 55*, 161–171.

Hindmarsh, P. C. (2009). Hyperplasia. *Best Practice & Research. Clinical Endocrinology & Metabolism, 23*, 193–208.

Houk, C. P., Rogol, A., & Lee, P. A. (2010). Fertility in men with Klinefelter syndrome. *Pediatric Endocrinology Reviews, 8*(Suppl 1), 182–186.

James, W. D. (2005). Clinical practice. Acne. *The New England Journal of Medicine, 352*, 1463–1472.

Kiess, W., Conways, G., Ritzen, M., et al. (2002). Induction of puberty in the hypogonadal girls—Practices and attitudes of pediatric endocrinologists in Europe. *Hormone Research, 57*, 66–71.

Lau, N. M., Huang, J. Y., MacDonald, S., Elizur, S., Gidoni, Y., Holzer, H., et al. (2009). Feasibility of fertility preservation in young females with Turner syndrome. *Reproductive Biomedicine Online, 18*, 290–295.

MacGillivray, M. H. (2004). Induction of puberty in hypogonadal children. *Journal of Pediatric*

Endocrinology & Metabolism, 17(Suppl 4), 1277–1287.

McCauley, E., Kay, T., Ito, J., & Treder, R. (1987). The Turner syndrome: Cognitive deficits, affective discrimination, and behavior problems. *Child Development, 58*, 464–473.

Meyer-Bahlburg, H. F. (2001). Gender and sexuality in classic congenital adrenal hyperplasia. *Endocrinology and Metabolism Clinics of North America, 30*, 155–171. viii.

Meyer-Bahlburg, H. F., Dolezal, C., Baker, S. W., & New, M. I. (2008). Sexual orientation in women with classical or non-classical congenital adrenal hyperplasia as a function of degree of prenatal androgen excess. *Archives of Sexual Behavior, 37*, 85–99.

Miller, W. L. (2005). Disorders of androgen synthesis–from cholesterol to dehydroepiandrosterone. *Medical Principles and Practice, 14*(Suppl 1), 58–68.

Miller, W. L., Achermann, J. C., & Flueck, C. E. (2008). The adrenal cortex and its disorders. In M. Sperling (Ed.), *Pediatric endocrinology* (pp. 444–529). Philadelphia: Saunders Elsevier.

Money, J., & Ehrhardt, A. A. (1972). Gender dimorphic behavior and fetal sex hormones. *Recent Progress in Hormone Research, 28*, 735.

Mouritsen, A., Jørgensen, N., Main, K. M., Schwartz, M., & Juul, A. (2010). Testicular adrenal rest tumours in boys, adolescents and adult men with congenital adrenal hyperplasia may be associated with the CYP21A2 mutation. *International Journal of Andrology, 33*, 521–527.

New, M. I. (2003). Inborn errors of adrenal steroidogenesis. *Molecular and Cellular Endocrinology, 211*, 75–83.

New, M. I. (2006). Extensive clinical experience: Nonclassical 21-hydroxylase deficiency. *Journal of Clinical Endocrinology and Metabolism, 91*, 4205–4214.

Otten, B. J., Stikkelbroeck, M. M., Claahsen-van der Grinten, H. L., & Hermus, A. R. (2005). Puberty and fertility in congenital adrenal hyperplasia. *Endocrine Development, 8*, 54–66.

Pasquino, A. M., Passeri, F., Pucarelli, I., Segni, M., & Municchi, G. (1997). Spontaneous pubertal development in Turner's syndrome. Italian Study Group for Turner's Syndrome. *Journal of Clinical Endocrinology and Metabolism, 82*, 1810–1813.

Prader, A. (1954). Genital findings in the female pseudohermaphroditism of the congenital adrenogenital syndrome; morphology, frequency, development and heredity of the different genital forms. *Helvetica Paediatrica Acta, 9*, 231–248.

Ranke, M. B., & Grauer, M. L. (1994). Adult height in Turner syndrome: Results of a multinational survey 1993. *Hormone Research, 42*, 90–94.

Ranke, M. B., Lindberg, A., Ferrández Longás, A., Darendeliler, F., Albertsson-Wikland, K., Dunger, D., et al. (2007). Major determinants of height development in Turner syndrome (TS) patients treated with GH: Analysis of 987 patients from KIGS. *Pediatric Research, 61*, 105–110.

Ranke, M. B., Lindberg, A., & on behalf of the KIGS International Board. (2011). Observed and predicted total pubertal growth (TPG) during treatment with growth hormone in adolescents with idiopathic growth hormone deficiency (GHD). Turner syndrome (TS). short stature born small for gestational age (SGA) and idiopathic short stature (ISS). KIGS analysis and review. *Hormone Research in Pædiatrics, 75*(6), 423–432.

Ranke, M. B., & Saenger, P. (2001). Turner's syndrome. *Lancet, 358*, 309–314.

Rao, E., Weiss, B., Fukami, M., et al. (1997). Pseudoautosomal deletions encompassing a novel homeobox gene cause growth failure in idiopathic short stature and Turner syndrome. *Nature Genetics, 16*, 54–63.

Reiter, E. O., Blethen, S. L., Baptista, J., & Price, L. (2001). Early initiation of growth hormone treatment allows age-appropriate estrogen use in Turner's syndrome. *Journal of Clinical Endocrinology and Metabolism, 86*, 1936–1941.

Rogol, A. D., & Tartaglia, N. (2010). Considerations for androgen therapy in children and adolescents with Klinefelter syndrome (47, XXY). *Pediatric Endocrinology Reviews, 8*(Suppl 1), 145–150.

Rosenfeld, R. G., Attie, K. M., Fr, J., Brasel, J. A., Burstein, S., Cara, J. F., et al. (1998). Growth hormone therapy of Turner's syndrome: Beneficial effect on adult height. *The Journal of Pediatrics, 132*, 319–324.

Rosenfield, R. L. (2005). Clinical practice. Hirsutism. *The New England Journal of Medicine, 353*, 2578–2588.

Ryan, S. (2010). The adolescent and young adult with Klinefelter syndrome:ensuring successful transitions to adulthood. *Pediatric Endocrinology Reviews, 8*(Suppl 1), 169–177.

Sheaffer, A. T., Lange, E., & Bondy, C. A. (2008). Sexual function in women with Turner syndrome. *Journal of Women's Health, 17*, 27–33.

Simpson, J. L., & Rajkovic, A. (1999). Ovarian differentiation and gonadal failure. *American Journal of Medical Genetics, 89*, 186–200.

Speiser, P. W., Azziz, R., Baskin, L. S., Ghizzoni, L., Hensle, T. W., Merke, D. P., et al. (2010). Congenital adrenal hyperplasia due to steroid 21-hydroxylase deficiency: An Endocrine Society clinical practice guideline. *Journal of Clinical Endocrinology and Metabolism, 95*, 4133–4160.

Thomsett, M. J. (2010). The spectrum of clinical paediatric endocrinology: 28 years of referrals to an individual consultant. *Journal of Paediatrics and Child Health, 46*, 304–309.

van Pareren, Y. K., de Muinck Keizer-Schrama, S. M., Stijnen, T., et al. (2003). Final height in girls with turner syndrome after long-term growth hormone treatment in three dosages and low dose estrogens. *Journal of Clinical Endocrinology and Metabolism, 88*, 1119–1125.

Venn, A., Hosmer, T., Hosmer, D., Bruinsma, F., Jones, P., Lumley, J., et al. (2008). Oestrogen treatment for tall stature in girls: Estimating the effect on height and the error in height prediction. *Clinical Endocrinology, 68*, 926–929.

Vidal, I., Gorduza, D. B., Haraux, E., Gay, C. L., Chatelain, P., Nicolino, M., et al. (2010). Surgical options in disorders of sex development (dsd) with ambiguous genitalia. *Best Practice & Research. Clinical Endocrinology & Metabolism, 24*, 311–324.

Walvoord, E. (2009). Sex steroid replacement for induction of puberty in multiple pituitary hormone deficiency. *Pediatric Endocrinology Reviews, 6*(Suppl 2), 298–305.

Wit, J., Ranke, M. B., & Kelnar, C. J. H. (2007). ESPE classification of paediatric endocrine diagnoses. *Hormone Research, 68*, 1–120.

Yin, A., & Swerdloff, R. (2010). Treating hypogonadism in younger males. *Expert Opinion on Pharmacotherapy, 11*, 1529–1540.

Musculoskeletal Injuries in Adolescents: A Sports Medicine Model

Asheesh Gupta, Ron Paik, Gloria Balague, John Coumbe-Lilley, and Mark R. Hutchinson

Introduction

It has been said that the best place to study trauma in adolescents is to witness an American high school football any Friday evening in the fall. In virtually every minute of the game, another collision is occurring that places the athlete at risk of musculoskeletal injury. This weekend observance for trauma is much more fruitful than sitting at the street corner waiting for the next car accident to occur. For the purposes of this chapter, a sports medicine model will be used to discuss common musculoskeletal injuries in adolescents ranging from acute traumatic injuries to chronic overuse injuries. The chapter will be broken into two sections: musculoskeletal injuries and the psychological basis of injury, recovery, and prevention. Special issues including musculoskeletal injuries related to child abuse as well as more classic traumatic injuries related to accidental falls and motor vehicle accident will be discussed in the context of epidemiological and prevention comparisons to the athletic population. The impact of musculoskeletal injury on the life of an adolescent will be emphasized in not only discussing the temporary physical challenges and impairments of specific injuries but also by the need for prevention. The final section of the chapter is dedicated to the psychological impact of overuse and traumatic musculoskeletal on the adolescent both in the short and long term as well as some clues regarding optimization of recovery for youth.

Section 1: Musculoskeletal Injuries in Youth

Epidemiology

In the United States an estimated 30 million youth participate in organized sports. The Youth Risk Behavior Survey was a large population-based study performed throughout the 1990s, enabling accurate measurement of the emerging trends in youth sports participation. Results from the 1997 survey reported that 62 % of US high school students participated in one or more sports teams, with most playing in a combination of both school and nonschool teams (Washington, Bernhardt, Gomez, et al., 2001). In addition, many more participate in recreational sports. Injuries are an inherent risk in sports, and approximately 80 % of sports injuries affect the musculoskeletal system. Many patients participate in multiple teams during a given sports season, the rest periods between seasons are short or nonexistent, and there is increasing demand for sporting success from par-

A. Gupta, M.D. (✉) • R. Paik, M.D.
M.R. Hutchinson, M.D.
Department of Orthopaedics, University of Illinois, 835 South Wolcott, 270 Medical Sciences Building, Chicago, IL 60612, USA
e-mail: mhutch@uic.edu

G. Balague, Ph.D. • J. Coumbe-Lilley, Ph.D.
University of Illinois at Chicago, 601 S. Morgan Street, Chicago, IL 60607, USA

W.T. O'Donohue et al. (eds.), *Handbook of Adolescent Health Psychology*,
DOI 10.1007/978-1-4614-6633-8_42, © Springer Science+Business Media New York 2013

ents, schools, and sporting establishments. In a survey of children and adolescents age 5–17 years, the estimated annual number of injuries resulting from participation in sports and recreational activities was 4,379,000 with 1,363,000 classified as serious (requiring hospitalization, surgical treatment, missed school, or a half day or more in bed). Up to 36 % of injuries may be directly related to sports participation in patients in these age groups (Bijur et al., 1995). While the definition of what constitutes a sports injury is varied, some common elements such as need for medical attention, time lost from practice or game, and decreased level of activity are widely used in different definitions. Injuries are commonly grouped into either acute or chronic which are designated macrotrauma and microtrauma, respectively.

One of the most commonly used measures in determining the severity of a sports injury is time lost from participation in the sport. The National Athletic Injury Reporting System (NAIRS) uses the following categories for severity: nonreportable, no time lost; minor, 1–7 days lost; moderate, 8–21 days lost; major, more than 21 days lost; and severe, resulting in permanent disability. Another important documented aspect of sports injuries is incidence of injuries. The two ways in which incidence of injuries are reported are cumulative incidence and incidence of first injury. Cumulative incidence reports the number of injuries sustained by a defined group of athletes. For example, cumulative incidence would record the incidence of injuries of football players over a set period of time. Cumulative incidence is useful because it provides information on an individual athlete's risk of injury. Incidence of first injury is the risk of any one athlete in a group of being injured.

From incidence studies, it is clear that chronic overuse injuries are far more prevalent than acute sports injuries in those 17 years old and younger. Not only is there a higher incidence of chronic injuries in adolescents but the severity as measured by time lost from sports is also greater. Of all injuries in adolescents, 30–50 % are due to chronic overuse in both sports-related and non-sports-related injuries.

The greatest source of available data on musculoskeletal sports injuries comes from those suffered during interscholastic high school sports. For boys in all sports combined, there is a yearly incidence of injury in high school sports of 27–39 %. Organized sports account for 25–30 % of total injuries, while non-organized sports account for 40 % of total injuries. As one would expect contact sports account for the greatest number of injuries in adolescents. In an 8-year longitudinal study of high school sports, researchers reported that 48 % of athletes sustained at least one injury during their season: 64.5 % of all injuries were minor (no days lost), 30.3 % were mild (1–7 days lost), 3.1 % were moderate (8–21 days lost), and 1.9 % were severe (22 days lost). A study by the American Academy of Pediatrics suggested that female athletes have higher rates of injuries when compared with male athletes (American Academy of Pediatrics: Committee on Sports Medicine and Fitness, 2000). A recent study looking at injury claims from an insurance provider for youth soccer leagues showed that knee and anterior cruciate ligament injuries in female youth soccer players age 12 through 15 were more common than ACL injuries in males of the same age (Shea, Pfeiffer, Wang, Curtin, & Apel, 2004).

Soft tissue injuries such as strains, sprains, and contusions are the most common types of acute injuries. In a national study on sports and recreational injuries, researchers found that 59 % of sprains, 48 % of fractures and dislocations, and 25.5 % of lacerations are caused by sports and recreational activities in those under the age of 18. Furthermore, 36 % of all injuries are from sports. Compared with other injuries, sports did not account for a disproportionate number of serious or repeat injuries. This could serve as an indication to use sports as a model for injuries in adolescents.

Why Are Adolescents Different?

There are a number of significant differences between the adult and adolescent musculoskeletal system. The most significant difference between an immature skeleton and the adult skeleton is the presence of growth plates. The growth plate, also known as the physis, is composed of four zones: the resting cartilage or reserve zone, the proliferating cartilage zone, the zone of hypertrophy, and the metaphysis. In bone, there is a diaphysis (middle part of long bone), an epiphysis (end part of long bone), and a metaphysis (between the diaphysis and epiphysis) components. The physis is wedged between the metaphysis and epiphysis. The cartilage of the physis is relatively weak and susceptible to injury, especially during periods of active growth. In particular, the zone of calcification within the physis is the weakest and most commonly injured area; however, fractures confined to this region typically heal without complication.

In adults, the fully grown calcified bone is significantly stronger than ligaments and other soft tissue around the joint. Consequently, in adults, ligaments and soft tissue are more susceptible to injury than bone. In contrast, during adolescence, the ligaments and other soft structures around the joint are two to five times stronger than the physis. Therefore, damage to the physis is more common than damage to ligaments in those with immature skeletons.

It is also important to note that adolescent bone is less dense, more porous, and more vascular than adult bone. Increased porosity contributes to prevent the spread of fractures. The pediatric skeleton has a number of other advantages including the capacity for rapid and predictable fracture healing, increased tolerance of long-term immobilization, and increased tendency to recover soft tissue mobility spontaneously following most injuries, and joint surfaces are generally more tolerant of irregularity than those of adults.

Not only is the skeleton growing during adolescence but there are profound changes in height, weight, muscle mass, motor skills, and coordination. The adolescent growth spurt is variable in its onset and duration. As a result, two individuals of the same size could have vastly different bone and muscle maturity leading to a size–size mismatch in sports. In collision sports such as football, size–size mismatch is magnified and leads to an increased risk and severity of injury for the less developed individual. Size–size mismatch is more pronounced in boys than girls because as girls experience only a slight increase in muscle strength after menarche boys continue to acquire muscle strength throughout adolescence. Similarly in girls, motor performance remains relatively constant throughout adolescence where as boys continue to see improved motor performance throughout adolescence. While there is no clear pattern of strength and motor skill development in girls, there appears to be a positive correlation between biological maturity and muscle strength and motor performance in boys. This positive correlation suggests that as an athlete matures, they acquire a greater skill level in their sport which can lead to a higher level of competition played at a higher intensity. Furthermore, as athletes mature, their maximal speed increases leading to more violent collisions with increased momentum. Both increased intensity and speed in collision sports add to the risk and severity of injury.

While the focus of this chapter has been the physical injuries adolescents' experience, equally important are the psychological aspects of sports and injuries. Youth play sports for a variety of reasons including social acceptance, love of the sport, and hope of obtaining an athletic scholarship to college. With much pressure on athletes to perform at a high level whether it is from self, coach, friends, or family injuries can often be unexpected, difficult, and stressful. Most athletes have the proper motivation and desire to go through rehabilitation and get back to their sport as soon as possible. However, some athletes stagnate and may become depressed and require extra support to get through their injury. Athletes may go through a series of reactions after an injury similar to the context of death or other loss. The stages go in order from disbelief, denial, isolation, anger, bargaining, depression, to acceptance, and resignation with hope. During the recovery process, the physician must continue to motivate the athlete, help the athlete understand realistic outcomes, and listen to and manage the patient's reactions.

Common Acute Trauma Injuries

It is estimated that 15–20 % of all injuries to long bone are acute injuries of the growth plate. A large number of these acute injuries happen during sports participation. Acute injuries of the growth plate in the upper extremity are twice as common compared to those of the lower extremity. Boys suffer more acute injuries, and the greatest number of injuries for boys occurs at the age of 12 and 13, whereas for girls, the greatest number of injuries occurs at the age of 11. A system called the Salter–Harris classification was developed to classify acute injuries to the growth plate in adolescents. The Salter–Harris scheme is the most widely used system and has practical use in treatment and prognosis.

There are five types of Salter–Harris fractures that increase in severity from 1 to 5. A Salter–Harris type 1 fracture is least severe and is a transverse fracture across the growth plate commonly through the hypertrophic zone. The metaphyseal and epiphyseal bones are spared from fracture. Since the normal osteogenesis in the reserve and proliferative zones remain undisturbed in a Salter–Harris type 1 fracture, the prognosis is good. Type 1 Salter–Harris fractures are known for their rapid healing time, and a gentle reduction followed by alignment to protect the bone and joint from displacement is usually satisfactory for treatment. With protection, only 4–6 weeks are needed for the fracture to heal.

A Salter–Harris type 2 fracture transverses the growth plate much like a type 1 fracture; however, the fracture also enters the metaphysis. As in type 1 fractures, the reserve zone and zone of proliferation are undamaged and therefore the treatment is the same as a type 1 fracture. Salter–Harris type 3 and 4 fractures occur from sheer forces and differ from less severe fractures in that the fracture crosses the epiphysis into the joint. The articular joint is disrupted as the proliferative zone is violated. Long-term problems associated with type 3 and 4 fractures are growth arrest and high risk of articular degeneration. Surgical intervention is often indicated for type 3 and 4 fractures. A Salter–Harris type 5 fracture results from a crush injury to the reserve or proliferative zones of the growth plate and can cause growth arrest.

Acute patellar dislocation is one of the most common causes of acute hemarthrosis in the young athlete. When comparing patellar dislocation in male and female patients, some studies have suggested similar rates (Hinton & Sharma, 2003), and others have demonstrated that females have higher dislocation rates in the under 18 age group (Fithian, Paxton, Stone, et al., 2004). Risk factors for patella dislocation include ligamentous laxity, increased genu valgum, patella alta, lower extremity version abnormalities such as femoral anteversion and external tibial torsion, trochlear dysplasia, increased quadriceps angle, foot pronation, and patellar tilt (Hinton & Sharma, 2003). Both the medial retinaculum and the medial patellofemoral ligament (MPFL) are primary restraints to patellar dislocation. The risk of recurrent patellar dislocations appears to be significantly higher in females. A prospective cohort study following 189 pts were followed for 2–5 years. The group with the highest risk of dislocation was females age 10–17 years; 61 % dislocations occurred during sports and 9 % during dancing (Fithian et al., 2004). Standard knee radiographs should be taken to evaluate for osteochondral injuries, avulsions of soft tissue fragments, patella height, and trochlear dysplasia. MRI is also useful to evaluate for significant soft tissue injuries. Initial treatment consists of a brief period of immobilization followed by early rehabilitation. A recent prospective study on surgical intervention for first-time dislocators in children/adolescents did not demonstrate better outcomes compared with nonsurgical management (Palmu, Kallio, Donell, Helenius, & Nietosvaara, 2008). For patients with recurrent symptomatic patellar instability, surgical intervention may be beneficial.

Traumatic shoulder dislocations occur primarily in collision and contact sports in young athletes. It has been estimated that around 40 % of shoulder dislocations occur in patients younger than 22 years of age. A significant challenge to treating physicians is the fact that athletes with a history of pediatric dislocation have a 90 % chance of recurrent dislocation (Bishop & Flatow, 2005; Deitch, Mehlman, Foad, Obbehat, & Mallory, 2003; Rowe, 1956). This is theorized to be due to the fact that pediatric dislocations are believed to stretch the capsule and diminishes its ability to provide support for the shoulder joint. Surgical treatment of shoulder instability has been shown to be generally successful in young patients (Chen, Diaz, Loebenberg, & Rosen, 2005). Physical examination in combination with diagnostic testing may demonstrate concurrent injuries of the anterior bony labrum or labral lesions (Bankart injury, superior labral anterior and posterior tear, Hill–Sachs lesions), rotator cuff tears, and subscapularis or lesser tuberosity avulsions. Three view radiographs of the shoulder including an anterior–posterior, Scapular-Y, and axillary lateral can help determine direction of dislocation and any other bony abnormalities. MRI arthrogram is useful for evaluating capsular and labral tissues. In the acute setting, immediate reduction of the dislocation shoulder be attempted. If successful, physical therapy protocol should be initiated for strengthening and range of motion. Treatment of first-time dislocation in high-risk athletes remains controversial, and there is some evidence that early surgery may play a role in reducing the risk of secondary dislocation (Bedi & Ryu, 2009). Families should be counseled about the high risk of recurrent instability episodes with possible surgical intervention if nonsurgical treatment fails.

The treatment of anterior cruciate ligament (ACL) injuries in skeletally immature patients remains controversial. Recent studies indicate that the incidence of this injury may be increasing, and young female athletes start sustaining these injuries in significant numbers around 12–13 years of age. Nonsurgical treatment has historically shown to have poor results due to inherent instability leading to meniscal (particularly medial) and chondral injuries (Graf, Lange, Fujisaki, Landry, & Saluja, 1992; McCarroll, Shelbourne, Porter, Rettig, & Murray, 1994). One of the most challenging aspects of surgical reconstruction involves prevention of physeal injury leading to growth disturbance (Kocher, Saxon, Hovis, & Hawkins, 2002). Several physeal sparing techniques have been described in patients with significant growth remaining. For older patients, different techniques using grafts crossing the physis have been described. A recent study of patients at Tanner stage 3 or 4 who underwent ACL reconstruction using transphyseal technique demonstrated no physeal complications with excellent clinical outcomes (Kocher, Smith, Zoric, Lee, & Micheli, 2007).

Tibial eminence fractures occur predominantly in the skeletally immature patient. The mechanism of injury is similar to that of the previously described ACL injury. They are classified into three types: type I, minimal displacement of tibial eminence; type II, displacement of anterior third to one half of the tibial eminence, producing a beak-like deformity on the lateral radiograph; and type III, the avulsed tibial eminence is completely lifted from the underlying bone (Meyers & McKeever, 1987). A rare fourth kind has been described with complete rotation of the fragment. Entrapment of the intermeniscal ligament or anterior meniscus is possible, which may be an impediment to reduction of these fractures (Kocher, Micheli, Gerbino, & Hresko, 2003). These fractures may be associated with other soft tissue injuries, including bone contusions, ligament injury, and meniscal tear (Monto, Cameron-Donaldson, Close, Ho, & Hawkins, 2006).

Fractures of the medial epicondyle of the elbow are more common than frank elbow dislocations and account for 10 % of elbow fractures in children. The ulnar collateral ligament may avulse the medial epicondyle during elbow trauma. Nearly 50 % of medial epicondyle fractures are associated with dislocation of the elbow; the displaced fragment can then become incarcerated in the joint, preventing a concentric reduction. Acute medial epicondyle fractures and dislocations of the elbow can occur in young gymnasts, and isolated medial epicondyle fractures are occasionally seen in adolescent pitchers (Caine & Nassar, 2005). Nondisplaced fractures are treated with casting. In athletes such as throwers, gymnasts, and wrestlers who place high physical demands on the elbow, anatomic reduction of medial epicondyle fractures may be important for future athletic performance.

Common Chronic Overuse Injuries

Overuse injuries are common in adolescents who participate in sports. Repetitive activities can lead to tendinopathies, many of which have terms related to various sports such as golfer's or tennis elbow (medial and lateral epicondylopathy, respectively). Tendinopathies can occur throughout the body. The histopathologic changes vary from the early stages of inflammation (tendinitis) to chronic noninflammatory, fatty degeneration (tendinosis). Treatment options start with conservative treatments such as rest, physical therapy, and anti-inflammatories. Individuals with symptoms refractory to more conservative treatment or those who need more aggressive therapy due to the need to perform at a high level such as professional or collegiate athletes can consider treatments such as ultrasound, steroid or platelet-rich plasma injections, or surgery.

Overuse can result in osteochondroses in adolescents due to their skeletal immaturity. These pathologic conditions involving the physis can occur in various area such as Osgood–Schlatter disease of the tibial tubercle apophysis, Sever's disease of the calcaneus, osteochondritis dissecans of the capitellum of the elbow, and Little Leaguer's elbow (medial epicondyle of the humerus). Treatment for these conditions primarily involves rest and anti-inflammatories/analgesics. If displaced or fragmented, surgery may be required.

Prevention has been more of a recent focus, especially in the case of Little League shoulder and elbow. In hopes of decreasing the incidence of these conditions, USA baseball released recommendations in the mid-1990s for youth pitchers limiting the number and types of pitches thrown depending on age (Benjamin & Briner, 2005). Pitchers 8–10 years old should be restricted to fastballs, 50 pitches per game, and 75 pitches per week (Benjamin & Briner, 2005). Pitchers 10–11 years old can start throwing changeups, 75 pitches per game, and 100 pitches per week. Pitchers 13–14 years old can start throwing curve balls and 125 pitches per week. They are still restricted to 75 pitches per game. Pitchers 15–16 years old can start throwing sliders, forkballs, splitters, and knuckleballs and 90 pitches per game. There are no restrictions for number of pitches per week starting at this age. Pitchers 17–18 years old can start throwing screwballs and 105 pitches per game.

Stress fractures are another type of injury that can result from overuse. Stress fractures are categorized into two groups depending on the etiology. Fatigue stress fractures are the result of abnormal stresses in normal bone (Dixon, Newton, & Teh, 2011). Insufficiency stress fractures occur due to normal stresses in abnormal bone such as those with anorexia or osteoporosis (Dixon et al., 2011). All young women who present with a stress fracture should be carefully screened for the female athlete triad which includes inadequate energy availability compared to energy used (formally defined as eating disorders such as anorexia), poor bone metabolism usually evidenced by the initial stress fracture (formally defined as osteoporosis), and hormonal imbalances leading to menstrual irregularities (formally defined as amenorrhea). The current thought is that the Triad is a continuum of these milder definitions up to and including the extreme definitions (see below).

Stress fractures can occur anywhere in the body but are most commonly in areas that provide support during weight-bearing activities such as the tibia, femoral neck, or pars interarticularis of the spine. This may also include the upper extremity in gymnasts. Runners are at increased risk of tibia and femoral neck stress fractures (Dixon et al., 2011; Harrast & Colonno, 2010). Spondylolysis, fracture of the pars interarticularis, is more common in wrestlers, gymnasts, and weightlifters (Dixon et al., 2011).

Images are needed to diagnose stress fractures. Radiographs often are nondiagnostic since the majority of stress fractures are nondisplaced and cannot be seen on normal X-ray films. Bone scans have been used historically to make the diagnosis; however, MRI is currently the gold standard since it may provide a better indication of the severity of injury and predict return to play.

Treatment of stress fractures depends on the nature and area of the injury. High-risk areas such as the femoral neck can have catastrophic consequences (i.e., displacement which may lead to necrosis of the femoral head) if not surgically stabilized. Stress fractures of the anterior tibia, proximal fifth metatarsal metadiaphyseal area, sesamoids, and navicular are at high risk of nonunion (Harrast & Colonno, 2010). Surgical stabilization should be considered. Otherwise, nonoperative treatment with rest or bracing can be implemented.

Special Issues in Musculoskeletal Injuries in Adolescents

Child abuse is an area that treating physicians should remain vigilant for when evaluating musculoskeletal injuries. Abuse in adolescents may not be as difficult to assess as it is in children who have limited speaking ability. Child abuse as described in "The Child Abuse Prevention and Treatment Act" (CAPTA) amended by the "Keeping Children and Families Safe Act of 2003" is any recent act or failure to act, on the part of the parent or caretaker which results in death, serious physical or emotional harm, sexual abuse or exploitation, or an act or failure to act which presents an imminent risk of serious harm (Sink, Hyman, Matheny, Georgopoulos, & Kleinman, 2011). A child is a person under the age of 18 years, unless the child protection law of the state in which the child resides specifies a younger age for cases not involving sexual abuse.

Skin injuries are the most common manifestation of physical abuse. Burns are present in 10–25 % of cases, and bruising is found in 50–75 % of abuse victims (McMahon, Grossman, Gaffney, & Stanitski, 1995; Sink et al., 2011). Bruising in different stages should increase suspicion for abuse. In adolescents, there are no classic injuries that are specific of physical abuse like metaphyseal corner fractures in younger children or femur fractures in children less than one.

As briefly mentioned above, adolescent girls especially those in aesthetic sports (ballet, rhythmic gymnastics, synchronized swimming, and figure skating) or those sports who have weight categories or in which weight plays a role (crew, ski jumping, wrestling) are at increased risk for a condition termed the female athlete triad. The American College of Sports Medicine (ACSM) in 1992 first developed a special task force to look into the relationship among disordered eating, amenorrhea, and osteoporosis in female athletes, termed the female athlete triad (Beals & Meyer, 2007). They later developed a position paper on the female athlete triad, calling for more research (Beals & Meyer, 2007; Otis, Drinkwater, Johnson, et al., 1997). The new ACSM definition has now replaced disordered eating with low energy availability, amenorrhea with hormonal dysfunction and menstrual irregularities, and osteoporosis with poor bone metabolism and osteopenia which often presents as a stress fracture (Hoch et al., 2009; Otis et al., 1997). One study found that 78 % of high school female athletes had at least one component of the disorder. Only 1 of the 80 athletes had all three components (Hoch et al., 2009). Due to the relative high mortality that occurs in the most severe cases, the clinician should carry a high sense of suspicion when evaluating female athletes with any or all of the components.

Weight training in adolescents anecdotally is thought to be a concern due to the risk of growth disturbances and injuries. However, studies have shown little to no evidence that resistance training will negatively impact growth or maturation (Faigenbaum et al., 2009; Malina, 2006). Resistance training programs are safe overall with low incidence of injury. In one study of 354 middle school and high school football players, the injury rate was 0.082 injuries per person-year (Risser, Risser, & Preston, 1990). Lower back strain is the most prevalent injury in adolescents participating in weight training (Faigenbaum et al., 2009; Risser et al., 1990).

Supervision, good technique, and safe training equipment are important measures to prevent injuries in adolescents (Faigenbaum et al., 2009; Malina, 2006; Risser et al., 1990). Studies have shown that there is an increased risk of injury when home exercise equipment is used (Faigenbaum et al., 2009).

Targeting Prevention of Musculoskeletal Injuries in Adolescents

Motor vehicle accidents are the leading cause of death in adolescents in the United States, comprising 32 % of all deaths and 70 % of unintentional deaths (Sleet, Ballesteros, & Borse, 2010). Fatal injuries are more likely to occur when seat belts are not used, the driver has been drinking, or an inexperienced driver is driving other teenagers (Chen, Baker, Braver, & Li, 2000; Quinlan, Brewer, Sleet, & Dellinger, 2000; Sleet et al., 2010). Proper use of a seat belt could prevent around 40–60 % of motor vehicle deaths (Cummins, Koval, Cantu, & Spratt, 2008; Sleet et al., 2010). Unfortunately, adolescents are among the highest demographic of people who do not wear seat belts. In 2007, 11.1 % of high school students reported never wearing seat belts (Eaton et al., 2008; Jones & Shults, 2009; Sleet et al., 2010). Nonuse was more prevalent in males and African American students. The good news is that in addition to preventing mortality, seat belts prevent morbidity in motor vehicle accidents. Seat belt use results in a reduction in maxillofacial and lower extremity injuries (Cox et al., 2004). Restrained occupants had relative risks of 0.42, 0.28, 0.35, and 0.49 compared unrestrained occupants for maxillofacial, pelvis, femur, and tibia/fibula fractures, respectively (Cox et al., 2004; Estrada, Alonso, McGwin, Metzger, & Rue, 2004).

Adolescents are at increased risk for unhealthy behaviors. Alcohol is the most commonly used drugs among teenagers (Sleet et al., 2010). People aged 12–20 years old drink 11 % of all alcohol consumed in the United States, of which 90 % is ingested while binge drinking (Sleet et al., 2010). Binge drinking is described as men consuming five or more drinks and women consuming four or more drinks within 2 h. In 2007, 75 % of high school students reported they had consumed alcohol during their lifetimes, 10 % reported they had driven a vehicle under the influence of alcohol within the past 30 days, and 29 % of students reported they had ridden with a driver who had been drinking alcohol within the past 30 days (Eaton et al., 2008; Jones & Shults, 2009; Sleet et al., 2010).

Other unsafe behaviors can also lead to catastrophic injuries such as diving accidents. Diving was the fourth most common cause of spinal cord injuries in the United States (Barss, Djerrari, Leduc, Lepage, & Dionne, 2008). Of all spinal cord injuries that are a result of diving accidents, 60 % occur in people younger than 24 years of age (Barss et al., 2008; National Spinal Cord Injury Statistical Center, 2006). These incidents occur from diving into shallow water, resulting in a flexion–compression injury to the spine. This can occur in the setting of recreational activities in the pool or any natural body of water. The injury typically occurs at C5–7 due to the greater mobility of these segments (Brown, Brunn, & Garcia, 2001; Korres et al., 2006). Quadriplegia is the most common result of these injuries (Barss et al., 2008).

Safe practices and education are important to prevent musculoskeletal injuries. Only 37 % of those with spinal cord injuries after diving accidents were aware of the hazard (Barss et al., 2008). Another example is with bicycle helmets, which reduce head injuries. It has been reported that 85.1 % of high school students rarely or never wear them (Sleet et al., 2010). Males are more likely than females to not wear helmets (Eaton et al., 2008; Jones & Shults, 2009; Sleet et al., 2010). Peer pressure, negative modeling by family members, and community climate are the most common reason given for not wearing helmets (Kakefuda, Henry, & Stallones, 2009; Liller, Morissette, Noland, & McDermott, 1998; Sleet et al., 2010).

Musculoskeletal injuries also may occur in sports due to athletes incorrectly wearing safety equipment. One example is in ice hockey players. Lacerations to the anterior tibial and extensor tendons occur from players folding down their boot tongue for comfort reasons (Simonet & Sim, 1995). Instead of acting as protection, the tongue becomes an aiming device to glide an inadvertent ice skating blade into the unprotected anterior ankle. Other examples include proper helmet fitting, the use of mouth guards, appropriately fitting shin guards in soccer, and the use of eye protection in high-risk sports.

As further studies on injuries are produced, sports governing organizations continue to adjust rules to protect players. In 1976, the National Collegiate Athletic Association and the National Federation of State High School Associations implemented major rule changes in football prohibiting the use of the head as the initial contact point when blocking and tackling in response to several studies on cervical spine injuries (Rihn et al., 2009). In the 1980s and 1990s, ice hockey governing bodies began to implement rules against checking from behind after studies showed the increased incidence of cervical spine injuries (Tator, Provvidenza, & Cassidy, 2009; Watson, Singer, & Sproule, 1996).

Safe training practices can reduce injuries such as overuse injuries. Injuries can be minimized with qualified supervision, appropriate program design, sensible progression, and careful selection of training equipment (Faigenbaum et al., 2009). In addition, the risk of injury can be minimized by limiting the number of heavy lifts during a workout, allowing for adequate recovery between training sessions, and listening to each child's or adolescent's questions and concerns (Faigenbaum et al., 2009).

In order to provide safe supervision of adolescents, the coaches need to stay up to date on safe practices and innovations. Rules are constantly being updated to address injury concerns. For example, the NFL is constantly changing rules on kickoffs to reduce injuries. In 2009, the number of players allowed to form a blocking wedge was reduced to 2. In 2011, they moved the kickoff to the 35-yard line to decrease the number of high-impact collisions (NFL moves kickoffs to 35-yard line, touchbacks unchanged, 2011).

Coaches can be used as great instruments to teach proper technique and disseminate new information to players. In 2002, the equipment manufacturer Riddell developed a new helmet that has an extended shell onto the mandible area and a face-mask system that claims to dampen impacts (Krauss, 2004). Additionally, it has changes in interior padding to improve energy attenuation in side and posterior impacts. This new helmet is widespread in the NFL and NCAA but is slowly filtering down to the high school level (Krauss, 2004). The news of this helmet could be spread more quickly if coaches stay educated on new innovations on the market and inform their players.

Section 2: Adolescent Sports Injuries—Psychological Aspects

We have seen in the previous section the specifics of getting injured and recovering from injury in an adolescent population. In this section, we will address the psychological aspects of sports injuries in adolescents. Four major aspects will be covered: vulnerability to injuries, psychological reactions to athletic injury, injury recovery, and finally prevention of future injuries. The model used to describe and explain the connection between psychological variables and injury will be the Shaffer's (1997) adaptation of Wiese-Bjornstal, Smith, & LaMott (1995). Figure 1 displays the main elements of the model which were supported in Shaffer's research.

Vulnerability to Injuries

One of the main variables consistently associated with injury vulnerability is stress. Stress is commonly defined as the response occurring when the perceived demands from the environment or situation cannot be met with the perceived resources one has (Lazarus & Folkman, 1984). Another definition of stress that fits very well the injury situation is the following: psychological stress is a reaction to an environment where there is a threat of loss of resources, an actual loss of resources, or a lack of gain after an investment (Hobfoll, 1988). *Resources* can be physical health, finances, mobility/independence, self-perception, achievements, and social roles. This model of stress incorporates six dimensions which help explain why different things are stressful for different people and even why the same person at different point in time will react differently to the same stressor.

Besides the above-mentioned resources, *strain* is defined as the negative consequences of stressful events which can be physical or psychological. In the case of athletic injuries, both types of effects occur, increasing the level of strain. *Needs* is another dimension of the model that refers to the biological, emotional, and cognitive requirements of the individual, and these needs interact with specific environments (such as family expectations and level of sports participation) to generate the demands which are perceived as pressure. *Time* is the next dimension because events have different impact at different points in the developmental process. Adolescence is a time for establishing one's identity, and some events become central to that definition. These dimensions of resources, needs, strain, and time are also framed within the global dimension of *values*.

Values are seen as the main criteria one uses to evaluate oneself and the environment. The model

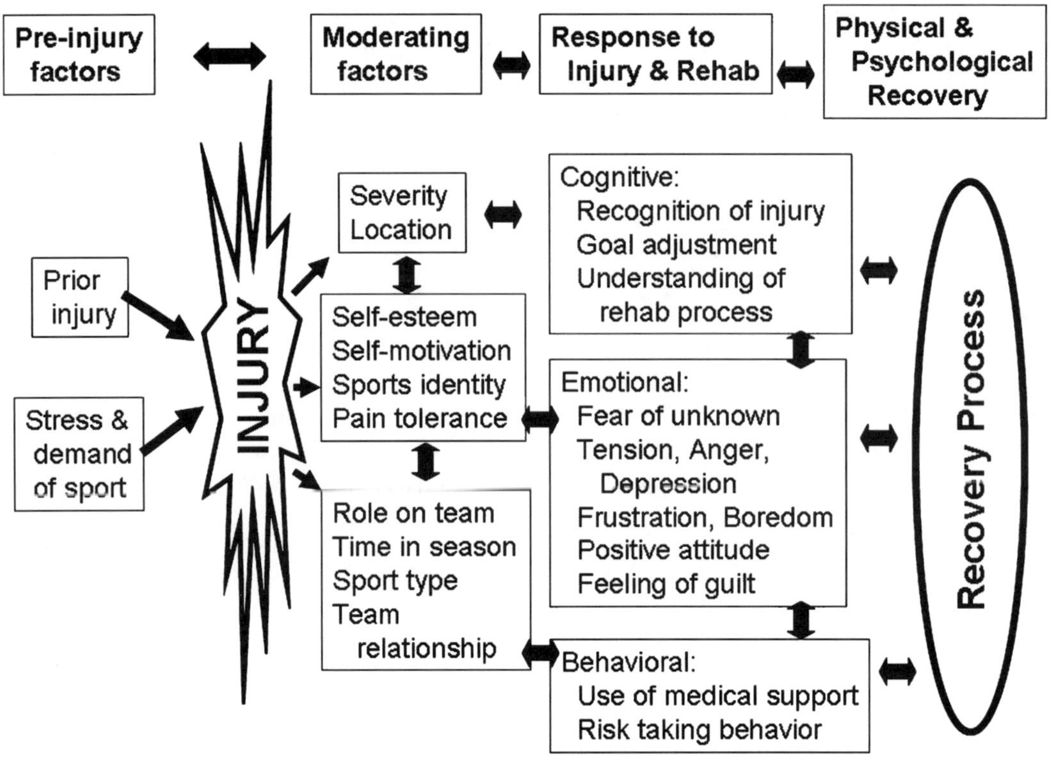

Fig. 1 Deductive analysis results supporting Wiese-Bjornstal et al.'s model

considers cultural and family values, personal values, and environmental constraints. We can agree that the value placed in athletic achievement has increased enormously in the last decades, and the specific values of the team or the family can significantly increase or decrease the stress level of an injured adolescent athlete. The final dimension of the model is *perception*, similar to what is described more commonly in the traditional stress literature. The difference here is that perception is just one of the dimensions, but it is tempered by actual events and objective environment situations. We can now look at the dimensions of the model in the context of vulnerability to injuries (Ford & Gordon, 1999).

Are There Some Athletes Who Are More at Risk of Athletic Injury than Others?

We can start with those who have been injured before and, therefore, are likely to worry more about reexperiencing the losses that accompany injury. This means that some of the cognitive resources are focused away from performance relevant cues, thus increasing the possibility of injury. Consistent with this are the results of Newcomer and Perna (2003), who found that athletes with a recent injury history exhibited a greater frequency of intrusive thoughts and avoidance behavior than did those without a recent injury history. The shift in attentional focus causes disruptions to the automaticity of the movement, changes in pace and rhythm, and even mechanical changes aimed at protecting the previously injured part, but that result in an inappropriate movement pattern. The same can be said of behaviors aimed at avoiding the conditions under which the original injury occurred, that is, a certain play or even competing, or running under specific weather conditions.

Are There Situational Factors that Can Place an Athlete at Risk of Injury?

Team culture that stresses that tolerating pain is not only acceptable but honorable and responding to it a weakness. Shaffer (1997) found that young wrestlers were willing to wrestle with pain and injury if they believed their coaches and/or parents would endorse that behavior and compliment them. The athletes' role on the team whether he is a starter or bench player may also play a role in injury risk. Evidence is mixed in this issue, with some studies showing that starters had higher levels of stress than nonstarters in a football study (Brewer, 2009), while some argue that players who come in from the bench are more likely to "try to prove themselves" and therefore at higher risk of injury. Finally, time in season may play a role (early versus postseason competition and championships). Early in the season, athletes may be forced through a period of double sessions and fitness training in large groups in which peer pressure pushes them beyond where the body would tell them to stop. Later in the season at what are considered "crucial" moments in the season, athletes are more willing to tolerate pain or to ignore warning signs of injury.

Can Individual Factors Play a Role in Predicting Risk of Injury?

Personal motivation and self-confidence clearly play a role in injury risk. There is likely to be an interaction between motivation, self-confidence, and climate of the team. In teams where there is a culture of "toughness," where paying attention to injury signs is considered a weakness, those athletes motivated by the approval of others and those athletes with lower levels of self-confidence are more likely to push themselves and put themselves at higher risk of injury.

Another factor related to injury is how much *being* an athlete is part of *who* the athlete defines they are. Athletic identity may be defined as the degree with which an individual identifies with the athlete role (Brewer, VanRaalte, & Linder, 1993). Vernau (2009) found that athletic identity significantly predicted injury both for males and females recreational basketball players. Griffith and Johnson (2002) found that athletic identity is independent of the level of sports performance, with Division III athletes showing levels of athletic identity as high as those of Division I players. The issue of athletic identity is complex. For those that felt it was a predominant part of who they were, they appeared to have a higher risk of injury; however, athletic identity also leads to a sense of social structure and support. To a limited degree, this may also have a protective effect based on the findings of Brewer (2009) that lack of social support is also one of the individual variables that seem to increase probability of athletic injury.

As we can see, the issue of vulnerability to injuries is a complex one, but integrating the concepts and results cited above, we can suggest the following Do's and Don'ts:

Decreasing vulnerability to injuries

The Do's	The Don'ts
Provide consistent support for the person, not just the athlete	Equate pain or injury with weakness and their tolerance with toughness
Encourage a broader identity	Reward results exclusively
Teach psychological skills, such as tension management, cognitive control, focusing and refocusing strategies	Expect the same from players of varied levels of skill or experience
Provide stress management tools	Ignore changes and pressures during the season

Recovering from Injury

Recovering from injury must extend beyond the physical and physiologic healing of the musculoskeletal injury but also include the whole athlete if the goal is to return them to full competitive play. This recovery will proceed through a series of expected phases and be dependent on the support network and social structure available to the individual athlete. Carrying on from the previous section, we will continue to show the typical responses that individuals experience during injury rehabilitation.

The First 24–48 h

In the 24–48 h following a moderately severe injury (defined as loss of play for 4–6 weeks), attention and help are often given to the individual, and there can be a period of enjoyment because of the assistance and attention received (Tracey, 2003). However, as distance grows from when the injury occurred, individuals experience a range of emotions that are heightened in intensity when the strength of their perceptions of their identity and self-worth are tied directly to their ability to perform. These emotions can range from despair, depression, anger, hostility, frustration, worry, and feeling sorry for oneself.

To mitigate the negative emotional affects that injury can cause. The key personnel involved in the adolescent's life following injury are critical to teaching and enabling them to return to play. At the time of the initial injury, the response of the medical staff is important because the child will read as much as they can from the first responders and who they perceive as the expert in the treatment to gain insight and confidence that the injury can be treated well. Secondly, the parental response is valuable because they can show caring for their child as a whole person without emphasizing the athletic identity to avoid heightening the negative influences of low self-esteem which is likely during injury rehabilitation and increases with long-term severe injuries that require months or longer periods of rehabilitation. Thirdly, coach and teammate responses are very important following an injury to show that the person is valuable to them whether they play or not. The last two points promote the concept that the child is more than a young athlete, they are a person that happens to play youth sports and treating them as more recognizes their whole self. These are positive attributes shown through social support.

Social Support

Social support has been found to be critical for injured athletes learning to cope, manage, and succeed through their injury experience. The sources of social support include medical staff, family, friends, coaches, teammates, and other injured athletes. The perception of the injured person determines the strength of the source of support. Which source means more? This depends on the value that person puts on that source, and it depends on the timing of the support, the manner in which it is shown and the consistency of its influence. This is a major source of self-efficacy and builds confidence through the rehabilitation process.

Tracey (2003) found that the sensory aspects of injury rehabilitation were very important to the growth of optimism and hope. Where movement was seen to improve, swelling and bruising reduced and pain felt to decrease. Positive thoughts and feelings increased and led to recommitment to adhering to the rehabilitation protocol which encouraged increased responsibility for self-care and self-management behaviors.

Educating

The individual should be informed, taught, and educated about their injury and how its optimal rehabilitation. Empowering the person by increasing self-awareness about the injury and instilling confidence by explaining the injury rehabilitation process has been found by Fisher, Domn, and Wuest (1988) and Duda, Smart, and Tappe (1989) to assist athletes tolerate pain and adhere better to rehabilitation protocols. This is important because the first hours of injury are critical to the emotional well-being of the person. When a rehabilitation plan is in place, this leads the use of psychological skills techniques outlined below that support the process and motivate adherence.

Psychological Skills Training

Goal setting has been shown to be influential on keeping energy and focus on adherence to treatment protocols (Evans & Hardy, 2002). Proximal short-term goals that concentrate effort on following the treatment protocol make the person more self-reliant especially when they are educated and trained to perform their own self-care.

Teaching young athletes visualization (imagery) skills and how to apply them to positive treatment and pain control outcomes has been found to be useful strategy to helping athletes cope and focus on the positive aspects of rehabilitation (Morris, Spittle, & Watt, 2005). Teaching imagery skills is linked directly with the sensory perceptions of athletes detailed above and helps to focus energy on productive thinking and future goals.

The following are our suggestions for more effective injury recovery:

The Do's of Injury Recovery

Educate and empower the child within the first 24–48 h after injury.
Promote consistent social support.
Emphasize the personally controllable aspects of the rehabilitation to the individual.
Plan the injury rehabilitation period: ensure that the individual feels in control of the plan.
Set return to proximal goals and monitor the rehabilitation plan.
Focus the possibilities child on future possibilities.

The Don'ts of Injury Recovery

Promote social isolation from family, teammates, and friends.
Emphasize the uncontrollable aspects.
Expect an adolescent to be completely responsible for their own rehabilitation.
Reinforce the loss of athletic performance.

The Psychological Approach to Injury Prevention and Supporting the Whole Young Athlete

Health professionals are encouraged to review the conceptual work and application of long-term athletic development (LTAD) pioneered by Istvan Balyi in Stafford (2005). The LTAD model has been accepted as an optimal way for children and adolescents to be trained in many countries with strong youth sports movements including Canada and the United Kingdom. The LTAD model has a strong science-based framework that concentrates parents, coaches, and medical professionals on the following aspects of child and adolescent growth and development:

Fundamental—basic movement literacy; emphasizes learning to move that include agility, balance, coordination, and speed. Girls 5–8, boys 6–9 years of age.

- Sports skills—building technique; focus on technical development for a given sport. Technical development is considered the primary concern of the child and adolescent. Girls 8–11, boys 9–12 years of age. Competition is still de-emphasized.
- Training to train—building the engine; boys and girls learn to condition themselves aerobically as their bodies manage aspects of physical, mental, and emotional growth and maturation. Competition is part of the environment, but training and improvement is the priority for participation. Girls 11–14, boys 12–15 years of age.
- Training to compete—optimizing the engine; youth sports participants focus on physical and technical conditioning and developing individual performance. The volume of training is high and the competition is low. Girls 14–16, boys 15–18 years of age.
- Training to win—maximizing the engine. This stage is about specializing performance for sport. Girls 16+, boys 18+ years of age.

The purpose of this model is to emphasize general sports preparation that develops into specialized sports performance as children develop. The benefits of this approach include but are not limited to the following:

- Increased enjoyment
- Reduced competitive stress and anxiety
- Fostered positive socialization in sport
- Improved technical ability
- Educated sports participants

These benefits mean that children are likely to be less vulnerable to injury when the focus is on personal growth and improvement and less on competition.

The Do's of Injury Prevention

- Educate the child about the demands and typical injuries associated with the sport.
- Promote personal improvement and growth.
- Encourage coaches and parents to ensure children are trained correctly.
- Emphasize effort goals over competitive goals.
- Refer parents to the best practices for injury prevention and conditioning provided by the National Strength and Conditioning Association and National Association of Athletic Trainers.

The Don'ts of Injury Prevention

- Emphasize competitive comparisons.
- Create unnecessary performance anxiety.
- Permit over training to go unchallenged.
- Use goals that the child has not control over.

In summary, this chapter has used a sports injury model in its approach to musculoskeletal injuries. This has allowed us to look at the incidence of musculoskeletal injuries in this age group, common musculoskeletal injuries in young athletes, as well as risk factors that place these young athletes at risk of injury. Perhaps, more importantly, the chapter has reviewed evidence-based injury prevention techniques regarding musculoskeletal injuries in youth sports. These interventions range from training techniques, early recognition and treatment of problems, and proper equipment, as well as proper coaching and parental feedback. The series of Do's and Don'ts guidelines on vulnerability to injury, injury recovery, and injury prevention can easily be extrapolated to musculoskeletal injuries in children who are not actively participating in sport but would benefit from a holistic approach to injury recovery and healing.

Acknowledgment Special acknowledgement to Neel Pancholi for his contributions to this chapter.

References

Section 1

American Academy of Pediatrics: Committee on Sports Medicine and Fitness. (2000). Injuries in youth soccer: A subjective review. *Pediatrics, 105*(3, pt1), 659–661.

Barss, P., Djerrari, H., Leduc, B. E., Lepage, Y., & Dionne, C. E. (2008). Risk factors and prevention for spinal cord injury from diving in swimming pools and natural sites in Quebec, Canada: A 44-year study. *Accident Analysis and Prevention, 40*(2), 787–797.

Beals, K. A., & Meyer, N. L. (2007). Female athlete triad update. *Clinics in Sports Medicine, 26*(1), 69–89.

Bedi, A., & Ryu, R. K. (2009). The treatment of primary anterior shoulder dislocations. *Instructional Course Lectures, 58*, 293–304.

Benjamin, H. J., & Briner, W. W., Jr. (2005). Little league elbow. *Clinical Journal of Sport Medicine, 15*(1), 37–40.

Bijur, P. E., Trumble, A., Harel, Y., Overpeck, M. D., Jones, D., & Scheidt, P. C. (1995). Sports and recreation injuries in US children and adolescents. *Archives of Pediatrics & Adolescent Medicine, 149*(9), 1009–1016.

Bishop, J. Y., & Flatow, E. L. (2005). Pediatric shoulder trauma. *Clinical Orthopaedics and Related Research, 423*, 41–48.

Brown, R. L., Brunn, M. A., & Garcia, V. F. (2001). Cervical spine injuries in children: A review of 103 patients treated consecutively at a level 1 pediatric trauma center. *Journal of Pediatric Surgery, 36*(8), 1107–1114.

Caine, D. J., & Nassar, L. (2005). Gymnastics injuries. *Medicine and Sport Science, 48*, 18–58.

Chen, L. H., Baker, S. P., Braver, E. R., & Li, G. (2000). Carrying passengers as a risk factor for crashes fatal to 16- and 17-year-old drivers. *Journal of the American Medical Association, 283*(12), 1578–1582.

Chen, F. S., Diaz, V. A., Loebenberg, M., & Rosen, J. E. (2005). Shoulder and elbow injuries in the skeletally immature athlete. *The Journal of the American Academy of Orthopaedic Surgeons, 13*, 172–185.

Cox, D., Vincent, D. G., McGwin, G., MacLennan, P. A., Holmes, J. D., & Rue, L. W., 3rd. (2004). Effect of restraint systems on maxillofacial injury in frontal motor vehicle collisions. *Journal of Oral and Maxillofacial Surgery, 62*(5), 571–575.

Cummins, J. S., Koval, K. J., Cantu, R. V., & Spratt, K. F. (2008). Risk of injury associated with the use of seat belts and air bags in motor vehicle crashes. *Bulletin of the NYU Hospital for Joint Diseases, 66*(4), 290–296.

Deitch, J., Mehlman, C. T., Foad, S. L., Obbehat, A., & Mallory, M. (2003). Traumatic anterior shoulder dislocation in adolescents. *The American Journal of Sports Medicine, 31*(5), 758–763.

Dixon, S., Newton, J., & Teh, J. (2011). Stress fractures in the young athlete: A pictorial review. *Current Problems in Diagnostic Radiology, 40*(1), 29–44.

Eaton, D. K., Kann, L., Kinchen, S., Shanklin, S., Ross, J., et al. (2008). Youth risk behavior surveillance—United States, 2007. *Morbidity and Mortality Weekly Report. Surveillance Summaries, 57*(4), 1–131.

Estrada, L. S., Alonso, J. E., McGwin, G., Jr., Metzger, J., & Rue, L. W., 3rd. (2004). Restraint use and lower extremity fractures in frontal motor vehicle collisions. *The Journal of Trauma, 57*(2), 323–328.

Faigenbaum, A. D., Kraemer, W. J., Blimkie, C. J., Jeffreys, I., Micheli, L. J., Nitka, M., et al. (2009). Youth resistance training: Updated position statement paper from the national strength and conditioning association. *Journal of Strength and Conditioning Research, 23*(5 Suppl), S60–S79.

Fithian, D. C., Paxton, E. W., Stone, M. L., et al. (2004). Epidemiology and natural history of acute patellar dislocation. *The American Journal of Sports Medicine, 32*(5), 1114–1121.

Graf, B. K., Lange, R. H., Fujisaki, C. K., Landry, G. L., & Saluja, R. K. (1992). Anterior cruciate ligament tears in skeletally immature patients: Meniscal pathology at presentation and after attempted conservative treatment. *Arthroscopy, 8*(2), 229–233.

Harrast, M. A., & Colonno, D. (2010). Stress fractures in runners. *Clinics in Sports Medicine, 29*(3), 399–416.

Hinton, R. Y., & Sharma, K. M. (2003). Acute and recurrent patellar instability in the young athlete. *The Orthopedic Clinics of North America, 34*(3), 385–396.

Hoch, A. Z., Pajewski, N. M., Moraski, L., Carrera, G. F., Wilson, C. R., Hoffmann, R. G., et al. (2009). Prevalence of the female athlete triad in high school athletes and sedentary students. *Clinical Journal of Sport Medicine, 19*(5), 421–428.

Jones, S. E., & Shults, R. A. (2009). Trends and subgroup differences in transportation-related injury risk and safety behaviors among US high school students, 1991–2007. *The Journal of School Health, 79*, 169–176.

Kakefuda, I., Henry, K. L., & Stallones, L. (2009). Associations between childhood bicycle helmet use, current use, and family and community factors among college students. *Family & Community Health, 32*(2), 159–166.

Kocher, M. S., Micheli, L. J., Gerbino, P., & Hresko, M. T. (2003). Tibial eminence fractures in children: Prevalence of meniscal entrapment. *The American Journal of Sports Medicine, 31*(3), 404–407.

Kocher, M. S., Saxon, H. S., Hovis, W. D., & Hawkins, R. J. (2002). Management and complications of anterior cruciate ligament injuries in skeletally immature patients: Survey of Herodicus Society and The ACL Study Group. *Journal of Pediatric Orthopedics, 22*(4), 452–457.

Kocher, M. S., Smith, J. T., Zoric, B. J., Lee, B., & Micheli, L. J. (2007). Transphyseal anterior cruciate ligament reconstruction in skeletally immature pubescent adolescents. *The Journal of Bone and Joint Surgery. American Volume, 89*(12), 2632–2639.

Korres, D. S., Benetos, I. S., Themistocleous, G. S., Mavrogenis, A. F., Nikolakakos, L., & Liantis, P. T. (2006). Diving injuries of the cervical spine in amateur divers. *The Spine Journal, 6*(1), 44–49.

Krauss, M. D. (2004). Equipment innovations and rules changes in sports. *Current Sports Medicine Reports, 3*(5), 27.

Liller, K. D., Morissette, B., Noland, V., & McDermott, R. J. (1998). Middle school students and bicycle helmet use: Knowledge, attitudes, beliefs, and behaviors. *The Journal of School Health, 68*, 325–338.

Malina, R. M. (2006). Weight training in youth-growth, maturation, and safety: An evidence-based review. *Clinical Journal of Sport Medicine, 16*(6), 478–487.

McCarroll, J. R., Shelbourne, K. D., Porter, D. A., Rettig, A. C., & Murray, S. (1994). Patellar tendon graft reconstruction for mid-substance anterior cruciate ligament rupture in junior high school athletes: An algorithm for management. *The American Journal of Sports Medicine, 22*(4), 478–484.

McMahon, P., Grossman, W., Gaffney, M., & Stanitski, C. (1995). Soft-tissue injury as an indication of child abuse. *The Journal of Bone and Joint Surgery. American Volume, 77*, 1179–1183.

Meyers, M. H., & McKeever, F. M. (1987). Fractures of the intercondylar eminence of the tibia. *The Journal of Bone and Joint Surgery. American Volume, 52*(8), 1677–1684.

Monto, R. R., Cameron-Donaldson, M. L., Close, M. A., Ho, C. P., & Hawkins, R. J. (2006). Magnetic resonance imaging in the evaluation of tibial eminence fractures in adults. *The Journal of Knee Surgery, 19*(3), 187–190.

National Spinal Cord Injury Statistical Center. (2006). *Facts and figures at a glance*. Birmingham: University of Alabama.

NFL moves kickoffs to 35-yard line; touchbacks unchanged. (2011) NFL.com. 2011-03-22. Retrieved May 23, 2011. http://www.nfl.com/news/story/09000d5d81ee38c1/article/.

Otis, C. L., Drinkwater, B., Johnson, M., et al. (1997). American college of sports medicine position stand: The female athlete triad: Disordered eating, amenorrhea, and osteoporosis. *Medicine and Science in Sports and Exercise, 29*(5), i–ix.

Palmu, S., Kallio, P. E., Donell, S. T., Helenius, I., & Nietosvaara, Y. (2008). Acute patellar dislocation in children and adolescents: A randomized clinical trial. *The Journal of Bone and Joint Surgery. American Volume, 90*(3), 463–470.

Quinlan, K. P., Brewer, R. D., Sleet, D. A., & Dellinger, A. M. (2000). Characteristics of child passenger deaths and injuries involving drinking drivers. *Journal of the American Medical Association, 283*(17), 2249–2252.

Rihn, J. A., Anderson, D. T., Lamb, K., Deluca, P. F., Bata, A., Marchetto, P. A., et al. (2009). Cervical spine injuries in American football. *Sports Medicine, 39*(9), 697–708.

Risser, W. L., Risser, J. M. H., & Preston, D. (1990). Weight-training injuries in adolescents. *American Journal of Diseases of Children, 144*(9), 1015–1017.

Rowe, C. R. (1956). Prognosis in dislocations of the shoulder. *The Journal of Bone and Joint Surgery. American Volume, 38*(5), 957–977.

Shea, K. G., Pfeiffer, R., Wang, J. H., Curtin, M., & Apel, P. J. (2004). Anterior cruciate ligament injury in pediatric and adolescent soccer players: An analysis of insurance data. *Journal of Pediatric Orthopedics, 24*(6), 623–628.

Simonet, W. T., & Sim, L. (1995). Boot-top tendon lacerations in ice hockey. *The Journal of Trauma, 38*(1), 30–31.

Sink, E. L., Hyman, J. E., Matheny, T., Georgopoulos, G., & Kleinman, P. (2011). Child abuse: The role of the orthopaedic surgeon in nonaccidental trauma. *Clinical Orthopaedics and Related Research, 469*(3), 790–797.

Sleet, D. A., Ballesteros, M. F., & Borse, N. N. (2010). A review of unintentional injuries in adolescents. *Annual Review of Public Health, 31*, 195–212.

Tator, C. H., Provvidenza, C., & Cassidy, J. D. (2009). Spinal injuries in Canadian ice hockey: An update to 2005. *Clinical Journal of Sport Medicine, 19*(6), 451–456.

Washington, R. L., Bernhardt, D. T., Gomez, J., et al. (2001). Organized sports for children and preadolescents. *Pediatrics, 107*, 1459–1462.

Watson, R. C., Singer, C. D., & Sproule, J. R. (1996). Checking from behind in ice hockey: A study of injury and penalty data in the Ontario University Athletic Association Hockey League. *Clinical Journal of Sport Medicine, 6*(2), 108–111.

Section 2

Brewer, B. W. (2009). *Sport psychology*. Oxford, UK: Wiley-Blackwell. doi:10.1002/9781444303650.

Brewer, B. W., VanRaalte, J. L., & Linder, D. E. (1993). Athletic identity: Hercules' muscles or Achilles heel? *International Journal of Sport Psychology, 24*, 237–254.

Duda, J., Smart, A., & Tappe, M. (1989). Predictors of adherence in the rehabilitation of athletic injuries: An application of personal investment theory. *Journal of Sport & Exercise Psychology, 11*, 367–381.

Evans, L. & Hardy, L. (2002). Injury rehabilitation: A goal setting intervention study. *Research Quarterly for Exercise and Sport, 73*(3), 310–319.

Fisher, A., Domn, M., & Wuest, D. (1988). Adherence to sports-injury rehabilitation programs. *The Physician and Sportsmedicine, 16*, 47–52.

Ford, U., & Gordon, S. (1999). Coping with sport injury: Resource loss and the role of social support. *Journal of Personal and Interpersonal Loss, 4*(3), 243–256.

Griffith, K., Johnson, C. (2002). Athletic identity and life roles of Division I and Division III collegiate athletes. *Journal of Undergraduate Research*, University of Wisconsin-La Crosse. Digital journal, http://murphylibrary.uwlax.edu/digital/jur/2002/griffith-johnson.pdf.

Hobfoll, S. E. (1988). *The ecology of stress*. Washington, D.C: Hemisphere.

Lazarus, R. S., & Folkman, S. (1984). *Stress, appraisal and coping*. New York, NY: Springer.

Morris, T., Spittle, M., & Watt, A. (2005). *Imagery in sport*. Champaign, IL: Human Kinetics Publishers.

Newcomer, R. R., & Perna, F. M. (2003). Features of posttraumatic distress among adolescent athletes. *Journal of Athletic Training, 8*(2), 163–166.

Shaffer, S. M. (1997). *Grappling with injury: What motivates young athletes to wrestle with pain*? ProQuest Information & Learning.

Stafford, I. (2005). *Coaching for long-term athlete development: To improve participation and performance in sport*. Leeds, England: Sports Coach UK.

Tracey, J. (2003). The emotional response to the injury and rehabilitation process. *Journal of Applied Sport Psychology, 15*, 279–293.

Vernau, D. P. (2009). *Gender, athletic identity, and playing through pain and injury in recreational basketball players*. Unpublished Doctoral Dissertation. Miami University.

Wiese-Bjornstal, D. M., Smith, A. M., LaMott, E. E. (1995). A model of psychological response to athletic injury and rehabilitation. *Athletic Training: Sports Health Care Perspectives, 1*(1), 17–30. Retrieved, from https://www.sportcentric.com/vsite/vfile/page/fileurl/0,11040,5157-184732-201954-124688-0-file,00.pdf, Amateur Swimming Association Technical Swimming Committee (2004).

Headache in Adolescence

Emily F. Law, Amy S. Lewandowski, and Gary A. Walco

Introduction

Headache is the most frequently reported recurrent pain problem among children and adolescents (Perquin et al., 2000). Epidemiological studies indicate that 26.2–31.8 % of youth ages 12–19 years report weekly head pain (Stanford, Chambers, Biesanz, & Chen, 2008). Migraine and tension-type headache (TTH) are the primary headache disorders experienced by adolescents, with 1-year prevalence being 7 % and 18 %, respectively (Zwart, Dyb, Holmen, Stovner, & Sand, 2004). During adolescence, headache can have a significant negative impact on physical and socioemotional functioning and is associated with poor quality of life, activity limitations, and poor school outcomes (Carlsson, Larsson, & Mark, 1996; Fichtel & Larsson, 2002; Powers, Patton, Hommel, & Hershey, 2004).

This chapter describes common headache disorders experienced by adolescents with a focus on migraine (with and without aura) and TTH. Information on diagnostic criteria and factors associated with headache etiology, physical symptoms, and impact of headache on physical and socioemotional functioning during adolescence are also presented. The conclusion of this chapter focuses on clinical assessment; pharmacological, psychological, lifestyle change; and physical approaches to headache treatment.

Headache Definitions and Subtypes

The International Classification of Headache Disorders (ICHD) criteria are used for headache diagnosis both in clinical and research settings. These criteria classify headache as either primary or secondary, with "primary headache" referring to headaches not associated with an underlying medical condition and "secondary headache" indicating the presence of a comorbid injury, disease, or disorder (e.g., brain tumor, head trauma). The ICHD criteria were updated in 2004, with a principal focus being to improve the validity of headache diagnosis in pediatric populations (International Classification of Headache Disorders (ICHD-2), 2004). The revisions include modified criteria for youth age 15 years and younger, particularly the frequency and duration of headache episodes.

E.F. Law, Ph.D. (✉)
Center for Child Health, Behavior and Development, Seattle Children's Research Institute, M/S CW8-6, P.O. Box 5371, Seattle, WA 98145, USA
e-mail: emily.law@seattlechildrens.org

A.S. Lewandowski, Ph.D. • G.A. Walco, Ph.D.
Department of Anesthesiology and Pain Medicine, Seattle Children's Hospital, University of Washington School of Medicine, M/SW-9824, P.O. Box 5371, Seattle, WA 98145, USA
e-mail: amy.lewandowski@seattlechildrens.org; gary.walco@seattlechildrens.org

W.T. O'Donohue et al. (eds.), *Handbook of Adolescent Health Psychology*,
DOI 10.1007/978-1-4614-6633-8_43, © Springer Science+Business Media New York 2013

Migraine

Migraine headaches are characterized by episodes of head pain accompanied by nausea, vomiting, photophobia (light sensitivity), and/or phonophobia (sensitivity to sound). These headaches include moderate or severe pain with a "pulsating quality" that is often aggravated by activity (ICHD-2, 2004). While often debilitating, by definition, migraine headaches alternate with pain-free periods. Many adolescents with migraine function normally during pain-free periods, attending school and participating in usual social and athletic activities with their peers.

Pediatric migraine is typically classified into two categories: migraine without aura and migraine with aura (ICHD-2, 2004). The term "aura" describes the addition of positive or negative visual symptoms (e.g., flickering lights, appearance of spots, reduced visual field), sensory symptoms (e.g., pins and needles sensation, numbness), or speech disturbance that precedes or develops in conjunction with headache pain. Auras last from a few minutes up to an hour and are fully reversible, meaning that symptoms are exclusive to migraine episodes alone. In adolescents, the majority of migraine episodes (approximately 65–80 %) occur without aura (Silberstein, Stiles, & Young, 2005). Diagnostic criteria also specify that pediatric migraines last between 1 and 48 h, and to receive the diagnosis of a migraine, adolescents must report having had five migraine attacks that are not attributed to another medical cause (ICHD-2, 2004). In contrast to diagnostic criteria for adults, pediatric migraine can be either unilateral or bilateral, with bilateral migraines common in youth.

Prevalence of migraine during adolescence varies by age and gender. Before puberty, migraines are more common in males than females, while after puberty, females are more commonly affected (Lipton et al., 2002). One study reported the 1-year prevalence of migraine was 5.0 % in boys and 7.7 % in girls, with more girls than boys affected after the age of 12 years (Bigal et al., 2007). Migraine prevalence increases during childhood and early adulthood, with the fastest rate of change occurring from age 3 years to the mid-20s (Victor, Hu, Campbell, Buse, & Lipton, 2010).

Children and adolescents with migraines commonly have an affected family member, with one study reporting that 65.8 % of children (ages 5–13 years) have a positive family history of migraine (Lee & Olness, 1997). In a 10-year longitudinal study of adolescents with migraine, a family history of migraines was associated with persistent migraine (Monastero, Camarda, Pipia, & Camarda, 2006). Genetic studies have shown a fourfold increased risk in relatives of people who have migraine with aura (Kors, Haan, & Ferrari, 1999). Other studies have looked at environmental and social factors associated with migraine onset. In a study of school children and early adolescents, first onset of migraine was associated with the timing of examinations (46.5 %) and was triggered by use of a computer (45.9 %), a loud noise (41.5 %), or a hot climate (37.1 %)(Bener et al., 2000).

Tension-Type Headache

TTH is the most common type of headache experienced by adolescents (Zwart et al., 2004). Like migraines, tension headaches are more common in females than males after puberty (Fillingim, King, Ribeiro-Dasilva, Rahim-Williams, & Riley, 2009). TTH is characterized by mild to moderate band-like pain or pressure that lasts from a half hour to several days. Tension headaches typically have a gradual pain onset and occur in the middle of the day. ICHD-2 criteria classifies TTH as one of three subtypes: infrequent (a minimum of 10 episodes of less than 1 day per month, averaging 12 headaches per year), frequent (a minimum of 10 episodes lasting 1–15 days per month for 3 months or less), and chronic (greater than 15 days per month for more than 3 months) (ICHD-2, 2004). In both frequent and infrequent tension headaches, duration may last 30 min to 7 days; for chronic tension headaches, length can be over several hours or be continuous. In all TTH subtypes, the headache must be bilateral, range in intensity from mild to moderate pain, and not be exaggerated by activity or accompanied by nausea or vomiting (ICHD-2, 2004).

TTH does not have a single etiological basis, and onset is thought to be associated with multiple factors, including muscle contraction in response to stress. Adolescents who report higher stress are at increased risk of TTH (Battistutta, Aliverti, Montico, Zin, & Carrozzi, 2009; Bruni et al., 1997). TTH is also associated with tightness in muscles in the back of the neck and scalp and may be exacerbated by poor posture. In contrast to migraine, hereditary factors have not been identified as playing a role in the pathogenesis of tension-type headaches.

Chronic Daily Headache

The term chronic daily headache (CDH) is used to describe a headache that persists for at least 15 days per month over a 3-month period (ICHD-2, 2004). Chronic daily headaches typically transform from other types of headache (e.g., episodic migraine, tension-type), with presence of headache during childhood or adolescence implicated in the development of CDH in adulthood (Spierings, Schroevers, Honkoop, & Sorbi, 1998). In terms of prevalence, 1–2 % of adolescents meet criteria for CDH, with the most common type being chronic TTH (Wang, Fuh, Lu, & Juang, 2006). Chronic daily headache is often viewed as the most disabling headache diagnosis due to the persistence of headache over time. Compared to adolescents with other headache diagnoses, those with chronic daily headache may report the most psychological symptoms and the poorest functioning due to the duration of pain. For example, studies have shown that children and adolescents with chronic daily headache frequently have sleep disturbance, school absences, and psychiatric comorbidity including anxiety and other mood disorders (Galli et al., 2004; Wang, Juang, Fuh, & Lu, 2007; Wiendels, van der Geest, Neven, Ferrari, & Laan, 2005).

Like other headache diagnoses, adolescents with CDH show differences by age and gender during childhood and adolescence. One study reporting the characteristics of a sample of youth with CDH found that the majority were female (61.8 %), with 10.5 years (SD = 3.1 years) being the average age at time of diagnosis (Cuvellier, Couttenier, Joriot-Chekaf, & Vallee, 2008). Studies examining risk factors associated with CDH have identified social stressors, psychological factors, and medication overuse as associated with pain reports and maintenance of symptoms. Wang and colleagues (Wang, Fuh, Lu, & Juang, 2007) followed youth with CDH for 2 years and found that the majority of adolescents continued to have frequent headaches at follow-up. In this study, independent predictors for CDH persistence were medication overuse and major depression. Other studies have also identified medication use as a factor. A study of adolescents with CHD found that youth who used analgesic medication greater three times per week were at risk for developing headaches secondary to the medication itself (Wang et al., 2006). In another study of youth with CDH, 82 % of the sample endorsed having associated stressors, with 52 % of youth also reporting frequent use of medication (Cuvellier et al., 2008).

Individual Difference Factors Related to Adolescent Headache

Specific etiological factors underlying headache have been difficult to ascertain. Certainly, a division has been espoused between those factors that are associated with migraine versus tension-type or chronic daily headaches, but in both instances, the role of central sensitization is becoming increasingly recognized. As described by Silberstein (2011), migraine headaches appear to arise from activation of nociceptors in the meninges and blood vessels. Stimulation of the trigeminal system leads to C-fiber-mediated release of substance P and calcitonin gene-related peptide (GCRP) as well as neurogenic inflammation. The latter causes peripheral sensitization of nerve fibers so that there is now a pain response to previously innocuous stimuli, such as blood vessel pulsations.

Formerly it was believed the contraction of the muscles in the neck and shoulders was the major nociceptive stimulus for tension-type headaches. Although myofascial elements, including pericranial tenderness and trigger point stimulation, remain a focus in current models, their specific roles and interplay with central elements are still being defined (Monteith & Sprenger, 2010). For example, there is evidence that bradykinin, serotonin, and substance P are released by nociceptive nerve endings in these processes. However, Fernandez-de-las-Penas, Cuadrado, Arendt-Nielsen, Simons, and Pareja (2007) go on to emphasize the significant interplay between peripheral and central pain mechanisms, concluding that the prolonged nociceptive input from muscle trigger points may lead to sensitization of nociceptive second-order neurons at the dorsal, cervical, and trigeminal levels. It is these central sensitization mechanisms that are thought to form the close links between headache, sleep problems, and psychiatric comorbidities. A review of this material is beyond the scope of this chapter (for more details, see de Tommaso et al., 2008; Woolf, 2011).

Psychological Factors

Depression and anxiety are widely recognized as correlates of headache in adolescents. Epidemiological data indicate that headache is twice as common among youth with major depressive disorder compared to youth who do not have major depression (Pine, Cohen, & Brook, 1996). Clinic-based studies indicate that 17–86 % of adolescents with headache report at least some symptoms of depression (Anttila et al., 2002; Kaiser, 1992). In a study of 123 clinic-referred youth with chronic daily headache, 9 % of the sample met diagnostic criteria for major depression (Seshia, 2004). Compared to their healthy peers, youth with headache typically report elevated symptoms of depression (Andrasik et al., 1988; Anttila et al., 2004; Martin-Herz, Smith, & McMahon, 1999; Mazzone, Vitiello, Incorpora, & Mazzone, 2006); however, rates of depressive symptoms in both the headache and non-headache groups typically fall within the normal range. These findings indicate that while youth with headache may have more depressive symptoms than their healthy peers, they are not more likely to meet diagnostic criteria for a depressive disorder.

Anxiety is also commonly reported by adolescents with headache. Epidemiological studies of nonclinical samples indicate greater anxiety symptoms among adolescents with frequent headaches compared to youth who have infrequent or no headache (Martin-Herz et al., 1999). Several studies have indicated that adolescents with migraine report greater anxiety symptoms than their healthy peers (Andrasik et al., 1988; Mazzone et al., 2006; Smith, Martin-Herz, Womack, & McMahon, 1999); however, anxiety symptoms were within the normal range for both the headache and non-headache groups in these studies. Several authors have proposed that the relation between anxiety and headache may be related to stress (Bjorling, 2009; Powers, Gilman, & Hershey, 2006; Seshia, Phillips, & von Baeyer, 2008). Youth with headache report higher levels of stress than their healthy peers (Carlsson et al., 1996) and often identify stress as a factor that precedes headache onset (Bjorling, 2009; Seshia et al., 2008). These findings suggest that youth with headache may have more difficulty coping with stress and anxiety than youth without headache or, at least at a minimum, that stressors have a negative impact on pain modulation networks and induce increased muscle tension.

Longitudinal studies have shown that anxiety and depressive symptoms are associated with headache persistence during adolescence (Stanford et al., 2008) and that children with headache have an increased risk of headache and psychiatric symptoms in adulthood (Fearon & Hotopf, 2001). The mechanisms underlying interrelations among depression, anxiety, and headache in adolescents are not well understood. For example, it is not clear whether psychiatric symptoms precede the onset of headache, if headache increases risk for psychiatric symptoms, or if this relationship is bidirectional. Prospective research is needed to evaluate the course and associations of depression, anxiety, and headache in childhood and adolescence.

Family Factors

Research has shown reciprocal influences between headache symptoms and family factors such as family functioning and family conflict during childhood and adolescence. Compromised family functioning and more family problems have been reported among children with headache (ages 8–9 years) compared to healthy controls (Anttila, Metsahonkala, Helenius, & Sillanpaa, 2000). Family conflict has been associated with higher reports of pain and headache-related disability among children and adolescents, and frequent quarreling was reported to increase the occurrence of weekly and monthly head pain (Kroner-Herwig, Heinrich, & Morris, 2007). In contrast, a positive family environment may be a protective factor for youth with headache. In a study of adolescents with recurrent headache, Palermo and colleagues (Palermo, Putnam, Armstrong, & Daily, 2007) found that adolescents with healthy family functioning had lower levels of depression, less functional impairment, and lower pain frequency and intensity compared to adolescents with unhealthy family functioning. While these studies do not suggest that family factors cause headache onset or associated disability, they indicate that family stress may be an important environmental trigger that should be assessed by clinicians working with these youth.

Lifestyle Factors

Sleep

Poor sleep is a common trigger of headache onset, as well as a consequence of headache pain. In a nonclinical sample of youth (age 8–15 years) with headache, Bruni et al. (2008) reported that poor sleep was the most frequent trigger of migraine and non-migraine headaches. Pain can also make it difficult for children and adolescents to fall asleep and stay asleep, with studies indicating that youth with headaches have difficulties falling asleep, with night awakenings, and daytime sleepiness. In one study of adolescents with head pain (90 % migraine; 10 % TTH), rates of self-reported sleep problems were striking, such that 65.7 % reported insufficient total sleep, 23.3 % daytime sleepiness, 40.6 % difficulty falling asleep, and 38 % night wakings (Gilman, Palermo, Kabbouche, Hershey, & Powers, 2007). This study also revealed significant relationships between headache characteristics and teen sleep behaviors, with poor sleep associated with greater headache frequency and intensity (Gilman et al., 2007). Headache during adolescence has also been associated with sleep disorders. Parasomnias and bedtime resistance have been linked to frequency and duration of migraines in children (Miller, Palermo, Powers, Scher, & Hershey, 2003). A thorough sleep assessment should be included in evaluations of adolescents with headache.

Diet

Research indicating that dietary factors precipitate headache in adolescents is mixed. In self-report studies, foods (e.g., processed meats, cheese, chocolate, citrus fruits), beverages (caffeinated drinks, alcohol), and additives (monosodium glutamate, aspartame) have been identified as triggering headache onset or worsening headache symptoms in both children and adults (for a review, see Millichap & Yee, 2003). It is hypothesized that foods and additives trigger headaches by impacting serotonin and norepinephrine levels which can subsequently lead to vasoconstriction, vasodilatation, or stimulation of other parts of the brain (e.g., brainstem, cortical neuronal pathways; see Millichap & Yee, 2003). While this theory is plausible, clinical research supporting the triggering effect of foods in pediatric populations is relatively small. Available research suggests that dietary factors have a more consistent impact on migraine compared to other headaches in youth (Karli, Akgoz, Zarifoglu, Akis, & Erer, 2006; Milde-Busch et al., 2010). Dietary triggers may be confounded by other factors including timing of meals and the combination of foods consumed together. For example, an adolescent who eats lunch late in the day may experience a headache due to delayed intake rather than the food itself. Beliefs about the associations between headache pain onset and certain food triggers may also confound the data. An adolescent may attribute their headache to a food they consumed rather than other predictive factors such as stress or muscle tension.

Other Health Behaviors

Other health behaviors, including physical activity and smoking, have been associated with adolescent headache. For example, one study of 10th and 11th graders found that physical inactivity, smoking, and high consumption of coffee and alcoholic drinks were associated with migraine and TTH, with physical inactivity alone associated with TTH (Milde-Busch et al., 2010). While inactivity has been associated with presence of headaches, excessive physical activity has also been identified as a trigger of headache, particularly migraine (Kelman, 2007).

Overweight or obese weight status has also been associated with headache morbidity in children and adolescents. In a longitudinal study of youth (ages 3–19 years, mean age 11.9 years) recruited from headache clinics, body mass index (BMI) was correlated with headache frequency and disability (Hershey et al., 2009). Change in BMI was associated with change in headache frequency at 3- and 6-month follow-ups such that reduction in BMI was associated with a reduction in headaches over time (Hershey et al., 2009). Studies have also examined headache prevalence in youth with multiple health-risk factors. In one large epidemiological study of Norwegian youth ages 13–18 years, 55 % of overweight, sedentary teens who smoked reported recent frequent headaches in comparison to 25 % of teens who did not report these health-risk behaviors (Robberstad et al., 2010). While these data indicate that health-risk behaviors are associated with headache in adolescence, it is not clear if these factors are a response to the headache and associated pain or if they are headache triggers in vulnerable teens. Longitudinal studies examining health behaviors in adolescents with headache are needed to answer this question.

Assessment

Accurate assessment of headache is critical for diagnosis and treatment. Evaluating a child who presents with headaches should not be targeted exclusively at identifying underlying organic pathology but should also look at additional factors that could be precipitating or intensifying pain symptoms (Palermo & von Baeyer, 2008). Headache assessment is often initially conducted by a pediatrician with a follow-up from a multidisciplinary team including neurologists and psychologists as indicated. Evaluation should begin with a thorough pain and medical history, psychiatric history, developmental history, and physical examination. Differential diagnosis is important for ruling out other medical conditions or presence of pathology (e.g., hypertension, deviations in cranial pressure, neoplasms) (Lewis, 2002). A comprehensive physical examination may also include an assessment of response to tender point stimulation, tenderness, and tension in the musculature of the neck, shoulders, and upper back. Given the psychosocial factors shown to be associated with headaches in adolescents, assessment should include questions about academic performance and cognitive functioning, coping style, and perceived stressors. Clinicians should also inquire about impact of headache pain across multiple settings including school, home, work, and the adolescent's social environment. Because there is some research that indicates headache onset may be triggered by dietary factors, it is important for these to be evaluated during the interview.

Headache diaries are often useful for tracking both the frequency and intensity of headache pain, as well as associated triggers, symptoms, and effectiveness of medications or strategies that the adolescent uses for pain relief. In addition, a variety of reliable and valid measures are available to assess headache-related disability in adolescents. The Pediatric Migraine Disability Scale (PedMIDAS) is a tool initially developed for adults that has recently been validated for use with children and adolescents aged 4–18 years (Hershey, Powers, Bentti, LeCates, & deGrauw, 2001). The questionnaire is a self-report measure completed by the patient or his or her parent regarding the impact of headache on school performance, headache-related disability at home, and limitations in social, athletic, and physical activities. Results provide a measure of headache-related disability ranging from "little to none" to "severe."

The PedsQL™ (Pediatric Quality of Life Inventory™) is another measure for assessing impact of headache on the quality of life of children and adolescents (Connelly & Rapoff, 2006). The measure is completed by children who report on their physical, emotional, social, and school functioning. Data can be examined as a total score or psychosocial and physical health summary scores. Current data show that the measure is valid for children and preadolescents with headache aged 7–12 years (Connelly & Rapoff, 2006). Other studies have used the measure and demonstrated that it is reliable for adolescents, but no specific validation studies have been conducted.

Pharmacologic Treatment

There have been many attempts to identify the specific mechanisms underlying migraine headaches, but the specific elements remain unclear. Although it is evident that certain neurotransmitters, such as serotonin, are central to the process, the debate wages on as to whether there are vascular or inflammatory elements operating. As summarized by Lewis (2010), it appears that there is an initial electrical phenomenon that begins in the cerebrum, triggering a cascade of events that impact the vasculature, releasing biochemical substances, which then lead to neurogenic inflammation. Thus, medications used to treat migraine have targeted one or more of these processes in order to prevent the characteristically episodic migraine pain (prophylactic medications) or treat symptoms once they occur (rescue medications). Although a comprehensive review of specific medications and their targets is beyond the scope of this chapter, a general overview will be provided. For more details the reader is referred to two reviews on the topic (Lewis, 2010; Sethna & LeBel, 2008).

With the premise that inflammation plays an important role in the cascade of events producing migraine headaches, medications that inhibit prostaglandin production, thereby reducing inflammation, should be front line. Thus, for mild to moderate pain, nonsteroidal anti-inflammatory drugs (NSAIDs), including over-the-counter preparations such as ibuprofen, naproxen, or acetaminophen, are often used, as well as prescribed NSAIDs, such as indomethacin and ketorolac (Waeber & Moskowitz, 2005). The second element, vasoconstriction, has been addressed with ergotamines (e.g., nasal dihydroergotamine; DHE) (Tfelt-Hansen & Koehler, 2008). Finally, triptans are being used with increasing frequency, which act on serotonin receptors, leading to decreases in neuropeptides, including substance P (Eiland & Hunt, 2010). These medications may be administered through multiple routes, such as orally (including rapidly disintegrating tablets), nasally, and subcutaneously. Most recently, a combination product of sumatriptan and naproxen has been released. Most of these medications have been studied minimally for specific use in children and adolescents, and while many have shown positive therapeutic benefit, each presents with its own array of side effects and idiosyncratic responses in individual patients. Finally, the phenomenon of "rebound headache," which can occur in the wake of frequent and excessive use of analgesics, triptans, and ergots, is of concern.

Prophylactic medications are intended to prevent headaches before they occur, a strategy that is especially useful for chronic daily headaches. Although operating through diverse mechanisms, the typical strategy involves relatively low doses and then titrating up to achieve clinical effect. Antidepressants, traditionally tricyclics (e.g., amitriptyline) and more recently selective serotonin and norepinephrine reuptake inhibitors (SSNRI, e.g., duloxetine), are employed, principally affecting the role of neuropeptides in the chain (Smitherman, Walters, Maizels, & Penzien, 2010). Beta blockers (e.g., propranolol), calcium channel blockers (e.g., verapamil), and anticonvulsants (e.g., topiramate, valproic acid) are also prescribed (Sethna & LeBel, 2008). Finally, partly to address allergies that may be impacting headaches, antihistamines may be used.

Psychological Treatment

Psychological interventions for pediatric headache can include self-regulatory strategies (e.g., relaxation training, self-hypnosis), biofeedback, cognitive strategies, and parent training in operant techniques. Training in self-regulatory strategies involves instruction in relaxation skills such as progressive muscle relaxation, guided imagery, autogenic training, and self-hypnosis. Several meta-analytic reviews have indicated that these psychological treatments are effective in reducing pain in adolescents with headache and that the benefits of these treatments appear to be maintained over time (Eccleston, Palermo, Williams, Lewandowski, & Morley, 2009; Hermann, Kim, & Blanchard, 1995; Trautmann, Lackschewitz, & Kroner-Herwig, 2006). Progressive muscle relaxation involves giving instructions to notice the feeling of tension in the muscles and then to release the tension and notice the relaxation in the muscle group. Progressive muscle relaxation is often combined with guided imagery, which involves describing images of relaxing situations as well as suggestions of relaxation and warmth. Autogenic training consists of suggestions of heaviness and warmth and positioning of the body to promote relaxation. Self-hypnosis typically involves a blend of progressive muscle relaxation techniques and guided imagery to achieve a sense of deep relaxation.

Relaxation training has been classified as a well-established and efficacious treatment for pediatric migraine and tension headache (Holden, Deichmann, & Levy, 1999). In this meta-analysis, Holden et al. (1999) included 11 studies that evaluated some form of relaxation training (i.e., deep breathing, progressive muscle relaxation, guided imagery, autogenic training, and/or self-hypnosis) for recurrent headaches. Results indicated that relaxation therapies are superior to self-monitoring and wait-list control conditions and that treatment gains are generally maintained over time. Relaxation training has been delivered in clinic-, home-, and school-based settings. Research indicates that relaxation training delivered to adolescents with headache at school resulted in significant reductions in headache activity immediately posttreatment and at 6–10-month follow-up (Larsson, Carlsson, Fichtel, & Melin, 2005). Beneficial effects have also been achieved via relaxation training programs that are administered by school nurses, which indicates that the school setting may be an ideal venue to reach large numbers of youth with headache pain (Larsson et al., 2005; Larsson & Carlsson, 1996).

Biofeedback is among the most widely studied treatments for pediatric headache (Eccleston et al., 2009). Biofeedback involves monitoring and providing feedback about physiological processes that are usually not thought to be under voluntary control. Electromyographic (EMG) and thermal biofeedback have been studied in the treatment of pediatric headache. EMG biofeedback for headache consists of monitoring auditory and/or visual signals generated by electrical signals in the frontalis muscles. Thermal biofeedback typically involves monitoring temperature changes in a thermistor placed on the fingers. Patients are taught self-control of the electrical signals (in EMG biofeedback) or skin temperature (in thermal biofeedback), typically in conjunction with relaxation techniques. Thermal biofeedback with autogenic training has received the most attention in the pediatric headache literature (Hermann & Blanchard, 2002).

Biofeedback alone has been classified as a "probably efficacious" treatment for pediatric headache (Holden et al., 1999). In their meta-analysis, Holden et al. (1999) reported that combined biofeedback and relaxation training results in significant improvement in headache with gains maintained up to 1 year posttreatment. A more recent review by Hermann and Blanchard (2002) indicated that biofeedback alone typically results in clinically significant improvement in headache symptoms (i.e., at least 50 % symptom reduction). Research comparing biofeedback to relaxation training is mixed; one study suggested relaxation training was more effective than biofeedback for vascular and migraine headache (Fentress, Masek, Mehegan, & Benson, 1986), while another indicated the two treatments were equally effective compared to a no-treatment control for youth with migraine (Labbe, 1995). Studies comparing biofeedback to a credible placebo condition are limited. Scharff, Marcus, and Masek (2002) compared hand-warming biofeedback plus stress management training to an attention control condition that consisted of hand-cooling biofeedback plus supportive therapy. Results indicated children who received hand-warming biofeedback were more likely to achieve clinical improvement in headache compared to those who received hand-cooling biofeedback, lending further support to the efficacy of biofeedback in the treatment of pediatric headache.

Significant reductions in headache activity have been reported for adolescents who receive biofeedback in both the clinic and home settings (Guarnieri & Blanchard, 1990; Hermann, Blanchard, & Flor, 1997). However, available data suggest that home-based biofeedback is generally less successful than clinician-administered biofeedback. For example, Guarnieri and Blanchard (1990) reported that 71 % of youth who received clinic-based treatment had significant improvement in headache activity compared to 33 % of those who received home-based treatment. The reason for the superior effects of clinic- versus home-based biofeedback training is unclear, although some authors have proposed that these findings may reflect differences in the amount of time spent practicing biofeedback and/or the effects of therapist contact (Hermann & Blanchard, 2002).

In addition to self-regulatory strategies and biofeedback, cognitive-behavioral treatment packages also typically include instruction in cognitive strategies and parent training in operant techniques. Cognitive strategies target negative thoughts and feelings that may be associated with the pain. For example, adolescents are taught to identify negative cognitions related to headache and other stressful events (e.g., "This pain will never go away!") and then replace them with more adaptive thoughts (e.g., "I can use my coping skills to help make my headache pain better."). Parent training in operant techniques is based on the principle that behaviors followed by positive outcomes will increase, while behaviors followed by undesirable outcomes will decrease (Fordyce, 1976). Typically, parents are taught operant strategies in order to address their child's pain-related disability. Parents are taught to increase desirable behaviors (e.g., participation in daily activities during a pain episode, school attendance) using praise and rewards and to decrease undesirable behaviors (e.g., staying in bed during a pain episode) by withholding rewards.

Operant training often involves having parents and adolescents create behavior contracts that specify targeted behaviors. For example, a behavior contract can be used to target school attendance for a teen who has been unable to attend school regularly due to headaches. The behavioral contract could specify that the adolescent must spend at least 4 h at school in order to have access to video games after school; if less than 4 h is spent at school, then video games after school are not available that day. It is important that adolescents are involved in creating behavioral contracts to ensure that salient rewards are selected to reinforce the targeted behaviors.

Allen and Shriver (1998) compared the efficacy of biofeedback only to biofeedback plus parent training in operant strategies for children and adolescents with migraine. Results indicated significant reductions in headache activity for both groups; however, the group who received parent training in operant strategies demonstrated significantly greater reductions in headache frequency. Furthermore, youth whose parents received operant training demonstrated better adaptive functioning than those who received biofeedback alone. These findings suggest that operant strategies may be a useful adjunct for psychological interventions targeting improvements in pain and daily functioning.

Several studies have examined the combined effect of relaxation training, biofeedback, and operant strategies (Mehegan, Masek, Harrison, Russo, & Leviton, 1987; Waranch & Keenan, 1985). Although these studies are limited by small sample size (i.e., *n*'s < 18), results indicate a decline in headache frequency and intensity immediately posttreatment and at 12-month follow-up. Research has also evaluated the efficacy of cognitive-behavioral treatment packages administered via distance formats. Significant improvements in headache activity have been reported by youth who received cognitive-behavioral intervention delivered via CD-ROM relative to wait-list control (Connelly, Rapoff, Thompson, & Connelly, 2006). A recent study evaluating an Internet-based cognitive-behavioral treatment for youth with headache demonstrated significant improvements in headache activity from pre- to posttreatment; however, youth who received Internet-based cognitive-behavioral therapy did not differ from those who received an active control condition that provided headache education (Trautmann & Kroner-Herwig, 2010).

Current understanding of the combined contributions of psychological treatment and pharmacotherapy for adolescents with headache is also limited. Available data suggest that significant improvement in tension headache can be achieved with home-based relaxation training with no further improvement in outcome associated with the addition of pharmacotherapy (Larsson, Melin, & Doberl, 1990). A double-blind cross-over trial comparing self-hypnosis and propranolol (acetaminophen) for adolescents with migraine indicated that self-hypnosis significantly lowered the frequency, but not intensity, of headache pain compared to propranolol (Olness, MacDonald, & Uden, 1987). More research is needed to elucidate the potential benefits of combining pharmacological and psychological interventions for treatment of headache in adolescents.

Adjunctive Lifestyle Interventions

Sleep

Although sleep deprivation is widely recognized as a headache trigger (Bruni et al., 2008; Connelly & Bickel, 2011; Kelman & Rains, 2005), little is known about the impact of targeted sleep interventions on headaches in youth and adults. One study indicated that psychoeducation in sleep hygiene practices resulted in reductions in headache frequency among youth with migraine compared to those youth who did not receive sleep hygiene education (Bruni, Falli, & Guidetti, 1999). The limited available data in the adult literature also suggest that sleep hygiene education is beneficial for individuals with migraine headache (Calhoun & Ford, 2007). Clearly, more research is needed to evaluate the impact of sleep interventions in people with headache.

Diet

As discussed above, scientific evidence to support the efficacy of dietary restrictions in the treatment of headache is limited. However, individual patients who report potential dietary triggers may benefit from dietary modification. In those cases, patients are typically instructed to eliminate all potential triggers and then reintroduce the foods one at a time to identify the foods that are most likely to be associated with headache. Some patients may report reductions in migraine frequency in response to eliminating foods that contain thiamine, gluten, sugar, or milk.

It is commonly recommended that adolescents with headache avoid caffeine because it can interfere with sleep, which may trigger headache episodes (Lewis, Yonker, Winner, & Sowell, 2005). Having a set time for meals can also prevent headaches that are triggered by low blood sugar (Powers & Andrasik, 2005). Drinking enough water during the day may also prevent headache episodes (Powers & Andrasik, 2005).

Physical Activity

Youth with headache are often encouraged to participate in regular aerobic activity (Gunner, Smith, & Ferguson, 2008); however, to our knowledge, no study to date has evaluated the effects of physical activity on headache pain in adolescents. It has been suggested that exercise may lead to improvements in pain and disability in youth with chronic pain conditions by causing changes in endorphins and other physiologic factors (e.g., increased blood flow) (Sherry, Wallace, Kelley, Kidder, & Sapp, 1999). Results from one adult study indicated that a 6-week aerobic exercise program was associated with significant reductions in pain severity among adults with migraines compared to participants who did not receive the exercise program (Lockett & Campbell, 1992). Of note, vigorous exercise can be a headache trigger particularly for those with migraine. Therefore, especially early on, patients should be encouraged to exercise at a moderate level to avoid an escalation in headache symptoms.

Physical Modalities

Physical Therapy

Muscle tightness, tenderness, and abnormalities in range of motion are common among individuals with migraine and tension-type headache (Kidd & Nelson, 1993; Lichstein et al., 1991). Physical therapy is recommended for adolescents with headache to correct posture, reduce muscle tension, and improve range of motion. Physical therapy techniques typically include postural correction, range of motion exercises, isometric strengthening exercises of the neck muscles, and whole-body stretching (e.g., Marcus, Scharff, Mercer, & Turk, 1998). Physical therapy may be particularly beneficial for individuals with tension-type headache by reducing muscle tension in the neck and shoulders (Hammill, Cook, & Rosecrance, 1996). Although the use of physical therapy as a stand-alone treatment for migraine is not well supported, it has been indicated as a useful adjunct to relaxation training and biofeedback (Marcus et al., 1998).

Acupuncture

Acupuncture has become an increasingly popular complementary and integrative intervention for headache in adolescents and adults. Research on the efficacy of acupuncture for treatment of headache is limited, and available results are mixed. A recent meta-analysis of eight randomized controlled trials comparing the efficacy of acupuncture with sham intervention indicated that acupuncture has limited efficacy for the reduction of headache frequency (Davis, Kononowech, Rolin, & Spierings, 2008). Research on the use of acupuncture for the treatment of headache in adolescents is even more limited. To our knowledge, only one randomized controlled study with a credible placebo condition has evaluated acupuncture in youth with headache (Gottschling et al., 2008). Results indicated that laser acupuncture for youth with headache resulted in significant reductions in headache frequency and severity compared to placebo laser. Despite the widespread use of acupuncture for headache, more rigorous study designs with larger sample sizes are needed to evaluate the potential benefits of acupuncture for adolescents with headache.

Conclusions and Recommendations

The purpose of this chapter was to describe common headache disorders experienced by adolescents and provide information regarding clinical assessment as well as pharmacological, psychological, lifestyle change, and physical approaches to headache treatment. Headaches are common during adolescence and when left untreated are associated with a host of negative consequences. Research supports the use of certain pharmacologic agents, behavioral, and cognitive-behavioral interventions to reduce headache activity in youth. However, the majority of studies that have examined treatment approaches for pediatric headache reflect less than optimal methodologies to test outcomes, including relatively small sample sizes and inadequate control groups.

More studies are needed to evaluate the safety and efficacy of medications for migraine and nonmigraine headache in younger patients. It is not sufficient to extrapolate findings from studies conducted on adults to assume similar outcomes in children and adolescents. Fortunately, as new products emerge, the United States Food and Drug Administration is working to acquire such data.

Likewise, little is known about the relative efficacy of cognitive-behavioral interventions for youth with headache compared to a credible placebo condition. Furthermore, the majority of these studies did not evaluate known correlates of headache pain such as psychiatric symptoms and functional disability. Given the known association between headache, psychiatric symptoms, and disability, the impact of interventions on these factors will be important to examine in future research. Finally, available data suggest that biofeedback and progressive muscle relaxation may be more effective than pharmacological treatment of adolescent headache; however, comparisons are limited by methodological flaws and small sample sizes (Hermann et al., 1995). Prospective randomized controlled trials are needed to compare the long-term efficacy of pharmacological and psychological interventions for pediatric headache.

In sum, headache in adolescents remains a challenging clinical problem. Although classification schemas help to differentiate the nature of the presenting condition and a good deal of research has helped identify contextual factors that may exacerbate and maintain pain and dysfunction, definitive treatment studies are few and far between. It appears at this juncture that an approach that combines pharmacological interventions to help prevent headache and treat acute exacerbations, along with psychological methods, lifestyle alterations, and physical modalities, is optimal.

References

Allen, K. D., & Shriver, M. D. (1998). Role of parent-mediated pain behavior management strategies in biofeedback treatment of childhood migraines. *Behavior Therapy, 29*, 477–490.

Andrasik, F., Kabela, E., Quinn, S., Attanasio, V., Blanchard, E. B., & Rosenblum, E. L. (1988). Psychological functioning of children who have recurrent migraine. *Pain, 34*, 43–52.

Anttila, P., Metsahonkala, L., Aromaa, M., Sourander, A., Salminen, J., Helenius, H., et al. (2002). Determinants of tension-type headache in children. *Cephalalgia, 22*, 401–408.

Anttila, P., Metsahonkala, L., Helenius, H., & Sillanpaa, M. (2000). Predisposing and provoking factors in childhood headache. *Headache, 40*, 351–356.

Anttila, P., Sourander, A., Metsahonkala, L., Aromaa, M., Helenius, H., & Sillanpaa, M. (2004). Psychiatric symptoms in children with primary headache. *Journal of the American Academy of Child and Adolescent Psychiatry, 43*, 412–419. doi:S0890-8567(09)61247-8 [pii]10.1097/00004583-200404000-00007.

Battistutta, S., Aliverti, R., Montico, M., Zin, R., & Carrozzi, M. (2009). Chronic tension-type headache in adolescents. Clinical and psychological characteristics analyzed through self- and parent-report questionnaires. *Journal of Pediatric Psychology, 34*, 697–706. doi:jsn102 [pii]10.1093/jpepsy/jsn102.

Bener, A., Uduman, S. A., Qassimi, E. M., Khalaily, G., Sztriha, L., Kilpelainen, H., et al. (2000). Genetic and environmental factors associated with migraine in schoolchildren. *Headache, 40*, 152–157.

Bigal, M. E., Lipton, R. B., Winner, P., Reed, M. L., Diamond, S., & Stewart, W. F. (2007). Migraine in adolescents: Association with socioeconomic status and family history. *Neurology, 69*, 16–25.

Bjorling, E. A. (2009). The momentary relationship between stress and headaches in adolescent girls. *Headache, 49*, 1186–1197. doi:HED1406 [pii]10.1111/j.1526-4610.2009.01406.x.

Bruni, O., Fabrizi, P., Ottaviano, S., Cortesi, F., Giannotti, F., & Guidetti, V. (1997). Prevalence of sleep disorders in childhood and adolescence with headache: A case–control study. *Cephalalgia, 17*, 492–498.

Bruni, O., Falli, F., & Guidetti, V. (1999). Sleep hygiene and migraine in children and adolescents. *Cephalalgia, 25*, 57–59.

Bruni, O., Russo, P. M., Ferri, R., Novelli, L., Galli, F., & Guidetti, V. (2008). Relationships between headache and sleep in a non-clinical population of children and adolescents. *Sleep Medicine, 9*, 542–548.

Calhoun, A. H., & Ford, S. (2007). Behavioral sleep modification may revert transformed migraine to episodic migraine. *Headache, 47*, 1178–1183. doi:HED780 [pii]10.1111/j.1526-4610.2007.00780.x.

Carlsson, J., Larsson, B., & Mark, A. (1996). Psychosocial functioning in schoolchildren with recurrent headaches. *Headache, 36*, 77–82.

Connelly, M., & Bickel, J. (2011). An electronic daily diary process study of stress and health behavior triggers of primary headaches in children. *Journal of Pediatric Psychology*. doi:jsr017 [pii]10.1093/jpepsy/jsr017.

Connelly, M., & Rapoff, M. A. (2006). Assessing health-related quality of life in children with recurrent headache: Reliability and validity of the PedsQLTM 4.0 in a pediatric headache sample. *Journal of Pediatric Psychology, 31*, 698–702. doi:jsj063 [pii]10.1093/jpepsy/jsj063.

Connelly, M., Rapoff, M. A., Thompson, N., & Connelly, W. (2006). Headstrong: A pilot study of a CD-ROM intervention for recurrent pediatric headache. *Journal of Pediatric Psychology, 31*, 737–747.

Cuvellier, J. C., Couttenier, F., Joriot-Chekaf, S., & Vallee, L. (2008). Chronic daily headache in French children and adolescents. *Pediatric Neurology, 38*, 93–98. doi:S0887-8994(07)00490-0 [pii]10.1016/j.pediatrneurol.2007.10.001.

Davis, M. A., Kononowech, R. W., Rolin, S. A., & Spierings, E. L. (2008). Acupuncture for tension-type headache: A meta-analysis of randomized, controlled trials. *The Journal of Pain, 9*, 667–677. doi:S1526-5900(08)00503-8 [pii]10.1016/j.jpain.2008.03.011.

de Tommaso, M., Sardaro, M., Vecchio, E., Serpino, C., Stasi, M., & Ranieri, M. (2008). Central sensitisation phenomena in primary headaches: Overview of a preventive therapeutic approach. *CNS and Neurological Disorders Drug Targets, 7*, 524–535.

Eccleston, C., Palermo, T. M., Williams, A. C., Lewandowski, A., & Morley, S. (2009). Psychological therapies for the management of chronic and recurrent pain in children and adolescents. *Cochrane Database Systematic Review* (2), Art. No.: CD007407. doi:007410.001002/14651858.CD14007407.pub14651852.

Eiland, L. S., & Hunt, M. O. (2010). The use of triptans for pediatric migraines. *Paediatric Drugs, 12*, 379–389. doi:10.2165/11532860-000000000-000005 [pii].

Fearon, P., & Hotopf, M. (2001). Relation between headache in childhood and physical and psychiatric symptoms in adulthood: National birth cohort study. *British Medical Journal, 322*, 1145.

Fentress, D. W., Masek, B. J., Mehegan, J. E., & Benson, H. (1986). Biofeedback and relaxation-response training in the treatment of pediatric migraine. *Developmental Medicine and Child Neurology, 28*, 139–146.

Fernandez-de-las-Penas, C., Cuadrado, M. L., Arendt-Nielsen, L., Simons, D. G., & Pareja, J. A. (2007). Myofascial trigger points and sensitization: An updated pain model for tension-type headache. *Cephalalgia, 27*, 383–393. doi:CHA1295 [pii]10.1111/j.1468-2982.2007.01295.x.

Fichtel, A., & Larsson, B. (2002). Psychosocial impact of headache and comorbidity with other pains among Swedish school adolescents. *Headache: The Journal of Head and Face Pain, 42*, 766–775. doi:10.1046/j.1526-4610.2002.02178.x.

Fillingim, R. B., King, C. D., Ribeiro-Dasilva, M. C., Rahim-Williams, B., & Riley, J. L., 3rd. (2009). Sex, gender, and pain: A review of recent clinical and experimental findings. *The Journal of Pain, 10*, 447–485. doi:S1526-5900(08)00909-7 [pii]10.1016/j.jpain.2008.12.001.

Fordyce, W. E. (1976). *Behavioral methods for chronic pain and illness*. St. Louis: Mosby.

Galli, F., Patron, L., Russo, P. M., Bruni, O., Ferini-Strambi, L., & Guidetti, V. (2004). Chronic daily headache in childhood and adolescence: Cinical aspects and a 4-year follow-up. *Cephalalgia, 24*, 850–858. doi:10.1111/j.1468-2982.2004.00758.xCHA758 [pii].

Gilman, D. K., Palermo, T. M., Kabbouche, M. A., Hershey, A. D., & Powers, S. W. (2007). Primary headache and sleep disturbances in adolescents. *Headache, 47*, 1189–1194.

Gottschling, S., Meyer, S., Gribova, I., Distler, L., Berrang, J., Gortner, L., et al. (2008). Laser acupuncture in children with headache: A double-blind, randomized, bicenter, placebo-controlled trial. *Pain, 137*, 405–412. doi:S0304-3959(07)00571-4 [pii]10.1016/j.pain.2007.10.004.

Guarnieri, P., & Blanchard, E. B. (1990). Evaluation of home-based thermal biofeedback treatment of pediatric migraine headache. *Applied Psychophysiology and Biofeedback, 15*, 179–184.

Gunner, K. B., Smith, H. D., & Ferguson, L. E. (2008). Practice guideline for diagnosis and management of migraine headaches in children and adolescents: Part two. *Journal of Pediatric Health Care, 22*, 52–59. doi:S0891-5245(07)00403-8 [pii]10.1016/j.pedhc.2007.10.009.

Hammill, J. M., Cook, T. M., & Rosecrance, J. C. (1996). Effectiveness of a physical therapy regimen in the treatment of tension-type headache. *Headache, 36*, 149–153.

Hermann, C., & Blanchard, E. B. (2002). Biofeedback in the treatment of headache and other childhood pain. *Applied Psychophysiology and Biofeedback, 27*, 143–162.

Hermann, C., Blanchard, E. B., & Flor, H. (1997). Biofeedback treatment for pediatric migraine: Prediction of treatment outcome. *Journal of Consulting and Clinical Psychology, 65*, 611–616.

Hermann, C., Kim, M., & Blanchard, E. B. (1995). Behavioral and prophylactic pharmacological intervention studies of pediatric migraine: An exploratory meta-analysis. *Pain, 60*, 239–255.

Hershey, A. D., Powers, S. W., Bentti, A. L., LeCates, S., & deGrauw, T. J. (2001). Characterization of chronic daily headaches in children in a multidisciplinary headache center. *Neurology, 56*, 1032–1037.

Hershey, A. D., Powers, S. W., Nelson, T. D., Kabbouche, M. A., Winner, P., Yonker, M., et al. (2009). Obesity in the pediatric headache population: A multicenter study. *Headache, 49*, 170–177.

Holden, E. W., Deichmann, M. M., & Levy, J. D. (1999). Empirically supported treatments in pediatric psychology: Recurrent pediatric headache. *Journal of Pediatric Psychology, 24*, 91–109.

International Classification of Headache Disorders (ICHD-2). (2004). The International Classification of Headache Disorders: 2nd edition. *Cephalalgia, 24*, 9–160.

Kaiser, R. S. (1992). Depression in adolescent headache patients. *Headache, 32*, 340–344.

Karli, N., Akgoz, S., Zarifoglu, M., Akis, N., & Erer, S. (2006). Clinical characteristics of tension-type headache and migraine in adolescents: A student-based study. *Headache, 46*, 399–412. doi:HED372 [pii]10.1111/j.1526-4610.2006.00372.x.

Kelman, L. (2007). The triggers or precipitants of the acute migraine attack. *Cephalalgia, 27*, 394–402. doi:CHA1303[pii]10.1111/j.1468-2982.2007.01303.x.

Kelman, L., & Rains, J. C. (2005). Headache and sleep: Examination of sleep patterns and complaints in a large clinical sample of migraineurs. *Headache, 45*, 904–910. doi:HED05159 [pii]10.1111/j.1526-4610.2005.05159.x.

Kidd, R. F., & Nelson, R. (1993). Musculoskeletal dysfunction of the neck in migraine and tension headache. *Headache, 33*, 566–569.

Kors, E. E., Haan, J., & Ferrari, M. D. (1999). Genetics of primary headaches. *Current Opinion in Neurology, 12*, 249–254.

Kroner-Herwig, B., Heinrich, M., & Morris, L. (2007). Headache in German children and adolescents: A population-based epidemiological study. *Cephalalgia, 27*, 519–527.

Labbe, E. E. (1995). Treatment of childhood migraine with autogenic training and skin temperature biofeedback: A component analysis. *Headache, 35*, 10–13.

Larsson, B., & Carlsson, J. (1996). A school-based, nurse-administered relaxation training for children with chronic tension-type headache. *Journal of Pediatric Psychology, 21*, 603–614.

Larsson, B., Carlsson, J., Fichtel, A., & Melin, L. (2005). Relaxation treatment of adolescent headache sufferers: Results from a school-based replication series. *Headache, 45*, 692–704. doi:HED05138 [pii]10.1111/j.1526-4610.2005.05138.x.

Larsson, B., Melin, L., & Doberl, A. (1990). Recurrent tension headache in adolescents treated with self-help relaxation training and a muscle relaxant drug. *Headache, 30*, 665–671.

Lee, L. H., & Olness, K. N. (1997). Clinical and demographic characteristics of migraine in urban children. *Headache, 37*, 269–276.

Lewis, D. W. (2002). Headaches in children and adolescents. *American Family Physician, 65*, 625–632.

Lewis, K. S. (2010). Pediatric headache. *Seminars in Pediatric Neurology, 17*, 224–229. doi:S1071-9091(10)00107-5 [pii]10.1016/j.spen.2010.10.004.

Lewis, D. W., Yonker, M., Winner, P., & Sowell, M. (2005). The treatment of pediatric migraine. *Pediatric Annals, 34*, 448–460.

Lichstein, K. L., Fischer, S. M., Eakin, T. L., Amberson, J. I., Bertorini, T., & Hoon, P. W. (1991). Psychophysiological parameters of migraine and muscle-contraction headaches. *Headache, 31*, 27–34.

Lipton, R. B., Scher, A. I., Kolodner, K., Liberman, J., Steiner, T. J., & Stewart, W. F. (2002). Migraine in the United States: Epidemiology and patterns of health care use. *Neurology, 58*, 885–894.

Lockett, D. M., & Campbell, J. F. (1992). The effects of aerobic exercise on migraine. *Headache, 32*, 50–54.

Marcus, D. A., Scharff, L., Mercer, S., & Turk, D. C. (1998). Nonpharmacological treatment for migraine: Incremental utility of physical therapy with relaxation and thermal biofeedback. *Cephalalgia, 18*, 266–272; discussion 242.

Martin-Herz, S. P., Smith, M. S., & McMahon, R. J. (1999). Psychological factors associated with headache in junior high school students. *Journal of Pediatric Psychology, 24*, 13–23.

Mazzone, L., Vitiello, B., Incorpora, G., & Mazzone, D. (2006). Behavioural and temperamental characteristics of children and adolescents suffering from primary headache. *Cephalalgia, 26*, 194–201.

Mehegan, J. E., Masek, B. J., Harrison, R. H., Russo, D. C., & Leviton, A. (1987). A multicomponent behavioral treatment for pediatric migraine. *The Clinical Journal of Pain, 2*, 191–196.

Milde-Busch, A., Blaschek, A., Borggrafe, I., Heinen, F., Straube, A., & von Kries, R. (2010). Associations of diet and lifestyle with headache in high-school students: Results from a cross-sectional study. *Headache, 50*, 1104–1114. doi:HED1706 [pii]10.1111/j.1526-4610.2010.01706.x.

Miller, V. A., Palermo, T. M., Powers, S. W., Scher, M. S., & Hershey, A. D. (2003). Migraine headaches and sleep disturbances in children. *Headache, 43*, 362–368.

Millichap, J. G., & Yee, M. M. (2003). The diet factor in pediatric and adolescent migraine. *Pediatric Neurology, 28*, 9–15. doi:S0887899402004666 [pii].

Monastero, R., Camarda, C., Pipia, C., & Camarda, R. (2006). Prognosis of migraine headaches in adolescents: A 10-year follow-up study. *Neurology, 67*, 1353–1356. doi:67/8/1353 [pii]10.1212/01.wnl.0000240131.69632.4f.

Monteith, T. S., & Sprenger, T. (2010). Tension type headache in adolescence and childhood: Where are we now? *Current Pain and Headache Reports, 14*, 424–430. doi:10.1007/s11916-010-0149-z.

Olness, K., MacDonald, J. T., & Uden, D. L. (1987). Comparison of self-hypnosis and propranolol in the treatment of juvenile classic migraine. *Pediatrics, 79*, 593–597.

Palermo, T. M., Putnam, J., Armstrong, G., & Daily, S. (2007). Adolescent autonomy and family functioning are associated with headache-related disability. *The Clinical Journal of Pain, 23*, 458–465.

Palermo, T. M., & von Baeyer, C. L. (2008). How to talk to parents about recurrent and chronic pain. In G. A. Walco & K. R. Goldschneider (Eds.), *Pediatric pain management in primary care: A practical guide* (pp. 125–132). Totowa, NJ: Humana.

Perquin, C. W., Hazebroek-Kampschreur, A. A., Hunfeld, J. A., Bohnen, A. M., van Suijlekom-Smit, L. W., Passchier, J., et al. (2000). Pain in children and adolescents: A common experience. *Pain, 87*, 51–58.

Pine, D. S., Cohen, P., & Brook, J. (1996). The association between major depression and headache: Results of a longitudinal epidemiologic study in youth. *Journal of Child and Adolescent Psychopharmacology, 6*, 153–164.

Powers, S. W., & Andrasik, F. (2005). Biobehavioral treatment, disability, and psychological effects of pediatric headache. *Pediatric Annals, 34*, 461–465.

Powers, S. W., Gilman, D. K., & Hershey, A. D. (2006). Headache and psychological functioning in children and adolescents. *Headache, 46*, 1404–1415. doi:HED583 [pii]10.1111/j.1526-4610.2006.00583.x.

Powers, S. W., Patton, S. R., Hommel, K. A., & Hershey, A. D. (2004). Quality of life in paediatric migraine: Characterization of age-related effects using PedsQL 4.0. *Cephalalgia, 24*, 120–127.

Robberstad, L., Dyb, G., Hagen, K., Stovner, L. J., Holmen, T. L., & Zwart, J. A. (2010). An unfavorable lifestyle and recurrent headaches among adolescents: The HUNT study. *Neurology, 75*, 712–717. doi:WNL.0b013e3181eee244 [pii]10.1212/WNL.0b013e3181eee244.

Scharff, L., Marcus, D. A., & Masek, B. J. (2002). A controlled study of minimal-contact thermal biofeedback treatment in children with migraine. *Journal of Pediatric Psychology, 27*, 109–119.

Seshia, S. S. (2004). Chronic daily headache in children and adolescents. *The Canadian Journal of Neurological Sciences, 31*, 319–323.

Seshia, S. S., Phillips, D. F., & von Baeyer, C. L. (2008). Childhood chronic daily headache: A biopsychosocial perspective. *Developmental Medicine and Child Neurology, 50*, 541–545. doi:DMCN3013 [pii]10.1111/j.1469-8749.2008.03013.x.

Sethna, N. F., & LeBel, A. A. (2008). Headaches. In G. A. Walco & K. R. Goldschneider (Eds.), *Pain in children: A practical guide for primary care* (pp. 173–183). Totowa, NJ: Humana.

Sherry, D. D., Wallace, C. A., Kelley, C., Kidder, M., & Sapp, L. (1999). Short- and long-term outcomes of children with complex regional pain syndrome type I treated with exercise therapy. *The Clinical Journal of Pain, 15*, 218–223.

Silberstein, S. D. (2011). Headache. In M. E. Lynch & K. D. Craig (Eds.), *Clinical pain management: A practical guide* (pp. 524–535). West Sussex: Wiley-Blackwell.

Silberstein, S., Stiles, A., & Young, W. B. (Eds.). (2005). *Atlas of migraine and other headaches*. London: Taylor & Francis.

Smith, M. S., Martin-Herz, S. P., Womack, W. M., & McMahon, R. J. (1999). Recurrent headache in adolescents: Nonreferred versus clinic population. *Headache, 39*(9), 616–624.

Smitherman, T. A., Walters, A. B., Maizels, M., & Penzien, D. B. (2010). The use of antidepressants for headache prophylaxis. *CNS Neuroscience and Therapeutics*. doi:CNS170 [pii]10.1111/j.1755-5949.2010.00170.x.

Spierings, E. L., Schroevers, M., Honkoop, P. C., & Sorbi, M. (1998). Presentation of chronic daily headache: A clinical study. *Headache, 38*, 191–196.

Stanford, E. A., Chambers, C. T., Biesanz, J. C., & Chen, E. (2008). The frequency, trajectories and predictors of adolescent recurrent pain: A population-based approach. *Pain, 138*, 11–21.

Tfelt-Hansen, P. C., & Koehler, P. J. (2008). History of the use of ergotamine and dihydroergotamine in migraine from 1906 and onward. *Cephalalgia, 28*, 877–886. doi:CHA1578 [pii]10.1111/j.1468-2982.2008.01578.x.

Trautmann, E., & Kroner-Herwig, B. (2010). A randomized controlled trial of Internet-based self-help training for recurrent headache in childhood and adolescence. *Behavior Research and Therapy, 48*, 28–37.

Trautmann, E., Lackschewitz, H., & Kroner-Herwig, B. (2006). Psychological treatment of recurrent headache in children and adolescents—a meta-analysis. *Cephalalgia, 26*, 1411–1426.

Victor, T. W., Hu, X., Campbell, J. C., Buse, D. C., & Lipton, R. B. (2010). Migraine prevalence by age and sex in the United States: A life-span study. *Cephalalgia, 30*, 1065–1072. doi:0333102409355601 [pii]10.1177/0333102409355601.

Waeber, C., & Moskowitz, M. A. (2005). Migraine as an inflammatory disorder. *Neurology, 64*, S9–S15. doi:64/10_suppl_2/S9 [pii].

Wang, S. J., Fuh, J. L., Lu, S. R., & Juang, K. D. (2006). Chronic daily headache in adolescents: Prevalence, impact, and medication overuse. *Neurology, 66*, 193–197. doi:66/2/193 [pii]10.1212/01.wnl.0000183555.54305.fd.

Wang, S. J., Fuh, J. L., Lu, S. R., & Juang, K. D. (2007). Outcomes and predictors of chronic daily headache in adolescents: A 2-year longitudinal study. *Neurology, 68*, 591–596. doi:01.wnl.0000252800.82704.62 [pii]10.1212/01.wnl.0000252800.82704.62.

Wang, S. J., Juang, K. D., Fuh, J. L., & Lu, S. R. (2007). Psychiatric comorbidity and suicide risk in adolescents with chronic daily headache. *Neurology, 68*, 1468–1473. doi:68/18/1468 [pii]10.1212/01.wnl.0000260607.90634.d6.

Waranch, H. R., & Keenan, D. M. (1985). Behavioral treatment of children with recurrent headaches. *Journal of Behavior Therapy and Experimental Psychiatry, 16*, 31–38.

Wiendels, N. J., van der Geest, M. C., Neven, A. K., Ferrari, M. D., & Laan, L. A. (2005). Chronic daily headache in children and adolescents. *Headache, 45*, 678–683. doi:HED05137[pii]10.1111/j.1526-4610.2005.05137.x.

Woolf, C. J. (2011). Central sensitization: Implications for the diagnosis and treatment of pain. *Pain, 152*, S2–S15. doi:S0304-3959(10)00584-1 [pii]10.1016/j.pain.2010.09.030.

Zwart, J. A., Dyb, G., Holmen, T. L., Stovner, L. J., & Sand, T. (2004). The prevalence of migraine and tension-type headaches among adolescents in Norway. The Nord-Trondelag Health Study (Head-HUNT-Youth), a large population-based epidemiological study. *Cephalalgia, 24*, 373–379. doi:10.1111/j.1468-2982.2004.00680.x.

Chronic Pain in Adolescents: Physiological and Psychological Bases for Pain

Anne M. Lynch-Jordan and Susmita Kashikar-Zuck

Chronic Pain in Adolescents: Physiological and Psychological Bases for Pain

Adolescence is a developmental period characterized by numerous biological, psychological, and interpersonal changes that are accompanied by an increased striving for independence. In the midst of these transitions and growth, over 30 % of adolescents are faced with the added challenge of coping with recurrent or chronic pain at some point during their teenage years. Pain is typically defined as "chronic" if it is present daily or recurrently for the duration of at least 3 months (Merskey & Bogduk, 1994). The etiology of chronic pain in adolescents is sometimes clearly identifiable when it is associated with a disease such as juvenile arthritis or sickle cell anemia. In other cases, pain can occur without a clear origin, as in the case of nonspecific back pain or abdominal pain, which can pose significant diagnostic and treatment challenges. Dealing with medically unexplained pain can be frustrating to adolescents, their parents, and medical providers alike. The objective of this chapter is to describe the prevalence of common, non-disease-based chronic pain conditions in adolescents and detail the physiological and psychological aspects of chronic pain. This will be followed by a more detailed discussion about three common conditions in adolescents, namely, chronic back pain, abdominal pain, and widespread musculoskeletal pain to give the reader a sense of the range of presenting problems, potential causes, and their impact on the lives of teenagers.

Prevalence

Chronic pain in children and adolescents is a surprisingly common problem. In a Dutch epidemiological study, the prevalence of chronic pain was reported to be 25 % across a community sample of children ages 0–18 years (Perquin et al., 2000). When segmented by age, prevalence rates highlight the significance of these problems in the adolescent years. Among younger adolescents (12–15 years), 35.7 % reported having chronic pain, with older adolescents (16–18 years) showing comparably high rates (31.2 %). As a follow-up to this 2000 study, those children and adolescents reporting chronic pain were reassessed for three consecutive years (Perquin et al., 2003). From the initial sample, 9.4 % of children and adolescents endorsed persistent chronic pain from baseline through

A.M. Lynch-Jordan, Ph.D. (✉)
S. Kashikar-Zuck, Ph.D.
Division of Behavioral Medicine and Clinical Psychology, Departments of Pediatrics and Anesthesia, Cincinnati Children's Hospital Medical Center, 3333 Burnet Avenue, ML 3015, Cincinnati, OH 45229, USA
e-mail: anne.lynch-jordan@cchmc.org; susmita.kashikar-zuck@cchmc.org

W.T. O'Donohue et al. (eds.), *Handbook of Adolescent Health Psychology*,
DOI 10.1007/978-1-4614-6633-8_44, © Springer Science+Business Media New York 2013

3 years post-baseline. Aside from headaches, abdominal, back, and other musculoskeletal (diffuse or localized) pains were most commonly reported (Huguet & Miro, 2008; Perquin et al., 2000, 2003; Roth-Isigkeit, Thyen, Raspe, Stoven, & Schmucker, 2004) [see separate chapter for in-depth discussion of headaches]. Additionally, the prevalence of multiple (vs. single) pain complaints increased with age as well. Thus, for some youth, pain becomes a way of life that may impact many domains of functioning.

As in adults, back pain is probably one of the most commonly encountered pain conditions in youth. The lifetime prevalence of low back pain ranged from about 30 % in US adolescents 11–17 years (Olsen et al., 1992) and Finnish schoolchildren aged 14 years (Salminen, Pentti, & Terho, 1992) to 50.4 % of English schoolchildren aged 15 years (Burton, Clarke, McClune, & Tillotson, 1996). In most cases, adolescents have an episode of pain that resolves relatively quickly (Salminen et al., 1992), but several studies reveal back pain of a chronic nature, with rates between 3 and 8.9 % among adolescents (Salminen et al., 1992; Taimela, Kujala, Salminen, & Viljanen, 1997; Viry, Creveuil, & Marcelli, 1999). However, few of these adolescents have back pain significant enough to merit medical intervention for pain management.

Another common pain condition is recurrent abdominal pain (RAP). In a landmark study of 1,000 English schoolchildren in 1957, Apley (Apley & Naish, 1958) reported the occurrence of RAP as 10.8 % across children 0–15 years. US and Spanish studies of schoolchildren replicate Apley's findings, with prevalence rates reported to be 11–17 % (Huguet & Miro, 2008; Hyams, Burke, Davis, Rzepski, & Andrulonis, 1996), although fewer had consulted a physician about these problems (Hyams et al., 1996). Among children and adolescents who do present to primary care offices for treatment, a significant percent report chronic symptoms severe enough to cause disruption to daily activities (Spee et al., 2010). Unlike previous studies of pediatric chronic pain, a Dutch study of schoolchildren ages 6–19 years found decreasing rates of abdominal pain with age, with only 5 % of youth reporting this pain complaint by the age of 16–17 (Oster, 1972).

Musculoskeletal pains, whether diffuse or localized, are another frequent pain complaint of youth. In a study of Spanish schoolchildren, the prevalence of chronic limb pain was 15.39 % (Huguet & Miro, 2008). In a Dutch study, by age 16–17 years, adolescents endorsed frequent "growing pains" approximately 15 % of the time (Oster, 1972). In Israel, Buskila (Buskila et al., 1993) found 6.2 % of schoolchildren ages 9–15 years met criteria for fibromyalgia, with a 4.0 % rate reported in the 13–15-year age group. In a younger sample (grades 3–5) of Finnish students, weekly musculoskeletal pain was reported 32.1 % of the time, with 7.5 % meeting criteria for diffuse, widespread pain problems (Mikkelsson, 1999). In a review of Spanish primary care visits from 1997 to 1999, 11.6 % of office visits were for adolescents with musculoskeletal pain (De Inocencio, 2004).

Although studies on the prevalence of chronic pain vary based upon the type of sample (community vs. clinical), the range of ages included, and the method of presentation of the data, it is clear from both community and clinical settings in studies from many different countries that chronic pain is a frequent phenomenon in adolescents.

Biopsychosocial Approach to Understanding Pain

Every adolescent has their own unique genetic predisposition, biological characteristics, emotional makeup, and social network of family and peers that serve as the backdrop to their pain experience. It is important to take into consideration all of these influences when describing the nature and impact of chronic pain in the lives of adolescents. The biopsychosocial approach first described by George Engel (1977) is the most comprehensive and widely used conceptualization of chronic pain. It contrasted the previous dualist model of pain whereby the mind and the body functioned separately from each other (Gatchel, Peng, Peters, Fuchs, & Turk, 2007). Instead, Engel and others described the pain experience as one that incorporates emotional and stress factors that contribute to pain perception. The current definition of pain developed by the International Association for the Study of Pain (IASP) is framed from this approach. Pain is described as "an unpleasant sensory and emotional experience associated with actual or potential tissue damage, or described in terms of such damage" (Merskey & Bogduk, 1994). Thus, the unique characteristics of the individual, both physical and emotional, can have an impact on pain perception. By including "actual or potential" tissue damage, this definition also includes the possibility that pain can exist without a clearly identifiable etiology.

Biological Aspects of Chronic Pain

Pain perception is also known as nociception, which is defined as "the neural process of encoding noxious stimuli" (Merskey & Bogduk, 1994). Nociception serves a protective role, alerting an organism to potentially dangerous or life-threatening conditions and resulting in both reflexive and behavioral responses that minimize further injury (Latremoliere & Woolf, 2009). For example, ankle pain serves as a warning to an adolescent athlete of a potential sprain or strain after a fall or being tripped by an opponent while playing soccer. Nociception involves the peripheral (sensory nerves and receptors) and central (spinal cord, brain) nervous systems. At a basic level, sensory receptors receive input from noxious physical stimuli that causes (or potentially causes) tissue damage. Receptor input is then transmitted to select areas of the spinal cord (spinal dorsal horn) via projecting nerve pathways in the peripheral nervous system. Noxious signals are further processed and modified in the spinal cord, before being relayed to a variety of brain structures that encode characteristics of the stimuli including intensity (how strong pain is), quality (sharp vs. aching pain), and emotional aspects (pain-related anxiety or worry) (Lee & Tracey, 2010; Thomas Cheng, 2010). In the 1960s, Melzack and Wall (1965) provided an initial description of this process via the Gate Control Theory of Pain. Their theory accounted for the role that cognitions (thoughts) and affect (emotions) played on the experience of pain, particularly in a loop pattern whereby descending neural pathways from the brain were identified as amplifying or dampening nociception based on organism-specific characteristics such as past pain history, attention to symptoms, and the emotional state of the individual (Melzack & Wall, 1965). The theory has undergone several transformations over the years, and with the advent of sophisticated research in neuroscience, genetics, and imaging, more elegant and complex models have been described. However, the Gate Control Theory of Pain provided a paradigm shift in the field of pain research with its focus on the multiple dimensions of pain and continues to inform pain conceptualization both in clinical and research settings.

The explosion of genetics research in pain has provided new insights into individual differences in pain perception and pain inhibition. As Mogil et al. (1996) noted, considerable variability has been found among people in overall sensitivity to pain as well as responsiveness to certain pain medications. These differences are in part found to be related to genetic makeup. To clarify these individual differences, researchers have used various methods such as studying people with a congenital insensitivity to pain [summary, Gatchel et al. (2007)] as well as family studies. Since pain problems have a tendency to aggregate in families (e.g., Arnold et al., 2004; Buskila & Neumann, 1997), studies have begun to elaborate on the shared genes that result in high heritability of pain conditions. Studies investigating these genetic factors can be done by looking at multiple generations of family members or twins (e.g., Yunus, 1998; Yunus et al., 1999) or by using animal models (mice and rat studies) in which genetic influences are easier to study in a controlled fashion (Mogil et al., 1996). Findings from genetic studies of pain were well summarized by Gatchel et al. (2007) who concluded that neural transmission of pain requires a variety of intricate processes, based upon the proteins and enzymes that form our genetic makeup. Disruption of any step of these processes in an individual can either amplify or reduce nociception, creating a genetic susceptibility to pain.

Identification of clear biomarkers or genetic vulnerability factors in chronic pain is challenging because of the complex and multifactorial nature of these disorders. For example, functional gastrointestinal disorders such as irritable bowel syndrome (IBS) often have a variety of biological mechanisms that are thought to contribute to the etiology, clinical symptoms can differ from one patient to the next, symptom severity can fluctuate over time, and family histories are positive for multiple pain syndromes, not just IBS (Saito, Mitra, & Mayer, 2010). IBS is therefore not considered to be a monogenic disease (a single gene defect), and dozens of genes have been investigated for their contribution to symptom presentation. Family and twin studies suggest that dual gene–environment influences are probably the best explanation for IBS. Thus, familial clustering of IBS may be related to genetic susceptibility as well as shared environmental factors such as similar eating habits, shared adverse life events, social modeling of adaptive or negative coping, and exposure to toxins or microorganisms (Saito et al., 2010). This type of complex relationship between an individual's genetic makeup and environmental expression of pain is most likely the reason why one adolescent with chronic pain complains of pain with even the lightest touch, yet another adolescent with the same pain condition may be very athletic and play competitive sports without complaining of much discomfort.

Technological advances in brain imaging have allowed a more in-depth exploration of the underlying brain structures and processes involved in the multidimensional experience of pain. Common imaging techniques used to study pain include functional magnetic resonance imaging (fMRI), positron emission tomography (PET), and scalp electroencephalography (EEG) (Lee & Tracey, 2010). In combination, these imaging techniques provide detailed information about neural activity in the brain, regional blood flow, brain structures and anomalies, and evoked potentials which clarify not only nociception but also the functional changes that happen in the brain during various emotional (anxiety) or coping (distraction) efforts. Several brain structures have been identified as centrally active and involved in pain processing including the somatosensory cortex, anterior insula, and anterior cingulate cortex (ACC) (Gatchel et al., 2007; Lee & Tracey, 2010). Moreover, additional involvement of brain regions including the hypothalamus, periaqueductal gray, prefrontal cortex, and cerebellum has been found. Even psychological processes such as catastrophizing, a negative thought process whereby an individual ruminates about pain, have been related to responses in the prefrontal cortex, insula, anterior cingulate cortex, and medial frontal cortex (Campbell & Edwards, 2009; Gracely et al., 2004; Gracely, McGrath, & Dubner, 1978; Seminowicz & Davis, 2006).

As one can surmise from the research discussed so far, there is not always a direct correlation between nociception and the presence of noxious stimuli. For adolescents with some pain conditions like chronic abdominal pain or fibromyalgia, no clear injury, illness, or other noxious trigger has been linked to their persistent, amplified pain. Pain hypersensitivity in these cases seems to result from a host of changes in neuronal pain pathways in the central nervous system and is known as "central sensitization." Central sensitization represents "an abnormal state of responsiveness to increased gain of the nociceptive system" (Latremoliere & Woolf, 2009, p. 896). In this state of hyperarousal, pain signals can spontaneously occur (with no clear triggering event), result from increasingly low levels of stimulation (minor events result in major pain), or result from an increasingly larger field of receptors to relay stimuli through pain pathways (the greater the number of receptors, the greater the ability to receive and transfer noxious stimuli). At the patient level, chronic pain stemming from central sensitization causes endless frustration for adolescents, who receive repeated negative results on standard medical tests, and their parents, who see their children continue to suffer from unrelenting symptoms.

In addition to genetic and neurological factors, the role of stress is becoming better understood as being an important factor in the onset and maintenance of persistent pain. Stress comes in many forms for adolescents—getting good grades, planning for college, parent–child conflict, peer relationship difficulties, and simply trying to juggle an increasingly busy schedule of activities. Not only can the psychological aspects of stress (tension, irritability, worry) impact the pain experience, but chronic pain by itself serves as a biological stressor which tends to disturb the body's natural state of homeostasis. This disturbance in homeostasis can cause a series of internal immune and hormonal reactions that attempt to rectify the disruption and restore balance (Melzack, 2005). These reactions include the release of substances to fight off infection and repair tissue damage, as well as the activation of the hypothalamic–pituitary–adrenal (HPA) system, resulting in a further cascade of chemical reactions that ultimately release cortisol, a stress hormone. In small doses, cortisol is an adaptive substance aimed at coping with a situation that threatens the integrity of the body. Prolonged cortisol exposure resulting from chronic stress becomes problematic as it has been shown to reduce immune system functioning and break down tissue in the body, all of which has implications for the maintenance of chronic pain (Bradley, Haile, & Jaworski, 1992). As Melzack (2005) noted, cortisol in and of itself may not be sufficient to trigger chronic pain but may be necessary to create the internal environment whereby chronic pain problems become possible.

Psychological Aspects of Pain

The second aspect of the biopsychosocial model of pain emphasizes the role of psychological factors in the pain experience. How adolescents cope with chronic pain varies greatly based upon their age, gender, psychosocial environment, and learning histories. For example, as they grow older, adolescents may use more positive self-talk (a more sophisticated cognitive technique) than younger children, reflective of their maturing cognitive skills. Also, adolescent males and females may differ in their methods of coping with their symptoms with girls showing a stronger tendency to seek social support (Hodgins & Lander, 1997; Lynch, Kashikar-Zuck, Goldschneider, & Jones, 2007; Spirito, Stark, Gil, & Tyc, 1995) and boys using more activity-oriented distraction (Lynch et al., 2007) and a greater number of techniques than girls (Holden, Gladstein, Trulsen, & Wall, 1994).

Both boys and girls report feeling greater efficacy related to pain coping the more frequently they engaged in adaptive coping such as using positive self-statements, behavioral distraction, and cognitive distraction (Lynch et al., 2007). In addition to positive strategies, adolescents can also engage in negative forms of coping (such as catastrophic thinking) that unintentionally worsen the pain experience. Research has shown a significant relationship between higher levels of pain intensity and catastrophizing about pain (Crombez et al., 2003) and generally using more emotion-focused strategies (Merlijn et al., 2003; Reid, Gilbert, & McGrath, 1998). Emotion-focused coping is described as excessive emotional expression or lack of effort to regulate the emotions that occur with the presence of pain (Reid et al., 1998). With their natural tendency of having more labile emotions, adolescents appear to have higher levels of emotion-focused coping than children, and this may be linked to greater functional disability associated with pain (Reid et al., 1998).

Recent studies of psychological coping have developed coping profiles based on the clinical presentation of youth with chronic pain related to their daily functioning, mood factors, and coping styles. "Avoidant copers" tended to catastrophize about their symptoms, avoided normal activities to prevent flare-ups, and showed significant mood problems (typically depression and anxiety symptoms) and higher disability in response to pain (Claar, Baber, Simons, Logan, & Walker, 2008; Walker, Baber, Garber, & Smith, 2008). These patients may be classified as distressed and low functioning (Scharff et al., 2005). Adolescents characterized as being "dependent copers" also reported higher catastrophizing and disability but sought social support and were less isolated. "Self-reliant and engaged copers" were described as more adaptive because they reported greater use of distraction and self-encouragement, less avoidance, and better problem solving. The more frequent use of these proactive techniques was in turn associated with lower levels of anxiety and depressive symptoms in "adaptive copers" (Claar et al., 2008). In other studies, these copers were also described as "high functioning" given their low levels of psychopathology and functional impairment (Scharff et al., 2005). Thus, coping style (adaptive or maladaptive) is one important factor that affects adolescents' psychological reactions to persistent pain problems.

For some adolescents, the emotional response to pain can be significant and associated with problematic levels of depressive or anxiety symptoms. Adolescents are at a vulnerable age for the development of mood problems in general, as depression tends to increase during this developmental period. The lifetime prevalence of depression in adolescents is 20 % based on findings from the National Longitudinal Study of Adolescent Health (Rushton, Forcier, & Schectman, 2002). Lifetime prevalence of anxiety disorders in the general population of children and adolescents ranges from 9.9 to 13 % (Costello, Mustillo, Erkanli, Keeler, & Angold, 2003; Shaffer et al., 1996). With the addition of a chronic medical problem, the risk for depression and anxiety may increase. In fact, studies have found increased depressive symptoms (Conte, Walco, & Kimura, 2003; Walker, Garber, & Greene, 1993) and generalized anxiety (Conte et al., 2003; Walker et al., 1993) among youth with chronic pain. In a US study investigating abdominal pain and depression in a representative sample of adolescents aged 13–18 years (Youssef, Atienza, Langseder, & Strauss, 2008), 16 % reported significant depressive symptoms based on a screening tool with clinical cutoffs to define cases of depression. The rate of depressive symptoms was significantly higher for adolescents having daily abdominal pain compared to those who experience it rarely (45 vs. 3.2 %). In a Dutch clinical sample of youth with unexplained chronic pain, the prevalence of comorbid psychiatric disorders was estimated using structured diagnostic interviews with parents and psychiatrists' clinical interviews with patients (Knook et al., 2011). Combining these two sources and using an impairment criterion, 35 % of the youth with chronic pain suffered from a DSM-IV psychiatric disorder. Anxiety disorders were diagnosed nearly as frequently (17.9 %) as depressive disorders (19.1 %) (Knook et al., 2011). The prevalence of concurrent psychiatric disorders is quite striking for adolescents diagnosed with fibromyalgia. In a clinical sample, 67.1 % of adolescents with fibromyalgia had a current DSM-IV diagnosis based on a semi-structured diagnostic interview, and 71.5 % had a lifetime diagnosis (Kashikar-Zuck, Parkins, et al., 2008). Current anxiety disorders were diagnosed more frequently (57.5 %) compared to mood disorders (22.0 %). Unfortunately, not only can anxiety and depression be a response to pain, but common shared brain structures and neurotransmitters, specifically norepinephrine and serotonin which are implicated in the mood–pain connection (Gatchel, 2004), may result in neurobiological changes that maintain both chronic mood and/or pain problems over time (Maletic & Raison, 2009).

Consideration of emotional factors has been found to be important for predicting the long-term trajectories of pain patients through the adolescent years. In a Canadian national sample of youth followed from ages 10–11 to 18–19 years, internalizing symptoms (anxiety/depression) at age 10–11 years predicted persistent high levels of pain at age 18–19, as well as increasing pain severity for headaches, abdominal pain, and back pain over the adolescent years (Stanford, Chambers, Biesanz, & Chen, 2008). Not all research, however, has found that children and adolescents with chronic pain suffer from significant emotional problems (e.g., Kashikar-Zuck, Goldschneider, Powers, Vaught, & Hershey, 2001; Reid, Lang, & McGrath, 1997). The ability to clarify why some adolescents with chronic pain develop mood problems and others do not is important for appropriate treatment planning. One potentially differentiating factor is the degree to which pain disrupts daily functioning and results in the inability to complete expected adolescent roles. Functional disability is characterized by the interruption in psychosocial functioning and physical activities due to pain symptoms (Walker & Greene, 1991). Impairments can occur in the domains of school attendance, academic performance, social life, athletic participation, and family expectations. Psychological factors may be the best predictors of pain-related functional disability (Kashikar-Zuck et al., 2001;

Lynch, Kashikar-Zuck, Goldschneider, & Jones, 2006), more so than actual physical damage or pain intensity. Among children and adolescents with chronic pain, depression has been repeatedly found to be strongly associated with and/or a predictor of functional disability (Balague et al., 1995; Claar & Walker, 2006; Gauntlett-Gilbert & Eccleston, 2007; Kashikar-Zuck et al., 2001; Reid et al., 1997). There is some evidence to suggest that this association may be more salient for girls, but not boys (Kaczynski, Claar, & Logan, 2009). Increased depressive symptoms also have been found to correlate with impaired school functioning (absences, school adjustment, scholastic competence, and grade decline) (Logan, Simons, & Kaczynski, 2009).

Overall, results from these studies strongly implicate the role of coping, psychological adjustment, and mood as being an integral aspect of the pain experience in adolescents. These psychological factors clearly contribute to impairments in functioning and must be properly assessed and treated in a comprehensive manner.

Social and Environmental Factors

The third aspect of the biopsychosocial model emphasizes the importance of the social environment and its impact on the pain experience. Since pain itself is invisible, adolescents must communicate about their pain in some overt form. Their expressions of pain in turn elicit responses from those in their immediate social environment (e.g., parents, teachers, and friends) which further influences the adolescents' experience of pain and their response to the pain.

Communication of the pain experience is typically done via pain behaviors, which are observable ways of showing pain (Fordyce, Fowler, & DeLateur, 1968; Tesler, Holzemer, & Savedra, 1998) and may be verbal (e.g., complaining, groaning) and/or nonverbal (e.g., limping, wincing, holding area of pain) (Revicki et al., 2009). Research examining the role of pain behavior in adolescents with chronic pain has shown that increased pain behaviors are related to depressive symptoms, functional disability, pain catastrophizing, and poor quality of life (Lynch-Jordan, Kashikar-Zuck, & Goldschneider, 2010), suggesting that persistent expressions of pain may keep adolescents focused on their symptoms. On the other hand, pain behaviors may also be an instrumental method of obtaining reassurance, intervention, or social support from others such as their caregivers (e.g., Hamers, Abu-Saad, van den Hout, Halfens, & Kester, 1996).

Parents are the primary caretakers of adolescents with chronic pain, and a great deal of research has focused on parental influences. Parents must make a host of decisions about how to respond to their adolescents' symptoms, such as whether or not to give pain medications, send them to school, or exempt them from chores when they are in pain. Palermo and Chambers (Palermo & Chambers, 2005) provided an excellent review in which they highlighted the complex interactive effects of family level variables on pediatric pain and accompanying functional disability. They noted that parent behaviors may both reward and discourage active coping in youth with pain. Reinforcement of poor functioning has been described as "illness behavior encouragement" or "solicitousness" and may have negative consequences for the adolescents who are recipients of this parenting style. Among children with chronic abdominal pain, mothers who self-described as "highly protective" had children with greater healthcare utilization and higher medical costs for gastrointestinal symptom management compared to mothers described as less protective (Walker, Levy, & Whitehead, 2006). In a study investigating a behavioral treatment intervention for headache, children who experienced more maternal rewarding of pain behaviors showed less improvement in headache reduction after treatment and at 1-year follow-up (Osterhaus, Lange, Linssen, & Passchier, 1997). Thus, some evidence suggests that children experience poorer outcomes with a parenting style that may undermine adaptive coping.

It is unclear, however, if solicitous behavior is uniformly associated with negative outcomes. Wall, Holden, and Gladstein (1996) studied parent responses to pain among children with headaches. Interestingly, higher levels of child-perceived parental solicitousness were correlated with fewer behavior problems (Wall et al., 1996). In another study of children with abdominal pain, Walker, Claar, and Garber (2002) hypothesized that parental responses would differentially affect pain symptoms, depending on the child's perceived self-worth and competence. As expected, children reporting lower global self-worth and academic competence showed more somatic symptoms at follow-up when receiving positive parental attention to symptoms. However, no such differences were noted for children with higher self-worth and academic competence, implying resilience to the sometimes negative influence of this parenting style. Similarly, higher levels of parental negative attention were associated with more symptoms at follow-up but only for children with low self-worth (Walker et al., 2002). In a different study, parent solicitousness was related to increased functional disability only among children with higher depression and anxiety. However, this relationship did not hold true for children with lower psychological distress (anxiety or depression) (Peterson & Palermo, 2004). Results from both of these studies provided evidence that parental responses to child pain may interact with individual personality characteristics to produce differential results and that solicitous behavior does not always produce a negative effect on children and adolescents with pain.

In keeping with findings about chronic pain clustering in families (Arnold et al., 2004; Buskila et al., 1993; Groholt, Stigum, Nordhagen, & Kohler, 2003; Merlijn et al., 2003), parents of adolescents with chronic pain often suffer from chronic pain themselves. When two family members share problems with chronic pain, the parent's ability to cope with their own health problems can have an impact on adolescent coping via social modeling. A parent who is receiving disability benefits due to pain, uses medication or other passive pain management strategies, and rarely engages in physical activity provides a much different model of coping compared to the parent who maintains but adjusts normal activities for pain, uses a variety of behavioral and life-style coping strategies, and rarely complains about health issues. A family pain history has been linked to offspring functional status and disability levels. Parents showing increased pain behaviors, disability, and distress tend to have children with more pain complaints (Jamison & Walker, 1992). Children having a parent with chronic pain report increased pain intensity and frequency (Jamison & Walker, 1992), greater pain-related impairment (Schanberg, Keefe, Lefebvre, Kredich, & Gil, 1998), more medication management of pain (Jamison & Walker, 1992), increased illness behaviors, greater school absences, and more visits to the nurses' office (Rickard, 1988) compared to offspring of healthy parents or parents with a non-pain chronic illness. Children with medically unexplained chronic pain identified more pain models in their environment and more reinforcing consequences to their pain than children with disease-related pain (Osborne, Hatcher, & Richtsmeier, 1989). These findings collectively reinforce the importance of environmental contributions to the expression of pain, whereby the manner in which parents cope and respond to adolescents' symptoms is as important as the shared genetic vulnerability for pain in the family.

The area of social adjustment and peer relationships of youth with chronic pain has received less empirical attention. In one Dutch study of children and adolescents with chronic pain, 40 % of youth reported impairment in social relationships (changed or less contact with peers) (Konijnenberg et al., 2005). Similar social problems have been noted in other pediatric studies of chronic pain (Kashikar-Zuck et al., 2007; Merlijn et al., 2003), but not all youth with chronic pain show substantial peer problems (Gauntlett-Gilbert & Eccleston, 2007; Guite, Logan, Sherry, & Rose, 2007). It is possible that for some adolescents, social reputation and adjustment may deteriorate over time secondary to pain-related school absences, mood problems, and fewer interpersonal interactions in class. In one study, poor social functioning was predicted by adolescents' reported functional disability and depressive symptoms but also by dysfunctional parent–child interactions (Gauntlett-Gilbert &

Eccleston, 2007). Thus, pain severe enough to disrupt daily functioning and mood may be more likely to have a broader social impact when accompanied by poor parent–child relationships.

Summary of the Biopsychosocial Model in Adolescent Pain. The biopsychosocial model illustrates the importance of considering more than the underlying disease process or pathology of chronic pain and highlights the contributions of adolescents' coping, psychological adjustment, and social environment. For these reasons, current treatment approaches to chronic pain in adolescents are multidisciplinary and include medication management (to reduce pain symptoms); psychological treatments such as cognitive behavioral therapy (CBT), biofeedback, hypnosis, and relaxation training (to modify the thoughts, feelings, and behaviors associated with chronic pain); and exercise-based interventions (to improve physical function and return to usual activities).

Common Chronic Pain Conditions

Three common pain conditions were selected as exemplars of adolescent chronic pain for further review because these are some of the most frequently seen in health care settings (e.g., Lynch-Jordan et al., 2010).

Recurrent Abdominal Pain

The criteria for diagnosing RAP were initially outlined by John Apley (Apley & Naish, 1958) and required at least three episodes of abdominal pain of sufficient intensity to impair functioning within a 3-month period of time. Recent work has attempted to classify youth with RAP into subtypes (e.g., IBS, functional dyspepsia, functional gastrointestinal disorders, and abdominal migraine) using a pediatric-derived version of the adult Rome criteria (Walker et al., 2004). However, RAP remains the most frequently used term to describe all types of RAP syndromes without clear medical etiology.

Most epidemiological studies report a peak prevalence of abdominal pain by about 10 years of age, with a steady decline thereafter (Apley & Naish, 1958; Chitkara, Rawat, & Talley, 2005; Oster, 1972). Females are more likely to experience RAP (Chitkara et al., 2005; Goodman & McGrath, 1991; Oster, 1972; Perquin et al., 2000; Stanford et al., 2008), particularly in the adolescent years (Goodman & McGrath, 1991; Perquin et al., 2000). Studies on younger children have typically found comparable rates of RAP among boys and girls, suggesting the importance of puberty on the divergence in prevalence by gender (Chitkara et al., 2005).

Like other pain conditions, RAP is frequently reported within family members. Apley and Naish (1958) found that children with chronic abdominal pain were significantly more likely to have other family members with RAP, along with a higher likelihood of family members with peptic ulcer, migraines, and emotional problems. This link between child and parent abdominal pain has been replicated in other studies (Groholt et al., 2003; Oster, 1972). RAP is also more likely to occur in patients from lower socioeconomic levels (Groholt et al., 2003) and in youth with more negative life events (Liakopoulou-Kairis et al., 2002). A prospective, longitudinal study of English children found that being diagnosed with RAP at age 6 was predicted by early life maternal (anxiety, somatic, depression, pain symptoms) and paternal (anxiety) factors and that maternal anxiety and child temperament were the strongest predictors of later RAP (Ramchandani, Stein, Hotopf, & Wiles, 2006).

Common symptoms associated with RAP are diarrhea, nausea, constipation, vomiting, fatigue, headache, and other body pains (Apley & Naish, 1958; Chitkara et al., 2005; Huertas-Ceballos, Logan, Bennett, & Macarthur, 2008; Kokkonen, Haapalahti, Tikkanen, Karttunen, & Savilahti, 2004). Due to the heterogeneity of symptoms, a myriad of mechanisms have been hypothesized to underlie RAP such as lactose intolerance, food allergies, fiber-deficient diets, and infections (such as H. pylori) (Huertas-Ceballos et al., 2008). Additional risk factors that have been associated with RAP are short duration of breastfeeding and colic in infancy, as well as the presence of atopic (e.g., asthma, atopic dermatitis) and chronic diseases (Kokkonen et al., 2004). While there appears to be relatively little consensus about the underlying physiological factors, there is converging evidence that psychological factors, particularly anxiety, contribute substantially to the presence of RAP (Apley & Naish, 1958; Campo et al., 2004; Chitkara et al., 2005; Huertas-Ceballos et al., 2008; Stanford et al., 2008). Apley's initial work found children with RAP to have more fears and sleep problems than pain-free children. They were described as significantly more "high-strung, excitable, and anxious" in their temperament (Apley & Naish, 1958). Among adolescents in middle and high school with IBS-like symptoms and pain, anxious personality traits and depressive symptoms were more frequently reported compared to peers without these symptoms. Higher anxiety scores were also correlated with increased pain intensity, frequency, and duration (Hyams et al., 1996). Additionally, youth with RAP presenting to primary care were more likely to be diagnosed with an anxiety or depressive disorder and have increased internalizing symptoms compared to pain-free control peers (Campo et al., 2004).

Treatment for RAP is usually begun after medical causes have been thoroughly investigated and ruled out. The physician needs to first reassure the family that no further medical tests are warranted and that it is important to focus on managing symptoms and resuming engagement in usual daily activities without fear of aggravating the condition. The rationale for how the original trigger for the pain may not be identifiable but that pain can take on "a life of its own" should be explained to the family. This understanding sets the stage for the introduction of behavioral and self-management approaches that have been found to be the cornerstone of successful treatment for RAP (Huertas-Ceballos et al., 2008; Robins, Smith, Glutting, & Bishop, 2005).

Back Pain

While receiving increasing empirical attention in recent years, back pain in young people remains an enigmatic diagnosis. Many studies focus on *low* back pain without any uniform criteria as to what constitutes this diagnosis, resulting in "low back pain" being a more generic term for any back pain arising from repetitive motion or overuse, mechanical problems, or a nonspecific origin (Davis & Williams, 2008). Review articles report a variety of prevalence rates (lifetime, point, chronic/recurrent) in youth (Balague, Troussier, & Salminen, 1999). As noted in the first section of this chapter, back pain in children and adolescents is typically limited, resolves independently, and is unlikely to require medical attention (Jones & Macfarlane, 2005). A relatively small proportion report recurrent or chronic symptoms (Balague et al., 1999).

Similar to other pain conditions, females appear more likely to experience back pain (Balague et al., 1999; Salminen et al., 1992; Troussier, Davoine, de Gaudemaris, Fauconnier, & Phelip, 1994; Viry et al., 1999) and also may be more likely to seek medical intervention for their pain (Jones, Stratton, Reilly, & Unnithan, 2004; Viry et al., 1999). There is a strong relationship between back pain and age (Balague et al., 1999), with the lifetime and recurrent prevalence rates significantly higher with advancement through adolescence (Jones et al., 2004; Taimela et al., 1997), again implicating this developmental period as a relative risk for the onset of pain problems. Adolescents with back pain tend to live in families where parents also have increased risk for back pain (Balague et al., 1995; Sjolie, 2002).

It is rare that severe underlying pathology (e.g., tumor) is found to explain adolescent back pain (Davis & Williams, 2008). Several structural changes can cause these pain problems, including spondylolysis (stress fracture of vertebrae) and spondylolisthesis (shifted vertebrae), curvature of the spine (including scoliosis or kyphosis), and disc degeneration whereby the discs between the vertebrae either bulge or break open and may press on nearby nerve roots causing pain, numbness, or tingling (Davis & Williams, 2008). Causes of these structural changes can be as benign as the normal wear and tear on the body due to repetitive "micro-trauma" through participation in athletics (Davis & Williams, 2008). Often, back pain is "nonspecific," meaning diagnostic tests can find no medical origin for symptoms. Unfortunately, the resulting limitations in physical functioning and lack of exercise can further decondition the body, resulting in persistent muscle tightness and spasms, poor posture, and compensatory body positioning that can perpetuate the pain (Davis & Williams, 2008).

Studies of risk factors for back pain have ranged from looking at body measures (height, weight, BMI) to psychological problems. Participation in competitive sports has been linked to low back pain (Balague et al., 1999; Kovacs et al., 2003), but many factors such as type of sports, level of competition, and intensity make a difference (Balague et al., 1999). Some studies have shown a link between back pain and carrying heavy schoolbags (Viry et al., 1999), but this finding has not been replicated. Youth with poorer emotional well-being (Sjolie, 2002), greater behavior problems (Jones, Watson, Silman, Symmons, & Macfarlane, 2003), and greater negative affect (Balague et al., 1995) show increased odds of having back pain. A few studies have reported a relationship between TV watching and back pain (Balague et al., 1995; Troussier et al., 1994). Presumably, engaging in increased sedentary behavior can lead to deconditioning and muscle weakness. This finding is intriguing given that current adolescent hobbies often include computer use and playing videogames for long periods of time. A school-based study of adolescents aged 12–16 years found no link between back, neck, or arm pain and computer use (Diepenmaat, van der Wal, de Vet, & Hirasing, 2006), while computer activities (such as using a joystick) or playing noneducational computer games was predictive of physical discomfort in a sample of youth from grades 1 to 12 (Burke & Peper, 2002). Few studies have investigated this topic, and more studies are needed in this area given the abundance of electronics and increasingly sedentary activities of adolescents.

Treatment for chronic back pain is frequently multidisciplinary in nature and takes a rehabilitation approach, including medications (nonsteroidal anti-inflammatory drugs, muscle relaxants), physical therapy and exercise, brace treatment, restriction or modification of activity, and behavioral medicine interventions (relaxation, distraction, cognitive therapy) (Davis & Williams, 2008). For adults with chronic pain, CBT shows positive effects on pain relief and physical functioning across multiple studies (Henschke et al., 2010; Hoffman, Papas, Chatkoff, & Kerns, 2007; van Tulder et al., 2001), although similar studies have not been done in the pediatric back pain population.

Widespread Musculoskeletal Pain/Fibromyalgia

In the literature, widespread pain conditions have been referred to by a variety of names including nonspecific or idiopathic musculoskeletal pain, juvenile fibromyalgia, or fibromyalgia syndrome. The cardinal feature of these syndromes is diffuse musculoskeletal pain in multiple body sites (three or more) for the duration of at least 3 months, as well as numerous painful tender points. The diagnosis of fibromyalgia syndrome in adults follows the American College of Rheumatology (ACR) criteria (Wolfe et al., 1990), while Yunus and Masi (1985) proposed different guidelines for children with juvenile fibromyalgia (JFM) emphasizing a constellation of associated symptoms in addition to diffuse pain based on the observation that adolescents may have fewer painful tender points than adults. Diagnosis is made based on physical examination and a tender point examination of 18 symmetric points on the upper and lower body that identifies sensitivity with palpation (Burckhardt et al., 2005). Youth with JFM show much lower thresholds for pain sensitivity compared to their healthy peers (Reid et al., 1997). Like other chronic pain conditions, diagnostic and laboratory tests are usually negative (Gedalia, Garcia, Molina, Bradford, & Espinoza, 2000; Reid et al., 1997). Sleep disturbance, fatigue, stiffness, and headaches are frequent comorbid symptoms (Gedalia et al., 2000; Reid et al., 1997; Siegel, Janeway, & Baum, 1998).

JFM is predominantly diagnosed in females (Gedalia et al., 2000; Siegel et al., 1998) during their adolescent years although onset of symptoms often occurs several years prior to diagnosis (Gedalia et al., 2000). Longitudinal studies of youth with fibromyalgia suggest that symptoms persist over time (Kashikar-Zuck et al., 2010; Malleson, al-Matar, & Petty, 1992; Siegel et al., 1998), even if all fibromyalgia criteria are not specifically met at follow-up assessments (Mikkelsson, 1999). Family studies have shown an aggregation of this syndrome in family members (Arnold et al., 2004; Buskila & Neumann, 1997), and adolescents diagnosed with JFM are more likely to have a parent diagnosed with fibromyalgia or another chronic pain condition (Kashikar-Zuck, Lynch, et al., 2008; Schanberg et al., 1998).

The impact of fibromyalgia on daily functioning and mood is significant, and adolescents with JFM report greater disability and poorer coping compared to healthy adolescents as well as those with other types of chronic pain (Kashikar-Zuck et al., 2001; Reid et al., 1997). Socially, these youth are viewed by their peers as more sensitive and isolated, are less well liked, and have fewer reciprocated friendships (Kashikar-Zuck et al., 2007). Symptoms of anxiety and depression are commonly present, compared to children and adolescents who are healthy or have other chronic medical conditions (Conte et al., 2003; Kashikar-Zuck, Lynch, et al., 2008). Using structured psychiatric interviews, one study found that over 70 % of adolescents with JFM met criteria for a lifetime DSM-IV diagnosis, with anxiety disorders (e.g., panic disorder, social phobia) most prevalent as a current or lifetime diagnosis (Kashikar-Zuck, Parkins, et al., 2008). Like their pain symptoms, psychiatric issues also appear to linger in adolescents diagnosed with juvenile-onset fibromyalgia. In a follow-up study of older adolescents (mean age 19) previously diagnosed with JFM, the youth continued to report significantly more symptoms of anxiety and depression than their matched healthy control peers (Kashikar-Zuck et al., 2010). Thus, comorbid psychiatric issues present a distinct vulnerability for adolescents coping with the board spectrum of symptoms encompassed by JFM.

Treatment for JFM has received little attention, and guidelines are generally derived from the treatment of adult patients with fibromyalgia (Burckhardt et al., 2005). The consensus for best outcomes appears to be a combination of pharmacological, physical, and psychological therapies (Burckhardt et al., 2005). Medication management usually includes low-dose tricyclic antidepressants to address sleep and pain, while selective serotonin reuptake inhibitors (SSRIs) may be prescribed to manage depression or other mood problems. Aerobic exercise is frequently recommended to prevent deconditioning and muscle weakness that could exacerbate pain intensity (Burckhardt et al., 2005). Cognitive behavioral interventions focus on enhancing pain coping skills and reducing functional disability. Two small-scale CBT studies showed promising results (Degotardi et al., 2006; Kashikar-Zuck, Swain, Jones, & Graham, 2005), and one recently completed randomized clinical trial showed that CBT is an effective treatment which resulted in significantly improved functioning and reduction in depressive symptoms (Kashikar-Zuck et al., 2012).

In this section, we discussed three of the more common chronic pain conditions in adolescents. Although the clinical presentation and associated symptoms vary, each of these conditions has been associated with significant impact on adolescents' daily functioning as well as changes in their emotional functioning. When viewed in the context of the biopsychosocial model, it is clear that there is a complex and bidirectional relationship between pain vulnerability, pain expression, adaptation to pain, and environmental factors that determine the ultimate experience of chronic pain for adolescents. It is only with continuing attention to the special developmental circumstances of this life stage including ongoing development of nervous systems, hormonal changes, family and peer relationships, and broader lifestyle factors that we can more fully explain the causes and maintenance of persistent symptoms and develop the best treatments for youth with chronic pain.

References

Apley, J., & Naish, N. (1958). Recurrent abdominal pains: A field survey of 1,000 school children. *Archives of Disease in Childhood, 33*(168), 165–170.

Arnold, L. M., Hudson, J. I., Hess, E. V., Ware, A. E., Fritz, D. A., Auchenbach, M. B., et al. (2004). Family study of fibromyalgia. *Arthritis and Rheumatism, 50*(3), 944–952.

Balague, F., Skovron, M. L., Nordin, M., Dutoit, G., Pol, L. R., & Waldburger, M. (1995). Low back pain in schoolchildren. A study of familial and psychological factors. *Spine, 20*(11), 1265–1270.

Balague, F., Troussier, B., & Salminen, J. J. (1999). Nonspecific low back pain in children and adolescents: Risk factors. *European Spine Journal, 8*(6), 429–438.

Bradley, L., Haile, J., & Jaworski, T. (1992). Assessment of psychological status using interviews and self-report instruments. In D. C. Turk & R. Melzack (Eds.), *Handbook of pain assessment* (pp. 193–213). New York: Guilford.

Burckhardt, C. S., Goldenberg, D. L., Crofford, L. J., Gerwin, R., Gowans, S., Jackson, K., et al. (2005). *Guidelines for the management of fibromyalgia syndrome pain in adults and children* (APS clinical practice guideline series, Vol. 4). Glenview, IL: American Pain Society.

Burke, A., & Peper, E. (2002). Cumulative trauma disorder risk for children using computer products: Results of a pilot investigation with a student convenience sample. *Public Health Reports, 117*(4), 350–357.

Burton, A. K., Clarke, R. D., McClune, T. D., & Tillotson, K. M. (1996). The natural history of low back pain in adolescents. *Spine (Phila Pa 1976), 21*(20), 2323–2328.

Buskila, D., & Neumann, L. (1997). Fibromyalgia syndrome (FM) and nonarticular tenderness in relatives of patients with FM. *Journal of Rheumatology, 24*(5), 941–944.

Buskila, D., Press, J., Gedalia, A., Klein, M., Neumann, L., Boehm, R., et al. (1993). Assessment of nonarticular tenderness and prevalence of fibromyalgia in children. *Journal of Rheumatology, 20*(2), 368–370.

Campbell, C. M., & Edwards, R. R. (2009). Mind-body interactions in pain: The neurophysiology of anxious and catastrophic pain-related thoughts. *Translational Research, 153*(3), 97–101.

Campo, J. V., Bridge, J., Ehmann, M., Altman, S., Lucas, A., Birmaher, B., et al. (2004). Recurrent abdominal pain, anxiety, and depression in primary care. *Pediatrics, 113*(4), 817–824.

Chitkara, D. K., Rawat, D. J., & Talley, N. J. (2005). The epidemiology of childhood recurrent abdominal pain in Western countries: A systematic review. *The American Journal of Gastroenterology, 100*(8), 1868–1875.

Claar, R. L., Baber, K. F., Simons, L. E., Logan, D. E., & Walker, L. S. (2008). Pain coping profiles in adolescents with chronic pain. *Pain, 140*(2), 368–375.

Claar, R. L., & Walker, L. S. (2006). Functional assessment of pediatric pain patients: Psychometric properties of the functional disability inventory. *Pain, 121*(1–2), 77–84.

Conte, P. M., Walco, G. A., & Kimura, Y. (2003). Temperament and stress response in children with juvenile primary fibromyalgia syndrome. *Arthritis and Rheumatism, 48*(10), 2923–2930.

Costello, E. J., Mustillo, S., Erkanli, A., Keeler, G., & Angold, A. (2003). Prevalence and development of psychiatric disorders in childhood and adolescence. *Archives of General Psychiatry, 60*(8), 837–844.

Crombez, G., Bijttebier, P., Eccleston, C., Mascagni, T., Mertens, G., Goubert, L., et al. (2003). The child version of the pain catastrophizing scale (PCS-C): A preliminary validation. *Pain, 104*(3), 639–646.

Davis, P. J., & Williams, H. J. (2008). The investigation and management of back pain in children. *Archives of Disease in Childhood. Education and Practice Edition, 93*(3), 73–83.

De Inocencio, J. (2004). Epidemiology of musculoskeletal pain in primary care. *Archives of Disease in Childhood, 89*(5), 431–434.

Degotardi, P. J., Klass, E. S., Rosenberg, B. S., Fox, D. G., Gallelli, K. A., & Gottlieb, B. S. (2006). Development and evaluation of a cognitive-behavioral intervention for juvenile fibromyalgia. *Journal of Pediatric Psychology, 31*(7), 714–723.

Diepenmaat, A. C., van der Wal, M. F., de Vet, H. C., & Hirasing, R. A. (2006). Neck/shoulder, low back, and arm pain in relation to computer use, physical activity, stress, and depression among Dutch adolescents. *Pediatrics, 117*(2), 412–416.

Engel, G. L. (1977). The need for a new medical model: A challenge for biomedicine. *Science, 196*(4286), 129–136.

Fordyce, W. E., Fowler, R. S., & DeLateur, B. (1968). An application of behavior modification technique to a problem of chronic pain. *Behaviour Research and Therapy, 6*(1), 105–107.

Gatchel, R. J. (2004). Comorbidity of chronic pain and mental health disorders: The biopsychosocial perspective. *The American Psychologist, 59*(8), 795–805.

Gatchel, R. J., Peng, Y. B., Peters, M. L., Fuchs, P. N., & Turk, D. C. (2007). The biopsychosocial approach to chronic pain: Scientific advances and future directions. *Psychological Bulletin, 133*(4), 581–624.

Gauntlett-Gilbert, J., & Eccleston, C. (2007). Disability in adolescents with chronic pain: Patterns and predictors across different domains of functioning. *Pain, 131*(1–2), 132–141.

Gedalia, A., Garcia, C. O., Molina, J. F., Bradford, N. J., & Espinoza, L. R. (2000). Fibromyalgia syndrome: Experience in a pediatric rheumatology clinic. *Clinical and Experimental Rheumatology, 18*(3), 415–419.

Goodman, J. E., & McGrath, P. J. (1991). The epidemiology of pain in children and adolescents: A review. *Pain, 46*(3), 247–264.

Gracely, R. H., Geisser, M. E., Giesecke, T., Grant, M. A., Petzke, F., Williams, D. A., et al. (2004). Pain catastro-

phizing and neural responses to pain among persons with fibromyalgia. *Brain, 127*(Pt 4), 835–843.
Gracely, R. H., McGrath, P., & Dubner, R. (1978). Validity and sensitivity of ratio scales of sensory and affective verbal pain descriptors: Manipulation of affect by diazepam. *Pain, 5*(1), 19–29.
Groholt, E. K., Stigum, H., Nordhagen, R., & Kohler, L. (2003). Recurrent pain in children, socio-economic factors and accumulation in families. *European Journal of Epidemiology, 18*(10), 965–975.
Guite, J. W., Logan, D. E., Sherry, D. D., & Rose, J. B. (2007). Adolescent self-perception: Associations with chronic musculoskeletal pain and functional disability. *The Journal of Pain, 8*(5), 379–386.
Hamers, J. P., Abu-Saad, H. H., van den Hout, M. A., Halfens, R. J., & Kester, A. D. (1996). The influence of children's vocal expressions, age, medical diagnosis and information obtained from parents on nurses' pain assessments and decisions regarding interventions. *Pain, 65*(1), 53–61.
Henschke, N., Ostelo, R. W. J. G., van Tulder, M. W., Vlaeyen, J. W. S., Morley, S., Assendelft, W. J. J., & Main, C. J. (2010). Behavioural treatment for chronic low-back pain. *Cochrane Database of Systematic Reviews, 7*, CD002014. doi:10.1002/14651858.CD002014.pub3.
Hodgins, M. J., & Lander, J. (1997). Children's coping with venipuncture. *Journal of Pain and Symptom Management, 13*(5), 274–285.
Hoffman, B. M., Papas, R. K., Chatkoff, D. K., & Kerns, R. D. (2007). Meta-analysis of psychological interventions for chronic low back pain. *Health Psychology, 26*(1), 1–9.
Holden, E. W., Gladstein, J., Trulsen, M., & Wall, B. (1994). Chronic daily headache in children and adolescents. *Headache, 34*(9), 508–514.
Huertas-Ceballos, A. A., Logan, S., Bennett, C., & Macarthur, C. (2008). Psychosocial interventions for recurrent abdominal pain (RAP) and irritable bowel syndrome (IBS) in childhood. *Cochrane Database of Systematic Reviews, 1*, CD003014. doi:10.1002/14651858.CD003014.pub2.
Huguet, A., & Miro, J. (2008). The severity of chronic pediatric pain: An epidemiological study. *The Journal of Pain, 9*(3), 226–236.
Hyams, J. S., Burke, G., Davis, P. M., Rzepski, B., & Andrulonis, P. A. (1996). Abdominal pain and irritable bowel syndrome in adolescents: A community-based study. *Journal of Pediatrics, 129*(2), 220–226.
Jamison, R. N., & Walker, L. S. (1992). Illness behavior in children of chronic pain patients. *International Journal of Psychiatry in Medicine, 22*(4), 329–342.
Jones, G. T., & Macfarlane, G. J. (2005). Epidemiology of low back pain in children and adolescents. *Archives of Disease in Childhood, 90*(3), 312–316.
Jones, M. A., Stratton, G., Reilly, T., & Unnithan, V. B. (2004). A school-based survey of recurrent non-specific low-back pain prevalence and consequences in children. *Health Education Research, 19*(3), 284–289.
Jones, G. T., Watson, K. D., Silman, A. J., Symmons, D. P., & Macfarlane, G. J. (2003). Predictors of low back pain in British schoolchildren: A population-based prospective cohort study. *Pediatrics, 111*(4 Pt 1), 822–828.
Kaczynski, K. J., Claar, R. L., & Logan, D. E. (2009). Testing gender as a moderator of associations between psychosocial variables and functional disability in children and adolescents with chronic pain. *Journal of Pediatric Psychology, 34*(7), 738–748.
Kashikar-Zuck, S., Goldschneider, K. R., Powers, S. W., Vaught, M. H., & Hershey, A. D. (2001). Depression and functional disability in chronic pediatric pain. *The Clinical Journal of Pain, 17*(4), 341–349.
Kashikar-Zuck, S., Lynch, A. M., Graham, T. B., Swain, N. F., Mullen, S. M., & Noll, R. B. (2007). Social functioning and peer relationships of adolescents with juvenile fibromyalgia syndrome. *Arthritis and Rheumatism, 57*(3), 474–480.
Kashikar-Zuck, S., Lynch, A. M., Slater, S., Graham, T. B., Swain, N. F., & Noll, R. B. (2008). Family factors, emotional functioning, and functional impairment in juvenile fibromyalgia syndrome. *Arthritis and Rheumatism, 59*(10), 1392–1398.
Kashikar-Zuck, S., Parkins, I. S., Graham, T. B., Lynch, A. M., Passo, M., Johnston, M., et al. (2008). Anxiety, mood, and behavioral disorders among pediatric patients with juvenile fibromyalgia syndrome. *The Clinical Journal of Pain, 24*(7), 620–626.
Kashikar-Zuck, S., Parkins, I. S., Ting, T. V., Verkamp, E., Lynch-Jordan, A., Passo, M., et al. (2010). Controlled follow-up study of physical and psychosocial functioning of adolescents with juvenile primary fibromyalgia syndrome. *Rheumatology (Oxford, England), 49*(11), 2204–2209.
Kashikar-Zuck, S., Swain, N. F., Jones, B. A., & Graham, T. B. (2005). Efficacy of cognitive-behavioral intervention for juvenile primary fibromyalgia syndrome. *Journal of Rheumatology, 32*(8), 1594–1602.
Kashikar-Zuck, S., Ting, T. V., Arnold, L. M., Bean, J., Powers, S. W., Graham, T. B., et al. (2012). A randomized clinical trial of cognitive behavioral therapy for the treatment of juvenile fibromyalgia. *Arthritis and Rheumatism, 64*(1), 297–305.
Knook, L. M., Konijnenberg, A. Y., van der Hoeven, J., Kimpen, J. L., Buitelaar, J. K., van Engeland, H., et al. (2011). Psychiatric disorders in children and adolescents presenting with unexplained chronic pain: What is the prevalence and clinical relevancy? *European Child & Adolescent Psychiatry, 20*(1), 39–48.
Kokkonen, J., Haapalahti, M., Tikkanen, S., Karttunen, R., & Savilahti, E. (2004). Gastrointestinal complaints and diagnosis in children: A population-based study. *Acta Paediatrica, 93*(7), 880–886.
Konijnenberg, A. Y., Uiterwaal, C. S., Kimpen, J. L., van der Hoeven, J., Buitelaar, J. K., & de Graeff-Meeder, E. R. (2005). Children with unexplained chronic pain: Substantial impairment in everyday life. *Archives of Disease in Childhood, 90*(7), 680–686.

Kovacs, F. M., Gestoso, M., Gil del Real, M. T., Lopez, J., Mufraggi, N., & Mendez, J. I. (2003). Risk factors for non-specific low back pain in schoolchildren and their parents: A population based study. *Pain, 103*(3), 259–268.

Latremoliere, A., & Woolf, C. J. (2009). Central sensitization: A generator of pain hypersensitivity by central neural plasticity. *The Journal of Pain, 10*(9), 895–926.

Lee, M. C., & Tracey, I. (2010). Unravelling the mystery of pain, suffering, and relief with brain imaging. *Current Pain and Headache Reports, 14*(2), 124–131.

Liakopoulou-Kairis, M., Alifieraki, T., Protagora, D., Korpa, T., Kondyli, K., Dimosthenous, E., et al. (2002). Recurrent abdominal pain and headache—psychopathology, life events and family functioning. *European Child & Adolescent Psychiatry, 11*(3), 115–122.

Logan, D. E., Simons, L. E., & Kaczynski, K. J. (2009). School functioning in adolescents with chronic pain: The role of depressive symptoms in school impairment. *Journal of Pediatric Psychology, 34*(8), 882–892.

Lynch, A. M., Kashikar-Zuck, S., Goldschneider, K. R., & Jones, B. A. (2006). Psychosocial risks for disability in children with chronic back pain. *The Journal of Pain, 7*(4), 244–251.

Lynch, A. M., Kashikar-Zuck, S., Goldschneider, K. R., & Jones, B. A. (2007). Sex and age differences in coping styles among children with chronic pain. *Journal of Pain and Symptom Management, 33*(2), 208–216.

Lynch-Jordan, A. M., Kashikar-Zuck, S., & Goldschneider, K. R. (2010). Parent perceptions of adolescent pain expression: The adolescent pain behavior questionnaire. *Pain, 151*(3), 834–842.

Maletic, V., & Raison, C. L. (2009). Neurobiology of depression, fibromyalgia and neuropathic pain. *Frontiers in Bioscience, 14*, 5291–5338.

Malleson, P. N., al-Matar, M., & Petty, R. E. (1992). Idiopathic musculoskeletal pain syndromes in children. *Journal of Rheumatology, 19*(11), 1786–1789.

Melzack, R. (2005). Evolution of the neuromatrix theory of pain. The Prithvi Raj Lecture: Presented at the third World Congress of World Institute of Pain, Barcelona 2004. *Pain Practice, 5*(2), 85–94.

Melzack, R., & Wall, P. D. (1965). Pain mechanisms: A new theory. *Science, 150*(699), 971–979.

Merlijn, V. P., Hunfeld, J. A., van der Wouden, J. C., Hazebroek-Kampschreur, A. A., Koes, B. W., & Passchier, J. (2003). Psychosocial factors associated with chronic pain in adolescents. *Pain, 101*(1–2), 33–43.

Merskey, H., & Bogduk, N. (Eds.). (1994). *Classification of chronic pain: Descriptions of chronic pain syndromes and definitions of pain terms* (2nd ed.). Seattle, WA: IASP Task Force on Taxonomy.

Mikkelsson, M. (1999). One year outcome of preadolescents with fibromyalgia. *Journal of Rheumatology, 26*(3), 674–682.

Mogil, J. S., Sternberg, W. F., Marek, P., Sadowski, B., Belknap, J. K., & Liebeskind, J. C. (1996). The genetics of pain and pain inhibition. *Proceedings of the National Academy of Sciences of the United States of America, 93*(7), 3048–3055.

Olsen, T. L., Anderson, R. L., Dearwater, S. R., Kriska, A. M., Cauley, J. A., Aaron, D. J., et al. (1992). The epidemiology of low back pain in an adolescent population. *American Journal of Public Health, 82*(4), 606–608.

Osborne, R. B., Hatcher, J. W., & Richtsmeier, A. J. (1989). The role of social modeling in unexplained pediatric pain. *Journal of Pediatric Psychology, 14*(1), 43–61.

Oster, J. (1972). Recurrent abdominal pain, headache and limb pains in children and adolescents. *Pediatrics, 50*, 429–436.

Osterhaus, S. O., Lange, A., Linssen, W. H., & Passchier, J. (1997). A behavioral treatment of young migrainous and nonmigrainous headache patients: Prediction of treatment success. *International Journal of Behavioral Medicine, 4*(4), 378–396.

Palermo, T. M., & Chambers, C. T. (2005). Parent and family factors in pediatric chronic pain and disability: An integrative approach. *Pain, 119*(1–3), 1–4.

Perquin, C. W., Hazebroek-Kampschreur, A. A., Hunfeld, J. A., Bohnen, A. M., van Suijlekom-Smit, L. W., Passchier, J., et al. (2000). Pain in children and adolescents: A common experience. *Pain, 87*(1), 51–58.

Perquin, C. W., Hunfeld, J. A., Hazebroek-Kampschreur, A. A., van Suijlekom-Smit, L. W., Passchier, J., Koes, B. W., et al. (2003). The natural course of chronic benign pain in childhood and adolescence: A two-year population-based follow-up study. *European Journal of Pain, 7*(6), 551–559.

Peterson, C. C., & Palermo, T. M. (2004). Parental reinforcement of recurrent pain: The moderating impact of child depression and anxiety on functional disability. *Journal of Pediatric Psychology, 29*(5), 331–341.

Ramchandani, P. G., Stein, A., Hotopf, M., & Wiles, N. J. (2006). Early parental and child predictors of recurrent abdominal pain at school age: Results of a large population-based study. *Journal of the American Academy of Child and Adolescent Psychiatry, 45*(6), 729–736.

Reid, G. J., Gilbert, C. A., & McGrath, P. J. (1998). The Pain Coping Questionnaire: Preliminary validation. *Pain, 76*(1–2), 83–96.

Reid, G. J., Lang, B. A., & McGrath, P. J. (1997). Primary juvenile fibromyalgia: Psychological adjustment, family functioning, coping, and functional disability. *Arthritis and Rheumatism, 40*(4), 752–760.

Revicki, D. A., Chen, W. H., Harnam, N., Cook, K. F., Amtmann, D., Callahan, L. F., et al. (2009). Development and psychometric analysis of the PROMIS pain behavior item bank. *Pain, 146*(1–2), 158–169.

Rickard, K. (1988). The occurrence of maladaptive health-related behaviors and teacher-rated conduct problems in children of chronic low back pain patients. *Journal of Behavioral Medicine, 11*(2), 107–116.

Robins, P. M., Smith, S. M., Glutting, J. J., & Bishop, C. T. (2005). A randomized controlled trial of a cognitive-behavioral family intervention for pediatric recurrent abdominal pain. *Journal of Pediatric Psychology, 30*(5), 397–408.

Roth-Isigkeit, A., Thyen, U., Raspe, H. H., Stoven, H., & Schmucker, P. (2004). Reports of pain among German children and adolescents: An epidemiological study. *Acta Paediatrica, 93*(2), 258–263.

Rushton, J. L., Forcier, M., & Schectman, R. M. (2002). Epidemiology of depressive symptoms in the National Longitudinal Study of Adolescent Health. *Journal of the American Academy of Child and Adolescent Psychiatry, 41*(2), 199–205.

Saito, Y. A., Mitra, N., & Mayer, E. A. (2010). Genetic approaches to functional gastrointestinal disorders. *Gastroenterology, 138*(4), 1276–1285.

Salminen, J. J., Pentti, J., & Terho, P. (1992). Low back pain and disability in 14-year-old schoolchildren. *Acta Paediatrica, 81*(12), 1035–1039.

Schanberg, L. E., Keefe, F. J., Lefebvre, J. C., Kredich, D. W., & Gil, K. M. (1998). Social context of pain in children with Juvenile Primary Fibromyalgia Syndrome: Parental pain history and family environment. *The Clinical Journal of Pain, 14*(2), 107–115.

Scharff, L., Langan, N., Rotter, N., Scott-Sutherland, J., Schenck, C., Tayor, N., et al. (2005). Psychological, behavioral, and family characteristics of pediatric patients with chronic pain: A 1-year retrospective study and cluster analysis. *The Clinical Journal of Pain, 21*(5), 432–438.

Seminowicz, D. A., & Davis, K. D. (2006). Cortical responses to pain in healthy individuals depends on pain catastrophizing. *Pain, 120*(3), 297–306.

Shaffer, D., Fisher, P., Dulcan, M. K., Davies, M., Piacentini, J., Schwab-Stone, M. E., et al. (1996). The NIMH Diagnostic Interview Schedule for Children Version 2.3 (DISC-2.3): Description, acceptability, prevalence rates, and performance in the MECA Study. Methods for the Epidemiology of Child and Adolescent Mental Disorders Study. *Journal of the American Academy of Child and Adolescent Psychiatry, 35*(7), 865–877.

Siegel, D. M., Janeway, D., & Baum, J. (1998). Fibromyalgia syndrome in children and adolescents: Clinical features at presentation and status at follow-up. *Pediatrics, 101*(3 Pt 1), 377–382.

Sjolie, A. N. (2002). Psychosocial correlates of low-back pain in adolescents. *European Spine Journal, 11*(6), 582–588.

Spee, L. A., van den Hurk, A. P., van Leeuwen, Y., Benninga, M. A., Bierma-Zeinstra, S. M., Passchier, J., et al. (2010). Childhood abdominal pain in primary care: Design and patient selection of the HONEUR abdominal pain cohort. *BMC Family Practice, 11*, 27.

Spirito, A., Stark, L. J., Gil, K. M., & Tyc, V. L. (1995). Coping with everyday and disease-related stressors by chronically ill children and adolescents. *Journal of the American Academy of Child and Adolescent Psychiatry, 34*(3), 283–290.

Stanford, E. A., Chambers, C. T., Biesanz, J. C., & Chen, E. (2008). The frequency, trajectories and predictors of adolescent recurrent pain: A population-based approach. *Pain, 138*(1), 11–21.

Taimela, S., Kujala, U. M., Salminen, J. J., & Viljanen, T. (1997). The prevalence of low back pain among children and adolescents. A nationwide, cohort-based questionnaire survey in Finland. *Spine (Phila Pa 1976), 22*(10), 1132–1136.

Tesler, M. D., Holzemer, W. L., & Savedra, M. C. (1998). Pain behaviors: Postsurgical responses of children and adolescents. *Journal of Pediatric Nursing, 13*(1), 41–47.

Thomas Cheng, H. (2010). Spinal cord mechanisms of chronic pain and clinical implications. *Current Pain and Headache Reports, 14*(3), 213–220.

Troussier, B., Davoine, P., de Gaudemaris, R., Fauconnier, J., & Phelip, X. (1994). Back pain in school children. A study among 1178 pupils. *Scandinavian Journal of Rehabilitation Medicine, 26*(3), 143–146.

van Tulder, M. W., Ostelo, R., Vlaeyen, J. W., Linton, S. J., Morley, S. J., & Assendelft, W. J. (2001). Behavioral treatment for chronic low back pain: A systematic review within the framework of the Cochrane Back Review Group. *Spine (Phila Pa 1976), 26*(3), 270–281.

Viry, P., Creveuil, C., & Marcelli, C. (1999). Nonspecific back pain in children. *Revue Du Rhumatisme [English Edition], 66*, 381–388.

Walker, L. S., Baber, K. F., Garber, J., & Smith, C. A. (2008). A typology of pain coping strategies in pediatric patients with chronic abdominal pain. *Pain, 137*(2), 266–275.

Walker, L. S., Claar, R. L., & Garber, J. (2002). Social consequences of children's pain: When do they encourage symptom maintenance? *Journal of Pediatric Psychology, 27*(8), 689–698.

Walker, L. S., Garber, J., & Greene, J. W. (1993). Psychosocial correlates of recurrent childhood pain: A comparison of pediatric patients with recurrent abdominal pain, organic illness, and psychiatric disorders. *Journal of Abnormal Psychology, 102*(2), 248–258.

Walker, L. S., & Greene, J. W. (1991). The functional disability inventory: Measuring a neglected dimension of child health status. *Journal of Pediatric Psychology, 16*(1), 39–58.

Walker, L. S., Levy, R. L., & Whitehead, W. E. (2006). Validation of a measure of protective parent responses to children's pain. *The Clinical Journal of Pain, 22*(8), 712–716.

Walker, L. S., Lipani, T. A., Greene, J. W., Caines, K., Stutts, J., Polk, D. B., et al. (2004). Recurrent abdominal pain: Symptom subtypes based on the Rome II criteria for pediatric functional gastrointestinal disorders. *Journal of Pediatric Gastroenterology and Nutrition, 38*(2), 187–191.

Wall, B. A., Holden, E. W., & Gladstein, J. (1996). Parent responses to pediatric headache. *Headache, 37*, 65–70.

Wolfe, F., Smythe, H. A., Yunus, M. B., Bennett, R. M., Bombardier, C., Goldenberg, D. L., et al. (1990). The American College of Rheumatology 1990 criteria for the classification of fibromyalgia. Report of the Multicenter Criteria Committee. *Arthritis and Rheumatism, 33*(2), 160–172.

Youssef, N. N., Atienza, K., Langseder, A. L., & Strauss, R. S. (2008). Chronic abdominal pain and depressive symptoms: Analysis of the national longitudinal study of adolescent health. *Clinical Gastroenterology and Hepatology, 6*(3), 329–332.

Yunus, M. B. (1998). Genetic factors in fibromyalgia syndrome. *Zeitschrift für Rheumatologie, 57*(Suppl 2), 61–62.

Yunus, M. B., Khan, M. A., Rawlings, K. K., Green, J. R., Olson, J. M., & Shah, S. (1999). Genetic linkage analysis of multicase families with fibromyalgia syndrome. *Journal of Rheumatology, 26*(2), 408–412.

Yunus, M. B., & Masi, A. T. (1985). Juvenile primary fibromyalgia syndrome. A clinical study of thirty-three patients and matched normal controls. *Arthritis and Rheumatism, 28*(2), 138–145.

Index

W.T. O'Donohue et al. (eds.), *Handbook of Adolescent Health Psychology*,
DOI 10.1007/978-1-4614-6633-8, © Springer Science+Business Media New York 2013

T

Printed by Printforce, the Netherlands